EMERGENCY
MEDICINE
MANUAL

EDITORS

O. John Ma, MD
Associate Professor of Emergency Medicine
University of Missouri-Kansas City School of Medicine
Vice Chair
Department of Emergency Medicine
Truman Medical Center
Kansas City, Missouri

David M. Cline, M.D.
Associate Professor
Research Director
Department of Emergency Medicine
Wake Forest University School of Medicine
Winston-Salem, North Carolina

Judith E. Tintinalli, M.D., M.S.
Professor and Chair
Department of Emergency Medicine
Adjunct Professor
Department of Health Policy and Administration
University of North Carolina at Chapel Hill
Chapel Hill, North Carolina

Gabor D. Kelen, M.D.
Professor and Chair
Department of Emergency Medicine
Johns Hopkins University
Baltimore, Maryland

J. Stephan Stapczynski, M.D.
Professor and Former Chair
Department of Emergency Medicine
University of Kentucky College of Medicine
Lexington, Kentucky

EMERGENCY MEDICINE MANUAL
sixth edition

O. John Ma, MD
Associate Professor of Emergency Medicine
University of Missouri-Kansas City School of Medicine
Vice Chair
Department of Emergency Medicine
Truman Medical Center
Kansas City, Missouri

David M. Cline, MD
Associate Professor
Research Director
Department of Emergency Medicine
Wake Forest University School of Medicine
Winston-Salem, North Carolina

American College of
Emergency Physicians®

McGraw-Hill
Medical Publishing Division
New York   Chicago   San Francisco   Lisbon   London   Madrid
Mexico City   Milan   New Delhi   San Juan   Seoul   Singapore
Sydney   Toronto

EMERGENCY MEDICINE MANUAL, 6TH EDITION

Copyright © 2004, 2000, 1996 by **The McGraw-Hill Companies, Inc.** All rights reserved. Printed in the United States of America. Except as permitted under the United States Copyright Act of 1976, no part of this publication may be reproduced or distributed in any form or by any means, or stored in a data base or retrieval system, without the prior written permission of the publisher.

1 2 3 4 5 6 7 8 9 0   DOC/DOC   0 9 8 7 6 5 4 3

ISBN: 0-07-141025-2

This book was set in Times Roman by ATLIS Graphics and Design.
The editors were Andrea Seils and Nicky Fernando.
The production supervisor was Catherine H. Saggese.
The cover designer was Aimee Nordin.
The index was prepared by Debbie Tourtlotte.
RR Donnelley was the printer and binder.

This book is printed on acid-free paper.

LIBRARY OF CONGRESS CATALOGING-IN-PUBLICATION DATA

Emergency medicine manual / edited by O. John Ma . . . [et al.]. — 6th ed.
    p. ; cm.
  Condensed version of: Emergency medicine. 6th ed., c2004.
  Includes bibliographical references and index.
  ISBN 0-07-141025-2
  1. Emergency medicine—Handbooks, manuals, etc.   2. Medical emergencies—Handbooks, manuals, etc.   3. Emergency medical services—Handbooks, manuals, etc.   I. Ma, O. John.
II. Emergency medicine.
  [DNLM: 1. Emergency Medicine—Handbooks.   WB 39 E5345 2004]
RC86.7.E574 2004
616.02′5—dc22
                                                                                2003061443

Contents

Contributors   *x*
Preface   *xiv*

Section 1 Resuscitative Problems and Techniques   1

1. Advanced Airway Support   *Robert J. Vissers*   3
2. Dysrhythmia Management   *James K. Takayesu*   9
3. Resuscitation of Children and Neonates   *Douglas K. Holtzman*   26
4. Fluids, Electrolytes, and Acid-Base Disorders   *David M. Cline*   32

Section 2 Shock   47

5. Therapeutic Approach to the Hypotensive Patient   *John E. Gough*   49
6. Septic Shock   *John E. Gough*   53
7. Cardiogenic Shock   *Rawle A. Seupaul*   57
8. Anaphylaxis and Acute Allergic Reactions   *Damian F. McHugh*   60
9. Neurogenic Shock   *Rawle A. Seupaul*   62

Section 3 Analgesia, Anesthesia, and Sedation   65

10. Acute Pain Management and Procedural Sedation   *Diamond Vrocher*   67
11. Management of Patients with Chronic Pain   *David M. Cline*   75

Section 4 Emergency Wound Management   81

12. Evaluating and Preparing Wounds   *Timothy Reeder*   83
13. Methods for Wound Closure   *David M. Cline*   87
14. Lacerations to the Face and Scalp   *Russel J. Karten*   94
15. Injuries of the Arm, Hand, Fingertip, and Nail   *David M. Cline*   99
16. Lacerations to the Leg and Foot   *David M. Cline*   106
17. Soft Tissue Foreign Bodies   *Rodney L. McCaskill*   109
18. Puncture Wounds and Mammalian Bites   *Chris Melton*   112
19. Post Repair Wound Care   *Eugenia B. Smith*   118

Section 5 Cardiovascular Diseases   121

20. Approach to Chest Pain and Ischemic Equivalents   *Thomas Rebbecchi*   123
21. Acute Coronary Syndromes: Management of Myocardial Infarction and Unstable Angina   *Jim Edward Weber*   129
22. Syncope   *Michael G. Mikhail*   137
23. Congestive Heart Failure and Acute Pulmonary Edema   *Chadwick D. Miller*   140
24. Valvular Heart Disease   *David M. Cline*   142
25. The Cardiomyopathies, Myocarditis, and Pericardial Disease   *N. Stuart Harris*   149
26. Pulmonary Embolism   *Christopher Kabrhel*   156
27. Hypertensive Emergencies   *Jonathan A. Maisel*   159
28. Aortic Dissection and Aneurysms   *David E. Manthey*   162
29. Peripheral Vascular Disorders   *Christopher Kabrhel*   166

Section 6 Pulmonary Emergencies   171

30	Respiratory Distress *Matthew T. Keadey*	173
31	Bronchitis, Pneumonia, and SARS *David M. Cline*	179
32	Tuberculosis *Amy J. Behrman*	184
33	Pneumothorax *Rodney L. McCaskill*	188
34	Hemoptysis *James E. Winslow*	190
35	Asthma and Chronic Obstructive Pulmonary Disease *Monika Ahluwalia*	192

Section 7 Gastrointestinal Emergencies   197

36	Acute Abdominal Pain *Peggy E. Goodman*	199
37	Gastrointestinal Bleeding *Mitchell C. Sokolosky*	204
38	Esophageal Emergencies *Mitchell C. Sokolosky*	206
39	Swallowed Foreign Bodies *Patricia Baines*	209
40	Peptic Ulcer Disease and Gastritis *Mark R. Hess*	212
41	Appendicitis *Peggy E. Goodman*	214
42	Intestinal Obstruction *Roy L. Alson*	217
43	Hernia in Adults and Children *N. Heramba Prasad*	219
44	Ileitis, Colitis, and Diverticulitis *Jonathan A. Maisel*	221
45	Anorectal Disorders *N. Heramba Prasad*	227
46	Vomiting, Diarrhea, and Constipation *Jonathan A. Maisel*	234
47	Jaundice, Hepatic Disorders, and Hepatic Failure *Gregory S. Hall*	239
48	Cholecystitis and Biliary Colic *Gregory S. Hall*	247
49	Acute Pancreatitis *Robert J. Vissers*	250
50	Complications of General Surgical Procedures *N. Heramba Prasad*	253

Section 8 Renal and Genitourinary Disorders   257

51	Acute Renal Failure *Marc D. Squillante*	259
52	Emergencies in Renal Failure and Dialysis Patients *Jonathan A. Maisel*	264
53	Urinary Tract Infections and Hematuria *Kama Guluma*	267
54	Male Genital Problems *Stephen H. Thomas*	271
55	Urologic Stone Disease *Geetika Gupta*	276
56	Complications of Urologic Devices *David M. Cline*	278

Section 9 Gynecology and Obstetrics   281

57	Vaginal Bleeding and Pelvic Pain in the Non-Pregnant Patient *Cherri Hobgood*	283
58	Ectopic Pregnancy *David M. Cline*	286
59	Comorbid Diseases in Pregnancy *Sally S. Fuller*	288
60	Emergencies during Pregnancy and the Postpartum Period *Sally S. Fuller*	294
61	Emergency Delivery *David M. Cline*	299
62	Vulvovaginitis *David A. Krueger*	302
63	Pelvic Inflammatory Disease and Tubo-Ovarian Abscess *Robert W. Shaffer*	305
64	Complications of Gynecologic Procedures *Debra Houry*	308

Section 10 Gynecology and Obstetrics   311

65	Fever *Douglas K. Holtzman*	313
66	Bacteremia, Sepsis, and Meningitis in Children *Milan D. Nadkarni*	315

67	Common Neonatal Problems *Lance Brown*	319
68	Pediatric Heart Disease *David M. Cline*	325
69	Otitis Media and Pharyngitis *David M. Cline*	330
70	Skin and Soft Tissue Infections in Children *David M. Cline*	334
71	Pneumonia *Lance Brown*	338
72	Asthma and Bronchiolitis *Douglas R. Trocinski*	340
73	Seizures and Status Epilepticus in Children *Michael C. Plewa*	344
74	Vomiting and Diarrhea *Debra G. Perina*	348
75	Pediatric Abdominal Emergencies *Debra G. Perina*	351
76	Diabetic Ketoacidosis in Children *David M. Cline*	355
77	Hypoglycemia in Children *Juan A. March*	357
78	Altered Mental Status and Headache in Children *Debra G. Perina*	359
79	Syncope and Sudden Death in Children and Adolescents *Debra G. Perina*	363
80	Fluid and Electrolyte Therapy *Lance Brown*	366
81	Upper Respiratory Emergencies *Juan A. March*	369
82	Pediatric Exanthems *Lance Brown*	374
83	Musculoskeletal Disorders in Children *David M. Cline*	383
84	Sickle Cell Anemia in Children *Douglas R. Trocinski*	391
85	Pediatric Urinary Tract Infections *Lance Brown*	397

Section 11 Infectious Diseases   399

86	Sexually Transmitted Diseases *Gregory S. Hall*	401
87	Toxic Shock *Kevin J. Corcoran*	407
88	Common Viral Infections *Matthew J. Scholer*	410
89	HIV Infections and AIDS *David M. Cline*	413
90	Infective Endocarditis *Chadwick D. Miller*	419
91	Tetanus and Rabies *C. James Corrall*	422
92	Malaria *Gregory S. Hall*	426
93	Infections from Helminths *Phillip A. Clement*	431
94	Zoonotic Infections *Gregory S. Hall*	437
95	Soft Tissue Infections *Chris Melton*	447
96	Bioterrorism *Roy Alson*	452
97	Management of the Transplant Patient *David M. Cline*	456

Section 12 Toxicology and Pharmacology   465

98	General Management of the Poisoned Patient *Sandra L. Najarian*	467
99	Anticholinergic Toxicity *O. John Ma*	476
100	Psychopharmacologic Agents *C. Crawford Mechem*	479
101	Sedatives and Hypnotics *Keith L. Mausner*	489
102	Alcohols *Michael P. Kefer*	494
103	Drugs of Abuse *Jeffrey N. Glaspy*	499
104	Analgesics *Keith L. Mausner*	505
105	Theophylline *Mark B. Rogers*	512
106	Cardiac Medications *C. Crawford Mechem*	514
107	Phenytoin and Fosphenytoin Toxicity *Mark B. Rogers*	521
108	Iron *O. John Ma*	524
109	Hydrocarbons and Volatile Substances *J. Christian Fox*	527
110	Caustics *Christian A. Tomaszewski*	530
111	Insecticides, Herbicides, and Rodenticides *Christian A. Tomaszewski*	533
112	Metals and Metalloids *Lance H. Hoffman*	538
113	Hazardous Materials *Christian A. Tomaszewski*	542
114	Herbals and Vitamins *Christian A. Tomaszewski*	546
115	Antimicrobials *Christian A. Tomaszewski*	549

116	Cyanide *Mark E. Hoffmann*	551
117	Dyshemoglobinemias *Howard E. Jarvis III*	553
118	Hypoglycemic Agents *Christian A. Tomaszewski*	555

Section 13 Environmental Injuries   559

119	Frostbite and Hypothermia *Mark E. Hoffmann*	561
120	Heat Emergencies *T. Paul Tran*	564
121	Bites and Stings *Burton Bentley II*	567
122	Trauma and Envenomation from Marine Fauna *Christian A. Tomaszewski*	575
123	High-Altitude Medical Problems *Keith L. Mausner*	578
124	Dysbarism and Complications of Diving *Christian A. Tomaszewski*	581
125	Near Drowning *Richard A. Walker*	584
126	Thermal and Chemical Burns *Robert J. French*	586
127	Electrical and Lightning Injuries *Howard E. Jarvis III*	593
128	Carbon Monoxide *Christian A. Tomaszewski*	598
129	Poisonous Plants and Mushrooms *Sandra L. Najarian*	601

Section 14 Endocrine Emergencies   605

130	Diabetic Emergencies *Michael P. Kefer*	607
131	Alcoholic Ketoacidosis *Michael P. Kefer*	612
132	Thyroid Disease Emergencies *Matthew A. Bridges*	614
133	Adrenal Insufficiency and Adrenal Crisis *Michael P. Kefer*	617

Section 15 Hematoloic and Oncologic Emergencies   619

134	Evaluation of Anemia and the Bleeding Patient *Sandra L. Najarian*	621
135	Acquired Bleeding Disorders *Matthew A. Bridges*	628
136	Hemophilias and von Willebrand Disease *Jeffrey N. Glaspy*	634
137	Hemolytic Anemias *Sandra L. Najarian*	641
138	Transfusion Therapy *Walter N. Simmons*	646
139	Exogenous Anticoagulants and Antiplatelet Agents *Robert A. Schwab*	653
140	Emergency Complications of Malignancy *T. Paul Tran*	656

Section 16 Neurology   665

141	Headache and Facial Pain *Jason Graham*	667
142	Stroke and Transient Ischemic Attack *J. Stephen Huff*	673
143	Altered Mental Status and Coma *C. Crawford Mechem*	679
144	Ataxia and Gait Disturbances *C. Crawford Mechem*	686
145	Vertigo and Dizziness *Andrew K. Chang*	688
146	Seizures and Status Epilepticus in Adults *C. Crawford Mechem*	693
147	Acute Peripheral Neurological Lesions *Howard E. Jarvis III*	699
148	Chronic Neurologic Disorders *Mark B. Rogers*	703
149	Meningitis, Encephalitis, and Brain Abscess *O. John Ma*	708

Section 17 Eye, Ear, Nose, Throat, and Oral Emergencies   713

150	Ocular Emergencies *Steven Go*	715
151	Face and Jaw Emergencies *Robert J. French*	724
152	Ear and Nose Emergencies *Jeffrey N. Glaspy*	728
153	Oral and Dental Emergencies *Steven Go*	734
154	Neck and Upper Airway Disorders *Robert J. French*	740

Section 18 Disorders of the Skin   745

155	Dermatologic Emergencies *Michael Blaivas*	747
156	Other Dermatologic Disorders *Michael Blaivas*	753

Section 19 Trauma   759

157	Initial Approach to the Trauma Patient *J. Christian Fox*	761
158	Pediatric Trauma *Charles J. Havel Jr*	764
159	Geriatric Trauma *O. John Ma*	768
160	Trauma in Pregnancy *C. Crawford Mechem*	771
161	Head Injury *O. John Ma*	774
162	Spine and Spinal Cord Injuries *Jeffrey N. Glaspy*	780
163	Maxillofacial Trauma *C. Crawford Mechem*	787
164	Neck Trauma *Walter N. Simmons*	792
165	Cardiothoracic Trauma *Jeffrey N. Glaspy*	795
166	Abdominal Trauma *O. John Ma*	803
167	Penetrating Trauma to the Flank and Buttock *Robert A. Schwab*	807
168	Genitourinary Trauma *C. Crawford Mechem*	810
169	Penetrating Trauma to the Extremities *C. Crawford Mechem*	814

Section 20 Injuries to the Bones, Joints, and Soft Tissue   817

170	Initial Evaluation and Management of Orthopedic Injuries *Michael P. Kefer*	819
171	Hand and Wrist Injuries *Michael P. Kefer*	822
172	Forearm and Elbow Injuries *Sandra L. Najarian*	826
173	Shoulder and Humerus Injuries *Robert French*	830
174	Pelvis, Hip, and Femur Injuries *E. Parker Hays Jr*	835
175	Knee and Leg Injuries *Jeffrey N. Glaspy*	840
176	Ankle and Foot Injuries *Michael C. Wadman*	844
177	Compartment Syndromes *Gary M. Gaddis*	848
178	Rhabdomyolysis *Gary M. Gaddis*	850

Section 21 Nontraumatic Musculoskeletal Disorders   853

179	Neck and Thoracolumbar Pain *Thomas K. Swoboda*	855
180	Shoulder Pain *Andrew D. Perron*	860
181	Acute Disorders of the Joints and Bursae *Andrew D. Perron*	862
182	Emergencies in Systemic Rheumatic Diseases *Michael P. Kefer*	867
183	Infectious and Noninfectious Disorders of the Hand *Michael P. Kefer*	869
184	Soft Tissue Problems of the Foot *Mark B. Rogers*	872

Section 22 Psychosocial Disorders   877

185	Clinical Features of Behavioral Disorders *Lance H. Hoffman*	879
186	Emergency Assessment and Stabilization of Behavioral Disorders *Lance H. Hoffman*	882
187	Panic and Conversion Disorders *Lance H. Hoffman*	885

Section 23 Abuse and Assault   889

188	Child and Elderly Abuse *Kristine L. Bott*	891
189	Sexual Assault and Intimate Partner Violence and Abuse *Stefanie R. Ellison*	894

Color plates fall between pages 754 and 755.

Index   899

Contributors

Monika Ahluwalia, M.D., Assistant Professor of Emergency Medicine, Emory University School of Medicine, Department of Emergency Medicine, Atlanta, Georgia [Chapter 35]

Roy L. Alson, M.D., Associate Professor of Emergency Medicine, Department of Emergency Medicine, Wake Forest University School of Medicine, Winston-Salem, North Carolina [Chapters 42 & 96]

Patricia Baines, M.D., Assistant Professor of Emergency Medicine, Department of Emergency Medicine, Emory University School of Medicine, Atlanta, Georgia [Chapter 39]

Amy J. Behrman, M.D., Associate Professor of Emergency Medicine, Department of Emergency Medicine, University of Pennsylvania Health System, Philadelphia, Pennsylvania [Chapter 32]

Burton Bentley II, M.D., Attending Staff Physician, Department of Emergency Medicine, Northwest Medical Center, Tucson, Arizona [Chapter 121]

Michael Blaivas, M.D., R.D.M.S., Associate Professor, Director of Emergency Ultrasound, Department of Emergency Medicine, Medical College of Georgia, Augusta, Georgia [Chapters 155 & 156]

Kristine L. Bott, M.D., Assistant Professor, Section of Emergency Medicine, University of Nebraska College of Medicine, Omaha, Nebraska [Chapter 188]

Matthew A. Bridges, M.D., Assistant Professor, University of Missouri—Kansas City School of Medicine, Department of Emergency Medicine, Truman Medical Center, Kansas City, Missouri [Chapters 132 & 135]

Lance Brown, M.D., M.P.H., Associate Professor of Emergency Medicine, Department of Emergency Medicine, Loma Linda University Medical Center and Children's Hospital, Loma Linda, California [Chapters 67, 71, 80, 82, & 85]

Andrew K. Chang, M.D., Assistant Professor, Department of Emergency Medicine, Albert Einstein College of Medicine, Montefiore Medical Center, Bronx, New York [Chapter 145]

Phillip A. Clement, M.D., Clinical Assistant Professor of Emergency Medicine, Department of Emergency Medicine, East Carolina University School of Medicine, Greenville, North Carolina [Chapter 93]

David M. Cline, M.D., Associate Professor of Emergency Medicine, Department of Emergency Medicine, Wake Forest University School of Medicine, Winston-Salem, North Carolina, [Chapters 4, 11, 13, 15, 16, 24, 31, 56, 58, 61, 68, 69, 70, 76, 83, 89, & 97]

Kevin J. Corcoran, D.O., Clinical Associate Professor of Emergency Medicine, Department of Emergency Medicine, East Carolina University School of Medicine, Greenville, North Carolina [Chapter 87]

C. James Corral, M.D., Staff Physician, Department of Emergency Medicine, Harrison Hospital, Bremerton, Washington [Chapter 91]

Stefanie R. Ellison, M.D., Assistant Professor, University of Missouri—Kansas City School of Medicine, Department of Emergency Medicine, Truman Medical Center, Kansas City, Missouri [Chapter 189]

J. Christian Fox, M.D., R.D.M.S., Assistant Clinical Professor, Director, Emergency Ultrasound Program, Department of Emergency Medicine, University of California, Irvine School of Medicine, Irvine, California [Chapters 109 & 157]

Robert J. French, D.O., Assistant Clinical Professor, Saint Luke's Hospital, Medical College of Wisconsin, Milwaukee, Wisconsin, [Chapters 126, 151, 154, & 173]

Sally S. Fuller, M.D., Clinical Assistant Professor of Emergency Medicine, Department of Emergency Medicine, University of North Carolina, Chapel Hill, North Carolina, Staff Physician, WakeMed, Department of Emergency Medicine, Raleigh, North Carolina [Chapters 59 & 60]

Gary M. Gaddis, M.D., Ph.D., Clinical Associate Professor, Saint Luke's Hospital,

---

* The numbers in brackets following the contributors' names indicate the chapters written by that contributor.

University of Missouri—Kansas City School of Medicine, Kansas City, Missouri, [Chapters 177 & 178]

Jeffrey N. Glaspy, M.D., Assistant Professor, University of Missouri—Kansas City School of Medicine, Associate Program Director, Department of Emergency Medicine, Truman Medical Center, Kansas City, Missouri [Chapters 103, 136, 152, 162, 165, & 175]

Steven Go, M.D., Assistant Professor, University of Missouri—Kansas City School of Medicine, Department of Emergency Medicine, Truman Medical Center, Kansas City, Missouri [Chapters 150 & 153]

John E. Gough, M.D., Associate Professor of Emergency Medicine, Department of Emergency Medicine, East Carolina School of Medicine, Greenville, North Carolina [Chapters 5 & 6]

Peggy E. Goodman, M.D., Associate Professor of Emergency Medicine, Department of Emergency Medicine, East Carolina School of Medicine, Greenville, North Carolina [Chapters 36 & 41]

Jason Graham, M.D., Assistant Professor, University of Missouri—Kansas City School of Medicine, Department of Emergency Medicine, Truman Medical Center, Kansas City, Missouri [Chapter 141]

Kama Guluma, M.D., Clinical Assistant Professor of Medicine, Division of Emergency Medicine, Department of Medicine, University of California, San Diego, San Diego, California [Chapter 53]

Geetika Gupta, M.D., Clinical Instructor of Emergency Medicine, Department of Emergency Medicine, University of Michigan, Staff Physician, Department of Emergency Medicine, St. Joseph Mercy Hospital [Chapter 55]

Gregory S. Hall, M.D., Assistant Professor of Emergency Medicine, Department of Emergency Medicine, University of Arkansas for Medical Science, Little Rock, Arkansas [Chapters 47, 48, 86, 92, & 94]

N. Stuart Harris, M.D., Clinical Instructor, Department of Emergency Medicine, Massachusetts General Hospital, Boston, Massachusetts [Chapter 25]

Charles J. Havel, Jr., M.D., Assistant Clinical Professor, Elmbrook Hospital, Medical College of Wisconsin, Milwaukee, Wisconsin [Chapter 158]

E. Parker Hays, Jr., M.D., Residency Program Director, Department of Emergency Medicine, Carolinas Medical Center, Charlotte, North Carolina [Chapter 174]

Mark R. Hess, M.D., Assistant Professor of Emergency Medicine, Department of Emergency Medicine, Wake Forest University School of Medicine, Winston-Salem, North Carolina [Chapter 40]

Cherri Hobgood, M.D., Assistant Professor of Emergency Medicine, Department of Emergency Medicine, University of North Carolina, Chapel Hill, North Carolina [Chapter 57]

Lance H. Hoffman, M.D., Assistant Professor, Section of Emergency Medicine, University of Nebraska College of Medicine, Omaha, Nebraska [Chapters 112 & 185–187]

Mark E. Hoffmann, M.D., Attending Staff Physician, Department of Emergency Medicine, St. Cloud Hospital, St. Cloud, Minnesota [Chapters 116 & 119]

Douglas K. Holtzman, M.D., Assistant Professor of Emergency Medicine, Department of Emergency Medicine, Wake Forest University School of Medicine, Winston-Salem, North Carolina [Chapters 3 & 65]

Debra Houry, M.D., Assistant Professor of Emergency Medicine, Department of Emergency Medicine, Emory University School of Medicine, Atlanta, Georgia [Chapter 64]

J. Stephen Huff, M.D., Associate Professor, Departments of Emergency Medicine and Neurology, University of Virginia School of Medicine, Charlottesville, Virginia, [Chapter 142]

Howard E. Jarvis III, M.D., Attending Staff Physician, Department of Emergency Medicine, Cox Medical Center, Springfield, Missouri [Chapters 117, 127, & 147]

Christopher Kabrhel, M.D., Clinical Instructor, Department of Emergency Medicine, Massachusetts General Hospital, Boston, Massachusetts, [Chapters 26 & 29]

Russel J. Karten, M.D., Assistant Professor of Emergency Medicine, Department of Emergency Medicine, University of Pennsylvania, Philadelphia, Pennsylvania [Chapter 14]

Matthew T. Keadey, M.D., Assistant Professor of Emergency Medicine, Department of Emergency Medicine, Emory University School of Medicine, Atlanta, Georgia [Chapter 30]

Michael P. Kefer, M.D., Attending Staff Physician, Department of Emergency Medicine, Oconomowoc Memorial Hospital, Oconomowoc, Wisconsin [Chapters 102, 130, 131, 133, 170, 171, 182, & 183]

David A. Krueger, M.D., Staff Physician, Department of Emergency Medicine, Appleton Medical Center, Appleton, Wisconsin [Chapter 62]

O. John Ma, M.D., Associate Professor, University of Missouri—Kansas City School of Medicine, Vice Chair, Department of Emergency Medicine, Truman Medical Center, Kansas City, Missouri [Chapters 99, 108, 149, 159, 161, & 166]

Jonathan A. Maisel, M.D., Clinical Assistant Professor of Surgery, Yale University School of Medicine, New Haven Connecticut, Associate Program Director for Emergency Medicine, Bridgeport Hospital, Bridgeport, Connecticut [Chapters 27, 44, 46, & 52]

David E. Manthey, M.D., Assistant Professor Emergency Medicine, Department of Emergency Medicine, Wake Forest University School of Medicine, Winston-Salem, North Carolina [Chapter 28]

Juan A. March, M.D., Professor of Emergency Medicine, Department of Emergency Medicine, East Carolina School of Medicine, Greenville, North Carolina [Chapters 77 & 81]

Keith L. Mausner, M.D., Attending Staff Physician, Waukesha Memorial Hospital, Waukesha, Wisconsin [Chapters 101, 104, & 123]

Rodney L. McCaskill, M.D., Clinical Assistant Professor of Emergency Medicine, Department of Emergency Medicine, University of North Carolina, Chapel Hill, North Carolina, Staff Physician, WakeMed, Department of Emergency Medicine, Raleigh, North Carolina [Chapters 17 & 33]

Damian F. McHugh, M.D., Staff Physician, Department of Emergency Medicine, Rex Hospital, Raleigh, North Carolina [Chapter 8]

C. Crawford Mechem, M.D., Associate Professor, Department of Emergency Medicine, University of Pennsylvania School of Medicine, Philadelphia, Pennsylvania [Chapters 100, 106, 143, 144, 146, 160, 163, 168, & 169]

Chris Melton, M.D., Assistant Professor of Emergency Medicine, Department of Emergency Medicine, University of Arkansas for Medical Science, Little Rock, Arkansas [Chapters 18 & 95]

Michael G. Mikael, M.D., Clinical Instructor of Emergency Medicine, Department of Emergency Medicine, University of Michigan, Ann Arbor, Michigan, Chairman of Emergency Medicine, Department of Emergency Medicine, St. Joseph Mercy Hospital, Ann Arbor, Michigan [Chapter 22]

Chadwick D. Miller, M.D., Assistant Professor Emergency Medicine, Department of Emergency Medicine, Wake Forest University School of Medicine, Winston-Salem, North Carolina [Chapters 23 & 90]

Milan D. Nadkarni, M.D., Assistant Professor Emergency Medicine and Pediatrics, Department of Emergency Medicine, Wake Forest University School of Medicine, Winston-Salem, North Carolina [Chapter 66]

Sandra L. Najarian, M.D., Assistant Professor, Case Western Reserve University School of Medicine, Department of Emergency Medicine, MetroHealth Medical Center, Cleveland, Ohio [Chapters 98, 129, 134, 137, & 172]

Debra G. Perina, M.D., Associate Professor of Emergency Medicine, Department of Emergency Medicine, University of Virginia Health Sciences, Charlottesville, Virginia [Chapters 74, 75, 78, & 79]

Andrew D. Perron, M.D., Assistant Professor, Departments of Emergency Medicine and Orthopedic Surgery, University of Virginia School of Medicine, Charlottesville, Virginia [Chapters 180 & 181]

Michael C. Plewa, M.D., Clinical Assistant Professor, Department of Surgery, Medical College of Ohio, Toledo, Ohio, Director of Research, Department of Emergency Medicine, Saint Vincent Mercy Medical Center, Toledo, Ohio [Chapter 73]

N. Heramba Prasad, M.D., Associate Professor of Emergency Medicine, Department of Emergency Medicine, State University of New York, Upstate Medical University, Syracuse, New York [Chapters 43, 45, & 50]

Thomas Rebbecchi, M.D., Assistant Professor of Emergency Medicine, University of Medicine Dentistry New Jersey, Robert Wood Johnson Medical School at Camden, Cooper Hospital/University Medical Center, Camden, New Jersey [Chapter 20]

Timothy J. Reeder, M.D., Assistant Professor of Emergency Medicine, Department of Emergency Medicine, East Carolina University School of Medicine, Greenville, North Carolina [Chapter 12]

Mark B. Rogers, M.D., Attending Physician, Breech Medical Center, Lebanon, Missouri [Chapters 105, 107, 148, & 184]

Robert A. Schwab, M.D., Professor and Chair, University of Missouri—Kansas City School of Medicine, Department of Emergency Medicine, Truman Medical Center, Kansas City, Missouri [Chapters 139 & 167]

Matthew J. Scholer, M.D., Ph.D., Assistant Professor of Emergency Medicine, Department of Emergency Medicine, University of North Carolina, Chapel Hill, North Carolina [Chapter 88]

Rawle A. Seupaul, M.D., Assistant Professor of Emergency Medicine, Department of Emergency Medicine, Indiana University School of Medicine, Indianapolis, Indiana [Chapters 7 & 9]

Walter N. Simmons, M.D., M.P.H., Assistant Professor, Department of Emergency Medicine, Rhode Island Hospital, Brown University, Providence, Rhode Island [Chapters 138 & 164]

Robert W. Shaffer, M.D., Staff Physician, Mount Auburn Hospital, Department of Emergency Medicine, Cambridge, Massachusetts [Chapter 63]

Eugenia B. Smith, M.D., Assistant Professor of Emergency Medicine, Department of Emergency Medicine, University of North Carolina, Chapel Hill, North Carolina [Chapter 19]

Mitchell C. Sokolosky, M.D., Assistant Professor Emergency Medicine, Department of Emergency Medicine, Wake Forest University School of Medicine, Winston-Salem, North Carolina [Chapters 37 & 38]

Marc D. Squillante, D.O., Program Director, Residency in Emergency Medicine, University of Illinois Collage of Medicine at Peoria, Peoria, Illinois [Chapter 51]

Thomas K. Swoboda, M.D., M.S., Assistant Professor, Louisiana State University Health Sciences Center, Department of Emergency Medicine, Shreveport, Louisiana [Chapter 179]

James Kimo Takayesu, M.D., Clinical Instructor, Department of Emergency Medicine, Massachusetts General Hospital, Boston, Massachusetts [Chapter 2]

Stephen H. Thomas, M.D., Assistant Professor, Department of Emergency Medicine, Massachusetts General Hospital, Boston, Massachusetts [Chapter 54]

Christian A. Tomaszewski, M.D., Associate Professor, Department of Emergency Medicine, Carolinas Medical Center, Charlotte, North Carolina [Chapters 110, 111, 113–115, 118, 122, 124, & 128]

T. Paul Tran, M.D., Assistant Professor, Section of Emergency Medicine, University of Nebraska College of Medicine, Omaha, Nebraska [Chapters 120 & 140]

Douglas R. Trocinski, M.D., Clinical Assistant Professor of Emergency Medicine, Department of Emergency Medicine, University of North Carolina, Chapel Hill, North Carolina, Associate Residency Director, WakeMed, Department of Emergency Medicine, Raleigh, North Carolina [Chapters 72 & 84]

Robert J. Vissers, M.D., Assistant Professor of Emergency Medicine, Department of Emergency Medicine, University of North Carolina, Chapel Hill, North Carolina [Chapters 1 & 49]

Diamond Vrocher, M.D., Assistant Professor of Emergency Medicine, Department of Emergency Medicine, University of Alabama at Birmingham, Birmingham, Alabama [Chapter 10]

Michael C. Wadman, M.D., Assistant Professor, Section of Emergency Medicine, University of Nebraska College of Medicine, Omaha, Nebraska [Chapter 176]

Richard A. Walker, M.D., Associate Professor, Section of Emergency Medicine, University of Nebraska College of Medicine, Omaha, Nebraska [Chapter 125]

Jim Edward Weber, D.O., Assistant Professor of Emergency Medicine, Department of Emergency Medicine, University of Michigan, Ann Arbor, Michigan, Director of Emergency Medicine Research, Hurley Medical Center, Flint, Michigan [Chapter 21]

James E. Winslow, M.D., Assistant Professor Emergency Medicine, Department of Emergency Medicine, Wake Forest University School of Medicine, Winston-Salem, North Carolina [Chapter 34]

Preface

The tremendous growth in the specialty of emergency medicine is reflected in the depth and breadth of the sixth edition of *Emergency Medicine: A Comprehensive Study Guide*. In 1996 and 2000, editions of the Companion Handbook were published as a clinical tool to guide clinicians with the diagnosis and management of patients in the emergency department. The Companion Handbook also has been published in English, Spanish, French, and Italian, which further reflects the growing number of emergency medicine practitioners worldwide.

The original goal of the Companion Handbook is preserved in this edition, which is now entitled Manual of Emergency Medicine. This handbook is written by and for health care workers who are engaged in the practice of clinical emergency medicine. Each chapter continues to emphasize the Clinical Features, Diagnosis and Differential, and Emergency Department Care and Disposition of the disease entity. In this edition, we have placed increased emphasis on key contemporary topics, including bioterrorism, SARS, West Nile virus, and toxicology. A new feature is the addition of color photographs that should assist clinicians with the diagnosis of certain challenging and unique disorders. We hope that this pocket-sized handbook will assist practitioners of emergency medicine with their primary endeavor: the skillful and timely care of their patients in the emergency department.

We would like to express our sincere appreciation to the Manual of Emergency Medicine chapter authors for their commitment and work ethic in helping to produce this handbook. We also are indebted to numerous individuals who assisted us with this project; in particular, we would like to thank Andrea Seils, Michelle Watt, Nicky Fernando, Catherine Saggese, and Martin Wonsiewicz at McGraw-Hill Medical Publishing. Finally, without the love, support, and encouragement of our families, this book would not have been possible. OJM would like to dedicate this book to Elizabeth for continually finding new ways to keep life interesting; DMC would like to dedicate this book to Lisa, the best teacher my children could hope for.

O. John Ma, MD
David M. Cline, MD

1 | RESUSCITATIVE PROBLEMS AND TECHNIQUES

1 | Advanced Airway Support

Robert J. Vissers

Control of the airway is the single most important task for emergency resuscitation. Indications for the airway management techniques described in this chapter include oxygenation, ventilation, protection of the airway, facilitation of therapy, and anticipation of a clinical course that requires preventative management (eg, burn victims).

INITIAL APPROACH

The initial approach to airway management is simultaneous assessment and management of the adequacy of airway patency (the A of the ABCs) and oxygenation and ventilation (the B of the ABCs).

1. The patient's color and respiratory rate must be assessed; respiratory or cardiac arrest may be an indication for immediate intubation.
2. The airway should be opened with head tilt-chin lift maneuver (jaw thrust should be used if C-spine injury is suspected). If needed, the patient should be bagged with the bag-valve-mask device, including an O_2 reservoir. For a good seal, the proper size mask should be ensured. This technique may require an oral or nasal airway or 2 rescuers to seal the mask (2 hands) and bag the patient.
3. The patient should be placed on a cardiac monitor, pulse oximetry, and possibly capnography (end-tidal CO_2), while the remaining vital signs, pulse, and blood pressure (temperature is important but can be delayed to ensure following the ABCs) can be collected.
4. The need for invasive airway management techniques must be determined and are described later. It is essential to not wait for arterial blood gas analyses if the initial assessment indicates the need for invasive airway management. If the patient does not require immediate airway or ventilation control, the patient should be administered oxygen by face mask, as necessary, to ensure an O_2 saturation of 95%. Laboratory studies should be collected as needed. Oxygen should not be removed from a patient to draw an arterial blood gas analysis unless deemed safe from the initial assessment.
5. If intubation is a possibility, all patients should be preoxygenated regardless of saturations, unless exacerbation of CO_2 retention is a concern. Assessment of airway difficulty must be considered before initiation of advanced airway techniques (see below).

OROTRACHEAL INTUBATION

The most common means used to ensure a patent airway, prevent aspiration, and provide oxygenation and ventilation is orotracheal intubation. This technique should be performed by using the method of rapid sequence intubation (RSI), described below, unless the patient's condition makes it unnecessary (ie, cardiac arrest) or it is contraindicated because of an anticipated difficult airway.

Emergency Department Care and Disposition

1. Preparation of equipment, personnel, and drugs should be done before proceeding with any attempts at intubation.

2. Adequate ventilation and oxygenation must be ensured while equipment is prepared. All patients should be preoxygenated with a non–re-breather oxygen mask at maximal oxygen flow rates or with a bag-valve-mask if the patient is not ventilating adequately. Vital signs must be monitored, and pulse oximetry should be used throughout the procedure. Intravenous access is desirable unless conditions preclude its immediate placement.

3. The blade type and size (usually a no. 3 or 4 curved blade or a No. 2 or 3 straight blade) should be selected; the blade light should be tested. The tube size (usually 7.5 to 8.0 mm in women, 8.0 to 8.5 mm in men) must be selected, and the balloon cuff should be tested. The end of the tube may be lubricated with lidocaine jelly or similar lubricant. The use of a flexible stylet is recommended. Suction should be assembled, functioning, and placed within easy reach. Personnel should be present at the bedside to pass equipment and provide cricoid pressure or bag the patient, if required.

4. The patient should be positioned with the head extended and neck flexed, possibly with a rolled towel under the occiput. If C-spine injury is suspected, the head and neck should be maintained in a neutral position with an assistant performing inline stabilization.

5. With the handle in the operator's left hand, the blade should be inserted to push the tongue to the patient's right and slowly advanced in search of the epiglottis. Suctioning may be required. It is not uncommon to go past the larynx into the esophagus. Gradual withdrawal of the blade will reveal the epiglottis. If the curved blade is used, the tip should be slid into the vallecula and lifted (indirectly lifting the epiglottis); if a straight blade is used, the epiglottis should be lifted directly. The direction of lift is along the axis of the laryngoscope handle. It is important to avoid levering the blade on the teeth to prevent dental trauma.

6. Once the vocal cords are visualized, the assistant should be asked to place the tube in the physician's hand. The tube is passed between the cords, avoiding force. The stylet should be removed, and the balloon cuff is inflated. The patient is ventilated with a bag-valve device and checked for bilateral breath sounds.

7. If the cords are not visualized, manipulation of the thyroid cartilage using backward, upward, and rightward pressure (the "burp" maneuver) may bring the cords into view. If unsuccessful, reoxygenation may need to be performed with bag-valve-mask device. Consider changing the blade, the tube size, or the position of the patient before further attempts. Three unsuccessful attempts defines a failed airway, and other rescue techniques must be considered.

8. Placement must be confirmed objectively with an end-tidal CO_2 detector (not reliable if the patient is in cardiac arrest), capnography, or an esophageal detection device. Tube length should be checked; the usual distance (marked on the tube) from corner of the mouth to 2 cm above the carina is 23 cm in men and 21 cm in women.

9. The tube should be taped in place and a bite block inserted. Correct intubation and tube placement can be verified with a portable radiograph.

Short-term complications from orotracheal intubation (trauma to surrounding structures) are unusual as long as correct position is confirmed. Failure to confirm the position immediately can result in hypoxia and neurologic injury. Endobronchial intubation is usually on the right side and is corrected by withdrawing the tube 2 cm and listening for equal breath sounds.

RAPID SEQUENCE INDUCTION

Orotracheal intubation is associated with a higher success rate and lower complication rate when performed with RSI. This technique couples sedation to induce unconsciousness (induction) with muscular paralysis. Intubation follows laryngoscopy while maintaining cricoid pressure to prevent aspiration. The principal contraindication is anticipated difficulty in mask ventilation or intubation.

1. Equipment, medication, and personnel should be prepared. Equipment should be checked, and medications should be available at the bedside before initiation of RSI.
2. The patient should be preoxygenated with 100% oxygen.
3. Pretreatment agents should be considered, depending on the underlying condition of the patient. To prevent reflex bradycardia, **atropine** 0.02 mg/kg intravenously may be beneficial in children younger than 5 years or younger than 10 years when also receiving succinylcholine. **Fentanyl** 3 mg/kg may be beneficial in those patients with possible raised intracranial pressure, cardiac ischemia, or aortic dissection.
4. An induction agent should be pushed intravenously. **Etomidate** 0.3 mg/kg is an excellent choice in most circumstances. **Thiopental** 3 to 5 mg/kg or **midazolam** 0.1 mg/kg also may be considered. Most induction agents should be used with caution in hypotensive patients, in particular barbiturates and benzodiazepines. **Ketamine** 1 to 2 mg/kg should be considered for the induction of a patient who has active bronchospasm for its bronchodilator properties but should be avoided in patients with elevated intracranial pressure. The induction agent should be given 3 minutes after any pretreatment agents.
5. A paralytic agent is pushed intravenously immediately after the induction dose. **Succinylcholine** 1.0 to 1.5 mg/kg is preferred in most cases because of its rapid onset and short duration of action; it should not be used in a patient with a neuromuscular disorder, a denervation injury older than 7 days, or severe burns older than 24 hours because hyperkalemia may occur. Nondepolarizing agents, such as **rocuronium** 0.6 mg/kg or **vecuronium** 0.08 to 0.15 mg/kg, may be used as alternatives; however, the onset of action and the duration of paralysis are increased considerably.
6. Cricoid pressure should be applied once paralysis begins and should be maintained until intubation is accomplished.
7. The trachea should be intubated and placement confirmed by using the techniques described above.
8. The physician should be prepared to bag the patient if intubation proves unsuccessful and saturations are less than 90%. Three unsuccessful attempts defines a failed airway, and other rescue techniques must be considered.

Before any attempt at RSI the patient should be assessed for possible difficult bag-valve-mask ventilation or intubation. The presence of 2 of the following 5 factors is predictive of possible difficulty with bagging: facial hair, obesity, no teeth, advanced age, or snoring. Multiple external features such as facial hair, obesity, short neck, short or long chin, and any airway deformity suggest possible difficulty with intubation. Adequacy of oral opening, neck mobility, and the amount of posterior pharynx that may be visualized are other factors to consider. If difficulty is anticipated, other methods of airway management should be considered such as a primary approach or an available rescue device.

NASOTRACHEAL INTUBATION

Nasotracheal intubation is indicated in situations where laryngoscopy is difficult, neuromuscular blockade is hazardous, or cricothyrotomy is unnecessary. Severely dyspneic, awake patients with congestive heart failure, chronic obstructive pulmonary disease, or asthma often cannot remain supine for other airway maneuvers but can tolerate nasotracheal intubation in the sitting position. Relative contraindications for this technique include complex nasal and massive midface fractures and bleeding disorders.

Emergency Department Care and Disposition

1. Both nares should be sprayed with a topical vasoconstrictor and anesthetic. Between 4% and 10% cocaine solution is an appropriate single agent but may cause unwanted systemic cardiovascular effects. Topical NeoSynephrine is an effective vasoconstrictor, and tetracaine is a safe and effective topical anesthetic.
2. The tube size must be chosen, usually between 7.0 mm and 7.5 mm in women and between 7.5 mm and 8.0 mm in men. The balloon cuff of the tube should be checked for leaks. The tube should be lubricated with lidocaine jelly or similar lubricant.
3. The largest nares should be used or the right side if the nares are equal. Some operators recommend dilating the nares with a lubricated nasal airway. The patient may be sitting up or supine.
4. An assistant can immobilize the patient's neck. The physician should stand to the patient's side, with 1 hand on the tube and with the thumb and index finger of the other hand straddling the larynx. The tube should be advanced slowly, with steady gentle pressure. The tube should be twisted to help move past obstructions in the nose and nasopharynx. The tube should be advanced until maximal airflow is heard through the tube; this means the larynx is now close by.
5. The physician should listen carefully to the rhythm of inspiration and expiration. The tube then should be gently but swiftly advanced during the beginning of inspiration. Entrance into the larynx may initiate a cough, and most expired air should exit the tube even though the cuff is not inflated. If the tube is foggy, the cuff should be inflated.
6. If intubation is unsuccessful, the physician should look carefully for a bulge lateral to the larynx (usually the tip of the tube is in the pyriform fossa on the same side as the nares used). If found, the tube must be retracted until maximal breath sounds are heard, and then intubation should be reattempted by manually displacing the larynx toward the bulge. If no bulge is seen, it is possible that the tube has gone posteriorly into the esophagus. In this case, the tube should be withdrawn until maximal breath sounds are heard. Intubation should be reattempted after the patient's head is extended, and a Sellick maneuver should be performed. Another option is to use a directional control tip (Endotrol) or fiberoptic laryngoscope. The head should not be moved if C-spine injury is suspected.

Complications other than local bleeding are rare. Occasionally, marked bleeding will prompt the need for orotracheal intubation or cricothyrotomy.

CRICOTHYROTOMY

Indications for immediate cricothyrotomy include severe, ongoing tracheo-bronchial hemorrhage, massive midface trauma, and inability to control the airway with the usual less invasive maneuvers. It is also used in the paralyzed patient who cannot be intubated or ventilated and other rescue techniques are unsuccessful. Cricothyrotomy is relatively contraindicated in patients with acute laryngeal disease due to trauma, infection, or recent prolonged intubation and should not be used in children younger than 12 years.

Emergency Department Care and Disposition

1. Sterile technique should be used. The cricothyroid membrane should be palpated with digital stabilization of the larynx (Fig. 1-1). With a No. 11 scalpel, a vertical, 3- to 4-cm incision should be started at the superior border of the thyroid cartilage and incised caudally toward the suprasternal notch.
2. The membrane should be re-palpated and a 1- to 2-cm horizontal incision should be made. The blade should be kept temporarily in place.
3. The larynx should be stabilized by inserting the tracheal hook into the cricothyroid space and retracting upon the inferior edge of the thyroid cartilage (an assistant should hold the hook after it is placed).
4. The scalpel should be removed and a dilator inserted (LaBorde or Trousseau).
5. A No. 4 tracheostomy tube should be introduced (or the largest tube that will fit). Alternatively, a small cuffed endotracheal tube may be used (No. 6 or the largest tube that will fit). The balloon should be inflated and the tube secured in place.
6. The physician should check for bilateral breath sounds. Once tube placement is confirmed, the hook may be removed. The presence of subcutaneous air suggests placement outside the trachea. Placement should be confirmed with an end-tidal CO_2 detector and radiogram.

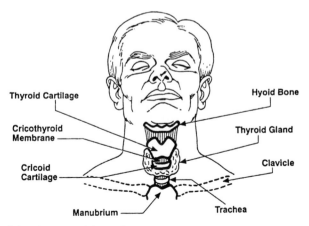

Thyroid Cartilage   **Hyoid Bone**

Cricothyroid Membrane —   **Thyroid Gland**

Cricoid Cartilage —   **Clavicle**

Manubrium —   **Trachea**

FIG. 1-1.   Anatomy of the neck.

Manufactured cricothyrotomy kits using a Seldinger technique are also available. Formal tracheostomy is not recommended as an emergency surgical airway technique due to increased technical difficulty and increased time required.

Alternative drugs for rapid sequence induction are listed in Chap. 19 of *Emergency Medicine: A Comprehensive Study Guide,* 6th ed. Airway management alternatives to the methods described earlier include retrograde tracheal intubation, translaryngeal ventilation, digital intubation, transillumination, fiberoptic assistance, and formal tracheostomy. Translaryngeal ventilation may be used to temporarily provide ventilation until a more definitive procedure is possible. When oral intubation is indicated but has been unsuccessful and the patient can be temporarily ventilated with a bag-valve-mask unit, the following assist methods are warranted: retrograde tracheal intubation, digital intubation, transillumination, or fiberoptic assistance may be helpful. These techniques are described in Chaps. 18, 19, and 20 of *Emergency Medicine: A Comprehensive Study Guide,* 6th ed.

For further reading in *Emergency Medicine: A Comprehensive Study Guide,* 6th ed., see Chap. 18, "Noninvasive Airway Management," by A. Michael Roman; Chap. 19, "Tracheal Intubation and Mechanical Ventilation," by Daniel F. Danzl and Robert J. Vissers; and Chap. 20, "Surgical Airway Management," by David R. Gens.

2 | Dysrhythmia Management

James K. Takayesu

SUPRAVENTRICULAR DYSRHYTHMIAS

Sinus Dysrhythmia

Some variation in the sinoatrial (SA) node discharge rate is common; however, if the variation exceeds 0.12 second between the longest and shortest intervals, sinus dysrhythmia is present. The Electrocardiogram (ECG) characteristics of sinus dysrhythmia are (*a*) normal sinus P waves and PR intervals, (*b*) 1:1 atrioventricular (AV) conduction, and (*c*) variation of at least 0.12 second between the shortest and longest P–P interval (Fig. 2-1). Sinus dysrhythmias are affected primarily by respiration and are most commonly found in children and young adults, disappearing with advancing age. Occasional junctional escape beats may be present during very long P–P intervals. No treatment is required.

Sinus Bradycardia

Clinical Features

Sinus bradycardia occurs when the SA node rate becomes slower than 60 beats/min. The ECG characteristics of sinus bradycardia are (*a*) normal sinus P waves and PR intervals, (*b*) 1:1 AV conduction, and (*c*) atrial rate slower than 60 beats/min. Sinus bradycardia represents a suppression of the sinus node discharge rate, usually in response to 3 categories of stimuli: (*a*) physiologic (vagal tone), (*b*) pharmacologic (calcium channel blockers, β-blockers, or digoxin), and (*c*) pathologic (acute inferior myocardial infarction [MI], increased intracranial pressure, carotid sinus hypersensitivity, hypothyroidism, or sick sinus syndrome).

Emergency Department Care and Disposition

Sinus bradycardia usually does not require specific treatment unless the heart rate is slower than 50 beats/min and there is evidence of hypoperfusion.

1. Symptomatic patients should receive **atropine** 0.5 mg intravenously (IV), which may be repeated every 3 to 5 minutes up to a total of 3 mg IV.
2. Transcutaneous cardiac pacing can be used in the patient refractory to atropine.
   a. The patient should be attached to the monitor leads of the external pacing device.
   b. The pacing pads should be attached to the patient. The anterior pad should be placed over the precordium, which may require retracting a

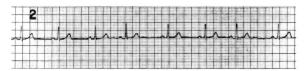

FIG. 2-1.   Sinus dysrhythmia.

woman's breast superiorly. The posterior pad should be placed at the level of the heart, between the spine and the left scapula. The multifunction pacing defibrillation pads should not be used unless the patient is unconscious because these pads cause more discomfort with pacing.

c. The pacing output should be slowly turned from 0 mA to the lowest point where continuous pacing is observed, usually in the range of 50 to 80 mA.

d. Electrical capture should be noted on the monitor, which can be recognized by a widened QRS after each pacing spike.

e. The patient may require sedation with lorazepam (1–2 mg IV) or a similar agent or pain control with morphine (2–4 mg IV) or a similar agent.

3. **Epinephrine** 2 to10 μg/min IV or **dopamine** 3 to 10 μg/kg/min IV may be used if external pacing is not available.

4. Internal pacing is rarely required in the patient with symptomatic recurrent or persistent sinus bradycardia due to sick sinus syndrome.

Sinus Tachycardia

Clinical Features

The ECG characteristics of sinus tachycardia are (*a*) normal sinus P waves and PR intervals and (*b*) an atrial rate usually between 100 and 160 beats/min. Sinus tachycardia is in response to 3 categories of stimuli: (*a*) physiologic (pain or exertion), (*b*) pharmacologic (sympathomimetics, caffeine, or bronchodilators), or (*c*) pathologic (fever, hypoxia, anemia, hypovolemia, pulmonary embolism, or hyperthyroidism). In many of these conditions, the increased heart rate is an effort to increase cardiac output to match increased circulatory needs.

Emergency Department Care and Disposition

The underlying condition should be diagnosed and treated.

Premature Atrial Contractions

Clinical Features

Premature atrial contractions (PACs) have the following ECG characteristics: (*a*) the ectopic P wave appears sooner (premature) than the next expected sinus beat; (*b*) the ectopic P wave has a different shape and direction; and (*c*) the ectopic P wave may or may not be conducted through the AV node (Fig. 2-2). Most PACs are conducted with typical QRS complexes, but some may be conducted aberrantly through the infranodal system. When the PAC occurs during the absolute refractory period, it is not conducted. The sinus node is often depolarized and reset so that, although the interval after the PAC is often slightly longer than the previous cycle's length, the pause is less than fully compensatory. PACs are associated with stress, fatigue, alcohol use, tobacco, coffee, chronic obstructive pulmonary disease (COPD), digoxin toxicity, coronary artery disease and may occur after adenosine-converted paroxysmal supraventricular tachycardia (PSVT). PACs are common in all ages and often seen in the absence of significant heart disease. Patients may complain of palpitations or an intermittent "sinking" or "fluttering" feeling in the chest.

Emergency Department Care and Disposition

1. Any precipitating drugs (alcohol, tobacco, or coffee) or toxins should be discontinued.

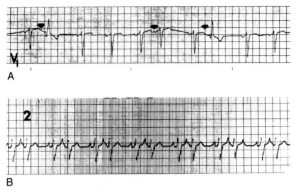

FIG. 2-2. Premature atrial contractions (PACs). **A.** Ectopic P′ waves (arrows). **B.** Atrial bigeminy.

2. Underlying disorders (stress or fatigue) should be treated.
3. PACs that produce significant symptoms or initiate sustained tachycardias can be suppressed with agents such as β-adrenergic antagonists (eg, metoprolol 25–50 mg orally 3 times daily), usually in consultation with a follow-up physician.

Multifocal Atrial Tachycardia

Clinical Features

Multifocal atrial tachycardia (MAT) is caused by at least 3 different sites of atrial ectopy. The ECG characteristics of MAT are (*a*) 3 or more differently shaped P waves; (*b*) changing PP, PR, and RR intervals; and (*c*) atrial rhythm usually between 100 and 180 beats/min (Fig. 2-3). Because the rhythm is irregularly irregular, MAT can be confused with atrial flutter or atrial fibrillation (AF). MAT is found most often in elderly patients with decompensated COPD, but it also may be found in patients with congestive heart failure (CHF), sepsis, methylxanthine toxicity, or digoxin toxicity.

Emergency Department Care and Disposition

1. Treatment is directed toward the underlying disorder.
2. Specific antidysrhythmic treatment is uncommonly indicated.
3. **Magnesium** sulfate 2 g IV over 60 seconds, followed by a constant infusion of 1 to 2 g/h, has been shown to decrease ectopy and convert MAT to sinus rhythm in many patients.

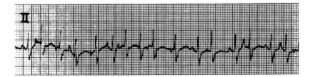

FIG. 2-3. Multifocal atrial tachycardia (MFAT).

4. Because COPD and CHF are relative contraindications to β-blockade, rate control may be achieved with **verapamil** 5 to 10 mg IV or diltiazem 10 to 20 mg IV.
5. Potassium levels should be repleted to greater than 4 mEq/L to increase myocardial membrane stability.

Atrial Flutter

Clinical Features

Atrial flutter is a rhythm that originates from a small area within the atria. The exact mechanism is not known; however, possible mechanisms include reentry, automatic focus, or triggered dysrhythmia. ECG characteristics of atrial flutter are (*a*) a regular atrial rate between 250 and 350 beats/min (most commonly between 280 and 320 beats/min); (*b*) "sawtooth" flutter waves directed superiorly and most visible in leads II, III, and aV_F; and (*c*) AV block, usually 2:1, but occasionally greater or irregular (Fig. 2-4). Carotid sinus massage or Valsalva maneuvers are useful techniques to slow the ventricular response by increasing the degree of AV block, which can unmask flutter waves in uncertain cases. Atrial flutter is seen most commonly in patients with ischemic heart disease. Less common causes include CHF, acute MI, pulmonary embolus, myocarditis, blunt chest trauma, and digoxin toxicity. Atrial flutter may be a transitional dysrhythmia between sinus rhythm and AF. Anticoagulation should be considered in patients with an unclear time of onset or duration longer than 48 hours before conversion to sinus rhythm due to increased risk of atrial thrombus and embolization.

Emergency Department Care

1. Unstable patients or patients with onset less than 48 hours before presentation or low-energy synchronized cardioversion (25–50 J).
2. Stable patients with atrial flutter for longer than 48 hours' duration should be anticoagulated with **heparin** (80 U/kg IV followed by an infusion at 18 U/kg/hr IV). A transesophageal echo can be performed to rule out atrial thrombus before early cardioversion in these patients. If this cannot be performed, patients should be anticoagulated for a minimum of 3 weeks before chemical or electrical cardioversion.
3. Rate control with **diltiazem** 20 mg (0.25 mg/kg) IV over 2 minutes is indicated for patients with normal or impaired (defined by current advanced cardiac life support (ACLS) guidelines as ejection fraction less than 40% or CHF) cardiac systolic function. A second dose of 25 mg (0.35 mg/kg) IV can be given in 15 minutes, if needed. Infusions of 5 to 15 mg/h may be necessary to maintain rate control.

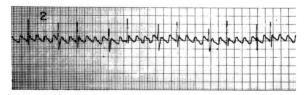

FIG. 2-4. Atrial flutter.

4. Alternative rate control agents for patients with normal cardiac function include **verapamil** 5 to 10 mg IV, **metoprolol** 5 to 10 mg IV, and **digoxin** 0.5 mg IV.

5. Alternative agents for patients with impaired cardiac function include **amiodarone** 150 mg IV over 10 minutes or digoxin 0.5 mg IV.

6. Patients with atrial flutter for less than 48 hours' duration can be considered for chemical or electrical cardioversion in the emergency department. Patients with normal cardiac function can be chemically cardioverted with amiodarone (as above) or **ibutilide** 0.01 mg/kg IV up to 1 mg infused over 10 minutes. A second ibutilide dose may be given if there is no response in 20 minutes. Because of the possibility of provoking torsade de pointes, ibutilide should not be administered to patients with known structural heart disease, hypokalemia, prolonged QTc intervals, hypomagnesemia, or CHF. Patients with impaired cardiac function may be cardioverted with amiodarone or electrically.

Atrial Fibrillation

Clinical Features

AF occurs when there are multiple, small areas of atrial myocardium continuously discharging in a disorganized fashion. This results in loss of effective atrial contraction and decreases left ventricular end-diastolic volume, which may precipitate CHF in patients with impaired cardiac function. The ECG characteristics of AF are (*a*) fibrillatory waves of atrial activity, best seen in leads V_1, V_2, V_3, and aV_F; and (*b*) an irregular ventricular response, usually between 170 to 180 beats/min in patients with a healthy AV node (Fig. 2-5). Predisposing factors for AF are increased atrial size and mass, increased vagal tone, and variation in refractory periods between different parts of the atrial myocardium. AF is can be idiopathic (lone AF) or may be found in association with longstanding hypertension, ischemic heart disease, rheumatic heart disease, alcohol use ("holiday heart"), COPD, and thyrotoxicosis.

Un-anticoagulated patients with AF have a yearly embolic event rate as high as 5% and a lifetime risk greater than 25%. Cardioversion from chronic AF to sinus rhythm carries a 1% to 2% risk of arterial embolism. Therefore, anticoagulation with heparin before conversion to sinus rhythm is recommended in patients with AF for longer than 48 hours' duration and in those patients with an uncertain time of onset.

Emergency Department Care and Disposition

1. Unstable patients should be treated with synchronized cardioversion (100–200 J).

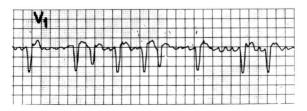

FIG. 2-5.   Atrial fibrillation.

2. Stable patients with AF for longer than 48 hours should be anticoagulated with **heparin** (80 U/kg IV followed by an infusion of 18 U/kg/hr IV) before cardioversion. A transesophageal echo should be considered to rule out atrial thrombus before cardioversion.

3. Rate control with **diltiazem** 20 mg (0.25 mg/kg) IV over 2 minutes is extremely effective for patients with normal or impaired (ejection fraction less than 40% or CHF) cardiac systolic function. A second dose of 25 mg (0.35 mg/kg) IV can be given in 15 minutes if rate control is not achieved. An infusion of 5 to 15 mg/h may be started after the initial dose to maintain rate control. Alternative rate control agents for patients with normal cardiac function include **verapamil** 5 to 10 mg IV, **metoprolol** 5 to 10 mg IV, and **digoxin** 0.5 mg IV.

4. Agents for patients with impaired cardiac function include **amiodarone** 150 mg IV over 10 minutes or **digoxin** 0.5 mg IV.

5. Patients with AF for shorter than 48 hours can be considered for chemical or electrical cardioversion in the emergency department. Patients with normal cardiac function can be electrically or chemically cardioverted with amiodarone, ibutilide (see comments for atrial flutter), procainamide, flecainide, or propafenone. Patients with impaired cardiac function may be electrically or chemically cardioverted with amiodarone.

Supraventricular Tachycardia

Clinical Features

Supraventricular tachycardia (SVT) is a regular, rapid rhythm that arises from impulse reentry or an ectopic pacemaker above the bifurcation of the His bundle. The reentrant variety is the most common (Fig. 2-6). These patients often present with acute, symptomatic episodes termed *paroxysmal supraventricular tachycardia.* In patients with atrioventricular bypass tracts, reentry can occur in either direction, usually (80–90% of patients) in a direction that goes down the AV node and up the bypass tract, thus producing a narrow QRS

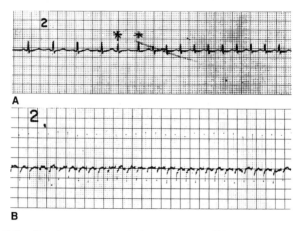

FIG. 2-6.   Reentrant supraventricular tachycardia (STV). **A.** 2nd (*) initiates run of PAT. **B.** SVT, rate 286.

complex (orthodromic conduction). In the remaining 10% to 20% of patients, reentry occurs in the reverse direction (antidromic conduction). Reentrant SVT can occur in a normal heart or in association with rheumatic heart disease, acute pericarditis, MI, mitral valve prolapse, or a preexcitation syndrome.

Ectopic SVT usually originates in the atria, with an atrial rate of 100 to 250 beats/min (most commonly 140–200 beats/min) (Fig. 2-7). This may be seen in patients with acute MI, chronic lung disease, pneumonia, alcohol intoxication, or digoxin toxicity.

Emergency Department Care and Disposition

1. Synchronized cardioversion (25–50 J) should be done in any unstable patient (eg, hypotension, pulmonary edema, or severe chest pain).
2. In stable patients, the first intervention should be vagal maneuvers, including:
   a. Carotid sinus massage: Listen to ensure that there is no carotid bruit and massage the carotid sinus against the transverse process of C6 for 10 seconds at a time, first on the side of the nondominant cerebral hemisphere. This should never be done simultaneously on both sides.
   b. Diving reflex: Have the patient immerse the face in cold water or apply a bag of ice water to the face for 6 to 7 seconds. This maneuver is particularly effective in infants.
   c. Valsalva maneuver: While in the supine position, ask the patient to strain for at least 10 seconds. The legs may be lifted to increase venous return and augment the reflex.
3. **Adenosine** 6 mg as a rapid IV push followed by a 20-mL normal saline rapid flush may be used. If there is no effect within 2 minutes, a second dose of 12 mg IV can be given. Most patients experience distressing chest pain, flushing, or anxiety lasting shorter than 1 minute during treatment. Ten percent of patients may experience transient AF or flutter after conversion.
4. In patients with narrow-complex SVT (orthodromic) and normal cardiac function, cardioversion can be achieved with:
   a. **Diltiazem** 20 mg (0.25 mg/kg) IV over 2 minutes or verapamil 0.075 to 0.15 mg/kg (3–10 mg) IV over 15 to 60 seconds with a repeat dose in 30 minutes, if necessary. Verapamil may cause hypotension that can be treated or prevented with calcium chloride 4 mL of a 10% solution.
   b. **Esmolol** 500 μg/kg IV, **metoprolol** 5 to 10 mg IV, or **propranolol** 0.5 to 1 mg IV.
   c. **Digoxin** 0.5 mg IV.
5. Patients with impaired cardiac function may be cardioverted with amiodarone 150 mg IV over 10 minutes, digoxin, or diltiazem.

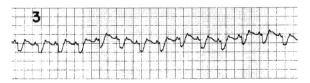

FIG. 2-7. Ectopic supraventricular, tachycardia (STV) with 2:1 AV conduction.

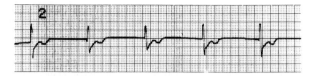

FIG. 2-8. Junctional escape rhythm, rate 42.

6. Patients with wide-complex SVT (antidromic) should be treated as presumed ventricular tachycardia (VT; see Ventricular Tachycardia).
7. Patients with digoxin toxicity can be treated with **phenytoin** (15–18 mg/kg IV infused at 50 mg/min) or **lidocaine** (1–1.5 mg/kg IV followed by an infusion at 1–4 mg/min) can be used for rate control. Patients unresponsive to these agents may require digoxin Fab fragments (empirically 10 vials IV).

Junctional Rhythms

Clinical Features

In patients with sinus bradycardia, SA node exit block or AV block, junctional escape beats may occur, usually at a rate between 40 and 60 beats/min, depending on the level of the rescue pacemaker within the conduction system. Junctional escape beats may conduct retrogradely into the atria, but the QRS complex usually will mask any retrograde P wave (Fig. 2-8). When alternating rhythmically with the SA node, junctional escape beats may cause bigeminal or trigeminal rhythms. Sustained junctional escape rhythms may be seen with CHF, myocarditis, acute MI (especially inferior MI), hyperkalemia, or digoxin toxicity ("regularized AF"). If the ventricular rate is too slow, myocardial or cerebral ischemia may develop. In cases of enhanced junctional automaticity, junctional rhythms may be accelerated (60–100 beats/min) or tachycardic ($\geq$100 beats/min), thus overriding the SA node rate.

Emergency Department Care and Disposition

1. Isolated, infrequent junctional escape beats usually do not require specific treatment.
2. If sustained junctional escape rhythms are producing symptoms, the underlying cause should be treated.
3. Unstable patients with junctional rhythms can be given **atropine** 0.5 mg IV every 5 minutes to a total of 0.04 mg/kg to accelerate the SA node discharge rate and enhance AV nodal conduction.
4. Transcutaneous or transvenous pacing is indicated in unstable patients not responsive to atropine.
5. Patients with digoxin toxicity should be managed as discussed for SVT.

VENTRICULAR DYSRHYTHMIAS

Aberrant Versus Ventricular Tachyarrhythmias

Clinical Features

In general, most patients with wide-complex tachycardia (WCT) have VT and should be approached as having VT until proven otherwise.

1. A preceding ectopic P wave favors aberrancy, although coincidental atrial and ventricular ectopic beats or retrograde conduction can occur in VT. During a sustained run of WCT, AV dissociation favors VT.
2. A changing bundle branch block pattern suggests aberrancy. The right bundle is the slowest to repolarize within the conduction system; therefore, aberrantly conducted beats tend to have right bundle branch block morphology.
3. Coupling intervals are usually constant with ventricular ectopic beats, unless parasystole is present. Changing coupling intervals suggest aberrancy.
4. Response to carotid sinus massage or other vagal maneuvers will slow conduction through the AV node and may abolish reentrant SVT with aberrancy and slow the ventricular response in other types of SVT. These maneuvers have essentially no effect on ventricular dysrhythmias.
5. Fusion beats favor VT but exceptions can occur.
6. A QRS duration longer than 0.14 second is usually found only in ventricular ectopy or VT.
7. Historical criteria are also useful in predicting VT: age older than 35 years or a history of MI, CHF, or coronary artery bypass grafting in a patient with WCT strongly suggests VT.

Emergency Department Care and Disposition

1. If pulseless, treat as VT with unsynchronized cardioversion (200–360 J) followed by epinephrine or vasopressin and ACLS management (see sections on VT and ventricular fibrillation [VF]).
2. Stable patients with WCT and normal cardiac function should be treated with **procainamide** (see Ventricular Tachycardia for dosing). Alternative agents include sotalol and amiodarone. Patients with impaired cardiac function should be treated with amiodarone or lidocaine followed by synchronized cardioversion (see section on VT).
3. **Adenosine** 6 mg IV push may be tried before procainamide in stable patients with suspected SVT with aberrancy without any historical criteria indicative of possible VT (see section on PSVT).

Premature Ventricular Contractions

Clinical Features

Premature ventricular contractions (PVCs) are due to impulses originating from single or multiple areas in the ventricles. The ECG characteristics of PVCs are: (*a*) a premature and wide QRS complex; (*b*) no preceding P wave; (*c*) the ST segment and T wave of the PVC are directed opposite the preceding major QRS deflection; (*d*) most PVCs do not affect the sinus node, so there is usually a fully compensatory post-ectopic pause, or the PVC may be interpolated between 2 sinus beats; (*e*) many PVCs have a fixed coupling interval (within 0.04 second) from the preceding sinus beat; and (*f*) many PVCs are conducted into the atria, thus producing a retrograde P wave (Fig. 2-9).

PVCs are very common, occurring in most patients with ischemic heart disease, and are almost universally found in patients with acute MI. Other common causes of PVCs include digoxin toxicity, CHF, hypokalemia, alkalosis, hypoxia, and sympathomimetic drugs. Ventricular parasystole occurs when the ectopic ventricular focus fires frequently enough to compete with the SA node.

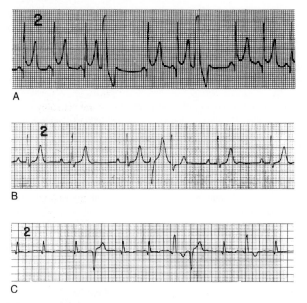

FIG. 2-9. Premature ventricular contractions (PVCs). **A.** Unifocal PVC. **B.** Interpolated PVC. **C.** Multifocal PVCs.

Emergency Department Care and Disposition

1. Stable patients require no treatment. Pooled data and meta-analysis have found no reduction in mortality from suppressive or prophylactic treatment of PVCs.
2. Patients with acute coronary syndromes and frequent PVCs should receive adequate β-adrenergic blockade to suppress ectopic rhythm generation with **metoprolol** 2.5 to 10 mg IV.
3. For hemodynamically unstable patients with PVCs, consider **lidocaine** 1 to 1.5 mg/kg IV (up to 3 mg/kg), although some patients may require procainamide.

Accelerated Idioventricular Rhythm

Clinical Features

The ECG characteristics of accelerated idioventricular rhythm (AIVR) are (*a*) wide and regular QRS complexes; (*b*) rate between 40 and 100 beats/min, often close to the preceding sinus rate; (*c*) most runs of short duration (3–30 beats/min); and (*d*) an AIVR often beginning with a fusion beat (Fig. 2-10). This condition is found most commonly with an acute MI.

Emergency Department Care and Disposition

1. Treatment is not necessary. On occasion, AIVR may be the only functioning pacemaker, and suppression with lidocaine can lead to cardiac asystole.

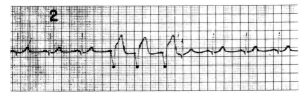

FIG. 2-10. Accelerated idioventricular rhythms (AIVRs).

Ventricular Tachycardia

Clinical Features

VT is the occurrence of 3 or more successive beats from a ventricular ectopic pacemaker at a rate faster than 100 beats/min. The ECG characteristics of VT are (*a*) a wide QRS complex, (*b*) a rate faster than 100 beats/min (most commonly 150–200 beats/min), (*c*) a regular rhythm, although there may be some beat-to-beat variation, and (*d*) a constant QRS axis (Fig. 2-11). The most common causes of VT are ischemic heart disease and acute MI. Other etiologies include hypertrophic cardiomyopathy, mitral valve prolapse, drug toxicity (digoxin, antiarrhythmics, or sympathomimetics), hypoxia, hypokalemia, and hyperkalemia. In general, all WCTs should be treated as VT. Adenosine appears to cause little harm in patients with VT; therefore, stable patients with WCT due to suspected SVT with aberrancy (see previous section) may be treated safely with adenosine when the diagnosis is in doubt.

Emergency Department Care and Disposition

1. Pulseless VT can be defibrillated with unsynchronized cardioversion starting at 200 J. Unstable patients who are not pulseless should be treated with synchronized cardioversion (200–360 J).
2. Hemodynamically stable patients with normal cardiac function should be treated with **procainamide** IV at 20 mg/min until 1 of the following occur: (*a*) the dysrhythmia converts, (*b*) the total dose reaches 15 to 17 mg/kg in healthy patients (12 mg/kg in patients with CHF), or (*c*) early signs of toxicity develop with hypotension or QRS prolongation greater than 50%. The loading dose should be followed by a maintenance infusion of 1 to 4 mg/min in normal subjects. Alternative agents include sotalol, amiodarone, and lidocaine.
3. Hemodynamically stable patients with impaired cardiac function (ejection fraction less than 40% or CHF) should be treated with **amiodarone** 150 mg IV over 10 minutes followed by a 6-hour infusion at 1 mg/min. Alternative therapy with **lidocaine** 75 mg (1.0–1.5 mg/kg) IV over 60 to 90 seconds, followed by a constant infusion at 1 to 4 mg/min (10–40 μg/kg/min) is also acceptable.

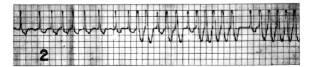

FIG. 2-11. Ventricular tachycardia.

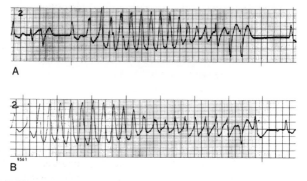

A

B

FIG. 2-12. Two examples of short runs of atypical ventricular tachycardia showing sinusoidal variation in amplitude and direction of the QRS complexes: "Le torsade de pointes" (twisting of the points). Note that the top example is initiated by a late-occurring PVC (lead II).

Torsade de Pointes

Clinical Features

Atypical VT (torsade de pointes, or twisting of the points) occurs when the QRS axis swings from a positive to a negative direction in a single lead (Fig. 2-12).

Drugs that further prolong repolarization—quinidine, disopyramide, procainamide, phenothiazines, and tricyclic antidepressants—exacerbate this dysrhythmia.

Emergency Department Care and Disposition

1. Overdrive pacing at 90 to 120 beats/min can terminate torsades.
2. Reports have shown that **magnesium** sulfate, 1 to 2 g IV over 60 to 90 seconds followed by an infusion of 1 to 2 g/h, is effective in abolishing torsades de pointes.

Ventricular Fibrillation

Clinical Features

VF is the totally disorganized depolarization and contraction of small areas of ventricular myocardium during which there is no effective ventricular pumping activity. The ECG shows a fine-to-coarse zigzag pattern without discernible P waves or QRS complexes (Fig. 2-13). VF is seen most commonly in patients with severe ischemic heart disease, with or without an acute MI. It also can be caused by digoxin or quinidine toxicity, hypothermia, chest

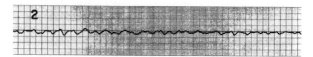

FIG. 2-13. Ventricular fibrillation.

trauma, hypokalemia, hyperkalemia, or mechanical stimulation (eg, catheter wire).

Primary VF occurs suddenly, without preceding hemodynamic deterioration, and usually is due to acute ischemia or peri-infarct scar reentry. Secondary VF occurs after a prolonged period of hemodynamic deterioration due to left ventricular failure or circulatory shock.

Emergency Department Care and Disposition

1. Immediate electrical defibrillation (unsynchronized) should be started at 200 J. If VF persists, defibrillation should be repeated immediately, with 200 to 300 J at the second attempt, and increased to 360 J at the third attempt. Defibrillation pads should be kept on the patient in the same location because, with successive countershocks, transthoracic impedance decreases.
2. If the initial 3 attempts at defibrillation are unsuccessful, cardiopulmonary resuscitation (CPR) and intubation should be initiated.
3. **Epinephrine** 1 mg IV push or **vasopressin** 40 U IV push (1 time only) should be followed by a 20-mL normal saline flush and a repeat countershock at 360 J.
4. Epinephrine 1 mg IV push may be repeated every 3 to 5 minutes, followed by a repeat countershock at 360 J. If this is not successful, high-dose epinephrine (0.1 mg/kg) may be considered.
5. Between successive countershocks, antidysrhythmics should then be administered. Preferred agents, in order of current ACLS recommendations, are **amiodarone** 300 mg IV push, **procainamide** 100 mg IV push every 5 minutes, and **lidocaine** 1.5 mg/kg IV.
6. **Magnesium sulfate** 2 g IV can be given in cases of presumed hypomagnesemia.

CONDUCTION DISTURBANCES

Atrioventricular Block

First-degree AV block is characterized by a delay in AV conduction, manifested by a prolonged PR interval ($\geq$0.2 second). It can be found in normal hearts and in association with increased vagal tone, digoxin toxicity, inferior MI, amyloid, and myocarditis. First-degree AV block needs no treatment and is not discussed further. Second-degree AV block is characterized by intermittent AV conduction: some atrial impulses reach the ventricles, whereas others are blocked, thereby causing "grouped beating." Third-degree AV block is characterized by complete interruption in AV conduction with resulting AV dissociation.

Second-Degree Mobitz I (Wenckebach) AV Block

Clinical Features

With this block there is progressive prolongation of conduction through the AV node itself until the atrial impulse is completely blocked. Usually, only 1 atrial impulse is blocked at a time. After the dropped beat, the AV conduction returns to normal and the cycle usually repeats itself with the same conduction ratio (fixed ratio) or a different conduction ratio (variable ratio).

The Wenckebach phenomenon has a seeming paradox. Although the PR intervals progressively lengthen before the dropped beat, the increments by which they lengthen *decrease* with successive beats. This produces a

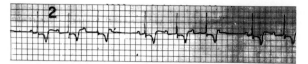

FIG. 2-14. Second-degree Mobitz I (Wenckebach) AV block 4:3 AV conduction.

progressive *shortening* of each successive R–R interval before the dropped beat (Fig. 2-14). This block is often transient and usually associated with an acute inferior MI, digoxin toxicity, or myocarditis or can be seen after cardiac surgery. Because the blockade occurs at the level of the AV node itself rather than at the infranodal conducting system, this is usually a stable rhythm.

Emergency Department Care and Disposition

1. Specific treatment is not necessary unless slow ventricular rates produce signs of hypoperfusion.
2. In cases associated with acute inferior MI, adequate volume resuscitation should be ensured before initiating further interventions to correct hypotension.
3. **Atropine** 0.5 mg IV repeated every 5 minutes as necessary may be given, titrated to the desired heart rate or until the total dose reaches 3.0 mg.
4. Although rarely needed, transcutaneous pacing may be used.

Second-Degree Mobitz II AV Block

Clinical Features

With this block, the PR interval remains constant before and after the non-conducted atrial beats (Fig. 2-15). One or more beats may be non-conducted at a single time. This block indicates significant damage or dysfunction of the infranodal conduction system; therefore, the QRS complexes are usually wide.

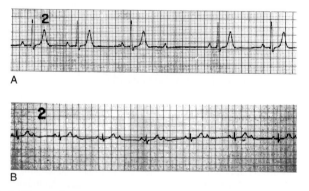

FIG. 2-15. **A.** Second-degree Mobitz II AV block. **B.** Second-degree AV block with 2:1 AV conduction.

Type II blocks are more dangerous than type I blocks because they are usually permanent and may progress suddenly to complete heart block, especially in the setting of an acute anterior MI. When second-degree AV block occurs with a fixed conduction ratio of 2:1, it is not possible to differentiate between a Mobitz type I (Wenckebach) and Mobitz type II block.

Emergency Department Care and Disposition

1. **Atropine** 0.5 to 1 mg IV push, repeated as needed up to 3.0 mg total dose, should be the first drug used, and pacing pads should be positioned on the patient ready for use in the case of further deterioration into complete heart block.
2. Transcutaneous cardiac pacing (see section on sinus bradycardia) is indicated in patients unresponsive to atropine.
3. Transvenous pacing (0.2–20 mA at 40–140 beats/min via a semi-floating or balloon-tipped pacing catheter) is indicated if transcutaneous pacing is unsuccessful. Balloon-tipped catheters are most common, and positioning the patient in the right decubitus position will assist passing the tip into the right ventricle.
4. Most cases, especially in the setting of acute MI, will require permanent cardiac pacemaker placement.

Third-Degree (Complete) AV Block

Clinical Features

In third-degree AV block, there is no AV conduction. The ventricles are paced by an escape pacemaker from the AV node or infranodal conduction system at a rate slower than the atrial rate (Fig. 2-16).

When third-degree AV block occurs at the AV node, a junctional escape pacemaker takes over with a ventricular rate of 40 to 60 beats/min; and, because the rhythm originates from above the bifurcation of the His bundle, the QRS complexes are narrow. Nodal third-degree AV block may develop in up to 8% of acute inferior MIs and it is usually transient, although it may last for several days.

When third-degree AV block occurs at the infranodal level, the ventricles are driven by a ventricular escape rhythm at a rate slower than 40 beats/min. Third-degree AV block located in the bundle branch or the Purkinje system invariably has an escape rhythm with a wide QRS complex. Like Mobitz type II block, this indicates structural damage to the infranodal conduction system and can be seen in acute anterior MIs. The ventricular escape pacemaker is usually inadequate to maintain cardiac output and is unstable with periods of ventricular asystole.

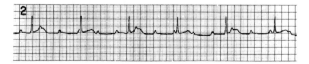

FIG. 2-16. Third-degree AV block.

Emergency Department Care and Disposition

1. Third-degree AV block should be treated the same as second-degree Mobitz II AV block, with atropine or a ventricular demand pacemaker, as required.
2. Transcutaneous cardiac pacing should be performed in unstable patients until a transvenous pacemaker can be placed.

PRETERMINAL RHYTHMS

Pulseless Electrical Activity

Pulseless electrical activity is the presence of electrical complexes without accompanying mechanical contraction of the heart. Potential mechanical causes should be diagnosed and treated, including severe hypovolemia, cardiac tamponade, tension pneumothorax, massive pulmonary embolus, MI, and rupture of the ventricular free wall. In addition, profound metabolic abnormalities such as acidosis, hypoxia, hypokalemia, hyperkalemia, and hypothermia also should be considered and treated.

After intubation and initiating CPR, stabilizing treatment includes **epinephrine** 1 mg IV push repeated every 3 to 5 minutes. This may be followed by high-dose epinephrine at 0.1 mg/kg IV if no response is seen. **Atropine** 1 mg IV, up to 3 mg total, is also acceptable therapy if the rhythm is slow (<60 beats/min).

Idioventricular Rhythm

Idioventricular rhythm is a ventricular escape rhythm at slower than 40 beats/min with a QRS wider than 0.16 second. It is associated with infranodal AV block, massive MI, cardiac tamponade, and exsanguinating hemorrhage.

After intubation and initiating CPR, stabilizing treatment includes identifying contributing mechanical factors (eg, volume resuscitation) and drug therapy with **epinephrine** 1 mg IV push every 3 to 5 minutes. One may also consider high-dose epinephrine at 0.1 mg/kg IV. Atropine has not been shown to be of benefit.

Asystole (Cardiac Standstill)

Asystole is the complete absence of cardiac electrical activity. Treatment is the same as that for pulseless electrical activity with the addition of transcutaneous pacing if the preceding measures fail (although this is rarely successful).

PREEXCITATION SYNDROMES

Clinical Features

Preexcitation occurs when an area of the ventricles is activated by an impulse from the atria sooner than would be expected if the impulse were transmitted down the normal conducting pathway. All forms of preexcitation are felt to be due to accessory tracts that bypass part or all of the normal conducting system, the most common form being Wolff-Parkinson-White (WPW) syndrome (Fig. 2-17). Activation via the AV node and myocardium causes initial fusion beat morphology with slurring of initial QRS complex, causing the pathognomonic delta wave.

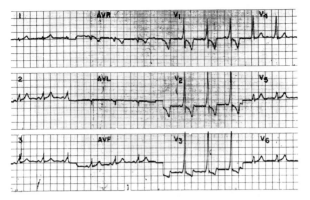

FIG. 2-17. Type A Wolff-Parkinson-White syndrome.

There is a high incidence of tachydysrhythmia in patients with WPW: atria flutter (about 5%), AF (10–20%), and paroxysmal reentrant SVT (40–80%). Among patients with WPW-PSVT, 80% to 90% will conduct in the orthodromic direction and the remaining 10% to 20% will conduct in the antidromic direction. ECG findings of AF or atrial flutter in patients with bypass tracts show a wide QRS complex that is irregular with a rate faster than 180 to 200 beats/min.

Emergency Department Care and Disposition

1. Reentrant SVT with a narrow QRS complex (orthodromic conduction) in WPW syndrome can be treated like other cases of reentrant SVT. **Adenosine** 6 mg IV or **verapamil** 5 to 10 mg IV is very successful at terminating this dysrhythmia in patients with WPW. β-Adrenergic antagonists usually are ineffective.
2. Reentrant SVT with a wide QRS complex in a patient with WPW syndrome usually is associated with a bypass tract with a short refractory period that permits antidromic conduction. Patients with this type of tachycardia are at risk for rapid ventricular rates and degeneration into VF. Unstable patients should be cardioverted at 50 to 100 J. Stable patients should be treated with **procainamide** 100 mg IV push every 5 minutes or an infusion at 20 mg/min to a total of 15 to 17 mg/kg. β-Adrenergic or calcium channel blockers (ie, verapamil) should be avoided.
3. Atrial flutter or AF with a rapid ventricular response and a wide QRS complex is best treated with cardioversion at 50 to 100 J. Stable patients can be treated with procainamide as above.

For further reading in *Emergency Medicine: A Comprehensive Study Guide,* 6th ed., see Chap. 28, "Disturbances of Cardiac Rhythm and Conduction," by Edmund Bolton; and Chap. 29, "Pharmacology of Antidysrhythmic and Vasoactive Medications," by Elizabeth A. Clements and Bryan R. Kuhn.

3 | Resuscitation of Children and Neonates

Douglas K. Holtzman

Children primarily develop cardiac arrest secondary to hypoxia from respiratory arrest or shock syndromes. Because of age and size differences among children, drug dosages, compression and respiratory rates, and equipment sizes differ considerably (Table 3-1).

PEDIATRIC CARDIOPULMONARY RESUSCITATION

Securing the Airway

The airway in infants and children is smaller, variable in size, and more anterior than that in the adult. The prominent occiput and relatively large tongue may lead to obstruction.

Mild extension of the head (sniffing position) opens the airway. Chin lift or jaw thrust maneuvers may relieve obstruction of the airway related to the tongue. Oral airways are not commonly used in pediatrics but may be useful in the unconscious child who requires continuous jaw thrust. Oral airways are inserted by direct visualization with a tongue blade.

A bag-valve-mask system is commonly used for ventilation. Minimum volume for ventilation bags for infants and children is 450 mL. The tidal volume necessary to ventilate children is 10 to 15 mL/kg. Observation of chest rise and auscultation of breath sounds will ensure adequate ventilation.

Endotracheal intubation usually is performed with a Miller (straight) blade in a properly sized tube. Resuscitation measuring tapes have been found to be the most accurate for determining tube size. The formula 16 plus age in years divided by 4 calculates approximate tube size. Uncuffed tubes are used in children up to 8 years. The position of the tube at the lip is 3 times the size of the tube.

Respiratory rates should be started at 20 breaths/min for infants, 15 breaths/min for young children, and 10 breaths/min for adolescents if hyperventilation is not required.

Rapid Sequence Induction

Rapid sequence induction is the administration of an intravenous (IV) anesthetic with a neuromuscular blocking agent to facilitate endotracheal intubation.

1. All equipment and supplies are prepared. A well-functioning IV line must be in place. A cardiac monitor and oximetry should be used. The laryngoscope light source should be checked. Suction equipment should be on and immediately available.
2. Preoxygenate with 100% oxygen.
3. Lidocaine 1 mg/kg IV may be considered in head trauma patients to prevent increased intracranial pressure (ICP), although efficacy recently has been questioned.
4. **Atropine** 0.02 mg/kg (minimum dose, 0.1 mg; maximum dose, 1 mg) should be used to prevent reflex bradycardia in children younger than 5 years.

TABLE 3-1 Length-Based Equipment Chart*

Item	Patient length (cm)						
	54–70	70–85	85–95	95–107	107–124	124–138	138–155
Endotracheal tube size (mm)	3.5	4.0	4.5	5.0	5.5	6.0	6.5
Lip-tip length (mm)	10.5	12.0	13.5	15.0	16.5	18.0	19.5
Laryngoscope	1 straight	1 straight	2 straight	2 straight or curved	2 straight or curved	2–3 straight or curved	3 straight or curved
Suction catheter	8 F	8–10 F	10 F	10 F	10 F	10 F	12 F
Stylet	6 F	6 F	6 F	6 F	14 F	14 F	14 F
Oral airway	Infant/small child	Small child	Child	Child	Child/small adult	Child/small	Medium adult
Bag-valve-mask	Infant	Child	Child	Child	Child	Child/adult	Adult
Oxygen mask	Newborn	Pediatric	Pediatric	Pediatric	Pediatric	Adult	Adult
Vascular access catheter/butterfly	22–24/23–25, intraosseous	20–22/23–25, intraosseous	18–22/21–23, intraosseous	18–22/21–23, intraosseous	18–20/21–23	18–20/21–22	18–20/18–21
Nasogastric tube	5–8 F	8–10 F	10 F	10–12 F	12–14 F	14–18 F	18 F
Urinary catheter	5–8 F	8–10 F	10 F	10–12 F	10–12 F	12 F	12 F
Chest tube	12–16 F	16–20 F	20–24 F	20–24 F	24–32 F	28–32 F	32–40 F
Blood pressure cuff	Newborn/infant	Infant/child	Child	Child	Child	Child/adult	Adult

*Directions for use: (a) measure patient length with centimeter tape; (b) using measured length in centimeters, access appropriate equipment column.

Source: Adapted from RD Luten, RL Wears, J Broselow, et al., Length-based endotracheal tube sizing and emergency equipment for pediatric resuscitation. Ann Emerg Med. 1992; 21:900.

5. Cricoid pressure should be applied before paralysis and maintained until intubation is confirmed.
6. Sedation is accomplished by using a variety of agents based on the clinical situation and the experience of the physician:
   a. **Midazolam** (0.1–0.2 mg/kg IV) has few side effects other than respiratory depression; it produces amnesia but has no analgesic properties.
   b. **Etomidate** (0.2–0.4 mg/kg IV) reduces ICP, is ultra short-acting, but may cause cardiovascular and respiratory depression.
   c. **Thiopental** (2–4 mg/kg IV) decreases ICP but has a negative inotropic effect and causes hypotension.
   d. **Ketamine** (1–2 mg/kg IV) is a bronchodilator, causes little respiratory depression, but increases ICP and blood pressure, and may cause laryngospasm.
   e. **Propofol** (2–3 mg/kg IV) is a rapid-acting, short-duration induction agent. It can cause hypotension and pain on injection and is expensive.
7. Neuromuscular blockade is accomplished by using succinylcholine, vecuronium, or rocuronium.
   a. **Succinylcholine** (2 mg/kg for infants, 1–1.5 mg/kg for children IV) is a depolarizing, rapid-onset (45 seconds), short-duration (3–5 minutes) agent. It has numerous disadvantages. Hyperkalemia (including life threatening); hypertension; rises in intracranial, intraocular, and intragastric pressures; muscle fasciculations; rhabdomyolysis; and malignant hyperthermia. It is relatively contraindicated in patients with burns older than 24 hours, crush injuries, glaucoma, open globe injuries, ICP, or conditions predisposing to hyperkalemia. It also causes bradycardia in young children, particularly infants.
   b. **Vecuronium** (0.1–0.2 mg/kg IV) is a nondepolarizing agent with an onset of 60 –to 90 seconds. It lasts 30 to 90 minutes.
   c. **Rocuronium** (0.6–1.2 mg/kg IV) has a rapid onset of action (45 seconds) and lasts 30 to 60 minutes.
8. The trachea should be intubated, placement confirmed, the tube secured, and cricoid pressure released.

Vascular Access

Vascular access is obtained in the quickest, least invasive manner possible; peripheral veins (arm, hand, foot, or scalp) are tried first. Intraosseous access is a quick, safe, and reliable route for resuscitation medications in the critically ill infant or child. Percutaneous access of the femoral vein or saphenous vein cutdowns also can be used but are more time consuming. Airway management is paramount in pediatric arrest and should not be delayed while obtaining vascular access.

The technique for insertion of the intraosseous line is as follows. The bone most commonly used is the proximal tibia. The anterior tibial tuberosity is palpated with the index finger. The cannulation site is 1 to 3 cm below this tuberosity and in the middle of the anteromedial surface of the tibia. A Jamshidi-type bone marrow needle is used most commonly; if a bone marrow needle is not available, an 18-gauge spinal needle can be used but is prone to bending. With sterile technique, the needle is inserted in a slightly caudal direction until the needle punctures the cortex. The stylet is removed, and marrow is aspirated to confirm placement. If no marrow is aspirated but the needle if thought to be in place, flush is attempted. Fluids or drugs (including glucose, epinephrine, dopamine, anticonvulsants, and antibiotics) may then be administered as they are through a normal IV line.

Fluids

In shock, IV isotonic fluid (ie, normal saline solution) boluses of 20 mL/kg should be given as rapidly as possible and should be repeated, depending on the clinical response. If hypovolemia has been corrected and shock or hypotension persist, a pressor agent should be considered.

Drugs

The indications for resuscitation drugs are the same for children as for adults; the exception is epinephrine, which is considered first-line therapy in children with bradycardia. Proper drug dosages in children require knowledge of the patient's weight. The use of a length-based system such as the Broselow tape for estimating the weight of a child in an emergency situation reduces dosage errors.

The rule of 6s may be used to quickly calculate continuous drug infusions of drugs such as dopamine and dobutamine. The calculation is 6 mg times weight in kilograms: fill to 100 mL with 5% dextrose in water. The infusion rate in milliliters per hour equals the microgram per kilogram per minute rate (ie, an infusion running at 1 mL/h = 1 μg/kg/min, or 5 mL/h = 5 μg/kg/min).

Epinephrine is the only drug proven effective in cardiac arrest. It is indicated in pulseless arrest and in hypoxia-induced slow (bradycardia) rates that are unresponsive to oxygenation and ventilation. The initial dose is 0.01 mg/kg (0.1 mL/kg of 1:10,000 solution) IV or intraosseously or 0.1 mg/kg (0.1 mL/kg of 1:1,000 solution, high dose) by endotracheal route. The second and subsequent doses for epinephrine are the same (0.01 mg/kg [0.1 mL/kg] of 1:10,000 solution), but higher doses (0.1–0.2 mg/kg [0.1–0.2 mL/kg] of 1:1,000) may be considered.

Sodium bicarbonate is no longer recommended as a first-line resuscitation drug. It is recommended only after effective ventilation is established, epinephrine given, and chest compressions to ensure adequate circulation. Calcium also is not recommended in routine resuscitation but may be useful in hyperkalemia, hypocalcemia, and calcium channel blocker overdose.

Dysrhythmias

Dysrhythmias in infants and children are most often the result of respiratory insufficiency or hypoxia, not of primary cardiac causes, as in adults. Careful attention to oxygenation and ventilation therefore are cornerstones of dysrhythmia management in pediatrics.

The most common rhythm seen in pediatric arrest situations is bradycardia leading to asystole. Oxygenation and ventilation are often sufficient in this situation; epinephrine may be useful if the condition is unresponsive to ventilation.

After the arrest situation, the most common dysrhythmia is supraventricular tachycardia (SVT). It presents with a narrow-complex tachycardia with rates between 250 and 350 beats/min. **Adenosine** 0.1 mg/kg given simultaneously with a saline flush as rapidly as possible through a well-functioning IV line as close to the central circulation as possible is the recommended treatment for stable SVT in children. Treatment of the unstable patient with SVT is synchronized cardioversion (0.25–0.5 J/kg).

It is sometimes difficult to distinguish between a fast sinus tachycardia and SVT. Small infants may have sinus tachycardia with rates faster than 200 beats/min. Patients with sinus tachycardia may have a history of fever, dehydration, or shock.

Defibrillation and Cardioversion

Ventricular fibrillation is rare in children but may be treated with defibrillation at 2 J/kg. If this attempt is unsuccessful, the energy is doubled to 4 J/kg. If 2 attempts at defibrillation at 4 J/kg are unsuccessful, epinephrine should be given and oxygenation and acid–base status should be reassessed. Cardioversion is used to treat unstable tachyarrhythmias at a dose of 0.25 to 0.5 J/kg.

The largest paddles that still allow contact of the entire paddle with the chest wall are used. Electrode cream or paste is used to prevent burns. One paddle is placed on the right of the sternum at the second intercostal space, and the other is placed at the left midclavicular line at the level of the xiphoid.

NEONATAL RESUSCITATION

Most newborns do not require specific resuscitation after delivery, but about 6% of newborns require some form of life support in the delivery room. Emergency departments, therefore, must be prepared to provide neonatal resuscitation in the event of delivery in the emergency department.

1. The first step in neonatal resuscitation is to maintain body temperature. The infant should be dried and placed in a radiant warmer.
2. The airway should be cleared by suctioning the mouth followed by the nose with a bulb syringe or mechanical suction device.
3. The examiner should then assess heart rate, respiratory effort, color, and activity quickly over the next 5 to 10 seconds. If the infant is apneic or the heart rate is slow (<100 beats/min), positive-pressure ventilation is administered with bag-valve-mask and 100% oxygen. The rate should be 40 breaths/min. In mildly depressed infants, a prompt improvement in heart rate and respiratory effort usually occur.
4. If no improvement is noted after 30 seconds or the infant's condition deteriorates, endotracheal intubation should be performed.
5. If the heart rate is still slower than 60 beats/min after intubation and assisted ventilation, cardiac massage should be started at 120 compressions per minute. Compressions and ventilations should be in a 3:1 ratio.
6. If there is no improvement in heart rate after these efforts, drug therapy may be used. Most neonates respond to appropriate airway management; therefore, drug therapy is rarely needed. Vascular access may be obtained peripherally or via the umbilical vein. The most expedient procedure in the neonate is to place an umbilical catheter in the umbilical vein and advance to 10 to 12 cm.
7. **Epinephrine** (0.01 mg/kg of 1:10,000 solution) may be used if the heart rate is still slower than 60 beats/min despite adequate ventilation and oxygenation.
8. **Naloxone** (0.1 mg/kg IV) may be useful to reverse narcotic respiratory depression.

9. **Sodium bicarbonate** during neonatal resuscitation remains controversial. A dose of 1 mEq/kg of a 4.2% solution 0.5 mEq/L IV may be given if there is a significant metabolic acidosis; this therapy should be guided by blood gas values.

Prevention of Meconium Aspiration

Aspiration of meconium-stained amniotic fluid is associated with high rates of morbidity and mortality. With proper perinatal management, it is almost entirely preventable. If meconium is noted at the time of delivery, the mouth, pharynx, and the nose, in that order, of the infant should be suctioned after delivery of the infant's head and before delivery of the shoulders. If the infant is vigorous after delivery, the mouth and nose should be suctioned again with no further intervention. If the infant is depressed after delivery, direct suctioning of the trachea should be performed by visualizing the trachea with a laryngoscope and suctioning via an endotracheal tube fitted with a meconium-suctioning adapter. If at any time during this procedure the heart rate decelerates to 100 beats/min or slower, positive pressure ventilation should be started.

For further reading in *Emergency Medicine: A Comprehensive Study Guide,* 6th ed., see Chap. 13, "Neonatal Resuscitation and Emergencies," by Eugene E. Cepeda and Mary P. Bedard; and Chap. 14, "Pediatric Cardiopulmonary Resuscitation," by William E. Hauda II.

4 | Fluids, Electrolytes, and Acid-Base Disorders

David M. Cline

FLUIDS

When altered, fluids and electrolytes should be corrected in the following order: (*a*) volume; (*b*) pH; (*c*) potassium, calcium, and magnesium; and (*d*) sodium and chloride. Reestablishment of tissue perfusion often equilibrates the fluid-electrolyte and acid-base balances. Because the osmolarity of normal saline (NS) matches that of serum, it is an excellent fluid for volume replacement. Hypotonic fluids such as 5% dextrose in water (D_5W) should never be used to replace volume. Lactated Ringer solution is commonly used for surgical patients or trauma patients; however, only NS can be given in the same line with blood components. D_5.45 NS, with or without potassium, is given as a maintenance fluid. The more concentrated dextrose solutions, $D_{10}W$ or $D_{20}W$, are used for patients with compromised ability to mobilize glucose stores, such as patients with hepatic failure, or as part of total parental nutrition solutions.

CLINICAL ASSESSMENT OF VOLUME STATUS

Volume loss and dehydration can be inferred by the patient history. Historical features include vomiting, diarrhea, fever, adverse working conditions, decreased fluid intake, chronic disease, altered level of consciousness, and reduced urine output. Tachycardia and hypotension are late signs of dehydration. On physical examination, one may find dry mucosa, shrunken tongue (excellent indicator), and decreased skin turgor. In infants and children, sunken fontanelles, decreased capillary refill, lack of tears, and decreased wet diapers are typical signs and symptoms of dehydration. Lethargy and coma are more ominous signs and may indicate a significant comorbid condition. Laboratory values are not reliable indicators of fluid status. Plasma and urine osmolarity are perhaps the most reliable measures of dehydration. Serum urea nitrogen (BUN), creatinine, hematocrit, and other chemistries are insensitive.

Volume overload is a purely clinical diagnosis and presents with edema (central or peripheral), respiratory distress (pulmonary edema), and jugular venous distention (in congestive heart failure). The significant risk factors for volume overload are renal, cardiovascular, and liver diseases. Blood pressure does not necessarily correlate with volume status alone; patients with volume overload can present with hypotension or hypertension.

MAINTENANCE FLUIDS

- Adult: D_5.45 NS at 75 to 125 mL/h + 20 mEq/L potassium chloride for an average adult (approximately 70 kg).
- Children: D_5.45 NS or D_{10}.45 NS, 100 mL/(kg · d) for the first 10 kg (of body weight) of the above solution, 50 mL/(kg · d) for the second 10 kg, and 20 mL/(kg · d) for every kilogram thereafter. (See Chap. 82 for further discussion of pediatric fluid management.)

ELECTROLYTE DISORDERS

Correcting a single abnormality may not be the only intervention needed because most electrolytes exist in equilibrium with others. Laboratory errors are common. Results should be double checked when the clinical picture and the laboratory data conflict. Abnormalities should be corrected at the same rate they developed; however, slower correction is usually safe unless the condition warrants rapid or early intervention (eg, hypoglycemia or hyperkalemia). Evaluation of electrolyte disorders frequently requires a comparison of the measured and calculated osmolarities (number of particles per liter of solution). To calculate osmolarity, measured serum values in milliequivalents per liter are used:

osmolarity (mosm/L)

$$= 2 \, [Na^+] + (glucose/18) + (BUN/2.8) + (ETOH/4.6)$$

Hyponatremia ($[NA^+] < 135$ mEq/L)

Clinical Features

The clinical manifestations of hyponatremia occur when the $[Na^+]$ drops below 120 mEq/L; they include abdominal pain, headache, agitation, hallucinations, cramps, confusion, lethargy, and seizures.

Diagnosis and Differential

The volume status and then the measured and calculated osmolarities are evaluated. True hyponatremia presents with a reduced osmolarity. Factitious hyponatremia presents with a normal to high osmolarity. The most common cause is dilutional. It may be brought on by trauma, sepsis, cardiac failure, cirrhosis, or renal failure. Hyponatremia also may be factitious (false measurement of the serum sodium) due to hyperglycemia, elevated protein, or hyperlipidemia. Extracellular fluid or volume status and urine sodium level can classify true hyponatremia (low osmolarity). The syndrome of inappropriate antidiuretic hormone is a diagnosis made by exclusion. Causes of hyponatremia are listed in Table 4-1.

Emergency Department Care and Disposition

1. The volume or perfusion deficit, if any, is corrected first with NS.
2. In stable normotensive patients, fluids are restricted (500–1,500 mL of water daily).
3. In severe hyponatremia ($[Na^+] < 120$ mEq/L) that has developed rapidly with central nervous system (CNS) changes such as coma or seizures, **hypertonic saline,** 3% NS (513 mEq/L), is given at 25 to 100 mL/h. Concomitant use of **furosemide** in small doses of 20 to 40 mg has been shown to decrease the incidence of central pontine myelinolysis.
4. The sodium deficit can be calculated as follows: weight (kg) $\times$ 0.6 $\times$ (140 $-$ measured $[Na^+]$) = sodium deficit (mEq).
5. Complications of rapid correction include congestive heart failure (CHF) and central pontine myelinolysis, which can cause alterations in consciousness, dysphagia, dysarthria, and paresis.

TABLE 4-1 Causes of Hyponatremia

Hypotonic (true) hyponatremia (P_{osm} <275)
  Hypovolemic hyponatremia
    Extrarenal losses (urinary [Na^+] >20 mEq/L)
      Volume replacement with hypotonic fluids
      Sweating, vomiting, diarrhea
      Third-space sequestration (burns, peritonitis, pancreatitis)
    Renal losses (urinary [Na+] >20 mEq/L)
      Loop or osmotic diuretics
      Aldosterone deficiency (Addison disease)
      Ketonuria
      Salt-losing nephropathies; renal tubular acidosis
      Osmotic diuresis (mannitol, hyperglycemia, hyperuricemia)
  Euvolemic hyponatremia (urinary [Na+] >20 mEq/L)
    Inappropriate ADH secretion (CNS, lung, or carcinoma disease)
    Physical and emotional stress or pain
    Myxedema, Addison disease, Sheehan syndrome
    Drugs, water intoxication
  Hypervolemic hyponatremia
    Urinary [Na+] >20 mEq/L
    Renal failure (inability to excrete free water)
    Urinary [Na+] >20 mEq/L
      Cirrhosis
      Cardiac failure
      Renal failure
Isotonic (pseudo) hyponatremia (P_{osm} 275–295)
  Hyperproteinemia, hyperlipidemia, hyperglycemia
Hypertonic hyponatremia (P_{osm} >295)
  Hyperglycemia, mannitol excess and glycerol use

Key: ADH = antidiuretic hormone, CNS = central nervous system.

Hypernatremia ([Na^+] >150 mEq/L)

Clinical Features

The symptoms of hypernatremia usually begin when the osmolarity is greater than 350. Irritability and ataxia occur at osmolarities above 375. Lethargy, coma, and seizures present with osmolarities above 400. Brain hemorrhage can be seen in neonates after rapid infusion of $NaHCO_3$. An osmolarity increase of 2% sets off thirst to prevent hypernatremia. Morbidity and mortality are highest in infants and the elderly who may be unable to respond to increased thirst.

Diagnosis and Differential

The most frequent cause of hypernatremia is a decrease in total body water due to decreased intake or excessive loss. Common causes are diarrhea, vomiting, hyperpyrexia, and excessive sweating. An important etiology of hypernatremia is diabetes insipidus, which results from loss of hypotonic urine. It may be central (no antidiuretic hormone secreted) or nephrogenic (unresponsive to antidiuretic hormone). The causes of hypernatremia are listed in Table 4-2.

Emergency Department Care and Disposition

1. Any perfusion deficits are treated with NS or lactated Ringer solution. Treatment then changes to 0.5 NS after a urine output of 0.5 mL/kg/h

TABLE 4-2 Causes of Hypernatremia

Loss of water
  Reduced water intake
    Defective thirst
    Unconsciousness
    Inability to drink water
    Lack of access to water
  Water loss in excess of sodium
    Vomiting, diarrhea
    Sweating, fever
    Diabetes insipidus
    Drugs including lithium, phenytoin
    Dialysis
    Osmotic diuresis
    Thyrotoxicosis
    Severe burns
Gain of sodium
  Increased intake
    Increased salt use, salt pills
    Hypertonic saline ingestion or infusion
    Sodium bicarbonate administration
  Mineralocorticoid or glucocorticoid excess
    Primary aldosteronism
    Cushing syndrome

is reached. Lowering the $[Na^+]$ more than 10 mEq/L per d should be avoided. Central venous pressure and pulmonary capillary wedge pressure are monitored.

2. Use the formula below to calculate the total body water deficit. As a rule, each liter of water deficit causes the $[Na^+]$ to increase 3 to 5 mEq/L: water deficit (L) = total body water $(1 -$ measured $[Na^+]$/desired $[Na^+]$).

3. If no urine output is observed after NS or lactated Ringer solution rehydration, rapidly switch to 0.5 NS: unload the body of the extra sodium by using a diuretic (eg, **furosemide** 20–40 mg intravenously [IV]).

4. Central diabetes insipidus is treated with **desmopressin** 0.05 mg orally (PO) every 12 hours (dose range is 0.1–1 mg/d divided 2–3 times daily).

5. In children with a serum sodium level higher than 180 mEq/L, peritoneal dialysis using high-glucose, low-$[Na^+]$ dialysate should be considered in consultation with a pediatric nephrologist.

Hypokalemia ($[K^+]$ <3.5 mEq/L)

Clinical Features

The signs and symptoms of hypokalemia occur usually at levels below 2.5 mEq/L and affect the following body systems: the CNS (weakness, cramps, hyporeflexia), gastrointestinal system (ileus), cardiovascular system (dysrhythmias, worsening of digoxin toxicity, hypotension or hypertension, U waves, ST-segment depression, and prolonged QT interval), and renal system (metabolic alkalosis and worsening hepatic encephalopathy); glucose intolerance also can develop.

Diagnosis and Differential

The most common cause is the use of loop diuretics. Table 4-3 lists the causes.

Emergency Department Care and Disposition

1. Replacement of $[K^+]$ at 20 mEq/h will raise the $[K^+]$ by 0.25 mEq/L.
2. Potassium chloride (KCl) 10 to 15 mEq is administered in 50 to 100 mL D_5W, piggybacked into saline over 3 to 4 h. In general, up to 10 mEq/h KCl can be given through a peripheral IV and up to 20 mEq/h can be given through a central line. No more than 40 mEq of KCl in 1 L IV fluids should be added. Patients should be monitored continuously for dysrhythmias.
3. Oral replacement (in the awake asymptomatic patient) is rapid and safer than IV therapy, and 20 to 40 mEq/L KCl or similar agent is used.

Hyperkalemia ($[K^+] > 5.5$ mEq/L)

Clinical Features

The most concerning and serious manifestations of hyperkalemia are the cardiac effects. At levels of 6.5 to 7.5 mEq/L, the electrocardiogram (ECG) shows peaked T waves (precordial leads) and prolonged PR and short QT intervals. At levels of 7.5 to 8.0 mEq/L, the QRS widens and the P wave flattens. At levels above 8 mEq/L, a sine-wave pattern, ventricular fibrillation, and heart blocks occur. Neuromuscular symptoms include weakness and paralysis. Gastrointestinal symptoms include vomiting, colic and diarrhea.

Diagnosis and Differential

Beware of pseudohyperkalemia, which is caused by hemolysis after blood draws. Renal failure with oliguria is the most common cause of true hyper-

---

TABLE 4-3 Causes of Hypokalemia

Shift into the cell
  Alkalosis and sodium bicarbonate
  β-Andrenergics
  Administration of insulin and glucose
Reduced intake
Increased loss
  Renal loss
  Primary hyperaldosteronism, osmotic diuresis
  Secondary hyperaldosteronism associated with diuretics
    Malignant hypertension, Bartter syndrome
    Renal artery stenosis
  Miscellaneous
    Licorice use
    Use of chewing tobacco
    Hypercalcemia
    Liddle syndrome
    Magnesium deficiency
    Renal tubular acidosis
    Acute myelocytic and monocytic leukemia
    Drugs and toxins (PCN, lithium, L-dopa, theophylline)
  GI loss (vomiting, diarrhea, fistulas)

Key: GI = gastrointestinal, PCN = penicillin.

kalemia. Appropriate tests for management include an ECG, electrolytes, calcium, magnesium, arterial blood gases (check for acidosis), urine analysis, and a digoxin level in appropriate patients. Causes of hyperkalemia are listed in Table 4-4.

Emergency Department Care and Disposition

1. Symptomatic patients are treated in a stepwise approach: the cardiac membrane is stabilized with $CaCl_2$ or Ca-gluconate and then the $[K^+]$ is shifted into the cell using glucose and insulin and/or bicarbonate. Potassium is excreted by using sodium polystyrene sulfonate (Kayexalate), diuretics, and dialysis in severe cases.
2. For levels over 7.0 mEq/L or if there are any ECG changes, IV **calcium chloride,** 5 mL of a 10% solution; or **calcium gluconate,** 10 to 20 mL IV, is given. In children calcium gluconate, 0.5 mL/kg of a 10% solution, is given.
3. The presence of digoxin toxicity with hyperkalemia is an indication for digoxin immune Fab therapy (see Chap. 106).
4. For levels above 5.5 mEq/L (especially in acidotic patients), 1 to 2 ampules of **sodium bicarbonate** is given. In children 1 to 3 mEq $NaHCO_2$ per kilogram is given.

TABLE 4-4 Causes of Hyperkalemia

Factitious
Laboratory error
Pseudohyperkalemia: hemolysis and leukocytosis
Metabolic acidemia (acute)
Increased intake into the plasma
Exogenous: diet, salt substitutes, low-sodium diet
Endogenous: hemolysis, GI bleeding, catabolic states, crush injury
Oliguric renal failure
Impaired renin-aldosterone axis
Addison disease
Primary hypoaldosteronism
Other (heparain, β-blockers, prostaglandin inhibitors, captopril)
Primary renal tubular potassium secretory defect
Sickle cell disease
Systemic lupus erythematosus
Postrenal transplantation
Obstructive uropathy
Inhibition of renal tubular secretion of potassium
Spironolactone
Digitalis
Abnormal potassium distribution
Insulin deficiency
Hypertonicity (hyperglycemia)
β-Adrenergic blockers
Exercise
Succinylcholine
Digitalis

Key: GI = gastrointestinal.

5. One ampule of **D$_{50}$W** with 10 to 20 U regular **insulin** IV push (5–10 U in dialysis patients) is given. In children, 0.5 to 1 g of glucose as D$_{10}$W plus insulin 0.5 U/kg is given.
6. Diuresis is maintained with **furosemide** 20 to 40 mg IV push (0.5– 1 mg/kg in children).
7. **Kayexalate** (PO or rectally [PR]) 1 g binds 1 mEq [K$^+$] over 10 minutes. Kayexalate 15 to 25 g PO with 50 mL 20% sorbitol is administered (sorbitol is used because Kayexalate is constipating). Per rectum, 20 g in 200 mL 20% sorbitol is administered over 30 minutes. Kayexalate can exacerbate CHF. In children Kayexalate 1 g/kg PO or PR is given.
8. In patients with acute renal failure, consult a nephrologist for emergent dialysis.
9. **Albuterol** (by nebulization) 0.5 mL 5% solution (2.5 mg) also may be used to lower [K$^+$] (transient effect).

Hypocalcemia ([Ca^{2+}] <8.5 mEq/L or ionized level <2.0 mEq/L)

Clinical Features

The signs and symptoms of hypocalcemia are usually seen with ionized [Ca^{2+}] levels below 1.5. Clinically patients have paresthesias, increased deep tendon reflexes (DTRs), cramps, weakness, confusion, and seizures. Patients also may demonstrate the Chvostek sign (twitch of the corner of mouth on tapping with finger over cranial nerve VII at the zygoma) or the Trousseau sign (more reliable; carpal spasm when the blood pressure cuff is left inflated at a pressure above the systolic blood pressure for longer than 3 minutes). If the patient is alkalotic, ionized calcium (physiologically active) may be very low, even with normal total calcium. In refractory CHF, [Ca^{2+}] may be low.

Diagnosis and Differential

Common causes are shock, sepsis, renal failure, pancreatitis, drugs (usually cimetidine), hypoparathyroidism, phosphate overload, vitamin D deficiency, fat embolism, strychnine poisoning, hypomagnesemia, and tetanus toxin. The ECG often shows prolonged QT.

Emergency Department Care and Disposition

1. If asymptomatic **calcium gluconate** tablets 1 to 4 g/d PO divided every 6 hours with or without **vitamin D** (calcitriol 0.2 µg twice daily) is used. Milk is not a good substitute (low [Ca^{2+}]).
2. In more urgent situations with symptomatic patients, calcium gluconate, or **calcium chloride,** 10 mL 10% solution can be given IV slowly over 10 minutes.

Hypercalcemia ([Ca^{2+}] >10.5 mEq/L or ionized [Ca^{2+}] >2.7 mEq/L)

Several factors affect the serum calcium level: parathyroid hormone increases calcium and decreases phosphate; calcitonin and vitamin D metabolites decrease calcium. Decreased [H$^+$] causes a decrease in ionized [Ca^{2+}]. Ionized [Ca^{2+}] is the physiologically active form. Each rise in pH of 0.1 lowers [Ca^{2+}] by 3% to 8%. A decrease in albumin causes a decrease in [Ca^{2+}] but not in the ionized portion. Most cases of hypercalcemia are due to hyperparathyroidism or malignancies. One third of the patients develop hypokalemia.

Clinical Features

Clinical signs and symptoms develop at levels above 12 mg/dL. A mnemonic to aid recall of common hypercalcemia symptoms is *stones* (renal calculi), *bones* (bone destruction secondary to malignancy), *psychic moans* (lethargy, weakness, fatigue, and confusion), and *abdominal groans* (abdominal pain, constipation, polyuria, and polydipsia).

Diagnosis and Differential

On the ECG depressed ST segments, widened T waves, shortened QT intervals, and heart blocks may be seen. Levels above 20 mEq/L can cause cardiac arrest. A mnemonic to aid recall of the common causes is *PAM P. SCHMIDT*: *p*arathyroid hormone, *A*ddison disease, *m*ultiple myeloma, *P*aget disease, *s*arcoidosis, *c*ancer, *h*yperthyroidism, *m*ilk-alkali syndrome, *i*mmobilization, excess vitamin *D*, and *t*hiazides.

Emergency Department Care and Disposition

1. Emergency treatment is important in the following conditions: a calcium level above 12 mg/dL, a symptomatic patient, a patient who cannot tolerate PO fluids, or a patient with abnormal renal function.
2. Correct dehydration with NS; 5 to 10 L may be required. Invasive monitoring might be considered.
3. **Furosemide** 40 mg may be administered, but dehydration, if present, should be exacerbated. The concurrent hypokalemia or hypomagnesemia should be corrected. Thiazide diuretics should be used because they worsen hypercalcemia.
4. If the above treatments are not effective, **calcitonin** 0.5 to 4 U/kg IV over 24 hours or intramuscularly divided every 6 hours with **hydrocortisone** 25 to 100 mg IV every 6 hours can be used.

Hypomagnesemia

Clinical Findings

$[Mg^{2+}]$, $[K^+]$, and $[PO_4^-]$ move together intra- and extracellularly. Hypomagnesemia can present with CNS symptoms (depression, vertigo, ataxia, seizures, increased DTR, or tetany) or cardiac symptoms (arrhythmias, prolonged QT and PR, or worsening of digitalis effects). Also seen are anemia, hypotension, hypothermia, and dysphagia.

Diagnosis and Differential

The diagnosis should not be based on $[Mg^{2+}]$ levels because total depletion can occur before any significant laboratory changes; it therefore must be suspected clinically. In the United States, the most common cause is alcoholism, followed by poor nutrition, cirrhosis, pancreatitis, correction of diabetic ketoacidosis (DKA), or excessive gastrointestinal losses.

Emergency Department Care and Disposition

1. Volume deficit and any decreased potassium, calcium or phosphate levels should be corrected first.
2. If the patient is an alcoholic in delirium tremens or pending delirium tremens, 2 g **magnesium sulfate** is administered in the first hour and then 6 g for the first 24 hours. DTRs are checked every 15 minutes. DTRs

disappear when the serum magnesium level rises above 3.5 mEq/L, at which time the magnesium infusion should be stopped.

Hypermagnesemia

Clinical Findings

Signs and symptoms manifest progressively; DTRs disappear with a serum magnesium level above 3.5 mEq/L, muscle weakness at a level above 4 mEq/L, hypotension at a level above 5 mEq/L, and respiratory paralysis at a level above 8 mEq/L.

Diagnosis and Differential

Hypermagnesemia is rare. Common causes are renal failure with concomitant ingestion of magnesium-containing preparations (antacids) and lithium ingestion. Serum levels are diagnostic. Coexisting increased potassium and phosphate should be suspected.

Emergency Department Care and Disposition

1. Rehydrate with NS and **furosemide** 20 to 40 mg IV (in the absence of renal failure).
2. Acidosis is corrected with ventilation and **sodium bicarbonate** 50 to 100 mEq, if needed.
3. In symptomatic patients, 5 mL (10% solution) of **calcium chloride** IV antagonizes the magnesium effects.

ACID-BASE PROBLEMS

Initial Assessment

Clinical Features

Several conditions should alert the clinician to possible acid-base disorders: history of renal, endocrine, or psychiatric disorders (drug ingestion); or signs of acute disease: tachypnea, cyanosis, Kussmaul respiration, respiratory failure, shock, changes in mental status, vomiting, diarrhea, or other acute fluid losses.

Acidosis is due to gain of acid or loss of alkali; causes may be metabolic (fall in serum [HCO_3^-]) or respiratory (rise in P_{CO_2}). Alkalosis is due to loss of acid or addition of base and is metabolic (rise in serum [HCO_3^-]) or respiratory (fall in P_{CO_2}). The lungs and kidneys primarily maintain the acid–base regulation. Metabolic disorders prompt an immediate compensatory change in ventilation, thereby venting CO_2 in cases of metabolic acidosis or retaining it in cases of metabolic alkalosis.

Diagnosis and Differential

The effect of the kidneys in response to metabolic disorders is to excrete the hydrogen ion (with chloride) and recuperate [HCO_3^-], a process that requires hours to days. The compensatory mechanisms of the lungs and kidneys will return the pH toward, but not to, normal. Diagnosis and differential must begin with defining the nature of the acid-base disorder (with the stepwise approach below) and then determining the most likely etiology from the differential listings in each section that follows. In a mixed disorder, the pH, P_{CO_2}, and [HCO_3^-] may be normal, and the only clue to a metabolic acidosis is a widened anion gap (AG; see step 4 below).

Stepwise Method of Acid-Base Clinical Problem Solving

1. If the patient's preillness values are known, they are used as a baseline; otherwise, a pH of 7.4, $[HCO_3]$ of 24 mm/L, and P_{CO_2} of 40 mm Hg can be considered normal.
2. If the pH indicates acidosis, the primary (or predominant) mechanism can be ascertained by examining the $[HCO_3^-]$ and P_{CO_2}. If not, see step 3.
3. If the $[HCO_3^-]$ is low (implying a primary metabolic acidosis), then the AG should be examined and, if possible, compared with a known prior steady-state value.
4. The AG is measured as follows: $AG = [Na^+] - ([Cl^-] + [HCO_3^-]) = $ approximately 10 to 12 mEq/L in the normal patient.
5. If the AG is increased as compared with the known previous value or greater than 15, then by definition a wide-AG metabolic acidosis is present. If the AG is unchanged, then the disturbance is a nonwidened (sometimes termed *unchanged* AG or hyperchloremic) metabolic acidosis.
6. The appropriateness of the ventilatory response is examined.
7. If the metabolic acidosis has been present for at least 24 hours, the expected P_{CO_2} can be calculated as $(1.5 \times [HCO_3^-] + 8) \pm 2$. However, if the disorder is acute, then the relationship is simpler: the expected fall in P_{CO_2} in response to a decrease in bicarbonate is the following: P_{CO_2} decreases by 1 mm Hg for every 1 mEq/dL decrease in bicarbonate. This relation holds true provided the bicarbonate level is higher than 8 mEq/dL.
8. If the respiratory change is acute (judged by history), the following formula is used to calculate the expected change in pH when P_{CO_2} changes: the change in $[H^+] = 0.8$ (change in P_{CO_2}). Thus, a 10-mm Hg increment in P_{CO_2} produces an 8-mmol increase in hydrogen ion concentration.
9. If the decrease in the P_{CO_2} equals the decrease in the $[HCO_3^-]$ (or as expected), there is appropriated respiratory compensation.
10. If the decrease in the P_{CO_2} is greater than the decrease in the $[HCO_3^-]$, there is a concomitant respiratory alkalosis. If the decrease in the P_{CO_2} is less than the decrease in $[HCO_3^-]$, there is also a concomitant respiratory acidosis.
11. If the P_{CO_2} is elevated (rather than the $[HCO_3^-]$ decreased), the primary disturbance is respiratory acidosis. The next step is to determine which type it is by examining the ratio of (the change in) $[H^+]$ to (the upward change in) the P_{CO_2}. If the ratio is 0.8, it is considered acute. If the ratio is 0.33, it is considered chronic.
12. If the pH is greater than 7.45, the primary or predominant disturbance is an alkalosis.
13. It is best to look at the $[HCO_3^-]$ first. If it is elevated, there is a primary metabolic alkalosis.
14. If the P_{CO_2} is low, there is a primary respiratory alkalosis.
15. See the sections below for determining the etiology and management.

Metabolic Acidosis

When considering metabolic acidosis, causes should be further divided into wide (elevated) and normal AG acidosis. The term *anion gap* is misleading because in serum there is no gap between total positive and negative ions; however, we commonly measure more positive than negative ions.

TABLE 4-5 Causes of High Anion-Gap Metabolic Acidosis

Lactic acidosis
Type A: Decrease in tissue oxygenation
Type B: No decrease in tissue oxygenation
Renal failure (acute or chronic)
Ketoacidosis
Diabetes
Alcoholism
Prolonged starvation (mild acidosis)
High-fat diet (mild acidosis)
Ingestion of toxic substances
Elevated osmolar gap
Methanol
Ethylene glycol
Normal osmolar gap
Salicylate
Paraldehyde
Cyanide

Clinical Features

No mater what the etiology, acidosis can cause nausea and vomiting, abdominal pain, change in sensorium, and tachypnea, sometimes a Kussmaul respiratory pattern. Acidosis also leads to decreased muscle strength and force of cardiac contraction, arterial vasodilatation, venous vasoconstriction, and pulmonary hypertension. Patients may present with nonspecific complaints or shock.

Diagnosis and Differential

Causes of metabolic acidosis can be divided into 2 main groups: (*a*) those associated with increased production of organic acids (increased anion gap metabolic acidosis; Table 4-5); and (*b*) those associated with a loss of bicarbonate or addition of chloride (normal AG metabolic acidosis; Table 4-6).

A mnemonic to aid the recall of the causes of increased AG metabolic acidosis is: *A MUD PILES: a*lcohol, *m*ethanol, *u*remia, *D*KA, *p*araldehyde, *i*ron and *i*soniazid, *l*actic *a*cidosis, *e*thylene *g*lycol, *s*alicylates, and *s*tarvation.

TABLE 4-6 Causes of Normal Anion Gap Metabolic Acidosis

With a tendency to hyperkalemia	With a tendency to hypokalemia
Subsiding DKA	Renal tubular acidosis—type I
Early uremic acidosis	(classical distal acidosis)
Early obstructive uropathy	Renal tubular acidosis—type II
Renal tubular acidosis—type IV	(proximal acidosis)
Hypoaldosteronism (Addison disease)	Acetazolamide
	Acute diarrhea with losses of HCO_3^- and K^+
Infusion or ingestion of HCl, NH_4Cl, lysine-HCl, or arginine-HCl	Ureterosigmoidostomy with increased resorption of H^+ and Cl^- and losses of HCO_3^- and K^+
Potassium-sparing diuretics	Obstruction of artificial ileal bladder
	Dilution acidosis

Key: DKA = diabetic ketoacidosis.

Caution should be used when applying the A MUD PILES mnemonic because the presence of alcohol in the patient's blood does not rule out a more serious cause of acidosis. Iron and isoniazid exert their effects on the AG due to lactic acidosis. A mnemonic that can aid the recall of normal AG metabolic acidosis is *USED CARP: u*reterostomy, *s*mall bowel fistulas, *e*xtra chloride, *d*iarrhea, *c*arbonic anhydrase inhibitors, *a*drenal insufficiency, *r*enal tubular acidosis, and *p*ancreatic fistula.

Emergency Department Care and Disposition

1. Supportive care is provided by improving perfusion, administering fluids as needed, and improving oxygenation and ventilation.
2. The underlying problem should be corrected. If the patient has ingested a toxin, activated charcoal is administered, the appropriate antidote is given, and dialysis is performed, as directed by the specific toxicology chapters in this handbook. If septic, cultures should be performed and antibiotics adminsitered, as directed by the appropriate chapters in this manual. If in shock, fluids and vasopressors are administered, as directed by the appropriate chapters in Section 2 of this book. If the patient is in DKA, treat as directed in Chap. 130 with IV fluids and insulin.
3. Indications for bicarbonate therapy are listed in Table 4-7.
4. When bicarbonate is given, 0.5 mEq/kg bicarbonate for each milliequivalents per liter desired rise in $[HCO_3^-]$ is recommended. The goal is to restore adequate buffer capacity ($[HCO_3^-] > 8$ mEq/dL) or achieve clinical improvement in shock or dysrhythmias.
5. Bicarbonate should be given as slowly as the clinical situation permits; 1.5 ampules of sodium bicarbonate in 500 mL D_5W produces a nearly isotonic solution for infusion.

Metabolic Alkalosis

The 2 most common causes of metabolic alkalosis are excessive diuresis (with loss of potassium, hydrogen ion, and chloride) and excessive loss of gastric secretions (with loss of hydrogen ion and chloride). Other causes of hypokalemia should be considered.

TABLE 4-7 Indications for Bicarbonate Therapy in Metabolic Acidosis

Indication	Rationale
Severe hypobicarbonatemia (<4 mEq/L)	Insufficient buffer concentrations may may lead to extreme increases in acidemia with small increases in acidosis
Severe acidemia (pH <7.20) with signs of shock or myocardial irritability that is not rapidly responsive to support measures	Therapy for the underlying cause of acidosis depends on adequate organ perfusion
Severe hyperchloremic acidemia*	Lost bicarbonate must be regenerated by kidneys and liver, which may require days

*No specific definition by pH exists. The presence of serious hemodynamic insufficiency despite supportive care should guide the use of bicarbonate therapy for this indication.

Clinical Features

Symptoms of the underlying disorder (usually fluid loss) dominate the clinical presentation, but general symptoms of metabolic alkalosis include muscular irritability, tachydysrhythmia, and impaired oxygen delivery. The diagnosis of metabolic alkalosis is made from laboratory studies showing a bicarbonate level above 26 mEq/L and a pH above 7.45. In most cases, there is also an associated hypokalemia and hypochloremia.

The differential diagnosis includes dehydration, loss of gastric acid, excessive diuresis, administration of mineralocorticoids, increased intake of citrate or lactate, hypercapnia, hypokalemia, and severe hypoproteinemia.

Emergency Department Care and Disposition

1. Fluids are administered in the form of NS in cases of dehydration.
2. Potassium is administered as KCl and no faster than 20 mEq/h, unless serum potassium is above 5.0 mEq/L.

Respiratory Acidosis

Clinical Features

Respiratory acidosis may be life threatening and a precursor to respiratory arrest. The clinical picture often is dominated by the underlying disorder. Typically, respiratory acidosis depresses the mental function, which may progressively slow the respiratory rate. Patients may be confused, somnolent, and, eventually, unconscious. Although frequently hypoxic, in some disorders the decrease in oxygen saturation may lag behind the elevation in Pco_2. Pulse oximetry may be misleading, making arterial blood gases essential for the diagnosis.

The differential diagnosis includes chronic obstructive pulmonary disease, drug overdose, CNS disease, chest wall disease, pleural disease, and trauma.

Emergency Department Care and Disposition

1. Ventilation is increased. In many cases, this requires intubation. The hallmark indication for intubation in respiratory acidosis is depressed mental status. Only in opiate intoxication is it acceptable to await treatment of the underlying disorder (rapid administration of naloxone) before reversal of the hypoventilation.
2. The underlying disorder is treated. High-flow oxygen therapy may lead to exacerbation of CO_2 narcosis in patients with chronic obstructive pulmonary disease and CO_2 retention. These patients should be monitored closely when administering oxygen and intubated, if necessary.

Respiratory Alkalosis

Clinical Features

Hyperventilation syndrome is a problematic diagnosis for the emergency physician because many life-threatening disorders present with tachypnea and anxiety: asthma, pulmonary embolism, diabetic ketoacidosis, and others. Symptoms of respiratory alkalosis often are dominated by the primary disorder promoting the hyperventilation. Hyperventilation by virtue of the reduction of Pco_2, however, lowers cerebral and peripheral blood flows, causing distinct symptoms. Patients complain of dizziness, painful flexion of the wrists, fingers, ankles and toes (carpal-pedal spasm), and, frequently, a chest pain described as tightness.

The diagnosis of hyperventilation due to anxiety is a diagnosis of exclusion. Arterial blood gases can be used to rule out acidosis and hypoxia. Causes of respiratory alkalosis to consider include hypoxia, pulmonary embolism, fever, hyperthyroidism, sympathomimetic therapy, aspirin overdose, progesterone therapy, liver disease, and anxiety.

Emergency Department Care and Disposition

1. The underlying cause is treated. Only when more serious causes of hyperventilation are ruled out should the treatment of anxiety be considered. Anxiolytics may be helpful, such as lorazepam 1 to 2 mg IV or PO.
2. Rebreathing into a paper bag can cause hypoxia; it is not recommended.

For further reading in *Emergency Medicine: A Comprehensive Study Guide,* 6th ed., see Chap. 25, "Acid-Base Disorders," by David D. Nicolaou and Gabor D. Kelen; Chap. 26, "Blood Gases: Pathophysiology and Interpretation," by Kelly Grogan and Peter J. Pronovost; and Chap. 27, "Fluid and Electrolyte Problems," by Michael Londner, Darcie Hammer, and Gabor D. Kelen.

2 | SHOCK

Therapeutic Approach to the Hypotensive Patient

John E. Gough

More than 1 million patients in shock present to emergency departments each year. Despite aggressive management, mortality remains high. Shock occurs when there is circulatory insufficiency between tissue oxygen supply and the resting metabolic demands of the tissues. Such tissue hypoperfusion is associated with decreased venous oxygen content and metabolic acidosis (lactic acidosis). Shock is classified into four categories based on etiology: (*a*) hypovolemic, (*b*) cardiogenic, (*c*) distributive (eg, neurogenic and anaphylactic), and (*d*) obstructive.

CLINICAL FEATURES

Factors that influence the clinical presentation of a patient in shock include the etiology, duration, and severity of the shock state and the underlying medical status of the patient. Often the precipitating cause of shock may be readily apparent (eg, acute myocardial infarction, trauma, gastrointestinal [GI] bleeding, or anaphylaxis). It is not uncommon for the patient to present with nonspecific symptoms (eg, generalized weakness, lethargy, or altered mental status). A targeted history of the presenting symptoms and previously existing conditions (eg, cardiovascular disease, GI bleeding, adrenal insufficiency, or diabetes) will aid in identifying the cause and guide the initial treatment of shock. Drug use (prescribed and non-prescribed) is an essential element of the initial history. Medication use may be the cause or a contributing factor to the evolution of shock. For example, diuretics can lead to volume depletion, and cardiovascular medications (eg, β-blockers and digoxin) can depress the pumping action of the heart. The possibility of drug toxicity and anaphylactic reactions to medications also should be considered.

Assessment of vital signs is a routine part of the physical examination; however, no single vital sign or value is diagnostic in the evaluation of the presence or absence of shock. The patient's temperature may be elevated or subnormal. The presence of hyper- or hypothermia may be a result of endogenous factors (eg, infections or hypometabolic states) or exogenous causes (eg, environmental exposures). The heart rate is typically elevated; however, bradycardia may be present with many conditions, such as excellent baseline physiologic status (young athletes), intraabdominal hemorrhage (secondary to vagal stimulation), cardiovascular medication use (eg, β-blockers and digoxin), hypoglycemia, and preexisting cardiovascular disease.

The respiratory rate is frequently elevated early in shock. Increased minute ventilation, increased dead space, bronchospasm, and hypocapnia may be seen. As shock progresses, hypoventilation, respiratory failure, and respiratory distress syndrome may occur.

Shock is usually, but not always, associated with systemic arterial hypotension, with a systolic blood pressure (BP) below 90 mm Hg. However, early in shock, the systolic and diastolic BPs may initially be normal or elevated in response to a compensatory mechanism such as tachycardia and vasoconstriction. As the body's compensatory mechanism fail, BP typically falls. Postural changes in BP, commonly seen with hypovolemic states, will precede overt hypotension. The pulse pressure, the difference between systolic and diastolic BP measurements, may be a more sensitive indicator. The pulse pressure usually rises early in shock and then decreases before a change in the systolic BP is seen. The shock index (heart rate/systolic BP; normal, 0.5–0.7) is related to left ventricular stroke work in acute circulatory failure. Persistent elevations (>1.0) of the shock index indicates impaired left ventricular function and is associated with increased mortality.

In addition to these vital sign abnormalities, other cardiovascular manifestations may include neck vein distention or flattening and cardiac dysrhythmias. A third heart sound (S_3) may be auscultated in high-output states. Decreased coronary perfusion pressures can lead to myocardial ischemia, decreased ventricular compliance, increased left ventricular diastolic pressures, and pulmonary edema.

Decreased cerebral perfusion leads to mental status changes such as weakness, restlessness, confusion, disorientation, delirium, syncope, and coma. Patients with longstanding hypertension may exhibit these changes without severe hypotension. Cutaneous manifestations may include pallor, pale or dusky skin, sweating, bruising, petechiae, cyanosis (may not be evident if the hemoglobin level is less than 5 g/dL), altered temperature, and decreased capillary refill.

GI manifestations resulting from low flow states may include ileus, GI bleeding, pancreatitis, acalculous cholecystitis, and mesenteric ischemia. To conserve water and sodium, levels of aldosterone and antidiuretic hormone are increased. This results in a reduced glomerular filtration rate, redistribution of blood flow from the renal cortex to the renal medulla, and oliguria. In sepsis, a paradoxical polyuria may occur and be mistaken for adequate hydration.

Early in shock a common metabolic abnormality is a respiratory alkalosis. As the shock state continues and compensatory mechanisms begin to fail, anaerobic metabolism occurs, leading to the formation of lactic acid and resulting in a metabolic acidosis. Other metabolic abnormalities that may be seen are hyperglycemia, hypoglycemia, and hyperkalemia.

DIAGNOSIS AND DIFFERENTIAL

The clinical presentation and presumed etiology of shock will dictate the diagnostic studies, monitoring modalities, and interventions used. The approach to each patient must be individualized; however, frequently performed laboratory studies include complete blood count; platelet count; electrolytes, serum urea nitrogen, and creatinine determinations; prothrombin and partial thromboplastin times; and urinalysis. Other tests commonly used are arterial blood gas, lactic acid, fibrinogen, fibrin split products, D-dimer, and cortisol determinations; hepatic function panel; cerebrospinal fluid studies; and cultures of potential sources of infection. A pregnancy test should be performed on all females of childbearing potential. Other common diagnostic tests include radiographs (chest and abdominal), electrocardiographs, ultrasound or computer tomography scans (chest, head, abdomen, and pelvis), and echocardiograms.

Continuous monitoring of vital signs should be instituted in all patients. In addition to commonly monitored parameters such as pulse, BP, respiratory rate, and temperature, modalities such as pulse oximetry, end-tidal CO_2, central venous pressure, central venous O_2 saturation, cardiac output, and calculation of systemic vascular resistance and systemic oxygen delivery may be indicated.

A search to determine the etiology of the shock must be undertaken. Lack of response to appropriate stabilization measures should cause the clinician to evaluate the patient for a more occult cause. First, the physician must be certain that the basic steps of resuscitation have been carried out appropriately. Consider whether or not the patient has been adequately volume resuscitated. Early use of vasopressors may elevate the central venous pressure and mask the presence of continued hypovolemia. Ensure that all equipment is connected and functioning appropriately. Carefully expose and examine the patient for occult wounds. Consider less commonly seen diagnoses, such as cardiac tamponade, tension pneumothorax, adrenal insufficiency, toxic or allergic reactions, and occult bleeding (eg, rupture ectopic pregnancy, or occult intraabdominal or pelvic bleeding) in the patient who is not responding as expected.

Please refer to the other chapters in this book regarding the evaluation of the specific forms of shock.

EMERGENCY DEPARTMENT CARE AND DISPOSITION

The goal of the interventions is to restore adequate tissue perfusion in concert with the identification and treatment of the underlying etiology.

1. Aggressive airway control, best obtained through endotracheal intubation, is indicated. Remember that associated interventions such as medications (ie, sedatives can exacerbate hypotension) and positive pressure ventilation may reduce preload and cardiac output and may contribute to hemodynamic collapse.

2. All patients should receive supplemental high-flow **oxygen.** If mechanical ventilation is used, neuromuscular blocking agents should be used to decrease lactic acidosis from muscle fatigue and increased oxygen consumption.

3. Early surgical consultation is indicated for internal bleeding. Most external hemorrhage can be controlled by direct compression. Rarely, clamping or tying off of vessels may be needed. All patients require adequate venous access. Cannulation of peripheral veins with large-bore catheters usually provides an adequate route to providing fluid resuscitation. For monitoring and treatment purposes (eg, long-term vasopressors, pacemakers), central venous access may be necessary.

4. The type, amount, and rate of fluid replacement remain areas of controversy. Most use **isotonic crystalloid** intravenous fluids (0.9% NaCl, Ringer lactate) in the initial resuscitation phase. Use of colloids (5% albumin, purified protein fraction, fresh-frozen plasma [FFP], and synthetic colloid solutions [hydroxyethyl starch or dextran 70]) continue to be advocated by some. Due to the increased cost, lack of proven benefit, and potential for disease transmission (with FFP), the routine use of colloids is questionable. Standard therapy in the hemodynamically unstable patient typically has been 20 to 40 mL/kg given rapidly (over 10 to 20 min). Because only about 30% of infused isotonic crystalloids remain in the intravascular space, it is recommended to infuse approximately 3 times the estimated blood loss. However, the benefits of early and aggressive fluid replacement in the emergency department or prehospital setting remain

unproven. Studies have suggested that rapid fluid administration may contribute to ongoing hemorrhage by mechanical effects and dilution of clotting factors. Although it is not appropriate to withhold fluids entirely, some amount of "hypotensive resuscitation" (ie, maintaining mean arterial BP near 60 mm Hg) may be beneficial until surgical control of the bleeding site can be accomplished.

5. **Blood** remains the ideal resuscitative fluid. When possible, fully cross-matched blood is preferred. If the clinical situation dictates more rapid intervention, type-specific, type O (rhesus negative to be given to females of childbearing years), or autologous blood may be used. The decision to use platelets or FFP should be based on clinical evidence of impaired hemostasis and frequent monitoring of coagulation parameters. Platelets are generally given if there is ongoing hemorrhage and the platelet count is 50 000 or lower; administer 6 U initially. FFP is indicated if the prothrombin time is prolonged beyond 1.5 seconds; administer 2 U initially.

6. Vasopressors are used after appropriate volume resuscitation has occurred and there is persistent hypotension. American Heart Association recommendations based on BP determinations are: **dobutamine** 2.0 to 20.0 µg/kg/min for systolic BP over 100 mm Hg, **dopamine** 5.0 to 20.0 µg/kg/min for systolic BP 70 to 100 mm Hg, and **norepinephrine** 0.5 to 30.0 µg/kg/min for systolic BP above 70 mm Hg.

7. Acidosis should be treated with adequate ventilation and fluid resuscitation. Sodium bicarbonate (1 mEq/kg) use is controversial. If it is used, it is given only in the setting of severe acidosis refractory to above-mentioned methods.

8. Early surgical or medical consultation for admission or transfer is indicated.

9. The pneumatic antishock garment is no longer recommended in the treatment of shock but may be used to splint and control bleeding of the lower extremities.

For further reading in *Emergency Medicine: A Comprehensive Study Guide,* 6th ed., see Chap. 30, "Approach to the Patient in Shock," by Emanuel P. Rivers, Ronny M. Otero, H. and Bryant Nguyen; and Chap. 31, "Fluid and Blood Resuscitation," by James E. Manning.

6 | Septic Shock

John E. Gough

Sepsis is a heterogeneous clinical syndrome that can be caused by any class of microorganism. A study from academic medical centers noted an incidence of 2 cases of sepsis per 100 hospital admissions. About 50% of these patients will develop shock, with an average mortality rate of 45%, ranging from 20% to 80% depending on comorbidities. The most frequent sites of infection are the lungs, abdomen, and urinary tract. The majority of sepsis occurs with gram-negative (55–60%) and gram-positive (35–40%) bacteria. Predisposing factors for gram-negative bacterial sepsis include diabetes mellitus, lymphoproliferative diseases, cirrhosis, burns, invasive procedures, and chemotherapy. Risk factors for gram-positive sepsis include vascular catheters, burns, indwelling mechanical devices, and intravenous (IV) drug use. Nonbacterial sepsis is more commonly seen in immunocompromised individuals.

CLINICAL FEATURES

Hyperpyrexia is commonly seen with infectious diseases; however, hypothermia is not uncommon with sepsis and septic shock (particularly with the extremes of age and immunocompromised patients). Other abnormalities concerning vital signs may include tachycardia, wide pulse pressure, tachypnea, and hypotension.

Mental status changes are commonly seen, ranging from mild disorientation to coma. Ophthalmic manifestations include retinal hemorrhages, cotton wool spots, and conjunctival petechiae.

Early cardiovascular manifestations include vasodilatation resulting in warm extremities. Cardiac output is initially maintained or increased through a compensatory tachycardia. Myocardial depression may occur early in sepsis. As sepsis progresses, hypotension may occur. Patients in septic shock may demonstrate a diminished response to volume replacement.

Respiratory symptoms include tachypnea and hypoxemia. Sepsis remains the most common condition associated with acute respiratory distress syndrome, which may occur within minutes to hours from the onset of sepsis.

Renal manifestations include acute renal failure with azotemia, oliguria, and active urinary sediment. Azotemia and oliguria are usually attributed to acute tubular necrosis. Although the exact pathogenesis of acute renal failure is unknown, predisposing factors include hypotension, dehydration, aminoglycoside administration, and pigmenturia.

Liver dysfunction is common, with the most frequent presentation being cholestatic jaundice. Increases in transaminases, alkaline phosphatase (up to 3 times that of normal levels), and bilirubin are often seen. Hyperbilirubinemia may be secondary to red blood cell hemolysis and hepatocellular dysfunction due to endotoxins, cytokines, or immune complex disease. Severe or prolonged hypotension may induce acute hepatic injury or ischemic bowel necrosis.

Major blood loss secondary to gastrointestinal (GI) bleeding occurs in only a small percentage of patients. However, minor blood loss from painless mucosal erosions in the stomach and/or duodenum predispose the patient to upper GI bleeds.

Frequent hematologic changes include neutropenia, neutrophilia, thrombocytopenia, and disseminated intravascular coagulation (DIC). A leukocytosis with a "left shift," resulting from de-margination and release of less mature granulocytes from the marrow, is common. Neutropenia, which occurs rarely, is associated with an increased mortality.

The hemoglobin and hematocrit are usually not affected unless the sepsis is prolonged or there is an associated GI bleed. Thrombocytopenia may be associated with DIC, although isolated thrombocytopenia may be present in more than 30% of patients with sepsis and may be an early clue to bacteremia. More commonly associated with gram-negative sepsis, DIC may have a *compensated* or *decompensated* form. Even though platelets and coagulation factors are consumed more rapidly than normal, bleeding is prevented in the compensated form due to increased coagulation factor production in the liver, release of platelets from storage sites, and increased synthesis of inhibitors. Decompensated DIC presents with clinical bleeding and/or thrombosis. Laboratory studies suggesting DIC include thrombocytopenia, prolonged prothrombin time (PT) and partial thromboplastin time, decreased fibrinogen level and antithrombin levels, and increased fibrin monomer, fibrin split values, and D-dimer values.

Hyperglycemia may be seen even without a history of diabetes, and uncontrolled glucose levels are associated with adverse outcomes. Hyperglycemia may result from increased catecholamines, cortisol, and glucagon. Increased insulin resistance, decreased insulin production, and impaired use of insulin may contribute to hyperglycemia. Rarely, depletion of glucagon and inhibition of gluconeogenesis leads to hypoglycemia.

Early in sepsis, blood gas determinations often show hypoxemia and a respiratory alkalosis. As perfusion worsens and glycolysis increases, a metabolic acidosis occurs from decreased tissue perfusion, glycolysis in peripheral tissues, and impaired hepatic clearance of lactate and pyruvate.

Cutaneous lesions may be (*a*) the result of direct invasion (cellulitis, erysipelas, or fasciitis), (*b*) a consequence of hypotension and/or DIC (acrocyanosis or necrosis of peripheral tissues), and (*c*) secondary to infective endocarditis (microemboli or immune complex vasculitis).

DIAGNOSIS AND DIFFERENTIAL

Septic shock should be suspected in any patient with a temperature above 38°C or below 36°C, systolic blood pressure below 90 mm Hg, and evidence of inadequate organ perfusion. Hypotension typically does not reverse with rapid volume replacement. Other clinical features include mental obtundation, hyperventilation, hot or flushed skin, and a widened pulse pressure. History and physical examination, coupled with other diagnostic modalities, often will aid in identifying the source of infection.

Many diagnostic tests are available to aid in the identification of the source of sepsis; however, septic shock remains a clinical diagnosis. Laboratory tests such as a complete blood count, platelet count, DIC panel (PT, partial thromboplastin time, fibrinogen, D-dimer, and antithrombin concentration), electrolyte levels, liver function tests, renal function tests, arterial blood gas analysis, and urinalysis are often used. Bacterial cultures of blood and urine should be obtained from all septic patients. In addition, cultures of cerebrospinal fluid, sputum, and other secretions should be obtained as indicated. A gram stain and counter immunoelectrophoresis can help quickly identify pathogens and guide initial therapy. Radiographs of suspected foci of infection (chest, abdomen, etc) should be obtained. Ultrasonography or computed tomography may help identify occult infections in the cranium, thorax, abdomen, and pelvis. Because acute meningitis is the most common central nervous system infection associated with septic shock, a lumbar puncture should be performed promptly when indicated. If meningitis is a serious consideration, empiric antibiotic therapy should be instituted as soon as possible. Differential diagnosis should include other noninfectious types of shock such as hypovolemic, cardiogenic, neurogenic, obstructive, endocrine, and anaphylactic.

EMERGENCY DEPARTMENT CARE AND DISPOSITION

1. The ABCs of resuscitation should be addressed. Aggressive airway management with high-flow oxygen (keeping oxygen saturation greater than 90%) through an endotracheal intubation may be necessary.
2. Hemodynamic stabilization is the second step. Rapid infusion of crystalloid IV fluid (lactate Ringer solution (LR) or normal saline) at 500 mL (20 mL/kg in children) every 5 to 10 minutes should be accomplished. Often, 4 to 6 L (60 mL/kg in children) is necessary. In addition to blood pressure, mental status, pulse, capillary refill, central venous pressure, pulmonary capillary wedge pressure, and urine output (>30 mL/h in adult, >1 mL/[kg · h] in children) should be monitored. If ongoing blood loss (eg, GI bleed) is suspected, blood replacement may be necessary.
3. If there is no response to fluid administration, **dopamine** 5 to 20 μg/kg/min titrated to response should be used.
4. If blood pressure remains below 70 mm Hg despite the preceding measures, **norepinephrine** 8 to 12 μg/min loading dose and 2 to 4 μg/min infusion to maintain mean arterial blood pressure of at least 60 mm Hg should be started. Norepinephrine may be more effective than dopamine.
5. The source of infection must be removed (eg, removal of indwelling catheters and incision and drainage (I&D) of abscesses).
6. Empiric antibiotic therapy is ideally begun after obtaining cultures, but administration should not be delayed. Dosages should be the maximum allowed and given intravenously. Initial and loading doses are listed below. When the source is unknown, therapy should be effective against gram-positive and gram-negative organisms. For antibiotic therapy in children, see Chap. 66. In adults a third-generation **cephalosporin** (eg, **ceftriaxone** 1 g IV, **cefotaxime** 2 g IV, or **ceftazidime** 2 g IV) or an antipseudomonal β-lactamase–susceptible penicillin (**imipenem** 750 mg IV) can be used. Also recommended is the addition of an aminoglycoside (**gentamicin** 2 mg/kg IV or **tobramycin** 2 mg/kg IV) to this regimen. In immunocompromised adults, **cetazidime** 2 g IV, **imipenem** 750 mg IV, or **meropenem** 1 g IV alone is acceptable. If there is high probability of gram-positive etiology (eg, illicit drug use), **oxacillin** 2 g IV or **vancomycin** 15 mg/kg IV should be added. If an anaerobic source is suspected (eg, intraabdominal, genital tract, odontologic, or necrotizing soft tissue infection), **metronidazole** 7.5 mg/kg IV or **clindamycin** 0.45 g IV also should be administered. If *Legionella* is a potential source, **erythromycin** 0.5 g IV can be added. **Vancomycin** 15 mg/kg IV can be administered if indwelling vascular devices are present.

7. Acidosis is treated with oxygen, ventilation, and IV fluid replacement. If severe, administration of sodium bicarbonate 1 mEq/kg IV is acceptable or as directed by arterial blood gases.

8. DIC should be treated with **fresh-frozen plasma,** 15 to 20 mL/kg initially, to keep PT at 1.5 to 2 times normal, and treated with a **platelet infusion** of 6 U, to maintain a serum concentration of at least $50,000/\mu L$.

9. If adrenal insufficiency is suspected, glucocorticoid (**hydrocortisone** 100mg IV) should be administered.

10. Tight glucose control (80–100 mg/dL) with intensive insulin therapy has demonstrated decreased mortality from multiorgan failure.

11. Multiple innovative therapies are currently under investigation. For more information, refer to Chap. 32 in *Emergency Medicine: A Comprehensive Study Guide,* 6th ed.

For further reading in *Emergency Medicine: A Comprehensive Study Guide,* 6th ed., see Chap. 32, "Septic Shock," by Jonathan Jui.

7 | Cardiogenic Shock

Rawle A. Seupaul

Cardiogenic shock occurs when there is insufficient cardiac output to meet the metabolic demands of the tissues. It usually results from an acute myocardial infarction (AMI) that affects greater than 40% of the left ventricular myocardium. Other etiologies include left ventricular aneurysm, cardiomyopathies, myocarditis, myocardial contusion, and drug or toxin effects. Mechanical impairments to systemic blood flow such as valvular dysfunctions, pulmonary embolism, wall rupture, tamponade, and aortic dissection also may play a role in the development of cardiogenic shock. Cardiogenic shock is the most common cause of in-hospital mortality from AMI, with an overall mortality of 40% to 50%. Most patients who develop cardiogenic shock will display symptoms within the first 8 hours.

CLINICAL FEATURES

The hallmark of all shock states is hypoperfusion. Cardiogenic shock commonly, but not always, presents with hypotension (systolic blood pressure < 90 mm Hg). Systolic blood pressure may be greater than 90 mm Hg if there is preexisting hypertension or compensatory increases in systemic vascular resistance. Other blood pressure parameters that may be more sensitive are a 30 mm Hg decrease in mean arterial blood pressure and a pulse pressure of less than 20 mm Hg. Sinus tachycardia is frequently seen, and treatment should be directed at the underlying cause. Other common findings include cool, clammy skin and oliguria. Decreased cerebral perfusion and hypoxemia may lead to mental status changes such as anxiety and confusion. Concomitant left ventricular failure frequently will present with tachypnea, rales, wheezing, and frothy sputum. Jugular venous distention without pulmonary edema in the setting of hypotension should raise the suspicion of right ventricular infarction, tamponade, or pulmonary embolus. Cardiac auscultation should be performed to identify the presence of a third (S_3) or fourth (S_4) heart sound. The presence of a murmur may represent valvular dysfunction or septal defects.

DIAGNOSIS AND DIFFERENTIAL

As with most patients encountered in the emergency department, a careful, directed history and physical examination are useful in the initial evaluation of a patient with suspected AMI and cardiogenic shock. Other clinical entities that may mimic cardiogenic shock include aortic dissection, pulmonary embolus, pericardial tamponade, acute valvular insufficiency, hemorrhage, and sepsis.

Perhaps the first and most important test to order is an electrocardiogram. The electrocardiogram will aid in the detection of ischemia or infarction, arrhythmias, electrolyte abnormalities, or drug toxicity. Care should be taken to look for evidence of right ventricular infarction that can be detected by ST-segment elevation in the right precordial leads. Right ventricular infarction increases mortality from approximately 6% to 31%. A chest radiogram also should be obtained to look for pulmonary edema, abnormally wide mediastinum, or other abnormalities of the cardiac silhouette.

57

Other ancillary tests are a complete blood count, coagulation profile, and chemistries. Cardiac markers such as troponin and creatine kinase-MB also should be obtained to establish the diagnosis of AMI. If available, B-type natruretic peptide also should be obtained. This marker has been shown to correlate with left ventricular end-diastolic pressure and is an excellent predictor of clinical development of heart failure after AMI.

Transthoracic echocardiography (TTE) is a useful bedside tool when evaluating a patient in cardiogenic shock. TTE can provide information on ventricular dysfunction and early myocardial dysfunction by visualizing a lack of compensatory hyperkinesis in the uninvolved myocardium. TTE also may aid in the diagnosis of other causes of cardiogenic shock including right ventricular dysfunction secondary to increased pulmonary hypertension as seen in pulmonary embolus, cardiac tamponade, and aortic root dissection.

EMERGENCY DEPARTMENT CARE AND DISPOSITION

For any patient in cardiogenic shock, close attention to the ABCs of resuscitation and established Advanced Cardiac Life Support (ACLS) guidelines are critical for immediate stabilization. Recent reports have emphasized the importance of thrombolytic therapy, intraaortic balloon counter pulsation, and early revascularization as methods to minimize morbidity and mortality in these patients. When appropriate, patients in cardiogenic shock should be transported to a facility with these capabilities if they do not exist at your venue.

1. Intravenous access, cardiac rhythm, and pulse oximetry monitoring should be initiated. Endotracheal intubation should be considered as needed.
2. Rhythm disturbances, hypoxemia, hypovolemia, and electrolyte abnormalities should be identified and treated.
3. The patient should chew and swallow **aspirin** 160 to 325 mg, unless there is an allergy or contraindication.
4. For chest pain, titrated intravenous **nitroglycerin** 5 to 100 μg/min or **morphine sulfate** given in 2-mg increments should be administered as needed. Hemodynamic parameters should be monitored.
5. For mild to moderate hypotension without hypovolemia, **dobutamine** 2.5 to 20.0 μg/kg/min should be administered. For severe hypotension, **dopamine** 2.5 to 20.0 μg/kg/min should be administered titrated to the desired effect with the lowest dose possible.
6. Intravenous **nitroglycerin** 5 to 100 μg/min and **sodium nitroprusside** 0.5 to 10.0 μg/kg/min should be administered to improve cardiac output through reduction of preload and afterload.
7. **Norepinephrine** may be used if there has been no or poor response to other pressors. An infusion should begin at 2 μg/min and titrated to the desired effect.
8. **Milrinone** may be used as a positive inotrope, but its use is best guided with a pulmonary artery catheter in place. Start with a loading dose of 50 μg/kg intravenously over 10 minutes followed by an infusion of 0.5 μg/kg/min.
9. As a temporizing measure, intraaortic balloon pump counter pulsation should be considered to decrease afterload and to augment coronary perfusion.

10. Thrombolytic therapy, percutaneous transluminal angioplasty, or emergent coronary artery bypass graft should be used as indicated or available.
11. Cardiology and cardiac surgery should be consulted early. Transfer should be arranged if indicated.

For further reading in *Emergency Medicine: A Comprehensive Study Guide,* 6th ed., see Chap. 33, "Cardiogenic Shock," by W. Frank Peacock IV and James Edward Weber.

8 | Anaphylaxis and Acute Allergic Reactions

Damian F. McHugh

Allergic reactions range from trivial urticaria to full-blown anaphylaxis. Although most acute allergic reactions are type I, in which the antigen interacts with immunoglobulin E (IgE) on mast cells and basophils, other hypersensitivity reactions include type II, the antigen interacting with IgG and IgM antibodies (eg, blood transfusion reaction and idiopathic thrombocytopenic purpura); type III, the deposition of antigen–antibody complexes (eg, serum sickness and poststreptococcal glomerulonephritis); and type IV, delayed hypersensitivity reaction from T lymphocytes (eg, poison ivy and the tuberculosis skin test).

CLINICAL FEATURES

Anaphylaxis may occur within seconds, but can be delayed an hour, after a sensitized individual is exposed to (*a*) drugs (penicillin and trimethoprim-sulfamethoxazole), (*b*) foods (shellfish, nuts, eggs, and preservatives such as sulfites and tetrazine dyes), and (*c*) stings, especially hymenoptera. Dextran, codeine, and radiocontrast material can cause an anaphylactoid reaction, which is non-IgE mediated and requires no sensitizing exposure. Aspirin and other nonsteroidal antiinflammatory drugs can cause anaphylactic symptoms through modulation of the cyclooxygenase–arachidonic acid pathway.

Clinical features of anaphylactic reactions range from local organ involvement to serious multisystem effects. Dermatologic features include pruritus, urticaria, and erythema multiforme (typical target skin lesions). Angioedema is a similar but deeper reaction, with dermal edema mostly affecting the face and neck and distal extremities; it can be seen as an isolated response (in 0.5%) to angiotensin-converting enzyme inhibitors. By definition, anaphylaxis includes respiratory compromise or cardiovascular collapse. Respiratory features may include laryngeal swelling, stridor, and wheeze. Gastrointestinal features include nausea, cramps, vomiting, and diarrhea. Untreated anaphylaxis causes shock with tachycardia and hypotension. Cardiac patients are susceptible to myocardial ischemia and an exaggerated allergic response if on β-blockers. If patients survive the initial insult, a second "biphasic" mediator release can occur at 4 to 8 hours in up to 20% of cases.

DIAGNOSIS AND DIFFERENTIAL

Diagnosis is based on symptoms. History may confirm exposure to a possible allergen, such as a new drug, food, or sting. There is no specific test available to confirm the diagnosis. Workup may be directed at ruling out other diagnoses or achieving patient stabilization. Differential diagnosis includes myocardial infarction, asthma, carcinoid, hereditary angioneurotic edema, and vasovagal reactions.

EMERGENCY DEPARTMENT CARE AND DISPOSITION

The airway is the primary concern. Patients with respiratory symptoms or abnormal vital signs should be placed on pulse oximetry and cardiac monitor with intravenous access. The combination of oxygen and epinephrine may reverse any impending respiratory compromise.

1. Oxygen should be administered as indicated by oximetry. Endotracheal intubation can be difficult because of angioedema or laryngeal spasm but should be anticipated. Preparations also should be made for "rescue" transtracheal jet insufflation or cricothyroidotomy.

2. Limit further exposure. This may be as simple as stopping an intravenous drug or removing a stinger. First aid measures, ice, and elevation may be helpful for local symptoms.

3. Patients with concerning airway symptoms should receive **epinephrine.** This should be given intramuscularly 0.3 to 0.5 mg (0.3 to 0.5 mL) of 1:1000 (pediatric dose, 0.01 mL/kg). Intramuscular administration has been shown to be superior to the subcutaneous route and should now be the initial treatment route of choice. The thigh achieves better peak blood levels than the deltoid.

4. Hypotensive patients require large volumes of crystalloid fluids due to the effects of distributive shock. If patients are still hypotensive after 1 to 2 L, then administer intravenous epinephrine. A bolus of 100 μg of 1:100,000 dilution (0.1 mL of 1:1000 in 10 mL normal saline) can be given over 5 to 10 minutes, with close observation for chest pain or arrhythmias.

5. Every patient with allergic symptoms requires antihistamines. **Diphenhydramine** can be given 25 to 50 mg (pediatric dose, 1 mg/kg), intravenously in serious cases. In addition, an H_2 blocker such as **ranitidine** 50 mg intravenously (pediatric dose, 0.5 mg/kg) may be helpful.

6. Bronchospasm can be treated with nebulized β-agonists such as **albuterol** 5% 0.5 mL in 3 mL saline. If refractory, consider inhaled anticholinergics or intravenous magnesium (2 g over 20–30 minutes in adults, 25–50 mg/kg in children).

7. Steroids are useful in controlling persistent or delayed allergic reactions. Severe cases can be treated with **methylprednisolone** 125 mg (pediatric dose, 1 to 2 mg/kg) intravenously. Milder reactions can be treated with oral **prednisone** 60 mg.

8. For patients on β-blockers, **glucagon** (1–2 mg every 5 minutes) can be used for hypotension refractory to epinephrine and fluids.

9. Patients with symptomatic hereditary angioneurotic edema should be treated with C1 esterase inhibitor replacement in consultation with an appropriate specialist.

After mild reactions, patients should be observed for 3 to 4 hours before discharge. Patients with angiotensin-converting enzyme inhibitor angioedema are often refractory to conventional therapy; patients with moderate to severe symptoms should be admitted for close observation. Discharge such patients on an antihistamine and prednisone for 4 days (the evidence for steroids is weak). Counsel all patients about the need to return to the emergency department in the event of late recurrence of symptoms. All serious cases deserve discussion of a self-administered epinephrine kit, Medic-Alert bracelets, and referral to an allergist. Unstable or refractory patients always merit admission to the intensive care unit.

For further reading in *Emergency Medicine: A Comprehensive Study Guide,* 6th ed., see Chap. 34, "Anaphylaxis and Acute Allergic Reactions," by Brian H. Rowe and Stuart Carr.

9 | Neurogenic Shock

Rawle A. Seupaul

Neurogenic shock is caused by an acute injury to the spinal cord, which is usually characterized by bradycardia and hypotension secondary to disruption of sympathetic outflow. This entity should not be confused with spinal shock, which is a temporary loss of spinal reflexes below the level of the injury. Most acute spinal cord injuries occur via blunt trauma, with penetrating injuries accounting for only 10% to 15% of cases. Approximately 10,000 cord injuries occur each year in the United States.

CLINICAL FEATURES

Patients with neurogenic shock are hypotensive, with warm, dry skin. These findings result from a loss of sympathetic tone disallowing redirection of blood volume from the periphery to the core. Most also will exhibit bradycardia due to increased vagal tone. These symptoms may last from 1 to 3 weeks.

The anatomic level of cord injury determines the severity of neurogenic shock. In general, the higher the injury, the more likely and severe symptoms may be. Injuries above T1 are more likely to result in a loss of sympathetic tone, and injuries from T1 to T3 may result in only a partial disruption.

DIAGNOSIS AND DIFFERENTIAL

The key to diagnosing neurogenic shock is to remember that it is a diagnosis of exclusion. Stringent adherence to a regimented and thorough evaluation of the traumatized patient is always recommended, beginning with the ABCDEs (see Chap. 157). It should be assumed that hypotension is the result of ongoing blood loss. Once other causes of hypotension have been excluded, the diagnosis of neurogenic shock can be safely made.

EMERGENCY DEPARTMENT CARE AND DISPOSITION

Adequate resuscitation should be accomplished quickly to minimize secondary cord injury from hypoperfusion or hypoxia (see Chap. 162).

1. The airway should be secured with inline spinal immobilization and protection.
2. **Intravenous fluids** should be administered to maintain a mean arterial pressure of 85 to 90 mm Hg. Excessive fluid resuscitation should be avoided to prevent heart failure and pulmonary edema. Use of a pulmonary artery catheter may be useful in preventing this iatrogenic complication. Although usually effective, if intravenous fluids do not suffice, pressor agents may be used to improve cardiac output and spinal cord perfusion pressure. Agents such as **dopamine** 2.5 to 20.0 μg/kg/min and **dobutamine** 2.0 to 20.0 μg/kg/min should be used and titrated to the desired effect.
3. Bradycardia may be treated with **atropine** 0.5 to 1.0 mg intravenously every 5 minutes for a total of 3 mg. If necessary, a pacemaker may be used.
4. Although this treatment is not without controversy, the current recommendation is high-dose **methylprednisolone** therapy instituted within the

first 8 hours of injury. A 30 mg/kg bolus over 15 minutes is followed by an infusion of 5.4 mg/kg/h for 23 hours.
5. Immediate consultation with trauma surgery, neurosurgery, and orthopedic surgery should be obtained if available, or the patient should be transferred to a regional spine or trauma center.

For further residing in *Emergency Medicine: A Comprehensive Guide,* 6th ed., see Chap. 35, "Neurogenic Shock," by Brian Euerle and Thomas Scalea.

3 | ANALGESIA, ANESTHESIA, AND SEDATION

10 | Acute Pain Management and Procedural Sedation

Diamond Vrocher

Acute pain is present in 50% to 60% of all emergency department (ED) patients. Factors that may contribute to the underuse of sedation and analgesia in the ED include communication barriers between patient and physician, lack of knowledge about sedative and analgesic agents, and fear of adverse events. Procedural sedation and analgesia (PSA) often is needed for painful interventions or diagnostic studies.

CLINICAL FEATURES

Physiologic responses to pain and anxiety include increased heart rate, blood pressure, and respiratory rate. Behavioral changes include facial expressions, posturing, crying, and vocalization. Because subjective impressions may be inaccurate, pain is best assessed with objective scales. Pain relief is a dynamic process, and reassessment is mandatory.

EMERGENCY DEPARTMENT CARE AND DISPOSITION

Pharmacologic and nonpharmacologic interventions may be helpful for treating anxiety and pain in the ED. Nonpharmacologic interventions, which may be used alone or adjunctively, include the application of heat or cold, immobilization and elevation of injured extremities, explanation and reassurance, music, biofeedback, guided imagery, and distraction. Communication with the patient in pain should be gentle, unhurried, and appropriate for the developmental stage of the patient. Discussing a painful intervention with a pediatric patient immediately before the procedure may decrease the anxiety created by anticipation. Parents should be included in pediatric interventions to help alleviate anxiety. If physical restraint is required for a child, the parents should not be responsible for restraining their child. When pharmacologic intervention is needed, the selection of agent should be guided by the need for sedation or analgesia, the route of delivery, and the desired duration of effects.

Systemic Analgesia and Sedation

The indications for PSA include abscess drainage, wound management, tube thoracostomy, orthopedic manipulation, cardioversion, and diagnostic studies. Analgesia is relief from the perception of pain. Minimal sedation is a drug-induced state characterized by normal responses to voice and normal cardiac and ventilatory functions. Moderate sedation and analgesia (conscious sedation) are characterized by responsiveness to voice or light tactile stimulation with normal cardiac and ventilatory functions. Deep sedation and analgesia are characterized by responsiveness to repeated or painful stimulation, potentially inadequate ventilation, and potential loss of protective reflexes.

Preparation

When PSA is performed, necessary equipment includes a continuous cardiac monitor and pulse oximetry, oxygen, suction, and immediate availability of

67

appropriate-size resuscitation equipment. The patient should be under constant observation by a provider trained in airway management. Informed consent should be obtained. Blood pressure, heart rate, respiratory rate, and level of consciousness should be assessed at baseline and every 5 to 10 minutes. The analgesic or sedative agents chosen should be individualized to the patient and the planned procedure. The agents used for PSA often have a narrow therapeutic index. Therefore, the agents should be administered in small, incremental intravenous doses, with adequate time between doses to determine peak effect. Other routes of administration may be appropriate (especially in children) but provide less ability to titrate the dose to produce the desired effect. All patients undergoing PSA should be reassessed continuously. Patients experiencing transient respiratory depression frequently can be managed by bag-mask-valve ventilation; however, some patients will require intubation.

Pre-calculated doses of reversal agents should be available: **naloxone** 0.1 mg/kg (up to 2 mg) every 2 to 3 minutes until the desired effect of reversing opiate-induced respiratory depression; and **flumazenil** 0.01 to 0.02 mg/kg (up to 0.2 mg) every 1 to 2 minutes until the desired effect of reversing benzodiazepine-induced respiratory depression. Because the half-lives of naloxone and flumazenil may be shorter than those of the drugs they reverse, patients who require reversal should be observed for a prolonged period to avoid rebound respiratory depression. Flumazenil should not be used in patients on chronic benzodiazepine or tricyclic antidepressant therapy due to the risk of seizure. Flumazenil is not recommended to routinely "wake up" patients from PSA.

Non-Opiate Analgesics

Acetaminophen is an anti-inflammatory and analgesic that can be used alone for mild pain or adjunctively with opiates for moderate to severe pain. **Acetaminophen** (15 mg/kg orally [PO] or rectally [PR] every 6 hours) dosing is not age dependent. Acetaminophen may be hepatotoxic above 140 mg/kg per d.

The nonsteroidal anti-inflammatory drugs (NSAIDS; aspirin, naproxen, indomethacin, ibuprofen, and ketorolac) are anti-inflammatory and analgesic agents with opiate-sparing effects. **Ketorolac** (0.5-1 mg/kg intramuscularly [IM], intravenously [IV], or PO, up to 60 mg) is the only parenteral NSAID available in the United States. **Ibuprofen** (10 mg/kg PO) is safe in children older than 6 months. Adverse effects of NSAIDS include renal dysfunction, platelet dysfunction, impaired coagulation, and gastrointestinal irritation. Aspirin should be avoided in children because of an association with Reye syndrome.

Opiates

Opiates are the agents of choice for moderate to severe pain and for procedural analgesia. Side effects of opiates include respiratory depression, nausea and vomiting, confusion, pruritus, and urinary retention. Opiates are relatively contraindicated in patients with hemodynamic instability, respiratory compromise, or altered mental status. **Morphine** is a naturally occurring opiate, with a peak effect at 15 to 30 minutes and a duration of 2 to 4 hours (Table 10-1). Morphine releases histamine and therefore may cause hypotension. Meperidine is a synthetic derivative of morphine whose use is no longer recommended in the ED for multiple reasons, including increased risk of hy-

TABLE 10-1 Initial Dosing of Common Analgesic and Sedative Agents

Drug	Adult dose	Pediatric dose
Morphine	0.05–0.1 mg/kg IV	0.05–0.1 mg/kg IV
Fentanyl	0.5–3 µg/kg IV	0.05–3 µg/kg IV
Hydromorphone	1–2 mg IV/IM	0.015 mg/kg IV
Oxycodone	5–10 mg PO	0.1 mg/kg PO
Hydrocodone	5–10 mg PO	0.1 mg/kg PO
Codeine	10–60 mg PO	0.5–2 mg/kg PO
Midazolam	0.02 mg/kg IV	0.05–0.1 mg/kg (2 mg max) IV 0.1–0.15 mg/kg IM 0.5 mg/kg (15 mg max) PR
Propofol	0.2 mg/kg/min infusion	
Etomidate	0.1–0.2 mg/kg IV	0.1–0.2 mg/kg IV
Ketamine	1–2 mg/kg IV	1–2 mg/kg IV 3–5 mg/kg IM 5–10 mg/kg PO/PR
Methohexital	0.5–1 mg/kg IV	1 mg/kg IV 20 mg/kg PR

Key: IM = intramuscularly, IV = intravenously, max = maximum, PO = orally, PR = rectally.

potension from histamine release, production of a metabolite (normeperidine) with central nervous system (CNS) toxicity, and potential for a fatal reaction when co-administered with monoamine oxidase inhibitors. The Demerol, Phenergan, and Thorazine cocktail, previously used for pediatric PSA, is no longer recommended because of its unreliable efficacy, the potential for respiratory depression, and a variable duration of action that may last several hours.

Fentanyl is a synthetic opiate with an almost immediate onset of action and a 30- to 90-minute duration (see Table 10-1). Its rapid onset makes it the opiate of choice for most brief PSA procedures. Fentanyl is less likely to cause respiratory depression and hypotension than are other opiates. Respiratory depression may be more common in patients with alcohol or benzodiazepine ingestion. Administering fentanyl slowly over 3 to 5 minutes can minimize respiratory depression. Chest wall rigidity unresponsive to naloxone may occur at higher doses (5–15 µg/kg), potentially necessitating neuromuscular blockade and mechanical ventilation.

Adjunctive agents such as **hydroxyzine** (0.5 mg/kg PO or IM) or benzodiazepines frequently are administered with opiates. These agents may have opiate dose-sparing effects, although the data are scant. The use of adjunctive agents should be used only to relieve symptoms such as nausea or anxiety.

Sedation

Benzodiazepines are the most commonly used sedative agents for PSA in the ED. Benzodiazepines provide sedation, anxiolysis, amnesia, and anticonvulsant effects. Side effects include cardiovascular and respiratory depression, especially when used in combination with alcohol or opiates and in the elderly. **Midazolam,** which has a 5-minute onset of effect and a 30- to 45-minute duration of effect, is the most commonly used benzodiazepine for PSA (see Table 10-1). The duration of effect may be increased substantially in obese patients, and children may develop paradoxical inconsolability that is reversed by flumazenil. Diazepam, a benzodiazepine with a duration of effect of 2 to 6 hours, may be useful for longer procedures.

Barbiturates are sedative agents without analgesic or amnestic properties. Side effects include laryngospasm, hypotension, respiratory depression, and CNS depression (especially when administered with opiates or benzodiazepines). Pentobarbital has a 30-second onset of effect and a 30- to 60-minute duration of effect when administered IV. **Methohexital** has a 30- to 60-second onset of effect and a 10-minute duration of effect when administered IV (see Table 10-1). Methohexital, which has been used PR in children, may precipitate seizures and should not be used in patients with a seizure disorder.

Propofol is an anesthetic agent with antiemetic properties administered by intravenous infusion (see Table 10-1). It has an onset of effect of 5 to 10 minutes and a duration of effect upon withdrawal of 5 to 10 minutes. Side effects include dose-related cardiovascular depression with decreases in systolic blood pressure of 25% to 40%. Because amnesia is not reliably produced in PSA doses of propofol, an adjunctive analgesic or amnestic agent may be needed.

Etomidate, which has a 20- to 30-second onset of effect and a 2- to 3-minute duration of effect, is a sedative agent with minimal cardiovascular depression (see Table 10-1). Side effects include nausea and vomiting, myoclonus, and adrenal insufficiency (with long-term infusion). Respiratory and CNS depressions may occur, especially when administered with opiates or benzodiazepines.

Chloral hydrate is a sedative agent that was used commonly in pediatric patients requiring painless diagnostic procedures (dose 25 to 75 mg/kg PO or PR). Side effects include nausea and vomiting, paradoxical delirium, airway obstruction, and death. Because of its delayed onset of effect (45–60 minutes) and its prolonged duration (several hours), it is no longer recommended for routine use in the ED.

Ketamine is a dissociative analgesic with sedative and amnestic properties that causes minimal respiratory depression (see Table 10-1). Ketamine may be administered IV, IM, PO, or PR. Ketamine may cause increased intracranial and intraocular pressure, hypersalivation, bronchorrhea, bronchodilation, laryngospasm, and a hallucinatory emergence reaction in older children and adults. It is a direct myocardial depressant and vasodilator, although its CNS effects usually result in mild tachycardia and vasoconstriction. **Atropine** (0.01 mg/kg IV or IM) may be used adjunctively to control hypersalivation. **Midazolam** (0.01 mg/kg IM or IV or 0.1 mg/kg PO) may attenuate the emergence reaction, but it may cause respiratory depression and delayed ketamine metabolism. Ketamine is contraindicated in children 3 months and younger and in those with airway abnormalities, a history of congestive heart failure or hypertension, acute closed head or eye injury, altered mental status or psychosis, CNS mass, poorly controlled seizure disorder, or glaucoma

Nitrous oxide is an inhaled agent with analgesic, sedative, and dissociative properties. It can be used alone or in conjunction with local anesthetics. **Nitrous oxide** is delivered as a 30% to 50% mixture with a minimum of 30% oxygen. It should be self-administered through a demand-valve apparatus with a scavenger device. Nitrous oxide has a 3- to 5-minute onset of effect and a duration of effect on withdrawal of 3 to 5 minutes. Nitrous oxide has minimal respiratory or cardiovascular effects but may cause nausea and vomiting. It is contraindicated in patients who have recently been sedated with another agent and those with altered mental status, balloon-tipped catheters, dyspnea, severe chronic obstructive pulmonary disease, pneumothorax, eye injury, middle ear effusion, or bowel obstruction.

Disposition

Patients are eligible for discharge only when fully recovered. When discharged, the patient must be accompanied by an adult and should not drive or operate machinery for 24 hours. Because many of the agents used for PSA produce anterograde amnesia, discharge instructions must be given to responsible accompanying adults.

Local and Regional Anesthesia

Local and regional anesthetics are essential tools for ED pain management. Agents can be administered topically, by infiltration directly into the area to be anesthetized or into the area of the peripheral nerves supplying the area to be anesthetized, and IV. This discussion focuses on topical and infiltrative anesthesia.

There are 2 classes of local anesthetics (LAs), amides and esters. The amides include prilocaine, lidocaine, bupivacaine, and mepivacaine. The esters include procaine and tetracaine. The toxicity of LAs is related to the total dose and the rate of plasma concentration increase and is increased in the setting of hypoxia, hypercarbia, and acidosis. The rate of plasma concentration increase is dependent on the vascularity of the site being infiltrated. Therefore, the maximum dose of LAs that can be administered for intercostal block is one tenth the subcutaneous dose. Toxic effects include confusion, seizures, coma, myocardial depression, and dysrhythmias. Allergic reactions to LAs are uncommon and usually due to a metabolite (in esters) or a preservative (in amides). If an allergy is suspected, the best approach is to use a preservative-free agent from the other class of LAs. Alternatively, diphenhydramine or benzyl alcohol may be used as an LA in the setting of a true allergy to conventional LAs.

LAs often cause pain during administration. Factors that may decrease the pain of infiltration include using slow injection through a 27- or 30-gauge needle, injecting through the wound margin, using warm solution, and using buffered (with bicarbonate) solution.

Epinephrine (1:100,000) is often added to LAs before administration. Addition of epinephrine increases the duration of anesthesia, provides wound hemostasis, and slows systemic absorption. Epinephrine causes vasoconstriction and therefore should be avoided in an end-arterial field such as the digits, pinna, nose, and penis.

Lidocaine, which is the most commonly used LA in the ED, has a 2- to 5-minute onset of effect and a 1- to 2-hour duration of effect. The maximum dose of infiltrative **lidocaine** is 4.5 mg/kg without or 7 mg/kg with epinephrine. Lidocaine is buffered to decrease the pain of injection by adding 1 mL $NaHCO_3$ to 9 mL lidocaine. Bupivacaine, which has an onset of effect of 3 to 7 minutes and a duration of effect of 90 minutes to 6 hours, is preferred for prolonged procedures. The maximum dose of infiltrative **bupivacaine** is 2 mg/kg without or 3 mg/kg with epinephrine. Buffering of bupivacaine is accomplished with 1 mL $NaHCO_3$ to 29 mL bupivacaine. Procaine and tetracaine are ester anesthetics most commonly used in patients with allergies to amide anesthetics.

Digital Blocks

Finger and toe blocks are advantageous because less anesthetic is needed, better anesthesia is obtained, and tissues are not distorted. The onset on anesthesia is delayed when compared with that of LA. Neurovascular status must be assessed and documented before the procedure. Lidocaine and bupivacaine are the most commonly used agents and depend on the time needed to perform the procedure. Epinephrine should not be used in these procedures. Complications include nerve injury and intravascular injection leading to systemic toxicity. Always aspirate before injecting to avoid inadvertent intravascular injection of LA.

The procedure for digital blocks involves sterile preparation of the skin, followed be the introduction of a 27-gauge or smaller needle into the skin (a skin wheal may be raised before deeper injection) and into one side of the extensor tendon of the affected finger just proximal to the web. After aspiration, approximately 1 mL LA is injected into the tissue on the dorsal surface of the extensor tendon. The needle is advanced toward the palm until its tip is seen beneath the volar skin at the base of the finger just distal to the web. After aspiration, 1 mL LA is injected. Before removing the needle, redirect it across the opposite side of the finger and inject approximately 1 mL across the dorsal digital nerve. Five minutes later, repeat the procedure on the opposite side of the finger (Fig. 10-1). An alternate method is to inject a 27-gauge needle into the web space between the affected and an adjacent finger while directing the needle to the metacarpal joint of the affected finger. After aspiration,

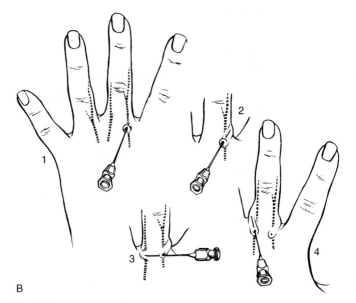

B

FIG. 10-1. Needle positions for digital nerve block.

inject 1 to 2 mL into the area of the digital nerve. Before removal of the needle, advance the needle first dorsally and then volarly, and inject 1 mL LA; repeat on the opposite side. Toes can be blocked in similar fashion. Great toes also can be blocked with a modified collar block. A 27-gauge needle is introduced to the dorsolateral aspect of the base of the toe until it blanches the plantar skin. As the needle is withdrawn, 1.5 mL LA is injected. Before the needle is removed, it is passed under the skin on the dorsal aspect of the toe, and 1.5 mL LA is injected as the needle is withdrawn. The needle is reintroduced through the anesthetized skin on the dorsomedial aspect of the toe and advanced until the plantar skin is blanched; as the needle is withdrawn, 1.5 mL LA is injected.

Local Anesthetic Infiltration

LAs can provide anesthesia at a site by infiltrating directly into the site or by infiltrating around the peripheral nerves supplying the site. The most common use of LA is infiltration for wound repair or invasive painful procedures. When repairing wounds, LA can be infiltrated into the wound margins or as a "field block" surrounding the wound. When infiltrating intact skin, raising a wheal may cause less pain on subsequent infiltration. LA also can be used in orthopedic procedures, such as fracture and joint reduction, by directly injecting the LA into the affected joint or fracture hematoma.

For some wounds, LA infiltration around the peripheral nerves is advantageous due to decreased total LA required and decreased pain at the site of injection. This is most commonly used for procedures involving the hand, digits, or foot. Before a regional block, it is imperative to assess neurovascular status. During administration, the syringe plunger must be drawn back to avoid intravascular injection of LA. Onset of effect of anesthesia with peripheral nerve blocks often is delayed (up to 15 minutes).

Topical Anesthetics

Topical anesthetics, which can eliminate the need for LA infiltration into some wounds, are applied painlessly, do not distort wound edges, and may provide hemostasis. Common preparations include tetracaine adrenaline cocaine (TAC), lidocaine epinephrine tetracaine (LET), lidocaine prilocaine (EMLA), and various preparations of lidocaine. TAC is no longer commonly used due to regularity issues and adverse effects such as seizures, respiratory arrest, and death. LET is applied by placing a LET-saturated cotton ball or gauze pad onto the wound for a minimum of 20 to 30 minutes. Neither TAC nor LET should be used on mucous membranes or in end-artery fields.

Topical lidocaine is marketed in a solution, cream, jelly, or ointment. Viscous lidocaine can be used for the temporary relief of inflamed mucous membranes. Lidocaine jelly can be used to facilitate the insertion of urinary catheters, nasogastric tubes, and fiberoptic scopes. As with infiltrative use of lidocaine, care must be taken not to exceed maximal doses.

EMLA is a cream composed of lidocaine and prilocaine used on intact skin to relieve the pain associated with venipuncture, arterial puncture, port access, and other superficial skin procedures. It has a 45- to 60-minute onset of effect and a 60-minute duration upon withdrawal. Because prilocaine may cause methemoglobinemia, EMLA should be used with caution in infants younger than 3 months and avoided in patients predisposed to methemoglobinemia.

For further reading in *Emergency Medicine: A Comprehensive Study Guide,* 6th ed., see Chap. 36, "Acute Pain Management in the Adult Patient," by Gary D. Zimmer; Chap. 38, "Procedural Sedation and Analgesia," by David D. Nicolaou; Chap. 134, "Acute Pain Management and Procedural Sedation in Children," by Michael N. Johnston and Erica Liebelt; and Chap. 37, "Local and Regional Anesthesia," by Eric Higginbotham and Robert J. Vissers.

11 | Management of Patients with Chronic Pain

David M Cline

Chronic pain is defined as a painful condition that lasts longer than 3 months. It also can be defined as pain that persists beyond the reasonable time for an injury to heal or a month beyond the usual course of an acute disease. Complete eradication of pain is not a reasonable endpoint in most cases. Rather, the goal of therapy is pain reduction and return to functional status.

CLINICAL FEATURES

Signs and symptoms of chronic pain syndromes are summarized in Table 11-1. Most of these syndromes will be familiar to emergency physicians.

Complex regional pain type I, also known as *reflex sympathetic dystrophy,* and complex regional pain type II, also known as *causalgia,* may be seen in the emergency department (ED) 2 weeks or more after an acute injury. These disorders should be suspected when a patient presents with classic symptoms: allodynia (pain provoked with gentle touch of the skin) and a persistent burning or shooting pain. Associated signs early in the course of the disease include edema, warmth, and localized sweating.

DIAGNOSIS AND DIFFERENTIAL

The most important task of the emergency physician is to distinguish chronic pain from acute pain that heralds a life- or limb-threatening condition. A complete history and physical examination should confirm the chronic condition or point to the need for further evaluation when unexpected signs or symptoms are elicited.

Rarely is a provisional diagnosis of a chronic pain condition made for the first time in the ED. The exception is a form of post nerve injury pain, complex regional pain. The sharp pain from acute injuries, including fractures, rarely continues beyond 2 weeks' duration. Pain in an injured body part beyond this period should alert the clinician to the possibility of nerve injury.

Definitive diagnostic testing of chronic pain conditions is difficult, requires expert opinion, and, often, expensive procedures such as magnetic resonance imaging, computed tomography, and thermography. Therefore, referral to the primary source of care and eventual specialist referral are warranted to confirm the diagnosis.

EMERGENCY DEPARTMENT CARE AND DISPOSITION

1. There are 2 essential points that affect the use of opioids in the ED: (*a*) opioids should be used only in chronic pain if they enhance function at home and at work, and (*b*) a single practitioner should be the sole prescriber of narcotics or be aware of their administration by others. A previous narcotic addiction is a relative contraindication to the use of opioids in chronic pain.
2. The management of chronic pain conditions is listed in Table 11-2. The need for longstanding treatment of chronic pain conditions may limit the safety of the nonsteroidal anti-inflammatory drugs.

TABLE 11-1 Signs and Symptoms of Chronic Pain Syndromes

Disorder	Pain symptoms	Signs
Myofascial headache	Constant dull pain, occasionally shooting pain	Trigger points on scalp, muscle tenderness and tension
Transformed migraine	Initially migraine-like, becomes constant, dull, nausea, vomiting	Muscle tenderness and tension, normal neurologic examination
Fibromyalgia	Diffuse muscular pain, stiffness, fatigue, sleep disturbance	Diffuse muscle tenderness, >11 trigger points
Myofascial chest pain	Constant dull pain, occasionally shooting pain	Trigger points in area of pain
Myofascial back pain syndrome	Constant dull pain, occasionally shooting pain, pain does not follow nerve distribution	Trigger points in area of pain, usually no muscle atrophy, poor ROM in involved muscle
Articular back pain	Constant or sharp pain exacerbated by movement	Local muscle spasm
Neurogenic back pain	Constant or intermittent, burning or aching, shooting or electric shock-like, may follow dermatome; leg pain > back pain	Possible muscle atrophy in area of pain, possible reflex changes
Complex regional pain type I (RSD)	Burning persistent pain, allodynia, associated with immobilization or disuse	Early: edema, warmth, local sweating Late: early signs alternate with cold; pale, cyanosis, eventually atrophic changes
Complex regional pain type II (causalgia)	Burning persistent pain, allodynia, associated with peripheral nerve injury	Early: edema, warmth, local sweating Late: early signs alternate with cold, pale, cyanosis, eventually atrophic changes
Postherpetic neuralgia	Allodynia, shooting, lancinating pain	Sensory changes in the involved dermatome
Phantom limb pain	Variable: aching, cramping, burning, squeezing or tearing sensation	None

Key: ROM = range of motion, RSD = reflex sympathetic dystrophy.

TABLE 11-2 Management of Selected Chronic Pain Syndromes

Disorder	Primary ED treatment	Secondary treatment*	Possible referral outcome
Cancer pain	NSAIDs, opiates	Long-acting opiates	Optimization of medical therapy
Myofascial headache	NSAIDs, cyclobenzaprine	Antidepressants, phenothiazine	Trigger point injections, optimization of medical therapy
Transformed migraine	NSAIDs, cyclobenzaprine	Antidepressants	Optimization of medical therapy, narcotic withdrawal
Fibromyalgia	NSAIDS	Antidepressants, exercise program	Optimization of medical therapy, dedicated exercise program
Myofascial chest pain	NSAIDs	Antidepressants	Trigger point injections, optimization of medical therapy
Myofascial back pain syndrome	NSAIDs, stay active	Antidepressants	Trigger point injections, optimization of medical therapy
Articular back pain	NSAIDs		Surgery, physical therapy
Neurogenic back pain	Acute: tapered prednisolone or prednisone	NSAIDs, muscle relaxants	Epidural steroids, surgery, exercise program
Complex regional pain types I and II (RSD and causalgia)	Prednisone 60 mg/d ×4 ds and then taper to include 3 wk of therapy	Calcitonin, antidepressants, anticonvulsants	Spinal cord stimulation, intrathecal baclofen, sympathetic nerve blocks, spinal analgesia
Postherpetic neuralgia	Simple analgesics	Gabapentin, antidepressants	Regional nerve blockade
Phantom limb pain	Simple analgesics	Antidepressants, anticonvulsants	TENS, sympathectomy

*If started in the ED, Consultation and/or follow-up with pain specialist or personal physician recommended.

Key: ED = emergency department, NSAIDs = nonsteroidal anti-inflammatory drugs, RSD = reflex sympathetic dystrophy, TENS = transcutaneous electrical nerve stimulation.

3. An evidence-based review found antidepressants effective in chronic low back pain, fibromyalgia, osteoarthritis, and neuropathic pain. A separate metaanalysis found tricyclic antidepressants more effective in states where symptoms were unexplained, such as fibromyalgia.
4. When antidepressants are prescribed in the ED, a follow-up plan should be in place. The most common drug and initial dose is **amitriptyline,** 10 to 25 mg, 2 hours before bedtime.
5. Gabapentin, a structural analog of γ-aminobutyric acid, has been shown to be effective in postherpetic neuralgia, painful diabetic neuropathy, and may have some benefit in complex regional pain syndromes. **Gabapentin** is started with an initial dose of 300 mg/d and is increased up to 1200 mg 3 times daily according to response.
6. A metaanalysis found calcitonin to be effective in the treatment of complex regional pain, type I (reflex sympathetic dystrophy). **Calcitonin** can be given at a dose of 100 IU/d as an intranasal spray.
7. Referral to the appropriate specialist is one of the most productive means to aid in the care of chronic pain patients who present to the ED. Chronic pain clinics have been successful at changing the lives of patients by eliminating opioid use, decreasing pain levels by one third, and increasing work hours 2-fold.

MANAGEMENT OF PATIENTS WITH DRUG-SEEKING BEHAVIOR

The spectrum of drug-seeking patients includes those who have chronic pain and have been advised to avoid taking narcotics, drug addicts who are trying to supplement their habit, and "hustlers" who are obtaining prescription drugs to sell on the street.

Clinical Features

Because of the spectrum of drug-seeking patients, the history given may be factual or fraudulent. Drug seekers may be demanding, intimidating, or flattering. In 1 ED study, the most common complaints of patients seeking drugs

TABLE 11-3 Characteristics of Drug Seeking Behavior

Behaviors predictive of drug-seeking behavior*
  Sells prescription drugs
  Forges/alters prescriptions
  Fictitious illness, requests narcotics
  Uses aliases to receive narcotics
  Admits to illicit drug addiction
  Conceals multiple physicians prescribing narcotics
  Conceals multiple visits to the emergency department to receive narcotics
Less predictive for drug-seeking behavior
  Admits to multiple doctors prescribing narcotics
  Admits to multiple prescriptions for narcotics
  Abusive when refused
  Multiple drug allergies
  Uses excessive flattery
  From out of town
  Asks for drugs by name

*Behaviors in this category are unlawful in many states.

were (in decreasing order) back pain, headache, extremity pain, and dental pain. Many fraudulent techniques are used, including "lost" prescriptions, "impending" surgery, fictitious hematuria with a complaint of kidney stones, self-mutilation, and fictitious injury.

Diagnosis and Differential

The diagnosis of drug-seeking behavior may not be possible in the ED. The medical record can provide a wealth of information regarding the patient, including documentation proving that the patient is supplying false information. Drug-seeking behaviors can be divided into 2 groups: predictive and less predictive (Table 11-3). The predictive behaviors are illegal in many states and form a solid basis to refuse narcotics to the patient.

Emergency Department Care and Disposition

The treatment of drug-seeking behavior is to refuse the controlled substance, consider the need for alternative medication or treatment, and consider referral for drug counseling.

For further reading in *Emergency Medicine: A Comprehensive Study Guide,* 6th ed., see Chap. 39, "Management of Patients with Chronic Pain," by David M. Cline.

4 | EMERGENCY WOUND MANAGEMENT

12 | Evaluating and Preparing Wounds

Timothy Reeder

CLINICAL FEATURES

Traumatic wounds are regularly encountered in the emergency department. It is important to document important historical information such as the mechanism, timing, and location of injury and the degree of contamination. Associated symptoms of pain, swelling, paresthesias, and loss of function should be identified. Ascertain factors will affect wound healing, such as the patient's age, location of injury, medications, chronic medical conditions (eg, diabetes, chronic renal failure, or immunosuppression), and previous scar formation (keloid). Patients with the sensation of a foreign body are much more likely to have retained a foreign body. Patient characteristics of handedness, occupation, tetanus status, and allergies (eg, to analgesics, anesthetics, antibiotics, or latex) should be documented. When caring for wounds, the ultimate goal is to restore the physical integrity and function of the injured tissue without infection.

When treating a wound, the emergency physician should consider the time and mechanism of injury and its location because these factors play a role in the potential for infection. Shear, compressive, or tensile forces cause acute traumatic wounds. Shear forces are produced by sharp objects with relatively low energy, resulting in a wound with a straight edge and little contamination that can be expected to heal with a good result. Wounds caused by compression forces crush the skin against underlying bone. These high-energy forces produce stellate lacerations. Tension forces produce flap-type lacerations. These wounds typically have surrounding devitalized tissue and result in a wound much more susceptible to infection than those caused by shear forces.

In addition to the mechanism of injury, the practitioner must thoroughly assess a wound's potential for infection. The risk of infection relates to the interaction of bacterial contamination, time to wound closure, and blood supply. The density of bacteria is quite low over the trunk and proximal arms and legs. Moist areas such as the axilla, perineum, and exposed hands and feet have a higher degree of colonization.

Wounds of the oral cavity are heavily contaminated with facultative and anaerobic organisms. Wounds sustained from contaminated objects or occurring in contaminated environments also have an increased risk of infection. Animal and human bites have an increased infection risk. Wounds contaminated with feces have a high risk of infection despite determined therapy. In general, the longer the time from injury to wound closure, the greater the risk of infection. Wounds in highly vascular areas such as the face and scalp are less likely to become infected. All of these factors must be considered in the evaluation and management of wounds.

DIAGNOSIS AND DIFFERENTIAL

Wound examination is greatly facilitated by a cooperative patient, good positioning, optimal lighting, and little or no bleeding. Universal precautions and adherence to strict sterile technique should be used and remain the standard of care. A thorough and compulsory examination will minimize the risk of missed foreign bodies and tendon and nerve injuries, a common cause of litigation.

Documentation of a wound should include the location, size, shape, margins, and depth. Pay particular attention to sensory, motor, tendon, vascular compromise, and injuries to specialized ducts. Careful palpation and inspection of the wound and surrounding area may show the presence of a foreign body or bony injury. Most foreign bodies and glass shards 2 mm or larger will be detected by routine radiographs. Foreign bodies with densities similar to those of soft tissue may require the use of computed tomography, magnetic resonance imaging, or ultrasound (see Chap. 17). Control of bleeding in an extremity can be accomplished by using a sphygmomanometer placed proximal to the injury and inflated to a pressure greater than the patient's systolic blood pressure. One should consider injecting joints with overlying wounds because the joint space could be violated.

EMERGENCY DEPARTMENT CARE AND DISPOSITION

Proper wound preparation is the most important step for adequate evaluation of the wound to restore the integrity and function of the injured tissue, prevent infection, and maximize cosmetic results.

ANESTHESIA

1. Pain control with consideration of local or regional anesthesia should be provided before any wound manipulation. This will enable better preparation and evaluation of the wound and a more relaxed, cooperative patient.
2. A careful neurovascular examination of the involved area should be performed and documented before anesthesia.

HEMOSTASIS

1. Control of bleeding is necessary for proper wound evaluation and treatment.
2. Direct pressure is the preferred method and is usually effective.
3. Epinephrine containing local anesthetics can be used except in distal anatomy such as fingers, nose, ear, and the penis.
4. Ligation of minor vessels in the extremity may be necessary and can be achieved by applying an absorbable suture material after isolating and clamping the involved vessel. Several chemical means of hemostasis such as epinephrine, absorbable gelation sponge (Gelfoam), and oxidized cellulose (Oxycel) or collagen sponge (Actifoam) are available. Gelfoam has no intrinsic hemostatic properties and works by the pressure it exerts as it becomes a fluid-filled sponge. Oxycel and Actifoam react with blood to form an artificial clot.

FOREIGN BODY AND HAIR REMOVAL

1. Visual wound inspection, down to the full depth and along the full course of the wound, is the most important method of detecting foreign bodies (see Chap. 17).
2. Hair, which can act as a foreign body, should be removed by clipping 1 to 2 mm above the skin with scissors. Shaving may damage the hair follicles,

thereby allowing bacterial invasion, and can increase the infection rate by 10-fold. Ointments can be used to clear hair away from the wound edges as an alternative to clipping.
3. Hair should never be removed from the eyebrows due to the potential for abnormal or lack of regeneration.

IRRIGATION

1. High-pressure irrigation decreases bacterial counts and helps to remove foreign bodies, thereby decreasing the risk of infection. Effective high-pressure irrigation can be achieved by using a 19-gauge needle or catheter attached to a 35- or 65-mL syringe. Although the precise volume of irrigant required is not known, 60 mL/cm of wound length is a useful guideline, with a 200 mL minimum.
2. Wound soaking is not effective in cleaning contaminated wounds and may increase wound bacterial counts. Sterile normal saline solution has the lowest toxicity. There is no added benefit to the addition of povidone iodine or hydrogen peroxide.

DEBRIDEMENT

Devitalized tissue may increase the risk of infection and delay healing. Debridement removes foreign matter, bacteria, and devitalized tissue and creates a sharp wound edge that is easier to repair.

1. Elliptical excision around the wound edges with a standard surgical blade is the most effective type of debridement. Tissue that has a narrow base or lacks capillary refill will require debridement.
2. Wounds with an extensive amount of nonviable tissue may require a large amount of tissue removal and will need more delayed wound closure or grafting. In general, a surgical specialist should be consulted to manage these wounds.

ANTIBIOTICS

Although there is no clear evidence that antibiotic prophylaxis prevents wound infection in most emergency department patients, there may be a role in selected high-risk wounds and populations.

1. When used, antibiotic prophylaxis should be (*a*) started rapidly, before significant tissue manipulation; (*b*) performed with agents that are effective against predicted pathogens; and (*c*) administered by routes that rapidly achieve desired blood levels. In general, the prophylaxis will require intravenous, broad-spectrum antibiotic. Oral administration also may work if given before wound manipulation.
2. Reasonable coverage can be expected from penicillinase-resistant penicillin (eg, **dicloxacillin** 12 to 25 mg/kg/day orally [PO] divided in 4 doses; 500 mg PO in 4 daily doses in adults) or a first-generation cephalosporin (eg, **cephalexin** 25 to 50 mg/kg/day PO divided in 4 doses; 500 mg PO in 4 daily doses in adults). Clindamycin may be used in penicillin-allergic patients. Antibiotics should be given for 3 to 5 days.
3. Human and mammalian bites should receive penicillin or amoxicillin-clavulanate for *Pasteurella* and *Eikenella,* respectively (see Chap. 18 for discussion).

4. Full-thickness oral lacerations should be treated for 3 to 5 days with **penicillin** (25 to 50 mg/kg/day PO divided in 4 doses; 500 mg PO in 4 daily doses in adults).

5. Wounds contaminated by fresh water and plantar puncture wounds through athletic shoes may require a fluoroquinolone (eg, **ciprofloxacin** 500 mg PO twice daily in adults only) to cover *Pseudomonas* for 3 to 5 days.

TETANUS PROPHYLAXIS

Guidelines for tetanus prophylaxis in wound management have been developed by several public and professional organizations. See Chap. 19 for the Centers for Disease Control and Prevention guidelines. Because the incubation period is 7 to 21 days, it is acceptable to give the absorbed tetanus toxoid days after injury. Immunization and immunoglobulin administration are safe during pregnancy.

For further reading in *Emergency Medicine: A Comprehensive Study Guide,* 6th ed., see Chap. 40, "Evaluation of Wounds," by Judd Hollander and Adam Singer; and Chap. 41, "Wound Preparation," by Susan C. Store and Wallace A. Carter.

13 | Methods for Wound Closure

David M. Cline

Wounds can be closed primarily in the emergency department (ED) by the placement of sutures, surgical staples, skin closure tapes, and adhesives. All wounds heal with some scarring; the goal is to use techniques that make the scar as small and invisible as possible. In closing a laceration, it is important to match each layer of a wound edge to its counterpart. Care must be taken to avoid having 1 wound edge rolled inward. The rolled-in edge occludes the capillaries, thereby promoting wound infection. The dermal side will not heal to the rolled epidermal side, thereby causing wound dehiscence when the sutures are removed, thus resulting in an inferior scar appearance. The techniques described are an overview of basic wound closure, which should aid the practitioner in achieving acceptable results.

SUTURES

Sutures are the strongest of all wound closure devices and allow the most accurate approximation of wound edges. Sutures are generally divided into 2 general classes, nonabsorbable and absorbable sutures, which lose all their tensile strength within 60 days. Monofilament synthetic sutures such as nylon or polypropylene have the lowest rates of infection and are the most commonly used suture material in the ED. Synthetic monofilament absorbable sutures (eg, Monocryl) are preferred for closure of deep structures such as the dermis or fascia because of their strength and low tissue reactivity. Rapidly absorbing sutures (eg, Vicryl Rapide) can be used to close the superficial skin layers or mucus membranes, especially when the avoidance of removal is desired.

Sutures are sized according to their diameter. For general ED use, the 6-0 suture is the smallest and is used for percutaneous closure on the face and other cosmetically important areas. Suture sizes 5-0 and 4-0 are progressively larger; 5-0 is commonly used for closure of hand and finger lacerations, and 4-0 is used to close lacerations on the trunk and proximal extremities. Very thick skin, as is found on the scalp and sole, may require closure with 3-0 sutures.

SUTURING TECHNIQUES

Percutaneous sutures that pass through the epidermal and dermal layers are the most common sutures used in the ED. Dermal, or subcuticular, sutures reapproximate the divided edges of the dermis without penetrating the epidermis. These 2 sutures may be used together in a layered closure as wound complexity demands. Sutures can be applied in a continuous fashion ("running" sutures) or as interrupted sutures.

Simple Interrupted Percutaneous Sutures

Percutaneous sutures should be placed to achieve eversion of the wound edges. To accomplish this, the needle should enter the skin at a 90° angle. The needlepoint also should exit the opposite side at 90°. The depth of the suture should be wider than the width. Sutures placed in this manner will encompass a portion of tissue that will evert when the knot is tied (Fig. 13-1). An

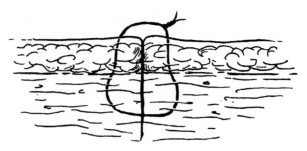

FIG. 13-1. A single interrupted percutaneous suture with everted edges.

adequate number of interrupted sutures should be placed so that the wound edges are closed without gaping. In general, the number of ties should correspond to the suture size (ie, 4 ties for 4-0 suture and 5 ties for 5-0 suture).

Straight, shallow lacerations must be closed with percutaneous sutures only, by sewing from 1 end toward the other and aligning edges with each suture bite. Deep, irregular wounds with uneven, unaligned, or gaping edges are more difficult to suture. Certain principles have been identified for these more difficult wounds:

1. Wounds in which the edges cannot be brought together without excessive tension should have dermal sutures placed to partly close the gap.
2. When wounds edges of different thicknesses are to be reunited, the needle should be passed through 1 side of the wound and then drawn out before reentry through the other side to ensure that the needle is inserted at a comparable level.
3. Uneven edges can be aligned by first approximating the midportion of the wound with the initial suture. Subsequent sutures are placed in the middle of each half, until the wound edges are aligned and closed.

Simple interrupted sutures are the most versatile and effective for realigning irregular wound edges and stellate lacerations (Fig. 13-2). An advantage of

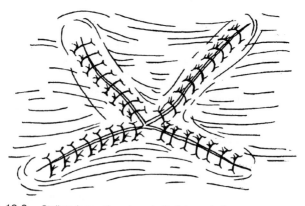

FIG. 13-2. Stellate laceration closed with interrupted sutures.

interrupted sutures is that only the involved sutures need to be removed in the case of wound infection.

Continuous "Running" Percutaneous Sutures

Continuous "running" percutaneous sutures are best when repairing linear wounds. An advantage of the continuous suture is that it accommodates to the developing edema of the wound edges during healing. However, a break in the suture may ruin the entire repair and may cause permanent marks if placed too tightly. Continuous suture closure of a laceration can be accomplished by 2 different patterns. In the first pattern, the needle pathway is at a 90° angle to the wound edges and results in a visible suture that crosses the wound edges at a 45° angle (Fig. 13-3A). In the other pattern, the needle pathway is at a 45° angle to the wound edges, so that the visible suture is at a 90° angle to the wound edges (Fig. 13-3B). In either case, the physician starts at the corner of the wound farthest away and sutures toward him- or herself.

Deep Dermal Sutures

The major role of these sutures is to reduce tension. They are also used to close dead spaces. However, their presence increases the risk of infection in contaminated wounds. Sutures through adipose tissues do not hold tension, increase infection rates, and should be avoided. With deep dermal sutures, the needle is inserted at the level of the mid dermis on 1 side of the wound and then exits more superficially below the dermal epidermal junction (Fig. 13-4). The

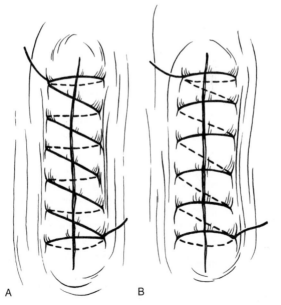

FIG. 13-3. **A.** Running suture crossing wound at 45°. **B.** Running suture crossing wound at 90°.

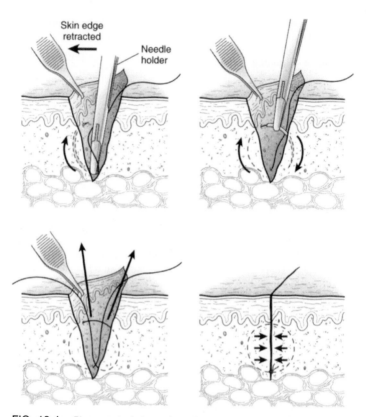

FIG. 13-4. Placement of deep dermal sutures. The needle is inserted at the depth of the dermis and directed upward, exiting beneath the dermal-epidermal junction. Then the needle is inserted across the wound and directed downward, exiting at the wound base. The suture knot is then placed deep in the wound. [Reproduced with permission from Singer AJ, Hollander JE (eds): *Lacerations and Acute Wounds. An Evidence-Based Guide.* Philadelphia, PA: FA Davis, 2003, p. 121.]

needle is then introduced below the dermal epidermal junction on the opposite side of the wound and exits at the level of the mid dermis. Thus the knot becomes buried in the depth of the tissue when tying of the suture is completed. The first suture is placed at the center of the laceration, and additional sutures sequentially bisect the wound. The number of deep sutures should be minimized.

Vertical Mattress Sutures

Vertical mattress sutures (Fig. 13-5) are used in certain situations. The vertical mattress suture is useful in areas of lax skin (elbow and dorsum of the hand) where the wound edges tend to fold into the wound. It can act as an "all-in-one" suture, thus avoiding the need for a layered closure.

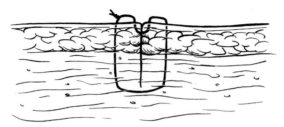

FIG. 13-5.   Vertical mattress suture.

Horizontal Mattress Sutures

Horizontal mattress sutures are faster and better at eversion than are vertical mattress sutures. These are especially useful in areas of increased tension such as the fascia, joints, and callus skin (Fig. 13-6). To avoid tissue strangulation, care must be taken not to tie the individual sutures too tightly.

Delayed Closure

Delayed primary closure is an option for wound closure suspected of contamination or for wounds presenting beyond 12 hours from injury. With this method, the wound is left open for 3 to 5 days, after which it may be closed if no infection supervenes. A study conducted in 2002 randomized patients to delayed primary closure or secondary closure (the wound is left open and allowed to close by intention). Healing times, appearance, and function were similar.

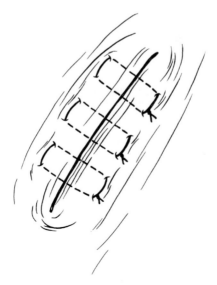

FIG. 13-6.   Horizontal mattress suture.

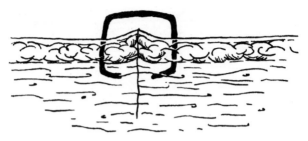

FIG. 13-7.   A cutaneous staple properly placed will evert the skin edges and not be in contact with the skin surface.

STAPLES

Skin closure by metal staples is quick and economical, with the advantage of low tissue reactivity. The skin staple, however, does not provide the same coaptation for lacerations with irregular skin edges that sutures can achieve and should be reserved for lacerations in areas where the healing scar is not readily apparent (eg, scalp). When placing staples, the wound edges should be held together with tissue forceps. The device should be placed gently against the skin, and the trigger should be squeezed slowly. A properly place staple should have its topside off the skin surface (Fig. 13-7).

ADHESIVE TAPES

Adhesive tapes are the least reactive of all wound closure devices. Skin closure tapes are used as an alternative to sutures and staples and for additional support after suture and staple removal. Tapes work best on flat, dry, nonmobile surfaces where the wound edges fit together without tension. Taped wounds are more resistant than sutured wounds to infection. They can be used for skin flaps, where sutures may compromise perfusion, and for lacerations with thin, friable skin that will not hold sutures. Adherence of tapes is enhanced by the use of benzoin to the skin surface 2 to 3 cm beyond the wound edges. Individual tapes are applied with some space between them but not so much that the wound edges gap open between the individual tapes. Tapes should stay in place about as long as an equivalent suture and will spontaneously detach as the underlying epithelium exfoliates.

CYANOACRYLATE TISSUE ADHESIVES

Cyanoacrylate tissues adhesives close wounds by forming an adhesive layer on top of intact epithelium. Cyanoacrylate adhesives should never be applied within wounds due to their intense inflammatory reaction with subcutaneous tissue. Adhesives should not be applied to mucous membranes, infected areas, joints, areas with dense hair (eg, scalp), or on wounds exposed to body fluids. Adhesives are most useful when they are used on wounds that close spontaneously, have clean or sharp edges, and are located on clean, nonmobile areas. Compared with sutured wounds, wound closure with adhesives is faster, less painful, has comparable rates of infection and optimal cosmetic appearance, and, when properly applied on selected wounds, has a similar dehiscence rate.

Wounds with edges separated by more than 5 mm are unlikely to stay closed with tissue adhesives alone. In this case, subcutaneous sutures can be inserted to relieve this tension. Tissue adhesives are equivalent in strength to 5-0 suture. Lacerations longer than 5 cm are prone to shear forces and unlikely to remain closed with tissue adhesives alone.

The adhesive is carefully expressed through the tip of the applicator and gently brushed over the wound surface in a continuous steady motion. The adhesive should cover the entire wound in addition to an area covering 5 to 10 mm on either side of the wound edges. After allowing the first layer of the adhesive to polymerize for 30 to 45 seconds, 2 to 3 additional layers of the adhesive are similarly brushed onto the surface of the wound, with pauses of 5 to 10 seconds between successive layers. Care should be taken to position the patient parallel to the floor, cover the eyes, and use gentle squeezing of the applicator to avoid problematic runoff.

Once applied, Cyanoacrylate should not be covered with ointment, bandage, or dressing. Patients should be instructed not to pick at edges of the adhesive. After 24 hours, the area can be gently washed with plain water but should not be scrubbed, soaked, or exposed to moisture for any length of time. The adhesive will spontaneously slough off in 5 to 10 days. Should a wound open, the patient should return immediately for closure.

For further reading in *Emergency Medicine: A Comprehensive Study Guide,* 6th ed., see Chap. 42, "Methods for Wound Closure," by Adam J. Singer and Judd E. Hollander.

14 | Lacerations to the Face and Scalp

Russell J. Karten

SCALP AND FOREHEAD

The scalp and forehead (which includes eyebrows) are parts of the same anatomic structure (Fig. 14-1). Eyebrows should never be clipped or shaved because their delicate contour and form are valuable landmarks for the meticulous reapproximation of the wound edges. After the wound has been cleaned and hemostasis achieved, the base of the wound always should be palpated for possible skull fracture. All depressed fractures should be evaluated by computed tomography.

When the edges of a laceration of the eyebrow or the scalp are devitalized, debridement is mandatory. The scalpel should cut an angle that is parallel to that of the hair follicles to prevent subsequent alopecia. In some cases, it may be necessary to control scalp hemorrhage by direct pressure or by clamping vessels at the wound edges. Wound closure should be initiated first with approximation of the galea aponeurotica with buried, interrupted absorbable 4-0 sutures. The divided edges of muscle and fascia also must be closed with buried, interrupted, absorbable 4-0 synthetic sutures to prevent further development of depressed scars. The skin can be closed by staples or by simple interrupted nylon sutures (sutures of a color different from the patient's hair should be considered).

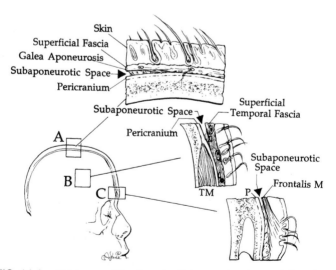

FIG. 14-1. The layers of the **A.** scalp, **B.** temporal region, and **C.** eyebrow. *Key:* TM = temporalis muscle.

The skin edges of anatomic landmarks on the forehead should be approximated first with key stitches by using interrupted, nonabsorbable monofilament 5-0 synthetic sutures. Accurate alignment of the eyebrow, transverse wrinkles of the forehead, and the hairline of the scalp is essential. It may be necessary to have younger patients raise their eyebrows to create wrinkles for accurate placement of the key stitches. A firm pressure dressing placed around the head can close any potential dead space, encourage hemostasis, and prevent hematoma formation. This pressure dressing should be left in place for 24 hours. Removal of scalp sutures and staples should occur in 7 to 10 days, whereas facial sutures should be removed in 3 to 5 days.

EYELIDS

A complete examination of the eye structure and function is essential, including an evaluation for foreign bodies (see Chap. 150). The lid should be examined for involvement of the canthi, the lacrimal system, the supraorbital nerve, and the infraorbital nerve or penetration through the tarsal plate or lid margin (Fig. 14-2). The following wounds should be referred to an ophthalmologist: (*a*) those involving the inner surface of the lid, (*b*) those involving the lid margins, (*c*) those involving the lacrimal duct, (*d*) those associated with ptosis, and (*e*) those extending into the tarsal plate. Failure to recognize and properly repair the lacrimal system can result in chronic tearing.

Uncomplicated lid lacerations can be readily closed by using nonabsorbable 6-0 suture, with removal in 3 to 5 days. Tissue adhesive is contraindicated near the eye.

NOSE

Lacerations of the nose may be limited to skin or involve the deeper structures (sparse nasal musculature, cartilaginous framework, and nasal mucous membrane). They are repaired by accurate reapproximation of each tissue layer. Inexperienced operators should refer such cases to an otolaryngologist or a plastic surgeon. Local anesthesia of the nose can be difficult because of the tightly adhering skin, and injection of epinephrine-containing anesthetics into the tip of the nose should be avoided. Topical anesthesia may be successful with lidocaine, epinephrine, and tetracaine.

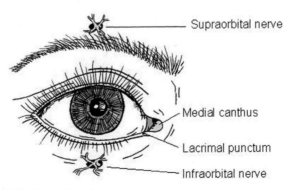

FIG. 14-2. External landmarks.

When the laceration extends through all tissue layers, closure should begin with a nonabsorbable, monofilament 5-0 synthetic suture that aligns the skin surrounding the entrances of the nasal canals to prevent malposition and notching of the alar rim. Traction on the long, untied ends of this suture approximates the wounds and aligns the anterior and posterior margins of the divided tissue layers. The mucous membrane then should be repaired with interrupted, braided, absorbable 5-0 synthetic sutures, with their knots buried in the tissue. The area is re-irrigated gently from the outside. The cartilage rarely may need to be approximated with a minimal number of 5-0 absorbable sutures. In sharply marked linear lacerations, closure of the overlying skin is usually sufficient. The cut edges of the skin, with its adherent musculature, are closed with interrupted, nonabsorbable, monofilament 6-0 synthetic sutures. Removal of the external sutures may take place in 3 to 5 days.

After any nasal injury the septum should be inspected for hematoma formation with a nasal speculum. The presence of bluish swelling in the septum confirms the diagnosis of septal hematoma. Treatment of the hematoma is evacuation of the blood clot. Drainage of a small hematoma can be accomplished by aspiration of the blood clot through an 18-gauge needle. A larger hematoma should be drained through a horizontal incision at the base. Bilateral hematomas should be drained in the operating room by a specialist. Reaccumulation of blood can be prevented by nasal packing. Antibiotic treatment is recommended to prevent infection that may cause necrosis of cartilage. An oral penicillin, cephalosporin, or macrolide is acceptable.

LIPS

The technique of closure will depend largely on the type of lip wound. Isolated intraoral lesions may not need to be sutured. Through-and-through lacerations that do not include the vermilion border can be closed in layers. A 5-0 absorbable suture should be used first for the mucosal surface, followed by reirrigation and closure of the orbicularis oris muscle with 5-0 absorbable suture. The skin should be closed with 6-0 nonabsorbable suture or tissue adhesive. Sutures should be removed in 5 days.

Closure of a complicated lip laceration should start at the junction between the vermilion and the skin with a nonabsorbable, monofilament 6-0 synthetic suture (Fig. 14-3). The orbicularis oris muscle is then repaired with interrupted, braided, absorbable 4-0 synthetic sutures. The junction between the vermilion and the mucous membrane is approximated with a braided, absorbable 5-0 synthetic suture. The divided edges of the mucous membrane and vermilion are then closed with interrupted, braided, absorbable 5-0 synthetic sutures in a buried knot construction. Skin edges of the laceration are usually jagged and irregular, but they can be fitted together as the pieces of a jigsaw puzzle by using interrupted, nonabsorbable, monofilament 6-0 synthetic sutures with their knots formed on the surface of the skin. Patients with sutured intraoral lacerations should receive prophylactic antibiotics.

EAR

Superficial lacerations of the ear can be closed with 6-0 nylon suture. Exposed cartilage should be covered. Debridement of the skin is not advisable because there is very little excess skin. In most through-and-through lacerations of the ear, the skin can be approximated and the underlying cartilage will be supported adequately (Fig. 14-4). After repair of simple lacerations,

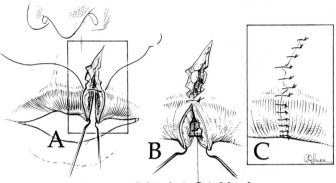

FIG. 14-3. Irregular-edged vertical laceration of the upper lip. **A.** Traction is applied to the lips and closure of the wound is begun first at the vermilion-skin junction. **B.** The orbicularis oris muscle is then repaired with interrupted, absorbable 4-0 synthetic sutures. **C.** The irregular edges of the skin are then approximated.

a small piece of nonadherent gauze may be applied over the laceration only and a pressure dressing applied. Gauze squares are placed behind the ear to apply pressure, and the head is wrapped circumferentially with gauze. Sutures should be removed in 5 days. An otolaryngologist or plastic surgeon should be consulted for more complex lacerations, ear avulsions, or auricular hematomas.

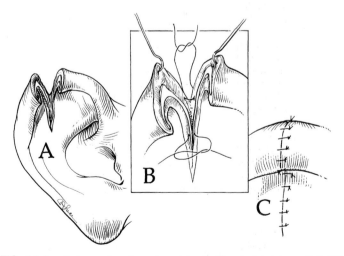

FIG. 14-4. **A.** Laceration through auricle. **B.** One or two interrupted, 6-0 coated nylon sutures will approximate divided edges of cartilage. **C.** Interrupted nonabsorbable 6-0 synthetic sutures approximate the skin edges.

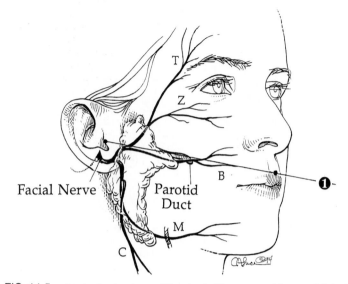

FIG. 14-5.   Anatomic structures of the cheek. The course of the parotid duct is deep to a line drawn from the tragus of the ear to the midportion of the upper lip. Branches of the facial nerve: temporal **(T)**, zygomatic **(Z)**, buccal **(B)**, mental **(M)**, and cervical **(C)**.

CHEEKS AND FACE

In general, facial lacerations are closed with 6-0 nonabsorbable, simple interrupted sutures and are removed after 5 days. Tissue adhesive is an alternative. Attention to anatomic structures including the facial nerve and parotid gland is necessary (Fig. 14-5). If these structures are involved, operative repair is indicated.

For further reading in *Emergency Medicine: A Comprehensive Study Guide*, 6th ed., see Chap. 43, "Lacerations to the Face and Scalp," by Wendy C. Coates.

15 | Injuries of the Arm, Hand, Fingertip, and Nail

David M. Cline

CLINICAL FEATURES

History should include occupation and hand dominance. Examination of arm and hand injuries includes inspection at rest, evaluation of motor nerve and tendon functions, evaluation of sensory nerve function, and evaluation of perfusion. The wound should be examined for evidence of potential artery, nerve, tendon, and bone injuries. The wound should be evaluated for foreign bodies, debris, or bacterial contamination. Examining active motion and resistance to passive movement assesses motor function (Table 15-1). Sensation should be assessed in the median, ulnar, and radial nerve distributions (Table 15-2).

DIAGNOSIS AND DIFFERENTIAL

For some injuries, a bloodless field may require a proximal tourniquet to temporarily halt arterial flow. A Penrose drain is commonly used for distal finger injures, and a manual blood pressure cuff is used for more proximal injures. Once adequate visualization is obtained, the injury can be examined for foreign bodies and tendon and joint capsule injuries. It is essential to examine the hand and arm in the position of injury to avoid missing deep structure injuries that may have moved out of the field of view when examined in a neutral position. Radiographic evaluation with anteroposterior and lateral films is indicated if bony injuries, retained radiopaque foreign bodies, or joint penetration are suspected.

EMERGENCY DEPARTMENT CARE AND DISPOSITION

1. All wounds require scrupulous cleaning and irrigation after adequate anesthesia, which may require a regional or digital nerve block.
2. Tetanus prophylaxis should be given as indicated (see Chap. 12).
3. Consultation with a plastic or hand surgeon is required with complex or extensive injuries, injuries requiring skin grafting, or injuries requiring technically demanding skills. Consultation with a specialist also is recommended if the hand is vital to patient's career (eg, a professional musician).
4. Management of individual wound types should be directed by the sections that follow.

TABLE 15-1 Motor Testing of the Peripheral Nerves of the Upper Extremity

Nerve	Motor examination
Radial	Dorsiflexion of wrist
	Extension of digits
Median	Thumb opposition
	Thumb abduction
	Thumb flexion
Ulnar	Adduction/abduction of digits
	Thumb adduction

TABLE 15-2 Sensory Testing of Peripheral Nerves in the Upper Extremity

Senory nerve	Area of test
Radial	First dorsal web space
Median	Volar tip of index finger
Ulnar	Volar tip of little finger

Forearm and Wrist Lacerations

1. Injury over the wrist raises the possibility of a suicide attempt, and the patient should be questioned about intent and a history of depression.
2. Tendons and distal nerves should be examined individually. The forearm has 6 extensor compartments located dorsally and innervated by the radial nerve (Table 15-3). Located on the volar surface of the forearm and crossing the wrist are the 12 flexor tendons innervated by the median and ulnar nerves (Table 15-4).
3. Injuries that involve more than 1 parallel laceration, classic for suicide attempts, may require horizontal mattress sutures to cross all lacerations for closure to prevent compromising the vascular supply of the island of skin located between incisions (Fig. 15-1).

Palm Lacerations

1. Injuries to the palm may require a regional anesthetic, eg, a median or ulnar nerve block.
2. Very careful exploration is mandatory. If no deep injury is suspected, the wound is closed, with particular attention to re-opposing the skin creases accurately.

TABLE 15-3 Extensor Compartments in the Forearm

Extensors in the forearm	Function
First compartment	
Abductor pollicis longus	Abduct thumb radially
Extensor pollicis brevis	Extends thumb at MCP joint
Second compartment	
Extensor carpi radialis longus	Extends wrist and
Extensor carpi radialis brevis	Radially deviates wrist (both)
Third compartment	
Extensor pollicis longus	Extends and adducts thumb
Fourth compartment	
Extensor digitorum communis	Splits into 4 tendons at wrist Joins with juncturae in dorsal hand, inserts to form extensors of index, ring, middle fingers
Extensor indicis proprius	Extensor for index finger
Fifth compartment	
Extensor digiti minimi	Extends MCP of little finger
Sixth compartment	
Extensor carpi ulnaris	Extends and ulnarly deviates wrist

Key: MCP = metacarpophalangea, carpometacarpal.

TABLE 15-4 Flexor Tendons in the Forearm

Flexor tendons	Function
Flexor carpi radialis	Flex wrist *plus* deviate radially
Flexor carpi ulnaris	Flex wrist *plus* deviate ulnarly
Palmaris longus	Flex wrist
Flexor pollicis longus	Thumb flexor
At index, middle, ring and little fingers	
Flexor digitorum superficialis	
Flexor digitorum profundus	Flex from wrist to PIP
	Flex from wrist to DIP

Key: DIP = distal interphalangeal joint, PIP = proximal interphalangeal joint.

3. Care should be taken to avoid using deep "bites" with the needle because this risks injury to the underlying tendons or tendon sheaths. Interrupted horizontal mattress sutures (see Chap. 13) with 5-0 monofilament suture are recommended to ensure these sutures do not pull through.
4. Deep injuries between the carpometacarpal joints and the distal creases of the wrist are considered to be in "no-mans' land" and should be referred to a specialist for exploration and repair.

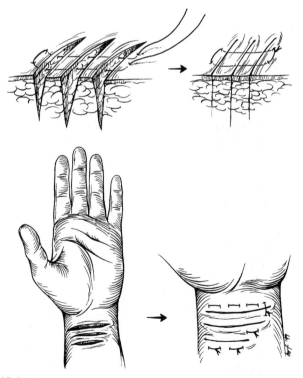

FIG. 15-1.   Horizontal mattress sutures for multiple parallel lacerations.

Dorsal Hand Lacerations

1. On the dorsum of the hand, lacerations over the metacarpophalangeal joint suggest a closed fist injury and require special care (see Chap. 18).
2. The pliable skin and extensive movements of the hand may hide tendon injuries; therefore, careful examination of the wound and hand function is essential.
3. Most dorsal hand lacerations can be repaired by emergency physicians using 5-0 nonabsorbable sutures.

Extensor Tendon Lacerations

1. Experienced emergency physicians may repair extensor tendon injuries over the dorsum of the hand, with the exception of the tendons to the thumb.
2. The tendon injury should be discussed with a hand specialist for preferred technique and to arrange follow-up.
3. Usually a figure-of-8 knot is used, with a 4-0 nonabsorbable suture material (Fig 15-2). The limb is then splinted.
4. Lacerations to the extensor tendons over the distal interphalangeal joint may produce a mallet deformity, whereas lacerations over the proximal interphalangeal joint may produce a boutonniere deformity. If the lacerations are open, they are surgically repaired; if closed, they are splinted for up to 6 weeks.

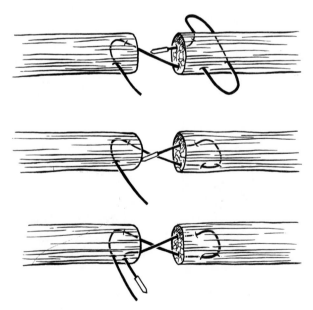

FIG. 15-2. Extensor tendon laceration repair with a figure-of-eight stitch.

Flexor Tendon Lacerations

1. Injuries to flexor tendons should be referred to a specialist. Some hand surgeons prefer to repair these injuries within 12 to 24 hours.
2. The repair can be delayed up to 7 days. In these cases, the wound should be cleaned, the skin repaired, the limb splinted in a position of function, and arrangements made for follow-up within 2 to 3 days with a hand surgeon.

Finger and Finger Tip Injuries

1. In general, finger lacerations are straightforward and can be repaired by using 5-0 nonabsorbable suture materials.
2. Digital nerve injuries should be suspected when static 2-point discrimination is distinctively greater on 1 side of the volar pad than on the other, or when it is greater than 10 mm. Digital nerve injuries can be repaired by using microvascular techniques acutely or days to weeks after the injury.
3. Successful repair of fingertip injuries requires knowledge of anatomy (Fig 15-3) and an understanding of techniques of reconstruction.
4. Distal fingertip amputations with skin or pulp loss only are best managed conservatively, with serial dressing change only, especially in children.
5. In cases with larger areas of skin loss (>1 cm^2), a skin graft using the severed tip itself or skin harvested from the hypothenar eminence may be required.
6. Complications of the skin graft technique include decreased sensation of the fingertip, tenderness at the injury and graft site, poor cosmetic result, and hyperpigmentation in dark-skinned patients.
7. Injuries with exposed bone are not amenable to skin grafting. Most of these injuries require specialist advice. If less than 0.5 mm of bone is exposed and the wound defect is small, the bone may be trimmed back and the wound left to heal by secondary intention. Injuries to the thumb or index finger with exposed bone nearly always require specialist attention.
8. Injuries to the nail bed require careful repair to reduce scar formation. They are associated with fractures of the distal phalanx in 50% of cases.

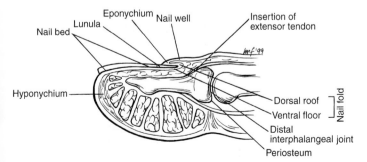

FIG. 15-3. Anatomy of the perionychium. [Reproduced with permission from Zook EG: The perionychium, in DP Green, (ed): *Operative Hand Surgery*, 2d ed. New York, NY: Churchill Livingstone, 1988, p. 1332.]

9. Subungual hematomas require decompression by simple trephination of the nail plate. Use of heated paper clip delays healing. Use of nail drill, scalpel, or 18-gauge needle is recommended.

10. Previously, it was recommended that, if a subungual hematoma occupied more than 50% of the nail bed area, the nail should be removed to inspect and repair a likely nail bed laceration. Two prospective studies have shown that, if other structures are intact, simple trephination produces an excellent result in patients with subungual hematoma regardless of size, injury mechanism, or presence of simple fracture.

11. Nail removal is needed if there is extensive crush injury, associated nail avulsion or surrounding nail fold disruption, or a displaced distal phalanx fracture on radiograph. The nail bed is inspected and repaired with 6-0 or 7-0 absorbable sutures. If the nail matrix is displaced from its anatomic position at the sulcus, the matrix should be carefully replaced and held in place with mattress sutures (Fig 15-4).

12. If there is extensive injury to the nail bed with avulsed tissue, specialist consultation is required.

13. In children with fractures of the distal phalanx, the nail plate may come to lie on the eponychium. After careful cleaning and adequate anesthesia, the nail plate should be replaced under the proximal nail fold.

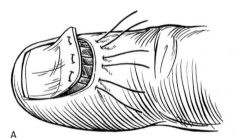

FIG. 15-4. Technique for repair of an avulsion of the germinal matrix using three horizontal mattress sutures. (Reproduced with permission from Chudnofsky CR, Sebastian S: Special wounds—Nail bed, plantar puncture, and cartilage. *Emerg Med Clin North Am.* 1992; 10:808.)

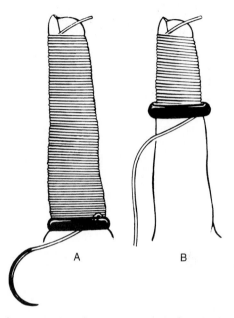

FIG. 15-5. String technique for ring removal. **A.** Completely wrapped. **B.** Unwrapping with ring advancing off with the string.

Ring Tourniquet Syndrome

1. Ring removal is required in all injured fingers. Swelling may require that the ring be cut off. If slower techniques are appropriate, simple lubrication may suffice.
2. The string technique is an alternative method (Fig 15-5).
   a. String, umbilical tape, or 0-gauge silk may be used.
   b. The string is passed under the ring and then wrapped firmly around the finger from proximal to distal.
   c. The proximal end of the string is then gently pulled, and the ring advances down the finger.

For further reading in *Emergency Medicine: A Comprehensive Study Guide,* 6th ed., see Chap. 44, "Injuries to the Arm, Hand, Fingertip and Nail" by Fiona E. Gallahue and Wallace A. Carter.

16 | Lacerations to the Leg and Foot

David M. Cline

CLINICAL FEATURES

The mechanism of the injury determines the likelihood of disruption to underlying tissue, the risk of a retained foreign body, and the degree of potential contamination. The following circumstances are associated with specific pathogens: (*a*) farming accidents (*Clostridium perfringens*), (*b*) wading in a freshwater stream *(Aeromonas hydrophila),* and (*c*) high-pressure water systems used for cleaning surfaces *(Acinetobacter calcoaceticus).* Evaluation of wounds in general is discussed in Chap. 12. It is important to determine the position of the limb at the time of injury, which will help to uncover occult tendon injuries.

DIAGNOSIS AND DIFFERENTIAL

Assessment for associated nerve, vessel, or tendon injury is mandatory. Before the use of anesthetic, the limb should be inspected for position at rest, and sensory neurologic function should be evaluated with light touch and 2-point discrimination testing. One side can be compared with the other. Motor function may be better assessed after the wound is anesthetized (Tables 16-1 and 16-2). At this time, the wound also can be explored. The limb should be moved through its full range of motion to exclude tendon injury. Each tendon function should be tested individually, but the tendon should be inspected visually to rule out a partial laceration.

Laboratory studies usually are not indicated. Radiology is required if there is a possibility of fracture or radiopaque foreign body. All injuries caused by glass should be radiographed unless physical examination can reliably exclude a foreign body (see Chap. 17).

EMERGENCY DEPARTMENT CARE AND DISPOSITION

General Recommendations

1. See Chap. 12 for discussion of wound preparation; thorough irrigation of lower extremity wounds is essential.
2. Wounds on the lower extremities are usually under greater tension than those on the upper limb. Consequently, a layered closure with 4-0 absorbable material to the fascia and interrupted 4-0 nonabsorbable sutures to the skin are preferred. The foot is an exception to this guideline.
3. Deep sutures should be avoided in diabetics and patients with stasis changes because of the increased risk of infection.
4. Tetanus immunization status should always be considered. The elderly are at particular risk for being nonimmunized.
5. Cyanoacrylate glue usually is not used on the lower extremities because of greater wound tension.
6. Lacerations involving the joint or tendons should be splinted in a position of function.

106

TABLE 16-1 Motor Function of Lower Extremity
Peripheral Nerves

Nerve	Motor function
Superficial peroneal	Foot eversion
Deep peroneal	Foot inversion
	Ankle dorsiflexion
Tibial	Ankle plantar flexion

Knee injuries

1. Wounds over the knee, as for all wounds over joints, should be examined throughout the range of movement.
2. Injuries over joints also should be evaluated for possible penetration of the joint capsule. If this is a consideration, radiography may show air in the joint.
3. An alternative approach to diagnose joint penetration is to inject 60 mL of sterile saline, with or without a few drops of sterile fluorescein, into the joint by using a standard joint aspiration technique at a site separate from the laceration. Leakage of the solution from the wound indicates joint capsule injury.
4. The popliteal artery, the popliteal nerve, and the tibial nerve are at risk around the knee: their integrity always should be ascertained.
5. After closure, the knee should be splinted to prevent excessive tension on the wound edges.

Ankle injuries

1. Lacerations to the ankle can easily damage underlying tendons. The joints should be moved through their full range, with direct inspection of the wound to ensure there is no partial injury to the tendon. Particularly at risk are the Achilles tendon, the tibialis anterior, and the extensor hallucis longus.
2. If any of these tendons are injured, they should be formally repaired.
3. The Achilles tendon can rupture without a penetrating injury when a tensed gastrocnemius is suddenly contracted. This injury is most common in an athletic middle-age male. The Thompson test can be used to assess the Achilles tendon. While kneeling on a chair, the patient's calf is gently squeezed at the midpoint. Absent plantar flexion of the foot indicates complete Achilles tendon laceration (a partial injury may yield plantar flexion).

Foot Injures

1. Lacerations of the sole of the foot must be explored carefully to ensure the absence of tendon injury and the absence of foreign bodies. The patient

TABLE 16-2 Tendon Function of the Lower Extremities

Tendon	Motor function
Extensor hallucis longus	Great toe extension with ankle inversion
Tibialis anterior	Ankle dorsiflexion and inversion
Achilles tendon	Ankle plantar flexion and inversion

lying prone, with the foot supported on a pillow or overhanging the bed, assists inspection.

2. Regional anesthesia is often best for exploration and repair of lacerations in this area.
3. Because of the high risk for infection, wounds older than 6 hours at presentation probably should not be repaired primarily.
4. Large needles are required to penetrate adequately the thick dermis of the sole. Absorbable material usually is avoided in the foot. Nonabsorbable 3-0 or 4-0 material is used. Injuries to the dorsum of the foot can be repaired with 4-0 or 5-0 nonabsorbable sutures.
5. Lacerations between the toes can be difficult to repair. The presence of an assistant who holds the toes apart can be a great help. An interrupted mattress suture often is required to ensure adequate skin apposition.
6. Crutches and a walking boot may be required after repair of any laceration on the foot.
7. Other potentially serious injuries to the foot may be caused by lawn mowers and by bicycle spokes. Extensive soft tissue injury can occur, in addition to underlying fractures and tendon lacerations. These severe injuries require the services of an orthopedic specialist.
8. Between 18% and 34% of foot lacerations become infected. Antibiotic prophylaxis should be considered for patients at risk by history or injury mechanism.
9. Wounds caused while wading in fresh water are prone to infection with *Aeromonas*. In these cases, a fluoroquinolone such as **ciprofloxacin** 500 mg twice daily is required. In children, **trimethoprim/sulfamethoxazole,** 5-mL suspension per 10 kg up to 20 mL twice daily, is used. *Aeromonas* should be considered in any rapidly progressive case of cellulitis in the foot after an injury.

Hair Tourniquet Syndrome

1. Hair tourniquet syndrome is an unusual type of injury seen in infants. A strand or strands of hair wrap around one of the toes, producing vascular compromise.
2. The hair must be completely cut to avoid compromising the neurovascular bundle to the toe.
3. This is best accomplished by making an incision on the extensor surface of the toe down to the extensor ligament.

Disposition

1. Patients should be instructed to keep wounds clean and dry.
2. Sutures should be removed in 10 to 14 days for the lower limb and in 14 days for lacerations over joints.
3. Patients should receive routine wound care instructions. Elevation of the affected limb will reduce edema and aid healing.
4. Wounds should be rechecked after 48 hours if they were heavily contaminated or if a complex repair was required.
5. Crutches can be used for 7 to 10 days, as needed, to prevent additional tension on the wound.

For further reading in *Emergency Medicine: A Comprehensive Study Guide,* 6th ed., see Chap. 45, "Lacerations of the Leg and Foot," by Earl J. Reisdorff.

17 | Soft Tissue Foreign Bodies

Rodney L. McCaskill

The potential exists for the presence of a foreign body in all wounds. Retained foreign bodies may lead to a severe inflammatory response (from wood, thorns, and spines), chronic local pain (from glass, metal, and plastic), local toxic reactions (from sea urchin spines, and catfish spines), systemic toxicity (from lead), or infection.

CLINICAL FEATURES

The mechanism of injury, composition, and shape of the wounding object and the shape and location of the resulting wound may increase the risk of a foreign body. Lacerating objects that splinter, shatter, or break increase the risk of a foreign body.

Because patients are often inaccurate in perceiving foreign bodies at the time of examination (43% sensitivity and 83% specificity), wound evaluation is critical. Careful exploration of the depths of all wounds increases the likelihood of finding a foreign body. Extending the edges of the wound is often necessary to thoroughly investigate for foreign bodies. Although puncture wounds and apparently superficial wounds can hold foreign bodies, wounds deeper than 5 mm and those whose depths cannot be investigated have a higher association with foreign bodies. Blind probing with a hemostat is less effective but may be used if the wound is narrow and deep and extending the wound is not desirable.

Patients returning to the emergency department with retained foreign bodies may complain of sharp pain at the wound site with movement, a chronically irritated nonhealing wound, or a chronically infected wound.

DIAGNOSIS AND DIFFERENTIAL

Imaging studies should be ordered if a foreign body is suspected. Most foreign bodies (80%-90%) can be seen on plain radiographs. Metal, bone, teeth, pencil graphite, certain plastics, glass, gravel, sand, and aluminum are visible on plain film. Using an under-penetrated soft tissue technique may increase the likelihood of identifying a foreign body by increasing the contrast between it and the surrounding tissue. Unfortunately, wood, thorns, cactus spines, some fish bones, most plastics, and other organic matter cannot be seen on plain film; however, because of its sensitivity in detecting different densities, computed tomography has been used successfully. Ultrasound is probably less accurate than computed tomography but it reportedly has a 90% sensitivity for detecting foreign bodies larger than 4 to 5 mm. Magnetic resonance imaging can detect radiolucent foreign bodies and is more accurate than the other modalities in identifying wood, plastic, spines, and thorns, but it is less available for emergency use.

EMERGENCY DEPARTMENT CARE AND DISPOSITION

General Principles

Not all foreign bodies need to be removed. Indications for foreign body removal include potential for infection, toxicity, functional problems, or

109

persistent pain. Radiopaque foreign bodies may be localized with skin markers and x-ray. Ultrasound may be used by experienced clinicians. Most busy emergency physicians will be able to dedicate only 15 to 30 minutes to removal procedures.

Specific Foreign Bodies and Removal Procedures

Metallic Needles

Needles may be difficult to locate. If the needle is superficial and can be palpated, an incision can be made over 1 end and the needle removed. If the needle is deeper, then the incision can be made at the midpoint of the needle and the needle grasped with a hemostat and pushed back out through the entrance wound. If the needle is perpendicular to the skin, the incision may need to be extended, and then pressure on the wound edges may demonstrate the needle so that it can be grasped and removed.

Wood Splinters and Organic Spines

Wooden splinters and organic spines are difficult to remove because of their tendency to break. Only splinters that are superficial should be removed by longitudinal traction. Otherwise the wound should be enlarged and the splinter lifted out of the wound intact. If the splinter is small and localization is difficult, then a block of tissue may be removed in an elliptical fashion and the remaining wound closed primarily. Because infection occurs frequently, subungual splinters should be removed with splinter forceps or by excising a portion of nail over the splinter and then removing the splinter intact. Cactus spines may be removed individually or with an adhesive such as facial gel, rubber cement, or household glue.

Fishhooks

Several techniques have been established to remove fishhooks. When using any of the techniques, anesthesia should be injected around the fishhook entry site. When using the string pull method, 1 hand depresses the shank of the hook to disengage the barb while the other gives a quick tug on a string that has been wrapped around the bend in the hook (Fig. 17-1). When using the needle cover technique, an 18-gauge needle is inserted beside the shank of the hook and attempts are made to sheath the barb of the hook. Once sheathed, the hook and needle are removed as 1 unit (Fig. 17-2). When the advance-and-cut technique is used, the point and the barb of the fishhook are pushed through the skin and clipped with wire cutters, and the remaining part of the

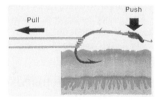

FIG. 17-1. String-pull technique. String or suture material is tied to the curve of the hook. The hook is positioned as described in the simple retrograde technique, and a quick pull on the string will dislodge the hook.

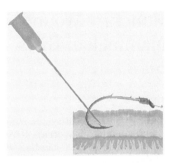

FIG. 17-2.   Needle-cover technique. The area is anesthetized, and an 18-gauge needle is inserted into the entrance wound along the hook. The lumen of the needle is placed over the barb to cover it, and both the hook and needle are backed out of the wound.

hook is threaded back through the original wound. The final technique involves enlarging the wound down to the barb and then removing the hook. This technique allows for easier wound exploration and cleaning.

Post-Removal Treatment

After removal of a foreign body, the wound should be adequately cleaned and irrigated, which may require extension of the incision. If the potential for infection is low, the wound may be closed primarily. If there is a significant risk of infection, delayed primary closure is preferred. If a foreign body is deliberately left in place, the patient should be informed and follow-up ensured.

Delayed Removal

If a foreign body is suspected or identified radiographically but cannot be located even after thorough wound evaluation, or if the foreign body is located in an area that prohibits removal, then the patient should be referred to a surgical specialist for delayed removal. If the foreign body is near a tendon or joint, the limb should be splinted. Prophylactic antibiotics, although widely prescribed, may not be necessary in wounds with no sign of infection.

For further reading in *Emergency Medicine: A Comprehensive Study Guide,* 6th ed. see
Chap. 42, "Soft Tissue Foreign Bodies," by Richard L. Lammers.

18 | Puncture Wounds and Mammalian Bites

Chris Melton

PUNCTURE WOUNDS

Puncture wounds may injure underlying structures, introduce a foreign body, and plant inoculum for infection. Infection occurs in 6% to 11% of puncture wounds, with *Staphylococcus aureus* predominating. *Pseudomonas aeruginosa* is the most frequent etiologic agent in post-puncture wound osteomyelitis, particularly when penetration occurs through the sole of an athletic shoe. Post-puncture wound infections and failure of an infection to respond to antibiotics suggests the presence of a retained foreign body. Organized evaluation and management is necessary to minimize complications.

Clinical Features (See Chap. 12)

Wounds older than 6 hours with large and deep penetration and obvious visible contamination, which occurred outdoors with penetration through footwear and involving the forefoot, carry the highest risk of infectious complications. Patients with a history of diabetes mellitus (DM), peripheral vascular disease (PVD), or immunosuppression are at increased risk of infection.

On physical examination, the likelihood of injury to structures beneath the skin must be determined. Distal function of tendons, nerves, and vessels should be assessed carefully. The site should be inspected for location, condition of the surrounding skin, and the presence of foreign matter, debris, or devitalized tissue. Infection is suggested when there is evidence of pain, swelling, erythema, warmth, fluctuance, decreased range of motion, or drainage from the site.

Diagnosis and Differential

A high index of suspicion must be maintained for a retained foreign body. Multiple view, "soft tissue," plain film radiographs should be obtained of all infected puncture wounds and of any wound suspicious for a retained foreign body (see Chap. 17 for recommendations on the diagnosis and management of retained foreign bodies).

Emergency Department Care and Disposition

Many aspects of the treatment of puncture wounds remain controversial.

1. Uncomplicated, clean punctures less than 6 hours after injury require only low-pressure irrigation and tetanus prophylaxis, as indicated. Soaking has no proven benefit. Healthy patients do not appear to require prophylactic antibiotics.
2. Prophylactic antibiotics "may" benefit patients with PVD, DM and immunosuppression. Plantar puncture wounds, especially those in high-risk patients, located in the forefoot, or through athletic shoes should be treated with prophylactic antibiotics. Fluoroquinolones (such as **ciprofloxacin** 500 mg twice daily) are broad-spectrum antibiotics that rapidly achieve high blood levels after an oral dose and are acceptable alternatives to par-

enteral administration of a cephalosporin and aminoglycoside. In general, prophylactic antibiotics should be continued for 5 to 7 days.

3. Ciprofloxacin is not recommended for routine use in children for prophylaxis. **Cephalexin** 25 to 50 mg/kg/d divided 4 times up to 500 mg can be used with close follow-up.

4. Wounds infected at presentation need to be differentiated into cellulitis, abscess, deeper spreading soft tissue infections, and bone or cartilage involvement. Plain radiographs are indicated to detect the possibility of radiopaque foreign body, soft tissue gas, or osteomyelitis.

5. Cellulitis usually is localized without significant drainage, developing within 1 to 4 days. There is no need for routine cultures, and antimicrobial coverage should be directed at gram-positive organisms, especially *S aureus*. Seven to 10 days of a first-generation cephalosporin is usually effective.

6. A local abscess may develop at the puncture site, especially if a foreign body remains. Treatment includes incision, drainage, and careful exploration for a retained foreign body. The wound should be rechecked in 48 hours. Serious, deep, soft tissue infections require surgical exploration and debridement in the operating room.

7. Any patient who relapses or fails to improve after initial therapy should be suspected of having osteomyelitis or septic arthritis. Radiographs, white blood cell count, erythrocyte sedimentation rate, and orthopedic consultation should be obtained. Definitive management frequently necessitates operative intervention for debridement. Pending cultures, antibiotics that cover *Staphylococcus* and *Pseudomonas* species are started. A reasonable regimen is parenteral **nafcillin** 1 to 2 g intravenously (IV) every 4 hours and **ceftazidime** 1 to 2 g IV every 8 hours.

8. Conditions for admission include wound infection in patients with DM, PVD, or other immunocompromised states; wounds with progressive cellulitis and lymphangitic spread; osteomyelitis; septic arthritis; and deep foreign bodies necessitating operative removal.

9. Tetanus prophylaxis should be provided according to guidelines (see Chap. 19). Outpatients should avoid weight bearing, elevate and soak the wound in warm water, and have follow-up within 48 hours.

NEEDLE-STICK INJURIES

Needle-stick injuries carry the risk of bacterial infection in addition to the risk of infection with hepatitis and human immunodeficiency virus (HIV). Each hospital should have a predesigned protocol developed by infectious disease specialists for the expeditious evaluation, testing, and treatment of needle-stick injuries, because recommendations in this area are complex and changing.

HIGH-PRESSURE-INJECTION INJURIES

High-pressure-injection injuries may present as puncture wounds, usually to the hand or foot. High-pressure-injection equipment is designed to force liquids (usually paint or oil) through a small nozzle under high pressure. These injuries are severe owing to intense inflammation incited by the injected liquid spreading along fascial planes. Patients have pain and minimal swelling. Despite an innocuous appearance, serious damage can develop. Pain control should be achieved with parenteral analgesics; digital blocks are contraindicated to avoid increases in tissue pressure with resultant further compromise in perfusion. An appropriate hand specialist should be consulted immediately, and early surgical debridement should be implemented for an optimal outcome.

HUMAN BITES

Human bites produce a crushing or tearing of tissue, with potential for injury to underlying structures and inoculation of tissues with normal human oral flora. Human bites are most often reported on the hands and upper extremities. Infection is the major serious sequelae.

Clinical Features (See Chap. 12)

Of particular concern is the clenched fist injury (CFI), which occurs at the metacarpophalangeal (MCP) region as the fist strikes the mouth and teeth of another individual. These hand injuries are at increased risk for serious infection, and any questionable injury in the vicinity of the MCP joint should be considered a CFI until proven otherwise.

The physical examination should include assessment of the direct injury and a careful evaluation of the underlying structures, including tendons, vessels, nerves, deep spaces, joints, and bone. Local anesthesia usually is required to perform a careful wound exploration. In a CFI, the wound must be examined through a full range of motion at the MCP joint to detect extensor tendon involvement, which may have retracted proximally in the unclenched hand. The examination also must assess a potential joint-space violation. Radiographs are recommended, particularly of the hand, to delineate foreign bodies and fractures.

Human bites to the hand frequently are complicated by cellulitis, lymphangitis, abscess formation, tenosynovitis, septic arthritis, and osteomyelitis. Infections from human bites are polymicrobial, with staphylococcal and streptococcal species being common isolates in addition to species-specific *Eikenella corrodens*.

Diagnosis and Differential

History and physical examination usually will indicate a straightforward diagnosis. There are times, however, when a patient may try to conceal or deny the true etiology of a human bite, and a high degree of suspicion is warranted, particularly when the wound is on the hand. It is important to keep in mind that viral diseases also can be transmitted by human bites (eg, herpes simplex, herpetic whitlow, and hepatitis B). The potential risk of acquiring HIV through a human bite appears to be negligible due to low levels of HIV in saliva.

Emergency Department Care and Disposition

1. Copious wound irrigation with a normal saline solution and judicious limited debridement of devitalized tissue are critical to initial management.
2. Human bites to the hand initially should be left open. Other sites can undergo primary closure unless there is a high degree of suspicion for infection.
3. Prophylactic antibiotics should be considered in all but the most trivial of human bites. **Amoxicillin/clavulanate** 500 to 875 mg orally (PO) twice daily is the antibiotic of choice.
4. Uncomplicated, fresh CFI wounds should be left open with an appropriate dressing. The hand should be immobilized and elevated for 24 hours, and

prophylactic antibiotics should be administered. The patient should be reevaluated in 1 to 2 days. If there is a laceration to the extensor tendon or joint capsule or radiographic findings, a hand specialist should be consulted for possible exploration in the operating room and admission for parenteral antibiotics.
5. Wounds that are infected at presentation require systemic antibiotics after cultures are obtained. Local cellulitis in healthy and reliable patients may be managed on an outpatient basis with immobilization, antibiotics, and close follow-up. Moderate to severe infections require admission for surgical consultation and parenteral antibiotics. Appropriate coverage includes **ampicillin/sulbactam** 3 g IV every 6 hours or **cefoxitin** 2.0 g IV every 8 hours. Penicillin-allergic patients may be treated with clindamycin plus ciprofloxacin.
6. All patients should receive tetanus immunization according to guidelines.

DOG BITES

Clinical Features

Dog bites account for 80% to 90% of reported animal bites, with school-age children sustaining the majority of reported bites. Infection occurs in approximately 5% of cases and is more common in patients older than 50 years, those with hand wounds or deep puncture wounds, and those who delay in seeking initial treatment over a 24-hour period. A thorough history and examination as outlined in the section on human bites are required to assess the extent of the wound and the likelihood of infection. Infections from dog bite wounds are often polymicrobial and include aerobic and anaerobic bacteria.

Diagnosis and Differential

Radiographs are recommended if there is evidence of infection, suspicion of a foreign body, bony involvement, or large dog intracranial penetration bites to the heads of small children.

Emergency Department Care and Disposition

1. All dog bite wounds require appropriate local wound care with copious irrigation and debridement of devitalized tissue.
2. Primary closure can be used in wounds to the scalp, face, torso, and extremities other than the feet and hands. Lacerations of the feet and hands should be left open initially. Large, extensive lacerations, especially in small children, are best explored and repaired in the operating room.
3. Puncture wounds, wounds to the hands and feet, and wounds in high-risk patients should receive 3 to 5 days of prophylactic antibiotics with **amoxicillin/clavulanate** 500 to 875 mg PO twice daily or clindamycin plus ciprofloxacin. In children, clindamycin plus trimethoprim-sulfamethoxazole should be used.
4. **Penicillin** (500 mg PO 4 times a day) is the drug of choice for *Capnocytophaga canimorsus* and should be used prophylactically in high-risk immunocompromised patients (ie, those with asplenia, alcoholism, or chronic lung disease). Cephalosporins, tetracycline, erythromycin, and clindamycin are reasonable alternatives.
5. Wounds obviously infected at presentation need to be cultured and antibiotics initiated. Reliable, low-risk patients with only local cellulitis and no

involvement of underlying structures can be managed as outpatients with close follow-up.

6. Infection developing within 24 hours after injury suggests *Pasteurella multocida,* and treatment with penicillin, ciprofloxacin, or trimethoprim-sulfamethoxazole is recommended. Wound infection developing beyond 24 hours after the bite implicates *Staphylococcus* and *Streptococcus,* and these patients should receive **dicloxacillin** (12 to 25 mg/kg/d divided 4 times daily; 500 mg 4 times daily in adults) or first-generation cephalosporin (eg, **cephalexin** 25 to 50 mg/kg/d divided 4 times daily; 500 mg 4 times daily in adults).

7. Significant wound infections require admission and parenteral antibiotics. Examples include infected wounds with evidence of lymphangitis, lymph-adenitis, tenosynovitis, septic arthritis, osteomyelitis, systemic signs, and injury to underlying structures, such as tendons, joints, or bones. Cultures should be obtained from deep structures, preferably during exploration in the operating room. Initial antibiotic therapy should begin with **ampi-cillin/sulbactam** 3 g IV every 6 hours or clindamycin plus ciprofloxacin. If the Gram stain reveals gram-negative bacilli, a third- or fourth-genera-tion cephalosporin or aminoglycoside should be added.

8. Tetanus prophylaxis should be provided according to standard guidelines.

CAT BITES

Cat bites account for 5% to 18% of reported animal bites, with the majority resulting in puncture wounds on the arm, forearm, and hand. Up to 80% of cat bites become infected.

Clinical Features

Pasteurella multocida is the major pathogen, isolated in 53% to 80% of in-fected cat bite wounds. *Pasteurella* causes a rapidly developing intense in-flammatory response with prominent symptoms of pain and swelling. It may cause serious bone and joint infections and bacteremia. Many patients with septic arthritis due to *P. multocida* have altered host defenses due to gluco-corticoids or alcoholism.

Diagnosis and Differential

Radiographs are recommended if there is evidence of infection, suspicion of a foreign body, or bony involvement.

Emergency Department Care and Disposition

Treatment for cat bite wounds is essentially the same as that for dog bite wounds.

1. All cat bite wounds require appropriate local wound care with copious ir-rigation and debridement of devitalized tissue.

2. Primary wound closure is usually indicated, except in puncture wounds and lacerations smaller than 1 to 2 cm, because they cannot be adequately cleaned. Delayed primary closure also can be used in cosmetically impor-tant areas.

3. Prophylactic antibiotics should be administered to high-risk patients in-cluding those with punctures of the hand; immunocompromised patients;

and patients with arthritis or prosthetic joints. The case can be made that all patients with cat bites should receive prophylactic antibiotics because of the high risk of infection. **Amoxicillin/clavulanate** 500 to 875 mg PO twice daily (45 mg/kg/d divided 2 times daily in children), **cefuroxime** 500 mg PO twice daily (20 to 30 mg/kg/d divided 2 times daily in children), or **doxycycline** 100 mg PO twice daily administered 3 to 5 days are appropriate.

4. For cat bites that develop infection, evaluation and treatment are similar to those for dog bite infections. Penicillin is the drug of choice for *P. multocida* infections.

5. Tetanus prophylaxis should be provided according to standard guidelines.

RODENTS, LIVESTOCK, EXOTIC AND WILD ANIMALS

Rodent bites are typically trivial, rodents are not known to carry rabies, and these bites have a low risk for infection. Livestock and large game animals can cause serious injury. There is also a significant risk of infection and systemic illness caused by brucellosis, leptospirosis, and tularemia. Aggressive wound care and broad-spectrum antibiotics are recommended.

For further reading in *Emergency Medicine: A Comprehensive Study Guide,* 6th ed., see Chap. 47, "Puncture Wounds and Mammalian Bites," by Robert A. Schwab and Robert D. Powers.

19 | Post Repair Wound Care

Eugenia B. Smith

USE OF DRESSINGS

Wound dressings provide a moist environment that promotes epithelialization and speeds healing. Semipermeable films such as OpSite are available in addition to conventional gauze dressings. The disadvantages of these materials are their inability to absorb large amounts of fluid. Alternatively, topical antibiotics may be used to provide a warm, moist environment. Topical antibiotics may reduce the rate of wound infection and also may prevent scab formation. Wounds closed with tissue adhesives should not be treated with topical antibiotic ointment because it will loosen the adhesive.

PATIENT POSITIONING AFTER WOUND REPAIR

The injured site should be elevated, if possible, to reduce edema around the wound and speed healing. Splints are useful for extremity injuries because they decrease motion and edema and increase attention paid to the body part. Pressure dressings minimize the accumulation of fluid and are most useful for ear and scalp lacerations. A pressure dressing on the ear decreases auricular hematoma formation, thereby reducing the likelihood of a cauliflower deformity (see Chap. 14).

PROPHYLACTIC ANTIBIOTICS

There is no benefit to prophylactic antibiotics for routine laceration repair. When deciding whether or not to prescribe antibiotics, consider the mechanism of injury (ie, crush injury), degree of bacterial or soil contamination, and host predisposition to infection. Prophylactic antibiotics are recommended for human bites, dog or cat bites on the extremities, intraoral lacerations, open fractures, and wounds with exposed joints or tendons. For most patients, a first-generation cephalosporin (eg, **cephalexin** 25 to 50 mg/kg divided in 4 daily doses, up to 500 mg per dose) or antistaphylococcal penicillin (eg, **dicloxacillin** 25 to 50 mg/kg divided in 4 daily doses, up to 500 mg per dose) is reasonable. **Penicillin** (25 to 50 mg/kg divided in 4 daily doses, up to 500 mg per dose), which is active against most oral pathogens, is recommended for intraoral wounds. **Amoxicillin/clavulanate** (20 to 40 mg/kg/d divided every 8 hours, up to 500 mg per dose) or a combination of penicillin and dicloxacillin is the preferred choice for high-risk mammalian bite wounds (see Chap. 18). For open fractures or joints, a parenteral antistaphylococcal agent and an aminoglycoside are recommended (see Chaps. 15 and 16). A 3- to 5-day course is adequate for non-bite injuries and a 5- to 7-day course is adequate for bite wounds.

TETANUS PROPHYLAXIS

The need for tetanus prophylaxis should be considered for every wounded patient. The only contraindication to tetanus toxoid is a history of neurologic or severe systemic reaction after a previous dose. Patients with clean minor wounds require tetanus prophylaxis if it has been longer than 10 years since the last dose. Tetanus prophylaxis is indicated for all other wounded patients if it has been longer than 5 years since the last dose. Administer tetanus-diphtheria (Td) 0.5 mL IM. Tetanus immune globulin 250 U, IM, should be administered to those without a history of a primary series of 3 tetanus immunizations. A second dose of tetanus immune globulin is required in 1 to 2 months and a third dose in 6 to 12 months.

PAIN CONTROL

Patients should be educated about the expected degree of pain and measures that might reduce pain. Splints can help reduce pain in extremity lacerations. Medications may be needed, but narcotic analgesia is rarely necessary after the first 48 hours.

WOUND CARE INSTRUCTIONS AND FOLLOW-UP

Standardized wound care instructions improve patient compliance and understanding. Sutured or stapled lacerations should be washed gently and cleaned as soon as 8 hours after closure. Patients with dressings should remove their dressings after 24 to 48 hours. Daily cleaning ensures that the patient examines the laceration for early signs of infection. Patients should be instructed to observe for redness, warmth, swelling, or drainage and to initiate contact with their provider if their observe these signs. Patients should be instructed about the timing of suture removal. Facial sutures should be removed in 3 to 5 days. Most other sutures can be removed in 7 to 10 days, except for sutures in the hands or over joints, which should remain for 10 to 14 days. Tissue adhesives will slough off within 5 to 10 days of application. In the case of high-risk wounds, patients may be instructed to return for a wound check, usually in 48 hours.

PATIENT EDUCATION ABOUT LONG-TERM COSMETIC OUTCOME

Patients should understand that all traumatic lacerations result in some scarring. They also should understand that the short-term cosmetic appearance is not highly predictive of the ultimate cosmetic outcome. Instruct patients to avoid sun exposure while their wounds are healing because it can cause permanent hyperpigmentation. Patients should wear sunblock for at least 6 to 12 months after injury.

5 | CARDIOVASCULAR DISEASES

20 | Approach to Chest Pain and Ischemic Equivalents

Thomas Rebbecchi

Patients with acute nontraumatic chest pain are among the most challenging patients cared for by emergency physicians. They may appear seriously ill or completely well and yet remain at significant risk for sudden death or an acute myocardial infarction (AMI).

CLINICAL FEATURES

The typical pain of myocardial ischemia has been described as retrosternal or epigastric squeezing, tightening, crushing, or pressure-like discomfort. The pain may radiate to the left shoulder, jaw, arm, or hand. In many cases, particularly in the elderly, the predominant complaint is not of pain, but of a poorly described visceral sensation with associated dyspnea, diaphoresis, nausea, lightheadedness, or profound weakness. The onset of symptoms may be sudden or gradual, and symptoms usually last minutes to hours. In general, symptoms that last less than 2 minutes or are constant over days are less likely to be ischemic in origin. Symptoms that are new or familiar to the patient but now occur with increasing frequency, severity, or at rest are called *unstable* and warrant urgent evaluation even if they are absent at the time of presentation. Cardiac risk factors should be used only to predict coronary artery disease within a given population and not in an individual patient. It should also be mentioned that women, diabetics, and patients with psychiatric disorders may have more subtle signs of ischemia.

PHYSICAL EXAMINATION

Patients with acute myocardial ischemia may appear clinically well or be profoundly hemodynamically unstable. The degree of hemodynamic instability is dependent on the amount of myocardium at risk, associated dysrhythmias, or preexisting valvular or myocardial dysfunction. Worrisome signs may be clinically subtle, particularly the presence of sinus tachycardia, which may be due to pain and fear or may be an early sign of physiologic compensation for left ventricular failure. Patients with acute ischemia often have a paucity of significant physical findings. Rales, a third or fourth heart sound, cardiac murmurs, or rub are clinically relevant and important findings. The presence of chest wall tenderness has been demonstrated in patients with AMI, so its presence should not be used to exclude the possibility of acute myocardial ischemia. Also, response to a particular treatment such as nitroglycerin or a "gastrointestinal (GI) cocktail" should not be taken as evidence of a certain disease.

DIAGNOSIS AND DIFFERENTIAL

Electrocardiography

Of all the diagnostic tools clinically used in assessing chest pain, the electrocardiogram (ECG) is the most reliable when used and interpreted correctly. Patients with acute infarctions may have ECG findings that range from acute

ST-segment elevations to completely normal. This range means that the ECG is useful only when it has a positive, or diagnostic, finding. New ST-segment elevations, Q waves, bundle branch block, and T-wave inversions or normalizations are strongly suggestive of ischemia and warrant aggressive management in the emergency department (ED). The presence of a normal or unchanged ECG does not rule out the diagnosis of acute myocardial ischemia.

Serum Markers

Serum markers, if positive, are highly specific for AMI. Myoglobin rises predictably in AMI but is found in all muscle tissue, making it less reliable in the setting of AMI. Creatinine phosphokinase and its MB isoenzyme constitute the historical gold standard for diagnosing AMI. Troponin I is not found in skeletal muscle, so it has a much greater sensitivity and specificity for AMI. The documentation of normal serum markers in the bloodstream does not exclude the diagnosis of AMI. In addition, these enzymes will not become elevated in serious disease conditions such as unstable angina. The use of these markers can aid the clinician in assessing risk for patients with chest pain, including disposition within the hospital. It must be remembered that a serial enzyme evaluation is needed to appropriately risk stratify individual patients (Fig. 20-1).

Echocardiography

Emergency 2-dimensional echocardiography may have value in the evaluation of chest pain when the ECG is nondiagnostic, eg, in patients with pacemakers, have a bundle branch block, or have a baseline abnormal ECG. The finding of regional wall motion abnormalities in the acutely symptomatic patient is strongly suggestive of active ischemia. Wall motion abnormality also may represent previous myocardial injury. Two-dimensional echocardiography also may aid in the diagnosis of other conditions that may mimic

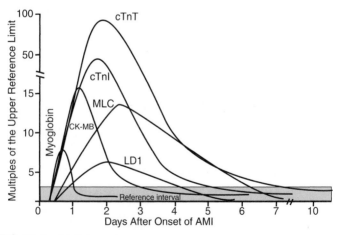

FIG. 20-1. Multiple marker curve.

ischemic disease, such as pericarditis, aortic dissection, or hypertrophic cardiomyopathy.

Provocative Tests

Many tests currently being performed in some EDs will unmask otherwise unrecognized, clinically significant ischemic disease. Patients with atypical chest pain and a normal stress thallium or technetium scan have a very low incidence of short- and long-term subsequent ischemic events. Thallium or sestamibi testing can be done in the ED to further risk stratify patients in the hospital and perhaps be used in consideration for patient discharge from the ED.

Differential Diagnosis

The priority must always be to exclude life-threatening conditions, and the ED physicians should organize their test-ordering strategies to screen for those conditions first. (Table 20-1 lists possible causes of nontraumatic chest pain.)

SPECIFIC CAUSES OF CHEST PAIN

Angina Pectoris

The pain of chronic stable angina is episodic and lasts 5 to 15 minutes. It is precipitated by exertion and relieved with rest or sublingual nitroglycerin within 3 minutes. The pain is typically visceral in nature (aching, pressure, and squeezing), with radiation to the neck, jaw, arm, or hand. In individual patients the character of each attack varies little with recurrent episodes. Most patients can differentiate their usual angina from other causes of pain. Physicians evaluating patients with stable angina should screen carefully for changes in the pattern that would suggest a shift from stable to unstable angina or even suggest a different diagnosis.

Unstable Angina

Patients who complain of recent onset of angina, changes in the character of the angina, or angina at rest are thought to have an unstable pattern of their angina. They are at risk for an AMI or sudden cardiac death (see Chap. 21 for management).

TABLE 20-1 Serious Causes of Chest Pain and Their Presentation

Diagnosis	Presentation
Pulmonary embolism (see Chap. 26)	Sudden onset, pleuritic pain, and dyspnea
Aortic dissection (see Chap. 28)	Tearing pain with radiation to back, neurologic symptoms
Pericarditis (see Chap. 25)	Positional ache, dyspnea
Pneumothorax (see Chap. 33)	Pleuritic pain and dyspnea
Acute coronary syndrome (see Chap. 21)	Vague, pressure-like pain, radiation to arm, neck, jaw
Esophageal rupture (see Chap. 38)	Constant retrosternal, epigastric pain, history of inciting event
Pneumonia (see Chap. 31)	Pleuritic pain, cough, dyspnea, chills

Variant (Prinzmetal) Angina

This form of angina is thought to be due to spasm of the epicardial vessels in patients with normal coronary arteries (one third of cases) or in patients with underlying atherosclerotic disease (two thirds of cases). Pain typically occurs at rest and may be precipitated by the use of tobacco or cocaine. The ECG typically shows ST-segment elevations during an acute attack.

Acute Myocardial Infarction

Ischemic pain that lasts longer than 15 minutes, is not relieved by nitroglycerin, or is accompanied by diaphoresis, dyspnea, nausea, or vomiting suggests the diagnosis of AMI. The clinician must understand the limitations of the screening tools used in the ED and should have a high level of suspicion for AMI in patients with risk factors and prolonged or persistent symptoms for whom there is no other clear diagnosis (see Chap. 21).

Aortic Dissection

This diagnosis should be suspected in the patient who complains of sudden onset of severe, tearing pain in the retrosternal or midscapular area. High-risk patients are also those at risk for AMI, specifically the middle-age hypertensive male. The patient may be hypertensive or hypotensive in shock. There may be a diastolic murmur of aortic regurgitation, indicating a proximal dissection, or distal pulse deficits, indicating a distal dissection. The dissection may occlude coronary ostia, resulting in myocardial infarction, or the carotids, resulting in cerebral ischemia and stroke. Chest x-ray, computed tomography, transesophageal echocardiography (TEE), and angiography can aid in the diagnosis of this condition (see Chap. 28 for a complete discussion of aortic dissection).

Pericarditis

The patient with pericarditis typically will complain of pain that is constant, retrosternal, and radiating to the back, neck, or jaw. Pain is classically worsened by lying supine and is relieved by sitting forward. The presence of a pericardial friction rub supports the diagnosis. ECG may show PR-segment depressions, diffuse ST-segment elevations, or T-wave inversions that are typically diffuse (see Chap. 25 for a complete discussion of pericarditis).

Acute Pericardial Tamponade

Patients with acute tamponade may complain of positional or pleuritic chest pain, dyspnea, and palpitations. Physical examination will show tachycardia, hypotension, jugular venous distention, and distant heart sounds. If cardiovascular collapse is imminent, emergent pericardiocentesis is indicated.

Pulmonary Embolus

Patients typically complain of sudden onset of pleuritic chest pain associated with dyspnea, tachypnea, tachycardia, or hypoxemia. The absence of any of these findings does not preclude the diagnosis, and a high index of suspicion is essential (see Chap. 26 for a complete discussion of pulmonary embolism).

Musculoskeletal Causes

Chest pain due to irritation or inflammation of structures in the chest wall is commonly seen in the ED. Possible causes include costochondritis, intercostal strain due to severe coughing, and pectoralis muscle strain in the setting of recent physical exertion. Patients will complain of sharp pain that is worsened with movement of the chest wall (eg, coughing, and some pain that can be elicited by palpation of the chest wall). These findings in patients without any other symptoms and no history of significant cardiac disease support the diagnosis of musculoskeletal pain. This pain is generally responsive to nonsteroidal anti-inflammatory drugs. It is important to emphasize that the presence of chest wall tenderness does not rule out the possibility of myocardial ischemia.

Gastrointestinal Causes

Esophageal reflux, dyspepsia syndromes, and esophageal motility disorders can produce chest pain that is difficult to distinguish from ischemic pain. Patients may complain of burning, gnawing pain associated with an acid taste radiating into the throat. Pain may be exacerbated by meals, worsen when supine, and may be associated with belching. Clinicians should determine whether the symptoms are due to a GI disorder based on the clinical presentation and the absence of findings and/or risk factors suggesting an ischemic cause. Diagnostic decisions should not be made on the basis of a response to a therapeutic trial of antacids, GI cocktails, or nitroglycerin (see Chaps. 36, 38, and 40 for more discussion of GI causes of chest pain).

EMERGENCY DEPARTMENT CARE AND DISPOSITION

It should be assumed that every patient complaining of chest pain might be having an AMI. Patients with suspicious histories should have a large-bore intravenous line established, a cardiac monitor, supplemental oxygen, and an ECG obtained as soon as possible. Vital signs and pulse oximetry should be monitored continuously.

1. Patients should be asked about cardiac risk factors, preexisting coronary artery disease, quality of chest pain, time of onset and duration of symptoms, and whether the pattern has been stable, unstable, continuous, or intermittent. Physicians should ask specifically for clues to noncardiac causes of chest pain: ability to elicit pain by movement or cough; the relation of pain to meals; or pain that is of sudden onset, referred to the back, or pleuritic in nature.
2. Patients should be examined while noting evidence of heart failure or valvular insufficiency, pericardial rubs, or tenderness of the chest wall. Specifically, physicians should ask whether pain elicited on palpation of the chest wall exactly reproduces the patient's pain.
3. An ECG should be obtained on all patients for whom there is a reasonable suspicion of myocardial ischemia. A normal ECG, although minimizing the likelihood of an AMI, does not definitively rule out the possibility of myocardial infarction (MI).
4. If the etiology of chest pain remains unclear in some patients, clinicians should consider more diagnostic tests as guided by clinical suspicion and findings.

5. Clinicians should not use patients' clinical response to GI cocktails, nitro-glycerin, or nonsteroidal anti-inflammatory drugs to exclude the possibility of myocardial ischemia.
6. In patients with nondiagnostic ECGs for whom there is a clinical suspicion for ischemia, clinicians should consider provocative testing, echocardiography, or admission and observation. Physicians should not rely on serum enzyme testing to rule out the possibility of clinically significant disease.

For further reading in *Emergency Medicine: A Comprehensive Study Guide*, 6th ed., see Chap. 49, "Approach to Chest Pain and Ischemic Equivalents," by Gary B. Green and Peter M. Hill.

21 | Acute Coronary Syndromes: Management of Myocardial Infarction and Unstable Angina

Jim Edward Weber

Ischemic heart disease is the leading cause of death among adults in the United States. Approximately 1.3 million nonfatal acute myocardial infarcts and 500,000 to 700,000 deaths occur yearly. Of these patients, 50% to 60% will die before hospital arrival. The majority of additional deaths will occur early during initial hospitalization. Currently, the greatest potential to decreasing mortality and morbidity is to minimize the time between injury and treatment.

CLINICAL FEATURES

Myocardial ischemia results from the imbalance between myocardial oxygen (O_2) supply and demand. Factors influencing O_2 supply include fixed or disrupted atherosclerotic lesions, vasospasm, platelet aggregation, and thrombus formation. Seven major risk factors for coronary artery disease (CAD) have been identified: age, male sex, family history, cigarette smoking, hypertension, hypercholesterolemia, and diabetes. However, cardiac risk factors are poor predictors of acute myocardial infarction (AMI) in emergency department (ED) patients. Cocaine is directly myotoxic, accelerates atherosclerosis and CAD, and may cause myocardial infarction (MI) in patients with or without CAD. The progression from ischemia to infarction (cell death) is a continuum. The degree and duration of the O_2 supply and demand mismatch determines whether the patient develops reversible ischemia without injury (angina) or with injury (MI).

Angina pectoris represents cardiac ischemia. Anginal pain is classically retrosternal and may radiate to the neck, jaw, shoulders, or the inside of the left or both arms. Anginal pain often is described as "discomfort." Patients may experience chest pressure, heaviness, fullness, squeezing, and sharp or stabbing pain. Reproducible chest wall tenderness is not uncommon. Associated symptoms include dizziness, palpitations, diaphoresis, dyspnea, nausea, fatigue, and vomiting. Stable angina is characterized by episodic chest pain, usually lasting 5 to 15 minutes. The pain is provoked by exertion, cold, or stress and relieved by rest or nitroglycerin (NTG). Stable angina is usually due to a fixed coronary lesion. Unstable angina represents a clinical state between stable angina and MI. Physiologically, unstable angina is due to plaque rupture and thrombosis. There are 3 forms of unstable angina: (*a*) new onset angina (within 2 months), (*b*) increasing angina (increased threshold, frequency, or duration), and (*c*) angina at rest (within 1 week).

Variant (Prinzmetal) angina occurs primarily at rest (without provocation) but can be provoked by cocaine or tobacco use. Coronary artery spasm is thought to cause variant angina.

MI patients usually present with more prolonged and severe anginal pain that is less responsive to NTG. Elderly patients and those with diabetes may have silent ischemia (painless) or atypical presentations (nonretrosternal

129

chest pain, atypical radiation, weakness, dizziness, or dyspnea). Patients with inferior MIs may have abdominal pain, nausea, or vomiting.

The major complications of cardiac ischemia or infarction are arrhythmias and impaired ventricular function. The major determinant of prognosis in MI is the amount of infarcted myocardium. In general, the more severe the degree of left ventricular (LV) dysfunction, the higher the mortality. Heart failure develops in up to 20% of patients with MI. One third of MI patients with acute heart failure have cardiogenic shock. Right ventricular (RV) MI occurs with approximately 30% of inferior MIs. RV MI may cause hypotension, which is worsened by NTG. Other complications of MI include mural thrombosis, systemic arterial embolism (strokes, etc), and rupture of the ventricular wall (cardiac rupture), ventricular septum, or papillary muscle (typically seen with inferior MI).

Dysrhythmic complications are frequent and can be fatal. The incidence of lethal dysrhythmias is greatest in the early phases of MI. Ventricular premature contractions are common in patients with MI but are not of prognostic significance. Sinus tachycardia is common in patients with anterior MI. Sinus bradycardia, first-degree atrioventricular blocks (AVBs), and Mobitz I AVBs are usually due to increased vagal tone, are more common in inferior MI, and rarely progress to higher AVB. Mobitz II and complete AVBs are usually due to structural damage to the conduction system seen in large anterior MI. Ventricular tachycardia and fibrillation occurring early in the setting of MI do not appear to have a great effect on prognosis. Delayed ventricular tachycardia and fibrillation are associated with significant mortality.

Pericarditis can occur during the first week after MI. Dressler syndrome occurs in the post-MI period and is characterized by chest pain, fever, pericarditis, and pleural effusions.

DIAGNOSIS AND DIFFERENTIAL

The diagnosis of angina is based on history. Physical examination of patients with ischemia or infarction is often unremarkable. The clinician must rapidly recognize the presence of complications: dysrhythmias, heart failure, and shock. New systolic murmurs may represent papillary muscle rupture (see Chap. 24). Friction rubs may be heard in the presence of pericarditis.

The most important diagnostic test in the ED is the electrocardiogram (ECG). However, only 50% of MI patients will have diagnostic changes on the initial ECG. A normal or nonspecific ECG does not rule out ischemia or negate the need for hospitalization. The diagnostic yield of ECGs can be im-

TABLE 21-1 Localization of Myocardial Infarction Based on Electrocardiographic Findings

Anterior	V_2–V_4
Inferior	II, III, aVF, V_5, V_6
Anteroseptal	V_1–V_3
Lateral	I, aVL, V_4–V_6
Anterolateral	V_1–V_6
Right ventricular	V_{4R}–V_{6R} (often associated with inferior)
Posterior MI	large R >0.04 mm, R/S >1, and ST depression in V_1 and V_2

Key: MI = myocardial infarction.

proved by recording additional leads (22 on the right side) and by obtaining serial or continuous recordings. Myocardial injury can be subendothelial (ST-segment depression) or transmural (ST-segment elevation). Ischemic T waves are deep, symmetrical, and inverted. After AMI, necrotic myocardium eventually produces Q waves. In the setting of MI, ST-segment changes are seen early, T-wave changes are variable, and Q waves take hours to develop. In general, the more elevated the ST segments and the more ST segments that are elevated, the more extensive the injury. Infarcts can be localized by determining the ECG leads affected (Table 21-1). ECG evaluation for ischemia can be difficult with paced rhythms or bundle branch block. MI in the setting of left bundle branch block or paced rhythms is suggested by (a) ST elevation greater than 1 mm concordant with the QRS complex; (b) ST depression greater than 1 mm in lead V_1, V_2, or V_3; and (c) discordant ST elevation of at least 5 mm.

Injured cardiac muscle cells release cardiac enzymes. Serial measurement of these enzymes is used to diagnose MI, but the role of these markers is limited in the ED. Many of these enzymes are not specific to myocardial injury (creatine phosphokinase, lactic acid dehydrogenase, myoglobin [MB], and troponin T). The cardiac isoform of troponin I is not found in skeletal muscle. Patients who are early in the course of MI may not have elevated creatine kinase (CK) MB, troponin I, or lactic acid dehydrogenase. The sensitivity of CK-MB immunoassays is 50% on presentation to the ED and rises to 90% if the duration of pain is longer than 9 hours. Troponin I has sensitivity and specificity similar to those of CK-MB. Troponin I is more sensitive for MI in the subset of patients with trauma, surgery, cocaine use, renal failure, or skeletal muscle disease. Myoglobin, troponin T, and CK-MB isoforms are released earlier than CK-MB. Patients with unstable angina will not show serial elevations in CK-MB. Elevations of troponins I and T are predictive of cardiovascular complications in patients with acute coronary syndromes (ACSs).

Echocardiography is useful in diagnosing impaired wall motion and anatomic complications of MI (ruptured papillary muscle or ventricular wall and pericardial effusion). Nuclear scans also may be used to diagnose MI. These modalities have been shown to be sensitive, but not specific, in the ED diagnosis of MI. Exercise stress testing can assist cardiovascular risk stratification in low to intermediate risk ED observation unit patients who have been ruled out for MI.

Differential diagnosis of cardiac ischemia or infarction includes pericarditis, cardiomyopathies, cardiac valvular disease, pulmonary embolism, pneumonia, pneumothorax, asthma or chronic obstructive pulmonary disease, gastrointestinal disorders (especially esophageal disease), chest trauma, chest wall disorders, hyperventilation, aortic aneurysm and dissection, and mediastinal disorders.

EMERGENCY DEPARTMENT CARE AND DISPOSITION

Treatment of ACS should be individualized based on symptoms, history physical examination, and ECG findings. Treatment strategies aim to achieve immediate patency and reperfusion to limit infarct size. Patency is established by medical (fibrinolytic therapy), mechanical (angioplasty), or surgical (coronary artery bypass graft [CABG]) means. Maintenance of patency is achieved by anticoagulation and antiplatelet agents. Protection of the myocardium is accomplished by reducing the heart's oxygen demand and increasing the oxygen delivery. Dysrhythmias should be treated if the effect on heart rate exacerbates oxygen supply or demand imbalance, or if the dysrhythmia seems capable of deteriorating into cardiac arrest (see Chap. 2).

1. All patients suspected of having cardiac pain should be placed on a cardiac monitor and receive an intravenous line and supplemental oxygen. A rapid screening, including risk factors, indications, and contraindications for thrombolytics, should be performed. ECGs should be obtained within 5 minutes of the patient's presentation to the ED. Treatment strategies to achieve immediate reperfusion and limit infarct size are listed in Table 21-2.

TABLE 21-2 Recommended Doses of Drugs Used in the Emergency Treatment of Acute Coronary Syndromes

Antiplatelet agents	
Aspirin	160–325 mg PO
Clopidogrel	Loading dose of 300 mg PO followed by 75 mg/d
Antithrombins	
Heparin	60–70 U/kg bolus (max, 5000 U) followed by infusion of 12–15 U/kg/h (max, 1000 U/h) titrated to a PTT 1.5–2.5 times control
Enoxaparin (LMWH)	1 mg/kg SC q12h
Fibrinolytic agents	
Streptokinase	1.5 million U over 60 min
Alteplase (tPA)	>67 kg: 15 mg initial IV bolus; 50 mg infused over next 30 min; 35 mg infused over next 60 min <67 kg: 15 mg initial IV bolus; 0.75 mg/kg infused over next 30 min; 0.5 mg/kg infused over next 60 min
Reteplase (rPA)	10-mg IV bolus followed by 10-mg IV bolus 30 min later
Tenecteplase (tPA)	Single bolus that is weight based, 30 to 50 mg
Glycoprotein IIb/IIIa inhibitors	
Abciximab	0.25 mg/kg bolus followed by infusion of 0.125 μg/kg/min (max, 10 μg/kg/min) for 12–24 h
Eptifibatide	180 μg/kg bolus followed by infusion of 2.0 μg/kg/min for 72–96 h
Tirofiban	0.4 μg/kg/min for 30 min followed by infusion of 0.1 μg/kg/min for 48–96 h
Other anti-ischemic therapies	
Nitroglycerin	SL: 0.4 mg q5 min × 3 PRN for pain IV: start at 10 μg/min, titrate to 10% reduction in MAP if normotensive, 30% reduction in MAP if hypertensive
Morphine	2–5 mg IV q5–15 min PRN for pain
Metoprolol	5 mg IV over 2 min q5 min up to 15 mg, followed by 50 mg PO q6h 15 min after last IV dose
Atenolol	5 mg IV over 5 min, repeat once 10 min later, followed with 50 mg PO

Key: IV = intravenously; LMWH = low-molecular-weight heparin; MAP = mean arterial pressure; max = maximum; PO = orally; PTT = partial thromboplastin time; q = every; rPA = recombinant plasminogen activator; SC = subcutaneously; SL = sublingual; tPA = tissue-type plasminogen activator.

2. **Aspirin** (ASA) has been shown to reduce cardiac deaths by up to 23%. ASA 160 to 325 mg should be given as soon as possible and chewed for more rapid onset. ASA and Indocin are also used to treat Dressler syndrome.

3. **Nitroglycerin** reduces cardiac mortality by up to 35%. Oral and transdermal NTG are useful in preventing angina. Sublingual NTG is usually effective for the treatment of acute anginal pain within 3 minutes. A sublingual dose should be repeated 3 times at 2- to 5-minute intervals. If there is no improvement with sublingual NTG, intravenous NTG should be started at 5 to 10 μg/min. Intravenous NTG is recommended for MI or recurrent ischemia. The dose should be titrated by 5- to 10-μg/min increments every 3 to 5 minutes to blood pressure reduction rather than to pain resolution. Doses above 100 μg/min have been associated with paradoxically increased ischemia. Such doses should be used cautiously in the setting of hypotension because they may further worsen perfusion to ischemic myocardium. NTG is not indicated in the setting of RV infarcts. A common side effect of NTG is headache.

4. **β-Blockers** can reduce the short- and long-term mortality in patients with MI. $β_1$-Blocking (cardioselective) agents are preferred (metoprolol). Indications for β-blockers include ST-segment elevation MI, recurrent ischemia, tachydysrhythmia, and non-ST-segment elevation MI (NSTEMI). Relative contraindications to the use of β-blockers are heart rate slower than 60 beats/min, systolic blood pressure below 100 mm Hg, moderate to severe congestive heart failure (CHF), signs of peripheral hypoperfusion, PR interval longer than 0.24 second, second- or third-degree AVB, severe chronic obstructive pulmonary disease, history of asthma, severe diabetes mellitus, and severe peripheral vascular disease. Used in the setting of MI, the greatest benefit is seen when treated within 8 hours. The targeted optimal heart rate is 60 to 90 beats/min in the setting of MI. Dosage of metoprolol is 5 mg given intravenously over 1 minute (smaller doses may be used in patients with relative contraindications). This bolus is repeated twice every 5 to 15 minutes, for a total of 15 mg. **Esmolol**, a short-acting β-blocker, also can be used. An initial 500-μg/kg bolus is infused over 1 minute, and a 50 μg/kg/min infusion is then titrated to a maximum dose of 200 μg/kg/min.

5. **Morphine sulfate** (2 to 10 mg intravenously, give in 2-mg increments) can be used to reduce anginal pain. Morphine has not been consistently shown to affect preload. Morphine may decrease cardiac output. Morphine should be used with caution in the presence of hypotension and in patients with inferior MI.

6. **Unfractionated heparin** (UFH) is used for its anticoagulative properties, which prevent the progression of coronary artery and mural thrombosis. UFH used in combination with ASA for patients with unstable angina (UA), reduces the risk of death or MI. The dose is 12,500 U twice a day. UFH requires close laboratory monitoring because of its unpredictable anticoagulant response. UFH use is associated with an increased risk of bleeding. Anticoagulation due to UFH can be reversed with protamine. The dosage is 1 mg of **protamine** per 100 U of UFH (UFH is given as a bolus or infused in the previous 4 hours).

7. **Low-molecular-weight heparins** have greater bioavailability, lower protein binding, longer half-life, and more reliable anticoagulative effect than their counterparts. They are administered in fixed subcutaneous

doses and do not require laboratory monitoring. Initial studies comparing low-molecular-weight heparin with UFH in ACS have demonstrated decreased ischemia and MI without increased bleeding complication. Enoxaparin is preferable over UFH in patients with UA/NSTEMI, unless CABG is planned in the next 24 hours.

8. **Fibrinolytics** are indicated for patients with symptoms compatible with MI, a time to treatment briefer than 6 to 12 hours, and ECG findings of at least 1-mm ST-segment elevation in 2 or more contiguous leads. The dosages of individual fibrinolytic agents are listed in Table 21-2. Because fibrinolytics have potentially fatal side effects, the appropriate selection of candidates for use is very important. Contraindications for fibrinolytics are listed in Table 21-3.

   a. The decision to administer fibrinolytics should be individualized. Elderly patients (>75 years) have more complications but benefit the most from fibrinolytics. There is evidence that treatment 6 to 12 hours after onset of symptoms may decrease mortality. However, the risk for intracerebral hemorrhage, CHF, and cardiac rupture is also increased. Intracerebral hemorrhage (occurring in approximately 1% of patients) is more common in patients older than 66 years, weighing less than 70 kg, and are hypertensive on presentation. Cardiology consultation before initiating thrombolytics in cases of delayed presentation is appropriate.

   b. Before administering thrombolytics, informed consent should be obtained (with particular attention paid to an understanding of the risks).

TABLE 21-3 Contraindications to Fibrinolytic Therapy in Acute Myocardial Infarction

Absolute contraindications
Previous hemorrhagic stroke at any time
Bland CVA in past year
Known intracranial neoplasm
Active internal bleeding (excluding menses)
Suspected aortic dissection
Relative contraindications
Severe uncontrolled blood pressure (>180/100 mm Hg)
History of chronic severe hypertension
History of prior CVA of known intracranial pathology not covered in contraindications
Current use of anticoagulants with known INR >2–3
Known bleeding diathesis
Recent trauma (past 2 wk)
Prolonged CPR (>10 min)
Major surgery (<3 wk)
Noncompressible vascular punctures (including subclavian and internal jugular central lines)
Recent internal bleeding (2–4 wk)
Prior streptokinase should not receive streptokinase
Pregnancy
Active peptic ulcer disease
Other medical conditions likely to increase risk of bleeding

Key: CPR = cardiopulmonary resuscitation; CVA = cerebral vascular accident; INR = international normalized ratio.

Arterial puncture should be avoided, as should venipuncture or central line placement in areas that are not readily compressible.

c. **Tissue plasminogen activator** (tPA) is a naturally occurring, human protein and is not antigenic. tPA is fibrin specific and has a half-life of 5 minutes. When compared with traditional dosing, front-loaded tPA has been shown to have superior 90-minute patency rates and reocclusion rates without increased bleeding risk.

d. **Reteplase** is a non–fibrin-specific deletion mutant of tPA with a prolonged half-life of 18 minutes versus 3 minutes. The GUSTO III study found similar mortality and stroke rates between the 2 agents. Reteplase may have a faster time to perfusion. The advantage of reteplase is that it is given in bolus rather than in infusion form. Intravenous heparin must be given simultaneously with tPA and reteplase.

e. **Tenecteplase** is a fibrin-specific substitution mutant of tPA that is given as a single bolus, but it requires weight-based dosing. tPA, reteplase, and tenecteplase have similar safety and efficacy profiles, so the choice of fibrinolytic is generally institutionally based.

f. **Streptokinase** (SK) activates circulating plasminogen and is not fibrin specific. It is derived from β-hemolytic streptococcus and is capable of generating an allergic reaction (minor, 5% to 5.7%; anaphylaxis <0.2% to 0.7%). Hypotension, usually responsive to fluids and slowing drug infusion, occurs in 13.3% to 15% of patients. Contraindications to the use of SK include the presence of hypotension, prior dose of SK in the past 6 months, and streptococcal infections in the past 12 months. The half-life of SK is 23 minutes, and systemic fibrinolysis persists for 24 hours. Heparin should be given within 4 hours of starting SK.

g. The most significant complication of thrombolytics is hemorrhage, especially intracranial bleeding. External bleeding usually can be controlled by prolonged external pressure. Significant bleeding, especially internal, requires cessation of thrombolytics, heparin, and ASA. Crystalloid and red blood cell infusion may be necessary. **Cryoprecipitate** and **fresh-frozen plasma** will reverse fibrinolysis due to thrombolytics. Initially, 10 U cryoprecipitate is given, and fibrinogen levels are obtained. If the fibrinogen level is lower than 1 g/L, the dose of cryoprecipitate should be repeated. If bleeding continues despite a fibrinogen level above 1 g/L, or if the fibrinogen level is less than 1 g/L after 20 U cryoprecipitate, then 2 U fresh-frozen plasma should be administered. If this does not control hemorrhage, then platelets or antifibrinolytic agents (aminocaproic acid or tranexamic acid) are indicated. Intracranial hemorrhage requires all of the preceding steps to be initiated.

9. Primary angioplasty refers to the practice of emergent coronary angiography followed by angioplasty (balloon, rotary, and laser), coronary artery stenting (bare or drug eluting), or atherectomy in lieu of fibrinolysis. In centers with significant expertise in direct angioplasty, primary angioplasty, as opposed to fibrinolytic therapy, reduces complications in patients with MI. There are 4 subsets of patients for which primary angioplasty is especially attractive: (*a*) patients with MI in cardiogenic shock, (*b*) patients with nondiagnostic ECG, (*c*) patients with contraindications to fibrinolysis, and (*d*) patients with refractory symptoms. Angiography also has the advantage of identifying patients who require bypass surgery.

10. **Clopidogrel,** when added to ASA, reduces the composite risk of cardio-vascular death, MI, or stroke. Clopidogrel should be considered in UA/NSTEMI patients with ASA allergy and in patients in whom noninvasive or percutaneous intervention (PCI) is planned. Clopidogrel increases risk of bleeding and should be withheld at least 5 days before CABG.

11. **Glycoprotein IIb/IIIa antagonists** are agents that bind to and inhibit platelet aggregation. Abciximab, eptifibatide, and tirofiban are currently available. These agents have been used: (*a*) adjuncts to angioplasty, (*b*) for medical stabilization of ACS, and (*c*) in combination with low-dose fibrinolytics. Abciximab with UFH and ASA, when used in conjunction with angioplasty, decreases mortality, MI, and urgent repeat intervention. An initial study has supported the same benefit with eptifibatide. Tirofiban and eptifibatide have demonstrated improved outcomes (composite death, MI, and recurrent ischemia) in medically treated patients with UA/NSTEMI. Abciximab did not demonstrate benefit in UA/NSTEMI patients who did not undergo PCI. Two, large, combination therapy trials (reduced dose lytic + IIb/IIIa) showed no mortality benefit in STEMI. Currently, combination therapy with IIb/IIIa inhibitors is unproven as a superior treatment to standard therapy.

12. **Angiotensin-converting enzyme** (ACE) inhibitors have been shown to decrease mortality when used in the setting of CHF and in the postinfarction period. Their efficacy in the acute treatment of UA has not been well studied. Oral ACE inhibitors should be started within the first 24 hours in patients with MI and ST elevation in 2 or more precordial leads or in the setting of heart failure. Intravenous enalapril increases hypotension and is not recommended for AMI. Bilateral renal artery stenosis, renal failure, cough, or angioedema due to ACE inhibitors in the past are other contraindications.

13. RV infarcts are treated somewhat differently than LV infarcts. Patients with RV infarcts are dependent on elevated RV filling pressures to maintain cardiac output. Diuretics and NTG should be avoided. Volume infusion should be used to increase cardiac output. Dobutamine is indicated if an inotropic agent is needed. Nitroprusside to decrease afterload or intraaortic balloon counterpulsation may be of benefit in refractory cases.

14. MI patients with continued hemodynamic instability and pain or those who have not reperfused after administration of thrombolytics are candidates for rescue angioplasty (see Chap. 7). Emergent coronary artery bypass surgery also may be indicated for these patients. Patients in refractory cardiogenic shock should undergo emergent angioplasty. Intraaortic balloon pump or other LV assisting devices also may be indicated for these patients.

15. Patients with acute MI or UA who have ongoing chest pain, ECG changes, dysrhythmias, or hemodynamic compromise require cardiac intensive care. Patients with UA and resolved chest pain, normal or nonspecific ECG changes, and no complications should be admitted to a monitored bed.

16. Chest-pain-free patients with normal or nonspecific ECGs can be admitted to a stepdown unit. Chest pain patients with low likelihood of MI can undergo serial ECG and cardiac enzyme rule out in a chest pain observation unit.

For further reading in *Emergency Medicine: A Comprehensive Study Guide,* 6th ed., see Chap. 50, "Acute Coronary Syndromes: Unstable Angina, Myocardial Ischemia, and Infarction," by Judd E. Hollander; and Chap. 51, "Intervention Strategies for Acute Coronary Syndrome," by Judd E. Hollander and Deborah B. Diercks.

22 | Syncope

Michael J. Mikhail

Syncope, which accounts for up to 3% of all emergency department visits, is a transient loss of consciousness accompanied by loss of postural tone. Although syncope typically is a benign vasovagal event, it may represent a life-threatening dysrhythmia, particularly in the elderly. Fifty percent of all patients will never have a definite etiology established for their syncopal episode.

CLINICAL FEATURES

The most common cause of syncope is reflex mediated, when a sympathetic response to stress is suddenly withdrawn leading to pronounced vagal tone with hypotension or bradycardia. The hallmark of vasovagal syncope is the prodrome of dizziness, nausea, diminished vision, pallor, and diaphoresis. In addition, the clinician should look for appropriate stimuli (ie, blood drawing, injury, and fear) in combination with standing before making the diagnosis of vasovagal syncope. An elderly patient may relate that he was wearing a tight collar, shaving, or turning his head immediately before fainting, thus suggesting carotid sinus hypersensitivity. In situational syncope, the autonomic reflexive response may result from a specific physical stimulus such as micturition, defecation, or extreme coughing.

A sudden change in posture after prolonged recumbence, with the inability to mount an adequate increase in heart rate or peripheral vascular resistance, results in orthostatic syncope. Often this is due to autonomic dysfunction, such as peripheral neuropathy, spinal cord injury, and Shy-Drager syndrome. More serious causes of orthostatic syncope are disorders that cause volume depletion, such as vomiting, diarrhea, bleeding, diuresis, and sepsis.

Cardiac syncope is due to a dysrhythmia or a structural cardiopulmonary lesion. Tachydysrhythmias, such as ventricular tachycardia, torsade de pointes, and supraventricular tachycardia, are common causes of syncope, but one is more likely to encounter incidental bradycardia on examination and electrocardiogram (ECG). Syncope from dysrhythmias is usually sudden, with a brief (<3 seconds) prodrome, if any. Structural abnormalities of the heart are unmasked as syncope during exertion or vasodilatory drugs. In the elderly, this is most commonly due to aortic stenosis. In the young patient, it is most commonly hypertrophic cardiomyopathy. Approximately 10% of patients with pulmonary embolism will have pulmonary outflow obstruction that leads to syncope.

Cerebrovascular disorders are rare as a cause of syncope. If brainstem ischemia is the cause, then usually the patient reports other posterior circulation deficits, such as diplopia, vertigo, and nausea, associated with the "drop attack." If patients report that upper extremity exercise preceded the event, then they may have obstruction of the brachiocephalic or subclavian artery (ie, subclavian steal syndrome). A transient rise in intracranial pressure with subarachnoid hemorrhage is suspected as the cause of syncope in patients with a severe "thunderclap" headache.

Because of poor autonomic responses and multiple medications, the elderly are particularly prone to syncope, usually due to cardiac causes.

137

Antihypertensive agents, such as β-blockers and calcium channel antagonists, blunt tachycardic reflexes to orthostatic or vasodilatory triggers. In addition, they may cause cardiac blocks and life-threatening dysrhythmias. Diuretics also contribute to orthostatic hypotension from volume depletion. Syncope is a dual threat to the elderly patients: it causes falls with orthopedic injuries and it portends sudden cardiac death in many cases.

DIAGNOSIS AND DIFFERENTIAL

Although an etiology for the syncopal episode may be difficult to establish, the most important tools in the workup of syncope are a comprehensive history, physical examination, and ECG. The history should be directed to high-risk factors, including age, medications, and prodromal events. Sudden events without warning suggest dysrhythmias; exertion may imply a structural cardiopulmonary lesion. Associated symptoms are helpful for detecting a cardiac (ie, palpitations and chest pain) or neurologic (ie, vertigo and focal weakness) cause for syncope. Back or abdominal pain may suggest a leaking abdominal aortic aneurysm or ruptured ectopic pregnancy. Trauma without defensive injuries or single-vehicle crashes may distract one from an initial syncopal event as the precipitating cause. In addition, the patient's medical history is useful in showing cardiac or psychiatric (eg, hyperventilation) causes for syncope.

Physical examination may show the ultimate cause of syncope. The cardiac examination may uncover a ventricular flow obstruction problem. A cardiac murmur may represent aortic stenosis or hypertrophic cardiomyopathy. An accentuated pulmonary gallop may be a clue to pulmonary embolism. A complete neurologic assessment and rectal examination may yield further secondary causes for syncope.

Although the yield is low, the ECG is useful in detecting ischemia and dysrhythmias. The ECG also can show a propensity to dysrhythmias such as a prolonged QT interval leading to torsade de pointes or shortening of the PR interval and a delta wave seen in Wolf-Parkinson-White syndrome. Prolonged monitoring may show a transient, but recurring, dysrhythmia.

Selected laboratory testing is the norm. A hematocrit or rectal examination for occult gastrointestinal bleeding may explain syncope associated with orthostatic hypotension. Women of childbearing potential warrant a pregnancy test. Although not recommended routinely, electrolytes may show a depressed bicarbonate after a seizure and are indicated in patients with weakness or irritable myocardium.

There are a variety of bedside tests that may provide clues in selected cases, such as reproducing presyncopal symptoms with hyperventilation. A blood pressure check in both arms with greater than a 20 mm Hg difference suggests subclavian steal syndrome. Carotid sinus massage can be performed in selected patients without bruits if one suspects carotid sinus hypersensitivity. Orthostatic hypotension (autonomic instability from drugs or disease) is defined as a systolic blood pressure drop of at least 20 mm Hg. The caveat of making this diagnosis is that symptoms should recur with standing.

Seizure is the most common disorder mistaken for syncope. The hallmarks of seizure (ie, tongue biting and incontinence) can also be seen with convulsive syncope, which are brief clonic jerks due to cerebral anoxia. The most helpful differentiating factor is that true seizures are followed by a postictal phase with disorientation and slow return to normal consciousness.

EMERGENCY DEPARTMENT CARE AND DISPOSITION

By definition, syncope results in spontaneous recovery of consciousness. Therefore, the main goal of emergency department care is to identify those patients at risk for further medical problems. Patients can be categorized into 1 of 3 classes after a careful history, physical examination, and ECG:

1. *If the diagnosis is established,* then the patient can be appropriately managed by directing attention to the underlying cause of the syncopal event. Patients with syncope in whom a life-threatening etiology is identified, including neurologic or cardiac causes, warrant admission. If the diagnosis is not established, then patients can be stratified further.
2. *High-risk patients* are those at risk for sudden cardiac death or ventricular dysrhythmia: abnormal ECG, age older than 45 years, or a history of ventricular dysrhythmia or congestive heart failure. With admission, the workup of these patients can be expedited to determine a possible structural or electrical cause of cardiac syncope.
3. *Low-risk patients* are those unlikely to have a cardiac etiology for their syncope. These patients are young (<45 years), have few comorbidities, and have a normal physical examination and ECG. Usually their syncope is due to vasovagal mechanisms, and they do not require further workup for an isolated episode. They can be discharged safely home with instructions to return if a recurrence of presyncopal symptoms. Worrisome or recurrent cases may benefit from further outpatient workup including Holter or loop-event monitoring. They also should be advised not to work at heights or drive their vehicles until a diagnosis is established.

For further reading in *Emergency Medicine: A Comprehensive Study Guide,* 6th ed., see Chap. 52, "Syncope," by Barbara K. Blok and Tina M. Newman.

23 | Congestive Heart Failure and Acute Pulmonary Edema

Chadwick Miller

Acute pulmonary edema is one of the most dramatic presentations of the many clinical effects of heart failure. The most common precipitating factors of heart failure are (*a*) cardiac tachyarrhythmias, such as atrial fibrillation; (*b*) acute myocardial infarction or ischemia; (*c*) discontinuation of medications, such as diuretics; (*d*) increased sodium load; (*e*) drugs that impair myocardial function; and (*f*) physical overexertion.

CLINICAL FEATURES

Patients with acute pulmonary edema usually present with symptoms of left ventricular heart failure, severe respiratory distress, frothy pink or white sputum, moist pulmonary rales, and a third heart sound (S_3) or fourth heart sound (S_4). Patients frequently are tachycardic, have cardiac dysrhythmias such as atrial fibrillation or premature ventricular contraction, and are hypertensive. There may be a history of exertional dyspnea, paroxysmal nocturnal dyspnea, and orthopnea. Patients with right ventricular heart failure have dependent edema of the extremities and may have jugular venous distention, hepatic enlargement, and a hepatojugular reflex.

DIAGNOSIS AND DIFFERENTIAL

The diagnosis of acute pulmonary edema is made with clinical findings and the chest x-ray. The severity of illness may demand that a portable anterior–posterior film be taken. Additional tests that should be ordered to help management include an electrocardiogram, electrolyte levels, serum urea nitrogen levels, creatinine level, complete blood cell count, arterial blood gas level, B-type natriuretic peptide level, and cardiac markers. The diagnosis of right-side heart failure is made clinically; if the cause is left-side heart failure, the heart will be enlarged on chest x-ray. In the differential diagnosis, consider the common causes of acute respiratory distress: asthma, chronic obstructive pulmonary disease, pneumonia, pulmonary embolus, allergenic reactions, and other causes of respiratory failure. Another consideration is causes of noncardiogenic pulmonary edema such as drug-related alveolar capillary damage or that seen with acute respiratory distress syndrome.

EMERGENCY DEPARTMENT CARE AND DISPOSITION

The treatment of patients in acute pulmonary edema includes oxygen, preload reducers, diuretics, afterload reducers, and inotropic agents.

1. One hundred percent oxygen by face mask must be administered to achieve an oxygen saturation of 95% by pulse oximetry.
2. If hypoxia persists despite oxygen therapy, continuous positive airway pressure or biphasic positive airway pressure should be applied via face mask.
3. Immediate intubation is indicated for unconscious or visibly tiring patients.

4. **Nitroglycerin** 0.4 mg must be administered sublingually (may be repeated every 1-5 minutes) or as a topical paste in 1 to 2 in. If the patient does not respond, or the electrocardiogram shows ischemia, nitroglycerin 10 μg/min should be initiated as an intravenous drip and titrated.
5. An alternative to a nitroglycerin infusion is **nesiritide,** with recommended dosing as an initial bolus of 2 μg/kg followed by a fixed infusion dose of 0.01 μg/kg/min. Nesiritide has properties of diuresis and of preload and afterload reduction. It is not recommended in cardiogenic shock.
6. After nitrates or nesiritide, a potent intravenous diuretic should be administrated, such as **furosemide** 40 to 80 mg intravenously or **bumetanide** 0.5 to 1 mg intravenously. Electrolytes should be monitored, especially serum potassium.
7. For patients with resistant hypertension or those who are not responding well to nitroglycerin, **nitroprusside** may be used, starting at 2.5 μg/kg/min and titrated.
8. For hypotensive patients or patients in need of additional inotropic support, **dopamine** should be started at 5 to 10 μg/kg/min and titrate to a systolic blood pressure of 90 to 100 mm Hg. Dobutamine can be given in combination with dopamine or as a single agent provided the patient is not in severe circulatory shock. **Dobutamine** should be started at 2.5 μg/kg/min and titrated to the desired response.

Some causes of acute pulmonary edema need to be determined rapidly because they require emergency intervention. Until excluded, acute myocardial infarction should be considered as the cause of exacerbation, and the initial electrocardiogram may fail to demonstrate ischemic changes. For those patients failing to improve, a repeat electrocardiogram is warranted. Acute mitral valve or aortic valve regurgitation should be considered, especially if the heart is of normal size, because the patient may need emergency surgery.

Coexisting dysrhythmias (see Chap. 2) or electrolyte disturbances (see Chap. 4) should be treated, and those therapies that impair the inotropic state of the heart should be avoided. **Morphine** can be given (2-5 mg intravenously) and repeated as needed. Its use is controversial, however, and may cause respiratory depression and add little to oxygen, diuretics, and nitrates. Digoxin acts too slowly to be of benefit in acute situations. For anuric (dialysis) patients, sorbitol and phlebotomy may have some benefit; however, dialysis is the treatment of choice in these patients who prove resistant to nitrates.

Patients with acute pulmonary edema may require admission to the intensive care unit and invasive hemodynamic monitoring. In the presence of new dysrhythmias, uncontrolled hypertension, or suspected myocardial infarction, the patient should be admitted to a telemetry bed for evaluation and optimization of drug therapy.

Long-term treatment of congestive heart failure includes dietary salt reduction, chronic use of diuretics such as furosemide, afterload reducers such as angiotensin-converting enzyme inhibitors, β-blockers, or digoxin. Patients with an exacerbation of chronic congestive heart failure without chest pain or complicating factors who respond to diuretics may be discharged home if close follow-up is arranged.

For further reading in *Emergency Medicine: A Comprehensive Study Guide,* 6th ed., see Chap. 53, "Congestive Heart Failure and Acute Pulmonary Edema," by W. Frank Peacock.

24 | Valvular Heart Disease

David M. Cline

Ninety percent of valvular disease is chronic, with decades between the onset of the structural abnormality and symptoms. Through chronic adaptation by dilation and hypertrophy, cardiac function can be preserved for years, which may delay the diagnosis for 1 to 2 decades until a murmur is detected on auscultation. The 4 heart valves prevent retrograde flow of blood during the cardiac cycle, thereby allowing efficient ejection of blood with each contraction of the ventricles. The mitral valve has 2 cusps, and the other 3 heart valves normally have 3 cusps. The right and left papillary muscles promote effective closure of the tricuspid and mitral valves, respectively.

MITRAL STENOSIS

Clinical Features

As with all valvular diseases, exertional dyspnea is the most common presenting symptom (80% of patients with mitral stenosis). In the past, hemoptysis was the second most common presenting symptom, but it is less common now with earlier recognition and treatment. Systemic emboli may occur and result in myocardial, kidney, central nervous system, or peripheral infarction. Most patients eventually develop atrial fibrillation because of progressive dilation of the atria. The classic murmur of mitral stenosis and associated signs are listed in Table 24-1.

Diagnosis and Differential

The electrocardiogram (ECG) may demonstrate notched or diphasic P waves and right axis deviation. On the chest radiography, straightening of the left heart border, indicating left atrial enlargement, is a typical early radiographic finding. Eventually, findings of pulmonary congestion are noted: redistribution of flow to the upper lung fields, Kerley B lines, and an increase in vascular markings. The diagnosis of mitral stenosis should be confirmed with echocardiography or consultation with a cardiologist. The urgency for an accurate diagnosis and appropriate referral depends on the severity of symptoms.

Emergency Department Care and Disposition

1. The medical management of mitral stenosis includes intermittent diuretics, such as **furosemide** 40 mg intravenously (IV), to alleviate pulmonary congestion, the treatment of atrial fibrillation (see Chap. 2), and anticoagulation for patients at risk for arterial embolic events.
2. Patients with mitral stenosis and paroxysmal or chronic atrial fibrillation or a history of an embolic event should be on long-term warfarin therapy with an international normalized ratio goal of 2 to 3.
3. Frank hemoptysis may occur in the setting of mitral stenosis and pulmonary hypertension. Bleeding may be severe enough to require blood transfusion, consultation with a thoracic surgeon, and emergency surgery.

TABLE 24-1 Comparison of Heart Murmurs, Sounds, and Signs

Valve disorder	Murmur	Heart sounds and signs
Mitral stenosis	Mid-diastolic rumble, crescendos into S_2	Loud snapping S_1, apical impulse is small, tapping due to under filled ventricle
Mitral regurgitation	Acute: harsh apical systolic murmur that starts with S_1 and may end before S_2 Chronic: high-pitched apical holosystolic murmur that radiates into S_2	S_3 and S_4 may be heard
Mitral valve prolapse	Click may be followed by a late systolic murmur that crescendos into S_2	Mid-systolic click; S_2 may be diminished by the late systolic murmur
Aortic stenosis	Harsh systolic ejection murmur	Paradoxic splitting of S_2; S_3 and S_4 may be present; pulse of small amplitude; pulse has a slow rise and sustained peak
Aortic regurgitation	High pitched blowing diastolic murmur immediately after S_2	S_3 may be present; wide pulse pressure

Key: S_1 = first heart sound, S_2 = second heart sound, S_3 = third heart sound, S_4 = fourth heart sound.

MITRAL INCOMPETENCE

Clinical Features

Acute mitral incompetence secondary to rupture of the chordae tendineae or papillary muscles presents with dyspnea, tachycardia, and pulmonary edema. Patients may quickly deteriorate to cardiogenic shock or cardiac arrest. Intermittent mitral incompetence usually presents with acute episodes of respiratory distress due to pulmonary edema and may be asymptomatic between attacks. Chronic mitral incompetence may be tolerated for years or even decades. The first symptom is usually exertional dyspnea, sometimes prompted by atrial fibrillation. If patients are not anticoagulated, systemic emboli occur in 20% and are often asymptomatic. The classic murmur and signs of mitral incompetence are listed in Table 24-1.

Diagnosis and Differential

In acute rupture, the ECG may show evidence of acute inferior wall infarction (more common than anterior wall infarction in this setting). On chest radiography, acute mitral incompetence from papillary muscle rupture may result in a minimally enlarged left atrium and pulmonary edema, with less cardiac enlargement than expected. In chronic disease, the ECG may demonstrate findings of left atrial and left ventricular hypertrophy (LVH). On chest radiography, chronic mitral incompetence produces left ventricular and atrial enlargements that are proportional to the severity of the regurgitant volume. Echocardiography is essential to make the diagnosis with certainty, and bedside technique may be mandatory in the acutely ill patient. However, trans-thoracic echocardiography may underestimate lesion severity, and the transesophageal technique should be undertaken as soon as the patient is adequately stable to leave the department. In stable patients, echocardiography can be scheduled electively.

Emergency Department Care and Disposition

1. Pulmonary edema should be treated initially with oxygen, intubation for failing respiratory effort, diuretics such as **furosemide** 40 mg IV, and nitrates as the patient tolerates.
2. Nitroprusside increases forward output by increasing aortic flow and partly restoring mitral valve competence as left ventricular size diminishes. **Nitroprusside** 5 μg/kg/min IV should be started unless the patient is hypotensive. There may be a subset of patients whose mitral regurgitation is worsened by nitroprusside (those patients who respond with a dilation of the regurgitant orifice); thus, careful monitoring is essential.
3. Hypotensive patients should receive inotropic agents such as **dobutamine** 2.5 to 20 μg/kg/min in addition to nitroprusside.
4. Aortic balloon counter pulsation increases forward flow and mean arterial pressure and diminishes regurgitant volume and left ventricular filling pressure and can be used to stabilize a patient while awaiting surgery.
5. Emergency surgery should be considered in cases of acute mitral valve rupture.

MITRAL VALVE PROLAPSE

Clinical Features

Most patients are asymptomatic. Symptoms include atypical chest pain, palpitations, fatigue, and dyspnea unrelated to exertion. The abnormal heart sounds are listed in Table 24-1. In patients with mitral valve prolapse without mitral regurgitation at rest, exercise provokes mitral regurgitation in 32% of patients and predicts a higher risk for morbid events.

Diagnosis and Differential

Echocardiography is recommended to confirm the clinical diagnosis of mitral valve prolapse and to identify any associated mitral regurgitation. Echocardiography or consultation with a cardiologist can be performed on an outpatient basis.

Emergency Department Care and Disposition

1. Initiating treatment for mitral valve prolapse is rarely required for patients seen in the emergency department. Patients with palpitations, chest pain, or anxiety frequently respond to β-blockers such as **atenolol** 25 mg daily.
2. Avoiding alcohol, tobacco, and caffeine also may relieve symptoms.

AORTIC STENOSIS

Clinical Features

The classic triad is dyspnea, chest pain, and syncope. Dyspnea is usually the first symptom, followed by paroxysmal nocturnal dyspnea, syncope on exertion, angina, and myocardial infarction. The classic murmur and associated signs of aortic stenosis are listed in Table 24-1. Blood pressure is normal or low, with a narrow pulse pressure.

Brachioradial delay is an important finding in aortic stenosis. The examiner palpates simultaneously the right brachial artery of the patient with the thumb and the right radial artery of the patient with the middle or index finger. Any palpable delay between the brachial artery and radial artery is considered abnormal.

Diagnosis and Differential

The ECG usually demonstrates criteria for LVH and, in 10% of patients, left or right bundle branch block. The chest radiograph is normal early, but eventually LVH and findings of congestive heart failure are evident if the patient does not have valve replacement. Echocardiography should be undertaken to confirm the suspected diagnosis of aortic stenosis and in the hospital if the murmur is associated with syncope.

Emergency Department Care and Disposition

1. Patients presenting with pulmonary edema can be treated with oxygen and diuretics such as **furosemide** 40 mg IV, but nitrates should be used with caution because reducing preload may cause significant hypotension. Nitroprusside is not well tolerated in patients with aortic stenosis.
2. New onset atrial fibrillation may severely compromise cardiac output and therefore require anticoagulation with heparin and cardioversion.
3. Patients with profound symptoms secondary to aortic stenosis such as syncope are usually admitted to the hospital.

AORTIC INCOMPETENCE

Clinical Features

In acute disease, dyspnea is the most common presenting symptom, seen in 50% of patients. Many patients have acute pulmonary edema with pink frothy sputum. Patients may complain of fever and chills if endocarditis is the cause. Dissection of the ascending aorta typically produces a "tearing" chest pain that may radiate between the shoulder blades. The classic murmur and signs of aortic incompetence are listed in Table 24-1. In the acute state, chest radiography demonstrates acute pulmonary edema with less cardiac enlargement than expected.

In the chronic state, about one third of patients will have palpitations associated with a large stroke volume and/or premature ventricular contractions. In the chronic state, signs include a wide pulse pressure with a prominent ventricular impulse, which may be manifested as head bobbing. "Water hammer pulse" may be noted; this is a peripheral pulse that has a quick rise in upstroke followed by a peripheral collapse. Other classic findings may include accentuated precordial apical thrust, pulsus biferiens, Duroziez sign (a to-and-fro femoral murmur), and Quincke pulse (capillary pulsations visible at the proximal nailbed while pressure is applied at the tip).

Diagnosis and Differential

ECG changes may be seen with aortic dissection, including ischemia or findings of acute inferior myocardial infarction, suggesting involvement of the right coronary artery.

In patients with acute regurgitation, the chest radiograph demonstrates acute pulmonary edema with less cardiac enlargement than expected. In chronic aortic incompetence, the ECG demonstrates LVH, and the chest radiograph shows LVH, aortic dilation, and possibly evidence of congestive heart failure. Echocardiography is essential for confirming the presence of and evaluating the severity of valvular regurgitation. Bedside transthoracic echocardiography should be undertaken in the unstable patient potentially in need of emergency surgery. Transesophageal echocardiography is recommended when aortic dissection is suspected but may not be possible in acutely unstable patients.

Emergency Department Care and Disposition

1. Pulmonary edema should be treated initially with oxygen and intubation for failing respiratory effort. Diuretics and nitrates can be used but cannot be expected to be effective.
2. **Nitroprusside** (start at 5 μg/kg/min) and inotropic agents such as **dobutamine** (start at 2.5 μg/kg/min) or **dopamine** (start 2 μg/kg/min) can be used to augment forward flow and reduce left ventricular end-diastolic pressure in an attempt to stabilize a patient before emergency surgery.
3. Intraaortic balloon counter pulsation is contraindicated.
4. Although β-blockers are often used in treating aortic dissection, these drugs should be used with great caution, if at all, in the setting of acute aortic valve rupture because they will block the compensatory tachycardia. When used, typically **labetalol** 20 mg IV is given.
5. Emergency surgery may be lifesaving.
6. Chronic aortic regurgitation is typically treated with vasodilators such as angiotensin-converting enzyme inhibitors or nifedipine (initiated by a patient's private physician).

PROSTHETIC VALVE DISEASE

Prosthetic valves are implanted in 40,000 patients per year in the United States. There are approximately 80 types of artificial valves, each with advantages and disadvantages. Patients who receive prosthetic valves are instructed to carry a descriptive card in their wallets.

Clinical Features

Many patients have persistent dyspnea and reduced effort tolerance after successful valve replacement. This is more common in the presence of preexisting heart dysfunction or atrial fibrillation. Large paravalvular leaks usually present with congestive heart failure. Patients with new neurologic symptoms may have thromboembolism associated with the valve thrombi or endocarditis. Patients with prosthetic valves usually have abnormal cardiac sounds. Mechanical valves have loud, metallic closing sounds. Systolic murmurs are commonly present with mechanical models. Loud diastolic murmurs are generally not present with mechanical valves. Patients with bioprostheses usually have normal S_1 and S_2, with no abnormal opening sounds. The aortic bioprosthesis is usually associated with short midsystolic murmur.

Diagnosis and Differential

New or progressive dyspnea of any form, new onset or worsening of congestive heart failure, decreased exercise tolerance, or a change in chest pain compatible with ischemia suggest valvular dysfunction. Persistent fever in patients with prosthetic valves should be evaluated with blood cultures for possible endocarditis. Blood studies that may be helpful include a blood count with red blood cell indices and coagulation studies if the patient is on warfarin. Emergency echocardiographic studies should be requested if there is any question about valve dysfunction. Ultimately, echocardiography and/or cardiac catheterization may be required for diagnosis.

Emergency Department Care and Disposition

1. It is critical that patients with suspected acute prosthetic valvular dysfunction have immediate referral to a cardiac surgeon for possible emergency surgery.
2. The need for the intensity of anticoagulation therapy varies with each type of mechanical valve, but its international normalized ratio goal ranges from 2 to 3.5.
3. Acute prosthetic valvular dysfunction due to thrombotic obstruction has

TABLE 24-2 Prophylaxis for Infective Endocarditis

Procedure	Standard regimen*	Alternate regimen
Dental procedure known to cause bleeding	Amoxicillin 2.0 g PO 1 h before procedure, or ampicillin 2.0 g IM or IV 30 min before procedure	Clindamycin 600 mg PO 1 h before procedure, or cephalexin 2.0 g PO 1 h before procedure, or cefadroxil 2.0 g PO 1 h before procedure, or azithromycin 500 mg PO 1 h before procedure, or clarithromycin 500 mg PO 1 h before procedure
Urethral catherization if infection is present; urethral dilatation	Ampicillin 2.0 g IV or IM plus gentamicin 1.5 mg/kg IV or IM (not to exceed 120 mg) 30 min before procedure followed by half the original dose of ampicillin 6 h later; or followed by amoxicillin 1.0 g PO	Vancomycin 1.0 g IV over 1 h plus gentamicin 1.5 mg/kg IV or IM (not to exceed 120 mg), complete infusion within 30 min of starting procedure; for moderate risk patients, amoxicillin 2.0 g PO 1 h before procedure
Incision and drainage of infected tissue	Cefazolin 1.0 g IV or IM 30 min before procedure, or cephalexin 2.0 g PO 1 h before procedure, or cefadroxil 2.0 g PO 1 h before procedure	Vancomycin 1.0 g IV over 1 h plus gentamicin 1.5 mg/kg IV or IM (not to exceed 120 mg), complete infusion within 30 min of starting procedure

*Includes patients with prosthetic heart valves and others at high risk. Initial pediatric doses are as follows: amoxicillin 50 mg/kg, ampicillin 50 mg/kg, cephalexin 50 mg/kg, cefadroxil 50 mg/kg, azithromycin 15 mg/kg, clarithromycin 15 mg/kg, clindamycin 20 mg/kg, gentamicin 2 mg/kg, and vancomycin 20 mg/kg. Pediatric doses should not exceed the listed adult doses.
Key: IM = intramuscularly, IV = intravenously, PO = orally.

been treated successfully with thrombolytic therapy, but the diagnosis generally requires consultation with a cardiologist. Lesser degrees of obstruction should be treated with optimization of anticoagulation.
4. Disposition of patients with worsening of symptoms can be problematic, and consultation with the patient's regular physician may be needed before consideration for discharge.

Prophylaxis for Infective Endocarditis

See Chapter 92 and Table 24-2 for recommendations on antibiotic prophylaxis before procedures performed in the emergency department.

For further reading in *Emergency Medicine: A Comprehensive Study Guide,* 6th ed., see Chap. 54, "Valvular Emergencies" by David M. Cline.

25 | The Cardiomyopathies, Myocarditis, and Pericardial Disease

N. Stuart Harris

THE CARDIOMYOPATHIES

Cardiomyopathies are the third most common form of heart disease in the United States and are the second most common cause of sudden death in the adolescent population. It is a disease process that directly affects the cardiac structure and alters myocardial function. Four types are currently recognized: (*a*) dilated cardiomyopathy (DCM), (*b*) hypertrophied cardiomyopathy (HCM), (*c*) restrictive cardiomyopathy, and (*d*) dysrhythmogenicity of right ventricular cardiomyopathy.

DILATED CARDIOMYOPATHY

Dilation and compensatory hypertrophy of the myocardium result in depressed systolic function and pump failure leading to low cardiac output. Eighty percent of cases of DCM are idiopathic. Idiopathic DCM is the primary indication for cardiac transplant in the United States. Blacks and males have a 2.5-fold increased risk as compared with whites and females. The most common age at the time of diagnosis is 20 to 50 years.

Clinical Features

Systolic pump failure leads to signs and symptoms of congestive heart failure (CHF) including dyspnea on exertion, orthopnea, and paroxysmal nocturnal dyspnea. Chest pain due to limited coronary vascular reserve also may be present. Mural thrombi can form from diminished ventricular contractile force, and there may be signs of peripheral embolization (eg, focal neurologic deficit, flank pain, hematuria, or pulseless, cyanotic extremity). Holosystolic regurgitant murmur of the tricuspid and mitral valve may be heard along the lower left sternal border or at the apex. Other findings include a summation gallop, an enlarged and pulsatile liver, bibasilar rales, and dependent edema.

Diagnosis and Differential

Chest x-ray usually shows an enlarged cardiac silhouette, biventricular enlargement, and pulmonary vascular congestion ("cephalization" of flow and enlarged hila). The electrocardiogram (ECG) shows left ventricular hypertrophy, left atrial enlargement, Q or QS waves, and poor R wave progression across the precordium. Atrial fibrillation and ventricular ectopy are frequently present. Echocardiography confirms the diagnosis and demonstrates ventricular enlargement, increased systolic and diastolic volumes, and a decreased ejection fraction. Differential diagnosis includes acute myocardial infarction, restrictive pericarditis, acute valvular disruption, sepsis, or any other condition that results in a low cardiac output state.

Emergency Department Care and Disposition

Patients with newly diagnosed, symptomatic DCM require admission to a monitored bed or intensive care unit. Initial management is directed by symptoms.

1. Intravenous access, supplemental oxygen, and continuous monitoring should be established.
2. Intravenous diuretics (eg, **furosemide** 40 mg intravenously) and **digoxin** (maximum dose, 0.5 mg intravenously) can be administered. These drugs have symptomatic benefit but have not been shown to increase survival.
3. Angiotensin-converting enzyme inhibitors (eg, **enalapril** 1.25 mg intravenously every 6 hours) and β-blockers (eg, **carvedilol** 3.125 mg orally) can be administered. These drugs have been shown to improve survival in DCM with CHF.
4. **Amiodarone** (loaded 150 mg intravenously over 10 minutes and then 1 mg/min for 6 hours) for complex ventricular ectopy can be administered.
5. Anticoagulation should be considered to reduce mural thrombus formation.

Patients with known DCM who present with mild to moderate exacerbations of their symptoms are most likely to be noncompliant with their medications or dietary restrictions. These patients often can be managed in the emergency department with intravenous diuretics, reinstitution of their medications, counseling, and prompt follow-up with their primary physicians. It is important to search for other causes of exacerbations of DCM such as myocardial ischemia or infarction, anemia, infection, new onset atrial fibrillation, bradydysrhythmia, valvular insufficiency, renal dysfunction, pulmonary embolism, or thyroid dysfunction.

HYPERTROPHIC CARDIOMYOPATHY

This illness is characterized by left ventricular and/or right ventricular hypertrophy that is usually asymmetric and involves primarily the intraventricular septum without ventricular dilatation. The result is decreased compliance of the left ventricle leading to impaired diastolic relaxation and diastolic filling. Cardiac output is usually normal. Fifty percent of cases are hereditary.

Clinical Features

Symptom severity progresses with age. Dyspnea on exertion is the most common symptom, followed by angina-like chest pain, palpitations, and syncope. Patients may be aware of forceful ventricular contractions and call these *palpitations.* Physical examination may show a fourth heart sound, hyperdynamic apical impulse, a precordial lift, and a systolic ejection murmur best heard at the lower left sternal border or apex. The murmur may be increased with the Valsalva maneuver or standing after squatting. The murmur can be decreased by squatting, forceful hand gripping, or passive leg elevation with the patient supine (see Chap. 24 for contrasting murmurs).

Diagnosis and Differential

The ECG demonstrates left ventricular hypertrophy in 30% of patients and left atrial enlargement in 25% to 50%. Large septal Q waves (>0.3 mV) are present in 25%. Another ECG finding is upright T waves in those leads with QS or QR complexes (T-wave inversion in those leads would suggest ischemia). Chest x-ray is usually normal. Echocardiography is the diagnostic study of choice and will demonstrate disproportionate septal hypertrophy.

Emergency Department Care and Disposition

Symptoms of HCM may mimic ischemic heart disease and treatment of those symptoms is covered in Chap. 21. Otherwise, general supportive care is indicated.

1. β-Blockers, such as **atenolol** 25 to 50 mg orally every day, are the mainstay of treatment for patients with HCM and chest pain.
2. Patients should be discouraged from engaging in vigorous exercise.
3. Those with suspected HCM who have syncope should be hospitalized and monitored.

RESTRICTIVE CARDIOMYOPATHY

This is one of the least common cardiomyopathies. In this form of the disease, the ventricular volume and wall thickness are normal, but there is decreased diastolic volume of both ventricles. Most causes are idiopathic, but systemic disorders have been implicated, such as amyloidosis, sarcoidosis, hemochromatosis, scleroderma, carcinoid, hypereosinophilic syndrome, and endomyocardial fibrosis.

Clinical Features

Symptoms of CHF predominate, including dyspnea, orthopnea, and pedal edema. Chest pain is uncommon. Physical examination may show third or fourth heart sound cardiac gallop, pulmonary rales, jugular venous distension, Kussmaul sign (inspiratory jugular venous distention), hepatomegaly, pedal edema, and ascites.

Diagnosis and Differential

The chest x-ray may show signs of CHF without cardiomegaly. Nonspecific ECG changes are most likely. However, in cases of amyloidosis or sarcoidosis, conduction disturbances and low-voltage QRS complexes are common.

Differential diagnosis includes constrictive pericarditis and diastolic left ventricular dysfunction (most commonly due to ischemic or hypertensive heart disease). Differentiating between restrictive cardiomyopathy and constrictive pericarditis (using echocardiography) is critical because constrictive pericarditis can be cured surgically.

Emergency Department Treatment and Disposition

1. Treatment is symptom directed with the use of diuretics and angiotensin-converting enzyme inhibitors.
2. Corticosteroid therapy is indicated for sarcoidosis.
3. Chelation is used for the treatment of hemochromatosis.
4. Admission is determined by the severity of the symptoms and the availability of prompt subspecialty follow-up.

DYSRHYTHMOGENICITY OF RIGHT VENTRICULAR CARDIOMYOPATHY

This is the most rare form of cardiomyopathy and is characterized by progressive replacement of the right ventricular myocardium with fibrofatty tissue. The typical presentation is that of sudden death or ventricular dysrhythmia in a young or middle-age patient. All these patients require extensive workup and hospitalization.

MYOCARDITIS

Inflammation of the myocardium may be the result of a systemic disorder or an infectious agent. Viral etiologies include coxsackie B, echovirus, influenza, parainfluenza, Epstein-Barr virus, and human immunodeficiency virus. Bacterial causes include *Corynebacterium diphtheria, Neisseria meningitides, Mycoplasma pneumoniae,* and β-hemolytic streptococci. Pericarditis frequently accompanies myocarditis.

Clinical Features

Systemic signs and symptoms predominate, including fever, tachycardia "out of proportion" to the fever, myalgias, headache, and rigors. Chest pain due to coexisting pericarditis is frequently present. A pericardial friction rub may be heard in patients with concomitant pericarditis. In severe cases, there may be symptoms of progressive heart failure (CHF, pulmonary rales, pedal edema, etc).

Diagnosis and Differential

Nonspecific ECG changes, atrioventricular block, prolonged QRS duration, or ST-segment elevation (in the setting of associated pericarditis) are seen. Chest x-ray is normal. Cardiac enzymes may be elevated. Differential diagnosis includes cardiac ischemia or infarction, valvular disease, and sepsis.

Emergency Department Care and Disposition

1. Supportive care is the mainstay of treatment.
2. If a bacterial cause is suspected, antibiotics are appropriate.
3. Many patients have progressive CHF; therefore, hospitalization in a monitored environment is usually indicated (see Chap. 23 for management of CHF).

ACUTE PERICARDITIS

Inflammation of the pericardium may be the result of viral infection (eg, Coxsackie virus, echovirus, and human immunodeficiency virus), bacterial infection (eg, *Staphylococcus, S pneumoniae,* β-hemolytic *Streptococcus,* and *Mycobacterium tuberculosis*), fungal infection (eg, *Histoplasmosis capsulatum*), malignancy (leukemia, lymphoma, melanoma, and metastatic breast cancer), drugs (procainamide and hydralazine), radiation, connective tissue disease, uremia, myxedema, or postmyocardial infarction (Dressler syndrome), or may be idiopathic.

Clinical Features

The most common symptom is sudden or gradual onset of sharp or stabbing chest pain that radiates to the back, neck, left shoulder or arm. Radiation to the left trapezial ridge (due to inflammation of the adjoining diaphragmatic pleura) is particularly distinctive. The pain may be aggravated by movement or inspiration. Typically, chest pain is made most severe by lying supine and often relieved by sitting up and leaning forward. Associated symptoms include low-grade intermittent fever, dyspnea, and dysphagia. A transient, intermittent friction rub heard best at the lower left sternal border or apex is the most common physical finding.

Diagnosis and Differential

ECG changes of acute pericarditis and its convalescence have been divided into 4 stages. During stage 1, or the acute phase, there is ST-segment elevation in leads I, V_5, and V_6, with PR-segment depression in leads II, aV_F and V_4 through V_6. As the disease resolves (stage 2), the ST segment normalizes and T-wave amplitude decreases. In stage 3, inverted T waves appear in leads previously showing ST elevations. The final phase, stage 4, is characterized by the resolution of repolarization abnormalities and a return to a normal ECG.

When sequential ECGs are not available, it can be difficult to distinguish pericarditis from the normal variant with "early repolarization." In these cases, the finding of a ST-segment/T-wave amplitude ratio greater than 0.25 in leads I, V_5, or V_6 is indicative of acute pericarditis. Pericarditis without other underlying cardiac disease does not typically produce dysrhythmias. Chest x-ray is usually normal but should be done to rule out other disease. Echocardiography is the best diagnostic test. Other tests that may be of value in establishing etiologic diagnosis include complete blood cell count with differential serum urea nitrogen and creatinine levels (to rule out uremia), streptococcal serology, appropriate viral serology, other serology (eg, antinuclear and anti-DNA antibodies), thyroid function studies, erythrocyte sedimentation rate, and creatinine kinase levels with isoenzymes (to assess for myocarditis).

Emergency Department Care and Disposition

1. Stable patients with idiopathic or presumed viral etiologies are treated as outpatients with nonsteroidal anti-inflammatory agents (eg, **ibuprofen** 400-600 mg orally 4 times daily) for 1 to 3 weeks.
2. Patients should be treated for a specific cause if one is identified.
3. Any patient with myocarditis, enlarged cardiac silhouette on chest x-ray, or hemodynamic compromise should be admitted into a monitored environment.

NONTRAUMATIC CARDIAC TAMPONADE

Tamponade occurs when the pressure in the pericardial sac exceeds the normal filling pressure of the right ventricle resulting in restricted filling and decreased cardiac output. Causes include metastatic malignancy, uremia, hemorrhage (excessive anticoagulation), idiopathic disorder, bacterial or tubercular disorder, chronic pericarditis, and others (eg, systemic lupus, postradiation, or myxedema).

Clinical Features

The most common complaints are dyspnea and decreased exercise tolerance. Other nonspecific symptoms include weight loss, pedal edema, and ascites.

Physical findings include tachycardia, low systolic blood pressure, and a narrow pulse pressure. Pulsus paradoxus (apparent dropped beats in the peripheral pulse during inspiration), neck vein distention, distant heart sounds, and right upper quadrant pain (due to hepatic congestion) also may be present. Pulmonary rales are usually absent.

Diagnosis and Differential

Low-voltage QRS complexes and ST-segment elevation with PR-segment depression may be present on the ECG. Electrical alternans (beat-to-beat variability in the amplitude of the P and R waves unrelated to inspiratory cycle) is a classic but uncommon finding (about 20% of cases). Chest x-ray may or may not show an enlarged cardiac silhouette. Echocardiography is the diagnostic test of choice.

Emergency Department Care and Disposition

Tamponade is a true emergency.

1. Standard supportive measures as previously discussed should be instituted promptly.
2. An intravenous fluid bolus of 500 to 1,000 mL normal saline will facilitate right heart filling and may temporarily improve the hemodynamics.
3. Pericardiocentesis is therapeutic and diagnostic.
4. These patients require admission to an intensive care unit or monitored setting.

CONSTRICTIVE PERICARDITIS

Constriction occurs when fibrous thickening and loss of elasticity of the pericardium results in interference of diastolic filling. Cardiac trauma, pericardiotomy (open heart surgery), intrapericardial hemorrhage, fungal or bacterial pericarditis, and uremic pericarditis are the most common causes.

Clinical Features

Symptoms develop gradually and mimic those of restrictive cardiomyopathy, including CHF, exertional dyspnea, and decreased exercise tolerance. Chest pain, orthopnea, and paroxysmal nocturnal dyspnea are uncommon. On physical examination patients may have pedal edema, hepatomegaly, ascites, jugular venous distention, and Kussmaul sign. A pericardial "knock" (an early diastolic sound) may be heard at the apex. There is usually no friction rub.

Diagnosis and Differential

The ECG usually is not helpful but may show low-voltage QRS complexes and inverted T waves. Pericardial calcification is seen in up to 50% of patients on lateral chest x-ray but is not diagnostic of constrictive pericarditis. Doppler echocardiography, cardiac computed tomography, and magnetic resonance imaging are diagnostic. Other diseases that should be considered include acute pericarditis or myocarditis, exacerbation of chronic ventricular dysfunction, or a systemic process resulting in decreased cardiac performance (eg, sepsis).

Emergency Department Care and Disposition

1. General supportive care is the initial treatment.
2. Symptomatic patients will require hospitalization and pericardiectomy.

For further reading in *Emergency Medicine: A Comprehensive Study Guide,* 6th ed., see Chap. 55, "The Cardiomyopathies, Myocarditis, and Pericardial Disease," by James T. Niemann.

26 | Pulmonary Embolism

Christopher Kabrhel

Pulmonary embolism (PE) is a common and deadly disease that accounts for more than 50,000 deaths each year in the United States. PE is a notoriously difficult diagnosis to make because its presentation is often nonspecific. Risk factors include hypercoagulable states such as malignancy, estrogen use, pregnancy or genetic conditions; venous stasis caused by trauma, surgery, paralysis, or debilitating illness; and endothelial damage from trauma, surgery, vascular access, indwelling catheters, or prior deep venous thrombosis (DVT).

CLINICAL FEATURES

The diagnosis of PE should be considered in any patient at risk who experiences acute dyspnea, chest pain, unexplained tachycardia or hypoxia, syncope, or shock. Common symptoms include dyspnea (the most common symptom), pleuritic chest pain, nonpleuritic chest pain, anxiety, cough, and syncope. Common signs include hypoxemia, tachypnea, tachycardia, hemoptysis, diaphoresis, fever. and signs of DVT. Clinical signs of DVT occur in about 50% of patients. Massive PE (5% of cases) can result in hypotension and severe hypoxia. Cardiac arrest occurs in about 2% of PE and usually presents as pulseless electrical activity (PEA) from massive PE. PE frequently presents atypically and may present without any symptoms or signs.

DIAGNOSIS AND DIFFERENTIAL

Once the clinician suspects PE, the pretest probability of PE should be determined. The patient's pretest probability of PE guides the clinician's choice of diagnostic testing and helps determine when to terminate ancillary testing. Pretest probability can be determined subjectively by the clinician, although accuracy requires clinical experience. Alternatively, clinical score systems and decision rules that incorporate symptoms, signs, and risk factors can categorize patients into large groups of low, intermediate, or high probability.

Disorders on the differential diagnosis include respiratory disorders such as asthma, chronic obstructive pulmonary disease, pneumonia, pneumothorax, pleural effusion, and pleurisy. Cardiac disorders that may mimic PE include myocardial infarction, supraventricular tachycardias, and pericarditis. Muscle strain and costochondritis can mimic the chest pain of PE. Anxiety and hyperventilation syndrome may mimic PE but should be considered a diagnosis of exclusion.

Studies such as chest radiography and electrocardiography should be ordered to direct further testing and to identify other diseases on the differential diagnosis. Blood tests including the hematocrit, prothrombin time and partial thromboplastin time, and serum creatinine may be necessary to determine the safety of testing and treatment for PE. However, none of these tests are sufficient to rule in or rule out PE.

Selective pulmonary angiography is the gold standard test for the diagnosis of PE. However, the test is invasive and has morbidity and mortality rates of 1% to 5%, and about 1% of patients will be diagnosed with PE within a few months after a normal pulmonary angiogram. Recent practice has shifted away from this invasive and difficult procedure.

D-dimer testing has become an important adjunct in the diagnosis or exclusion of PE. It is important to understand the type of D-dimer assay being used in the hospital laboratory because the sensitivity of qualitative D-dimers such as the erythrocyte agglutination assay is about 85%, whereas the sensitivity of quantitative D-dimers such as enzyme-linked immunosorbent assay and the turbidimetric assay is about 95%. Most published research has restricted the use of D-dimer assays to patients with low pretest probability. There are many conditions other than PE (pregnancy, trauma, infection, malignancy, inflammatory conditions, recent surgery, and advanced age) that can elevate the D-dimer. The specificity of all D-dimer assays is therefore low. Regardless of the assay used, a positive D-dimer should be followed by confirmatory testing for PE.

Ventilation/perfusion (V/Q) scanning traditionally has been the first diagnostic imaging modality used in the diagnosis of PE. A normal V/Q scan effectively excludes PE. A high-probability V/Q scan effectively confirms the diagnosis of PE for patients with intermediate and high pretest probabilities. Patients with low pretest probability and high-probability scans and all patients with indeterminate scans should go on to further testing such as computed tomography (CT) or pulmonary angiography.

CT recently has emerged in some centers as the imaging test of choice for the initial evaluation of PE. Recent studies have shown sensitivity of 70% to 90%. Sensitivity is highest for large central PE and lowest for small subsegmental PE. One advantage to CT its ability to identify alternative diagnoses that may explain the patient's symptoms.

EMERGENCY DEPARTMENT CARE AND DISPOSITION

The treatment of PE consists of initial stabilization, anticoagulation with heparin, and thrombolytic therapy in severe cases. All patients suspected of having PE should have their cardiac rhythm, blood pressure, and pulse oxygenation measured continuously.

1. Patients should be placed on supplemental oxygen to maintain a pulse oximetry reading greater than 95%.
2. Intravenous access should be secured, and crystalloid intravenous fluids should be given to augment preload and correct hypotension.
3. Anticoagulation with a heparin is standard treatment for acute PE. Dosing of **unfractionated heparin** should be weight based, with 80 U/kg given as an initial bolus followed by 18 U/kg/h. Low-molecular-weight heparin has been shown to be safe and effective for the treatment of PE. Examples include **enoxaparin** 1 mg/kg subcutaneously as the initial dose in the emergency department. There are few absolute contraindications to anticoagulation with heparin for acute PE, although patients with recent intracranial hemorrhage or active gastrointestinal hemorrhage may have anticoagulation withheld. For patients with high pretest probability and no contraindications, heparin therapy should be initiated before diagnostic testing.
4. Thrombolytic therapy should be considered for patients who require more aggressive treatment for PE. Currently, the only patients who have been shown to clearly benefit from thrombolytic therapy are those with hemodynamic instability. Patients with echocardiographic evidence of right ventricular dysfunction may benefit from thrombolytic therapy, although evidence is conflicting as to whether the benefits outweigh the risks of

hemorrhage in these patients. The US Food and Drug Administration has approved 3 regimens for treatment of PE: streptokinase, urokinase, and tissue plasminogen activator. Approved dosing is similar to that used in myocardial infarction. The most common regimen is **tissue plasminogen activator** 50 to 100 mg infused over 2 to 6 hours, although it may be given as a bolus in the case of severe shock.

5. Stable patients with PE can be admitted to a telemetry bed. Patients who exhibit signs of circulatory compromise and all patients who receive thrombolytic therapy should be admitted to an intensive care unit.

For further reading in *Emergency Medicine: A Comprehensive Study Guide,* 6th ed., see Chap. 56. "Pulmonary Embolism," by Jeffrey A. Kline.

27 | Hypertensive Emergencies

Jonathan A. Maisel

Although hypertension (HTN) is defined as a systolic blood pressure (SBP) above 140 mm Hg or a diastolic blood pressure (DBP) above 90 mm Hg, management depends more on the patient's clinical condition than on absolute systolic or diastolic values. Classification of HTN into 4 categories facilitates management:

1. Hypertensive emergency: elevated blood pressure (BP) associated with target organ (central nervous system, cardiac, or renal) dysfunction. Immediate recognition and treatment are required.
2. Hypertensive urgency: elevated BP associated with risk for imminent target organ dysfunction. Decreasing the BP over 24 to 48 hours and follow-up the next day are recommended.
3. Acute hypertensive episode: SBP above 180 mm Hg and DBP above 110 mm Hg without signs or symptoms. Usually no immediate treatment is required, but the patient should have follow-up the next day.
4. Transient HTN: elevated BP associated with another condition (eg, anxiety, alcohol withdrawal, or cocaine abuse). Patients usually become normotensive once the precipitating event resolves.

The clinician must ensure that the BP cuff size is appropriate for the patient's size; a small cuff produces a falsely elevated BP reading.

CLINICAL FEATURES

Essential historic features include a prior history of HTN; noncompliance with BP medications; cardiovascular, renal, or cerebrovascular disease; diabetes; hyperlipidemia; chronic obstructive pulmonary disease or asthma; and a family history of HTN. Precipitating causes such as pregnancy, illicit drug use (cocaine and methamphetamines), monoamine oxidase inhibitor, or decongestants should be considered. Patients should be asked about central nervous system symptoms (headaches, visual changes, weakness, seizures, and confusion), cardiovascular symptoms (chest pain, palpitations, dyspnea, pedal edema, or tearing pain radiating to the back or abdomen), and renal symptoms (anuria, edema, or hematuria). The patient should be examined for evidence of papilledema, retinal exudates, neurologic deficits, seizures, meningismus, or encephalopathy; the presence of any findings constitutes a hypertensive emergency. The patient also should be assessed for carotid bruits, heart murmurs, gallops, symmetrical pulses (coarctation vs aortic dissection), pulsatile abdominal masses, and pulmonary rales. In the pregnant (or postpartum) patient, the clinician should look for hyperreflexia and peripheral edema, suggesting preeclampsia.

DIAGNOSIS AND DIFFERENTIAL

Renal impairment may present as hematuria, proteinuria, red cell casts, or elevations in serum urea nitrogen, creatinine, and potassium levels. An electrocardiogram may show ST- and T-wave changes consistent with coronary ischemia, electrolyte abnormalities, strain, or left ventricular hypertrophy. A chest x-ray may help identify congestive heart failure, aortic dissection, or coarctation. In patients with neurologic compromise, computed tomography of the head may show ischemic changes, edema, or blood. A urine or serum drug screen may identify illicit drug use. A pregnancy test should be done on all hypertensive women of childbearing potential.

EMERGENCY DEPARTMENT CARE AND DISPOSITION

Patients with hypertensive emergencies require O_2 supplementation, cardiac monitoring, and intravenous access. After attention to the ABCs of resuscitation, the treatment goal is to reduce mean arterial pressure (DBP + 1/3 [SBP − DBP]) by 20% over 60 minutes by using the following regimens.

1. For hypertensive encephalopathy, use **sodium nitroprusside,** beginning at 0.3 μg/kg/min and titrating to a maximum of 10 μg/kg/min. Avoid rapid correction of BP to prevent cerebral ischemia secondary to hypoperfusion. Its onset of action occurs within seconds. An arterial line should be placed to closely monitor the BP, and the solution and tubing should be wrapped in aluminum foil to prevent degradation by light.

2. **Labetalol** is a second-line agent for hypertensive encephalopathy. Its onset of action is 5 to 10 minutes. Treatment should begin with incremental boluses of 20 to 40 mg intravenously (IV), and repeated every 10 minutes until the target BP is achieved, or a total of 300 mg is administered. Alternatively, after an initial bolus, a continuous infusion at 2 mg/min can be used. The clinician should avoid using it in patients with reactive airway disease or heart block.

3. **Fenoldopam,** a new selective postsynaptic dopaminergic receptor agonist, is as effective as nitroprusside for hypertensive emergencies, with no effect on heart rate. It is given IV at a dose of 0.05 to 0.1 mg/kg/min and increased by 0.1 mg/kg/min to a maximum of 1.6 mg/kg/min.

4. HTN associated with stroke is often a physiologic response to the stroke itself and not its immediate cause. When DBP is above 140 mm Hg, it should be reduced slowly by up to 20% using 5-mg increments of IV **labetalol.** With hemorrhagic strokes, oral **nimodipine** (60 mg every 4 hours) or **nicardipine** (2 mg IV bolus, followed by 4 to 15 mg/h infusion) can reverse vasospasm associated with subarachnoid hemorrhage.

5. For HTN associated with pulmonary edema, intravenous **nitroglycerin** (begin at 5-20 μg/min and titrate to symptom relief by 5 μg/min every 5 minutes) or **nitroprusside** (started at 0.3 μg/kg/min) should be used. Diuretics, morphine sulfate, and **enalaprilat** (0.625-1.25 mg IV every 6 hours) also can be used.

6. For HTN associated with myocardial ischemia, **nitroglycerin** (5-20 μg/min) is first-line therapy. β-Blockers and morphine can be added.

7. For HTN associated with aortic dissection, reducing the BP and ventricular ejection force may limit the dissection. **Labetalol** alone (given in 20-mg increments as described earlier) or a combination of **nitroprusside** (started at 0.3 μg/kg/min) and **esmolol** (500 μg/kg over 1 minute, followed by an infusion of 50-300 μg/kg/min) can be used. Propranolol and metoprolol are alternatives.

8. For HTN associated with renal failure, **nitroprusside** 0.3 to 10 μg/kg/min is the preferred agent. Diuresis, **nitroglycerin,** clonidine (dose given later), and emergency dialysis are other options.

9. For HTN associated with pregnancy, including eclampsia, **hydralazine** can be given as a 10- to 20-mg IV dose or a 10- to 50-mg intramuscular dose, and can be repeated at 30-minute intervals.

10. For hypertensive urgency, useful agents include oral **labetalol** 200 to 400 mg, repeated every 2 to 3 hours; oral captopril 25 mg every 4 to 6 hours; sublingual **nitroglycerin** spray or tablets (0.3-0.6 mg); or **clonidine**, 0.2 mg oral loading dose, followed by 0.1 mg/h until the DBP is below 115 mm Hg, or a maximum of 0.7 mg. Because of the potential for serious adverse reactions (eg, stroke), oral or sublingual **nifedipine** is not recommended.

11. For non-emergent, nonurgent HTN, the choice of the oral agent should be based on coexisting conditions, if any. Diuretics, such as **hydrochlorothiazide** 25 mg/d, should be used in most patients with uncomplicated HTN (the clinician should consider an oral potassium supplement). For patients with angina, postmyocardial infarction, migraines, or supraventricular arrhythmias, a β-blocker should be considered, such as **metoprolol** 50 mg orally 2 times daily. Angiotensin-converting enzyme inhibitors such as **captopril** 25 mg 2 to 3 times daily can be used in those with congestive heart failure, renal disease, recurrent strokes, or diabetes mellitus. In addition, restarting a noncompliant patient on a previously established regimen is an acceptable strategy.

CHILDHOOD HYPERTENSIVE EMERGENCIES

Children often will have nonspecific complaints such as throbbing frontal headache or blurred vision. Physical findings associated with HTN are similar to those found in adults.

The most common etiologies in this age group are renovascular lesions and pheochromocytoma. The decision to treat a hypertensive emergency in a child is based on the BP and associated symptoms. Urgent treatment is required if the BP exceeds prior measurements by 30%. The goal is to reduce the BP by 25% within 1 hour. **Nitroprusside** (0.3-8.0 μg/kg/min) and **labetalol** (1-3 mg/kg/h) are the agents of choice. Nicardipine by continuous infusion is an excellent alternative. The treatment of pheochromocytoma is sur-gical excision and managing the BP with α-adrenergic blockers such as phentolamine. Pediatric HTN that requires intervention in the emergency department will likely require admission.

For further reading in *Emergency Medicine: A Comprehensive Study Guide,* 6th ed., see Chap. 57, "Hypertension," by Melissa M. Wu and Arjun Chanmugam.

| Aortic Dissection
and Aneurysms

David E. Manthey

Aortic dissection and abdominal aortic aneurysms (AAAs) are important causes of morbidity and death that require rapid diagnosis and frequently require prompt operative repair to offer the patient any chance of survival. Diagnosing these conditions can be challenging and carries a high risk of misdiagnosis.

ABDOMINAL AORTIC ANEURYSMS

Clinical Features

Four clinical scenarios arise regarding AAAs: acute rupture, aortoenteric fistula, chronic contained rupture, and an incidental finding.

Acute rupturing AAA is a true emergency that, if not rapidly identified and repaired, will lead to death. The classic presentation is of an older (>60 years) male smoker with atherosclerosis who presents with sudden onset severe back or abdominal pain, hypotension, and a pulsatile abdominal mass. Patients may present with syncope or some variation of unilateral flank pain, groin pain, hip pain, or pain localizing to 1 quadrant of the abdomen.

Fifty percent of patients describe a ripping or tearing pain that is severe and abrupt in onset. Patients may have a tender pulsatile abdominal mass on physical examination, but the absence of pain does not imply an intact aorta. Obesity may mask a pulsatile abdominal mass. Nausea and vomiting are commonly present.

Shock may persist through presentation or may transiently improve due to compensatory mechanisms. Femoral pulsations are typically normal. Retroperitoneal hemorrhage may be appreciated as periumbilical ecchymosis (Cullen sign), flank ecchymosis (Grey-Turner sign), or scrotal hematomas. If blood compresses the femoral nerve, a neuropathy of the lower extremity may be present.

Aortoenteric fistulas, although rare, present as gastrointestinal bleeding, either a small sentinel bleed or massive life-threatening hemorrhage. A history of previous aortic grafting (eg, AAA repair) increases the suspicion. Because the duodenum is the usual site of the fistula, the patient may present with hematemesis, melenemesis, melena, or hematochezia.

Chronic contained rupture of AAA is an uncommon presentation. If an AAA ruptures into the retroperitoneum, there may be significant fibrosis and a limiting of blood loss. The patient typically appears quite well and may complain of pain for an extended period.

Discovering a previously undiagnosed asymptomatic AAA on physical or radiologic examination can be lifesaving. Those aneurysms larger than 5 cm in diameter are at a greater risk for rupture, but all should be referred to a vascular surgeon.

Diagnosis and Differential

Although the diagnosis may be relatively straightforward in the setting of syncope, back pain, and shock with a tender pulsatile abdominal mass, the differential diagnosis varies depending on the presentation. Missed AAAs are most frequently misdiagnosed as renal colic. This life-threatening disease process should be considered in the differential diagnosis for any patient that presents with back pain, an intraabdominal process (pancreatitis, diverticulitis, mesenteric ischemia, etc), possible testicular torsion, or gastrointestinal bleeding disorders (eg, esophageal varices, tumors, or ulcers).

If the diagnosis of rupturing AAA is clear on clinical grounds, the operating vascular surgeon should immediately evaluate the patient. However, when the diagnosis is not entirely clear, confirming studies may be required. In the unstable patient, technically adequate bedside abdominal ultrasound has virtually 100% sensitivity for identifying AAA and can measure the diameter of the aneurysm. Be aware that aortic rupture cannot be reliably identified with ultrasound. Obesity and bowel gas technically may limit the study. In the stable patient, computed tomography (CT) can identify the AAA and delineate the anatomic details of the aneurysm and any associated rupture. The role of plain radiography in the diagnosis of rupturing AAA in unclear because a calcified bulging aortic contour is present in only 65% of patients with symptomatic AAA.

Emergency Department Care and Disposition

The primary role of the emergency physician is in identifying AAA.

1. For suspected rupturing AAA or aortoenteric fistula, prompt surgical consultation in anticipation of emergency surgery is critical. No diagnostic testing should delay surgical repair.
2. The patient is stabilized with large-bore intravenous access, judicious fluid administration for hypotension, treatment of hypertension (see Chap. 27), and typing and cross-matching of several units of packed red blood cells, with transfusion as needed. Because patients may rapidly deteriorate, those who undergo diagnostic testing should not be left unattended in the radiology department.
3. For chronic contained rupturing AAA, consultation with a vascular surgeon for urgent repair and intensive care unit admission should be sought.
4. For AAA identified as an incidental finding, the patient potentially can be discharged home, depending on the aneurysmal size and comorbid factors. Telephone consultation with a vascular surgeon for admission or close office follow-up is usually adequate.

AORTIC DISSECTION

Clinical Features

Aortic dissection typically presents (>85% of patients) with acute onset of pain that is most severe at onset located in the chest and radiating to the back. The location of the pain may indicate the area of the aorta that is involved. Seventy percent of patients with ascending involvement have anterior chest pain, and 63% of patients with involvement of the descending aorta have back pain. The pain pattern may change as the dissection progresses from one anatomic area to another. The pain is described as ripping or tearing by 50% of patients. Accompanying nausea, vomiting, and diaphoresis are common.

Most patients are male (66%), older than 50 years (mean age, 63), and have a history of hypertension (72%). Another group of patients are younger with identifiable risk factors such as connective tissue disorders, congenital heart disease, and pregnancy. Up to 30% of patients with Marfan syndrome will develop a dissection. Iatrogenic induced aortic dissection may occur after aortic catheterization or cardiac surgery.

To communicate more effectively with the surgeons, the emergency department physician should classify aortic dissections in 1 of 2 ways. The Stanford classification divides dissections into those that involve the ascending aorta (type A) and those that are restricted to the descending aorta (type B). The DeBakey classification divides dissections into 3 groups: involvement of the ascending and descending aortas (type I), involvement of only the ascending aorta (type II), or involvement of only the descending aorta (type III).

As the dissection progresses, seemingly unrelated symptom complexes may present themselves. Presentations include aortic valve insufficiency, coronary artery occlusion with myocardial infarction, carotid involvement with stroke symptoms, occlusion of vertebral blood supply with paraplegia, cardiac tamponade with shock and jugular venous distention, compression of the recurrent laryngeal nerve with hoarseness of the voice, and compression of the superior cervical sympathetic ganglion with Horner syndrome. The dissection may open back into the true aortic lumen with a marked decrease in symptoms, leading to a false sense of security.

The patient's physical examination findings will depend on the location and progression of the dissection. A diastolic murmur of aortic insufficiency may be heard. Hypertension and tachycardia are common, but hypotension also may be present. Fifty percent of patients have decreased pulsation in the radial, femoral, or carotid arteries. Although one might expect a difference in extremity blood pressures, no specific threshold values have been defined. Forty percent of patients have neurologic sequelae.

Diagnosis and Differential

The differential diagnosis to be considered depends on the location and progression of the dissection. Other causes of aortic insufficiency, myocardial infarction, esophageal rupture, other causes of strokes, spinal injury or tumor, vocal cord tumors, and other causes of cardiac tamponade, including pericardial disease, may need to be considered. An electrocardiogram would help demonstrate disruption of a coronary artery, most commonly the right.

The diagnosis of aortic dissection depends on radiographic confirmation once the diagnosis is suspected. The chest x-ray is abnormal in 88% of patients with aortic dissection. The abnormality may be an abnormal aortic contour; widening of the mediastinum; deviation of the trachea, mainstem bronchi, or esophagus; apical capping; or pleural effusion. The "calcium sign" may be present, with intimal calcium deposits seen distant from the edge of the aortic contour. CT is 83% to 100% sensitive and 87% to 100% specific for the diagnosis of dissection. Spiral CT with rapid contrast boluses is the most sensitive. Angiography, although considered the gold standard, is invasive and has a specificity of 94% and a sensitivity of 88%. It may better define the anatomy, extent, and complications of a dissection. Transesophageal echocardiograms, in experienced hands, are 97% to 100% sensitive and 97% to 99% specific. The use of these studies is institutionally dependent, and they should be ordered in conjunction with the consulting vascular or thoracic surgeon.

Emergency Department Care and Disposition

All patients with aortic dissection or strongly suspected aortic dissection require emergent vascular or thoracic surgical consultation and prompt radiographic confirmation of the diagnosis, which is best directed by the operating surgeon. In general, patients with dissection of the ascending aorta require prompt surgical intervention. The operative care of dissection of only the descending aorta is controversial and should be evaluated on a case-by-case basis.

1. Stabilization of the patient typically requires large-bore intravenous access with availability of type and cross-matched blood in case of free rupture.
2. Management of hypertension is best done with β-blockers because these decrease the blood pressure and the shear force (see Chap. 27).
3. Vasodilators, such as nitroprusside, should be used only after adequate inotropic blockade has been made with β-receptor or calcium-channel blockers (see Chap. 27).

For further reading in *Emergency Medicine: A Comprehensive Study Guide,* 6th ed., see Chap. 58, "Aortic Dissection and Aneurysms," by Louise A. Prince and Gary A. Johnson.

29 | Peripheral Vascular Disorders

Christopher Kabrhel

DEEP VENOUS THROMBOSIS AND THROMBOPHLEBITIS

Deep venous thrombosis (DVT) is a common condition with an estimated annual incidence of 2 million cases in the United States. DVT is part of the spectrum of venous thromboembolic disease that also includes pulmonary embolism (PE; see Chap. 26). Most (90%) cases of DVT occur in the lower extremities, although thrombosis of the upper extremities can occur, especially in the presence of an indwelling venous catheter.

Clinical Features

Superficial thrombophlebitis is a common, self-limiting condition that presents with pain, redness, and tenderness along a superficial vein. The incidence of DVT from extension of superficial thrombophlebitis is about 3%.

DVT forms at sites of endothelial injury and venous stasis and is augmented by hypercoagulable states. Thrombus is composed mostly of erythrocytes, fibrin, and platelets. The most significant risk factors for DVT are major surgery or trauma, prolonged immobilization, malignancy or other hypercoagulable state (factor V Leiden being the most common), and prior thromboembolic disease. Pregnancy, the immediate postpartum state, estrogen use, congestive heart failure, inflammatory conditions, and prolonged travel are other significant risk factors.

Unfortunately, the clinical examination is unreliable for DVT. The classic constellation of calf or leg pain, redness, swelling, tenderness, and warmth is present in fewer than 50% of patients with confirmed lower extremity DVT. Homan sign (ie, pain in the calf with forced dorsiflexion of the ankle with the leg straight) is unreliable for DVT. Several decision instruments have been developed to categorize patients as having low, moderate, or high probability of DVT before diagnostic testing. One scoring system developed by Wells and associates is presented in Table 29-1. The analysis is as follows: a score of at least 3 indicates high probability, a score of 1 to 2 indicates moderate probability, and a score of 0 or lower indicates low probability.

Uncommon but severe presentations of DVT include *phlegmasia cerulea dolens* and *phlegmasia alba dolens*. Phlegmasia cerulea dolens is a high-grade obstruction that elevates compartment pressures and can compromise limb perfusion. It presents as a massively swollen, cyanotic limb. Phlegmasia alba dolens is usually associated with pregnancy and has a similar pathophysiology but presents as a pale limb secondary to arterial spasm.

Diagnosis and Differential

The history and physical examination are unreliable for DVT. Similar presentations can be seen with congestive heart failure, cellulitis, venous stasis without thrombosis, and musculoskeletal injuries. Therefore, some type of objective testing for DVT is necessary. Assessing clinical probability with an objective and validated instrument can help guide the type and extent of objective testing necessary (see Table 29-1).

TABLE 29-1 Predictors of Deep Venous Thrombosis

Clinical feature	Score
Active cancer (treatment ongoing, palliative)	1
Paralysis, paresis, or recent plaster immobilization of lower extremities	1
Recently bedridden >3 d or major surgery within 4 wk	1
Localized tenderness along the distribution of the deep venous system	1
Entire leg swollen	1
Calf swelling >3 cm on asymptomatic side (10 cm below tibial tuberosity)	1
Pitting edema confined to the symptomatic leg	1
Collateral superficial veins (nonvaricose)	1
Alternative diagnosis as likely or greater than that of deep venous thrombosis	−2

Source: Adapted with permission from Wells PS, Anderson DR, Ginsberg J. Assessment of deep vein thrombosis or pulmonary embolism by the combined use of clinical model and noninvasive diagnostic tests. *Semin Thromb Hemos.* 2000; 26:643–656.

A rapid enzyme-linked immunosorbent assay D-dimer has high sensitivity (97% to 99%) for DVT and can be used to exclude the diagnosis in low- to moderate-probability patients. The use of latex D-dimer assays to exclude DVT is not recommended due to their low (80%) sensitivity for DVT. Erythrocyte agglutination D-dimer assays have a sensitivity of 84% to 94%, and the use of these tests to rule out DVT is controversial.

Duplex ultrasonography (real-time B-mode imaging combined with Doppler flow imaging) is the test of choice for evaluating DVT in the emergency department (ED). Duplex ultrasonography has high sensitivity (97%) and specificity (94%) for DVT. Sensitivity is lower for pelvic and isolated calf DVT (73%). Some algorithms recommend serial ultrasonography for patients with high clinical probability of DVT and negative initial ultrasound. Two negative duplex scans 1 week apart carries less than 1% risk of symptomatic DVT or PE in 3 months. For patients with suspected upper extremity DVT, duplex ultrasound has a sensitivity of 56% to 100%.

Impedance plethysmography measures changes in electrical resistance in response to changes in calf volume secondary to venous obstruction. Sensitivity is 73% to 96% and specificity is 83% to 97%. However, due to its lower sensitivity, this technique has been largely supplanted by duplex ultrasonography.

The traditional gold standard for DVT has been contrast venography. However, the technique is invasive and impractical, so it is rarely performed. Magnetic resonance imaging may represent a new gold standard for diagnosing DVT, but its application to the ED is unclear.

Emergency Department Care and Disposition

Treatment of superficial thrombophlebitis is conservative. Mild cases can be treated with warm compresses, analgesia, and elevation. Antibiotics and anticoagulants are of no proven benefit in superficial thrombophlebitis, although it may be necessary to rule out associated DVT, especially in cases of proximal disease.

Treatment of DVT centers on aggressive anticoagulation to prevent the extension of clot, allow for its lysis by the intrinsic fibrinolytic system, and prevent PE. Any patient with documented DVT on duplex ultrasonography should receive immediate anticoagulation with heparin and eventually warfarin.

1. Low-molecular-weight heparins (LMWHs) are safe and effective for the treatment of DVT. The 3 most commonly used LMWHs are dalteparin (200 U/kg subcutaneously every 24 hours; maximum, 18,000 U), enoxaparin (1.5 mg/kg subcutaneously every 24 hours; maximum, 180 mg), and tinzaparin (175 U/kg subcutaneously every 24 hours; maximum, 18,000 U).
2. When LMWH is unavailable or contraindicated, unfractionated heparin therapy should be initiated. Dosing is weight based at 80 U/kg as an intravenous bolus followed by 18 U/kg/h infusion. The activated partial thromboplastin time should be maintained between 55 and 80 seconds (1.5 to 2.5 times normal).
3. For patients with documented heparin-induced thrombocytopenia, a thrombin inhibitor such as lepirudin can be given as a 0.4 mg/kg slow bolus up to 44 mg followed by an infusion of 0.1 to 0.15 mg/kg/h.
4. Oral anticoagulation with warfarin can be initiated simultaneously with heparin therapy. Usual initial dosing is 5 mg/d with a target international normalized ratio of 2 to 3.
5. An inferior vena cava filter can be placed to prevent PE when anticoagulation is contraindicated, a major complication occurs, or DVT continues to propagate despite adequate anticoagulation.
6. Many patients can be discharged from the ED after a dose of LMWH if appropriate follow-up is arranged and more invasive therapy is not required. However, hospital admission should be considered for complicated cases or when appropriate follow-up cannot be arranged.
7. Patients with high clinical probability of DVT and negative initial ultrasound should be considered for referral for repeat scanning in 1 week.

ACUTE ARTERIAL OCCLUSION

Acute arterial occlusion secondary to thrombosis or embolism is less common than venous occlusion but is potentially life threatening and carries a mortality of 25%. In survivors of this condition, limb amputation is necessary in 20%. The most frequently involved arteries, in descending order, are the femoropopliteal, tibial, aortoiliac, and brachiocephalic.

Clinical Features

Patients with acute arterial limb ischemia typically present with 1 of the "six Ps": pain, pallor, polar (coldness), pulselessness, paresthesias, and paralysis. Pain is the earliest symptom and may increase with elevation of the limb. Changes in skin color and temperature are common. A decreased pulse distal to the obstruction is an unreliable finding for early ischemia, especially in patients with peripheral vascular disease and well-developed collateral circulation.

Diagnosis and Differential

A history of an abruptly ischemic limb in a patient with atrial fibrillation or recent myocardial infarction is strongly suggestive of an embolus. A history of claudication suggests a thrombosis.

For more objective testing, a handheld Doppler can document blood flow or its absence in the affected limb, whereas Duplex ultrasonography can detect an obstruction to flow with a sensitivity greater than 85%. In addition, the ankle-brachial index should be determined. It is the ratio of the systolic blood pressure measured just above the malleoli to the brachial pressure in the arm. With arterial occlusion, the ankle-brachial index usually is markedly diminished (<0.5). A pressure difference greater than 30 mm Hg between any 2 adjacent levels can localize the site of obstruction. The diagnostic gold standard is the arteriogram, which can define the anatomy of the obstruction and direct treatment.

Emergency Department Care and Disposition

1. Patients with acute arterial occlusion should be stabilized, and fluid resuscitation should be initiated as needed.
2. It is standard procedure to initiate anticoagulation with unfractionated heparin (as above), although there is no equivocal evidence demonstrating the benefit of this practice. Dosing is weight based at 80 U/kg intravenous bolus followed by 18 U/kg/h infusion. The activated partial thromboplastin time should be maintained between 55 and 80 seconds (1.5 to 2.5 times normal).
3. Definitive treatment should be performed in consultation with a vascular surgeon. Catheter embolectomy using a Fogarty balloon is the preferred method. Other options include thrombolysis and standard surgery.
4. All patients with an acute arterial occlusion should be admitted to a telemetry bed or to the intensive care unit depending on the stability of the patient and the planned course of therapy.

For further reading in *Emergency Medicine: A Comprehensive Study Guide,* 6th ed., see Chap. 59, "Peripheral Vascular Disorders (Nontraumatic)," by Anil Chopra.

6 | PULMONARY EMERGENCIES

30 | Respiratory Distress

Matthew T. Keadey

Respiratory distress is a common finding in many patients who present to the emergency department. Causes are multifactorial and include the findings of dyspnea, hypoxia, hypercapnia, and cyanosis. Despite the increasing reliance on ancillary studies and technology, the evaluation of respiratory distress depends on a careful history and physical examination.

DYSPNEA

Dyspnea is the subjective feeling of difficult, labored, or uncomfortable breathing. There is no single pathophysiologic mechanism that causes dyspnea. However, 66% of patients with dyspnea have a cardiac or a pulmonary cause.

Clinical Features

The initial assessment of any patient with dyspnea should be directed toward identifying respiratory failure. Dyspnea is a subjective complaint and often difficult to measure. Vital signs including pulse oximetry and general impression of the patient will identify those in significant distress. Tachycardia, tachypnea, stridor, and the use of accessory respiratory muscles point to significant respiratory distress. Other significant signs include the inability to speak from breathlessness, altered mental status, lethargy, and agitation. In patients with any of these signs or symptoms, oxygen should be administered immediately. With no improvement, the need for aggressive airway management and mechanical ventilation should be anticipated. Lack of these signs and symptoms indicates a lesser degrees of distress, thereby allowing for a detailed history and physical examination that often can help identify the etiology of dyspnea.

Diagnosis and Differential

The history and physical examination should be the primary aids in identifying the etiology of dyspnea; however, ancillary testing may aid in determining the severity and specific cause (Table 30-1). Pulse oximetry is a rapid but insensitive screen for disorders of gas exchange. Arterial blood gas (ABG) analysis has improved sensitivity but does not take into account work of breathing. ABG analysis may also show a metabolic acidosis, which can be a common cause of hyperpnea. A chest radiograph may identify pulmonary and cardiac causes of dyspnea. In addition, an abnormal electrocardiogram or abnormal cardiac enzymes may point to a cardiac cause of dyspnea. A peak expiratory flow rate may indicate reactive airway disease. Laboratory tests that may prove helpful include a complete blood count, B-type natriuretic peptide, and D-dimer assay. Uncommonly, the cause of dyspnea may not be identified. Specialized testing that may be indicated include computed tomography of the chest, echocardiography, pulmonary function testing, cardiac stress testing, nuclear medicine scans, or combined cardiopulmonary exercise testing.

TABLE 30-1 Causes of Dyspnea

Most common causes	Most immediately lifethreatening
Obstructive airway disease; asthma, COPD	Upper airway obstruction: foreign body, angioedema, hemorrhage
Congestive heart failure/cardiogenic pulmonary edema	Tension pneumothorax
Ischemic heart disease: unstable angina and myocardial infarction	Pulmonary embolism
Pneumonia Psychogenic	Neuromuscular weakness: myasthenia gravis, Guillain-Barré syndrome, botulism

Key: COPD = chronic obstructive pulmonary disease.

Emergency Department Care and Disposition

Just as there is no single cause of dyspnea, there is no single treatment.

1. Patients identified with impending respiratory failure will need aggressive airway management and mechanical ventilation. Noninvasive positive pressure ventilation techniques such as continuous positive airway pressure and biphasic positive airway pressure should be considered.
2. The goal of therapy is to maintain the Pao_2 above 60 mm Hg or oxygen saturation above 90%. The goals can be lowered in those with chronic obstructive pulmonary disease or chronic lung disease.
3. After oxygenation has been ensured, disorder-specific treatment can be provided.
4. The disposition of patients with dyspnea is disorder specific. Any patient with hypoxia and an unclear cause of dyspnea requires hospital admission.

HYPOXEMIA

Hypoxia is the inadequate delivery of oxygen to the tissues. Oxygen delivery is mainly a function of cardiac output, hemoglobin concentration, and oxygen saturation. Hypoxemia is arbitrarily defined as a Pao_2 below 60 mm Hg. Hypoxemia results from a combination of 5 distinct mechanisms: (*a*) hypoventilation hypoxia in which lack of ventilation increases $Paco_2$, thereby displacing it from the alveolus and lowering the amount delivered to the alveolar capillaries; (*b*) right-to-left shunt in which blood bypasses the lungs, thereby increasing the amount of unoxygenated blood entering the systemic circulation; (*c*) ventilation/perfusion mismatch in which areas of the lung are perfused but not ventilated from a variety of conditions; (*d*) diffusion impairment in which alveolar–blood barrier abnormality causes impairment of oxygenation; and (*e*) low inspired oxygen, which occurs at high altitude.

Clinical Features

Signs and symptoms of hypoxemia are nonspecific. Acute physiologic responses to dyspnea include an increase in minute ventilation, pulmonary arterial vasoconstriction, and an increase in sympathetic tone. These physiologic responses result in tachypnea, tachycardia, and an initial hyperdynamic cardiac state. Changes in mental status may predominate, including headache, somnolence, lethargy, anxiety, agitation, coma, or seizures. Chronic hypoxemia may result in polycythemia, clubbing of the digits, cor pulmonale, and changes in body habitus (the "pink puffer or blue bloater"). Cyanosis may be present but is not a sensitive or specific indicator of hypoxemia.

Diagnosis and Differential

The diagnosis of hypoxemia requires clinical suspicion and objective measurement. Formal diagnosis requires ABG analysis, but pulse oximetry may be useful for gross abnormalities. The exact etiology of hypoxemia can be multifactorial and similar to that of dyspnea (see Table 30-1). Determination of the exact cause is thorough, careful history and physical examination. Quantification of the arterial-alveolar oxygen gradient may further quantitate the degree of hypoxemia and give clues to the etiology.

$$\text{arterial-alveolar oxygen gradient} = (Fio_2 - [1.2 \times Paco_2]) - Pao_2$$
$$Fio_2 = \text{fraction of inspired oxygen concentration}$$
$$Paco_2 = \text{arterial partial pressure of } CO_2$$

Emergency Department Care and Disposition

Regardless of the specific cause of hypoxemia, the initial approach remains the same.

1. Supplemental oxygen is administered to achieve an O_2 saturation greater than 90%.
2. The airway is managed aggressively (see Chap. 1).
3. Cause-specific treatment is administered.
4. All patients with new hypoxemia should be admitted and monitored until their condition is stabilized.

HYPERCAPNIA

Hypercapnia is arbitrarily defined as a $Paco_2$ above 45 mm Hg and is exclusively due to alveolar hypoventilation. Factors that affect alveolar ventilation include respiratory rate, tidal volume, and dead space volume. Because CO_2 easily diffuses across the pulmonary membrane, intrinsic lung disease (unless from an increase in anatomic dead space) and increased CO_2 production almost never cause hypercapnia.

Clinical Features

The signs and symptoms of hypercapnia depend on the rate of change and the absolute value of $Paco_2$. Acute elevations result in increased intracranial pressure, with patients complaining of headache, confusion, and lethargy. In severe cases in which the $Paco_2$ is above 80 mm Hg, coma, encephalopathy, and seizures may present. If changes in $Paco_2$ are chronic, large variations may be tolerated.

Diagnosis and Differential

The diagnosis requires clinical suspicion and ABG analysis. In some cases, pulse oximetry can be completely normal. In acute cases, the ABG will demonstrate respiratory acidosis with minimal metabolic compensation. Table 30-2 shows common causes of hypercapnia.

TABLE 30-2 Causes of Hypercapnia

Depressed central respiratory drive
Structural CNS disease: brainstem lesions
Drug depression of respiratory center: opioids, sedatives, anesthetics
Endogenous toxins: tetanus
Thoracic cage disorders
Kyphoscoliosis
Morbid obesity
Neuromuscular impairment
Neuromuscular disease: myasthenia gravis, Guillain-Barré syndrome
Neuromuscular toxin: organophosphate poisoning, botulism
Intrinsic lung disease associated with increased dead space
COPD
Upper airway obstruction

Key: CNS = central nervous system, COPD = chronic obstructive pulmonary disease.

Emergency Department Care and Disposition

Treatment of acute hypercapnia requires aggressive measures to increase minute ventilation.

1. Airway maintenance is crucial and mechanical ventilation may be indicated (see Chap. 1).
2. A trial of biphasic positive airway pressure or continuous positive airway pressure may prove helpful and improve minute ventilation.
3. Disposition depends on etiology, but many patients with hypercapnia require hospital admission and monitoring.

WHEEZING

Wheezes are described as "musical," high-pitched, adventitious lung sounds produced by the airflow through central and lower airways. They are produced from airway flutter and vortex shedding that is more pronounced in obstructed airways. Airway obstruction may result from increased secretions, smooth muscle constriction, muscular hypertrophy, and peribronchial inflammation.

Clinical Features

Wheezing is not synonymous with airway obstruction and asthma. Conversely, patients with severe airflow obstruction may not have any wheezing secondary to lack of airflow. Duration of the expiratory phase has been used to quantify the severity of airflow obstruction. Most patients with bronchospastic disease report recurrent episodes of dyspnea and wheezing.

Diagnosis and Differential

Cardiovascular and intrinsic lung diseases can cause wheezing, and distinguishing one from the other is often difficult. Table 30-3 lists common causes of wheezing. Airflow obstruction can be assessed by bedside spirometry or peak expiratory flow, but neither is possible in the severely dyspneic patient. Chest x-ray may be important to exclude cardiac or infectious causes of

TABLE 30-3 Causes of Wheezing

Upper airway (more likely to be stridor, may have element of wheezing)
  Angioedema: allergic, ACE inhibitor, idiopathic
  Foreign body
  Infection: croup, epiglottitis, tracheitis
Lower airway
  Asthma
  Transient airway hyperreactivity (usually due to infection or irritation)
  Bronchiolitis
  COPD
  Foreign body
Cardiovascular
  Cardiogenic pulmonary edema ("cardiac asthma")
  Noncardiogenic pulmonary edema (adult respiratory distress syndrome)
  Pulmonary embolus (rare)
Psychogenic

Key: ACE = angiotension-converting enzyme, COPD = chronic obstructive pulmonary disease.

wheezing. ABG analysis may be helpful if the examination suggests hypoxemia, hypercapnia, or acidosis.

Emergency Department Care and Disposition

1. Treatment of wheezing is directed at the underlying disorder.
2. Patients with reactive airway disease typically require bronchodilator and steroid therapy (see Chap. 35).
3. Disposition is dependent on response to therapy and the underlying etiology.

CYANOSIS

Cyanosis is a bluish color of the skin or mucous membranes and results from an increased amount of deoxyhemoglobin. The detection of cyanosis is highly subjective and not a sensitive indicator of arterial oxygenation. Traditional teaching purports that cyanosis develops when the deoxyhemoglobin level exceeds 5 mg/dL, but this is greatly variable.

Clinical Features

The presence of cyanosis suggests tissue hypoxia. The presence of cyanosis with a normal Pao_2 suggests an abnormal hemoglobin such as methemoglobin. Cyanosis is divided into central and peripheral. Central cyanosis is more common with low Pao_2 or abnormal hemoglobins, whereas peripheral cyanosis is associated with poor perfusion of the extremities. Central cyanosis is observed most reliably under the tongue.

Diagnosis and Differential

The causes of cyanosis may be multifactorial (Table 30-4). The differentiation between central and peripheral cyanosis may be difficult if the cyanosis is severe. Pulse oximetry is easily available for continuous monitoring, but ABG analysis is the gold standard for diagnosis of hypoxia. Abnormal hemoglobins may skew the ABG results. Methemoglobinemia and carboxyhemoglobinemia may cause cyanosis with a normal Pao_2. Methemoglobinemia yields

TABLE 30-4 Causes of Cyanosis

Central cyanosis	Peripheral cyanosis

Hypoxemia
  Decreased Fio$_2$: high altitude
  Hypoventilation
  Ventilation-perfusion mismatch
  Right-to-left shunt: congential
  heart disease, pulmonary
  arteriovenous fistulas, multiple
  intrapulmonary shunts
	Reduced cardiac output
	Cold extremities
	Maldistribution of blood flow:
	distributive forms of shock
	Arterial or venous obstruction

Hemoglobin abnormalities
  Methemoglobinemia: hereditary,
  acquired
  Sulfhemoglobinemia: acquired
  Carboxyhemoglobinemia (not
  true cyanosis)	

Key: Fio$_2$ = fraction of inspired oxygen concentration.

blood that has been described as chocolate brown and does not change with exposure to room air. Carboxyhemoglobin produces a cherry red cyanosis. A hematocrit may demonstrate polycythemia vera or severe anemia, both of which can be culprits of cyanosis.

Emergency Department Care and Disposition

1. Patients with cyanosis require aggressive treatment and rapid identification of the underlying etiology.
2. Patients should be started on supplemental oxygen to achieve an oxygen saturation greater than 90%. Those with central cyanosis should improve rapidly. If they do not, abnormal hemoglobins or pseudo-cyanosis should be suspected.
3. Peripheral cyanosis should respond to therapy directed at the specific condition.

For further reading in *Emergency Medicine: A Comprehensive Study Guide,* 6th ed., see Chap. 62, "Respiratory Distress," by J. Stephen Stapczynski.

31 | Bronchitis, Pneumonia, and SARS

David M. Cline

BRONCHITIS

Uncomplicated acute bronchitis (UAB) is an infection of the conducting airways of the lung. Respiratory viruses cause the vast majority of UAB cases. Influenzae B and A, parainfluenza, and respiratory syncytial virus are implicated most often.

Clinical Features

The cough of UAB is commonly productive and may last up to 2 months. The presence of purulent sputum is unimportant in diagnosing or treating UAB unless other symptoms and signs suggest pneumonia. Fever higher than 38°C (100.4°F), heart rate faster than 100 beats/min, respiratory rate faster than 24 breaths/min, and chills suggest pneumonia; fewer than 10% of patients with UAB are febrile. The strongest independent predictors of UAB are cough and wheezing; nausea is the strongest negative predictor of UAB. Approximately 33% of patients presenting with symptoms of UAB may have asthma.

Diagnosis and Differential

Clinical diagnosis of UAB is made with the following criteria: (*a*) acute cough (shorter than 2 weeks' duration), (*b*) no prior lung disease, and (*c*) no auscultatory abnormalities that suggest pneumonia. Pulse oximetry is indicated if the patient describes dyspnea or appears short of breath. Bedside peak flow testing is indicated if wheezing is heard on examination. A chest radiograph is not required in patients who appear nontoxic. Studies have found pertussis in up to 20% of patients with cough persisting for 2 to 3 weeks.

Emergency Department Care and Disposition

1. Unless pertussis is a consideration, antibiotics do not improve the cough of UAB but commonly produce side effects including nausea, vomiting, or vaginitis.
2. Patients with evidence of airflow obstruction should be treated with bronchodilators. **Albuterol** by metered dose inhaler, 2 puffs every 4 to 6 hours, is usually effective. Otherwise, supportive treatment is the rule.
3. Cough suppression with a non-narcotic or narcotic agent should be considered on an individual basis after considering comorbidities, sleep patterns, and potential side effects.

PNEUMONIA

Pneumonia is the sixth leading cause of death in the United States. Bacterial causes are the most common. Pneumococcus is responsible for up to 90% of all bacterial pneumonias, with *Escherichia coli, Pseudomonas aeruginosa, Klebsiella pneumoniae, Staphylococcus aureus, Haemophilus influenzae,* and group A streptococci accounting for most of the rest. *Legionella* species and anaerobes are less frequent causes of bacterial pneumonia, with the latter being primarily the result of aspiration. Respiratory viruses, *Mycoplasma,* and *Chlamydia* account for the bulk of atypical pneumonia, which account for 33% or more of all cases of pneumonia. Patients with chronic diseases, such as congestive failure, cancer, bronchiectasis, chronic obstructive pulmonary disease, diabetes, sickle cell anemia, acquired immunodeficiency syndrome, and other immunodeficiencies, are at greater risk for pneumonia, as are smokers and postsplenectomy patients. Aspiration pneumonia occurs more frequently in alcoholics and patients with seizures, stroke, or other neuromuscular diseases. *Pneumocystis pneumonia* is a common complication of infection with the human immunodeficiency virus and is discussed in Chap. 89.

Clinical Features

Patients with bacterial pneumonia generally present with some combination of fever, dyspnea, cough, pleuritic chest pain, and sputum production. Pneumococcus classically presents abruptly with fever, rigors, and rusty brown sputum; *H influenzae* is more common in smokers and the elderly. *Staphylococcus aureus* frequently follows a viral respiratory illness, especially influenza and measles. Pneumonia due to *Legionella* is spread via airborne, aerosolized water droplets rather than by person-to-person contact. This form of pneumonia presents, as do *Mycoplasma, Chlamydia,* and viral pneumonia, with fever, chills, malaise, dyspnea, and a nonproductive cough. *Legionella* also commonly causes gastrointestinal symptoms of anorexia, nausea, vomiting, and diarrhea. Mental status changes also may be present.

Physical findings of pneumonia vary with the offending organism and the type of pneumonia each causes, although most are associated with some degree of tachypnea and tachycardia. Lobar pneumonias, such as those caused by pneumococcus and *Klebsiella,* exhibit signs of consolidation, including bronchial breath sounds, egophony, increased tactile and vocal fremitus, and dullness to percussion. A pleural friction rub and cyanosis may be present. Bronchopneumonias, such as those caused by *H influenzae,* present with rales and rhonchi on examination without signs of consolidation. A parapneumonic pleural effusion may occur in either setting; empyemas are most common with *S aureus, Klebsiella,* and anaerobic infections. *Legionella,* which begins with findings of patchy bronchopneumonia and progresses to signs of frank consolidation, has other common signs, including a relative bradycardia and confusion. Interstitial pneumonias, such as those caused by viruses, *Mycoplasma,* and *Chlamydia,* may exhibit fine rales, rhonchi, or normal breath sounds. Bullous myringitis, when present in this setting, is pathognomonic for *Mycoplasma* infection.

Clinical features of aspiration pneumonitis depend on the volume and pH of the aspirate, the presence of particulate matter in the aspirate, and bacterial contamination. Although acid aspiration results in the rapid onset of symptoms of tachypnea, tachycardia, and cyanosis and often progresses to frank pulmonary failure, most other cases of aspiration pneumonia progress more insidiously. Physical signs develop over hours and include rales, rhonchi, wheezing, and copious frothy or bloody sputum. The right lower lobe is most commonly involved due to the anatomy of the tracheobronchial tree and to gravity.

Diagnosis and Differential

The differential diagnosis includes acute tracheobronchitis; pulmonary embolus or infarction; exacerbation of chronic obstructive pulmonary disease;

pulmonary vasculitides, including Goodpasture disease and Wegener granulomatosis; bronchiolitis obliterans; and endocarditis. The diagnosis of pneumonia is made on the presenting signs and symptoms, examination of the sputum, and chest radiograph. Other tests include a white blood count with differential count, pulse oximetry analysis, blood cultures, and pleural fluid examination. Arterial blood gas analysis may be performed in ill-appearing patients. If *Legionella* is being considered, serum chemistry studies and liver function tests should be performed because hyponatremia, hypophosphatemia, and elevated liver enzymes are commonly found. Also when appropriate, urine should be tested for *Legionella* antigen, and serologic testing for *Mycoplasma* can be performed, although these tests will have no impact on the emergency management of the patient. Results of bedside cold agglutinin tests may be positive in cases of *Mycoplasma* but are nonspecific.

Emergency Department Care and Disposition

The emergency department treatment and disposition of pneumonia depend primarily on the severity of the clinical presentation and radiographic findings. Sputum Gram stain results are also useful.

1. Oxygen should be administered as needed, and antibiotic treatment should be initiated.
2. Outpatient management is standard in otherwise healthy patients who are nontoxic and without significant comorbid diseases. Antibiotic choices include **azithromycin** 500 mg on day 1 followed by 250 mg daily for 4 additional days, **clarithromycin** 500 mg twice daily for 10 days, **cefpodoxime** 200 mg twice daily for 10 days, or **amoxicillin/clavulanate** 875 mg orally (PO) twice daily for 10 days. **Doxycycline** 100 mg twice daily for 10 days is a low-cost alternative.
3. Oral fluoroquinolones, such as **levofloxacin** 500 mg daily, **moxifloxacin** 400 mg daily, or **gatifloxacin** 400 mg daily for 10 to 14 days, are highly effective; however, because their overuse may promote fluoroquinolone-resistant pneumonia, the Centers for Disease Control and Prevention (CDC) recommends reserving these agents for those who cannot tolerate or have failed other agents.
4. For outpatient management of patients older than 60 years or those with comorbid diseases, **levofloxacin** is a good choice as a single agent. Otherwise, **azithromycin** or **clarithromycin** in combination with **cefuroxime** 500 mg PO daily for 10 days or **amoxicillin/clavulanate** 875 mg PO twice a day for 10 days are excellent dual-drug regimens.
5. Close follow-up is necessary to monitor response to therapy.
6. Hospital admission should be reserved for patients at the extremes of life, patients with immunocompromise, pregnant women, and those with clinical signs of toxicity (ie, respiratory rate faster than 30 breaths/min, heart rate faster than 125 beats/min, systolic blood pressure below 90 mm Hg, hypoxemia, altered mental status, or volume depletion) or serious comorbid conditions (eg, neoplastic disease, renal failure, diabetes, cardiac disease, or debilitated state).
7. Patients requiring admission generally also receive empiric antibiotic therapy. Early antibiotic administration in the emergency department may shorten the patient's hospital stay. Recommended treatments include **ceftriaxone** 1 to 2 g intravenously (IV) daily, **levofloxacin** 500 mg IV

daily, **cefotaxime** 1 to 2 g IV every 8 hours, **ampicillin/sulbactam** 3 g IV every 6 hours, **piperacillin/tazobactam** 3.375 g every 6 hours, or **cefepime** 1 to 2 g every 12 hours.

8. Patients at high risk for gram-negative pneumonia or *Legionella* (eg, alcoholics, diabetics, and institutionalized or intubated patients) should be treated with **levofloxacin** as monotherapy or with a combination of a macrolide such as **erythromycin** 1 g IV every 6 hours and **ampicillin/ sulbactam** 3 g IV every 6 hours or **ceftriaxone** 1 to 2 g IV daily.

9. If *Pseudomonas* is suspected, double coverage with an antipseudomonal penicillin (eg, ticarcillin) or cephalosporin (eg, ceftazidime) plus an antipseudomonal aminoglycoside (eg, tobramycin) or a fluoroquinolone (eg, ciprofloxacin) is recommended.

10. Local antibiotic sensitivities and resistance patterns in addition to local standards of care should help determine final antibiotic selection.

11. Aspiration pneumonitides require a different therapeutic approach. Witnessed aspirations should be treated with immediate tracheal suctioning, and the pH of the aspirate should be ascertained. Bronchoscopy is indicated for the removal of large particles and for further clearing of the airways. Patients requiring intubation also should be treated with positive end-expiratory pressure. Oxygen should be administered, but steroids and prophylactic antibiotics are of no value and should be withheld. For patients at risk of aspiration who present with signs and symptoms of infection, antibiotics are indicated. **Levofloxacin** 500 mg/d IV or PO or **ceftriaxone** 1 to 2 g/d IV or intramuscularly are sufficient for most cases of aspiration. In cases of severe periodontal disease, putrid sputum, or alcoholism, **piperacillin/tazobactam** 3.375 g every 6 hours, **imipenem** 500 mg every 8 hours, or a fluoroquinolone plus **clindamycin** 600 mg every 8 hours can be considered.

12. Failure of outpatient therapy generally requires hospital admission and broader-spectrum IV antibiotics. Patients with hypoxemia despite oxygen therapy or those with impending respiratory failure should be treated with endotracheal intubation and mechanical ventilation.

SEVERE ACUTE RESPIRATORY SYNDROME

Severe acute respiratory syndrome (SARS) came to worldwide attention in the winter of 2003. Numerous deaths were reported in Asia, North America, and Europe. The etiologic agent is a coronavirus, SARS-CoV. Up-to-date information regarding SARS can be found at the CDC Web site (http://www.cdc.gov/ncidod/sars/) or by telephone (770-488-7100).

Clinical Features

SARS should be considered in symptomatic individuals who have traveled to an area with current or previously documented or suspected community transmission of SARS. Currently those areas are China (mainland), Hong Kong, Hanoi, Singapore, Toronto, Taiwan, and Beijing. SARS also should be considered in symptomatic individuals with close contact within 10 days of symptom onset with a person known or suspected to have SARS. Moderate disease is defined as temperature higher than 100.4°F (38°C) and 1 or more findings of cough, shortness of breath, difficulty breathing, or hypoxia. Severe respiratory illness plus radiographic evidence of pneumonia, respiratory distress syndrome, or findings at autopsy are considered criteria for moderate disease.

Diagnosis or Differential

Initial diagnostic testing for suspected SARS patients should include chest radiograph, pulse oximetry, blood cultures, sputum Gram stain and culture, and testing for viral respiratory pathogens, notably influenzae A and B and respiratory syncytial virus. Any patient who meets exposure and clinical criteria for SARS should be reported to local health agencies and have confirmatory testing. At this time, the recommendation is for the testing of nasopharyngeal, oropharyngeal, and serum samples. Local health agencies and the CDC can provide additional information concerning testing and isolation procedures.

Emergency Department Care and Disposition

1. No specific treatment recommendations can be made at this time.
2. Clinicians evaluating suspected cases should use standard precautions (eg, hand hygiene) in addition to airborne (eg, N-95 respirator) and contact (eg, gowns and gloves) precautions. Eye protection also should be considered.
3. Empiric therapy should include coverage for organisms associated with any community-acquired pneumonia of unclear etiology, including agents with activity against typical and atypical respiratory pathogens. Treatment choices may be influenced by severity of the illness. See section above.
4. Infectious disease consultation is recommended.

For further reading in *Emergency Medicine: A Comprehensive Study Guide,* 6th ed., see Chap. 63, "Bronchitis, Pneumonia, and Pleural Empyema" by Donald A. Moffa Jr and Charles L Emerman; and Chap. 64, "Aspiration Pneumonia and Lung Abscess," by Eric Anderson.

32 | Tuberculosis

Amy J. Behrman

The incidence of tuberculosis (TB) rose sharply in the United States between 1984 and 1992, driven by factors including rising rates of incarceration, human immunodeficiency virus (HIV) infection, drug-resistant TB strains, and immigration from areas with endemic TB. Stronger TB control programs targeting high-risk groups have reversed this trend since 1993. However, TB remains an important public health problem, particularly among foreign-born persons. Patients with undiagnosed TB frequently present to the emergency department (ED) for evaluation and care.

CLINICAL FEATURES

Primary TB

Primary TB infection is usually asymptomatic, presenting most frequently with only a new positive reaction to TB skin testing. Some patients may, however, present with active pneumonitis or extra-pulmonary disease. Immunocompromised patients are much more likely to develop rapidly progressive primary infections.

Reactivation TB

Latent tuberculosis infections are asymptomatic with positive tuberculin skin tests. Latent tuberculosis infections will progress to active disease in 5% of cases within 2 years of primary infection; an additional 5% will reactivate over their lifetimes. Reactivation rates are higher in the young, the elderly, persons with recent primary infection, those with immune deficiency (in particular HIV), and those with chronic diseases such as diabetes and renal failure. Most patients present subacutely with fever, cough, weight loss, fatigue, and night sweats.

Most patients with active TB have pulmonary involvement characterized by constitutional symptoms and (usually productive) cough. Hemoptysis, pleuritic chest pain, and dyspnea may develop. Rales and rhonchi may be found, but the pulmonary examination is usually nondiagnostic.

Extra-pulmonary TB develops in up to 15% of cases. Lymphadenitis, with painless enlargement and possible draining sinuses, is the most common presentation. Symptomatic pleural effusion, pericarditis, peritonitis, or meningitis may be the presentation of TB. The course is often more acute in children.

Miliary TB is a multisystem disease caused by massive hematogenous dissemination. It is most common in immunocompromised hosts and children. Symptoms and findings may include fever, cough, weight loss, adenopathy, hepatosplenomegaly, and cytopenias. Extrapulmonary TB also may involve bone, joints, skin, kidneys, and adrenals.

HIV and TB

Immunocompromised patients and HIV patients in particular are extremely susceptible to TB and far more likely to develop active infections with atypical presentations. TB should be considered in any HIV patient with respiratory symptoms, even if chest radiographs (CXRs) are normal. Disseminated extra-pulmonary TB is also more common in HIV patients and should be considered in the evaluation of nonpulmonary complaints.

Multidrug-Resistant TB

Multidrug-resistant TB (MDR-TB) peaked during the recent resurgence of TB in this country, particularly among HIV patients. It remains a large problem among foreign-born persons who accounted for 72% of MDR-TB cases in 2000. It should be considered whenever TB is diagnosed, especially among those with suboptimal prior care such as immigrants from endemic areas, prisoners, homeless persons, and drug users. MDR-TB is still more common in HIV patients than in the general population and has a high fatality rate in this group.

DIAGNOSIS AND DIFFERENTIAL

Consider the diagnosis of TB in any patient with respiratory or systemic complaints to facilitate early diagnosis, protect hospital staff, and make appropriate dispositions.

CXRs are the most useful diagnostic tool for active TB in the ED. Active primary TB usually presents with parenchymal infiltrates in any lung area. Hilar and/or mediastinal adenopathy may occur with or without infiltrates. Lesions may calcify. Reactivation TB typically presents with lesions in the upper lobes or superior segments of the lower lobes. Cavitation, calcification, scarring, atelectasis, and effusions may be seen. Cavitation is associated with increased infectivity. Miliary TB may cause diffuse, small (1–3 mm) nodular infiltrates. Patients co-infected with HIV and TB are particularly likely to present with atypical CXRs.

Acid fast staining of sputum can detect mycobacteria in 60% of patients with pulmonary TB, although the yield is less in HIV patients. Atypical mycobacteria can yield false positives. Many patients will have false negatives on a single sputum sample. Microscopy of non-sputum samples (eg. pleural fluid and cerebrospinal fluid) is even less sensitive. Definitive cultures generally take weeks, but new genetic tests using DNA probes or polymerase chain reaction technology can confirm the diagnosis in hours.

Mantoux testing (intradermal tuberculin skin testing with purified protein derivative [PPD]) identifies most patients with *latent, prior,* or *active* TB infection. Results are read 48 to 72 hours after placement, thus limiting the usefulness of this test for ED patients. Patients with HIV or other immunosuppressive conditions and patients with disseminated TB may have false negative skin tests even if not fully anergic.

EMERGENCY DEPARTMENT CARE AND DISPOSITION

1. Initial therapy should include at least 4 drugs until susceptibility profiles are available for a patient. Beginning therapy usually includes isoniazid (INH), rifampin, pyrazinamide, and streptomycin or ethambutol for 2 months. At least 2 drugs (usually INH and rifampin) are continued for 4 more months. Patients with immune compromise or MDR-TB may require more drugs for longer periods. Table 32-1 summarizes usual initial daily drug doses and side effects. Medications can be tailored to culture and sensitivity results when known.
2. Admission is indicated for clinical instability, diagnostic uncertainty, unreliable outpatient follow-up or compliance, and active known MDR-TB.

TABLE 32-1 Dosages and Common Side Effects of Some Drugs Used in Tuberculosis

Drug/route	Daily dose (maximum)	Potential side effects
Isoniazid/PO	Adult: 5 mg/kg (300 mg) Child: 10–20 mg/kg (300 mg)	Hepatitis, neuritis, abdominal pain, acidosis, drug interactions
Rifampin/PO	Adult: 10 mg/kg (600 mg) Child: 10–20 mg/kg (600 mg)	Hepatitis, thrombocytopenia, GI disturbance, fever, drug interactions
Pyrazinamide/PO	Adult: 15–30 mg/kg (2 g) Child: same	Hepatitis, rash, arthralgia, GI disturbance, hyperuricemia
Ethambutol/PO	Adult: 15–25 mg/kg (2.5 g) Child: same	Optic neuritis, headache, peripheral neuropathy, GI disturbance
Ciprofloxacin/PO	Adult: 750 mg bid Child: contraindicated	Arthropathy, GI disturbance, CNS disturbance
Streptomycin/IM	Adult: 15 mg/kg (1 g) Child: 20–30 mg/kg (1 g)	Eighth cranial neuropathy, rash, renal failure proteinuria

Key: bid = twice daily, CNS = central nervous system, GI = gastrointestinal, IM = intramuscularly, PO = orally.

186

Physicians should know local laws regarding involuntary hospitalization and treatment. Admission to respiratory or "droplet" isolation is mandatory for all cases of suspected TB.

3. Patients with active TB who are discharged from the ED must have documented immediate referral to a physician or the local public health department for long-term treatment. Patients should be educated about home isolation, follow-up, and screening of household contacts. Daily and intermittent regimens are available. Some patients require directly observed therapy to ensure compliance. Persons with positive PPDs and no active TB disease should be evaluated for prophylactic treatment with INH to prevent reactivation TB.

4. The ED staff should be trained to identify patients at risk for active TB as soon as possible in their ED and prehospital course. Patients with suspected TB should be masked or placed in respiratory isolation rooms in the ED. They should be transported while wearing masks and admitted to respiratory isolation areas. Staff caring directly for patients with suspected TB should wear protection approved by the Occupational Safety and Health Administration, usually N-95 respirators. Engineering controls in the ED can minimize transmission from undiagnosed cases. The ED staff should receive regular PPD skin testing to detect new primary infections, rule out active disease, and consider INH prophylaxis.

For further reading in *Emergency Medicine: A Comprehensive Study Guide,* 6th ed., see Chap. 65, "Tuberculosis," by Janet M. Poponick.

33 | Pneumothorax

Rodney L. McCaskill

Pneumothorax occurs when air enters the potential space between the parietal and visceral pleura, leading to partial lung collapse. Primary pneumothorax occurs most frequently in male smokers, with a large height-to-weight ratio, and seems to result from bleb rupture. Secondary pneumothorax occurs most often in patients with chronic obstructive pulmonary disease, but other underlying diseases such as asthma, cystic fibrosis, interstitial lung disease, cancer, and *Pneumocystis carinii* pneumonia have been implicated. Iatrogenic pneumothorax occurs secondary to invasive procedures such as needle biopsy of the lung, placement of a subclavian line, nasogastric tube placement, or positive pressure ventilation. Tension pneumothorax results from positive pressure in the pleural space leading to decreased venous return, hypotension, and hypoxia.

CLINICAL FEATURES

Symptoms resulting from a pneumothorax are directly related to its size, rate of development, and the health of the underlying lung. Acute onset of pleuritic pain is found in 95% of patients, whereas dyspnea occurs in 80% and predicts a larger pneumothorax. Decreased breath sounds on the affected side are present 85% of the time. Only 5% have tachypnea with rates faster than 24 breaths/min or tachycardia with rates faster than 120 breaths/min.

DIAGNOSIS AND DIFFERENTIAL

The diagnosis of tension pneumothorax is based on clinical features, including hypoxia, hypotension, distended neck veins, displaced trachea, and unilaterally decreased breath sounds, and should be treated immediately. In stable patients, an upright posteroanterior chest x-ray is the "gold standard," but it is only 83% sensitive. Expiratory films may slightly improve visualization. Chest computed tomography likely is more sensitive. Recent studies have shown ultrasound to be almost 100% sensitive in diagnosing pneumothorax. Differential diagnosis of suspected pneumothorax includes costochondritis, myocardial infarction or ischemia, pulmonary embolus, pericarditis, pleurisy, and pneumonia.

EMERGENCY DEPARTMENT CARE AND DISPOSITION

1. In patients with unstable vitals signs and clinical features suggestive of tension pneumothorax, immediate needle thoracostomy followed by tube thoracostomy is indicated. X-rays should not be obtained before treatment.
2. In stable patients, oxygen 2 to 4 L/min by nasal canula helps increase resorption of intrapleural air.
3. Patients with small primary pneumothoraces may be observed for 6 hours and discharged with surgical follow-up if there is no enlargement on repeat x-ray; however, 23% to 40% eventually require tube thoracostomy.
4. A catheter may be used to aspirate a small pneumothorax, and the patient can be discharged with surgical follow-up at 6 hours if there is no recurrence.

5. Tube thoracostomy and admission is indicated for failed aspiration, recurrent pneumothorax, severe underlying pulmonary disease, and in patients with abnormal vital signs. Tube thoracostomy also should be considered in patients undergoing general anesthesia, mechanical ventilation, or helicopter transport.

For further reading in *Emergency Medicine: A Comprehensive Study Guide,* 6th ed., see Chap. 66, "Spontaneous and Iatrogenic Pneumothorax," by William Franklin Young, Jr. and Roger Loyd Humphries.

34 | Hemoptysis

James E. Winslow

Hemoptysis is the expectoration of blood from the bronchopulmonary tree. Massive hemoptysis is an emergency and is defined as greater than 600 mL per 24 hours and requires prompt intervention to prevent asphyxiation from impaired gas exchange. Minor hemoptysis is the production of smaller quantities of blood, often mixed with mucus, and also requires careful emergency department management.

CLINICAL FEATURES

Hemoptysis may be the presenting symptom for many different diseases. A careful history should be conducted to evaluate for any underlying lung disease or history of tobacco use. The acute onset of fever, cough, and bloody sputum may indicate pneumonia or bronchitis. An indolent productive cough can indicate bronchitis or bronchiectasis. Dyspnea and pleuritic chest pain are often markers of pulmonary embolism. Tuberculosis should be considered if there is a history of fever or night sweats. Bronchogenic carcinoma may present with chronic weight loss and a change in cough. Chronic dyspnea and minor hemoptysis may indicate mitral stenosis or alveolar hemorrhage syndromes. Alveolar hemorrhage syndromes are often associated with renal disease.

The physical examination is aimed at assessing the severity of hemoptysis and the underlying disease process but is usually not helpful in localizing the site of bleeding. Common signs include fever and tachypnea. Tachypnea may be a sign of respiratory compromise with hypoxemia. Hypotension is an ominous sign because it is common only in massive hemoptysis. The cardiac examination may show valvular heart disease (ie, diastolic murmur of mitral stenosis). Auscultation of the lungs may show inspiratory crackles due to blood in the alveoli or expiratory crackles from secretions or blood in the airways. The nasal and oral cavities should be inspected carefully to help rule out an extra pulmonary source of bleeding (pseudohemoptysis).

DIAGNOSIS AND DIFFERENTIAL

A careful history and physical examination may suggest a diagnosis. Pulse oximetry and a chest x-ray are often the most helpful tests. Posteroanterior and lateral chest radiographs should be obtained unless the patient is unstable. The clinical picture determines whether other tests may be helpful. Some of these supplemental tests may include arterial blood gas, hemoglobin and hematocrit levels, platelet count, coagulation studies, urinalysis, and electrocardiogram. Chest computed tomography should be considered if there is hemoptysis with an abnormal chest radiograph. The differential diagnosis includes infectious, neoplastic, and cardiac etiologies. Infectious etiologies include bronchitis, bronchiectasis, bacterial pneumonia, tuberculosis, fungal pneumonia, and lung abscess. Neoplastic etiologies include bronchogenic carcinoma and bronchial adenoma. Cardiogenic etiologies include mitral stenosis and left ventricular failure. Trauma, foreign body aspiration, pulmonary embolism, primary pulmonary hypertension, pulmonary vasculitis, and bleeding diathesis are other potential causes. There is no definitive diagnosis in 28% of cases.

EMERGENCY DEPARTMENT CARE AND DISPOSITION

1. Supplemental oxygen should be given to maintain adequate oxygenation.
2. Normal saline or lactated Ringer solution should be administered initially for hypotension.
3. Blood should be typed and cross-matched if transfusion might be necessary. Packed red blood cells should be transfused as needed.
4. Fresh frozen plasma (2 U) should be administered to patients with coagulopathies; platelets should be given for thrombocytopenia (see Chap. 138).
5. Patients with continuing massive hemoptysis should be placed in the decubitus position with the bleeding lung down.
6. **Codeine** (15–30 mg) or other opioids may be helpful in cough suppression.
7. Endotracheal intubation with a large diameter (8.0 mm) tube should be done if there is respiratory failure or if the patient cannot clear blood or secretions from the airway. A larger tube will allow for better suctioning and permit bronchoscopy.
8. Any patient with moderate to severe hemoptysis requires admission to the hospital, and strong consideration should be given to placement in the intensive care unit. Patients with mild hemoptysis who have conditions that predispose them to severe bleeding also should be considered for admission to an intensive care unit. The input of a pulmonologist or thoracic surgeon is required for decisions as to whether bronchoscopy, computed tomography, or angiography for bronchial artery embolization might be needed. If the appropriate specialists are not available, the patient should be stabilized and then transferred to the appropriate facility.
9. Patients who are discharged home should be treated for several days with cough suppressants (ie, **codeine** 15–30 mg every 4 to 6 hours), inhaled β-agonist bronchodilators as needed, and antibiotics if bacterial infection is thought to be the cause. Close follow-up is essential.

For further reading in *Emergency Medicine: A Comprehensive Study Guide,* 6th ed., see Chap. 67, "Hemoptysis," by William Franklin Young Jr and Michael W. Stava.

35 | Asthma and Chronic Obstructive Pulmonary Disease

Monika Ahluwalia

Asthma and chronic obstructive pulmonary disease (COPD) are worldwide respiratory health problems. Although most asthmatic attacks are mild and reversible, severe attacks can be fatal. COPD is the sixth leading cause of death in the world and has been increasing in prevalence over the past 2 decades.

CLINICAL FEATURES

Asthma is reversible airway obstruction associated with hyperresponsiveness of the tracheobronchial tree. There are 2 dominant clinical forms of COPD: (*a*) pulmonary emphysema, characterized by abnormal, permanent enlargement and destruction of the air spaces distal to the terminal bronchioles; and (*b*) chronic bronchitis, a condition of excess mucous secretion in the bronchial tree, with a chronic productive cough occurring on most days for at least 3 months in the year for at least 2 consecutive years. Elements of both forms are often present, although 1 predominates.

Acute exacerbations of asthma and COPD are usually triggered by smoking, exposure to noxious stimuli (eg, pollutants, cold, stress, antigens, or exercise), adverse response to medications (eg, antihistamines, decongestants, β-blockers, nonsteroidal anti-inflammatory drugs, sulfating agents, food additives and preservatives, hypnotics, and tranquilizers), allergic reactions, and noncompliance with prescribed therapies. Respiratory infection, pneumothorax, myocardial infarction, dysrhythmias, pulmonary edema, chest trauma, metabolic disorders, and abdominal processes are triggers and complications of asthma and COPD.

Classically, patients with exacerbations of asthma or COPD present complaints of dyspnea, chest tightness, wheezing, and cough. Physical examination shows wheezing with prolonged expiration. Wheezing does not correlate with degree of airflow obstruction. A "quiet chest" may indicate severe airflow restriction. Patients with severe attacks may demonstrate sitting up and forward posturing, pursed-lip exhalation, accessory muscle use, paradoxical respirations, and diaphoresis. Pulsus paradoxus of 20 mm Hg or higher may be noted. Severe airflow obstruction and ventilation perfusion imbalance can cause hypoxia and hypercapnia. Hypoxia is characterized by tachypnea, cyanosis, agitation, apprehension, tachycardia, and hypertension. Signs of hypercapnia include confusion, tremor, plethora, stupor, hypopnea, and apnea. Alteration in mental status, lethargy, quiet chest, acidosis, worsening hypoxia, and hypercapnia are indicative of impending respiratory failure.

DIAGNOSIS AND DIFFERENTIAL

Emergency department diagnosis of asthma or COPD usually is made clinically. The clinician should attempt to determine the severity of the attack, the cause for the decompensation, and the presence of complications. Objective measurements of airflow obstruction, such as sequential peak expiratory flow rate, have been shown to be more accurate than clinical judgment in determining the severity of the attack and the response to therapy. Chest x-ray is used to diagnose complications such as pneumonia and pneumothorax. Pulse oximetry is a fast, easy, and noninvasive means for assessing and monitoring oxygen saturation during treatment, but it does not aid in predicting clinical outcomes. Although pulse oximetry can provide information regarding hypoxia, it cannot predict acid-base disturbances or hypercapnia. Arterial blood gas (ABG) serves primarily to evaluate hypercapnia and acidosis in moderate to severe attacks. Compensated hypercapnia and hypoxia is common in COPD patients; therefore, comparison with previous ABG values is helpful. Normal P_{CO_2} in the setting of an acute asthmatic attack is an ominous finding if the patient is doing poorly. An arterial pH below that consistent with renal compensation implies acute hypercarbia or metabolic acidosis. Electrocardiograms are useful to identify dysrhythmias or suspected ischemic injury.

The differential diagnosis of decompensated asthma and COPD includes congestive heart failure ("cardiac asthma"), interstitial lung diseases, pulmonary embolism, pulmonary neoplasia, aspirated foreign bodies, pleural effusions, and exposure to asphyxiants.

EMERGENCY DEPARTMENT CARE AND DISPOSITION

Although patients with COPD often have more underlying illnesses than do asthmatics, the therapy for acute bronchospasm and that for inflammation are similar. Treatment should precede history taking in acutely dyspneic patients because patients may decompensate rapidly. These patients should be placed on a cardiac monitor and a noninvasive blood pressure device and have continuous pulse oximetry. An intravenous line should be started in patients with moderate and severe attacks. The primary goal of therapy is to correct tissue oxygenation.

1. Empiric supplemental oxygen should be administered. The need for supplemental oxygen in the setting of COPD must be balanced against progressive hypercarbia and suppression of hypoxic ventilatory drive. Arterial saturation should be corrected to above 90%.
2. β-Adrenergic agonists are first-line agents used to treat acute bronchospasm in COPD and asthma. Aerosolized or parenteral forms should be used in critical settings. Aerosol therapy minimizes systemic toxicity and is preferred. **Albuterol sulfate** 1.25 to 5 mg and metaproterenol 10 to 15 mg are the most β_2-specific agents. Delivering doses in rapid succession or continuously maximizes results. Frequency of dosing depends on clinical response and signs of drug toxicity. Metered dose inhalers with spacer devices may be reasonable to use in less ill patients. Subcutaneous **terbutaline sulfate** (0.25-0.5 mL) or **epinephrine** 1:1,000 (0.1-0.3 mL) also may be administered. Epinephrine should be avoided in the first trimester of pregnancy and possibly in patients with underlying cardiovascular disease. β-Adrenergic agonists may inhibit uterine contractions when used near term.
3. Steroids should be given immediately to patients with severe attacks and to patients who are currently taking, or have recently taken, these drugs. Although their use is well established in asthma and severe COPD, there is a lack of supporting evidence for the use of steroids in the treatment of chronic compensated or mild to moderate exacerbations of COPD. The optimal daily dose is the equivalent of 60 to 180 mg/d of **prednisone,**

with an initial dose being the equivalent of 40 to 80 mg of prednisone. The choice of steroid is not critical. If the patient is unable to take oral medication, intravenous **methylprednisolone** 60 to 125 mg may be used. Additional doses may be given every 4 to 6 hours. Inhaled steroids are extremely useful in the treatment of chronic asthma and COPD but should not be used for the treatment of acute symptoms. A 3- to 10-day course of oral steroids (**prednisone** 40-60 mg/d) is beneficial for discharged patients who have previously been on steroids, are high-risk patients, or were placed on steroids during their emergency department care.

4. Anticholinergics are useful adjuvants when given with other therapies. Nebulized **ipratropium** (500 mg = 2.5 mL) may be administered alone or mixed with albuterol. The effects of ipratropium peak in 1 to 2 hours and last 3 to 4 hours. Dosages may be repeated every 1 to 4 hours. When used with β-agonist agents, effects may be additive.

5. Broad-spectrum antibiotics (trimethoprim-sulfamethoxazole DS, doxycycline, macrolides, cephalosporins, and newer fluoroquinolones) are indicated for treatment of bacterial respiratory infections. Preventive polyvalent pneumococcal and trivalent influenza vaccination may be administered to stable COPD patients.

6. Intravenous **magnesium sulfate** (1-2 g over 30 minutes) is used in the management of severe asthma exacerbation due to its bronchodilating properties. However, it is not currently recommended for mild to moderate asthma exacerbations and should not be substituted for standard regimens.

7. Several studies have demonstrated that an 80%:20% mixture of helium and oxygen (Heliox) can lower airway resistance and aid in drug delivery in the patient with very severe asthma exacerbation. Care must be taken with use of this therapy in the oxygen-dependent patient.

8. **Ketamine** 1 to 2 mg/kg intravenously as the initial dose has been used successfully in cases of refractory asthma. The bronchodilatory properties of ketamine make it a good choice, especially in combination with a low-dose benzodiazepine for sedation of mechanically ventilated patients with bronchospasm.

9. In selected cooperative patients, noninvasive, positive pressure ventilation (intermittent, continuous or biphasic) may avert artificial ventilation.

10. Assisted mechanical ventilation is indicated for inability to maintain O_2 saturation above 90% or severe hypercarbia associated with stupor, altered mental status, exhaustion, narcosis, or acidosis. Oral intubation is preferred because larger endotracheal tubes can be used. Larger tubes facilitate suctioning, fiberoptic bronchoscopy, and ventilator weaning. Initially, high inspired oxygen concentrations may be used. A volume-cycled ventilator should always be used. Excessive tidal volumes ($\geq$15 mL/kg ideal body weight) and air trapping (due to bronchospasm) can cause barotrauma and hypotension. Using rapid inspiratory flow rates at a reduced respiratory frequency (12-14 breaths/min) allows for adequate expiration. The goal of this approach, referred to as *controlled mechanical hypoventilation,* is to maintain adequate oxygenation with little regard for hypercarbia. Therapy should be guided by pulse oximetry and ABG results. Sedation and continued therapy for bronchospasm should continue after the patient has been placed on artificial ventilation.

11. Criteria for admission of patients with asthma include failure of outpatient treatment, persistent and worsening dyspnea, forced expiratory vol-

ume in 1 second or peak expiratory flow rate of less than 50% of predicted, comorbid diseases, hypoxia, hypercarbia, and altered mental
status. Patients with acute exacerbations of COPD are more likely to require admission. Indications for admission are severe dyspnea, failure of
therapy, significant comorbid diseases, arrhythmias, older age, insufficient home support, worsening hypoxia and hypercapnia with acidosis,
and impaired mental status.

In the absence of intubation, sedatives, hypnotics, and other medications that
depress respiratory drive are generally contraindicated. The role of methyl-
xanthines in the treatment of acute asthma and COPD has been seriously
challenged. β-Blockers may exacerbate bronchospasm. Antihistamines and
decongestants also should be avoided because they diminish the ability to
clear respiratory secretions. Mucolytics may provoke further bronchospasm.
Mast cell and leukotriene modifiers have no role in the treatment of acute exacerbations of asthma or COPD. Many asthmatics respond poorly to ultra-
sonic nebulization and intermittent positive pressure breathing.

Close follow-up care must be arranged for discharged patients to ensure
resolution of the exacerbation and review the management plan. Despite appropriate therapy, these patients have high relapse rates. Education of the
asthma and COPD patients before discharge (ie, review of medications, inhaler techniques, use of peak flow measurements, avoidance of noxious stimuli, and need to follow-up) should be an integral part of emergency department care.

For further reading in *Emergency Medicine: A Comprehensive Study Guide,* 6th ed., see
   Chap. 68, "Acute Asthma in Adults," by Rita K. Cydulka; and Chap. 69, "Chronic
   Obstructive Pulmonary Disease," by Rita K. Cydulka and Mohak Dave.

7 | GASTROINTESTINAL EMERGENCIES

36 | Acute Abdominal Pain

Peggy E. Goodman

Acute abdominal pain or nontraumatic abdominal pain in postpubescent patients shorter than 1 week's duration is one of the most common and most challenging complaints to evaluate in the emergency department. It may be due to numerous etiologies including gastrointestinal, genitourinary, cardiovascular, pulmonary, and other sources.

There are 3 categories of pain: poorly localized, visceral pain due to stimulation of autonomic nerve fibers; parietal pain caused by local irritation of peritoneal nerve fibers; and referred pain, which occurs at a location distant from the affected organ. Pain is then classified according to intraabdominal or extraabdominal sources. Intraabdominal sources of pain include peritonitis due to disease or injury of the abdominal or pelvic viscera; obstruction of the intestine, ureter, or biliary tree; gynecologic disorders; and vascular disorders, such as bowel infarction and aortic dissection, leakage, or rupture. Other sources of pain perceived as abdominal can be extraabdominal, metabolic, or neurogenic. Extraabdominal sources of pain include abdominal wall, thoracic, and pelvic pain. Abdominal wall pain is usually traumatic in origin. Vague abdominal distress, nausea, vomiting, and diaphoresis may accompany intrathoracic disease, including pneumonia, pulmonary embolism, pneumothorax, esophageal disease, and acute myocardial ischemia. Pelvic sources of pain, such as salpingitis, tubo-ovarian abscess, ovarian cyst torsion or rupture, abortion, and ectopic pregnancy also need to be considered in the differential diagnosis. Metabolic disorders, including diabetic ketoacidosis, sickle cell crisis, porphyria, spider and scorpion bites, heavy metal intoxication, autoimmune disease, and neurogenic disorders, such as preeruptive herpes zoster and spinal disk disease, may be interpreted as abdominal pain. The most common causes of abdominal pain are listed in Table 36-1.

CLINICAL FEATURES

When evaluating a patient with abdominal pain, it is important to consider immediate life threats that might require emergency intervention. Important aspects of the patient's history include time of onset of pain; character, severity, location of pain and its referral; aggravating and alleviating factors; and any changes in these symptoms. Cardiorespiratory symptoms, such as chest pain, dyspnea, and cough; genitourinary symptoms, such as urgency, dysuria, and vaginal discharge; and any history of trauma should be elicited. In older patients it is also important to obtain a history of myocardial infarction, other ischemic states, dysrhythmias, coagulopathies, and vasculopathies. Past medical and surgical histories should be elicited, and a list of medications, particularly steroids, antibiotics, or nonsteroidal anti-inflammatory drugs (NSAIDs), should be noted. A thorough gynecologic history is indicated in female patients.

The physical examination should include the patient's general appearance. Patients with visceral pain tend to move about, whereas patients with peritonitis tend to lie still. The skin should be evaluated for pallor or jaundice. The vital signs should be inspected for signs of hypovolemia due to blood loss or dehydration. Due to medications or the physiology of aging, tachycardia may

199

TABLE 36-1 Most Common Causes of Acute Abdominal Pain

Final Diagnosis	Proportion of >10,000 Patients	
Nonspecific abdominal pain (NSAP)	34%	
Appendicitis	28%	
Biliary tract disease	10%	
Small bowel obstruction	4%	
Acute gynecologic disease	4%	
	Salpingitis	68%
	Ovarian cyst	21%
	Ectopic	6%
	Incomplete abortion	5%
Pancreatitis	3%	
Renal colic	3%	
Perforated peptic ulcer	3%	
Cancer	2%	
Diverticular disease	2%	
Other (<1% each)	6%	

not always occur in the face of hypovolemia. A core temperature should be obtained; however, absence of fever does not rule out infection, particularly in the elderly.

The abdomen should be inspected for contour, scars, peristalsis, masses, distention, and pulsation. Contrary to conventional teaching, absent or diminished bowel sounds provide little clinically useful information. The presence of hyperactive or high-pitched or tinkling bowel sounds are somewhat more helpful, thereby increasing the likelihood of small bowel obstruction.

Palpation is the most important aspect of the physical examination. The abdomen and genitals should be assessed for tenderness, guarding, masses, organomegaly, and hernias. "Rebound" tenderness, often regarded as the clinical criterion standard of peritonitis, has several important limitations. In patients with peritonitis, the combination of rigidity, referred tenderness, and, especially, "cough pain" usually provides sufficient diagnostic confirmation; false positive rebound tenderness occurs in about 1 patient in 4 without peritonitis. This has led some investigators to conclude that rebound tenderness, in contrast to cough pain, is of "no predictive value."

A useful and underused test to diagnose abdominal wall pain is the sit-up test, also known as the *Carnett sign*. After identification of the site of maximum abdominal tenderness, the patient is asked to fold his or her arms across the chest and sit up halfway. The examiner maintains a finger on the tender area, and if palpation in the semisitting position produces the same or increased tenderness, the test is said to be positive for an abdominal wall syndrome.

Retroperitoneal disorders may exhibit no "classic" abnormalities on examination. A pelvic examination is recommended in all postpubertal females. During the rectal examination, the lower pelvis should be assessed for tenderness, bleeding, and masses.

Elderly patients with abdominal pain present significant challenges in diagnosis and management. Causes of abdominal pain stratified by age are listed in Table 36-2. It can be difficult to obtain an accurate history from the

TABLE 36-2 Causes of Acute Abdominal Pain Stratified by Age

Final Diagnosis	≥50 Years (N = 2406)	<50 Years (N = 6317)
Biliary tract disease	21%	6%
Nonspecific abdominal pain (NSAP)	16%	40%
Appendicitis	15%	32%
Bowel obstruction	12%	2%
Pancreatitis	7%	2%
Diverticular disease	6%	<.1%
Cancer	4%	<.1%
Hernia	3%	<.1%
Vascular	2%	<.1%
Gynecologic	<.1%	4%
Other	13%	13%

patient or from caregivers, and there may be delays in presentation. Elderly patients often fail to manifest the same signs and symptoms as younger patients, with decreased pain perception and decreased febrile or muscular response to infection or inflammation. Hypotension from volume contraction, hemorrhage, or sepsis can be missed if a normally hypertensive patient appears normotensive. Comorbid diagnoses such as cardiovascular, pulmonary, or renal disease are more common. Older patients are generally at higher initial operative risk, so that observation is more likely if the diagnosis is unclear. As a result, emergent surgical intervention for deterioration, such as sepsis, perforation, or rupture, has much higher complication and mortality rates than in younger patients. Conditions more common in the elderly include biliary tract disease, sigmoid volvulus, diverticulitis, acute mesenteric ischemia, and abdominal aortic aneurysm. Mesenteric ischemia should be considered in any patient older than 50 years with abdominal pain out of proportion to physical findings; it can be due to arterial or venous occlusion and has a very high morbidity due to short warm ischemia time in the bowel, delays in diagnosis, and patient comorbidities. Angiography is the diagnostic test of choice, and aggressive surgical intervention may be lifesaving.

DIAGNOSIS AND DIFFERENTIAL

Laboratory evaluation is supplementary to a careful history and physical examination. Complete blood count values can be normal in the presence of disease; however, an elevated white blood cell count should alert the clinician, and a source should be sought more diligently. Serial hematocrits may be of value in patients with acute blood loss, although it may take several hours for a change to be evident. Urinalysis may show hematuria in cases of renal colic or pyuria in urinary tract infection or other intraabdominal inflammation near the urinary tract. A pregnancy test should be obtained in women of childbearing potential and is useful in the assessment for ectopic pregnancy. Serum amylase elevation and electrolyte abnormalities are neither specific nor sensitive diagnostic tools. Persistently normal serial serum lactate levels markedly reduce the likelihood of mesenteric ischemia, although elevated serum lactate is too nonspecific to reliably confirm a specific diagnosis. An electrocardiogram should be considered, particularly in patients older than 40 years or with upper abdominal or nonspecific symptoms.

Imaging studies used as adjuncts to diagnosis include plain abdominal radiographs (PARs), ultrasound, and computed tomography (CT). PARs provide nonspecific assessment for calculi and calcifications and for air and fluid patterns and continue to be markedly overused. Studies have suggested that restriction of the PAR to patients with suspected obstruction, perforation, ischemia, peritonitis, or renal colic would markedly reduce imaging, with no impact on management. Ultrasonography is useful for the diagnosis of cholelithiasis, choledocholithiasis, cholecystitis, biliary duct dilatation, pancreatic masses, hydroureter, intrauterine or ectopic pregnancies, ovarian and tubal pathologies, free intraperitoneal fluid, suspected appendicitis, and abdominal aortic aneurysm. They are also useful in some cases when CT is contraindicated due to dye allergy or renal insufficiency. Disadvantages include variations in the performance and interpretation of the study and can be limited by patient factors such as bowel gas and obesity. CT is the preferred imaging method for pancreatitis, biliary obstruction, aneurysm, appendicitis, and urolithiasis and is markedly superior for identifying virtually any abnormality that can be seen on plain films. Limitations include availability of equipment and interpretation of studies. Barium contrast and radioisotope studies are rarely available or useful in the emergent setting and may limit the ability to perform other, more definitive tests.

EMERGENCY DEPARTMENT CARE AND DISPOSITION

Resuscitative and stabilizing measures should be instituted as appropriate. Unstable patients should be diagnosed clinically, with immediate intervention and surgical consultation.

1. During the initial evaluation, the patient should have nothing by mouth. Consider intravenous hydration with normal saline or lactated Ringer solution.
2. The judicious use of analgesics is appropriate and may facilitate the ability to obtain a better history and more accurate physical examination from a more comfortable patient. Opiates in appropriate doses (eg, **morphine** 0.1 mg/kg intravenously) may decrease guarding and improve localization of abdominal pain; if necessary, the effects can be reversed by naloxone. NSAIDs may be of use in patients with renal colic, but their use in other conditions is controversial. NSAIDs may cause additional gastrointestinal irritation, and their anti-inflammatory effects may mask diagnostic signs and symptoms. Antiemetics, such as intravenous **metoclopramide** 10 to 20 mg, also increase the patient's comfort and facilitate assessment of the patient's signs and symptoms (see Chap. 46). When appropriate, antibiotic treatment with combined therapy or monotherapy should be initiated, depending on the suspected source of infection. See specific chapters that follow in this section for additional guidelines.
3. Surgical or obstetric and gynecologic consultation should be obtained for patients with suspected acute abdominal or pelvic pathology requiring immediate intervention, including, but not limited to, abdominal aortic aneurysm, intraabdominal hemorrhage, perforated viscus, intestinal obstruction or infarction, and ectopic pregnancy.

Despite these measures, approximately 40% of patients presenting to the emergency department for acute abdominal pain will receive no definitive diagnosis. Indications for admission (or continued observation with serial examinations) include toxic appearance, unclear diagnosis in elderly or immunocompromised patients, inability to reasonably exclude serious etiologies, intractable pain or vomiting, altered mental status, and inability to follow discharge or follow-up instructions. Many patients with nonspecific abdominal pain can be discharged safely with 24 hours of follow-up and instructions to return immediately for increased pain, vomiting, fever, or failure of symptoms to resolve.

For further reading *Emergency Medicine: A Comprehensive Study Guide,* 6th ed., see Chap. 72, "Acute Abdominal Pain," by E. John Gallagher; and Chap. 73, "Abdominal Pain in the Elderly," by Robert McNamara.

37 | Gastrointestinal Bleeding

Mitchell C. Sokolosky

Gastrointestinal (GI) bleeding is a common problem in emergency medicine and should be considered life threatening until proven otherwise. Acute upper GI bleeding is more common than lower GI bleeding. Upper GI bleeding is defined as that originating proximal to the ligament of Treitz. Peptic ulcer disease is the most common cause of upper GI bleeding, followed by erosive gastritis and esophagitis, esophageal and gastric varices, and Mallory-Weiss syndrome. The most common cause of apparent lower GI bleeding is upper GI bleeding. Hemorrhoids are the most common cause of actual lower GI bleeding, followed by diverticular disease, arteriovenous malformations, inflammatory disease, and polyps.

CLINICAL FEATURES

Most patients present complaints of hematemesis, hematochezia, or melena. Some will have more subtle presentations of hypotension, tachycardia, angina, syncope, weakness, and confusion. Hematemesis or coffee-ground emesis suggests a source proximal to the right colon. Hematochezia indicates a more distal colorectal lesion. Weight loss and changes in bowel habits are classic symptoms of malignancy. Vomiting and retching, followed by hematemesis, is suggestive of a Mallory-Weiss tear. A history of medication or alcohol use should be sought. This history may suggest peptic ulcer disease, gastritis, or esophageal varices. Spider angiomata, palmar erythema, jaundice, and gynecomastia suggest underlying liver disease. Ingestion of iron or bismuth can simulate melena, and certain foods, such as beets, can simulate hematochezia; however, stool guaiac testing will be negative.

DIAGNOSIS AND DIFFERENTIAL

The diagnosis may be obvious with the finding of hematemesis, hematochezia, or melena. A careful ear, nose, and throat (ENT) examination can exclude swallowed blood as a source. Nasogastric tube placement and aspiration may detect occult upper GI bleeding. A rectal examination is mandatory to detect the presence of blood, its appearance (bright red, maroon, or melanotic), and the presence of masses. In patients with significant GI bleeding, the most important laboratory test is the typed and crossmatched blood. Other important tests include a complete blood count, electrolytes, serum urea nitrogen, creatinine, glucose, coagulation studies, and liver function tests. The initial hematocrit level often will not reflect the actual amount of blood loss. Upper GI bleeding may elevate the serum urea nitrogen level. Routine abdominal radio-graphs, including barium contrast studies, are of limited value in the emergency setting. Controversy remains as to whether scintigraphy, angiography, or colonoscopy, and in which order, should be the initial diagnostic procedure in the evaluation of lower GI bleeding.

EMERGENCY DEPARTMENT CARE AND DISPOSITION

1. Emergency stabilization evaluating the airway, breathing, and circulation is foremost.

2. Oxygen, large-bore intravenous catheters, and monitors should be applied.
3. Replace volume loss immediately with crystalloids. The decision to start blood should be based on clinical factors (no improvement in perfusion after 2 L crystalloids) rather than on initial hematocrit values.
4. A nasogastric tube should be placed in all patients with significant bleeding, regardless of the presumed source. Concerns that a nasogastric tube passage may provoke bleeding in patients with varices are unwarranted.
5. Early therapeutic endoscopy, where available, should be considered the treatment of choice for significant upper GI bleeding.
6. Consider infusing **octreotide** 25 to 50 μg/h intravenously for esophageal varices.
7. Balloon tamponade with the Sengstaken-Blakemore tube or its variants can control documented variceal hemorrhage but, because of adverse reactions, should be considered an adjunctive or temporizing measure only.
8. With patients who do not respond to medical therapy and in whom endoscopic hemostasis, if available, fails, emergency surgical intervention is indicated.
9. Patients with GI hemorrhage will require hospital admission, and early referral to an endoscopist is advisable if it was not done previously.

38 | Esophageal Emergencies

Mitchell C. Sokolosky

Patients develop a wide variety of problems related to the esophagus. The complaints of dysphagia, odynophagia, or ingested foreign body immediately implicate the esophagus. The esophagus also is often the site of pathology in patients presenting with chest pain, upper gastrointestinal (GI) bleeding, malignancy, and mediastinitis. Many diseases of the esophagus can be evaluated over time in an outpatient setting, but several, such as variceal bleeding and esophageal perforation, can be fulminant and rapidly fatal.

DYSPHAGIA

Clinical Features

Historical information is the key to the diagnosis of dysphagia.

Transport dysphagia that is present for solids only generally suggests a mechanical or obstructive process. Motility disorders typically cause transport dysphagia for solids and liquids. A poorly chewed meat bolus may obstruct the esophagus and be the presenting sign for a variety of underlying esophageal pathologies. These patients are often unable to swallow their own secretions on presentation.

Diagnosis and Differential

The diagnosis of the underlying pathology of dysphagia is most often made outside the emergency department. Initial evaluation may include anteroposterior and lateral neck and chest x-rays. Barium swallow is usually the first test for patients with transport dysphagia. Direct laryngoscopy can be used to identify structural lesions. Oropharyngeal dysphagia is best worked up by video esophagography. Structural or obstructive causes of dysphagia include neoplasms (squamous cell is most common), esophageal strictures and webs, Schatzki ring, and diverticula. Motor lesions causing dysphagia include neuromuscular disorders (cerebrovascular accident is most common), achalasia, and diffuse esophageal spasm. Physical examination of patients with dysphagia should focus on the head and neck and the neurologic examination. Unfortunately, the examination is often normal, despite the high-yield nature of this complaint.

Emergency Department Care and Disposition

1. Protection of the airway and breathing is vital because aspiration is a major concern with most causes of dysphagia.
2. Most causes of dysphagia can be further evaluated and managed in the outpatient setting.
3. Many of the structural lesions ultimately will require dilatation as definitive therapy.

GASTROESOPHAGEAL REFLUX DISEASE

Clinical Features

Heartburn is the classic symptom of gastroesophageal reflux disease (GERD). Chest discomfort may be the sole manifestation of the disease. The association of pain with meals, postural changes, and relief of symptoms with antacids are more consistent with GERD. Less obvious presentations of GERD also occur, such as pulmonary symptoms, especially asthma exacerbations, and multiple ear, nose, and throat symptoms. GERD also has been implicated in the etiology of dental erosion, vocal cord ulcers and granulomas, laryngitis with hoarseness, chronic sinusitis, and chronic cough. Over time, GERD can cause complications such as strictures, inflammatory esophagitis, and Barrett's esophagus (a premalignant condition).

Diagnosis and Differential

Diagnosis often is made by history and favorable response to antacid treatment.

Unfortunately, like cardiac pain, GERD pain may be squeezing or pressure-like and include a history of onset with exertion or rest. Both types of pain may be accompanied by diaphoresis, pallor, radiation, and nausea and vomiting.

Emergency Department Care and Disposition

1. Comprehensive treatment of reflux disease involves decreasing acid production in the stomach, enhancing upper tract motility, and eliminating risk factors for the disease.
2. Mild disease often is treated empirically with an H_2 blocker or proton pump inhibitor.
3. A prokinetic drug also may greatly decrease symptoms.
4. Patients should avoid agents that exacerbate GERD (ethanol, caffeine, nicotine, chocolate, or fatty foods), sleep with the head of the bed elevated (30°), and avoid eating within 3 hours of going to bed at night.

ESOPHAGEAL PERFORATION

Clinical Features

Pain is classically described as acute, severe, unrelenting, and diffuse and is reported in the chest, neck, and abdomen. Pain can radiate to the back and shoulders, or back pain may be the predominant symptom. Swallowing often exacerbates pain. Physical examination varies with the severity of the rupture and the elapsed time between the rupture and presentation. Abdominal rigidity with hypotension and fever often occur early. Tachycardia and tachypnea are common. Mediastinal emphysema takes time to develop. It is less commonly detected by examination or radiography in lower esophageal perforation, and its absence does not rule out perforation. Hammon crunch, caused by air in the mediastinum being moved by the beating heart, sometimes can be auscultated.

Pleural effusions develop in 50% of patients with intrathoracic perforations and are uncommon in cervical perforations.

Diagnosis and Differential

Chest radiography and contrast esophagography with water-soluble contrast most often make the diagnosis. Endoscopy, computed topography of the chest, and thoracentesis can be useful adjuncts. Endoscopy often is done after negative esophagography in penetrating trauma with suspicion of esophageal perforation. Esophageal perforation often is ascribed to acute myocardial infarction, pulmonary embolus, peptic ulcer disease, aortic catastrophe, or acute abdomen, resulting in critical delays in diagnosis, the most important factor in determining morbidity and mortality.

Emergency Department Care and Disposition

1. Rapid, aggressive management is the key to minimizing the morbidity and mortality associated with esophageal perforation.
2. In the emergency department, resuscitation of shock (see Chaps. 5 and 6), and broad-spectrum parental antibiotics to cover aerobic and anaerobic organisms. Examples include single drug coverage such as **piperacillin/tazobactam** 3.375 g intravenously (IV) or double drug coverage with **cefotaxime** 2 g IV or **ceftriaxone** 2 g IV plus **clindamycin** 600 mg IV or **metronidazole** 1 g IV.
3. Emergent surgical consultation should be obtained as soon as the diagnosis is seriously entertained.
4. All of these patients require admission to the hospital.

ESOPHAGEAL BLEEDING

Clinical Features

Acute onset of upper GI bleeding is the usual presentation, although some patients may present with melena or hematochezia. The spectrum of severity of bleeding is broad. Fewer than 50% of patients with Mallory-Weiss tears will report a history of vomiting before hematemesis.

Diagnosis and Differential

Diagnosis is made by history and the presence of acute upper GI bleeding.

Gastric aspiration may aid in the diagnosis. Endoscopy may be diagnostic and therapeutic. Esophageal cancer often results in heme-positive stools but is an uncommon cause of significant upper or lower GI bleeding.

Emergency Department Care and Disposition

1. Resuscitation proceeds concurrently with the diagnostic effort of history, physical examination, and laboratory evaluation.
2. Definitive airway control should be used as needed.
3. Oxygen, large-bore intravenous catheters, and monitors should be applied.
4. Replace volume loss immediately with crystalloids.
5. The decision to start blood should be based on clinical factors (no improvement in perfusion after 2 L crystalloids) rather than on initial hematocrit values.
6. Gastroenterology should be consulted early.
7. Gastric lavage through a nasogastric tube is generally accepted.
8. Consider infusing **octreotide** 25 to 50 μg/h IV for varices.
9. Balloon tamponade to control documented variceal bleeding should be considered only as an adjunctive or temporizing measure.
10. Surgical intervention may be necessary for those who fail medical and endoscopic hemostatic measures.
11. Patients should be admitted to an appropriate facility and level of care.

39 | Swallowed Foreign Bodies

Patricia Baines

Foreign body ingestion occurs in all age groups. Most cases occur in children, who swallow coins, toys, and other small objects. Many of the remaining cases occur in edentulous adults, psychiatric patients, or prisoners. Adults generally ingest meat or bones, and psychiatric and prison inmates ingest atypical foreign bodies, such as toothbrushes, spoons, and razor blades. Objects lodge in areas of physiologic narrowing, where they can cause airway obstruction, stricture, or perforation, with infection, abscess, and fistula. Once an object has passed through the pylorus, it generally will pass without difficulty.

CLINICAL FEATURES

Objects lodged in the esophagus can produce anxiety, retrosternal discomfort, retching, vomiting, dysphagia, coughing, choking, or aspiration, and the patient may be unable to swallow secretions. The adult patient usually can provide an accurate history regarding the type of foreign body and the time of its impaction. In the pediatric patient it may be necessary to rely on clues such as refusal to eat, vomiting, gagging, choking, stridor, neck or throat pain, dysphagia, and increased salivation.

DIAGNOSIS AND DIFFERENTIAL

Physical examination includes evaluation of the entire upper airway, including the neck and subcutaneous tissues. Direct or indirect laryngoscopy should be performed; in the absence of a foreign body, findings consistent with foreign body ingestion, particularly in the pediatric age group, consist of red throat, palatal abrasion, temperature elevation, and peritoneal signs. Radiopaque objects can be visualized on standard x-rays of the neck, chest, or abdomen, or visualized by laryngoscopy or endoscopy. Differential diagnosis includes dysphagia, esophageal carcinoma, and gastrointestinal (GI) reflux disease.

EMERGENCY DEPARTMENT CARE AND DISPOSITION

General Care

1. Aspiration of the foreign body or built-up secretions should be prevented. If necessary, a tube should be placed proximal to the foreign body to remove un-swallowed fluids or secretions.
2. Serial abdominal examinations should be performed to detect early signs of developing peritonitis secondary to perforation.
3. The progression of the foreign body through the GI tract can be monitored with the use of serial x-ray films or hand-held metal detectors.

Food Impaction

1. If the patient is able to manage secretions, conservative treatment is appropriate.
2. If the food does not pass within 12 hours or the patient is unable to swallow fluids, intervention is necessary.

209

3. Lower esophageal sphincter relaxation, to facilitate bolus passage, can be attempted by the administration of **glucagon** 1 mg, sublingual **nitroglycerin** 0.3 to 0.4 mg, or sublingual **nifedipine** 10 mg, while monitoring carefully for hypotension.
4. Endoscopy is the preferred method of bolus removal; therefore, esophagogram, which impairs visualization, should be avoided if possible.
5. Use of proteolytic enzymes (eg, papain) should be avoided due to risks of esophageal perforation.
6. Most patients with an impacted food bolus have an esophageal lesion that will require elective specialist referral for further evaluation.

Coin Ingestion

1. Approximately 33% of children with a coin lodged in the esophagus will be asymptomatic.
2. Radiographs should be performed on all children suspected of swallowing coins to determine the presence and location of the object.
3. Coins in the esophagus lie in the frontal plane, whereas coins in the trachea lie in the sagittal plane. Coins usually pass spontaneously but can be removed endoscopically if lodged in the esophagus.

Button Battery Ingestion

1. Button battery ingestion is a true emergency because of its rapid caustic action. Esophageal burns have occurred within 4 hours, with perforation within 6 hours. Lithium cells have a high incidence of adverse outcomes, and mercuric oxide cells fragment more frequently than do other cells, although heavy metal poisoning does not appear to be a significant complication.
2. Blood and mercury levels should be monitored if a mercury-containing cell has opened while in the GI tract.
3. If the button battery is suspected in the esophagus, the location should be documented by radiograph, followed by emergent endoscopy.
4. Button batteries that have passed the esophagus in an asymptomatic patient may be treated conservatively, unless the battery has not passed the pylorus after 48 hours of observation. Most batteries pass through the body within 48 to 72 hours.
5. Symptomatic patients should have early surgical consultation due to risks of mucosal damage and perforation.
6. Battery identification assistance is available from the National Button Battery Ingestion Hotline (202-625-3333).

Ingestion of Sharp Objects

1. Management is controversial. Objects longer than 5 cm and wider than 2 cm rarely pass the stomach, and objects with extremely pointed edges, such as open safety pins or razor blades, may cause intestinal perforation, most commonly at the ileocecal valve.
2. For children who have swallowed sharp objects, an initial radiograph and examination should be performed.
3. Asymptomatic children can be managed conservatively with serial radiographs.

Cocaine Ingestion

1. Cocaine packet ingestion is used for drug concealment. Multiple small packets of cocaine may be contained within a condom.
2. Conservative treatment and full bowel irrigation have been used.

Foreign Body Retrieval

1. Endoscopy is the procedure of choice for foreign body retrieval, except for cocaine, due to risks of packet rupture. It should be performed for objects lodged in the esophagus, heavy objects, sharp objects, coins, batteries that do not pass through the pylorus within 48 hours, open batteries, and in all other symptomatic patients.
2. Fewer than 1% of ingested foreign bodies require surgical treatment. Surgical intervention is the safest method of cocaine packet recovery and may be necessary in cases of GI obstruction or perforation.

For further reading in *Emergency Medicine: A Comprehensive Study Guide*, 6th ed., see Chap. 76, "Swallowed Foreign Bodies," by Wade R. Gaasch and Robert A. Barish.

40 | Peptic Ulcer Disease and Gastritis

Mark R. Hess

Peptic ulcer disease (PUD) is a chronic affliction marked by recurrent gastroduodenal ulcerations affecting up to 10% of the population at any time. The 2 independent risk factors for PUD are nonsteroidal anti-inflammatory drug (NSAID) use and *Helicobacter pylori* infection. Associated disorders are gastritis (ie, inflammation of the gastric mucosal) and dyspepsia (ie, upper abdominal discomfort).

CLINICAL FEATURES

PUD classically presents with burning epigastric pain, usually after meals, and often awakening the patient at night. Pain is typically relieved by food, milk, or antacids but then recurs hours later. Elderly patients may have less pain associated with their ulcers and instead have nausea, vomiting, anorexia, weight loss, and bleeding.

A history of frequent vomiting, weight loss, early satiety, or nausea should suggest gastric outlet obstruction. Hemodynamic instability, hematemesis, or melena confirm hemorrhagic complications. Although not commonly bleeding, a perforation usually will present with severe pain or peritoneal signs. Sudden mid-back pain may signify pancreatitis from posterior perforation.

DIAGNOSIS AND DIFFERENTIAL

Typically, the diagnosis of PUD is based on history and examination. The patient may have very mild epigastric tenderness. A succussion splash (shake the patient's abdomen by holding 1 side of the pelvis to elicit sounds) in the presence of excessive vomiting suggests gastric outlet obstruction. Directed laboratory work, such as complete blood cell count, lipase levels, and liver function tests, may confirm associated illness. Rectal examination and nasogastric aspiration may aid in diagnosing bleeding complications. In the presence of bleeding, one should consider clotting studies. Radiologic studies that might be useful include an upright chest (or left lateral decubitus) radiogram to detect free air, and an ultrasound or helical computed tomography of the abdomen to rule out cholelithiasis or aortic aneurysm.

The definitive diagnosis of PUD can be made only with an upper gastrointestinal series using barium or direct endoscopic visualization. Such tests are usually reserved for patients with severe pain or bleeding. Because of the prevalence of infection as an etiology of PUD, most clinicians advocate testing for *H pylori*. The easiest test in the emergency department is a rapid serologic detection of immunoglobulin G antibodies with sensitivity and specificity approaching 90%. Although the test may be useful in patients with severe or refractory symptoms, it is not a test of cure because antibodies can remain for years.

Many disorders mimic PUD in pattern and location of pain. Pancreatitis is usually associated with worse pain and more commonly radiates to the back. Similarly, the pulsatile epigastric mass representative of an abdominal aortic aneurysm may present with back pain. With gastroesophageal reflux the patient

212

may relate positional pain originating substernally. Clues to biliary colic include a history of fatty food intolerance (rather than relief of pain with food), typically in a middle-age, obese female. In addition to cholecystitis, right upper quadrant pain may signify hepatitis. The most serious diagnosis confused with PUD is myocardial ischemia or infarction, which should be considered in any patient older than 40 years or with cardiac risk factors. Other gastrointestinal disorders that mimic PUD include gastroesophageal reflux disease, with burning into the chest, and gastric cancer, with chronic pain and weight loss.

EMERGENCY DEPARTMENT CARE AND DISPOSITION

The treatment of PUD is done primarily on an outpatient basis unless complications exist. Traditional treatment has been simply to promote healing through decreasing or neutralizing hydrochloric acid in the gut with antacids or H_2-receptor antagonists. However, actual cure of this disease requires eradication of *H pylori* infection. Any NSAID use must be discontinued to prevent further recurrence.

1. Pain can be relieved with **liquid antacids** (eg, magnesium or aluminum hydroxide gel) 15 mL 1 and 3 hours after each meal and at bedtime.
2. PUD is most conveniently treated with H_2-receptor antagonists: **cimetidine** (may cause drug interactions) 300 mg intravenously or 800 mg orally at bedtime; **ranitidine** 50 mg intravenously or 300 mg orally at bedtime; **famotidine** 20 mg intravenously or 20 to 40 mg orally at bedtime; and **nizatidine** 300 mg orally at bedtime.
3. **Sucralfate** 1 g 4 times daily heals ulcers but may interfere with absorption of other medications.
4. In cases of resistant ulcers, one can use proton pump inhibitors such as **omeprazole** (may cause drug interactions) 20 mg daily or **lansoprazole** 15 mg daily.
5. Patients with positive serological testing require eradication of *H pylori* with 1 of several combination therapies for 10 to 14 days: (*a*) bismuth subsalicylate 2 tablets 4 times daily with meals and at bedtime plus metronidazole 500 mg with meals plus tetracycline 500 mg 4 times daily with meals and at bedtime with or without omeprazole 20 mg every day; (*b*) Helidac 4 times daily; or (*c*) Prevpac 2 times daily.
6. Patients who demonstrate any complication of PUD should be stabilized and admitted to the hospital. For the treatment of hemorrhage, see Chap. 37. Perforation requires nasogastric suction, broad-spectrum antibiotics, and surgical consultation. Gastric outlet obstruction requires correction of fluid and electrolyte abnormalities, with referral for possible surgical correction.
7. Stable patients with benign examination can be discharged on antacids or H_2-receptor antagonists. They should be referred for definitive diagnosis if symptoms persist.
8. Worrisome patients with anorexia, dysphagia, anemia, or weight loss or who are elderly will require early endoscopy to rule out cancer.
9. All patients require counseling against the use of aspirin, NSAIDs, tobacco, and alcohol. In addition, they should be told to return for worsening and confounding symptoms (eg, vomiting, bleeding, syncope, chest pain, or fever) or lack of improvement in 24 to 48 hours.

For further reading in *Emergency Medicine: A Comprehensive Study Guide,* 6th ed., see Chap. 77, "Peptic Ulcer Disease and Gastritis," by Matthew C. Gratton.

41 Appendicitis

Peggy E. Goodman

Appendicitis is a relatively common disorder that affects approximately 6% of the population. Newer imaging techniques are improving the ability to diagnose appendicitis more accurately and decrease the number of unnecessary appendectomies; however, there are still many cases in which some or all of the "classic" signs and symptoms are absent, leading to continued difficulty in diagnosis. Complications from misdiagnosis of appendicitis include intraabdominal abscess, wound infection, adhesion formation, bowel obstruction, and infertility.

CLINICAL FEATURES

Abdominal pain is the most reliable symptom in appendicitis. The visceral innervation of the inflamed appendix results in dull pain originating in the periumbilical or epigastric region with localization to the right lower quadrant as peritoneal irritation occurs. Other symptoms classically associated with appendicitis include anorexia, nausea, and vomiting, which occur after the onset of abdominal pain. Although 60% of patients will have some combination of these symptoms, they are by themselves neither specific nor sensitive for appendicitis. The symptoms generally increase over approximately a 24-hour period and also may be accompanied by dysuria, tenesmus, or other symptoms related to irritation of the abdominal or pelvic viscera. The McBurney point is the classic location of maximal tenderness, just below the middle of a line connecting the umbilicus and the anterior superior iliac spine. Palpation of the left lower quadrant with pain referred to the right lower quadrant is referred to as the Rovsing sign. The psoas sign is elicited by placing the patient in the left lateral decubitus position and extending the right leg at the hip. The obturator sign is elicited by passively flexing the right hip and knee and internally rotating the hip. If the psoas muscle or obturator muscle is irritated by an inflamed appendix, these maneuvers will be painful. Patients with a pelvic appendix may be most tender on rectal examination, and patients with a retrocecal appendix may have more prominent right flank pain than abdominal pain. Fever is a relatively late finding in appendicitis and rarely exceeds 39°C (102.2°F), unless rupture or other complications occur.

DIAGNOSIS AND DIFFERENTIAL

The diagnosis of acute appendicitis is primarily clinical. Factors that increase the likelihood of appendicitis, listed in decreasing order of importance, are right lower quadrant pain, rigidity, migration of pain to the right lower quadrant, pain before vomiting, positive psoas sign, rebound tenderness, and guarding. Additional studies, such as complete blood count, urinalysis, pregnancy test, and imaging studies, may be performed if the diagnosis is unclear. Elevation of the white blood cell count is sensitive but has very low specificity and is of limited value. Urinalysis is useful to help rule out other diagnoses, such as urolithiasis or urinary tract infection, but pyuria and hematuria can occur when an inflamed appendix overlies the ureter. A pregnancy test should be obtained as part of the evaluation of abdominal pain in any fertile female.

The role of imaging studies in the diagnosis of appendicitis has recently gained increased significance, particularly when the diagnosis is uncertain. Plain radiographs of the abdomen are often abnormal but are not specific; even if a fecalith or an ileus is noted, correlation to the patient's acute presentation is unclear. Ultrasonography has a high sensitivity but is limited in evaluating a ruptured appendix or an abnormally located (eg, retrocecal) appendix.

Computed tomography (CT) is now considered the imaging study of choice. It is more sensitive than ultrasound, with comparable specificity, is widely available, and can provide alternate diagnoses. Current debate exists regarding whether focused appendiceal CT or traditional non-focused abdominal CT is the better choice. CT findings suggesting acute appendicitis include pericecal inflammation, abscess, and periappendiceal phlegmon or fluid collections.

Patients with atypical presentations can be observed with serial abdominal examinations to avoid premature surgical intervention or discharge of the patient with an uncertain diagnosis.

Certain patient populations have higher rates of misdiagnosis of appendicitis, with increased morbidity and mortality rates. Patients younger than 6 years have a high misdiagnosis rate due to poor communication skills and the association of many nonspecific symptoms, such as lethargy, upper respiratory symptoms, and urinary symptoms. Elderly patients may have decreased perceptions of symptoms due to the physiology of aging, medications, and comorbid conditions. The most significant predictors of acute appendicitis in the elderly are tenderness, rigidity, pain at diagnosis, fever, and previous abdominal surgery.

Pregnant patients are at risk for misdiagnosis because nausea and vomiting may be incorrectly attributed to the pregnancy, and appendiceal displacement by the gravid uterus may result in tenderness and pain in the right upper quadrant. Appendicitis is the most common extrauterine surgical emergency in pregnancy, and fetal mortality rates are high if perforation and peritonitis occur. Ultrasound is the preferred diagnostic aid due to risks of radiation from CT.

Patients with acquired immunodeficiency syndrome are susceptible to complications from appendicitis because of delays in diagnosis due to their frequently preexisting gastrointestinal symptoms and their immunocompromised state.

EMERGENCY DEPARTMENT CARE AND DISPOSITION

Before surgery, patients should have nothing by mouth and should have intravenous (IV) access, analgesia, and institution of antibiotic therapy.

1. Short-acting narcotic analgesics, such as **fentanyl** 0.01 to 0.02 mg/kg, are preferred because they can be reversed by naloxone if needed.
2. Antibiotics are most effective when given before surgery, thereby decreasing the incidence of postoperative wound infection or, in cases of perforation, postoperative abscess formation. Several antibiotic regimens to cover anaerobes, enterococci and gram-negative intestinal flora have been recommended, including **piperacillin/tazobactam** 3.375 g IV or **ampicillin/ sulbactam** 3 g IV.
3. Patients with abdominal pain generally can be stratified into 4 groups: (*a*) patients with "classic" appendicitis requiring surgical consult and appendectomy; (*b*) patients with signs and symptoms suspicious for appendicitis

who would benefit from imaging studies and/or serial examinations, with surgical consult when appropriate; (*c*) patients previously discussed as high risk (pediatric, geriatric, pregnant, or immunocompromised) who require a high index of clinical suspicion and a low threshold for surgical consultation; and (*d*) patients in whom appendicitis is considered unlikely.

4. If no precise diagnosis is determined after evaluation and observation, the patient should be diagnosed as having "nonspecific abdominal pain" rather than given a more specific diagnosis. These patients may be discharged if they have appropriate medical follow-up and specific discharge instructions. They should be seen within 24 hours by their primary care physicians or another primary care provider to evaluate the course of their illness, should avoid strong analgesics, and should return if they develop increased pain, fever, nausea, or other signs or symptoms of illness that are worsening or not resolving.

For further reading in *Emergency Medicine: A Comprehensive Study Guide,* 6th ed., see Chap. 78, "Acute Appendicitis," by Denis J. FitzGerald and Arthur M. Pancioli.

42 | Intestinal Obstruction

Roy L. Alson

Intestinal obstruction results from mechanical blockage or the loss of normal peristalsis. The latter (adynamic or paralytic ileus) is more common and usually self-limiting. Mechanical bowel obstruction has intrinsic or extrinsic mechanisms. Most commonly, mechanical small bowel obstruction (SBO) results from adhesions due to previous surgical procedures or inflammatory diseases. Incarcerated inguinal hernia is the second most common cause of SBO. Other hernias (obturator, femoral, or umbilical) may incarcerate and cause obstruction. Intraluminal masses are rarely causes of SBO. Other causes to consider are inflammatory bowel diseases, congenital anomalies, and foreign bodies. Fecal impaction and carcinomas are common problems causing large bowel obstruction in the elderly. Intussusception in children and volvulus in the elderly should be kept in mind.

CLINICAL FEATURES

Abdominal pain and inability to have a bowel movement or to pass flatus are often presenting complaints. Crampy, intermittent, progressive abdominal pain is the main feature of intestinal obstruction. Vomiting, bilious in early stages and feculent in late stages, is usually present. Physical signs vary, ranging from abdominal distention, localized or general tenderness, to obvious signs of peritonitis. Localization of pain may provide clues as to the site of obstruction. Most small intestinal disorders tend to cause periumbilical pain initially, whereas colonic diseases localize in the hypogastric region. Active, high-pitched bowel sounds can be heard in mechanical SBO. Presence of abdominal surgical scars, hernias, and other mass lesions should be noted. Rectal examination may demonstrate fecal impaction, rectal carcinoma, or occult blood. Empty rectal ampulla may be strongly suggestive of intestinal obstruction. Patients with partial SBO can still pass flatus. Presence of preexisting stool in the rectum does not rule out obstruction. Systemic symptoms and signs will depend on the extent of dehydration and the presence of bowel necrosis or infection. Patients may be septic and acutely dehydrated. Pelvic examination may show a gynecologic process causing obstruction.

DIAGNOSIS AND DIFFERENTIAL

Intestinal obstruction should be suspected in any patient with abdominal pain, distention, and vomiting, especially in those with previous abdominal surgery or groin hernias. X-rays are helpful in localizing the site of obstruction to the large or small bowel. Flat and upright abdominal radiographs and an upright chest x-ray should be obtained (left lateral decubitus film in patients who cannot be upright). Distended intestines in the flat plate and stepladder patterns of air-fluid levels in the upright or decubitus film will confirm the diagnosis. Films should be examined closely for the presence of free air from perforation, pneumonitis, pleural effusion, presence of gallstones, and mass lesions such as enlarged viscera or phlegmon from inflammatory processes.

Laboratory tests should include a complete blood count, electrolytes, serum urea nitrogen, creatinine, serum amylase, and lipase levels and a urinalysis. Liver function tests and typing and cross-matching for blood products may be

217

required. Extreme dehydration from vomiting and fluid sequestration in the bowel may cause hematocrit and serum urea nitrogen levels to be elevated. Leukocytosis with left shift may suggest abscesses, gangrene, or peritonitis. High white blood cell counts may suggest mesenteric vascular occlusion. High urine-specific gravity, ketonuria, and metabolic acidosis may indicate the severity of the obstruction. Sigmoidoscopy and barium enema may be necessary to determine the site and etiology of obstruction. Some have advocated contrast-enhanced computed tomography to differentiate between partial and complete obstruction. This may not be clinically indicated.

EMERGENCY DEPARTMENT CARE AND DISPOSITION

Once the diagnosis of mechanical obstruction is established, surgical intervention is usually necessary.

1. Surgical consultation should be obtained without delay. In the emergency department, the bowel should be decompressed with a nasogastric tube.
2. Intravenous crystalloid replacement should be initiated. The patient's response to fluid therapy should be monitored closely with the blood pressure, pulse, and urine output. Impending shock should be recognized, and the patient should be vigorously resuscitated.
3. Most patients will need broad-spectrum antibiotic coverage (such as **piperacillin/tazobactam** 3.375 g or **ampicillin/sulbactam** 3.0 g intravenously). When the diagnosis is uncertain or if adynamic ileus is suspected, conservative measures, such as nasogastric decompression, intravenous fluids, and observation without surgical intervention, may be appropriate.

Pseudoobstruction commonly occurs in the low colonic region. Depression of intestinal motility from medications such as anticholinergic agents or tricyclic antidepressants will cause large amounts of gas to be retained in the large intestine. Colonoscopy will be diagnostic and therapeutic. Surgery is not indicated.

For further reading in *Emergency Medicine: A Comprehensive Study Guide,* 6th ed., see Chap. 79, "Intestinal Obstruction," by Salvator J. Vicario and Timothy G. Price.

43 | Hernia in Adults and Children

N. Heramba Prasad

A hernia is an external or internal protrusion of a body part from its normal cavity. Typically, *hernia* is most commonly used to describe a protrusion of bowel or other body parts externally through the abdominal wall. The most common types of abdominal hernias are inguinal, femoral, umbilical, and anterior abdominal wall (Fig. 43-1).

Predisposing factors include family history, lack of developmental maturity, undescended testes, genitourinary abnormalities, conditions that increase intraabdominal pressure (eg, ascites or pregnancy), chronic obstructive pulmonary disease, and surgical incision sites.

CLINICAL FEATURES

Most hernias are detected on routine physical examination or inadvertently by the patient. When the contents of a hernia can be easily returned to the original cavity by manipulation, it is defined as *reducible;* when it cannot, it is *irreducible* or *incarcerated. Strangulation* refers to vascular compromise of the incarcerated contents. Incarcerated hernias may have acute inflammation and edema, leading to bowel obstruction and/or strangulation. When not relieved, strangulation may produce gangrene. Perforation, peritonitis, or septic shock may occur as a complication of strangulation.

Symptoms other than an obvious protruding mass from the abdominal wall include localized pain, nausea, and vomiting. Children may exhibit irritability. Careful evaluation for obstruction is essential.

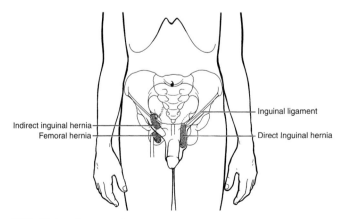

Indirect inguinal hernia
Femoral hernia

Inguinal ligament
Direct Inguinal hernia

FIG. 43-1. Groin hernias.

DIAGNOSIS AND DIFFERENTIAL

Physical examination is the predominate means of diagnosis. Laboratory testing has no reliable indicators; however, leucocytosis and acidosis may be indicative of ischemic bowel. An upright chest x-ray should be obtained to detect free air if perforation is suspected. Flat and upright abdominal films may be helpful in evaluation for obstruction. Occasionally, loops of bowel may be seen entering the hernial sac. Internal hernias may be diagnosed by the use of computed tomography or abdominal ultrasound.

The differential diagnosis of groin masses includes direct or indirect hernias, testicular torsion, tumor, lymph node, epididymitis, groin abscesses, retracted or undescended testes, and hydrocele. Lymph nodes are generally multiple, firm, and movable. Hydroceles will transilluminate. Incarcerated hernias do not transilluminate and may be tender. In children, retracted or undescended testes may be mistaken for inguinal hernias.

EMERGENCY DEPARTMENT CARE AND DISPOSITION

1. If there is a history consistent with recent incarceration, an attempt to reduce the hernia should be made. If there is a question of the duration of the incarceration, no attempt to reduce should be made. The goal is to not introduce dead bowel into the abdomen. To reduce a hernia, (*a*) place the patient in the Trendelenburg position, (*b*) give sedation or anxiolytics (see Chap. 10), (*c*) place a warm compress on the area, and (*d*) gently compress the hernia, avoiding prolonged use of excessive force.

2. Because inguinal hernias have a high risk of incarceration in the first year of life, infants with inguinal hernias reduced in the emergency department generally should have repair within 24 hours.

3. Umbilical hernias in children are common. Unless there is evidence of obstruction or incarceration, immediate treatment is not recommended. These patients should be followed longitudinally by their primary care providers. Referral for surgical evaluation is recommended in children older than 4 years or with hernias greater than 2 cm in diameter.

4. In adults with reducible hernias, refer for outpatient surgical evaluation and repair. Discharge instructions should include avoidance of heavy lifting and return to the emergency department if the hernia could not be reduced promptly. Signs of obstruction also should be discussed.

5. Emergent surgical intervention is the treatment of choice for incarcerated hernias that are tender and cannot be reduced or are strangulated. Patients should be monitored closely, given nothing by mouth, and have intravenous (IV) fluid replacement. In these cases, insertion of a nasogastric tube is indicated. Broad-spectrum antibiotics are indicated if there is evidence of perforation or strangulation. Examples include single drug coverage such as **piperacillin/tazobactam** 3.375 g IV or double drug coverage with **cefotaxime** 2 g IV or **ceftriaxone** 2 g IV plus **clindamycin** 600 mg IV or **metronidazole** 1 g IV. Vigorous fluid resuscitation may be necessary in the case of shock.

For further reading in *Emergency Medicine: A Comprehensive Study Guide*, 6th ed., see Chap. 80, "Hernia in Adults and Children," by Frank W. Lavoie and Mary Harkins Becker.

44 | Ileitis, Colitis, and Diverticulitis

Jonathan A. Maisel

CROHN DISEASE

Crohn disease, also described as regional enteritis, terminal ileitis, and granulomatous ileocolitis, is an idiopathic gastrointestinal (GI) tract disease. Segmental involvement of any part of the GI tract from the mouth to the anus by a nonspecific granulomatous inflammatory process characterizes the disease.

Clinical Features

Abdominal pain, anorexia, diarrhea, and weight loss are present in up to 80% of cases, although the clinical course is variable and unpredictable. Patients commonly report a history of recurring fever, abdominal pain, and diarrhea over several years without a definitive diagnosis. One third of patients develop perianal fissures or fistulas, abscesses, or rectal prolapse. Fistulas occur between the ileum and sigmoid colon, the cecum, another ileal segment, or the skin. Obstruction, hemorrhage, and toxic megacolon also occur. Half of all cases of toxic megacolon, frequently associated with massive GI bleeding, occur in patients with Crohn disease.

Up to 30% of patients develop extraintestinal manifestations, including arthritis, uveitis, and skin disease (eg, erythema nodosum or pyoderma gangrenosum). Hepatobiliary disease, including gallstones, pericholangitis, and chronic active hepatitis, is commonly seen, as is pancreatitis. Hyperoxaluria causes nephrolithiasis in up to 25% of patients. Some patients develop thromboembolic disease as a result of a hypercoagulable state and have a 25% mortality rate. Malabsorption, malnutrition, and chronic anemia develop in long-standing disease, and the incidence of GI tract malignant neoplasm is triple that of the general population. The recurrence rate for those with Crohn disease is 25% to 50% when treated medically and higher for patients treated surgically.

Diagnosis and Differential

The definitive diagnosis of Crohn disease usually is established months or years after the onset of symptoms. Common misdiagnoses are appendicitis and pelvic inflammatory disease. A careful and detailed history for previous bowel symptoms that preceded acute presentation may provide clues for correct diagnosis. The absence of true guarding or rebound is noted. Peritonitis and leukocytosis can be masked in patients taking glucocorticoids.

Laboratory evaluation should include complete blood count, chemistries, and type and crossmatch when indicated. Plain abdominal x-rays may identify obstruction, perforation, and toxic megacolon, which may appear as a long, continuous segment of air-filled colon greater than 6 cm in diameter. Computerized tomography of the abdomen is the most useful test to identify intra- and extraintestinal manifestations of Crohn disease. A definitive diagnosis is confirmed by an upper GI series, an air-contrast barium enema, and colonoscopy.

The differential diagnosis of Crohn disease includes lymphoma, ileocecal amebiasis, sarcoidosis, tuberculosis, Kaposi sarcoma, *Campylobacter* enteritis, and *Yersinia* ileocolitis. Most of these conditions are uncommon, and the last two can be differentiated by stool cultures.

Emergency Department Care and Disposition

Initial evaluation should determine the severity of the attack and identify significant complications such as hemorrhage, obstruction, abscess, or toxic megacolon. The goal of therapy includes relief of symptoms, suppression of the inflammatory disease, avoidance or management of complications, and maintenance of hydration and nutrition. Available pharmacologic agents are as follows:

1. **Sulfasalazine** 3 to 4 g/d is effective for mild to moderate active Crohn disease but has multiple toxic side effects, including GI and hypersensitivity reactions. **Mesalamine,** up to 4 g/d, is equally effective, with fewer side effects.
2. Glucocorticoids (**prednisone**) 40 to 60 mg/d are reserved for severe small intestine disease and ileocolitis.
3. Immunosuppressive drugs, **6-mercaptopurine** 1 to 1.5 mg/kg/d or **azathioprine** 2 to 2.5 mg/kg/d, are used as steroid-sparing agents in healing fistulas and in patients with serious surgical contraindications.
4. **Metronidazole** 10 to 20 mg/kg/d or **ciprofloxacin** 500 to 750 mg twice daily is useful in patients with perianal complications and fistulous disease.
5. Patients with medically resistant, moderate to severe Crohn disease may benefit from the anti–tumor necrosis factor antibody **infliximab** 5 mg/kg intravenously.
6. Diarrhea can be controlled by **loperamide** 4 to 16 mg/d, **diphenoxylate** 5 to 20 mg/d, or **cholestyramine** 4 g 1 to 6 times daily.

Patients who should be admitted to the hospital include those who demonstrate signs of fulminant colitis, peritonitis, obstruction, significant hemorrhage, severe dehydration, or electrolyte imbalance and those with less severe disease who fail outpatient management. Surgical intervention is indicated in patients with intestinal obstruction or hemorrhage, perforation, abscess or fistula formation, toxic megacolon, or perianal disease, and in some patients who fail medical therapy. When patients can be discharged from the hospital, alterations in therapy should be discussed with a gastroenterologist, and close follow-up is recommended.

ULCERATIVE COLITIS

Ulcerative colitis is an idiopathic chronic inflammatory and ulcerative disease of the colon and rectum characterized clinically most often by bloody diarrhea.

Clinical Features

Ulcerative colitis is commonly characterized by intermittent attacks of acute disease with complete remission between bouts. Patients with mild disease (60% of cases) have fewer than 4 bowel movements per day, no systemic symptoms, and few extraintestinal manifestations. Severe disease (15% of cases) is associated with frequent daily bowel movements, weight loss, fever, tachycardia, anemia, and more frequent extraintestinal manifestations, including peripheral arthritis, ankylosing spondylitis, episcleritis, uveitis, pyoderma gangrenosum, and erythema nodosum. Ninety percent of deaths from ulcerative colitis occur in patients with severe disease.

The most serious complication is toxic megacolon, which may lead to perforation and peritonitis. Abscess and fistula formation, which are much more common in patients with Crohn disease, occur in 20% of patients with ulcerative colitis. GI hemorrhage (most common), obstruction secondary to stricture formation, and acute perforation are other complications. There is a 10- to 30-fold risk of developing colon carcinoma.

Diagnosis and Differential

The diagnosis of ulcerative colitis may be considered for patients with a history of abdominal cramps, diarrhea, and mucoid stools. Laboratory findings are nonspecific and may include leukocytosis, anemia, thrombocytosis, decreased serum albumin levels, abnormal liver function test results, and negative stool studies for ova, parasites, and enteric pathogens. Abdominal computed tomography may suggest the diagnosis, and barium enema can confirm the diagnosis and defines the extent of colonic involvement. Colonoscopy is the most sensitive diagnostic method. The differential diagnosis includes infectious, ischemic, irradiation, anti-neoplastic agent induced, pseudomembranous, and Crohn colitis. When the disease is limited to the rectum, consider sexually acquired diseases, such as rectal syphilis, gonococcal proctitis, lymphogranuloma venarum, and inflammation caused by herpes simplex virus, *Entamoeba histolytica, Shigella,* and *Campylobacter.*

Emergency Department Care and Disposition

Severe Disease

Patients with severe disease should be admitted for intravenous fluid replacement, correction of electrolyte abnormalities, and the following treatment:

1. Intravenous antibiotics, active against coliforms and anaerobes, such as **ampicillin** (2 g every 6 hours), **gentamicin** (1.5 mg/kg every 8 hours), and **clindamycin** (300-600 mg every 6 hours) or **metronidazole** (500 mg every 8 hours) should be initiated.
2. Patients on steroids should receive **hydrocortisone** 300 mg/d, **methylprednisolone** 48 mg/d, or **prednisone** 60 mg/d.
3. **Cyclosporine** 4 mg/kg/d has been advocated for cases of fulminant colitis that have failed treatment with intravenous steroids.

Complete bowel rest and parenteral nutrition remains controversial in patients with fulminant disease. Patients with significant GI hemorrhage, toxic megacolon, and bowel perforation should be admitted with consultation to a gastroenterologist and a surgeon.

Mild to Moderate Disease

Most patients with mild and moderate disease can be treated as outpatients. Therapies listed below should be discussed with a gastroenterologist, and close followup must be ensured.

1. **Prednisone** 40 to 60 mg/d is usually sufficient and can be adjusted depending on the severity of the disease. Once clinical remission is achieved,

steroids should be slowly tapered and discontinued because there is no evidence that maintenance dosages of steroids reduce the incidence of relapses.

2. **Sulfasalazine** 1.5 to 2 g/d is inferior to steroids in treating acute attacks and is most useful as maintenance therapy by reducing the recurrence rate. Newer 5-aminosalicylic derivatives, such as **mesalamine** 800 mg orally twice daily, are quite effective in inducing and maintaining remission, with fewer side effects.

3. In patients with active proctitis, 5-aminosalicylic enemas and topical steroid preparations, such as beclomethasone, hydrocortisone, tixocortol, or budesonide, can be used acutely and to maintain remission, with fewer side effects.

4. In refractory cases, a combination of glucocorticoids and an immunomodulator such as **6-mercaptopurine** 1 to 1.5 mg/kg/d or **azathioprine** 1 to 2 mg/kg/d should be considered.

5. Supportive measures include replenishment of iron stores, dietary elimination of lactose, and addition of bulking agents such as psyllium (Metamucil). Antidiarrheal agents can precipitate toxic megacolon and should be avoided.

PSEUDOMEMBRANOUS COLITIS

Pseudomembranous colitis is an inflammatory bowel disorder in which membrane-like yellowish plaques of exudate overlay and replace necrotic intestinal mucosa. Broad-spectrum antibiotics, most notably clindamycin, cephalosporins, and ampicillin/amoxicillin, alter the gut flora in such a way that toxin-producing *Clostridium difficile* can flourish within the colon and produce clinical manifestations of pseudomembranous colitis.

Clinical Features

Clinical manifestations can vary from frequent, watery, mucoid stools to a toxic picture, including profuse diarrhea, crampy abdominal pain, fever, leukocytosis, and dehydration. Examination of the stool may show fecal leukocytes.

Diagnosis and Differential

The disease typically begins 7 to 10 days after the institution of antibiotics, but the range is from a few days up to 8 weeks. The diagnosis is confirmed by the demonstration of *C difficile* in the stool and by the detection of toxin in stool filtrates. Colonoscopy is not routinely needed to confirm the diagnosis.

Emergency Department Care and Disposition

The treatment of pseudomembranous colitis includes discontinuing antibiotic therapy, initiating intravenous fluid replacement, and correcting electrolyte abnormalities. This is effective without additional treatment in 25% of patients.

1. Oral **metronidazole** 250 mg 4 times daily is the treatment of choice in patients with mild to moderate disease who do not respond to supportive measures. **Vancomycin** 125 to 250 mg 4 times daily should be reserved for patients who have not responded to or are intolerant of metronidazole and for children and pregnant patients.

2. Patients with severe diarrhea, those with a systemic response (eg, fever, leukocytosis, or severe abdominal pain), and those whose symptoms persist despite appropriate outpatient management must be hospitalized and should receive vancomycin 125 to 250 mg 4 times daily for 10 days. The symptoms usually resolve within a few days.
3. Antidiarrheal agents may prolong or worsen symptoms and should be avoided.

Relapses occur in 10% to 20% of patients.

DIVERTICULITIS

Diverticulitis is caused by bacterial proliferation within an existing colonic diverticulum, leading to microperforation and inflammation of pericolonic tissue. Clinical diverticulitis occurs in 10% to 25% of patients with diverticulosis. One third of the US population will have acquired diverticulosis by age 50 years and two thirds by 85 years. Only 2% to 4% of patients with diverticulitis are younger than 40 years, but the younger age group tends to have a more virulent form of the disease, with frequent complications requiring earlier surgical intervention.

Clinical Features

The most common symptom is a steady, deep discomfort in the left lower quadrant of the abdomen. Other symptoms include tenesmus and changes in bowel habits, such as diarrhea or increasing constipation. The involved diverticulum can irritate the urinary tract and cause frequency, dysuria, or pyuria. If a fistula develops between the colon and the bladder, the patient may present with recurrent urinary tract infections or pneumaturia. Paralytic ileus with abdominal distention, nausea, and vomiting may develop secondary to intraabdominal irritation and peritonitis. Small bowel obstruction and perforation also can occur. Right lower quadrant pain, which may be indistinguishable from acute appendicitis, can occur with ascending colonic diverticular involvement and in patients with a redundant right-side sigmoid colon.

Physical examination frequently demonstrates a low-grade fever, but the temperature may be higher in patients with generalized peritonitis and in those with an abscess. The abdominal examination demonstrates localized tenderness, often with voluntary guarding and rebound tenderness. A fullness or mass may be appreciated over the affected area of colon. Occult blood may be present in the stool. A pelvic examination should be performed in female patients to exclude a gynecologic source of symptoms.

Diagnosis and Differential

The differential diagnosis includes appendicitis, peptic ulcer disease, pelvic inflammatory disease, endometriosis, ischemic colitis, aortic aneurysm, renal calculus, irritable bowel syndrome, lactate intolerance, colon carcinoma, intestinal lymphoma, Kaposi sarcoma, sarcoidosis, collagen vascular disease, irradiation colitis or proctosigmoiditis, fecal impaction, foreign body granuloma, and any bacterial, parasitic, or viral infectious cause.

Laboratory studies should include routine screening blood tests, urinalysis, and an abdominal radiographic series. Leukocytosis is present in only 36% of patients with diverticulitis. The abdominal series may be normal or may demonstrate an associated ileus; partial small bowel obstruction; colonic obstruction; free air indicating bowel perforation; or extraluminal collections of air, suggesting a walled-off abscess. Computerized tomography of the abdomen is the diagnostic procedure of choice and may demonstrate diverticula, inflammation of pericolic fat, bowel wall thickening, or peri-diverticular abscess.

Emergency Department Care and Disposition

Initial resuscitation of patients should include appropriate fluid and electrolyte replacement and focus on determining the severity of the illness. If a patient has systemic signs and symptoms of infection, has failed outpatient management, or demonstrates signs of peritonitis, hospitalization and surgical consultation are indicated.

1. Inpatient treatment includes intravenous antibiotics, usually an aminoglycoside, such as **gentamicin** or **tobramycin** 1.5 mg/kg every 8 hours and **metronidazole** 500 mg every 8 hours or **clindamycin** 300 to 600 mg every 6 hours, for aerobic and anaerobic organism coverage. Ticarcillin-clavulanic acid or imipenem has been used as an alternate agent.
2. The patient is placed on bowel rest, nothing by mouth is given, and intravenous fluids are administered. Nasogastric suction may be indicated in patients with bowel obstruction or adynamic ileus.
3. Outpatient management is acceptable for patients with localized pain without signs and symptoms of local peritonitis or systemic infection. Treatment consists of bowel rest and broad-spectrum oral antibiotic therapy. Common agents effective against aerobic organisms include **ampicillin** 500 mg every 6 hours, **trimethoprim/sulfamethoxazole** 2 tablets every 12 hours, **ciprofloxacin** 500 mg every 12 hours, or **cephalexin** 500 mg every 6 hours. One of these medications is taken in combination with an agent effective against anaerobic organisms, such as **metronidazole** 500 mg every 6 to 8 hours or **clindamycin** 300 mg every 6 hours. Patients should limit activity and maintain a liquid diet for 48 hours. If symptoms improve, low-residue foods are added to the diet. Patients are advised to contact their physicians or return to the emergency department if they develop increasing abdominal pain or fever or are unable to tolerate oral intake.

For further reading in *Emergency Medicine: A Comprehensive Study Guide,* 6th ed., see Chap. 80, "Ileitis, Colitis, and Diverticulitis," by Howard A. Werman, Hagop, S. Mekhjian, and Douglas A. Rund.

45 | Anorectal Disorders

N. Heramba Prasad

Anorectal disorders may be due to local disease processes or underlying serious systemic disorders. Whenever a patient has rectal bleeding or pain, the following disorders should be considered. (Anorectal manifestations of sexually transmitted diseases are discussed in Chap. 86.)

ANATOMY

The entodermal rectum begins at the third sacral level and is about 15 cm long. It joins the ectodermal anal canal at the dentate line, at approximately 4 cm from the anal verge. The rectal ampulla narrows proximal to the dentate line, causing the mucosa to form 8 to 14 pleated columns of Morgagni. At the dentate line, the columns form small anal crypts. These crypts sometimes contain small anal glands that extend through the internal sphincter. The submucosa of the rectum contains blood vessels that thicken at the dentate line, forming the internal hemorrhoidal plexus. The inner circular muscle layer of the rectum forms the internal sphincter. Voluntary muscles of the pelvic floor, levator ani, and puborectalis form the external sphincter (Fig. 45-1).

Examination

After a detailed history, a digital examination of the rectum should be performed, followed by anoscopy or rectosigmoidoscopy. Patients should be placed in 1 of 3 positions for anoscopy:

1. The left lateral or Sim position, with the left leg extended and the right leg flexed at the knee and hip, is probably the most common position used in the emergency department (ED).
2. The supine or lithotomy position should be used for debilitated patients.
3. The knee-to-chest position in patients who are cooperative provides for a thorough examination.

HEMORRHOIDS

Engorgement, prolapse, or thrombosis of the internal hemorrhoidal veins or the external hemorrhoidal veins is termed *hemorrhoids*. Internal hemorrhoids are not readily palpable and are best visualized through an anoscope. They are constant in location and are found at 2, 5, and 9 o'clock positions when patients are prone. Constipation and straining at stool, pregnancy, ascites, ovarian tumors, radiation fibrosis, and increased portal venous pressure are some of the common causes of hemorrhoids. Tumors of the rectum and sigmoid colon should be considered in patients older than 40 years.

Clinical Features

Painless, self-limited, bright red rectal bleeding is the usual symptom in uncomplicated hemorrhoids. Pain usually is associated with thrombosed hemorrhoids. Large hemorrhoids may result in prolapse that may spontaneously reduce or require periodic manual reduction by patients (second- and third-degree hemorrhoids, respectively). They may become incarcerated and

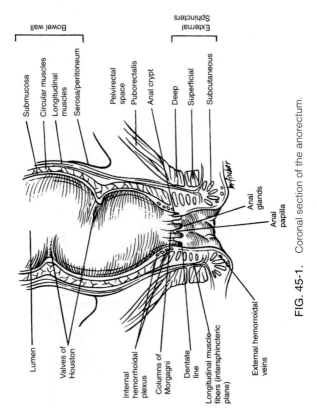

FIG. 45-1.   Coronal section of the anorectum.

gangrenous, requiring surgical intervention. Prolapse may cause mucous discharge and pruritus. Strangulation, severe bleeding, and thrombosis are common complications.

Emergency Department Care and Disposition

Unless a complication is present, management is usually nonsurgical.

1. Hot sitz baths for at least 15 minutes, 3 times per day, and after each bowel movement will ameliorate pain and swelling. After the sitz baths, the anus should be gently but thoroughly dried. Use of topical steroids and analgesics may provide temporary relief.
2. Bulk laxatives, such as psyllium seed compounds or stool softeners, should be used after the acute phase has subsided. Laxatives causing liquid stool are best avoided because they may result in cryptitis and sepsis.
3. Surgical treatment for hemorrhoids is indicated for severe, intractable pain, continued bleeding, incarceration, or strangulation.
4. Acute and recently thrombosed painful hemorrhoids should he treated with excision of the clots. After analgesia with appropriate conscious sedation and local infiltration with 1% lidocaine, an elliptical skin incision is made over the hemorrhoids and the thrombosed vein is removed with the elliptical skin (Fig. 45-2). Packing and a pressure dressing usually will control the bleeding. The pressure dressing may be removed after about 6 hours, when the patient takes the first sitz bath.

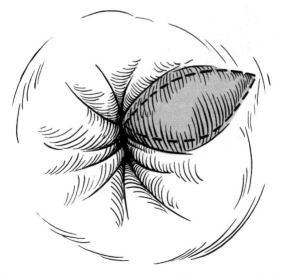

FIG. 45-2. Elliptical excision of thrombosed external hemorrhoid. (From Goldberg SM et al: *Essentials of Anorectal Surgery.* Philadelphia, Lippincott, 1980. With permission.)

CRYPTITIS

Sphincter spasm and repeated trauma from large hard stools cause breakdown of the mucosa over the crypts. This may lead to inflamed anal glands and abscess formation, fissures, and fistulae.

Clinical Features

Anal pain, especially with bowel movements, and itching, with or without bleeding, are the usual symptoms of cryptitis. Diagnosis is confirmed by palpation of tender, swollen crypts with associated hypertrophied papillae. The anoscope provides definitive diagnosis. The crypts commonly involved are in the posterior midline of the anal ring.

Emergency Department Care and Disposition

Bulk laxatives, additional roughage, hot sitz baths, and warm rectal irrigations will enhance healing. Surgical treatment may he needed in refractory cases.

FISSURE IN ANO

Anal fissures are superficial linear tears of the anal canal and are the most common cause of painful rectal bleeding. Swelling of the surrounding tissues produces hypertrophied papillae proximally and sentinel pile distally. Most anal fissures occur in the midline posteriorly. A fissure not in the midline should alert the physician for other potentially life-threatening causes, such as Crohn disease, ulcerative colitis, carcinomas, lymphomas, syphilis, acquired immunodeficiency syndrome, tuberculosis, and other sexually transmitted diseases such as gonorrhea, chlamydia, and lymphogranuloma venereum.

Clinical Features

Sharp cutting pain occurs with defecation and subsides between bowel movements, which distinguishes fissures from other anorectal disorders. Bleeding is bright and in small quantities. Rectal examination is very painful and often not possible without application of topical anesthetic agents. In many instances, sentinel pile and the distal end of the fissure can be seen after gently retracting the buttocks, and further rectal examination may be deferred.

Emergency Department Care and Disposition

Treatment is aimed at relieving sphincter spasm and pain and preventing stricture formation. Hot sitz baths and the addition of bran (fiber) to the diet are helpful. Use of topical analgesics or steroids may be temporarily helpful. Surgical excision of the fissure may be required if the area does not heal after adequate treatment.

ANORECTAL ABSCESSES

Abscesses start from the anal crypts and spread to involve the perianal, intersphincteric, ischiorectal, or deep perianal space. Perianal abscess is the most common form seen at the anal verge. When not associated with any other perirectal infection or systemic symptoms, perianal abscess is the only one that may be safely incised in the ED. Perirectal abscesses such as supralevator or ischiorectal abscesses should be drained in the operating room.

Clinical Features

Pain can be dull, aching, or throbbing and becomes worse before defecation, but persists between bowel movements. Fever and leukocytosis may be present.

Emergency Department Care and Disposition

Most abscesses should be drained in the operating room. Simple perianal abscesses may be drained in the ED if surgical consultation is not readily available. After adequate local analgesia with conscious sedation, a cruciate incision is made over the abscess, and the "dog ears" are excised. Packing usually is not required. Sitz baths should be started the next day. Antibiotics usually are not necessary unless systemic infection or toxicity is present.

FISTULA IN ANO

Fistulae commonly result from perianal or ischiorectal abscess. Crohn disease, ulcerative colitis, tuberculosis, gonococcal proctitis, and carcinomas should be considered in the etiology. Persistent bloody, malodorous discharge occurs as long as the fistula remains open. Blockage of the tract causes recurrent bouts of abscess formation. Ultrasonography with a 7-MHz endoprobe may aid in the diagnosis.

Emergency Department Care and Disposition

Surgical excision is the definitive treatment. Sitz baths and local cleaning will temporize the condition before surgery.

RECTAL PROLAPSE

Prolapse (procidentia) may involve the mucosa alone or all layers of the rectum. In addition, intussusception of the rectum may present as a prolapse.

Clinical Features

Most patients will complain of protruding mass, mucous discharge, associated bleeding, and pruritus.

Emergency Department Care and Disposition

In children, under proper analgesia and sedation, the prolapse can be gently reduced. Every effort should be made to prevent the child from being constipated. Surgical correction is usually necessary in all other age groups unless the prolapse is minimal.

RECTAL FOREIGN BODIES
Emergency Department Care and Disposition

Some rectal foreign bodies, if they are low lying, can be removed in the ED. All others require surgical intervention. If the size and shape are such that perforation is suspected, a follow-up proctoscopy or x-ray may be required. Adequate sphincter relaxation is essential for removal of foreign bodies. Local infiltration anesthesia injected through a 30-gauge needle into the internal sphincter muscle circumferentially will provide good relaxation. The examiner's finger in the rectum will help guide the needle into the sphincter.

Intravenous sedation also may be considered. Large bulbar objects may create a vacuum-like effect proximally, making removal by simple traction impossible. In these cases, the vacuum can be overcome by passing a catheter around the foreign body into the ampulla and injecting air. Occasionally, passing a Foley catheter proximal to the foreign body, inflating the balloon, and applying gentle traction may help maneuver the foreign body into a more desirable position for ease of removal.

PILONIDAL SINUS

These cysts occur in the midline in the upper part of the natal cleft. Pilonidal abscesses may be mistaken for perirectal abscesses. Pilonidal sinus is considered to be an acquired problem. It is caused by foreign body granuloma reaction to ingrown hair. It most commonly occurs in white males before the fourth decade of life.

Clinical Features

Swelling, pain, and persistent discharge are the usual complaints. An abscess may present as a tender indurated mass with different degrees of fluctuation.

Emergency Department Care and Disposition

Acute infections may be drained in the ED and packed. The patient is placed prone and the buttocks are retracted. After appropriate sedation and local anesthesia, the abscess is drained and loculations are gently broken. The wound is packed loosely with gauze, and a bulky dressing is applied. The patient is advised to start sitz baths the following day. Antibiotics or cultures usually are not necessary, unless the patient is immunocompromised.

ANORECTAL TUMORS

The most common (80%) and most aggressive anorectal tumor is the anal canal tumor located proximal to the dentate line and including the transitional zone of epithelium. Neoplasms that occur in this group include adenocarcinoma, malignant melanoma, and Kaposi sarcoma.

Clinical Features

Patients present with nonspecific symptoms including sensation of a mass, pruritus, pain, and blood on the stool. Constipation, anorexia, and weight loss, narrowing of the stool caliber, and tenesmus eventually develops. An anal margin neoplasm frequently will present as an ulcer that fails to heal in a timely manner.

Diagnosis and Differential

Tumors may be misdiagnosed as hemorrhoids. Complications of anorectal tumors include rectal prolapse, prolonged blood loss, perirectal abscesses, or fistulas.

Emergency Department Care and Disposition

Referral for proctoscopic or sigmoidoscopic examination and biopsy is mandatory.

PRURITUS ANI

Although primary or idiopathic pruritus does occur, other causes should be ruled out. These include fissures, fistulae, hemorrhoids, and prolapse; dietary factors such as caffeine, milk, chocolate, tomatoes, citrus fruits; and pin-worms, *Candida trichophyton,* and local irritants. Treatment will depend on the underlying condition.

For further reading in *Emergency Medicine: A Comprehensive Study Guide,* 6th ed., see Chap. 82, "Anorectal Disorders," by Brian E.Burgess and James K Bouzoukis.

Jonathan A. Maisel

Although vomiting, diarrhea, and constipation are typically due to gastrointestinal disorders, the clinician also must consider systemic causes. Careful evaluation will allow the clinician to determine the presence of a benign condition requiring symptomatic relief or an emergent condition requiring surgical intervention.

VOMITING AND DIARRHEA

Clinical Features

Vomiting

History is essential in determining the cause of vomiting. Vomiting with blood could represent gastritis, peptic ulcer disease, or carcinoma. However, aggressive nonbloody vomiting followed by hematemesis is more consistent with a Mallory-Weiss tear. The presence of bile rules out gastric outlet obstruction, such as from pyloric stenosis or strictures. An associated symptom such as fever would direct one to an infectious or inflammatory cause. Vomiting with chest pain suggests myocardial infarction or pneumonia. Vomiting with back pain may be seen with aortic aneurysm or dissection, pancreatitis, pyelonephritis, or renal colic. Headache with vomiting suggests increased intracranial pressure, such as with subarachnoid hemorrhage or head injury. Vomiting in a pregnant patient is consistent with hyperemesis gravidarum in the first trimester; but in the third trimester it could represent preeclampsia if accompanied by hypertension. Associated medical conditions are also useful in discerning the cause of vomiting: diabetes mellitus suggests ketoacidosis, peripheral vascular disease suggests mesenteric ischemia, previous abdominal surgery suggests intestinal obstruction, and medication use (eg, lithium or digoxin) suggests toxicity.

The physical examination in a vomiting patient includes a careful assessment of the gastrointestinal, pelvic, and genitourinary systems. In addition, assessment of hydration status is important. Other clues to specific causes for vomiting may come from the dermal examination (eg, hyperpigmentation with Addison disease) or pulmonary examination (eg, signs of consolidation suggesting pneumonia).

Diarrhea

By definition, diarrhea represents a daily stool output larger than 200 g but generally refers to any increase in frequency or liquidity. Other important historical factors include duration of illness and presence of blood. Acute diarrhea briefer than 2 to 3 weeks' duration is more likely to represent a serious cause, such as infection, ischemia, intoxication, or inflammation. Associated factors, such as fever, pain, presence of blood, or type of food ingested, may help in the diagnosis of infectious gastroenteritis or diverticulitis. Neurologic symptoms may be seen in certain diarrheal illnesses, such as seizure with shigellosis or theophylline toxicity or paresthesias with ciguatoxin.

Details about the host also can better define the diagnosis. Malabsorption from pancreatic insufficiency or bowel disorders related to the human immunodeficiency virus need not be considered in a healthy host. Dietary practices, including frequent restaurant meals, exposure to day care centers, consumption of street-vendor food or raw seafood, overseas travel, and camping with the ingestion of lake or stream water, may isolate the vector and narrow the differential diagnosis for infectious diarrhea (eg, oysters suggest *Vibrio;* rice suggests *Bacillus cereus;* eggs suggest *Salmonella;* and meat suggests *Campylobacter, Staphylococcus, Yersinia, Escherichia coli,* or *Clostridium*). Certain medications, particularly antibiotics, colchicine, lithium, and laxatives, can contribute to diarrhea. Travel may predispose the patient to enterotoxigenic *E coli* or *Giardia.* Social history, such as sexual preference, drug use, and occupation, may suggest diagnoses such as illness related to the human immunodeficiency virus or organophosphate poisoning.

The physical examination initially usually concentrates on assessment of hydration status. Abdominal examination can narrow the differential diagnosis and show the need for surgical intervention. Even appendicitis can present with diarrhea in up to 20% of cases. Rectal examination can rule out impaction or presence of blood, with the latter suggesting inflammation, infection, or mesenteric ischemia.

Diagnosis and Differential

A mnemonic to prompt the physician's recall of disease groupings causing vomiting and diarrhea is GASTROENTERITIS: gastrointestinal diseases, appendicitis or aorta, specific disease (eg, glaucoma), trauma, medications (Rx), obstetric and gynecologic disorders, endocrine disorders, neurologic disease, toxicology, environmental disorders, renal disease, infection, tumors, ischemia, and supratentorial.

Vomiting

All women of childbearing potential warrant a pregnancy test. In vomiting associated with abdominal pain, liver function tests, urinalysis, and lipase or amylase determinations may be useful. Electrolyte determinations and renal function tests are usually of benefit only in patients with severe dehydration or prolonged vomiting. In addition, they may confirm Addisonian crisis with hyperkalemia and hyponatremia. The electrocardiogram and chest radiograph can be reserved for patients with suspected ischemia or pulmonary infection. An acute abdominal series can be used to confirm the presence of obstruction.

Diarrhea

The most specific tests in diarrheal illness involve examination of the stool in the laboratory. Wright stain for fecal leukocytes has an 82% sensitivity and 83% specificity for the presence of invasive bacterial pathogens. Current therapeutic strategies, however, suggest that this test is no longer useful. Stool culture is expensive and labor intensive. To limit cost and increase yield, testing should be limited to severely dehydrated or toxic patients, children, immunocompromised patients, and those with diarrhea lasting longer than 3 days. In addition, it may be useful for patients involved in public health–sensitive occupations. In patients with chronic persistent diarrhea, an examination for ova and parasites may be useful to rule out *Giardia* or *Cryptosporidium.* Assay for *Clostridium difficile* toxin may be useful in ill patients with antibiotic-associated diarrhea. Because of the low sensitivity and delay in results, laboratory testing in routine diarrheal cases is not indicated.

General laboratory testing in patients with diarrhea is usually unnecessary. However, in extremely dehydrated or toxic patients, electrolyte determinations and renal function tests may be useful. (Hemolytic-uremic syndrome, characterized by acute renal failure, thrombocytopenia, and hemolytic anemia, may complicate *E coli* 0157:H7 infections in children and the elderly.) If toxicity is suspected, tests for levels for theophylline, lithium, or heavy metals will aid in the diagnosis. Radiographs are reserved for ruling out intestinal obstruction or pneumonia, in particular *Legionella*. In addition, angiography may be indicated in acute mesenteric ischemia.

Emergency Department Care and Disposition.

The treatment of vomiting and diarrhea consists of correcting fluid and electrolyte problems. In addition, one must initiate specific therapy for any life-threatening cause identified in the initial workup of vomiting and diarrhea.

1. Replacement of fluids can be intravenous (IV; bolus 500 mL IV in adults, 10–20 mL/kg in children), with normal saline solution in seriously ill patients. Mildly dehydrated patients may tolerate an oral rehydrating solution containing sodium (at least 45 mEq/L in children) and glucose to enhance fluid absorption. The World Health Organization advocates a mixture of 1 c (0.24 L) orange juice, 4 tsp (20 mL) sugar, 1 tsp (5 mL) baking powder, and 3/4 tsp (3.75 mL) salt in 1 L boiled water. The goal is 50 to 100 mL/kg over the first 4 hours.

2. Nutritional supplementation should be started as soon as nausea and vomiting subside. Patients can quickly advance from clear liquids to solids, such as rice and bread. Patients may benefit from avoiding raw fruit, caffeine, and lactose- and sorbitol-containing products.

3. Antibiotics are recommended for adult patients with severe or prolonged diarrhea. In addition, they are indicated for travelers from tropical or Third World countries. Although single-dose fluoroquinolones show some effectiveness, **ciprofloxacin** 500 mg orally (PO) twice daily for 3 days is recommended. Although inferior, **trimethoprim-sulfamethoxazole** (TMP-SMX), TMP:SMX 10:50 mg/kg/d (maximum dose, TMP:SMX 160:800 mg) for 3 days is indicated for children or nursing mothers, if antibiotics are truly necessary. It should be noted that antibiotics are of questionable value in infectious diarrhea from *E coli* O157:H7.

4. **Metronidazole** 250 to 750 mg PO 3 times daily for 5 to 14 days is indicated for *C difficile*, *Giardia*, or *Entamoeba* infection. Antibiotics are especially indicated in patients or workers in the food industry or institutional settings, such as day care centers and nursing homes.

5. Antidiarrheal agents, especially in combination with antibiotics, have been shown to shorten the course of diarrhea. **Loperamide** is given 4 mg PO initially and then 2 mg PO after each diarrheal stool, to a maximum of 16 mg/d (for children older than 2 years, 1–2 mg 2–3 times daily on day 1 and then 0.1 mg/kg after each loose stool). **Diphenoxylate and atropine** 1 to 2 tablets PO every 6 hours for 2 days or less may be helpful for more severe diarrhea.

6. Antiemetic agents are useful in actively vomiting patients with dehydration (see Chap. 74 for recommendations in children). **Promethazine** 25 mg intramuscularly (IM) or rectally (PR) every 6 hours is prescribed.

Prochlorperazine 5 to 10 mg IV or IM or 25 mg PR every 6 to 8 hours is effective. **Metoclopramide** 5 to 10 mg IV or IM every 6 to 8 hours is useful and can be given in pregnancy (category B). For severe or refractory cases, **ondansetron** 4 to 8 mg IV may be used.

Patients with a life-threatening cause of vomiting or diarrhea require admission. In addition, toxic or severely dehydrated patients, in particular infants and the elderly, or those still intolerant of oral fluids after hydration warrant admission. Patients with an unclear diagnosis but favorable examination findings after hydration can be discharged home safely with antiemetics. Work excuses are indicated for patients in the food, day care, and health care industries.

CONSTIPATION

Clinical Features

Constipation is the most common digestive complaint in the United States. Constipation is demonstrated by the presence of hard stools that are difficult to pass. Acute onset implies obstruction until proven otherwise. Chronic constipation is less ominous and can be managed on an outpatient basis. Associated symptoms such as vomiting and inability to pass flatus confirm obstruction. Associated illnesses can help disclose the underlying diagnosis: cold intolerance (hypothyroidism), diverticulitis (inflammatory stricture), or nephrolithiasis (hyperparathyroidism).

Physical examination should focus on detection of hernias or abdominal masses. Rectal examination will detect masses such as fecal impaction, anal fissures, or fecal blood. Fecal blood accompanied by weight loss or decreasing stool caliber suggests colon carcinoma. Fecal impaction can cause rectal bleeding from stercoral ulcers. The presence of ascites in postmenopausal women raises suspicion of ovarian or uterine carcinoma.

Diagnosis and Differential

Directed testing in acute constipation, based on suspicion, can include a complete blood count (to rule out anemia), thyroid panel (to rule out hypothyroidism), and electrolyte determinations (to rule out hypokalemia or hypercalcemia). Flat and erect abdominal films may be useful in confirming obstruction or assessing stool burden.

The differential diagnosis for constipation is extensive, reflecting issues related to diet, exercise, disability, medications, and gastrointestinal and systemic illness. Chronic constipation is a functional disorder that can be worked up on an outpatient basis. Nevertheless, complications of chronic constipation, such as fecal impaction and intestinal pseudoobstruction, will require manual, colonoscopic, or surgical intervention.

Emergency Department Care and Disposition

Treatment of functional constipation is directed at symptomatic relief and addressing lifestyle issues. Occasionally, specific treatment is required for complications of constipation or for underlying disorders that can lead to organic constipation.

1. The most important prescription for functional constipation is a dietary and exercise regimen that includes fluids (1.5 L/d), fiber (10 g/d), and

exercise. Fiber in the form of bran, 1 c/d, or **psyllium,** 1 tsp 3 times daily, increases stool volume and gut motility.

2. Medications can provide temporary relief for this chronic problem. Stimulants can be given PO, as with an **anthraquinone** (eg, **Peri-Colace** 1-2 tablets PO at bedtime), or PR, as with **bisacodyl,** 10 mg 3 times daily in adults or children. In the absence of renal failure, saline laxatives such as **milk of magnesia** 15 to 30 mL PO 1 to 2 times daily or **magnesium citrate** 200 mL PO once are useful. Hyperosmolar agents, such as **lactulose or sorbitol** 15 to 30 mL PO twice daily also may be helpful. In children, **glycerin rectal suppositories or mineral oil** (age 5-11 years: 5-15 mL PO daily; age >12 years: 15-45 mL PO daily) have been advocated.

3. **Enemas of soapsuds** 1,500 mL PR or **phosphate** (eg, **Fleets** 1 U PR; 1 oz [30 mL]/10 kg in children) are generally reserved for severe cases or after fecal disimpaction. Use care to avoid rectal perforation.

4. Fecal impaction should be removed manually by using local anesthetic lubricant. In female patients, transvaginal pressure with the other hand may be helpful. An enema or suppositories to complete evacuation can follow.

All patients with apparent functional constipation can be managed as outpatients. Early follow-up is indicated in patients with recent severe constipation or systemic symptoms, such as weight loss, anemia, or change in stool caliber. Patients with organic constipation from obstruction require hospitalization and surgical evaluation. Intestinal pseudoobstruction and sigmoid volvulus sometimes can be corrected colonoscopically.

For further reading in *Emergency Medicine: A Comprehensive Study Guide,* 6th ed., see Chap. 79, "Vomiting, Diarrhea, and Constipation," by Annie Tewel Sadosty and Brain J. Browne.

47 | Jaundice, Hepatic Disorders, and Hepatic Failure

Gregory S. Hall

JAUNDICE

Jaundice, a yellowish discoloration of the skin, sclerae, and mucous membranes, results from hyperbilirubinemia (breakdown of hemoglobin) and thus the deposition of bile pigments. It has many etiologies (Table 47-1). Hyperbilirubinemia can be divided into 2 types. The unconjugated form results from increased bilirubin production or a liver defect in its uptake or conjugation. The conjugated form occurs in the setting of intra- or extrahepatic cholestasis, resulting in decreased excretion of conjugated bilirubin. The total serum bilirubin should be elevated in a jaundiced patient. Clinically, jaundice usually becomes noticeable at a serum bilirubin level of 2.0 to 2.5 mg/dL and is often first seen in the sclera. An indirect fraction of serum bilirubin of 85% or higher is consistent with the unconjugated type, whereas a direct fraction of 30% or above indicates the conjugated form. Conjugated bilirubin is water soluble and is detectable in the urine even with low serum levels.

Clinical Features

Sudden onset of jaundice in a previously healthy young person and a prodrome of fever, malaise, myalgias, and a tender enlarged liver point to hepatitis (probably viral) as a likely cause. Heavy ethanol use suggests alcoholic hepatitis. In the setting of alcoholic liver disease and cirrhosis, jaundice usually develops gradually. A family history of jaundice or a history of recurrent mild jaundice that spontaneously resolves usually accompanies inherited causes of jaundice such as Gilbert syndrome. Cholecystitis may not cause jaundice unless there is acute biliary obstruction present, such as with a retained common bile duct gallstone. Painless jaundice in an older patient classically suggests pancreatic or hepatobiliary malignancy. Patients with a known prior malignancy and a hard, nodular liver accompanied by jaundice are likely to be found to have liver metastases. Biliary tract scarring or strictures always must be suspected as a cause of jaundice in patients with a prior history of biliary tract surgery, pancreatitis, cholangitis, or inflammatory bowel disease. Hepatomegaly with jaundice, accompanied by pedal edema, jugular venous distention, and a gallop rhythm suggest chronic heart failure.

Diagnosis and Differential

Initial laboratory tests that should be obtained in the workup of a jaundiced patient include serum bilirubin level (total and direct fractions; indirect fraction can be deduced by simple subtraction), serum aminotransferases and alkaline phosphatase levels, urinalysis to check for bilirubin and urobilinogen, and a complete blood count (CBC). Additional laboratory tests may be indicated based on the clinical setting (serum amylase and lipase levels, prothrombin time [PT], electrolytes and glucose levels, serum urea nitrogen [BUN] and creatinine levels, viral hepatitis panels, drug levels, and pregnancy test). With normal liver enzyme levels, the jaundice is more likely to be

TABLE 47-1 Causes of Jaundice
Disorders of bilirubin metabolism
Neonatal jaundice
Hemolysis
Hemoglobinopathy
Transfusion reaction
Inborn errors of metabolism
Hepatocellular causes
Infections
Viral hepatitis
Leptospirosis
Infectious mononucleosis
Drugs and toxins
Ethanol
Acetaminophen
Amanita toxin
Carbon tetrachloride
Anabolic steroids
Chlorpromazine
Isoniazid
Metabolic
Wilson disease
Reye syndrome
Hemachromatosis
Granulomatous
Wegener granulomatosis
Sarcoidosis
Lymphoma
Mycobacterial
Miscellaneous
Fatty liver of pregnancy
Ischemia
Primary biliary cirrhosis
Benign recurrent intrahepatic cholestasis
Postoperative cholestasis
Amyloidosis
Bile duct obstruction
Gallstones
AIDS cholangiopathy
Primary sclerosing cholangitis
Bile duct stricture
Pancreatic tumors or cysts
Pancreatitis
Cholangiocarcinoma

Key: AIDS = acquired immunodeficiency syndrome.

caused by sepsis or systemic infection, inborn errors of metabolism, or pregnancy, rather than by primary hepatic disease. With abnormally elevated liver enzymes, the pattern of abnormalities may suggest the etiology. Aminotransferase elevation, if predominant, suggests hepatocellular diseases such as viral or toxic hepatitis or cirrhosis, whereas markedly elevated alkaline phosphatase levels (2 to 3 times that of normal levels) and gamma-glutamyl transferase (GGT) points to intra- or extrahepatic obstruction (gallstones, stricture, or malignancy). A Coombs test and hemoglobin electrophoresis may be useful if anemia is present, in addition to normal liver aminotransferase levels (hemolysis and hemoglobinopathy). If clinical features and initial laboratory results indicate conjugated hyperbilirubinemia, ultrasound studies of the biliary tract, liver, and pancreas should be performed to rule out gallstones, dilated extrahepatic biliary ducts, or mass or tumor in the liver, pancreas, and portal region. Computed tomography also may be considered but is often more costly and not as sensitive as ultrasound for detection of gallstones in the gallbladder.

Emergency Department Care and Disposition

1. Jaundice by itself is not an adequate justification for hospital admission.
2. In some situations, discharge from the emergency department pending further outpatient workup may be appropriate, if a patient is hemodynamically stable with new onset jaundice and has no evidence of liver failure or acute biliary obstruction, and if appropriate laboratory studies have been ordered, timely follow-up is available, and the patient is reliable and has adequate social support.
3. If extrahepatic biliary obstruction is suspected, surgical consultation should be obtained in the emergency department.

HEPATITIS

Hepatitis is defined by liver inflammation with hepatocellular necrosis. In the United States, it is commonly associated with viral infection or ethanol use (and other toxins; see Chapters 98-118 on toxicology). Risk factors for viral hepatitis include male homosexuality, hemodialysis, intravenous (IV) drug abuse, raw seafood ingestion, blood product transfusion, tattoos or body piercing, needle punctures, foreign travel, or close contact with an infected source patient. Viral- and toxin-induced hepatitis may lead to fulminant hepatic failure, chronic liver disease, cirrhosis, and end-stage liver disease. In the United States, the majority (50%) of cases of end-stage liver disease results from alcohol abuse. The remainder of this section focuses on viral hepatitis, and the next section deals with alcohol hepatitis and cirrhosis.

Clinical Features

Viral hepatitis may range in severity from asymptomatic infection to fulminant hepatic failure to chronic cirrhosis. Symptomatic patients usually report sudden or insidious onset of prodrome of anorexia, nausea, emesis, fatigue, malaise, and altered taste. Low-grade fever, accompanied by pharyngitis, coryza, and headache, may confuse the picture and lead to an initial misdiagnosis of upper respiratory infection or flulike illness. A few days of generalized pruritus and dark urine may precede the onset of gastrointestinal (GI) symptoms and jaundice. Malaise usually persists, whereas the other prodromal symptoms resolve. Right upper quadrant pain with an enlarged tender liver and splenomegaly may be found. Many patients do *not* become clinically jaundiced, and most will recover gradually over the ensuing 3 to 4 months. Rarely, fulminant hepatic failure develops with a clinical picture of encephalopathy, coagulopathy, and rapidly worsening jaundice. Chronic persistent infection (usually with hepatitis B or C) can lead to the development of cirrhosis with gradual jaundice, ascites, peripheral edema, and liver failure over a period of 10 to 20 years.

Hepatitis A is transmitted predominantly by the fecal oral route and is commonly seen in Americans. Hepatitis B is acquired primarily via a percutaneous exposure to infected blood or body fluids. An effective vaccine against hepatitis B has resulted in a decline in the prevalence of hepatitis in the US population. Hepatitis C is the most common of all blood-borne infections in the United States and may be contracted via parenteral, sexual, and perinatal contacts. Unfortunately, chronic hepatitis C infection occurs in 85% of patients and up to 70% progress to cirrhosis and end-stage liver disease.

Diagnosis and Differential

Establishment of a diagnosis of viral hepatitis depends primarily on liver function abnormalities coupled with the clinical picture. Serum transaminase levels (GGT, aspartate aminotransferase [AST], and alanine aminotransferase [ALT]) should be checked because elevations are suggestive of hepatitis. Values in the hundreds of units per liter are consistent with viral inflammation, but elevations into the thousands suggest hepatocellular necrosis, extensive liver injury, and more fulminant disease. In acute and chronic viral hepatitis, the ratio of AST to ALT is usually less than 1 (whereas a ratio greater than 2 is more suggestive of alcoholic hepatitis). Serum alkaline phosphatase level also should be determined; if elevated more than 3-fold above normal, cholestasis should be suspected (a concurrently elevated GGT supports this suspicion). Total serum bilirubin level and its direct fraction (indirect fraction can be deduced by simple subtraction) also may be useful because a conjugated (direct) fraction of 30% or higher is consistent with viral hepatitis. However, the magnitude of transaminase elevation is not a reliable marker of disease severity, but a persistent total bilirubin level above 20 mg/dL or a PT prolonged by more than a few seconds indicates a poor prognosis (hence, PT time should be checked). Serum electrolytes, BUN, and creatinine levels should be checked if there is clinical suspicion of volume depletion or electrolyte abnormalities. Abnormal mental status should prompt an immediate determination of serum glucose level, which may be low due to poor oral intake or hepatic failure. (Other causes of abnormal mental status such as hypoxia, sepsis, intoxication, structural intracranial process, or encephalopathy must be considered.) A CBC may be useful because an early transient neutropenia followed by a relative lymphocytosis with atypical forms is often seen with viral hepatitis. Anemia, if present, may be more suggestive of alcoholic hepatitis, decompensated cirrhosis, GI bleeding, or a hemolytic process. Serologic studies to determine the specific viral agent responsible may be ordered in the emergency department to facilitate the final diagnosis, but these results are rarely immediately available and thus play no significant role in emergency department management. Important differential diagnoses include alcohol- or toxin-induced hepatitis, infectious mononucleosis, cholecystitis, ascending cholangitis, sarcoidosis, lymphoma, liver metastases, and pancreatic or biliary tumors.

Emergency Department Care and Disposition

Supportive care is the mainstay of therapy for acute viral hepatitis.

1. Most patients can be managed successfully as outpatients with emphasis on rest, adequate oral intake, strict personal hygiene, and avoidance of hepatotoxins (ethanol and drugs). Patients should be instructed to return for worsening symptoms, in particular vomiting, fever, jaundice, or abdominal pain. Follow-up arrangements should be made.

2. There is no antiviral therapy recommended for acute viral hepatitis. Patients with chronic viral hepatitis B are treated with lamivudine or interferon. Patients with chronic viral hepatitis C may be treated with pegylated interferon or standard interferon plus ribavirin.
3. Patients with any of the following should be admitted to the hospital: encephalopathy, PT prolonged by more than a few seconds, intractable vomiting, hypoglycemia, bilirubin level above 20 mg/dL, age older than 45 years, immunosuppression, or suspected toxin-induced hepatitis.
4. Volume depletion and electrolyte imbalances should be corrected with IV crystalloid. Hypoglycemia should be treated initially with 1 ampule of 50% dextrose in water IV followed by the addition of dextrose to IV fluids and careful monitoring.
5. Fulminant hepatic failure should warrant admission to the intensive care unit, with aggressive support of circulation and respiration, monitoring and treatment of increased intracranial pressure if present, correction of hypoglycemia and coagulopathy, administration of oral lactulose or neomycin, and a protein-restricted diet (see the following section on treatment of cirrhosis). Consultations with a hepatologist and liver transplant service are indicated.
6. Glucocorticoid therapy has no value in acute viral hepatitis, even with fulminant hepatic failure, and should be avoided.

ALCOHOLIC LIVER DISEASE AND CIRRHOSIS

Three clinical syndromes best describe liver injury secondary to alcohol: hepatic steatosis (fatty liver), alcoholic hepatitis, and alcoholic cirrhosis. An enlarged, non- or mildly tender liver from steatosis is usually seen in a relatively asymptomatic alcoholic patient. Alcohol-induced hepatitis may present as a very mild or severe acute illness in a chronic alcohol user, whereas cirrhosis from alcohol abuse or other causes represents a chronic process with intermittent exacerbations or associated complications, which usually prompt most emergency department visits.

Clinical Features

Alcoholic hepatitis is typically found in the chronic alcoholic who has gradual onset of anorexia, nausea, fever, dark urine, jaundice, weight loss, abdominal pain, and generalized weakness. Physical examination demonstrates a tender, enlarged liver, low-grade fever, and icteric mucous membranes, sclera, or skin. Patients with cirrhosis generally report a gradual deterioration in their health, with anorexia, muscle loss (often masked by edema or ascites), fatigue, nausea, emesis, diarrhea, and increasing abdominal girth (ascites). Low-grade intermittent or continuous fever also may be present, whereas hypothermia may be seen at end-stage disease. Abdominal palpation may demonstrate a small, firm liver and possibly splenomegaly. Jaundice, pedal edema, ascites, and spider angiomata are also common. Hepatic encephalopathy, characterized by a fluctuating level of consciousness and confusion and, possibly, hyperreflexia, spasticity, and generalize seizures, also may be present. Asterixis ("liver flap") is characteristic but not specific for encephalopathy due to liver failure. Patients with cirrhosis often come to the emergency department because of worsening ascites or edema, complications such as GI or variceal bleeding (see Chap. 37), encephalopathy, spontaneous bacterial peritonitis (abdominal pain), and various concurrent infections (urinary tract infection, pneumonia, etc).

Diagnosis and Differential

Alcoholic hepatitis and cirrhosis may be diagnosed by their clinical features and laboratory findings. Laboratory studies that should be checked include levels of serum transaminases (GGT, ALT, and AST), serum alkaline phosphatase, total bilirubin (and its fractions), serum albumin, serum glucose and electrolytes, BUN and creatinine, CBC, and PT. In the setting of alcoholic hepatitis, serum transaminase levels are usually elevated to a range of 2 to 10 times that of normal, with a AST-to-ALT ratio of 1.5 to 2.0 (AST production is stimulated by ethanol). With cirrhosis, transaminase levels are often only mildly elevated. Alkaline phosphatase and bilirubin levels are usually only mildly elevated with alcoholic hepatitis and cirrhosis. Anemia, leukopenia, and thrombocytopenia are commonly seen in chronic ethanol abusers. If concurrent pancreatitis is suspected, serum lipase and amylase levels should be checked. Fever with or without leukocytosis in a chronic alcoholic warrants a chest radiograph to rule out pneumonia; cultures of blood, urine, and ascitic fluid; and a thorough search for other sources of sepsis (meningitis, cholecystitis, cellulitis, perirectal abscess, etc). Elevated serum ammonia level unfortunately does not correlate well with acute deterioration of liver function due to cirrhosis and, although it may be checked as a marker of encephalopathy, it cannot be used as an index of its severity or response to treatment.

Spontaneous bacterial peritonitis (SBP), the most common complication of cirrhotic ascites, should be suspected in any cirrhotic patient with fever, abdominal pain or tenderness, worsening ascites, subacute functional decline, or encephalopathy. Other subtle clues to SBP include deteriorating renal function, hypothermia, and diarrhea. SBP may be confirmed through sampling of ascitic fluid by paracentesis, ideally under ultrasound guidance to minimize the risk of bowel puncture. Culture results from ascitic fluid are often negative, but placing 10 mL ascitic fluid in a blood culture bottle may improve the yield. Ascitic fluid should be tested for total protein and glucose level, lactate dehydrogenase, Gram stain, and white blood cell count (WBC) with differential. A total WBC larger than $1,000/\mu L$ or neutrophil count larger than $250/\mu L$ is diagnostic for SBP. (A total WBC $>10,000/\mu L$, total protein >1 g/dL, glucose <50 mg/dL, or elevated lactate dehydrogenase point to the possibility of generalized peritonitis due to a local focus of infection, eg, cholecystitis or appendicitis.) Culture results from ascitic fluid are often negative, but placing 10 mL ascitic fluid in a blood culture bottle may improve the yield. Gram-negative Enterobacteriaceae (*Escherichia coli, Klebsiella,* etc) account for 63% of SBP cases, followed by the pneumococcus (15%) and the enterococcus (6% to 10%).

Hepatorenal syndrome, a refractory form of acute renal failure that occurs in cirrhotic patients, may develop in the setting of sepsis, acute dehydration, overzealous diuresis, or high-volume paracentesis. The differential diagnosis includes other forms of hepatitis (drugs, toxins, etc) and other causes of upper abdominal pain (cholecystitis, biliary colic, gastritis or peptic ulcer disease, pancreatitis, etc).

Cirrhosis is often caused by ethanol or chronic viral hepatitis; uncommon causes include drugs or toxins, hemochromatosis, Wilson disease, and primary (idiopathic) biliary cirrhosis.

Emergency Department Care and Disposition

Alcoholic Hepatitis

1. Hospital admission is required for all but the mildest cases of alcoholic hepatitis.
2. Fluid therapy with dextrose-containing IV fluids should be given with the goal of maintaining adequate intravascular volume and avoiding fluid overload in the edematous or ascitic patient. In some cases, central venous pressure monitoring may be needed to help guide fluid therapy. **Thiamine** (100 mg) should always be given with initial IV fluids and dextrose. Vitamin supplements also should be given to any malnourished alcoholic. Correction of electrolyte abnormalities should be initiated (many alcoholic patients will require supplemental magnesium and potassium).
3. Careful attention to any additional drug therapies must be maintained to avoid the use of any hepatotoxic agents and to account for possible alterations in normal drug metabolism. The patient will have to abstain from alcohol and should be monitored for withdrawal symptoms and given prophylactic treatment with a long-acting benzodiazepine such as lorazepam.
4. Identified bacterial coinfections should be treated promptly with appropriate parenteral antibiotics, and broad-spectrum coverage should be initiated in any alcoholic with suspected sepsis, pending culture results (see Chap. 6).

Cirrhosis and Liver Failure

1. Abstinence from alcohol and other hepatotoxins (drugs, etc) is essential for outpatient management. Adjunctive measures may include salt and water restriction, cautious diuretic use (spironolactone), a protein-restricted diet, and therapeutic paracentesis for relief of abdominal distention.
2. Emergency management often includes changing diuretic dosage, correction of fluid or electrolyte abnormalities, and blood transfusion for symptomatic anemia.
3. New onset or worsening encephalopathy warrants hospital admission.
   a. Management includes supplemental oxygen, support of perfusion and respiration, as needed, and supplemental dextrose in IV fluids.
   b. Precipitating factors such as a coexisting infection, GI bleeding, or renal failure must be carefully investigated and aggressively treated.
   c. Lactulose (30 mL syrup or 20 g in water or fruit juice) may be given orally by nasogastric tube or by enema (300 mL syrup diluted with 700 mL water and retained for 30 minutes) up to 3 times a day until 1 to 2 soft stools per day are produced.
   d. Although not necessary in the emergency department, neomycin may be given to help clear the gut of bacteria and nitrogenous products. Rifaximin is an alternative to neomycin and may have less nephrotoxicity and ototoxicity.
4. **Cefotaxime** 2 g IV followed by 1 to 2 g IV every 4 to 6 hours, or **piperacillin-tazobactam** 3.375 g IV every 6 hours, or **ampicillin-sulbactam** 3 g IV every 6 hours, or **ticarcillin-clavulanate** 3.1 g IV every 6 hours, or **ceftriaxone** 2 g IV every 24 hours are acceptable empiric antimicrobial choices for SPB pending culture results. Patients may have had prior infections, and prior culture results with antimicrobial sensitivities should be reviewed if available. If a resistant *E coli* or *Klebsiella* is

suspected, imipenem, meropenem, or a fluoroquinolone should be added to 1 of the above regimens. In addition, albumin 1.5 g/kg IV may be given at the time of diagnosis (and again at 1 g/kg IV on day 3) to stabilize intravascular volume because it may reduce renal failure and hospital mortality.

5. *Gastroesophageal variceal bleeding* should be suspected in any chronic liver patient with hematemesis, melena, or even hematochezia (see Chap. 37 for management).

6. Acute liver failure from any cause (with prolonged PT, hypoglycemia, co-agulopathy, encephalopathy, marked jaundice, etc) should warrant admission to the intensive care unit, aggressive treatment, and consultation with a hepatologist and transplant team, if available.

7. Any cirrhotic patient whose clinical stability is in doubt always should be considered for admission. All patients with clearly decompensated cirrhosis, fever, hypothermia, or complications such as concurrent infection, SBP, GI bleeding, encephalopathy, and acute or worsening renal function should be admitted.

8. Discharged patients should have timely follow-up arranged with their primary care provider and should be given careful instructions to return for any worsening of their baseline status or for symptoms such as abdominal pain, fever, melena, hematemesis, vomiting, worsening diarrhea, or mental status changes.

9. Large-volume paracentesis may be required for patients with cirrhosis or other forms of chronic liver disease who present with tense ascites. This measure may temporarily relieve abdominal pain, anorexia, and dyspnea. Volumes as large as 6 to 9 L have been removed without complication. Ultrasound-guided technique may reduce complications, but this technique is not mandatory.

For further reading in *Emergency Medicine: A Comprehensive Study Guide,* 6th ed., see Chap. 84, "Jaundice," by Richard O. Shields Jr; and Chap. 86, "Hepatic Disorders and Hepatic Failure," by Joshua S. Broder and Rawden Evans.

48 | Cholecystitis and Biliary Colic

Gregory S. Hall

Biliary tract emergencies most often result from obstruction of the gallbladder or biliary duct by gallstones. The 4 most common biliary tract emergencies caused by gallstones are biliary colic, cholecystitis, gallstone pancreatitis, and ascending cholangitis. Biliary colic and cholecystitis are more frequently encountered in patients at emergency departments. Gallstones, although common in the general population, remain asymptomatic in some patients. Classically, the patient with symptomatic gallstone disease is an obese, fertile female between 20 and 40 years of age. Biliary disease, however, affects all age groups, especially diabetics and the elderly. Common risk factors associated with gallstones and cholecystitis include advanced age, female sex and parity, obesity, rapid weight loss or prolonged fasting, familial tendency, oral contraceptive use, clofibrate, ceftriaxone, Asian descent, chronic liver disease, and hemolytic disorders (eg, sickle cell disease).

CLINICAL FEATURES

Patients with acute biliary colic may have a wide range of symptoms; unfortunately, the location, radiation, and duration of the abdominal pain are not reliable guides to the presence of gallbladder disease. Biliary colic may present with epigastric or right upper quadrant pain, may range from mild to severe, and, although classically described as intermittent or colicky, is often constant. Nausea and vomiting are usually present. Pain may be referred to the right shoulder or left upper back. It may begin after eating but bears no association to meals in at least 33% of patients. Acute episodes of biliary colic typically last for 2 to 6 hours, followed by a gradual or sudden resolution of symptoms. Recurrent episodes are usually infrequent, generally at intervals longer than 1 week. Biliary colic seems to follow a circadian pattern, with highest incidence of symptoms between 9 PM and 4 AM. At presentation, physical examination commonly demonstrates right upper quadrant or epigastric tenderness without findings of peritonitis. Volume depletion due to emesis may be evident. Symptoms and findings are easy to confuse with dyspepsia, peptic ulcer disease, gastritis, and esophageal reflux.

Acute cholecystitis presents with pain similar to that of biliary colic that persists for longer than the typical 6 hours of colic. Fever, chills, nausea, emesis, and anorexia are common. Past history of similar attacks or known gallstones may be reported. As the gallbladder becomes progressively inflamed, the initial poorly localized upper abdominal pain often becomes sharp and localized to the right upper quadrant. The patient may have moderate to severe distress and may appear toxic. Other findings may include abdominal distention, hypoactive bowel sounds, and the Murphy sign, ie, increased pain or inspiratory arrest during deep subcostal palpation of the right upper quadrant during deep inspiration. Generalized abdominal rigidity, although rare, suggests perforation and diffuse peritonitis, if present. Volume depletion is common, but jaundice is unusual. Acalculous cholecystitis occurs in 5% to 10% of patients with cholecystitis, has a more rapid, aggressive clinical course, and

247

occurs more frequently in patients with diabetes, the elderly, trauma or burn victims, after prolonged labor or major surgery, or with systemic vasculitides.

The clinical presentation of gallstone pancreatitis will be similar to those of other forms of pancreatitis (see Chap. 49). Ascending cholangitis, a life-threatening condition with high mortality, results from complete biliary obstruction (often a common duct stone; less commonly a tumor) with bacterial superinfection and septicemia. Patients often present in extremis with jaundice, fever, mental confusion, and shock. The Charcot triad of fever, jaundice, and right upper quadrant pain is suggestive, but all 3 features may be present in only 25% of patients.

DIAGNOSIS AND DIFFERENTIAL

Suspicion of gallbladder or biliary tract disease must be maintained in any patient at risk who presents with upper abdominal pain. Patients with uncomplicated biliary colic usually have normal laboratory findings. Laboratory studies that may aid in diagnosis include a white blood cell count; leukocytosis with left shift suggests acute cholecystis, pancreatitis, or cholangitis, but a normal white blood cell count does not exclude them. With biliary colic or cholecystitis, serum bilirubin and alkaline phosphatase levels may be normal or mildly elevated. Serum amylase and/or lipase levels should be checked to help exclude pancreatitis. Urinalysis should be performed to rule out urinary tract infection, and all women of childbearing potential require a serum or urine pregnancy test to rule out obstetric causes of abdominal pain. Levels of serum electrolytes, glucose, serum urea nitrogen, and creatinine should be obtained to exclude diabetic ketoacidosis and may aid evaluation of the patient's volume status. Plain x-ray films of the abdomen may visualize other causes of upper abdominal pain (eg, bowel obstruction), but gallstones will be radiopaque in only 10% to 20%. Chest x-ray may aid in excluding right lower lobe pneumonia or pleural effusion. A 12-lead electrocardiogram should be considered in older patients to rule out myocardial infarction or ischemia.

Ultrasound of the hepatobiliary tract is presently the initial diagnostic study of choice for patients with suspected biliary colic or obstruction. It can detect stones as small as 2 mm and signs of cholecystitis: thickened gallbladder wall, gallbladder distention, and pericholecystic fluid. A positive sonographic Murphy sign, if elicited during the scan, is highly suggestive of cholecystitis.

Computed tomography of the abdomen is most useful when other intraabdominal processes are suspected in the differential diagnosis. Unfortunately, computed tomography has only 50% sensitivity for cholecystitis. Radionuclide cholescintigraphy (technetium-iminodiacetic acid [HIDA]) or diisopropyl iminodiacetic acid ([DISIDA] scans) offers a sensitivity of 97% and a specificity of 90% for cholecystitis. A reasonable emergency department approach to suspected cholecystitis would be to obtain an ultrasound scan and then a radionuclide scan only if ultrasound fails to establish the diagnosis.

The differential diagnosis of patients with upper abdominal pain should include gastritis, peptic ulcer, hepatitis or hepatic abscess, pancreatitis, Fitz-Hugh-Curtis syndrome, pelvic inflammatory disease, pyelonephritis, pleurisy or pneumonia, acute myocardial infarction, and diabetic ketoacidosis.

EMERGENCY DEPARTMENT CARE AND DISPOSITION

Emergency department management of any patient with abdominal pain always should begin with the ABCs of resuscitation and supportive care. Uncomplicated biliary colic should resolve spontaneously over a few hours, whereas cholecystitis, pancreatitis, and cholangitis require admission.

1. Isotonic crystalloid intravenous fluids should be given to correct volume deficits and electrolyte imbalances. Septic shock, if present, should be aggressively resuscitated with crystalloids and intravenous vasopressors, if necessary, to support perfusion (see Chap. 6).

2. Symptomatic treatment for emesis is best achieved with antiemetics (**promethazine** 12.5-25 mg intravenously) or antispasmodics (**glycopyrrolate** 0.1 mg intravenously). Gastric decompression with nasogastric tube suctioning may be instituted if vomiting is intractable.

3. For analgesia, **meperidine** 0.5 to 1.0 mg/kg intravenously or intramuscularly is preferred over other opiates because it causes less spasm of the sphincter of Oddi. **Ketorolac tromethamine** 15 to 30 mg intravenously or 30 to 60 mg intramuscularly may help relieve the pain of gallbladder distention in patients with biliary colic, but it is less effective in cholecystitis.

4. Early antibiotic therapy should be initiated in any patient with suspected cholecystitis or cholangitis. Single-agent therapy with a parenteral third-generation cephalosporin (**cefotaxime or ceftazidime** 1-2 g intravenously every 8 hours, **ceftizoxime** 1-2 g intravenously every 8-12 h, or **ceftriaxone** 1-2 g intravenously every 12-24 hours) may be adequate for patients without sepsis. Those with sepsis or obvious peritonitis are best managed with triple coverage by using **ampicillin** (0.5-1.0 g intravenously every 6 hours), **gentamicin** (3 mg/kg/d intravenously divided every 8 hours), and **clindamycin** (1,200-2,700 mg/d intravenously divided into 2, 3, or 4 equal doses), or the equivalent substitutes (eg, metronidazole for clindamycin, third-generation cephalosporins or piperacillin/tazobactam, or a quinolone for ampicillin).

5. Patients diagnosed with acute cholecystitis, gallstone pancreatitis, or ascending cholangitis require immediate surgical consultation with hospital admission. Signs of systemic toxicity or sepsis warrant admission to the intensive care unit pending surgical treatment.

6. Patients accurately diagnosed with uncomplicated biliary colic whose symptoms abate with supportive therapy within 4 to 6 hours of onset can be discharged home if they are able to maintain oral hydration. Oral narcotic-acetaminophen analgesics may be prescribed for the next 24 to 48 hours for the common residual abdominal aching. Timely outpatient follow-up should be arranged with a surgical consultant or the patient's primary care physician. The patient should be carefully instructed to return to the emergency department if fever develops, abdominal pain worsens, intractable vomiting returns, or another significant attack occurs before follow-up.

For further reading in *Emergency Medicine: A Comprehensive Study Guide,* 6th ed., see Chap. 85, "Cholecystitis and Biliary Colic," by Tom P. Aufderheide, William J. Brady, and Judith E. Tintinalli.

49 | Acute Pancreatitis

Robert J. Vissers

Acute pancreatitis (AP) is a common cause of abdominal pain, and the diagnosis is based primarily on clinical presentation. The severity of the disease may range from mild local inflammation to multisystem organ failure due to a systemic inflammatory response. Alcohol abuse and cholelithiasis are the most common causes, but there are many potential etiologies (Table 49-1).

CLINICAL FEATURES

The most common symptom is a midepigastric, constant, boring pain radiating to the back, which is often associated with nausea, vomiting, abdominal distention, and exacerbation in the supine position. Low-grade fevers, tachycardia, and hypotension may be present. Epigastric tenderness is common, whereas peritonitis is a late finding. Refractory hypotensive shock, renal failure, and respiratory failure may accompany the most severe forms.

DIAGNOSIS AND DIFFERENTIAL

The diagnosis should be suspected by the history, physical examination, and presence of elevated pancreatic enzymes. Serum amylase and lipase are the most common tests used to assist in the diagnosis. There are many sources of extra pancreatic amylase, making this a relatively nonspecific test. Conversely, AP also may occur with a normal amylase. Amylase appears to be most useful at a cutoff of 3 times the upper limit of normal, which has a specificity of 75% and a sensitivity of 80% to 90%. Lipase has a longer half-life than does amylase (7 vs 2 hours); at a cutoff of 2 times the upper limit of normal, it is as sensitive and more specific (90%) than amylase. There is no benefit to ordering both tests. The absolute levels do not correlate with severity. Leukocytosis is usually present. An elevated alkaline phosphatase level suggests biliary disease. Persistent hypocalcemia (<7 mg/100 mL), hypoxia, increasing serum urea nitrogen, and metabolic acidosis are associated with a potentially complicated course.

Plain radiographs play a small role in the diagnosis of AP, although calcification, when present, suggests preexisting pancreatic disease. Patients with AP may have a partial ileus or gaseous distention of the colon with a distally collapsed colon. The hypoxic patient may show signs of adult respiratory distress syndrome or a left pleural effusion. Ultrasound may identify diagnostic gallstones or biliary tree dilation, but it lacks diagnostic value in other etiologies of AP. Computed tomography may show edema indicative of AP and local complications such as phlegmon, abscesses, and pseudocysts but lacks sensitivity in mild or early disease.

The differential diagnosis of AP includes left lower lobe pneumonia, rupture of a pseudocyst, gallbladder disease (cholecystitis or choledocholithiasis), peritonitis (appendicitis, diverticulitis, or perforated viscus), peptic ulcer disease (gastritis or gastric outlet obstruction), small bowel obstruction, renal colic, dissecting aortic aneurysm, diabetic ketoacidosis, and gastroenteritis. AP may be a difficult diagnosis to establish, and repeated evaluations and surgical consultation are often necessary.

TABLE 49-1 Common Etiologic or Contributing Factors in Acute Pancreatitis

Ethanol ingestion

Biliary tract disease

Trauma, penetrating or blunt

Penetrating peptic ulcer

Following endoscopic procedures

Obstruction secondary to neoplasms, diverticula, and polyps

Metabolic disturbances
 Hyperlipemia (Frederickson types I, IV, V)
 Hypercalcemia
 Diabetes mellitus, diabetic ketoacidosis
 Uremia

Viral Infections
 Viral hepatitis
 Infectious mononucleosis
 Coxsackie group B
 Human immunodeficiency virus

Pregnancy—any trimester, postpartum

Collagen vascular disease

Liver disease

Generalized infections

Drugs
 Oral contraceptives
 Azathioprine
 Glucocorticoids
 Tetracyclines
 Isonazid
 Indomethacin
 Thiazides
 Salicylates
 Calcium
 Warfarin

EMERGENCY DEPARTMENT CARE AND DISPOSITION

Treatment of AP revolves around fluid resuscitation, prevention of vomiting, pain control, and pancreatic rest (nothing orally).

1. Fluid resuscitation with crystalloid intravenous fluids is the mainstay of treatment to maintain blood pressure and ensure adequate urine output. Pressors are indicated for hypotension not responsive to adequate fluid resuscitation.
2. Oxygen should be administered to maintain a pulse oximetry reading of 95% oxygen saturation. Respiratory failure is a rare but well-described complication of AP.
3. A nasogastric tube to low suction should be considered if the patient is distended or actively vomiting. The nasogastric tube theoretically reduces pancreatic stimulation and prevents vomiting, although no controlled trial has shown its value.
4. Parenteral analgesia is should be given as necessary for patient comfort. Intravenous narcotics such as **morphine** 0.1 mg/kg are often required,

5. Antiemetics, such as **promethazine** 12.5 to 25 mg intravenously, may be helpful to reduce vomiting (see Chap. 46).
6. Empirical antibiotics, steroids, and H2 blockers have no proven benefit in isolated AP.
7. Patients with acute biliary obstruction may require urgent decompression via endoscopic sphincterotomy of the ampulla of Vater.
8. Prophylaxis for alcohol withdrawal with benzodiazepines such as **chlordiazepoxide** 25 to 50 mg orally, intravenously, or intramuscularly in the appropriate setting is indicated.
9. Patients with severe systemic disease will require intubation, intensive monitoring, Foley catheterization, and transfusion of blood and blood products as needed. Laparotomy may be indicated for hemorrhage or abscess drainage.

Patients with mild AP may be managed as outpatients with close follow-up, provided they can tolerate clear liquids and oral analgesics. Most patients will require hospital floor admission to a medical or surgical service. Patients who demonstrate poor prognostic signs (dropping hemoglobin, poor urine output, persistent hypotension, hypoxia, acidosis, or hypocalcemia) despite aggressive early treatment should be admitted to the intensive care unit with surgical consultation.

For further reading in *Emergency Medicine: A Comprehensive Study Guide,* 6th ed., see Chap. 87, "Acute and Chronic Pancreatitis," by Robert J. Vissers and Riyad B. Abu-Laban.

50 | Complications of General Surgical Procedures

N. Heramba Prasad

Outpatient surgical procedures are becoming increasingly common. Emergency physicians, therefore, will see more and more postoperative complications. Fever, respiratory complications, genitourinary complaints, wound infections, vascular problems, and complications of drug therapy are some common postoperative disorders seen in the emergency department. Most of these are discussed elsewhere in this book; certain specific problems are mentioned here.

CLINICAL FEATURES

Fever

The causes of postoperative fever are listed as the 5 Ws: wind (respiratory), water (urinary tract infection [UTI]), wound, walking (deep venous thrombosis [DVT]), and wonder drugs (pseudomembranous colitis [PMC]). Fever in the first 24 hours is usually due to atelectasis, necrotizing fasciitis, or clostridial infections. Between 24 and 72 hours, pneumonia, atelectasis, intravenous catheter–related thrombophlebitis, and infections are the major causes. UTIs are seen 3 to 5 days postoperatively. DVT typically occurs 5 days after the procedure, and wound infections generally manifest 7 to l0 days after surgery. Antibiotic-induced PMC is seen 6 weeks after surgery.

Respiratory Complications

Postoperative pain and inadequate clearance of secretions contribute to the development of atelectasis. Fever, tachypnea, tachycardia, and mild hypoxia are usually seen. Pneumonia may develop 24 to 96 hours later. Hypoxia-widened A-a gradient and respiratory distress should point to the diagnosis of pulmonary embolism (see Chap. 26 for diagnosis and management).

Genitourinary Complications

UTIs are more common after instrumentation of the urinary tract. Urinary retention occurs in 4% of all surgical patients and in 60% of patients after urethral surgery. It is more common in elderly males, especially after excessive fluid administration and after spinal anesthesia. Lower abdominal pain, urgency, and inability to void should alert the clinician to suspect urinary retention. Oliguria or anuria commonly results from volume depletion. Intrinsic factors such as acute tubular necrosis, drug nephrotoxicity, and postrenal obstructive uropathy also may lead to acute renal failure.

Wound Complications

Hematomas result from inadequate hemostasis. Careful evaluation to rule out infections must he undertaken. Seromas are collections of clear fluid under the wound. Extremes of age, diabetes, poor nutrition, necrotic tissue, poor perfusion, foreign bodies, and wound hematomas contribute to the development of wound infections. Necrotizing fasciitis is characterized by extremely painful, erythematous, swollen, and warm areas without sharp margins. This staphylococcal infection spreads rapidly. The patient will exhibit marked systemic toxicity; and crepitance and bullae may be present. Wound dehiscence can occur due to diabetes, poor nutrition, chronic steroid use, and inadequate or improper closure of the wound. Dehiscence of an abdominal wound may result in evisceration of abdominal organs.

Vascular Complications

Superficial thrombophlebitis usually occurs in the upper extremities after intravenous catheter insertion or in the lower extremities because of stasis and varicosity of veins. DVT commonly occurs in the lower extremities. Swelling and pain of the calf are commonly encountered (see Chap. 29 for diagnosis and management).

Drug Therapy Complications

Many drugs are known to cause fever and antibiotic-induced diarrhea. PMC, a dreaded complication, is caused by *Clostridium difficile* toxin. Bloody, watery diarrhea, fever, and crampy abdominal pain are the usual complaints.

DIAGNOSIS AND DIFFERENTIAL

Patients with suspected respiratory complications should have chest x-rays. They may show platelike or discoid atelectases, pneumonia, or pneumothorax. Pneumothorax occurs early after certain surgical procedures or catheter insertion, and chest x-ray will help confirm the diagnosis.

Patients with oliguria or anuria should be evaluated for signs of hypovolemia or urinary retention. Diagnosis of PMC is established by demonstrating *C difficile* cytotoxin in the stool. Nevertheless, in 27% of cases, the assay may be negative.

EMERGENCY DEPARTMENT CARE AND DISPOSITION

Always discuss patients and proposed treatment with the surgeon who initially cared for the patient. Although debilitated patients may need hospitalization, many patients with atelectasis can be treated as outpatients.

1. Postoperative pneumonia is polymicrobial, and an anti-*Pseudomonas* antibiotic with an aminoglycoside is usually recommended. Most patients with UTI can be managed as outpatients with oral antibiotic therapy (see Chap. 53).
2. Insertion of a Foley catheter and prompt drainage will alleviate urinary retention (see Chap. 56). There is no need for periodic clamping of the catheter. Prophylactic antibiotics are reserved for patients who have had urinary tract instrumentation, those with prolonged retention, and those at risk for infection.
3. Wound hematomas may require removal of some sutures and evacuation. Surgical consultation before treatment is appropriate. Seromas can be treated with needle aspiration and wound cultures. Admission may not be necessary.
4. Most wound infections can be treated with oral antibiotics (usually the surgeon's choice) unless the patient manifests systemic symptoms and signs. Perineal infections usually require hospital admission and parenteral an-

tibiotics. Surgical debridement and parenteral antibiotics are indicated for necrotizing fasciitis, so physicians should start clindamycin 900 mg and penicillin G 6 million U intravenously.

5. Most patients with superficial thrombophlebitis can be treated with local heat and elevation of the affected area, if there is no evidence of cellulitis or lymphangitis. Patients with suppurative thrombophlebitis, characterized by erythema, lymphangitis, fever, and severe pain, should be hospitalized and treated with excision of the affected vein.

6. Fluid resuscitation, oral vancomycin, and oral or intravenous metronidazole are currently available treatment modalities for drug-induced PMC (see Chap. 44).

SPECIFIC CONSIDERATIONS

Complications of Breast Surgery

Wound infections, hematomas, pneumothorax, necrosis of the skin flaps, and lymphedema of the arms after mastectomy are common problems seen after breast surgery. Lymphedema of the arm occurs in 5% to 10% of patients. Elevation and minor activity restriction will help reduce swelling.

Complications of Gastrointestinal Surgery

With regard to *intestinal obstruction,* neuronal dysfunction after any surgery in which the peritoneum is entered causes paralytic ileus. After gastrointestinal surgery, small bowel tone returns to normal within 24 hours, gastric function within 2 days, and colonic function within 3 days.

Prolonged ileus should alert the clinicians to peritonitis, abscesses, hemoperitoneum, pneumonia, sepsis, and electrolyte imbalance. Clinical features include nausea, vomiting, obstipation, constipation, abdominal distention, and pain.

Abdominal x-rays; complete blood cell count; electrolytes, serum urea nitrogen, and creatinine levels; and urinalysis should be obtained. Treatment of adynamic ileus consists of nasogastric suction, bowel rest, and hydration. Mechanical obstruction is usually due to adhesions and may require surgical intervention.

Intraabdominal abscesses are caused by preoperative contamination or postoperative anastomotic leaks. Diagnosis can be confirmed by computed tomography or ultrasonography. Surgical exploration, evacuation, and parenteral antibiotics will be required.

Pancreatitis occurs especially after direct manipulation of the pancreatic duct. Patients typically present with nausea, vomiting, abdominal pain, and leukocytosis. Lumbar pain, left pleural effusion, Turner sign (discoloration of the flank), and Cullen sign (periumbilical ecchymosis) may be present. Serum amylase and lipase levels are usually elevated (see Chap. 49 for management).

Cholecystitis and biliary colic have been reported as postoperative complications. Elderly patients are more prone to develop acalculous cholecystitis (see Chap. 48 for management).

Fistulas, internal or external, may result from direct bowel injury and require surgical consultation and hospitalization. *Anastomotic leaks* are especially devastating after esophageal or colon surgery. Esophageal leaks occur 10 days after the procedure. Dramatic presentation with shock, pneumothorax, and pleural effusion is usually seen.

Dumping syndrome is noticed in gastric bypass procedures. It is due to the sudden influx of hyperosmolar chyle into the small intestine resulting in fluid sequestration and hypovolemia. Patients experience nausea, vomiting, epigastric discomfort, palpitations, dizziness, and sometimes syncope.

Alkaline reflux gastritis is caused by the reflux of bile into the stomach. Endoscopic evaluation will establish the diagnosis. Postvagotomy diarrhea and afferent loop syndrome are seen in some patients.

Complications of transabdominal feeding tubes and *percutaneous endoscopic gastrostomy* tubes include infections, hemorrhage, peritonitis, aspiration, wound dehiscence, sepsis, and obstruction of the tube. The tube should be replaced with the appropriately sized tube of the same type, if possible. Stomas close quickly, so the stoma should be kept open with a largest possible catheter until the proper replacement tube can be obtained.

Complications arising from stomas are due to technical errors or from underlying disease such as Crohn disease and cancer. Ischemia, necrosis, bleeding, hernia, and prolapse are sometimes seen.

Colonoscopy may cause hemorrhage, perforation, retroperitoneal abscesses, pneumoscrotum, pneumothorax, volvulus, and infection.

Rectal surgery complications include urinary retention, constipation, prolapse, bleeding, and infections.

Tetanus has been known to occur after surgical wounds.

For further reading in *Emergency Medicine: A Comprehensive Study Guide,* 6th ed., see
Chap. 88, "Complications of General Surgical Procedures," by Edmond A. Hooker;
and Chap. 89, "Complications of Gastrointestinal Devices," by Edmond A. Hooker.

8 | RENAL AND GENITOURINARY DISORDERS

51 | Acute Renal Failure

Marc D. Squillante

Renal dysfunction and acute renal failure (ARF) present with a wide variety of manifestations, depending on the underlying etiology. Although the initial symptoms may be those of the primary cause, ultimately patients will develop deterioration of renal function. Risk factors include hypovolemia from any cause, cardiac disease, vascular or thrombotic disorders, glomerular diseases, diseases affecting the renal tubules, use of nephrotoxic drugs, and a variety of anatomic problems of the genitourinary tract.

CLINICAL FEATURES

Deterioration in renal function leads to excessive accumulation of nitrogenous waste products in the serum. ARF can be classified as *oliguric* (<400 mL urine/24 h) and *nonoliguric* (>400 mL/24 h); nonoliguric ARF has improved mortality and renal function recovery. Patients usually have signs and symptoms of their underlying causative disorder but eventually develop stigmata of renal failure. Volume overload, hypertension, pulmonary edema, mental status changes or neurologic symptoms, nausea and vomiting, bone and joint problems, anemia, and increased susceptibility to infection (a leading cause of death) can occur as patients develop more chronic uremia.

DIAGNOSIS AND DIFFERENTIAL

History and physical examination usually provide clues to etiology. Signs and symptoms of the underlying causative disorder (Table 51-1) should be vigorously sought. Physical examination should assess vital signs, volume status, establish urinary tract patency and output, and search for signs of chemical intoxication, drug usage, muscle damage, infections, or associated systemic diseases. Diagnostic studies include urinalysis, serum urea nitrogen and creatinine levels, serum electrolytes, urinary sodium and creatinine levels, and urinary osmolality. Analysis of these tests allows most patients to be categorized as prerenal, renal, or postrenal. Fractional excretion of sodium and the renal failure index can be calculated to help in this categorization (Table 51-2). Normal urinary sediment may be seen in prerenal and postrenal failure, hemolytic-uremic syndrome, and thrombotic thrombocytopenic purpura. The presence of albumin may indicate glomerulonephritis or malignant hypertension. Granular casts are seen in acute tubular necrosis (ATN). Albumin and red blood cell casts are found in glomerulonephritis and malignant hypertension. White blood cell casts are seen in interstitial nephritis and pyelonephritis. Crystals can be present with renal calculi and certain drugs (sulfas, ethylene glycol, and radiocontrast agents). Ultrasonography is the radiologic procedure of choice in most patients with ARF when hydronephrosis is suspected.

Prerenal failure is produced by conditions that decrease renal perfusion (see Table 51-1) and is the most common cause of community-acquired ARF (40–80% of cases). It also is a common precursor to ischemic and nephrotoxic causes of intrinsic renal failure. *Intrinsic renal failure* has vascular and ischemic etiologies; glomerular and tubulointerstitial diseases are also causative. ATN due to severe and prolonged prerenal etiologies causes most cases of intrinsic renal failure. Nephrotoxins are the second most common

TABLE 51-1 Common Causes of Acute Renal Failure

Prerenal	Renal (intrinsic)	Postrenal
Decreased cardiac output	Vascular/ischemia	Penile lesions
Myocardial ischemia/infarction	Renal vasculature thrombosis, TTP, DIC,	Phimosis
Valvular heart disease	NSAIDs, severe hypertension, hemolytic-	Meatal stenosis
Cardiomyopathy	uremic syndrome	Urethral stricture
Pericardial tamponade	Glomerular	
High-output failure	Primary glomerular diseases (acute	Prostatic enlargement
Hypovolemia	glomerulonephritis) or systemic disease with	Benign prostatic enlargement
Blood loss/hemorrhagic shock	glomerular involvement (SLE, vasculitis, HSP,	Prostate cancer
Vomiting/diarrhea	endocarditis)	Upper urinary tract/ureteral diseases (usually
Diuretics	Tubulointerstitial	requires bilateral involvement/
Obstructive diuresis	Ischemic ATN, rhabdomyolysis, toxin-induced	obstruction)
Fluid sequestration	tubular damage (aminoglycosides,	Calculi, tumors, blood clots
Cirrhosis	radiocontrast, solvents, heavy metals, ethylene	Papillary necrosis
Pancreatitis	glycol, myoglobin/ hemoglobin), acute	Vesicoureteral reflux
Burns	interstitial nephritis, infiltrative and	Stricture
General anesthesia	autoimmune diseases, infectious agents	Abdominal aortic aneurysm
Septic shock		Retroperitoneal fibrosis

Key: ATN = acute tubular necrosis, DIC = disseminated intravascular coagulation, HSP = Henoch-Schönlein purpura, NSAIDs = nonsteroidal anti-inflammatory drugs, SLE = systemic lupus erythematosus, TTP = thrombotic thrombocytopenic purpura.

TABLE 51-2 Laboratory Studies Aiding in the Differential Diagnosis of Acute Renal Failure

Test employed	Prerenal	Renal*	Postrenal†
Urine sodium (mEq/L)	<20	>40	>40
FE_{Na} (%)‡	<1	>1	>1
RFI#	<1	>1	>1
Urine osmolality (mOsm/L)	>500	<350	<350
Urine:serum creatinine	>40:1	<20:1	<20:1
Serum urea nitrogen:creatinine	>20:1	10:1	>10:1

*FE_{Na} may be less than 1 in patients with intrinsic renal failure plus glomerulonephritis, hepatorenal syndrome, radiocontrast acute tubular necrosis, myoglobinuric and hemoglobinuric acute renal failure, renal allograft rejection, and certain drugs (angiotensin-converting enzyme inhibitors and nonsteroidal antiinflammatory agents).

†One can see indices similar to prerenal early in the course of obstruction. With continued obstruction, tubular function is impaired and indices mimic those of renal causes.

‡FE_{Na} = ([urine sodium/serum sodium] ÷ [urine creatinine/serum creatinine]) × 100.

#RFI = (serum sodium ÷ [urine creatinine/serum creatinine]) × 100.

Key: FE_{Na} = fractional excretion of sodium, RFI = renal failure index.

cause of ATN. *Postrenal azotemia* occurs primarily in elderly men with high-grade prostatic obstruction. Lesions of the external genitalia (ie, strictures) are also common causes.

EMERGENCY DEPARTMENT CARE AND DISPOSITION

Initial care of patients with ARF focuses on treating the underlying cause and correcting fluid and electrolyte derangements. Efforts should be made to prevent further renal damage and provide supportive care until renal function has recovered (see Chap. 4 for treatment of electrolyte and acid-base disorders).

Prerenal Failure

1. Effective intravascular volume should be restored with isotonic fluids (normal saline or lactated Ringer solution) at a rapid rate in appropriate patients; resuscitation is the first priority.
2. If cardiac failure is causing prerenal azotemia, cardiac output should be optimized to improve renal perfusion, and reduction in intravascular volume (ie, with diuretics) may be appropriate.

Renal Failure (Intrinsic)

Adequate circulating volume must be restored first; hypovolemia potentiates and exacerbates all forms of ARF. Ischemia or nephrotoxic agents are the most common causes of intrinsic ARF. History, physical examination, and baseline laboratory tests should provide clues to the diagnosis. Nephrotoxic agents (drugs and intravenous contrast) should be avoided.

1. The use of diuretics to "convert" oliguric to nonoliguric ARF is not beneficial.

2. Low-dose dopamine (1 to 5 μg/kg/min) may improve renal blood flow and urine output, but it does not lower mortality rates or improve recovery. It is probably best used in ARF patients with congestive heart failure.
3. Mannitol may be protective against myoglobinuric ARF in early rhabdomyolysis.
4. Large-volume crystalloid infusions are the primary treatment; urinary alkalinization with sodium bicarbonate is also recommended. A bolus of 1 to 2 mEq/kg of **sodium bicarbonate** is administered. Then 100 to 150 mEq sodium bicarbonate is added to 1 L 5% dextrose in water and infused at 1.5 to 2.0 times the patient's maintenance rate; the infusion is adjusted to maintain urine pH above 7.5. Serum electrolyte levels and fluid status should be monitored; potassium chloride is added as needed (see Chap. 4) to maintain a pH level of 4.0 or higher.

Renally excreted drugs (digoxin, magnesium, sedatives, and narcotics) should be used with caution because therapeutic doses may accumulate to excess and cause serious side effects. Fluid restriction may be required. Interventions useful in the prevention of radiocontrast nephropathy include acetylcysteine, fenoldopam, and crystalloid infusions.

Postrenal Failure

Appropriate urinary drainage should be established; the exact procedure depends on the level of obstruction.

1. A Foley catheter should be placed to relieve obstruction caused by prostatic hypertrophy. There is no support for the practice of intermittent catheter clamping to prevent hypotension and hematuria; urine should be completely and rapidly drained.
2. Percutaneous nephrostomy may be required for ureteral occlusion until definitive surgery to correct the obstruction can take place once the patient is stabilized.
3. For the acutely anuric patient, obstruction is the major consideration. If no urine is obtained on initial bladder catheterization, emergency urologic consultation should be considered.
4. With chronic urinary retention, postobstructive diuresis may occur due to osmotic diuresis or tubular dysfunction. Patients may become suddenly hypovolemic and hypotensive. Urine output must be closely monitored, with appropriate fluid replacement.

Dialysis

If treatment of the underlying cause fails to improve renal function, hemodialysis or peritoneal dialysis should be considered.

1. The nephrology consultant usually makes decisions about dialysis. Dialysis often is initiated when the serum urea nitrogen is greater than 100 mg/dL or serum creatinine is greater than 10 mg/dL.
2. Patients with complications of ARF such as cardiac instability (due to metabolic acidosis and hyperkalemia), intractable volume overload, hyperkalemia, and uremia (ie, encephalopathy, pericarditis, and bleeding diathesis) not easily corrected by other measures should be considered for emergency dialysis. However, morality in ARF has changed little since the advent of dialysis.

Disposition

Patients with new onset ARF usually require hospital admission, often to an intensive care unit. Transferring patients to another institution should be considered if nephrology consultation and dialysis facilities are not available.

For further reading in *Emergency Medicine: A Comprehensive Study Guide,* 6th ed., see Chap. 92, "Acute Renal Failure," by Richard Sinert and Peter R. Peacock, Jr.

52 | Emergencies in Renal Failure and Dialysis Patients

Jonathan A. Maisel

Patients with end-stage renal disease (ESRD) may sustain multiple complications of their disease process and treatment (see the appropriate chapters for discussion on the management of hypertension, heart failure, bleeding disorders, and electrolyte disorders).

CARDIOVASCULAR COMPLICATIONS

Creatine kinase (and the MB fraction), troponin I, and troponin T are not significantly elevated in ESRD patients and have been shown to be specific markers of myocardial ischemia in these patients. Hypertension occurs in 80%–90% of patients starting dialysis. Management includes control of blood volume, followed by use of adrenergic-blocking drugs, angiotensin-converting enzyme inhibitors, or vasodilating agents.

Congestive heart failure may be caused by hypertension, coronary ischemia, and valvular disease and by uremic cardiomyopathy, fluid overload, and arteriovenous fistulas (high-output failure). Treatment is similar to that in non-ESRD patients. Diuretics (eg, furosemide 60-100 mg) are useful, even in oliguric patients, because they cause pulmonary vessel vasodilatation. Preload can be reduced by inducing diarrhea with sorbitol and with phlebotomy (minimum, 150 mL). Hemodialysis (HD) is the definitive treatment.

Pericarditis in ESRD patients is usually due to worsening uremia. Electrocardiographic changes typical of acute pericarditis are not seen. Pericardial friction rubs are louder than in most other forms of pericarditis, often palpable, and frequently persist after the metabolic abnormalities have been corrected. Uremic pericarditis is treated with intensive dialysis therapy. Cardiac tamponade is the most serious complication of uremic pericarditis. It presents with changes in mental status, hypotension, or dyspnea. An enlarged heart on chest x-ray may suggest the diagnosis, which can be confirmed with echocardiography. Hemodynamically significant pericardial effusions require pericardiocentesis under fluoroscopic or ultrasonographic guidance.

NEUROLOGIC COMPLICATIONS

Uremic encephalopathy presents with cognitive defects, memory loss, slurred speech, and asterixis. The progressive neurologic symptoms of uremia are the most common indications for initiating HD. It should remain a diagnosis of exclusion until structural, vascular, infectious, toxic, and metabolic causes of neurologic dysfunction have been ruled out.

Peripheral neuropathy, manifested by impaired vibration sense and "stocking glove" pain or anesthesia, occurs in more than 50% of patients with ESRD. Autonomic dysfunction, characterized by impotence, postural dizziness, gastric fullness, bowel dysfunction, and reduced sweating, is common in ESRD patients but is not responsible for intradialytic hypotension.

Subdural hematoma is seen in 3.5% of HD patients, presumably related to trauma, anticoagulation, excessive ultrafiltration, or hypertension. It should be considered in any ESRD patient presenting with a change in mental status.

Dialysis disequilibrium, generally occurring at the end of dialysis, is characterized by nausea, vomiting, and hypertension, which can progress to seizures, coma, and death. Treatment consists of terminating dialysis and administering mannitol intravenously to increase serum osmolarity. This syndrome should be distinguished from other neurologic disorders, such as subdural hematoma, stroke, hypertensive crisis, hypoxia, and seizures.

GASTROINTESTINAL COMPLICATIONS

Anorexia, nausea, and vomiting are common symptoms of uremia and are used as an indication to initiate dialysis and assess its efficacy (see Chap. 46 for management).

HEMATOLOGIC COMPLICATIONS

Abnormal hemostasis in ESRD is multifactorial in origin, resulting in an increased risk of gastrointestinal tract bleeding, subcapsular liver hematomas, subdural hematomas, and intraocular bleeding. Immunologic compromise, caused by impaired leukocyte chemotaxis and phagocytosis, leads to high mortality rates from infection. Dialysis therapy does not appear to improve immune system function.

COMPLICATIONS OF HEMODIALYSIS

Hypotension is the most frequent complication of HD. Excessive ultrafiltration from underestimation of the patient's ideal blood volume (dry weight) is the most common cause of intradialytic hypotension. Cardiac compensation for fluid loss may be compromised by diastolic dysfunction common in ESRD patients. Other causes of intradialytic hypotension include myocardial dysfunction from ischemia, hypoxia, arrhythmias, and pericardial tamponade; abnormalities of vascular tone secondary to sepsis, overproduction of nitric oxide, and antihypertensive medications; and volume loss from vomiting, diarrhea, gastrointestinal bleeding, or blood tubing or filter leaks. Treatment consists of Trendelenberg positioning, oral salt solution, or infusion of parenteral normal saline solution.

COMPLICATIONS OF VASCULAR ACCESS

Complications of vascular access account for more inpatient hospital days than any other complication of HD. Thrombosis and stenosis are the most common complications, presenting with loss of the bruit and thrill over the access. These need to be treated within 24 hours with angiographic clot removal or angioplasty.

Vascular access infections often present with signs of systemic sepsis, including fever, hypotension, and an elevated white blood cell count. Classic signs of pain, erythema, swelling, and discharge are often missing. *Staphylococcus aureus* is the most common infecting organism, followed by gram-negative bacteria. Patients usually require hospitalization, and treatment with vancomycin (1 g intravenously) and an aminoglycoside (eg, gentamicin 100 mg intravenously initially and after each dialysis).

Potential life-threatening hemorrhage from a vascular access may result from a ruptured aneurysm or anastomosis or overanticoagulation. Bleeding often can be controlled with 5 to 10 minutes of pressure at the puncture site. Life-threatening hemorrhage may require placement of a tourniquet proximal to the access and vascular surgery consultation. If the etiology is excessive anticoagulation, the effects of heparin can be reversed with protamine 0.01 mg/IU heparin dispensed during dialysis (10-20 mg protamine if the heparin dose is unknown). If a newly inserted vascular access continues to bleed, desmopressin acetate (0.3 μg/kg intravenously) can be given as an adjunct to direct pressure.

COMPLICATIONS OF PERITONEAL DIALYSIS

Peritonitis is the most common complication of peritoneal dialysis. Signs and symptoms are similar to those seen in other patients with peritonitis and include fever, abdominal pain, and rebound tenderness. A cloudy effluent supports the diagnosis. Laboratory evaluation should include complete blood cell count and analysis of peritoneal fluid for cell count, Gram stain, culture, and sensitivity. In the setting of peritonitis, cell counts usually exceed 100 leukocytes, with more than 50% neutrophils. Gram stain is positive in only 10% to 40% of culture-proven peritonitis. Organisms isolated include *Staphylococcus epidermidis, S aureus, Streptococcus* species, gram-negative bacteria, anaerobes, and fungi. Empiric therapy begins with a few rapid exchanges of dialysate to decrease the number of inflammatory cells within the peritoneum. The addition of heparin (500-1,000 IU/L dialysate) decreases fibrin clot formation. Next, empiric antibiotics, covering gram-positive organisms (eg, cephalothin or vancomycin 500 mg/L dialysate) and gram-negative organisms (eg, gentamicin 100 mg/L dialysate), are added to the dialysate.

Inpatient versus outpatient treatment of peritonitis related to peritoneal dialysis should be based on clinical presentation.

For further reading in *Emergency Medicine: A Comprehensive Study Guide,* 6th ed., see Chap. 93, "Emergencies in Renal Failure and Dialysis Patients," by Richard Sinert.

53 Urinary Tract Infections and Hematuria

Kama Guluma

Urinary tract infection, defined as a symptomatic and significant bacteriuria, is a common precipitant of a visit to emergency department (ED). There are 4 groups of patients at risk for urinary tract infection (UTI): neonates, girls, young women, and older men. In neonates, UTI affects slightly more males than females and may occur as part of a gram-negative sepsis syndrome. With age, the incidence in girls rises in relation to that in boys, with girls being affected 10 times as often as boys in preschool, and a 5% incidence being almost exclusively in girls by school age. In young adult women, the incidence of UTI rises with commencement of sexual activity and increases with age after menopause as, under the influence of decreased estrogen, *Escherichia coli* replaces vaginal lactobacilli. The incidence of UTI in males older than 50 years approaches and eventually exceeds that of females due to the increasing prevalence of prostate hypertrophy and related instrumentation.

At least 1 episode of painless hematuria, a complaint that may or may not be related to a concurrent UTI, is reported by approximately 3% of the general population. The incidence is higher in women (because of UTI) and older patients (because of malignancy and, in men, benign prostate hypertrophy).

CLINICAL FEATURES

UTIs presenting to the ED are categorized into 2 major clinical syndromes: acute cystitis and acute pyelonephritis. Patients with acute cystitis, in which infection is localized to the bladder, typically will present with dysuria, frequency, and suprapubic discomfort. In the young male, however, dysuria is likely to represent urethritis or prostatitis. Patients with acute pyelonephritis, in which infection has spread to the kidney, typically present with localized kidney pain, fever, chills, nausea, vomiting, malaise, and costovertebral angle tenderness, in addition to the preceding symptoms of cystitis.

Subclinical pyelonephritis, a syndrome in which infection has spread to the kidneys without overt symptoms and signs beyond those of cystitis, is clinically indistinguishable from acute cystitis without specialized diagnostic techniques and is estimated to be present in about 25% to 30% of patients diagnosed with cystitis. Epidemiologic risk factors include lower socioeconomic status, pregnancy, structural urinary tract abnormality, history of UTI relapse after treatment, prior history of acute pyelonephritis, frequent UTIs, symptoms for longer than 7 days, or diabetes or immunosuppressing infections.

Hematuria may be microscopic or gross (visible). Microscopic hematuria, which is primarily a laboratory entity, suggests, although not exclusively, a renal source. Gross hematuria, which presents in a spectrum from discoloration of the urine to passage of frank blood and clots, suggests a lower tract source.

DIAGNOSIS AND DIFFERENTIAL

The differential diagnosis of UTI includes vulvovaginitis, cervicitis, mechanical or chemical urethritis, and urolithiasis. A mid-stream urine specimen or a sample from urethral catheterization, if otherwise necessary, should be analyzed for nitrite and leukocyte esterase reactions, pyuria, bacteriuria, and hematuria.

The urine nitrite reaction has a high specificity but a low sensitivity for UTI; a positive result strongly suggests the diagnosis, but a negative result does not rule it out. A positive urine leukocyte esterase reaction from pyuria, although marginally sensitive as an indicator of UTI in ED patients in general, is relatively sensitive in symptomatic women with high levels of pyuria. Abnormal pyuria in women is defined as 2 to 5 leukocytes (white blood cells) per high power field ($\times 400$) from a centrifuged specimen. In men, more than 1 to 2 white blood cells per high power field in the presence of bacteriuria is significant. False negatives can occur with large, dilute urine volumes, partly treated UTI, renal obstruction, or systemic leukopenia. Bacteriuria may be absent in women with low-grade, noncoliform or chlamydial UTIs but is a specific marker for detection of UTI. More than 15 bacteria per oil power field in a centrifuged specimen is significant, but false positives can occur with vaginal or fecal contamination. In a male with dysuria, a Gram stain of urethral discharge may show evidence suggestive of a gonococcal or chlamydial urethritis or another sexually transmitted infection.

Urine cultures should be sent in the following settings of UTI: acute pyelonephritis, patients needing to be hospitalized, patients with chronic indwelling urinary catheters, pregnant women, children, and adult males. Asymptomatic bacteriuria, defined as a urine culture with more than $10^5/mL$ of a single bacterial species in an asymptomatic patient, occurs in up 5% of women ages 18 to 40 years and even more frequently in female nursing home residents and patients with indwelling urinary catheters.

Elderly, diabetic, or severely ill patients with acute pyelonephritis that has been poorly responsive to therapy should undergo imaging with renal ultrasound or other modalities to evaluate for obstruction.

The differential diagnosis of apparent gross hematuria includes myoglobinuria, hemoglobinuria, porphyruria, pigmenturia from various foods, and medication metabolite excretion. True hematuria may result from infection, inflammation trauma, or uroepithelial breakdown in any part of the genitourinary tract, from kidneys to urethra. Etiologies include UTI, nephrolithiasis, autoimmune or immune-mediated disease (eg, Henoch-Schönlein purpura, immunoglobulin A nephropathy, and post streptococcal glomerulonephritis), shistosomiasis, renal vein thrombosis, malignant hypertension, sickle cell anemia, strenuous exercise (a common benign cause in younger patients) and urogenital malignancy (typically in older patients), and coagulopathy or anticoagulant use.

In the urinalysis for hematuria, free hemoglobin, myoglobin, porphyrins, or povidone-iodine in urine may lead to a false positive urine test strip reaction for blood, so confirmatory microscopic analysis is helpful. Microscopic hematuria is defined as more than 5 red blood cells (RBCs) per high power field in centrifuged urine. Abnormal RBC morphology, RBC casts, and proteinuria suggest glomerular disease.

EMERGENCY DEPARTMENT CARE AND DISPOSITION

Urinary Tract Infection

The most common urinary pathogen in UTI is *E coli,* accounting for up to 80% of cases, with *Klebsiella, Proteus, Enterobacter,* and *Pseudomonas*

species, *Chlamydia trachomatis,* and *Staphylococcus saprophyticus* constitut-
ing the remainder.

1. Adult females with a diagnosis of simple cystitis and few prior episodes of
   UTI, brief duration of symptoms, no risk factors for subclinical pyelonephritis, and good available follow-up should be treated with a 3-day course of
   oral antibiotic therapy with 1 of the following: a fluoroquinolone such as
   ciprofloxacin 250 to 500 mg twice daily (bid), **levofloxacin** 250 mg every
   24 hours, or **ofloxacin** 200 to 400 mg bid; **co-trimoxazole,** 1 double-
   strength tablet bid or **trimethoprim** 200 mg bid. **Amoxicillin/clavulanate**
   250/125 mg bid or **nitrofurantoin** macrocrystals 100 mg 4 times daily can
   be used, especially in pregnant patients (who also can be treated with
   cephalexin 500 mg 4 times daily for 7 days or **amoxicillin** 250 mg 3 times
   daily for 7 days), but may require 5 to 7 days of treatment. Emerging resistance to these routinely used antibiotics, with the exception of the
   quinolones, has made quinolone therapy a first-line treatment choice.
2. Adult females with risk factors for subclinical pyelonephritis and a low
   likelihood of compliance with follow-up should receive a 10- to 14-day
   course of 1 of the above-mentioned antibiotics because they are likely to
   respond poorly to a shorter course of therapy.
3. Adult males with lower UTI also should receive a 10-day course of antibiotics, once urethritis and prostatitis are ruled out, and referred to a urologist for evaluation of a suspected underlying anatomic abnormality.
4. Asymptomatic bacteriuria poses a special problem in pregnancy; if untreated, it has a significantly higher likelihood of progression to symptomatic UTI or pyelonephritis than in nonpregnant patients, leading to
   subsequent complications including miscarriage. Treatment of asymptomatic bacteriuria in pregnancy, with a 7-day course, is therefore unequiv-
   ocally indicated (see Chap. 59).
5. The decision to admit the patient with acute pyelonephritis is based on age,
   host factors, comorbidity, and response to initial ED interventions. Adequate
   intravenous fluid should be administered to dehydrated or vomiting patients.
   Urine cultures should be analyzed. A dose of an oral or intravenous antibiotic should be administered. Intravenous options include a fluoroquinolone
   such as **ciprofloxacin** 400 mg every 12 hours or **levofloxacin** 250 mg every
   24 hours, **ampicillin** 1 g plus **gentamicin** 2 mg/kg, or a third-generation
   cephalosporin such as **ceftriaxone** 1 g every 12 hours.
6. Young patients with no comorbidity who are able to take oral fluids and
   antibiotics can be discharged on a 10- to 14-day course of a fluoroquinolone or 1 of the oral regimens described above if available culture
   sensitivities suggest susceptibility.
7. Patients with intractable nausea and vomiting, unremitting fever, and loss
   of vasomotor tone should be admitted.
8. Additional indications for admission involve factors associated with an un-
   favorable prognosis, such as advanced age, debility, renal calculi or obstruction, a history of recent hospitalization or instrumentation, diabetes
   mellitus, chronic nephropathy, sickle cell anemia, underlying carcinoma,
   or intercurrent cancer chemotherapy.

Hematuria

Causes of hematuria include UTI, nephrolithiasis, autoimmune or immune-
mediated disease (eg, Henoch-Schönlein purpura, immunoglobulin A

nephropathy, and post streptococcal glomerulonephritis), shistosomiasis, renal vein thrombosis, malignant hypertension, sickle cell anemia, strenuous, urogenital malignancy, and anticoagulants or coagulopathy. Treatment of hematuria should be directed at the underlying cause, if known and amenable. The crux of subsequent ED management is the minimization of complications and appropriate referral or admission for additional evaluation.

1. In patients with gross hematuria likely to lead to bladder outlet obstruction by coagulated blood, insertion of a triple lumen urinary catheter and bladder irrigation with saline until clearing will facilitate drainage.

2. Patients younger than 40 years with painless hematuria, which is usually benign and transient, may be referred to a primary care provider for a repeat urinalysis.

3. Patients older than 40 years, especially with risk factors for urogenital malignancy, should be referred to a urologist for a timely outpatient evaluation.

4. All patients with hematuria and significant proteinuria (which implies glomerular disease) require a referral for an expeditious outpatient work-up.

5. Patients with bladder outlet obstruction, pregnancy, or new diagnosis of frank glomerulonephritis (especially with evidence of pulmonary edema, volume overload, or renal dysfunction) should be admitted.

For further reading in *Emergency Medicine: A Comprehensive Study Guide,* 6th ed., see Chap. 94, "Urinary Tract Infections," and Chap. 97, "Hematuria and Hematospermia," by David S. Howes and Mark P. Bogner.

54 | Male Genital Problems

Stephen H. Thomas

From the patient's perspective, few problems match the anxiety of a male with acute genital pain. The extensive sensory innervation of the perineal structures combines with the psychological impact of genital pain to pose a unique challenge for the emergency physician.

TESTICULAR TORSION

Clinical Features

Testicular torsion must be the primary consideration in any male (in any age group) complaining of testicular pain. Pain usually occurs suddenly, is severe, and is felt in the lower abdominal quadrant, the inguinal canal, or the testis. The pain may be constant or intermittent but is not positional because torsion is primarily an ischemic event. Although symptom onset tends to occur after exertion, the testicle also may twist from unilateral cremasteric muscle contraction during sleep.

Diagnosis and Differential

In indeterminate cases, color-flow duplex ultrasound and, less commonly, radionuclide imaging may be helpful. In addition, urinalysis is typically ordered, but pyuria does not rule out testicular torsion.

Torsion of the appendages is more common than testicular torsion but is not dangerous because the appendix testis and appendix epididymis have no known function. If the patient is seen early, diagnosis can be supported by the following: pain is most intense near the head of the epididymis or testis; there is an isolated tender nodule; or the pathognomonic blue dot appearance of a cyanotic appendage is illuminated through thin prepubertal scrotal skin. If normal intratesticular blood flow can be demonstrated with color Doppler, immediate surgery is not necessary because most appendages calcify or degenerate over 10 to 14 days and cause no harm.

The differential for testicular torsion also includes epididymidis, inguinal hernia, hydrocele, and scrotal hematoma.

Emergency Department Care and Disposition

1. When the diagnosis is obvious, urologic consultation is indicated for exploration because imaging tests can be too time-consuming.
2. The emergency physician can attempt manual detorsion. Most testes twist in a lateral to medial direction, so detorsion is performed in a medial to lateral direction, similar to the opening of a book. The endpoint for successful detorsion is pain relief; urologic referral is still indicated.
3. Urology is consulted early in the patient's course even when confirmatory testing is planned. When the diagnosis of testicular torsion cannot be ruled out by diagnostic studies or examination, urologic consultation is indicated.

EPIDIDYMITIS AND ORCHITIS

Clinical Features

Epididymitis is characterized by gradual onset of pain due to inflammatory causes. Bacterial infection is the most common, with infecting agents dependent on the patient's age. In patients younger than 40 years, epididymitis is due primarily to sexually transmitted diseases; culture or DNA probe for gonococcus and *Chlamydia* is indicated in males younger than 40 years even in the absence of urethral discharge. Common urinary pathogens predominate in older men. Epididymitis causes lower abdominal, inguinal canal, scrotal, or testicular pain alone or in combination. Due to the inflammatory nature of the pain, patients with epididymitis may note transient pain relief when elevating the scrotal contents while recumbent (positive Prehn sign).

Diagnosis and Differential

Initially, when tenderness is well localized to the epididymis, the clinical diagnosis is clear. However, progression of inflammation results in the physical examination finding of a single, large testicular mass (epididymoorchitis), which is difficult to differentiate from testicular torsion or carcinoma. Testicular malignancy should be suspected in patients presenting with asymptomatic testicular mass, firmness, or induration. Ten percent of tumors present with pain due to hemorrhage within the tumor. Orchitis in isolation is rare; it usually occurs with viral or syphilitic disease.

Emergency Department Care and Disposition

1. If the patient appears toxic, admission for intravenous antibiotics (eg, **ceftriaxone** 1 to 2 g every 12 hours or **trimethoprim/sulfamethoxazole** 5 mg/kg of trimethoprim component every 6 hours) is indicated.
2. Outpatient treatment is the norm in patients who do not appear toxic; urologic follow-up within 1 week is indicated. Oral antibiotic regimens should include 10 days of therapy with 1 of the following: **doxycycline** 100 mg twice daily or **ofloxacin** 300 mg twice daily for patients younger than 40 years; for patients 40 years or older, **trimethoprim/sulfamethoxazole,** 1 double-strength tablet twice daily, or a quinolone, such as **levofloxacin** 250 mg daily, is indicated.
3. In addition, scrotal elevation, ice application, nonsteroidal anti-inflammatory drugs, opioids for analgesia, and stool softeners are indicated.
4. Orchitis is treated with disease-specific therapy, symptomatic support, and urologic follow-up. (Patients at risk for syphilitic disease should be treated as directed in Chap. 86.)

SCROTUM

Scrotal abscesses may be localized to the scrotal wall or may arise from extensions of infections of intrascrotal contents (ie, testis, epididymis, and bulbous urethra). A simple hair follicle scrotal wall abscess can be managed by incision and drainage; no antibiotics are required in immunocompetent patients. When a scrotal wall abscess is suspected of coming from an intrascrotal infection, ultrasound and retrograde urethrography may demonstrate pathology in the testis and/or epididymis and in the urethra, respectively. Definitive care of any complex abscess calls for a urology consultation.

Fournier gangrene is a polymicrobial infection of the perineal subcutaneous tissues. Diabetic males are at highest risk, but any immunocompromise can be associated with the disease. Prompt diagnosis is essential to prevent extensive tissue loss. Early surgical consultation is recommended for at-risk patients who present with scrotal, rectal, or genital pain. Treatment mainstays include aggressive fluid resuscitation with normal saline solution; broad-spectrum antibiotics to cover gram-positive, gram-negative, and anaerobic organisms, such as **ampicillin/sulbactam** 3 g intravenously; surgical debridement; and hyperbaric oxygen therapy.

PENIS

Balanoposthitis is inflammation of the glans (balanitis) and foreskin (posthitis). Upon foreskin retraction, the glans and prepuce appear purulent, excoriated, malodorous, and tender. Treatment consists of cleaning with mild soap, ensuring adequate dryness, application of antifungal creams (**nystatin** 4 times daily or **clotrimazole** twice daily) and an oral azole (**fluconazole** daily), and urologic referral for follow-up and possible circumcision. An oral cephalosporin (eg, **cephalexin** 500 mg 4 times a day) should be prescribed in cases of secondary bacterial infection.

Phimosis is the inability to retract the foreskin proximally. Hemostatic dilation of the preputial ostium relieves the urinary retention until definitive dorsal slit or circumcision can be performed. Topical steroid therapy, such as **hydrocortisone** 1% cream for 4 to 6 weeks, reduces the rate of required circumcision.

Paraphimosis is the inability to reduce the proximal edematous foreskin distally over the glans. Paraphimosis is a true urologic emergency because resulting glans edema and venous engorgement can progress to arterial compromise and gangrene. If surrounding tissue edema can be successfully compressed, as by wrapping the glans with 2 × 2-in. elastic bandages for 5 minutes, the foreskin may be reduced. Making several puncture wounds with a small (22- to 25-gauge) needle may help with expression of glans edema fluid. Local anesthetic block of the penis is helpful if patients cannot tolerate the discomfort associated with edema compression and removal. If arterial compromise is suspected or has occurred, local infiltration of the constricting band with 1% plain lidocaine followed by superficial vertical incision of the band will decompress the glans and allow foreskin reduction.

Penile entrapment injuries occur when various objects are wrapped around the penis. Such objects should be removed, and urethral integrity (retrograde urethrogram) and distal penile arterial blood supply (Doppler studies) should be confirmed when indicated.

Penile fracture occurs when there is an acute tear of the penile tunica albuginea. The penis is acutely swollen, discolored, and tender in a patient with history of intercourse-associated trauma accompanied by a snapping sound. Urologic consultation is indicated.

Peyronie disease presents with patients noting sudden or gradual onset of dorsal penile curvature with erections. Examination shows a thickened plaque on the dorsal penile shaft. Assurance and urologic follow-up are indicated.

Priapism is a painful pathologic erection that may be associated with urinary retention. Infection and impotence are other complications. In most cases, the initial therapy for priapism is **terbutaline** 0.25 to 0.5 mg (repeated in 20 minutes, if needed) subcutaneously in the deltoid area. If patients present early (within 4 hours), oral **pseudoephedrine** (60 to 120 mg) may be effective. Patients with priapism from sickle cell disease are usually treated with simple or exchange transfusion. Corporal aspiration and irrigation with normal saline solution or an α-adrenergic antagonist is the next step and may need to be performed by the emergency physician when urologic consultation is not available. Even when emergency physicians provide stabilizing care, urologic consultation is indicated in all cases.

URETHRA

Urethral stricture is becoming more common due to the high incidence of sexually transmitted diseases. If a patient's bladder cannot be cannulated with a 14- or 16-French Foley or Coudé catheter, the differential diagnosis includes urethral stricture, voluntary external sphincter spasm, bladder-neck contracture, or benign prostatic hypertrophy. Retrograde urethrography can be performed to delineate the location and extent of urethral stricture. Endoscopy is necessary to confirm bladder neck contracture or define the extent of an obstructing prostate gland. Suspected voluntary external sphincter spasm can be overcome by holding the patient's penis upright and encouraging him to relax his perineum and breathe slowly during the procedure. After no more than 3 gentle attempts to pass a 12-French Coudé catheter into a urethra prepared with anesthetic lubricant, urologic consultation should be obtained. In an emergency situation, suprapubic cystotomy can be performed. The infraumbilical and suprapubic areas are prepped with povidone-iodine solution. A 25- to 27-gauge spinal needle is used to locate the bladder (emergency department ultrasound can facilitate this), followed by placement of the cystotomy with the Seldinger technique. Urologic follow-up should occur within 48 hours.

Urethral foreign bodies are associated with bloody urine and slow, painful urination. Radiography of the bladder and urethral areas may disclose a foreign body. Removal of the foreign body may be achieved with a gentle milking action; retrograde urethrography or endoscopy is required in such cases to confirm an intact urethra. Often, urologic consultation for endoscopy or open cystotomy is required for foreign body removal.

URINARY RETENTION

Clinical Features

Urinary retention syndromes can range from overt retention to insidious overflow incontinence. A detailed history, including over-the-counter cold and diet aids, may indicate the cause of urinary retention. Men do not void as completely when sitting down, and infrequent ejaculation may lead to a secondary prostatic congestion and symptoms of outlet obstruction. An intact sensory examination, anal sphincter examination, and bulbocavernosus reflex test differentiate chronic outlet obstruction from the sensory or motor neurogenic bladder and spinal cord compression.

Diagnosis and Differential

Physical examination should include search for meatal stenosis, palpation of urethral length for masses or fistulae consistent with urethral stricture disease or abscess formation, lower abdominal examination for palpation of suprapubic mass, and rectal examination to evaluate anal sphincter tone and prostate size and consistency.

Emergency Department Care and Disposition

1. Most patients with bladder outlet obstruction are in distress, and passage of a urethral catheter alleviates their pain and their urinary retention. Copious intraurethral lubrication including a topical anesthetic should be used, and a 16-French Coudé catheter is recommended if straight catheters fail. The catheter should be passed to its fullest extent to obtain free urine flow before inflating the balloon. The catheter should be left indwelling and connected to a leg drainage bag.
2. **Belladonna** and **opium** suppositories (1 every 4 to 6 hours) can be prescribed to alleviate the constant urge to void secondary to bladder spasm, which frequently accompanies an indwelling catheter.
3. In patients whose bladder catheter will be left in longer than 5 to 7 days, prophylactic antibiotics (eg, **trimethoprim** 100 mg/d) should be instituted. Otherwise, antibiotics are indicated only if urinalysis is consistent with urinary tract infection.
4. If urinary retention has been chronic, postobstructive diuresis may occur even in the presence of normal serum urea nitrogen and creatinine levels. In such patients, close monitoring of urinary output is indicated, and they should be observed for 4 to 6 hours after catheterization.
5. In all cases of urinary retention, urologic follow-up is indicated for a complete genitourinary evaluation.

For further reading in *Emergency Medicine: A Comprehensive Study Guide,* 6th ed., see Chap. 95, "Male Genital Problems," by Robert E. Schneider.

55 | Urologic Stone Disease

Geetika Gupta

The acute phenomenon of renal stones migrating down the ureter is referred to as *renal colic*. Adults and children present with kidney stones. In adults, the condition is 3 times more common in males than in females, and kidney stones usually occur in the third to fifth decade of life. Children constitute 7% of cases seen, with the distribution being equal between the sexes.

CLINICAL FEATURES

Patients usually present with an acute onset of severe pain, which may be associated with nausea, vomiting, and diaphoresis. The pain is sharp and episodic in nature due to the intermittent obstruction and is relieved after the stone passes. The pain typically originates in either flank, radiating around the abdomen toward the groin; however, as the stone passes distally, it may become anterior abdominal or suprapubic in nature. Vesicular stones may present with intermittent dysuria and terminal hematuria. Patients are frequently anxious, pacing, or writhing and are unable to hold still or converse. Children may present in a similar fashion, but up to 30% have only painless hematuria. Vital signs may demonstrate tachycardia and an elevated blood pressure, which are secondary to pain. Pyrexia may be present if there is a concomitant urinary tract infection. Examination may show costovertebral tenderness or abdominal tenderness over the site of the impacted stone.

DIAGNOSIS AND DIFFERENTIAL

Upon clinical suspicion of a kidney stone, an initial dipstick urine test and complete urinalysis expedites the differential diagnosis and rules out infection. Microscopic hematuria is present 90% of cases. Plain abdominal films have poor sensitivity and specificity for detecting renal calculi.

The use of noncontrast helical computed tomography is the mainstay of diagnosis in the emergency department (ED). Positive findings include ureteral caliber changes, suspicious calcifications, stranding of perinephric fat, and dilation of the collecting system. Disadvantages are that it does not evaluate renal function or define the degree of obstruction. For this purpose, the intravenous pyelogram (IVP) is still useful.

The IVP provides functional and anatomical information. Before obtaining an IVP, the patient's potential for an allergic reaction or nephrotoxicity in response to the contrast agent should be assessed by review of the patient's history, comorbidities, hydration status, and a current serum urea nitrogen and creatinine level. Appropriate materials for managing allergic reactions should be readily available. Positive findings include distention of the renal pelvis, calyceal distortion, dye extravasation, hydronephrosis, ureteral column dye cutoff, and a delay in appearance of a nephrogram. Postvoid films are useful in diagnosing distal stones. False negative IVP can occur in the radiolucent, partly obstructing stone.

Ultrasound, an anatomic rather than a functional test, is useful in patients who are not candidates for IVP or computed tomography. It detects hydronephrosis and larger stones but is not sensitive for midureteral stones or small stones (<5 mm).

A differential diagnosis for renal stone includes a symptomatic abdominal aortic aneurysm, incarcerated hernia, epididymitis, testicular torsion, ectopic pregnancy, salpingitis, pyelonephritis, papillary necrosis (sickle cell disease, diabetes, nonsteroidal analgesic abuse, or infection), renal infarction, appendicitis, herpes zoster, drug-seeking behavior, and musculoskeletal strain. A right ureteral stone can resemble cholecystitis. Patients receiving outpatient extracorporeal shock wave lithotripsy for urolithiasis may present to the ED with renal colic because the resulting "sludge" is passed in the urine.

EMERGENCY DEPARTMENT CARE AND DISPOSITION

In most cases the diagnosis of urologic stones and renal colic is clinical. Management consists of excluding infection and other diagnoses, supportive care, analgesia, and appropriate referral.

1. Aggressive titration of analgesia is required. Narcotics, such as **morphine** 8 to 10 mg intravenously or **hydromorphone** 1 to 2 mg intravenously, may be accompanied by nonsteroidal anti-inflammatory drugs (NSAIDs) but should not be their replacement, because the onset of pain relief with NSAIDs is much slower. NSAIDs also should be used with caution in patients with suspected compromise of overall renal function.
2. It is controversial as to which patients require ED imaging. For healthy young patients in whom the diagnosis is very straightforward, it may be appropriate to delay workup to an outpatient basis. For older patients with a more complicated differential diagnosis, the diagnosis should be confirmed by some imaging modality.
3. While the patient is in the ED, all urine should be collected and strained for pathologic analysis of collected stones. In cases of complicating urinary tract infection, antibiotics (eg, **ciprofloxacin** 500 mg orally twice daily) should be started.
4. Discharge is appropriate for patients with small unilateral stones (<6 mm), no infection, and pain controlled by oral analgesics. Patients may be given a urinary strainer, prescriptions for oral narcotics, and urologic follow-up within 7 days. If the stone is passed in the ED, no treatment is necessary other than elective urologic follow-up. Patients should be instructed to return if they develop fever, persistent vomiting, or uncontrolled pain.
5. Urologic consultation on an emergent basis is prudent in the patient with infection and concurrent obstruction. Disposition should be discussed with a urologist in patients with a stone larger than 6 mm, renal insufficiency, severe underlying disease, IVP with extravasation or complete obstruction, or failed outpatient management.
6. Hospitalization is indicated if the patient has an infection with concurrent obstruction, solitary kidney and complete obstruction, uncontrolled pain, intractable emesis, and large or proximal stones.

For further reading in *Emergency Medicine: A Comprehensive Study Guide,* 6th ed., see Chap. 96, "Urologic Stone Disease," by Rakesh Engineer and W. F. Peacock, IV.

56 | Complications of Urologic Devices

David M. Cline

COMPLICATIONS OF URINARY CATHETERS

Infection is the most common complication of urinary catheters, and management is discussed in Chap. 53. Minor traumatic complications of urinary catheters may require no therapy, whereas major complications (eg, bladder perforation) require consultation with a urologist.

Nondraining Catheter

Obstruction is suggested when the catheter does not easily flush or when there is no return of the irrigant. Obstruction of the catheter by blood clots often creates a situation in which the catheter is easily flushed, but little or no irrigant is returned. If this occurs, the catheter can be replaced with a triple lumen catheter so that the bladder can be easily irrigated. If, after clearing the bladder of all clots, evidence of continued bleeding is present, urologic consultation is recommended for possible cystoscopy. Some physicians advocate the use of single lumen catheters to lavage the bladder because its larger lumen may aid in the evacuation of larger clots.

Nondeflating Retention Balloon

If the obstruction is distal, the result of a crushed or defective valve, the catheter can be cut proximal to the defect. If this does not deflate the balloon, a lubricated guidewire can be introduced into the cut inflation channel in an attempt to clear the obstruction. The balloon can be ruptured within the bladder. However, urologic consultation should be considered before rupturing the balloon because overinflation (using sterile water) often requires 10 to 20 times the normal balloon volume. Urologic consultation will be required if simple measures are not successful.

COMPLICATIONS OF PERCUTANEOUS NEPHROSTOMY TUBES

Percutaneous nephrostomy is a urinary drainage procedure used for supravesical or ureteral obstruction secondary to malignancy, pyonephrosis, genitourinary stones, or ureteral strictures. Bleeding may occur, and most episodes can be managed with irrigation to clear the nephrostomy tube of clots. In resistant cases, check the complete blood cell count, renal function, and coagulation studies (as indicated by comorbidities). The patient should be treated for hemodynamic instability and consult urology.

Infectious complications of nephrostomy tubes range from simple bacteriuria, pyelonephritis, renal abscess, bacteremia, and urosepsis. Any wound drainage should be checked, an antibiotic, such as ciprofloxacin 400 mg intravenously, should be started, and urology should be consulted.

Mechanical complications, such as catheter dislodgement and tube blockage, can occur with these devices. The urologist has several techniques available to reestablish access to an obstructed nephrostomy tube.

COMPLICATIONS OF URETERAL STENTS

Dysuria, urinary urgency, frequency, and abdominal and flank discomfort are common complaints in patients with ureteral stents. The baseline discomfort in a functioning, well-positioned stent can range from minimal to debilitating. However, an abrupt change in the character, location, or intensity of the pain requires further evaluation for stent malposition, malfunction, and infection.

Ureteral stents may remain in place for weeks to months and often function with no complication during the entire period. However, stents often can become encrusted with mineral deposits and may obstruct. Complete obstruction of urine flow is possible, although this tends to occur more often in patients with stents in place for long-term use. These patients may require urologic consultation and in some cases may require stent replacement.

URINARY TRACT INFECTION VERSUS STENT MIGRATION AND MALFUNCTION

Changing abdominal or flank pain or bladder discomfort may be indicative of stent migration. X-ray examination is indicated with comparison with a previous film to evaluate stent position, and urologic consultation with further studies to evaluate stent position eventually may be necessary.

When a urinary tract infection occurs in the presence of a stent, stent removal is not mandatory because most infections can be managed with outpatient antibiotics. If pyelonephritis or systemic infection is evident, then further evaluation and emergent intervention are indicated. Plain x-ray examination to check for stent migration and urologic consultation for evaluation of stent migration and malfunction are indicated, as is initiation of antibiotic therapy.

For further reading in *Emergency Medicine: A Comprehensive Study Guide,* 6th ed., see Chap. 98, "Complications of Urologic Procedures and Devices," by Elaine B. Josephson and Jatinder Singh.

9 | GYNECOLOGY AND OBSTETRICS

57

Vaginal Bleeding and Pelvic Pain in the Non-Pregnant Patient

Cherri Hobgood

PREPUBERTAL CHILDREN

In prepubertal girls, vaginitis is the most common cause of pelvic pain and bleeding. Candidiasis is the most common pathogen and can be treated with topical creams (see Chap. 62). Vaginal bleeding can be secondary to maternal estrogen withdrawal in neonates. Trauma to the genital area must alert physicians to the possibility of sexual assault. Vaginal foreign bodies may present with intermittent bloody, foul-smelling discharge. Other conditions to consider are congenital vaginal abnormalities, precocious puberty and menarche, urethral prolapse, and dermatologic lesions.

VAGINAL BLEEDING IN ADOLESCENTS AND ADULTS

Clinical Features and Diagnosis

Once pregnancy is excluded, consider structural and traumatic causes of bleeding. A thorough pelvic examination may show the source. Bleeding can arise from the uterus or cervix and may be due to cervicitis, endometrial or cervical polyps, cervical or endometrial (especially in older women) cancer, submucosal fibroids, local trauma to the genitalia, or retained foreign body. In postmenopausal women the most common causes of vaginal bleeding are exogenous estrogens, atrophic vaginitis, and endometrial lesions including cancer, with each accounting for approximately 30% of cases. Other tumors such as vulvar, vaginal, and cervical compose approximately 10% of cases. Most of these patients can be referred for definitive gynecologic care.

Dysfunctional uterine bleeding (anovulatory), which yields irregular shedding of a thickened endometrium, is a likely cause if the findings on pelvic examination are normal. Anovulation is especially common in peri-menarcheal girls and perimenopausal women, although in the latter malignancy is the most worrisome concern. Patients with anovulatory cycles present with prolonged menses, irregular cycles, or intermenstrual bleeding. Usually the bleeding is painless and minimal, but severe bleeding can occur, resulting in anemia and iron depletion. In these cases coagulopathy must be excluded. Coagulopathy is considered a cause of vaginal bleeding, especially in young women with menorrhagia. Primary coagulation disorders account for 19% of menorrhagia in teenagers, including von Willebrand disease, myeloproliferative disorders, and immuno-thrombocytopenia. Skin signs such as petechiae may be absent.

Emergency Department Care and Disposition

Most patients with vaginal bleeding require no immediate interventions. Hemodynamically unstable patients require standard resuscitation, and prompt dilation and curettage usually is indicated. Intravenous (IV) conjugated estrogens may be administered in the unstable patient. Hemodynamically stable patients thought to have anovulatory dysfunctional uterine bleeding can be managed medically with hormonal manipulation.

1. For patients with severe bleeding, IV conjugated **estrogen** 25 mg may be given every 2 to 4 hours for 24 hours until bleeding slows. More commonly, oral (PO) therapy is given: conjugated **estrogen** 2.5 mg 4 times daily. **Medroxyprogesterone** 10 mg/d is added when the bleeding subsides; both drugs are continued for 7 to 10 days

2. **PO contraceptive** is given: ethinyl estradiol 35 μg and norethindrone 1 mg, 4 tablets/d for 7 days. A slow taper may be given: ethinyl estradiol 35 μg and norethindrone 1 mg, 4 tablets for 2 days, 3 tablets for 2 days, 2 tablets for 2 days, and then 2 tablets for 3 days.

3. **Medroxyprogesterone** (Provera) 10 mg/d PO for 10 days also can be used to stabilize the endometrium.

With all therapies, withdrawal bleeding occurs 3 to 10 days after stopping progesterone and may be heavy. Older patients in whom there is concern about underlying malignancy should not be started on hormones in the emergency department (ED) but should be referred to a gynecologist for biopsy. Nonsteroidal anti-inflammatory drugs are useful adjuncts to decrease bleeding in most patients. In patients with bleeding dyscrasias or known fibroid disease, these drugs should be used with caution, if at all.

PELVIC PAIN

Although most female patients with pelvic pain have a gynecologic etiology, consideration must be given to nongynecologic conditions such as inflammatory bowel disease, gastroenteritis, diverticulitis, urinary tract infection or obstruction, and, in particularly appendicitis. Pelvic inflammatory disease, a serious and common cause of pelvic pain, is covered in detail in Chap. 63.

Ovarian Cysts

A common noninfectious cause of pelvic pain is ovarian cysts. Ovarian cysts occur in women with normal menstrual cycles. Ovarian enlargement is initially asymptomatic or causes poorly defined visceral pain due to poor afferent innervation. When leakage or rupture occurs, acute pain results from irritation of the parietal peritoneum from the cyst or mass contents. There may be associated peritoneal signs due to irritation from cystic fluid or blood. Pregnancy must be excluded because rupture of a cyst can mimic ectopic pregnancy. Transvaginal ultrasound is the most useful test for detection of adnexal pathology and free fluid. Patients with unruptured cysts smaller than 8 mm can be treated with pain medication, typically nonsteroidal anti-inflammatory agents, and should be referred for gynecologic follow-up. If a cyst has ruptured and the patient is hemodynamically stable, she may be discharged with analgesics and follow-up. Rupture of a hemorrhagic corpus luteum cyst may cause hemoperitoneum with hypotension and require surgical intervention (but abdominal pain without significant bleeding is more likely). Rupture is most common in the second half of the menstrual cycle.

Ovarian Torsion

Ovarian torsion and adnexal torsion are rare but serious causes of pelvic pain in women. Torsion often occurs in ovaries that are enlarged or abnormal due to cyst or tumor. The ovary twists on its pedicle, with compromise of its blood supply and necrosis. Torsion of tubal masses and pedunculated fibroids can present similarly. Patients have sudden onset of severe pelvic pain. Many patients have nausea and vomiting. There may be a history of previous similar episodes. On pelvic examination, patients have unilateral adnexal tenderness, pain, and usually a mass. Ultrasound, in particular Doppler flow ultrasound, may be helpful, but often the diagnosis is not made until the time of surgery. When this diagnosis is suspected, urgent gynecologic consultation and preparation for surgery are warranted. Laparoscopic ovarian or adnexal detorsion or removal is the treatment of choice.

Endometriosis

In this disease, normal endometrium occurs in ectopic locations. Most commonly, pelvic structures, including the gutters, cul-de-sac, ligaments, and pelvic peritoneum, are affected, but distant extrapelvic endometrium also occurs.

After primary dysmenorrhea, this is the most common cause of mid-cycle pain. Symptoms include pelvic pain, usually at menses; dyspareunia; and dysmenorrhea. Pelvic examination is most commonly normal or may demonstrate pain and tenderness. Rupture of an ovarian endometrioma may present with acute, severe pain with peritoneal signs. Ultrasound may show endometriomas, but the definitive diagnosis is rarely made in the ED and must be confirmed at laparoscopy. The most appropriate ED management is analgesia and referral.

Leiomyomas

Commonly called fibroids, leiomyomas are benign muscle tumors. They are the most common pelvic tumor, occurring in 1 in 4 women by the age of 40 years. They are often multiple. Up to 30% of women with fibroids have associated pelvic pain and bleeding. Acute pain is rare, but severe pain may be associated with torsion of a pedunculated fibroid or fibroid degeneration. In pregnant women, fibroids may degenerate (infarct) due to rapid growth with outstripping of the blood supply, causing acute severe pain. The diagnosis usually is suggested on pelvic examination by an enlarged uterus or palpable uterine masses. Ultrasound is confirmatory. With degeneration, an acute abdomen may occur, but most patients can be managed with analgesia and referral. Nonsteroidal anti-inflammatory treatment is not useful in the treatment of pain associated with fibroids.

Complications of In Vitro Fertilization

Ovarian hyperstimulation syndrome resulting in ovarian enlargement and fluid loss occurs in up to 10% of patients undergoing in vitro fertilization. Mild forms present with weight gain, thirst, and abdominal pain. Severe forms present with hypovolemia, hypotension, and acute respiratory distress. Physical manifestations may include pericardial effusion, ascites, hydrothorax, hepatorenal failure, and thromboembolism. Patients should be evaluated with liver and renal function tests, coagulation screens, and chest radiograph. Treatment is standard resuscitation with IV fluids, avoidance of diuretic therapy, and heparin when indicated.

For further reading in *Emergency Medicine: A Comprehensive Study Guide,* 6th ed., see Chap. 101, "Vaginal Bleeding and Pelvic Pain in the Nonpregnant Patient," by Laurie Morrison and Julie Spence; and Chap 102, "Abdominal and Pelvic Pain in the Nonpregnant Patient," by Reb Close.

58 | Ectopic Pregnancy

David M. Cline

Ectopic pregnancy (EP) occurs in 2% of all pregnancies and is the leading cause of maternal death in the first trimester. Twenty percent of EPs are ruptured at the time of presentation. Major risk factors include history of pelvic inflammatory disease; surgical procedures on the fallopian tubes, including tubal ligation; previous EP; diethylstilbestrol exposure, intrauterine device use; and assisted reproduction techniques. This diagnosis must be considered in every woman of childbearing age presenting with abdominal pain.

CLINICAL FEATURES

The classic triad of abdominal pain, vaginal bleeding, and amenorrhea used to describe EP may be present, but many cases occur with more subtle findings. Presenting signs and symptoms may be different in ruptured versus nonruptured EP. Only 90% of women with EP complain of abdominal pain; 80% have vaginal bleeding; and only 70% give a history of amenorrhea. The pain described may be sudden, lateralized, extreme, or relatively minor and diffuse. The presence of hemoperitoneum causing diaphragmatic irritation may cause pain to be referred to the shoulder or upper abdomen. Vaginal bleeding is usually light; heavy bleeding is more commonly seen with threatened abortion or other complications of pregnancy. Presenting vital signs may be entirely normal even with a ruptured ectopic pregnancy or may indicate advanced hemorrhagic shock. There is poor correlation with the volume of hemoperitoneum and vital signs in EP. Relative bradycardia may be present even in cases with rupture and intraperitoneal hemorrhage. Physical examination findings are highly variable. The abdominal examination may show signs of localizing or diffuse tenderness with or without peritoneal signs. The pelvic examination findings may be normal but more often shows cervical motion tenderness, adnexal tenderness with or without a mass, and possibly an enlarged uterus. Fetal heart tones are only rarely audible.

DIAGNOSIS AND DIFFERENTIAL

Urine pregnancy testing (for urinary β-human chorionic gonadotropin [β-hCG]) should be performed immediately. Dilute urine may result in a false negative result; serum testing will produce a more definitive result in such situations. Transvaginal ultrasound is the test of choice to identify EP. If an intrauterine pregnancy is identified, the chance of a coexisting EP is extremely small in most patients. However, if a patient has been on fertility drugs, has had in vitro fertilization, or has multiple risk factors for EP, further evaluation for EP is warranted. A progesterone level of 5 ng/mL or lower with an empty uterus or nonspecific fluid collection in the uterus determined by ultrasound is highly suggestive of EP, but a progesterone level cannot be used to exclude EP.

Sonographic findings of an empty uterus with adnexal mass (other than a simple cyst) with or without free fluid in the abdomen are highly suggestive of EP. Sonographic findings of empty uterus without an adnexal mass or free fluid in a woman with a positive pregnancy test result is considered indeterminate. In such situations, the findings must be evaluated in context with the patient's quantitative β-hCG level. A high β-hCG level (>6,000 mIU/mL) with an empty uterus is suggestive of EP. If the β-hCG is low (<1,000 mIU/mL), then the pregnancy may indeed be intrauterine or ectopic but too small to be visualized on ultrasound. In this situation, repeat quantitative β-hCG testing in 2 days must be performed. A normal intrauterine pregnancy should show at least a 66% increase in the β-hCG level in that period; EP would show a slower rate of increase. Levels between 1,000 and 6,000 mIU/mL may warrant dilation and curettage or laparoscopy to diagnose EP after evaluation by an obstetric-gynecologic consultant. Individual hospitals may vary in the expertise of the sonographers available, and levels other than 1,000 and 6,000 mIU/mL may be reasonable guidelines in certain institutions.

Differential diagnosis in the patient presenting with abdominal pain, vaginal bleeding, and early pregnancy includes threatened, incomplete, or missed abortion; recent elective abortion; or endometritis.

EMERGENCY DEPARTMENT CARE AND DISPOSITION

Treatment of patients with suspected EP depends on the patient's vital signs, physical signs, and symptoms. Close communication with the obstetric-gynecologic consultant is essential.

1. For unstable patients, 2 large-bore intravenous lines are started for rapid infusion of crystalloid and/or packed red blood cells to maintain blood pressure.
2. Bedside urine pregnancy test is performed.
3. An obstetric-gynecologic consultant is notified immediately for the unstable patient, even before laboratory and diagnostic tests are complete.
4. Blood is drawn for complete blood count, blood typing, and rhesus (Rh) factor determination (or crossmatching for the unstable patients), quantitative β-hCG determination (if indicated), and serum electrolytes determination, as required.
5. If the patient is stable, the diagnostic workup, including transvaginal ultrasound, in continued. Reliable patients with indeterminate ultrasound results and a β-hCG level below 1,000 mIU/mL are discharged with ectopic precautions and arranged follow-up in 2 days for repeat β-hCG determination, and obstetric-gynecologic reevaluation is appropriate.
6. Definitive treatment, as determined by the obstetric-gynecologic consultant, may involve laparoscopy, dilation and curettage, or medical management with methotrexate.

For further reading in *Emergency Medicine: A Comprehensive Study Guide,* 6th ed., see Chap. 103, "Ectopic Pregnancy," by Richard S. Krause and David M. Janicke.

59 | Comorbid Diseases in Pregnancy

Sally S. Fuller

DIABETES

Diabetics are at increased risk for hypertensive diseases, preterm labor, spontaneous abortion, pyelonephritis, fetal demise, hypoglycemia, and diabetic ketoacidosis (DKA). For those diabetics whose blood sugar is not controlled with diet, insulin is required (oral hypoglycemic agents are contraindicated). Insulin requirements increase throughout pregnancy, from 0.7 to 1.0 U/(kg · d) at term. Typically, two thirds of the insulin is given in the morning (two thirds NPH and one third regular) and one third is given in the evening (one half NPH and one half regular). DKA tends to occur more rapidly and at lower glucose levels than in a non-pregnant patient and has a high rate of fetal mortality. DKA is treated with continuous insulin infusion. Oxygen and left lateral positioning to improve uterine blood flow is also recommended. Hypoglycemia management is unchanged in pregnancy. Mild hypoglycemia is treated with a snack of milk and crackers, with care to avoid overcorrection of the blood sugar. Intravenous (IV) dextrose and/or intramuscular glucagon is used in the obtunded patient.

HYPERTHYROIDISM

Hyperthyroidism in pregnancy increases the risk of preeclampsia and neonatal morbidity. Clinical features may be subtle and may include hyperemesis gravidarum. Propylthiouracil is the treatment of choice.

Thyroid storm has a high mortality rate and presents with fever, volume depletion, and cardiac decompensation. Propylthiouracil, sodium iodide, and propranolol (unless cardiac failure is present) can control symptoms. Radioactive iodine is not used. (For further information, see Chap. 132.)

DYSRHYTHMIAS

Dysrhythmias, rare in pregnancy, are treated with lidocaine, digoxin, procainamide, and verapamil in the usual doses. β-Blockers may be used acutely for control but not for long-term use. Cardioversion has not been shown to be harmful to the fetus. For anticoagulation with atrial fibrillation, heparin or enoxaparin is used.

THROMBOEMBOLISM

Factors associated with increased risk of thromboembolism include advanced maternal age, increasing parity, multiple gestations, operative delivery (13- to 16-fold increase compared with vaginal delivery), bedrest, obesity, and hypercoagulable states. Clinical features of deep venous thrombosis (DVT) and pulmonary embolism (PE) are similar in pregnant and non-pregnant patients. Diagnosis of DVT may be made by duplex Doppler studies, impedance plethysmography, or technetium 99m radionuclide venography. To diagnose PE, ventilation and perfusion scanning or pulmonary angiography may be performed. Iodine 125 fibrinogen scanning should not be used. Spiral computed tomography for PE has not been studied in pregnancy.

DVT and PE are treated with heparin (to maintain a partial thromboplastin time of 1.5 to 2 times normal) or enoxaparin 1 mg/kg twice daily. Warfarin is contraindicated (see Chap. 29).

ASTHMA

Clinical presentation of cough, wheezing, and dyspnea is similar in pregnant and non-pregnant patients. Peak expiratory flow rates are unchanged in pregnancy. However, the normal Pco_2 on the arterial blood gas is 27 to 32, with a normal pH of 7.40 to 7.45.

Acute therapy includes β_2-agonists such as albuterol via nebulizer. IV methylprednisolone, oral prednisone, and subcutaneous epinephrine can be used in pregnancy. Oxygen should be administered to maintain a Po_2 greater than 65 mm Hg. As in any potentially serious medical condition, the patient in the third trimester should be positioned with a left-leaning tilt to maximize uterine blood flow and oxygen delivery. Fetal monitoring should be done after 20 weeks' gestation. Criteria for intubation or admission are similar in pregnant and non-pregnant patients; standard agents for rapid sequence intubation are used.

URINARY TRACT INFECTIONS

Urinary tract infection is the most common bacterial infection in pregnancy. Clinical features are similar in pregnant and non-pregnant women. Simple cystitis may be treated for 3 days with **nitrofurantoin** slow release 100 mg orally (PO) twice daily (first choice), **amoxicillin** 500 mg PO 3 times daily, or **cephalexin** 500 mg PO 4 times daily. Patients with pyelonephritis are treated more aggressively in the pregnant population because of increased risk of preterm labor and sepsis. Admission for IV hydration and antibiotics (**cefazolin** 1-2 g IV, or **ampicillin** 1 g IV plus **gentamicin** 1 mg/kg IV) should be arranged. After treatment for pyelonephritis, antibiotic suppression should continue for the remainder of the pregnancy. Quinolones are contraindicated during pregnancy. Sulfonamides should be avoided close to term. Trimethoprim may be used after the first trimester.

INFLAMMATORY BOWEL DISEASE

The general treatment of the pregnant patient with inflammatory bowel disease is the same as that of the non-pregnant patient. Antidiarrheal drugs including codeine and Lomotil may be used safely. Sulfasalazine, in combination with folic acid supplements, also may be used.

SICKLE CELL DISEASE

Women with sickle cell disease are at higher risk for miscarriage, preterm labor, and vasoocclusive crises. Clinical features, evaluation, and treatment are similar in pregnant and non-pregnant patients. Management includes aggressive hydration and analgesic therapy. Narcotics should be used; nonsteroidal anti-inflammatory agents should be avoided after 32 weeks' gestation. Hydroxyurea should be discontinued in pregnancy. Aplastic crises occur rarely and are associated with parvovirus infection (Fifth disease) and hydrops fetalis.

MIGRAINE

Classic migraine headaches usually improve during pregnancy. Treatment includes acetaminophen and narcotics. Ergot alkaloids and Triptan should not be used.

SEIZURE DISORDERS

Management of a pregnant patient with a known seizure disorder is similar to that of a non-pregnant patient. Valproic acid is avoided because of an association with neural tube defects. Other anticonvulsants also have associated risks to the fetus; therefore, management with a single drug is desirable. Isolated seizures usually cause no apparent harm to the fetus. However, status epilepticus with prolonged maternal hypoxia and acidosis has a high mortality rate for the mother and infant. Status epilepticus should be treated aggressively with early intubation and ventilation. Fetal oxygenation should be optimized by placing the patient in the left lateral position and administering supplemental oxygen.

INFECTION WITH HUMAN IMMUNODEFICIENCY VIRUS

All pregnant women with the human immunodeficiency virus beyond 14 weeks' gestation should be on zidovudine therapy to reduce the risk of transmission to the fetus.

Patients with CD4 counts lower than 200 should be on prophylaxis for *Pneumocystis carinii;* trimethoprim-sulfamethoxazole or aerosolized pentamidine may be used, although trimethoprim-sulfamethoxazole should be discontinued close to term. Treatment of opportunistic infections is unchanged in pregnancy (see Chap. 89 for more information).

SUBSTANCE ABUSE

Cocaine use is associated with increased incidence of fetal death in utero, placental abruption, preterm labor, premature rupture of membranes, spontaneous abortion, intrauterine growth restriction, and fetal cerebral infarcts. Benzodiazepines should be avoided in early pregnancy; otherwise, treatment of toxicity is unchanged in pregnancy. Opiate withdrawal in pregnant women is treated with methadone or clonidine (0.1–0.2 mg every hour until signs of withdrawal resolve; up to 0.8 mg total). Alcohol use contributes to increased rates of spontaneous abortion; low-birthweight, preterm deliveries; and fetal alcohol syndrome. Acute withdrawal is treated with short-acting barbiturates; benzodiazepines are avoided in early pregnancy.

DRUG USE IN PREGNANCY

Table 59-1 provides general recommendations regarding drug use in pregnancy. For any drug not listed in the table, the manufacturer's recommendations should be checked before administration.

DOMESTIC VIOLENCE

Approximately 15% of pregnant women are victims of domestic violence. They are at risk for placental abruption, uterine rupture, preterm labor, and fetal fractures. Rhesus immune globulin (RhoGAM) 300 μg intramuscularly should be considered after blunt abdominal trauma in rhesus-negative patients.

TABLE 59-1 Drug Use in Pregnancy*

Drug	Category†	Comments
Antibiotic		
Cephalosporins	B	
Penicillins	B	
Erythromycin	B	Estolate salt contraindicated due to hepatotoxicity, otherwise may use
Azithromycin	B	
Clarithromycin	C	
Nitrofurantoin	B	
Clindamycin	B	
Metronidazole	B	Should be avoided in first trimester
Ethambutol	B	
Quinolones	C, D	Toxicity to fetal cartilage
Aminoglycosides	C, D	Some of this class cause ototoxicity
Isoniazid	C	In TB, benefit may outweigh risk
Clavulanate combos	B	
Sulfonamides	C	Avoid close to term due to hyperbilirubinemia
Tetracycline	D	Not recommended in second half of pregnancy due to tooth discoloration
Trimethoprin	C	
Antivirals		
Acyclovir	B	
Zidovudine	C	Recommended in HIV-infected patients to prevent fetal transmission
Antihypertensives		
α-Methyldopa	B	
β-Blockers	C	
Calcium channel blockers	C	
Hydralazine	C	Frequently used
ACE inhibitors	D, X	Contraindicated due to occurrence of fetal death, oligohydramnios
Anticonvulsants		
Valproic acid	X	2–3% incidence of neural tube defects reported
Phenytoin	C, D	Congenital malformations have been reported, but benefits may outweigh risks, folic acid 1 mg/d may help prevent teratogenesis
Carbamazepine	C, D	
Corticosteroids	C	May be used for serious maternal conditions, gestational diabetes may develop

(*continued*)

TABLE 59-1 Drug Use in Pregnancy* *(continued)*

Drug	Category†	Comments
Anticoagulants		
Heparin	C	
Enoxaparin	B	
Warfarin	X	Contraindicated due to birth defects and bleeding complications
Analgesics		
Acetaminophen	A	
Propoxyphene	C	Caution advised when used close to term, neonatal withdrawal may occur
Opiates	C	
Ibuprofen	B	Frequently used for short duration, should not be used after 32 wk
Naproxen		
Other NSAIDs	C, D	
Sumatriptan	C	
Ergot alkaloids	X	Potential for fetal death and abortion
Antiemetics		
Meclizine	B	
Diphenhydramine	B	
Metoclopramide	B	
Phenothiazine	C	Widely used
Ondansetron	B	
Vaccines		
Live vaccines (measles/mumps/rubella)	X	Potential exists for fetal transmission
Inactivated viral vaccines-rabies, hepatitis B, influenza	C	Commonly given in pregnancy
Pneumococcal vaccine	C	Avoid using in first trimester
Tetanus and diphtheria	C	Commonly given in pregnancy
Tetanus immune globulin	C	Commonly given in pregnancy

*Few studies have been done on pregnant women, therefore any medication should be used only if clearly necessary. Consult drug reference for more information.

†A = safe, B = presumed safe, C = possible adverse effect, D = unsafe but use may be justifiable in certain circumstances, X = contraindicated.

Key: ACE = angiotensin-converting enzyme, HIV = human immunodeficiency virus, NSAIDs = nonsteroidal anti-inflammatory drugs, TB = tuberculosis.

DIAGNOSTIC IMAGING IN PREGNANCY

The threshold for teratogenesis from ionizing radiation is 0.1 Gy, with 8 to 15 weeks' gestation being the most vulnerable period. The effects of radiation exposure change with gestational age. The second to the eighth week post conception is the period of organogenesis, when the fetus is most at risk for birth defects. Mental retardation and other problems may occur with significant x-ray exposure between 8 and 25 weeks. No single test exceeds the teratogenic threshold, but the effects are cumulative, and multiple tests may exceed the threshold. Ultrasound, ventilation/perfusion scanning, and magnetic resonance imaging have not shown any teratogenic effects.

For further reading in *Emergency Medicine: A Comprehensive Study Guide,* 6th ed., see Chap. 105, "Comorbid Diseases in Pregnancy," by Jessica L. Bienstock and Harold E. Fox.

60 | Emergencies during Pregnancy and the Postpartum Period

Sally S. Fuller

THREATENED ABORTION AND ABORTION

Clinical Features

The different stages of abortion are distinguished by history and physical examination. Vaginal bleeding in the first 20 weeks, with a closed cervical os, benign examination, and no passage of tissue, is termed *threatened abortion.* When the cervix is dilated, the likelihood of abortion becomes much greater, hence, the term *inevitable abortion. Incomplete abortion* is defined as partial passage of the conceptus and is more likely between 6 and 14 weeks of pregnancy. The patient may report passage of grayish white products of conception (POC), or the POC may be evident on pelvic examination. *Complete abortion* is passage of all fetal tissue before 20 weeks' gestation. In general, an ultrasound is necessary to confirm that all POC have passed. All recovered POC should be sent for pathologic examination. *Missed abortion* is fetal death at less than 20 weeks without passage of fetal tissue noted by the patient or on pelvic examination. *Septic abortion* implies evidence of infection during any stage of abortion, with signs and symptoms of pelvic pain, fever, cervical motion or uterine tenderness, or purulent or foul-smelling drainage.

Diagnosis and Differential

A pelvic examination is performed, and a complete blood count (CBC), blood typing and rhesus (Rh) factor determination, quantitative β-human chorionic gonadotropin (β-hCG), and urinalysis are obtained. The differential diagnosis includes ectopic pregnancy (see Chap. 58) and gestational trophoblastic disease (GTD). GTD is a neoplastic disease of trophoblastic tissue and is usually distinguished from threatened abortion by ultrasound. It may be noninvasive (hydatidiform mole) or invasive (choriocarcinoma).

Emergency Department Care and Disposition

1. Hemodynamic instability is managed with rapid infusion of intravenous (IV) crystalloid or packed red blood cells. The gynecologist is consulted emergently in the unstable patient.
2. Rh-negative women should receive 300 μg **Rh (D) immune globulin.**
3. Vaginal ultrasound should show a gestational sac in a normal pregnancy, with a β-hCG level higher than 1,000 mIU/mL. Absence of a gestational sac with a β-HCG higher than 1,000 mIU/mL suggests complete abortion or ectopic pregnancy.
4. Incomplete abortion or GTD requires dilatation and curettage. GTD patients must receive close follow-up until quantitative β-hCG has returned to 0. Failure of the hCG to return to normal may indicate choriocarcinoma.
5. Septic abortion requires gynecologic consultation and broad-spectrum antibiotics such as **ampicillin/sulbactam** 3.0 g IV or **clindamycin** 600 mg plus **gentamicin** 1 to 2 mg/kg IV.

6. Patients with threatened abortion or complete abortion may be discharged with close follow-up arranged. Discharge instructions include pelvic rest (no intercourse or tampons) and instructions to return for heavy bleeding, fever, or pain.

NAUSEA AND VOMITING OF PREGNANCY

Clinical Features

Hyperemesis gravidarum (intractable nausea and vomiting without significant abdominal pain) can cause hypokalemia or ketonemia and may result in a low-birthweight infant. Diagnostic workup should include a CBC, electrolyte panel, and urinalysis.

Emergency Department Care and Disposition

1. Rehydration should begin with IV fluid, 5% dextrose in normal saline, or 5% dextrose in lactate Ringer solution. Failure to include dextrose may result prolonged ketosis.
2. Frequently used antiemetics are **metoclopramide** 10 mg IV, **promethazine** 25 mg IV (pregnancy class C, but widely used), and **odansetron** 4 mg IV.
3. If the patient improves in the emergency department (urine ketones clearing and tolerating oral liquids), she may be discharged with prescription for antiemetics.
4. Admission is indicated for persistent ketonuria, electrolyte abnormalities, or weight loss greater than 10% of prepregnancy weight.

VAGINAL BLEEDING DURING THE SECOND HALF OF PREGNANCY

Abruptio placentae, placenta previa, and preterm labor are the most common causes. Speculum and digital pelvic examinations are contraindicated until ultrasound has been obtained to rule out placenta previa.

Clinical Features and Diagnosis

Abruptio Placentae

Abruptio placentae is the premature separation of the placenta from the uterine wall. Clinical features include vaginal bleeding, abdominal pain, uterine tenderness, hypertonic contractions, increased uterine tone, fetal distress, and, in severe cases, disseminated intravascular coagulation (DIC) and fetal and/or maternal death. Vaginal bleeding may be mild or severe, depending on whether the area of abruption communicates to the cervical os. Abruption of greater than 50% of the placenta usually results in fetal demise. Emergency delivery may be needed to save the life of the fetus or mother.

Placenta Previa

Placenta previa is the implantation of the placenta over the cervical os. Clinical features include painless, bright red vaginal bleeding. The amount of bleeding is frequently large as opposed to normal "bloody show," when a small amount of bright red blood and mucous are passed. Diagnosis is made by abdominal ultrasound, and pelvic examinations are contraindicated due to the potential for causing catastrophic bleeding.

Premature Rupture of Membranes

Premature rupture of membranes (PROM) is rupture of membranes before the onset of labor. Clinical presentation is a rush of fluid or continuous leakage of fluid from the vagina. Diagnosis is confirmed by finding a pool of fluid in the posterior fornix with pH greater than 6.5 (dark blue on Nitrazine paper) and ferning pattern on smear. Sterile speculum examinaiton may be done; however, digital pelvic examination should be deferred, if possible, or done with sterile gloves. Tests for chlamydia, gonorrhea, bacterial vaginosis, and group B streptococcus should be performed.

Emergency Department Care and Disposition

1. Hemodynamic instability is managed with IV normal saline or packed red blood cells.
2. Emergent obstetric consultation, CBC, type and crossmatching, and electrolyte studies on all patients and a DIC profile on the patient with suspected abruptio placentae should be obtained.
3. Transabdominal pelvic ultrasound is used to determine whether placenta previa is present.
4. **Rh (D) immune globulin** 300 µg intramuscularly should be given to Rh-negative patients.
5. Patients with abruptio placentae or placenta previa may need emergent caesarean delivery. Patients with suspected PROM should be admitted.
6. Tocolytics should not be used in patients with suspected abruption.

PRETERM LABOR

Clinical Features and Diagnosis

Preterm labor is defined as labor before 37 weeks' gestation. Clinical features include regular uterine contractions with effacement of the cervix. The diagnosis is made by observation with external fetal monitoring and serial sterile speculum examinations. Digital pelvic examination should be avoided, if possible, or performed with sterile gloves. Tests for chlamydia, gonorrhea, bacterial vaginosis, and group B streptococci should be obtained. Cervical fluid should be examined for possible PROM.

Emergency Department Care and Disposition

1. Mother and fetus are monitored.
2. An obstetrician is consulted for admission and decision regarding tocolytics.
3. If tocolytics are initiated, the mother should receive glucocorticoids to hasten fetal lung maturity.
4. Tocolytics are not used if abruptio placenta is suspected.
5. Gestational age younger than 34 weeks is associated with poorer outcomes; if possible, the patient should be transferred to a tertiary care center with a high-risk intensive care unit.

HYPERTENSION, PREECLAMPSIA, AND RELATED DISORDERS

Hypertension with pregnancy is associated with preeclampsia, eclampsia, HELLP (hemolysis, elevated liver enzymes, and low platelets) syndrome, abruptio placenta, preterm birth, and low-birthweight infants. Hypertension in pregnancy is defined as a blood pressure higher than 140/90 mm Hg, a rise of 20 mm Hg in systolic blood pressure, or a rise of 10 mm Hg in diastolic blood pressure above the prepregnancy level. Hypertension in pregnancy may be chronic due to preexisting hypertension, transient, or preeclampsia.

Clinical Features

Preeclampsia is characterized by hypertension, proteinuria, and usually edema in patient of 20 or more weeks of gestation through the postpartum period. It rarely presents before 20 weeks in patients with GTD. Patients may present with headache, visual disturbances, edema, or abdominal pain. Eclampsia is preeclampsia with seizures. The HELLP syndrome is a clinical variant of preeclampsia. The usual presenting complaint is abdominal pain, especially epigastric and right upper quadrant pain. Because the blood pressure is not always elevated, HELLP syndrome should be considered in the evaluation of all pregnant women (>20 weeks' gestation) with abdominal pain (Table 60-1).

Diagnosis and Differential

Preeclampsia is a clinical diagnosis based on the definition above. The HELLP variant is diagnosed by laboratory tests: schistocytes on peripheral smear, platelet count lower than 150 000/mL, elevated aspartate aminotransferase and alanine aminotransferase levels, and abnormal coagulation profile.

Emergency Department Care and Disposition

1. CBC, urinalysis, electrolyte panel, liver panel, and coagulation profile should be otained.
2. Severe preeclampsia or eclampsia is treated with a **magnesium sulfate** loading dose of 4 to 6 g in 100 mL fluid over 20 minutes, followed by a maintenance infusion of 1 to 2 g/h to prevent seizure. Serum magnesium and reflexes must be monitored.
3. Hypertension is treated with **hydralazine** 2.5 mg initially, followed by 5 to 10 mg IV every 10 minutes; or with **labetalol** 20 mg IV as the initial bolus, with repeat boluses of 40 to 80 mg, if needed, to a maximum of 300 mg for blood pressure control. Nitroglycerin or nitroprusside infusions also may be used.
4. An obstetrician is consulted emergently for severe preeclampsia or eclampsia. Definitive treatment requires delivery of the fetus.

TABLE 60-1 Criteria for Hypertension, Preeclampsia, and Eclampsia

Hypertension	BP >140/90 mm Hg measured twice at least 6 h apart
Transient hypertension	BP >140/90 mm Hg without other signs of preeclampsia or eclampsia
Preeclampsia	BP >140/90, >20 mm Hg rise in systolic, or >10 mm Hg rise in diastolic BP Proteinuria (300 mg/24 h or 1 g/mL) Generalized or pedal edema or weight gain of at least 5 lb over 1 wk
Eclampsia	Above findings plus generalized seizure

Key: BP = blood pressure.

5. All patients with a sustained blood pressure of 140/90 mm Hg or higher plus any symptoms of preeclampsia should be hospitalized.
6. Definitive treatment requires delivery of the fetus.

POSTPARTUM HEMORRHAGE

The differential diagnosis of hemorrhage in the first postpartum day includes uterine atony (most common), uterine rupture, laceration of the lower genital tract, retained placental tissue, uterine inversion, and coagulopathy. After the first 24 hours, retained POC, uterine polyps, or coagulopathy such as von Willebrand disease are the more likely causes. Diagnosis is by physical examination: the uterus is enlarged and "doughy" with uterine atony; a vaginal mass is suggestive of an inverted uterus. Bleeding despite good uterine tone and size may indicate retained POC or uterine rupture. Vaginal or cervical lacerations must be assessed for size, location, and severity. The first priority of emergency department management is stabilization of the patient with crystalloid IV fluids and/or packed red blood cells, if needed. CBC, clotting studies, and type and crossmatching must be obtained. Uterine atony is treated with **oxytocin** 20 U in 1 L intravenous fluids (IVF) at 200 mL/h. Minor lacerations may be repaired when using local anesthetic. Extensive lacerations, retained POC, uterine inversion, or uterine rupture require emergency operative treatment by the obstetrician.

POSTPARTUM ENDOMETRITIS

Postpartum endometritis is most common after caesarean delivery. The etiology is usually polymicrobial. Clinical features include fever, lower abdominal pain, and foul-smelling lochia. Diagnosis is made by physical examination showing uterine or cervical motion tenderness and discharge. Discharge may be minimal in group B streptococcal infections. CBC, urinalysis, and cervical cultures should be obtained. Admission for antibiotic treatment (**cefoxitin** 1-2 g IV every 6 hours or combination therapy with **ampicillin** 1 g IV every 6 hours and **gentamicin** 1.5 mg/kg IV every 8 hours) is appropriate for all but the mildest cases.

MASTITIS

Mastitis is cellulitis of the periglandular breast tissue. Clinical features include swelling, redness, and tender engorgement of the involved portion of the breast. Treatment is with **dicloxacillin** 500 mg orally 4 times daily or **cephalexin** 500 mg orally 4 times daily. Patients should continue nursing on the affected breast.

AMNIOTIC FLUID EMBOLISM

Amniotic fluid embolism is a sudden, catastrophic illness with mortality rates of 60% to 80%. Clinical features include sudden cardiovascular collapse with hypoxemia, seizures, and DIC. Intensive management for cardiovascular collapse and DIC is indicated.

For further reading in *Emergency Medicine: A Comprehensive Study Guide*, 6th ed., see Chap. 106, "Emergencies During Pregnancy and the Postpartum Period," by Gloria J. Kuhn.

61 | Emergency Delivery

David M. Cline

CLINICAL FEATURES

Every patient presenting with signs of active labor should receive immediate monitoring of maternal vital signs and fetal heart rate. Maternal blood pressure should be monitored, and Doppler heart tones are helpful to confirm normal fetal heart rate (120-160 beats/min). A persistently slow fetal heart rate (fewer than 100 beats/min) is an indicator of fetal distress, and emergent obstetric consultation is necessary.

False labor is characterized by irregular, brief contractions usually confined to the lower abdomen. These contractions, commonly called Braxton-Hicks contractions, are irregular in intensity and duration. True labor is characterized by painful, regular contractions of steadily increasing intensity and duration leading to progressive cervical dilatation. True labor typically begins in the fundal region and upper abdomen and radiates into the pelvis and lower back.

DIAGNOSIS AND DIFFERENTIAL

Patients without vaginal bleeding should be examined bimanually and with a sterile speculum. Patients presenting with vaginal bleeding should be evaluated initially with ultrasound before any speculum or bimanual examination to rule out placenta previa. If spontaneous rupture of membranes (SROMs) is suspected, examination with a sterile speculum should be performed and digital examination avoided because studies have shown an increased risk of infection after a single digital examination.

Determining whether membranes have ruptured is an important predictor of the likelihood of imminent labor and the potential for complications such as infection or cord prolapse. SROM occurs during the course of active labor in most patients, although it may occur before the onset of labor in 10% of third-trimester patients. SROM typically occurs with a gush of clear or blood-tinged fluid. It can be confirmed by using Nitrazine paper to test residual fluid in the fornix or vaginal vault while a sterile speculum examination is performed. Amniotic fluid has a pH of 7.0 to 7.4 and will turn Nitrazine paper dark blue. Vaginal fluid typically has a pH of 4.5 to 5.5 and will make the Nitrazine strip remain yellow.

EMERGENCY DEPARTMENT CARE AND DISPOSITION

Emergency Delivery

1. The use of routine episiotomy for a normal spontaneous vaginal delivery has been discouraged in recent years because it increases the incidence of third- and fourth-degree lacerations at the time of delivery.
2. If an episiotomy is necessary, it may be performed as follows.
   a. A solution of 5 to 10 mL of 1% **lidocaine** is injected with a small-gauge needle into the posterior fourchette and perineum.
   b. While protecting the infant's head, a 2- to 3-cm cut is made with scissors to extend the vaginal opening.
   c. The incision must be supported with manual pressure from below, taking care not to allow the incision to extend into the rectum.

3. Control of the delivery of the neonate is the major challenge. As the infant's head emerges from the introitus, the physician should support the perineum with a sterile towel placed along the inferior portion of the perineum with 1 hand while supporting the fetal head with the other. Mild counterpressure is exerted to prevent the rapid expulsion of the fetal head, which may lead to third- or fourth-degree perineal tears.

4. As the infant's head presents, the left hand may be used to control the fetal chin while the right remains on the crown of the head, supporting the delivery. This controlled extension of the fetal head will aid in the atraumatic delivery.

5. The mother is then asked to breathe through contractions rather than bearing down and attempting to push the baby out rapidly.

6. Immediately after delivery of the infant's head, the infant's nose and mouth should be suctioned. This is particularly important in infants presenting with meconium to prevent aspiration. A simple bulb will assist in the routine clearing of the infant's nose and mouth.

7. After suctioning, the neck should be palpated for the presence of a nuchal cord. This is a common condition, found in 25% of all cephalad-presenting deliveries. If the cord is loose, it should be reduced over the infant's head; the delivery may then proceed as usual. If the cord is tightly wound, it may have to be clamped in the most accessible area by 2 clamps in close proximity and cut to allow delivery of the infant.

8. After delivery of the head, the head will restitute or turn to 1 side or the other. As the head rotates, the physician's hands are placed on either side of it, providing gentle downward traction to deliver the anterior shoulder. The physician's hand then gently guides the fetus upward, delivering the posterior shoulder and allowing the remainder of the infant to be delivered.

9. It is useful to prepare for the delivery by placing the posterior (left) hand underneath the infant's axilla before delivering the rest of the body. The anterior hand may then be used to grasp the infant's ankles and ensure a firm grip.

10. The infant is then loosely wrapped in a towel and stimulated as it is dried. The umbilical cord is double clamped and cut with sterile scissors.

11. The infant is then further dried and warmed in an incubator, where postnatal care may be provided and Apgar scores calculated at 1 and 5 minutes after delivery.

12. Scoring includes general color, tone, heart rate, respiratory effort, and reflexes.

Cord Prolapse

1. In the event that the bimanual examination shows a palpable, pulsating cord, the examiner's hand should not be removed, but rather should be used to elevate the presenting fetal part to reduce compression of the cord.

2. Immediate obstetric assistance is then necessary, as a cesarean section is indicated.

3. The examiner's hand should remain in the vagina while the patient is transported and prepped for surgery to prevent further compression of the cord by the fetal heat.

Shoulder Dystocia

1. Shoulder dystocia is first recognized after the delivery of the fetal head, when routine downward traction is insufficient to deliver the anterior shoulder.
2. After delivery of the infant's head, the head retracts tightly against the perineum (the "turtle sign").
3. Upon recognizing shoulder dystocia, the physician should suction the infant's nose and mouth and call for assistance to position the mother in the extreme lithotomy position, with legs sharply flexed up to the abdomen (the McRoberts maneuver) and held by the mother or an assistant.
4. The bladder should be drained if this has not already been done.
5. A generous episiotomy also may facilitate delivery.
6. Next, an assistant should apply suprapubic pressure to disimpact the anterior shoulder from the pubic symphysis.
7. One should never apply fundal pressure because this will further force the shoulder against the pelvic rim.

Breech Presentation

1. Breech presentations may be classified as frank, complete, incomplete, or footling.
2. The frank breech and the complete breech presentations serve as a dilating wedge nearly as well as the fetal head, and delivery may proceed in an uncomplicated fashion.
3. The main point in a frank or complete breech presentation is to allow the delivery to progress spontaneously. This lets the presenting portion of the fetus to dilate the cervix maximally before the presentation of the fetal head. It is recommended that the examiner refrain from touching the fetus until the scapulae are visualized.
4. Footling and incomplete breech positions are not considered safe for vaginal delivery because of the possibility of cord prolapse or incomplete dilatation of the cervix. In any breech delivery, immediate obstetric consultation should be requested.

Postpartum Care

1. The placenta should be allowed to separate spontaneously and assisted with gentle traction. Aggressive traction on the cord risks uterine inversion, tearing of the cord, or disruption of the placenta, which can result in severe vaginal bleeding.
2. After removal of the placenta, the uterus should be gently massaged to promote contraction. **Oxytocin** 20 U in 1 L of 0.9 normal saline is infused at a moderate rate to maintain uterine contraction.
3. Episiotomy or laceration repair may be delayed until an experienced obstetrician is able to close the laceration and inspect the patient for forth-degree (rectovaginal) tears.

62 | Vulvovaginitis

David A. Krueger

Vulvovaginitis is a common problem whose causes include infections, irritants and allergies, foreign bodies, and atrophy. The normal vaginal flora helps maintain an acidic pH between 3.5 and 4.1, which decreases pathogen growth. (For coverage of genital herpes, see Chap. 86.)

BACTERIAL VAGINOSIS

Bacterial vaginosis (BV) is the most common cause of vaginal discharge and odor in women, although many women who meet the clinical criteria described below are asymptomatic. BV occurs when vaginal lactobacilli are replaced by anaerobes, *Gardnerella vaginalis,* and *Mycoplasma hominis.*

Clinical Features

When symptomatic, women with BV have vaginal discharge and may have itching. Examination findings range from mild vaginal redness to a frothy gray-white discharge.

Diagnosis and Differential

The diagnostic criteria of the Centers for Disease Control and Prevention include 3 of the following: (*a*) discharge, (*b*) pH higher than 4.5, (*c*) fishy odor when 10% KOH is added to the discharge (positive amine test result), or (*d*) clue cells, which are epithelial cells with clusters of bacilli stuck to the surface, seen on saline wet preparation. Often, however, the diagnosis of BV is suspected from a compatible presentation in addition to absence of *Candida* and *Trichomonas.*

Emergency Department Care and Disposition

Metronidazole 500 mg orally (PO) twice daily for 7 days is standard treatment of BV. **Clindamycin** 300 mg PO twice daily for 7 days is an alternative. Treatment is not recommended for male partners or asymptomatic women. Routine treatment of asymptomatic pregnant women with BV is not recommended. Pregnant women at high risk of preterm labor should be treated. During the first trimester, metronidazole 0.75% is used in 1 applicator intravaginally twice daily for 5 days.

CANDIDA VAGINITIS

Candida albicans is a normal vaginal commensal in up to 20% of women, and candidiasis is not considered a sexually transmitted disease, although it can be transmitted sexually. Conditions that promote candida vaginitis include systemic antibiotics, diabetes, pregnancy, birth control pills, and the postmenopausal state.

Clinical Features

Symptoms of candidal vaginitis include vaginal discharge, itching, dysuria, and dyspareunia. Signs include vulvar and vaginal edema, erythema, and a thick "cottage cheese" discharge.

Diagnosis and Differential

Vaginal secretions are examined microscopically in a few drops of saline solution or KOH preparation. Ten percent KOH dissolves vaginal epithelial cells, leaving yeast buds and pseudohyphae intact and easier to see. The sensitivity of the KOH technique is 80%.

Emergency Department Care and Disposition

The imidazoles are the drugs of choice. **Clotrimazole** can be given as a 1% to 2% cream or 100 mg to 200 mg vaginal suppository for 3 to 7 days. **Butoconazole** can be given daily as 2% cream with a vaginal applicator for 3 days. **Miconazole** can be given as a 1,200 mg vaginal suppository once daily. **Fluconazole** 150 mg PO is an alternative in the nonpregnant patient. Treatment of sexual partners is not necessary unless candidal balanitis is present.

TRICHOMONAS VAGINITIS

Trichomoniasis, caused by a protozoan, *Trichomonas vaginalis,* is almost always a sexually transmitted disease. However, up to 25% of women harboring the organism are asymptomatic.

Clinical Features

Most patients have vaginal discharge. Other symptoms include perineal irritation, dysuria, spotting, and pelvic pain. Discharge may be frothy and malodorous. Vaginal erythema and irritation are common.

Diagnosis and Differential

Saline wet prep shows motile, pear-shaped, flagellated trichomonads that are slightly larger than leukocytes. The sensitivity of this test is 40% to 80%.

Emergency Department Care and Disposition

One 2-g PO dose of **metronidazole** is the drug of choice. For treatment failures, metronidazole 500 mg twice daily for 7 days is recommended. Concomitant alcohol use may induce a disulfiram-like reaction. Most infected men are asymptomatic; male partners need treatment to avoid retransmission of disease. Metronidazole can be used in pregnancy, with a single dose recommended, but it is not approved until the second trimester. Topical clotrimazole is less effective but safe. If symptoms persist and are severe, metronidazole can be given after the first trimester. During lactation, the single 2-g oral dose is recommended, with no breastfeeding for 24 hours.

CONTACT VULVOVAGINITIS

Common causes of contact vulvovaginitis include douches, soaps, bubble baths, deodorants, perfumes, feminine hygiene products, topical antibiotics, and tight undergarments. Patients complain of perineal burning, itching, swelling, and often dysuria. The examination shows a red and swollen vulvovaginal area. In severe cases, there may be vesicles and ulceration. Vaginal pH changes may promote overgrowth of *Candida,* thus obscuring the primary problem.

The precipitating agent should be identified and infectious causes ruled out. Most cases resolve spontaneously when the precipitant is withdrawn. For more severe reactions, cool sitz baths, compresses with Burrow solution, and topical corticosteroids may help. Oral antihistamines are drying but may be helpful if a true allergy is identified.

VAGINAL FOREIGN BODIES

In younger girls, common items are toilet paper, toys, and small household objects. Later, a forgotten or irretrievable tampon or diaphragm is often the culprit. Patients present with a foul-smelling or bloody discharge. Removal of the object is usually curative without other therapy.

ATROPHIC VAGINITIS

After menopause, the lack of estrogen stimulation leads to vaginal mucosal atrophy. The epithelium becomes pale, thin, and less resistant to minor trauma or infection. Bleeding can occur. The vaginal pH also increases, and subsequent changes in the vaginal flora can predispose to bacterial infection with purulent discharge. Treatment is a topical vaginal **estradiol** cream (0.1 mg/g cream). Treatment begins with 1 to 2 g or the cream per vagina daily for 1 week and then tapers gradually to 1 g/wk. A sulfa cream should be used for secondary infection. Estrogen creams should not be prescribed in the emergency department for women with prior reproductive tract cancer or postmenopausal bleeding. Because carcinoma is a major concern, such patients should be referred to a gynecologist.

For further reading in *Emergency Medicine: A Comprehensive Study Guide,* 6th ed., see Chap. 108, "Vulvovaginitis," by Gloria J. Kuhn.

63 | Pelvic Inflammatory Disease and Tubo-Ovarian Abscess

Robert W. Shaffer

Pelvic inflammatory disease (PID) is the most common serious infection occurring in reproductive-age women in the United States. PID occurs when an infection ascends from the lower genital tract into the normally sterile endometrium, adnexa, or peritoneal cavity. This may lead to salpingitis, endometritis, tubo-ovarian abscess (TOA), perihepatitis, or focal pelvic peritonitis. The disease is almost always caused by *Neisseria gonorrhea* or *Chlamydia trachomatis;* however, 30% to 40% of infections are polymicrobial. Risk factors include multiple sexual partners, sexual abuse, adolescence, presence of other sexually transmitted diseases, douching, and intrauterine device use. PID occurs less commonly in pregnancy, but first-trimester infections can lead to fetal loss. Long-term sequelae include ectopic pregnancy, infertility, and chronic pain.

CLINICAL FEATURES

Lower abdominal pain is usually present. Other symptoms include vaginal discharge, vaginal bleeding, dyspareunia, urinary discomfort, fever, nausea, and vomiting. Peritoneal signs may be present. Occasionally, symptoms are minimal. The presence of right upper quadrant tenderness, especially with associated jaundice, may suggest Fitz-Hugh-Curtis syndrome (perihepatitis).

DIAGNOSIS AND DIFFERENTIAL

Diagnostic criteria are listed in Table 63-1. A pregnancy test, wet prep, and endocervical swabs for gonorrhea and chlamydia are obtained. Elevations in

TABLE 63-1 Treatment Guidelines for Pelvic Inflammatory Disease Based on Diagnostic Criteria

Group 1: Minimum criteria; empirical treatment indicated if no other etiology explains findings
  Uterine or adnexal tenderness
  Cervical motion tenderness

Group 2: Additional criteria improving diagnostic specificity
  Oral temperature >101°F (38.3°C)
  Abnormal cervical or vaginal mucopurulent secretions
  Elevated erythrocyte sedimentation rate
  Elevated C-reactive protein
  Laboratory evidence of cervical infection with *Neisseria gonorrhea* or *Chlamydia trachomatis* (ie, culture or DNA probe techniques)

Group 3: Specific criteria for PID based on procedures that may be appropriate for some patients
  Laparoscopic confirmation
  Transvaginal ultrasound (or MRI) showing thickened, fluid-filled tubes with or without free pelvic fluid or tuboovarian complex
  Endometrial biopsy showing endometritis

Key: MRI = magnetic resonance imaging, PID = pelvic inflammatory disease.
Source: Adapted for *MMWR.* 2002;51(R-6):1.

TABLE 63-2 Parenteral Treatment Regimens for Pelvic Inflammatory Disease

1. Cefotetan 2 g IV q12h *or* cefoxitin 2 g IV q6h
   +
   Doxycycline 100 mg IV/PO q12h
2. Clindamycin 900 mg IV q8h
   +
   Gentamicin 2 mg/kg IV loading dose followed by 1.5 mg/kg q8h
3. Ofloxacin 400 mg IV q12h *or* Levofloxacin 500 mg IV q24h
   +
   Doxycycline 100 mg PO or IV q12h
   ±
   Metronidazole 500 mg IV q8h *or* ampicillin-sulbactam 3 g IV q6h

Key: IV = intravenously, PO = orally, q = every.
Source: Adapted from *MMWR.* 2001; 51(RR-6):1.

white blood cell count, erythrocyte sedimentation rate, and C-reactive protein may help support the diagnosis. A pelvic ultrasound will help detect TOA. PID may mimic surgical conditions such as appendicitis, cholecystitis, and ovarian torsion, and further testing or imaging should be implemented if any of these conditions are suspected. Other differential diagnoses include gastroenteritis, diverticulitis, ectopic pregnancy, spontaneous or septic abortion, ovarian cyst, pyelonephritis, and renal colic.

EMERGENCY DEPARTMENT CARE AND DISPOSITION

1. Treatment guidelines of the Centers for Disease and Control Prevention are outlined in Tables 63-2 and 63-3. Adequate analgesia and hydration should be provided as needed.
2. The decision for inpatient management should be guided by toxic appearance, inability to tolerate oral medication, inability to exclude alternative diagnoses, pregnancy, adolescence, immunosuppression, fertility issues, concern for noncompliance, or suspected anaerobic infection (intrauterine device use, suspected abscess, or recent instrumentation).
3. Sixty percent to 80% of TOAs respond to antibiotics alone; the remainder require drainage.

TABLE 63-3 Oral and Outpatient Treatment Regimens for Pelvic Inflammatory Disease

1. Ofloxacin 400 mg PO BID for 14 d *or* levofloxacin 500 mg PO qd for 14 d
   ±
   Metronidazole 500 mg PO BID for 14 d
2. Ceftriaxone 250 mg IM × 1 *or* cefoxitin 2 g IM × 1 *and* probenecid 1 g PO × 1
   +
   Doxycycline 100 mg PO BID for 14 d
   ±
   Metronidazole 500 mg PO BID for 14 d

Key: BID = twice daily, IM = intramuscularly, PO = orally, qd = daily.
Source: Adapted from *MMWR.* 2002;51(RR-6):1.

4. Outpatients should always follow up within 72 hours. The patient and the sexual partner(s) must complete the full treatment course before resuming sexual activity to prevent reinfection. Preventative counseling and referral for testing for the human immunodeficiency virus should be provided.

For further reading in *Emergency Medicine: A Comprehensive Study Guide,* 6th ed., see Chap 109, "Pelvic Inflammatory Disease," by Amy J. Behrman, William Shoff, and Suzanne M. Shepherd.

64 | Complications of Gynecologic Procedures

Debra Houry

The most common reasons for emergency department visits during the post-operative period after gynecologic procedures are pain, fever, and vaginal bleeding. A focused but thorough evaluation should be performed including sterile speculum and bimanual examination. (Complications common to gynecologic and general surgeries are covered in Chap. 50.)

COMMON COMPLICATIONS OF ENDOSCOPIC PROCEDURES

Laparoscopy

The major complications associated with the use of the laparoscope are: (*a*) thermal injuries to the bowel; (*b*) bleeding at the site of tubal interruption or sharp dissection; (*c*) incisional hernia; and (*d*) rarely, ureteral or bladder injury, large bowel injury, and pelvic hematoma or abscess. Of these complications, the most serious is thermal injury to the bowel. These patients generally appear 3 to 7 days postoperatively, depending on the degree of necrosis, with signs and symptom of peritonitis, including bilateral lower abdominal pain, fever, elevated white blood cell count, and direct and rebound tenderness. X-rays show an ileus or free air under the diaphragm. Although gas has been used to insufflate the abdomen, it should be absorbed totally within 3 postoperative days. Patients who have increasing pain after laparoscopy, either early or late, have a bowel injury until proved otherwise. If thermal injury is a serious consideration and cannot be distinguished from other causes of peritonitis, it is best to err on the side of early laparotomy.

Hysteroscopy

Complications of hysteroscopy include (*a*) reaction to the distending media, (*b*) uterine perforation, (*c*) cervical laceration, (*d*) anesthesia reaction, (*e*) intraabdominal organ injury, (*f*) infection, and (*g*) postoperative bleeding. Postoperative bleeding will be the most likely cause of hospital revisit. After hemodynamic stabilization of the patient, the gynecologist can insert a pediatric Foley or balloon catheter to tamponade the bleeding. Infection as a result of the hysteroscopic procedure is uncommon. Treatment should be commensurate with presentation and symptoms.

MISCELLANEOUS COMPLICATIONS OF MAJOR GYNECOLOGIC PROCEDURES

Cuff Cellulitis

Cuff cellulitis refers to infections of the contiguous retroperitoneal space immediately above the vaginal apex and the surrounding soft tissue. It is a common complication after abdominal and vaginal hysterectomies. It usually produces a fever between postoperative days 3 and 5. These patients complain of fever, pelvic pain, and abnormal vaginal discharge. Pelvic tenderness and induration are prominent during the bimanual examination. A vaginal cuff abscess may be palpable. The treatment of choice is readmission, drainage, and intravenous antibiotics as determined by the gynecologist.

Post-Conization Bleeding

The most common complication associated with loop electrocautery and cold-knife conization of the cervix is bleeding. If delayed hemorrhage occurs, it usually occurs 7 days postoperatively. Bleeding after this procedure can be rapid and excessive. Visualization of the cervix is the key to controlling such bleeding. Application of Monsel solution or cauterization with silver nitrate is a reasonable first step. Suturing of the bleeding arteriole may be necessary. Usually, the patient must be taken to the operating room for repair secondary to poor visualization.

Induced Abortion

Retained products of conception and a resulting endometritis are the most common delayed complications. Patients usually complain of excessive bleeding, fever, and abdominal pain 3 to 5 days posttermination, but patients may not return with complaints for up to 2 weeks. Pelvic examination will show a sub-involuted tender uterus with foul-smelling blood vaginally. An elevated white blood cell count is common. Treatment must include evacuation of intrauterine contents and intravenous antibiotic therapy. If the patient has pain, bleeding, or both but without fever, missed ectopic pregnancy must be ruled out.

Assisted Reproductive Technology/Ovarian Hyperstimulation Syndrome

Although complications related to ultrasound-guided retrieval of oocytes are rare, patients may present with ovarian hyperstimulation syndrome, pelvic infections, intraperitoneal bleeding, and adnexal torsion. Ovarian hyperstimulation syndrome can be life-threatening and occurs in 1% to 2% after assisted reproductive technology. Early symptoms include abdominal distention, ovarian enlargement, and weight gain. In severe form, patients have massive third spacing of fluids into the abdominal cavity, which can progress to ascites, electrolyte imbalances, pleural effusions, and hypovolemia. Abdominal and pelvic examinations are contraindicated due to extremely fragile ovaries that are at high risk of rupture or hemorrhage. The gynecologist should be consulted early for admission.

For further reading in *Emergency Medicine: A Comprehensive Study Guide,* 6th ed., see Chap. 112, "Complications of Gynecologic Procedures," by Michael A. Silverman and Karen M. Hardart.

10 | PEDIATRICS

65 | Fever

Douglas K. Holtzman

Fever is the most common chief complaint presenting to an emergency department and accounts for 30% of outpatient visits each year. Fever is the result of the body's thermostat being reset by exogenous and endogenous pyrogens. It has long been argued that "fever is good" and should be allowed to persist. Most children, however, feel uncomfortable, and certain children are at risk for febrile seizures, so fever is generally treated.

CLINICAL FEATURES

Present pediatric guidelines consider any rectal temperature of at least 38°C (100.4°F) to be a fever and warrants an evaluation. In general, higher temperatures are associated with a higher incidence of bacteremia.

DIAGNOSIS AND DIFFERENTIAL

Infants up to 3 Months

Early studies suggested that infants younger than 3 months were at high risk of a serious bacterial illness (SBI). Current practice guidelines use 0 to 8 weeks of age, with some clinicians using an upper limit of 6 weeks. Febrile infants younger than 1 month are at the greatest risk of bacteremia (an average of 13%), with a bacteremia risk of 10% during their second month of life. The birth history is vital because certain etiologies of infection may be related to that time.

The young infants are especially problematic in assessing severity of illness. Immature development and immature immunity make reliable examination findings difficult. Persistent crying, inability to console, poor feeding, or temperature instability may be the only findings suggestive of an SBI. A history of cough, tachypnea, or hypoxia should alert the examiner to a possible lower respiratory tract infection.

Criteria used to help define the infant at low risk for an SBI include well appearance without a history of prematurity, white blood cell count (WBC) between 5,000 and 15,000/mm^3, absolute neutrophil count of less than 10,000/μL, urinalysis with fewer than 10 WBCs per high powered field (HPF), cerebral spinal fluid with fewer than 5 WBCs/HPF, and stool with fewer than 5 WBCs/HPF in infants with diarrhea. Infants with a suggestion of lower respiratory tract disease should have a chest x-ray.

Any infant with abnormal criteria should receive parenteral antibiotic therapy and be admitted to the hospital. Management of low-risk infants remains a subject of significant debate. In general, all infants younger than 1 month should be started on parenteral antibiotics (**ceftriaxone** 50 mg/kg or **cefotaxime** 50 mg/kg if younger than 1 week) and admitted to the hospital regardless of low-risk findings because of their immature immune status. Infants older than 4 weeks at low risk may be managed conservatively as inpatients with **ceftriaxone** 50 mg/kg pending cultures; as inpatients without antibiotics; as outpatients with **ceftriaxone** 50 mg/kg or **amoxicillin** 45 mg/kg twice daily; or as outpatients without antibiotics. The key deciding factor should be the physician's comfort level and the ability for close follow-up, typically within 24 hours.

Infants 3 to 24 Months

Physical examination findings appear to be more reliable in this age group. The history and physical examination often will lead the clinician to the diagnosis. Viral illnesses including pneumonia account for most febrile illnesses in this age group. The most common bacterial etiology is *Streptococcus pneumoniae.* Other etiologies for otitis media include nontypeable *Haemophilus influenza* and *Moraxella catarrhalis.* Of those children ages 3 to 36 months with *S pneumoniae* bacteremia, only 0.019% develop meningitis. Urinary tract infections are a significant source in females and uncircumcised males younger than 2 years and all males younger than 1 year.

The typical meningitic symptoms of nuchal rigidity, Kernig or Brudzinski signs, may not be apparent in children younger than 2 years. A high index of suspicion should occur in children presenting with new seizure activity, inability to be consoled, bulging fontanelle, or severe irritability.

Current recommendations for treating suspected occult bacteremia include **ceftriaxone** (50 mg/kg) or **amoxicillin** (45 mg/kg twice daily) with a 24-hour follow-up regardless of therapy chosen. Ceftriaxone should never be initiated without appropriate antecedent or coincident diagnostic studies.

Older Febrile Children

The risk for bacteremia in children older than 3 years is significantly low. Etiologies to consider include streptococcal pharyngitis, pneumonia, and mononucleosis.

EMERGENCY DEPARTMENT CARE AND DISPOSITION

Although fever makes children uncomfortable and may potentiate seizures, it typically is not harmful to children. The physician can use several methods to reduce fever.

1. Removing excessive clothing and blankets can increase heat loss through radiation.
2. **Acetaminophen** 10 to 15 mg/kg can be given every 4 hours (maximum of 5 doses in 24 hours). Some clinicians advocate the use of 40 to 45 mg/kg as an initial loading dose when using it rectally.
3. **Ibuprofen** 5 to 10 mg/kg can be given every 6 hours (maximum of 40 mg/kg in 24 hours). Some clinicians recommend caution when patients have a known streptococcal pharyngitis because of the increased association with toxin-mediated disease.
4. All children with positive blood cultures should be recalled for a repeat evaluation. If the patient is afebrile and clinically well, that patient should complete a 10-day course of antibiotic therapy (typically **amoxicillin** 40 to 45 mg/kg twice daily).
5. If the child with a positive blood culture remains febrile or continues to appear ill, a full septic workup (complete blood cell count, repeat blood culture, lumbar puncture, urine culture, and chest x-ray) should be performed. The patient should be hospitalized and receive parenteral antibiotics.

For further reading in *Emergency Medicine: A Comprehensive Study Guide,* 6th ed., see Chap. 115, "Fever," by Carol D. Berkowitz.

66 | Bacteremia, Sepsis, and Meningitis in Children

Milan D. Nadkarni

OCCULT BACTEREMIA

Children ages 3 to 36 months are at increased risk of occult bacteremia (OB), which occurs in approximately 2.8% of patients with rectal temperatures of 39°C (102.2°F) or higher. *Streptococcus pneumoniae* accounts for more than 90% of OB cases, with *Neisseria meningitidis,* group A streptococcus, and *Salmonella* responsible for the remainder.

Clinical Features

The hallmark symptom of OB is fever, and the incidence rises incrementally with rectal temperatures above 39°C (102.2°F). The child appears relatively well, exhibiting fever alone or in combination with signs of minor infection, such as upper respiratory infection, vomiting, or diarrhea. Because children with OB do not appear toxic, clinical signs are not reliable indicators of this condition.

Diagnosis and Differential

Children between 3 and 36 months of age have the highest incidence of OB but the lowest rate of serious bacterial illness. Evaluation of fever in this age group is also dependent on the extent of the fever, the presence of risk factors, focus of infection, and the ability to ensure adequate and timely follow-up. Focus of infection is defined as an identifiable source of infection; examples include bronchiolitis, gastroenteritis, gingivostomatitis, moderate to severe upper respiratory infection, and otitis media. Children between the ages of 3 and 36 months without a focus of infection may need a bacteremia workup, which includes a complete blood count (CBC), blood culture, urine analysis and urine culture, and a chest radiograph (only if respiratory signs and symptoms are present). Definitive diagnosis of OB is made by blood culture. Predictors of OB include temperature above 39°C (102.2°F), white blood cell count (WBC) above 15,000/μL or below 5,000/μL, absolute neutrophil count above 10,000/μL, or larger than 10% band count (regardless of total WBC).

Emergency Department Care and Disposition

1. All febrile infants younger than 6 weeks should undergo a septic workup, be given intravenous (IV) antibiotics (Table 66-1), and be admitted to the hospital.
2. Febrile infants 6 to 12 weeks may not require a full septic evaluation if they have no risk factors, have reliable caretakers, and follow-up can be arranged within 12 hours. Acceptable options follow.
   a. CBC, blood culture, catheter urinalysis, and culture and sensitivities are collected, but antibiotics are not given and follow-up is within 12 hours.
   b. A complete septic workup is done, and **ceftriaxone** 50 mg/kg intramuscularly is administered, with follow-up in 12 hours.
   c. A complete septic workup is done; antibiotics are withheld and follow-up is in 12 hours.

TABLE 66-1 Initial Intravenous Antibiotic Therapy for Sepsis and Meningitis

Age	Sepsis*	Meningitis
<60 d	Ampicillin 100 mg/kg plus	Ampicillin 100 mg/kg plus
	Cefotaxime 50 mg/kg consider	Cefotaxime 50 mg/kg consider
	Acyclovir 20–30 mg/kg†	Acyclovir 20–30 mg/kg
2 mo and older children	Cefotaxime 50 mg/kg or	Cefotaxime 100 mg/kg or
	Ceftriaxone 50 mg/kg plus consider	Ceftriaxone 100 mg/kg plus
	Vancomycin 15 mg/kg‡	Vancomycin 15 mg/kg

*Use meningitis doses if the patient is considered too unstable for lumbar puncture.

†Consider acyclovir for patients with cerebrospinal fluid pleocytosis or neonatal seizures.

‡Consider addition of vancomycin in sepsis with critical illness.

  d. A complete septic workup with admission to the hospital and IV antibiotics is performed.
3. Indications for empiric antibiotic treatment for OB are temperature above 39°C (102.2°F) in children ages 3 to 36 months, WBC above 15,000/μL or below 5,000/μL, absolute neutrophil count above 10,000/μL (regardless of total WBC), and larger than 10% band count (regardless of total WBC).
4. There is considerable debate about the choice of empiric antibiotic treatment of OB. Options include:
  a. **Ceftriaxone** 50 mg /kg IV or intramuscularly once, which effectively covers the patient until culture results are available. There is good evidence that this action prevents sequelae.
  b. Ceftriaxone as above plus **amoxicillin** 80 mg/kg/d divided 2 times a day for 7 days. This action provides presumptive treatment because cultures may be negative even if bacteremia is present.
  c. Oral **amoxicillin** only, 80 mg/kg/d divided 2 times daily. There is debate about whether this prevents meningitis and other sequelae.
5. All children who are presumptively treated for OB should have a follow-up at 24 and 48 hours.
6. If the child appears toxic at follow-up, a lumbar puncture and repeat blood cultures should be obtained and the child should be admitted for IV antibiotics.
7. If the child appears nontoxic but febrile at follow-up, a second dose of ceftriaxone is given with another follow-up appointment in 24 hours.
8. If the child appears nontoxic and afebrile, no further treatment may be required, or a second dose of ceftriaxone may be administered while awaiting cultures.

SEPSIS

Sepsis is bacteremia with clinical evidence of systemic infection can rapidly progress to multiorgan failure and death. Risk factors include prematurity, immunoincompetence, recent invasive procedures, and indwelling foreign objects such as catheters. Sepsis in children tends to have age-related causes, often with common organisms (Table 66-2).

TABLE 66-2 Common Organisms Causing Sepsis and Meningitis

Age	Organisms
0–2 mo	Group B *Streptococcus* *Escherichia coli* *Listeria monocytogenes*
2 mo to 5 y	*Streptococcus pneumoniae* *Neisseria meningitidis* β-Hemolytic *Streptococcus* *Haemophilus influenzae* b* *Rickettsia rickettsii*† *Salmonella* sp (gastroenteritis) *E. coli* (pyelonephritis)

*Marked decline in cases since the introduction of the *Haemophilus influenzae* vaccine; consider in those unimmunized.

†Etiologic agent for Rocky Mountain spotted fever; seen in endemic areas after tick bites, with summer or fall predominance.

Clinical Features

Clinical signs may be vague and subtle in the young infant, including lethargy, poor feeding, irritability, or hypotonia. Fever is common; however, very young infants may be hypothermic. Tachypnea and tachycardia are usually present as a result of fever but also may be secondary to hypoxia and metabolic acidosis. Sepsis can rapidly progress to shock manifest as prolonged capillary refill, decreased peripheral pulses, altered mental status, and decreased urinary output. Hypotension is usually a very late sign of septic shock in children and, in conjunction with respiratory failure and bradycardia, indicates a grave prognosis.

Diagnosis and Differential

Diagnosis is based on clinical findings and confirmed by positive blood culture results. All infants who appear toxic should be considered septic. The workup of a child with presumed sepsis should include a CBC, blood culture, catheterized urinalysis with culture and sensitivities, chest radiograph, lumbar puncture, and stool studies in the presence of diarrhea. A serum glucose level should be performed on any critically ill child with cardiorespiratory instability.

Emergency Department Care and Disposition

1. Administration of high-flow oxygen, cardiac monitoring, and securing IV access are first steps. Endotracheal intubation should be performed in the presence of respiratory failure.
2. Shock is treated with 20-mL/kg boluses of **normal saline** solution with serial assessments of perfusion.
3. If fluid resuscitation fails, **dopamine** 5 to 10 μg/kg/min or **epinephrine** 0.1 μg/kg/min may be necessary.
4. Hypoglycemia is corrected with 0.5-g/kg IV boluses of 25% **dextrose.** In general, the concentration of glucose administered to neonates should not exceed 12.5%.

5. Antibiotic therapy should begin as soon as IV access is achieved and should not be delayed due to difficulty with procedures such as lumbar puncture. Empiric antibiotic coverage is chosen based on the age of the patient (see Table 66-1).

Consider the presence of drug-resistant organisms or immunoincompetence and infection with unusual or opportunistic organisms.

MENINGITIS

Meningitis is usually a complication of a primary bacteremia and has a peak incidence in children between birth and 2 years of age. Prematurity and immunoincompetence put children at higher risk. Organisms responsible for meningitis are essentially the same as those that cause sepsis (see Table 66-2).

Clinical Features

Meningitis may present with the subtle signs that accompany less serious infections, such as otitis media or sinusitis. Typical of these are irritability, inconsolability, hypotonia, and lethargy. In young infants, suspicion should be especially strong due to the often nonspecific presentation of the illness. Older children may complain of headache, photophobia, nausea, and vomiting and exhibit the classic signs of meningismus with complaints of neck pain. Occasionally, meningitis presents as a rapidly progressive, fulminant disease characterized by shock, seizures, or coma.

Diagnosis and Differential

Diagnosis is made by lumbar puncture and analysis of the cerebrospinal fluid (CSF). The CSF should be examined for white blood cells, glucose, and protein and undergo Gram stain and culture. Herpes encephalitis should be considered in the seizing neonate and any child with CSF pleocytosis. In the presence of immunoincompetence, infections with opportunistic or unusual viral organisms should be considered. Cranial computed tomography should be performed before lumbar puncture in the presence of focal neurologic signs or increased intracranial pressure.

Emergency Department Care and Disposition

1. Treatment should always begin with the ABCs and restoration of oxygenation and perfusion (see specific treatment recommendations under Sepsis, above).
2. Empiric antibiotic therapy is based on the patient's age (see Table 66-1).
3. Antibiotic administration should not be deferred or delayed when meningitis is strongly suspected. The role of steroids in the management of meningitis is highly controversial.

For further reading in *Emergency Medicine: A Comprehensive Study Guide,* 6th ed., see Chap. 116, "Bacteremia, Sepsis, and Meningitis in Children," by Peter Mellis.

67 | Common Neonatal Problems

Lance Brown

In general, the signs and symptoms of illness are vague and nonspecific in neonates (ie, infants in the first month of life), thus making the identification of specific diagnoses very challenging (Table 67-1). The survival of premature infants has produced a population of children whose corrected gestational age (chronological age since birth in weeks minus the number of weeks of prematurity) makes them similar to neonates. Some of these children have multiple medical problems and may become frequent visitors to the emergency department. Neonates present to the emergency department with a range of conditions that span from normal to critical.

NORMAL VEGETATIVE FUNCTIONS

Bottle-fed infants generally will take 6 to 9 feedings per 24-hour period, with a relatively stable pattern developing by the end of the first month of life. Breast-fed infants generally will prefer feedings every 2 to 4 hours. Infants typically lose 5% to 10% of their birth weight during the first 3 to 7 days of life. After this time, infants are expected to gain about 1 oz/d (20–30 g) during the first 3 months of life. The number, color, and consistency of stool in the same infant changes from day to day and certainly among infants. Normal breast-fed infants may go 5 to 7 days without stooling or have 6 to 7 stools per day. Color has no significance unless blood is present. Respiratory rates in newborns can vary, with normal ranges from 30 to 60 breaths/min. Periodic breathing with brief (<5–10 seconds) pauses in respiration may be normal. Normal newborns awaken at variable intervals that can range from about 20 minutes to 6 hours. Neonates and young infants tend to have no differentiation between day and night until approximately 3 months of age.

ACUTE, UNEXPLAINED, EXCESSIVE CRYING (INCONSOLABILITY)

There are multiple causes of prolonged crying in infants (Table 67-2). These causes range from the relatively benign to the life threatening. True inconsolability represents a serious condition in most infants and should be investigated. If, after a thorough emergency department evaluation, a cause for excessive crying has not been identified and the child continues to have

TABLE 67-1 Nonspecific Signs and Symptoms of Neonatal Illness

Fever or hypothermia
Abnormal tone (limp or stiff)
Weak suck
Poor feeding
Jaundice
Grunting respirations
Cyanosis or mottling
Vomiting

TABLE 67-2 Conditions Associated With Acute, Unexplained, Excessive Crying in Neonates

Corneal abrasion

Hair tourniquet (finger, toe, penis)

Stomatitis

Subdural hematoma (nonaccidental trauma)

Fracture (nonaccidental trauma)

Dehydration

Inborn error of metabolism

Acute infections (sepsis, urinary tract infection, meningitis)

Congenital heart disease (including supraventricular tachycardia)

Encephalitis (herpes)

its only awake state be that of inconsolability, admission to the hospital is warranted.

INTESTINAL COLIC

Intestinal colic is the most common cause of excessive (but not inconsolable) crying. The cause is unknown. The incidence is about 13% of all neonates. The formal definition includes crying for at least 3 hours per day for at least 3 days per week over a 3-week period. Intestinal colic seldom lasts beyond age 3 months. In general, the initial diagnosis of colic is not made in the emergency department.

NONACCIDENTAL TRAUMA (CHILD ABUSE)

A battered child may present with unexplained bruises at different ages, skull fractures, intracranial injuries identifiable on computed tomography of the head, extremity fractures, cigarette burns, retinal hemorrhages, unexplained irritability, lethargy, or coma.

FEVER AND SEPSIS

Fever in the neonate (age 28 days or younger) is defined as the history of (temperature taken by parent) or presence of a rectal temperature of 38°C (100.4°F) or higher. Fever in the neonate must be taken seriously, and at this point in time the proper management includes a septic workup (complete blood count, urinalysis, blood culture, urine culture, lumbar puncture and analysis of cerebrospinal fluid, cerebrospinal fluid culture, chest x-ray if respiratory symptoms are present, stool culture if diarrhea is present), the administration of parenteral antibiotics, and admission. Appropriate intravenous antibiotics include **ampicillin** (50 mg/kg per dose) **plus gentamicin** (2.5 mg/kg per dose) or **cefotaxime** (50 mg/kg per dose). Well appearance on clinical examination and initial tests with results available in the emergency department cannot reliably rule out serious bacterial infection in the neonate. The signs and symptoms of neonatal sepsis are typically nonspecific (see Table 67-1).

GASTROINTESTINAL SYMPTOMS

Surgical Lesions

Surgically correctable abdominal emergencies in neonates are uncommon, may present with nonspecific symptomatology, and, when suspected, require prompt consultation with an experienced pediatric surgeon. The most common signs and symptoms are nonspecific and include irritability and crying, poor feeding, vomiting, constipation, and abdominal distention. Bilious vomiting is suggestive of malrotation with midgut volvulus and requires emergent surgical consultation. A groin mass may represent an incarcerated hernia, although inguinal hernias are usually seen in older infants.

Feeding Difficulties

An emergency department visit may arise when there is a parental perception that an infant's food intake is inadequate. If the patient's weight gain is adequate (see Normal Vegetative Functions) and the infant appears satisfied after feeding, parental reassurance is appropriate. A successful trial of feeding in the emergency department can reassure parents, emergency department nurses, and physicians alike. When there is an underlying anatomic abnormality interfering with feeding or swallowing (eg, esophageal stenosis, esophageal stricture, laryngeal clefts, compression of the esophagus, or trachea by a double aortic arch), the infant typically has had trouble feeding since birth and usually presents with malnourishment and dehydration. Infants with a recent and true decrease in intake usually have an acute disease, most commonly an infection.

Regurgitation

Regurgitation is due to reduced lower esophageal sphincter pressure and relatively increased intragastric pressure in neonates. Regurgitation is typically a self-limited condition and, if an infant is thriving and gaining weight appropriately, reassurance is appropriate.

Vomiting

Vomiting is differentiated from regurgitation by forceful contraction of the diaphragm and abdominal muscles. Vomiting has a variety of causes and is rarely an isolated symptom. Vomiting from birth is usually due to an anatomic anomaly and usually inhibits an infant from being discharged from the newborn nursery. Vomiting is a nonspecific but serious symptom in neonates. Etiologies are diverse and include increased intracranial pressure (eg, shaken-baby syndrome), infections (eg, urinary tract infections, sepsis, or gastroenteritis), hepatobiliary disease (usually accompanied by jaundice), and inborn errors of metabolism (usually accompanied by hypoglycemia and metabolic acidosis). Bilious vomiting in a neonate should be considered a surgical emergency (malrotation should be assumed until proven otherwise).

Diarrhea

Although bacterial diarrhea is a cause of bloody diarrhea, it is rare in neonates. The most common causes of blood in the stool in infants younger than 6 months are cow's milk intolerance and anal fissures. Breast-fed infants may have heme-positive stool from swallowed maternal blood due to bleeding nipples. Necrotizing enterocolitis may present as bloody diarrhea and usually presents with other signs of sepsis (eg, jaundice, lethargy, fever, poor feeding, or abdominal distention). Abdominal radiography may demonstrate pneumatosis intestinalis or free air. Dehydrated neonates (and neonates with impending dehydration from rotavirus) should be admitted for rehydration.

Abdominal Distention

Abdominal distention can be normal in the neonate and is usually due to lax abdominal muscles and relatively large intraabdominal organs. In general, if the neonate appears comfortable, is feeding well, and the abdomen is soft, there is no need for concern.

Constipation

Infrequent bowel movements in neonates do not necessarily mean that the infant is constipated. Stool patterns can be quite variable and breast-fed infants may go 1 week without passing stool and then pass a normal stool. If an infant has never passed stool, the differential diagnosis includes intestinal stenosis or atresias, Hirschsprung disease, and meconium ileus or plug. Constipation that develops later in the first month of life suggests Hirschsprung disease, hypothyroidism, or anal stenosis. Laxatives and enemas are contraindicated in neonates.

CARDIORESPIRATORY SYMPTOMS

Noisy Breathing and Stridor

Noisy breathing in a neonate is usually benign. Infectious causes of stridor seen commonly in older infants and young children (eg, croup) are rare in neonates.

Stridor in a neonate is often due to a congenital anomaly, with laryngomalacia being the most common. Other include webs, cysts, atresias, stenoses, clefts, and hemangiomas. Nasal congestion from a mild upper respiratory tract infection may cause significant problems in a neonate. Neonates are obligate nasal breathers and feed for relatively prolonged periods while breathing only through their noses (having the bottle or breast occlude the mouth). The use of **saline drops** and suctioning is typically effective.

Apnea and Periodic Breathing

Periodic breathing may be normal in neonates. *Apnea* is formally defined as a cessation of respiration for longer than 10 to 20 seconds with or without bradycardia and cyanosis. Apnea generally signifies a critical illness, and prompt investigation (especially for sepsis) and admission for monitoring and therapy (including empiric antibiotics) should be initiated. Apnea may be the first sign of bronchiolitis with respiratory syncytial virus in neonates and occur before wheezing.

Cyanosis and Blue Spells

Many disorders may present with cyanosis, and differentiating them may present quite a diagnostic challenge. However, some symptom patterns may help differentiate various causes and assist in suggesting the correct diagnosis and course of action. Rapid, unlabored respirations and cyanosis suggest cyanotic heart disease with right-to-left shunting. Irregular, shallow breathing and cyanosis suggest sepsis, meningitis, cerebral edema, or intracranial hemorrhage. Labored breathing with grunting and retractions is suggestive of pulmonary disease such as pneumonia or bronchiolitis. All cyanotic neonates should be admitted to the hospital for monitoring, therapy, and further investigation.

Bronchopulmonary Dysplasia

Premature infants who have survived the neonatal intensive care unit may have residual lung injury and bronchopulmonary dysplasia (BPD). Young infants with BPD may be on home oxygen, diuretics, bronchodilators, or steroids. Infants with BPD may have respiratory deterioration due to acute illnesses, including bronchiolitis, pneumonia, dehydration, sepsis, gastroesophageal reflux and aspiration, and congestive heart failure. The most common cause of acute respiratory deterioration in an infant with BPD is a lower respiratory tract infection. Respiratory syncytial virus infections are particularly common and may be quite severe. Basic treatment for BPD exacerbations includes oxygenation and bronchodilators (nebulized **albuterol** 5 mg in 6 mL normal saline delivered as blow by). Antibiotics, admission, and mechanical ventilation may be required based on the clinical presentation.

JAUNDICE

There are multiple causes of jaundice, and the likelihood of these causes is based on the age at which the patient has the onset of jaundice. Jaundice that occurs within the first 24 hours of life tends to be serious in nature and usually is addressed while the patient is in the newborn nursery. Jaundice that develops during the second or third day of life is usually physiologic; if the neonate is gaining weight, feeding well, is not anemic, and does not have a bilirubin approaching 20 mg/dL, reassurance and close follow-up are appropriate. Jaundice that develops after the third day of life is generally serious. Causes include sepsis, congenital infections, congenital hemolytic anemias, breast milk jaundice, and hypothyroidism. Workup of these infants usually includes a septic workup, including a lumbar puncture, a peripheral blood smear, direct and total bilirubin levels, reticulocyte count, and a Coombs test. Empiric antibiotics (see Fever and Sepsis) are generally administered when sepsis is suspected.

ORAL THRUSH

Intraoral lesions due to *Candida* are typically white and pasty and cover the tongue, lips, gingiva, and mucous membranes. The presence of oral thrush may prompt a visit to the emergency department because the parent notices "something white" in the mouth or because the discomfort of extensive lesions interferes with feeding. Treatment consists of the topical application of oral **nystatin** suspension 4 times a day.

APPARENT LIFE-THREATENING EVENTS

An *apparent life-threatening event* (ALTE) is defined as an episode that is frightening to the observer and involves a period of apnea, transient color change (pale or cyanotic), a transient change in tone (limp or stiff), and a period of choking or gagging. According to the conventional use of *ALTE,* these children appear well on presentation to the emergency department and all abnormal behaviors have stopped. The presentation of a child with ALTE is nonspecific. Once it is determined that an ALTE has occurred, the workup typically includes pulse oximetry; complete blood count; glucose, electrolyte, calcium, phosphorous, magnesium, and ammonia levels; chest x-ray; electrocardiogram; and a septic workup, including blood, urine, and cerebrospinal fluid. Currently, these patients are typically admitted to the hospital for further workup and apnea monitoring. The utility of apnea monitoring (particularly in the home) has been questioned recently. At the conclusion of hospitalization, diagnoses of infants with ALTE may remain elusive. When identified, diagnoses may include inborn errors of metabolism, seizure, gastroesophageal reflux, lower respiratory tract infection, pertussis, gastroenteritis, asthma, head injury, feeding difficulties, and urinary tract infections. There appears to be a relation between ALTEs and sudden infant death syndrome, but the nature of this relation is not clear.

For further reading in *Emergency Medicine: A Comprehensive Study Guide,* 6th ed., see Chap. 117, "Common Neonatal Problems," by Tonia J. Brousseau and Niranjan Kissoon; Chap 118, "The NICU Graduate," by Daniel G. Batton; and Chap 119 "Sudden Infant Death Syndrome and Apparent Life-Threatening Event," by Carol D. Berkowitz.

68 | Pediatric Heart Disease

David M. Cline

There are 6 common clinical presentations of pediatric heart disease: cyanosis, congestive heart failure (CHF), pathologic murmur in an asymptomatic patient, abnormal pulses, hypertension, and syncope. Table 68-1 lists the most common lesions in each category. Congenital heart disease also may present with shock. Pediatric heart disease is frequently misdiagnosed as a viral upper respiratory tract illness or feeding intolerance. In fact, feeding intolerance may be the first symptom of congenital heart disease. This chapter focuses on conditions producing cardiovascular symptoms seen in the emergency department (ED). These conditions require immediate recognition, therapeutic intervention, and prompt referral to a pediatric cardiologist. Treatment of dysrhythmias is discussed in Chap. 3. Pediatric hypertension is discussed in Chap. 27. Syncope is discussed in Chap. 79.

Evaluation of an asymptomatic murmur is an elective diagnostic workup that can be done on an outpatient basis. The Still murmur, which is the most common innocent murmur, is early systolic in timing, located at the apex or the left sternal border, and does not radiate. Common pathologic murmurs in children are holosystolic, continuous, or diastolic in timing and usually radiate.

CYANOSIS AND SHOCK

Determining the cause of cyanosis and respiratory distress in the critically ill neonate is difficult. The clinician should consider congenital heart disease, respiratory disorders, central nervous system disease, and sepsis. The hyperoxic test helps to differentiate respiratory disease from cyanotic congenital heart disease (although imperfectly). The infant should be placed on 100% oxygen. Persistence of hypoxemia suggests the presence of a shunt from congenital heart disease.

TABLE 68-1 Clinical Presentation of Pediatric Heart Disease

Cyanosis	TGA, TOF, TA, Tat, TAVR
Congestive heart failure	See Table 68-2
Murmur/symptomatic patient	Shunts: VSD, PDA, ASD
	Obstructions
	Valvular incompetence
Abnormal pulses	
Bounding	PDA, AI, AVM
Decreased with prolonged amplitude	Coarctation, HPLV
Hypertension	Coarctation
Syncope	
Cyanotic	TOF
Acyanotic	Critical AS

Key: AI = aortic insufficiency; AS = aortic stenosis; ASD = atrial septal defect; AVM = arteriovenous malformation; HPLV = hypoplastic left ventricle; PDA = patent ductus arteriosus; TA = truncus arteriosus; Tat = tricuspid atresia; TAVR = total anomalous venous return; TGA = transposition of the great arteries; TOF = tetralogy of Fallot; VSD = ventricular septal defect.

325

Clinical Features

An accurate set of vital signs including pulse oximetry and blood pressure is essential. Cyanosis associated with a heart murmur strongly suggests congenital heart disease, but the absence of a murmur does not exclude a structural heart lesion. Early signs of inadequate cardiac output in the neonate may be suggested by slow feeding or tachypnea, diaphoresis, or staccato cough with feeding.

Shock with or without cyanosis, especially during the first 2 weeks of life, should alert the clinician to the possibility of congenital heart disease associated with closure of a patent ductus arteriosus. Neonates with shunt-dependent lesions will experience profound symptoms with closure of the ductus. Shock in the neonate is recognized by inspection of the patient's skin for pallor, cyanosis, and skin mottling and assessment of the mental status appropriate for age. Mental status changes may be fluctuating signs of apathy, irritability, or failure to respond to pain or parents. Tachycardia and tachypnea are commonly present as the initial signs. Tachypnea associated with congenital heart disease is typically effortless, without accessory muscle use commonly seen with respiratory disease. Distal pulses should be assessed for quality, amplitude, and duration, (see Table 68-1).

Diagnosis and Differential

The workup for congenital heart disease begins with chest radiogram and electrocardiogram (ECG) with pediatric analysis. Chest radiogram should be assessed for heart size, shape, and pulmonary blood flow. An abnormal right position of the aortic arch may be a clue to the diagnosis of congenital cardiac lesion. Increased pulmonary vascularity may be seen with significant left-to-right shunting or left-side failure. Echocardiography is generally required to define the diagnosis.

The differential diagnosis for cyanosis or shock due to congenital heart disease typically includes cyanotic lesions: transposition of the great vessels, tetralogy of Fallot, and other forms of right ventricular outflow tract obstruction or abnormalities of right heart formation. Typically, acyanotic lesions that can present with shock include severe coarctation of the aorta, critical aortic stenosis, and hypoplastic left ventricle. It should be noted that cyanosis may accompany shock of any cause.

Transposition of the great vessels represents the most common cyanotic defect presenting with symptoms during the first week of life. This entity is easily missed due to the absence of cardiomegaly or murmur. Symptoms (before shock) include dusky lips, increase respiratory rate, and/or feeding difficulty. ECG may show right-side force dominance.

Tetralogy of Fallot produces the following features: a holosystolic murmur of ventricular septal defect, a diamond-shape murmur of pulmonary stenosis, and cyanosis. The toddler may relieve symptoms by squatting. Chest radiogram may show a boot-shape heart with decreased pulmonary vascular markings or a right-side aortic arch. The ECG may show right ventricular hypertrophy and right axis deviation.

Hypercyanotic episodes, or "*tet spells,*" may bring children with tetralogy of Fallot to the ED with dramatic presentations. Symptoms include paroxysmal dyspnea, labored respiration, increased cyanosis, and possibly syncope. If the condition is accompanied by polycythemia, the patient may suffer seizures, cerebrovascular accidents, or death. These episodes frequently fol-

low exertion due to feeding, crying, or straining at stool and last from minutes to hours.

Left ventricular outflow obstruction syndromes may present with shock,
with or without cyanosis. Several congenital lesions fall into this category, but
in all these disorders, systemic blood flow is dependent on a large contribu-
tion of shunted blood from a patent ductus arteriosus. When the ductus closes,
these infants present with decreased or absent perfusion, hypotension, and severe acidosis.

Emergency Department Care and Disposition

1. Cyanosis and respiratory distress are first managed with high-flow oxygen, cardiac and **oxygen** monitoring, and a stable intravenous line.
2. Noncardiac causes of symptoms should be considered and treated appropriately, including a fluid challenge of 20 mL/kg of **normal saline** solution, as indicated.
3. Immediate consultation should be obtained with a pediatric cardiologist
   and, if the patient is in shock, a pediatric intensivist.
4. Management of hypercyanotic spells consists of positioning the patient in
   the knee-to-chest position and administration of **morphine** sulfate
   0.2 mg/kg subcutaneously or intramuscularly. Resistant cases should
   prompt immediate consultation with a pediatric cardiologist for consideration of phenylephrine for hypotension or propranolol for tachycardia.
5. For severe shock in infants suspected of having shunt-dependent lesions,
   prostaglandin E$_1$ can be given in an attempt to reopen the ductus. Treatment begins with 0.05 to 0.1 µg/kg/min; this may be increased to
   0.2 µg/kg/min if there is no improvement. Side effects include fever, skin
   flushing, diarrhea, and periodic apnea. Intubation and ventilation are often
   required.
6. Epinephrine is the initial drug of choice for hypotension. An infusion
   is started at 0.05 to 0.5 µg/kg/min and titrated to the desired blood
   pressure.

By definition, these children are critically ill and require admission, usually
to the pediatric intensive care unit.

CONGESTIVE HEART FAILURE

Clinical Features

The distinction between pneumonia and CHF in infants requires a high index
of clinical suspicion and is a difficult one to make. Pneumonia can cause a
previously stable cardiac condition to decompensate; thus, both problems can
present simultaneously. The predominant symptoms include poor feeding, diaphoresis, irritability or lethargy with feeding, weak cry, and, in severe cases,
grunting and nasal flaring. Note that the tachypnea associated with CHF in infants is typically "effortless" and the first manifestation of decompensation,
followed by rales on examination.

Diagnosis and Differential

Cardiomegaly evident on chest radiogram is universally present except in
constrictive pericarditis. A cardiothoracic index greater than 0.6 is abnormal. The primary radiographic signs of cardiomegaly on the lateral chest

TABLE 68-2 Differential Diagnosis of Congestive Heart Failure Based on Age of Presentation

Age	Spectrum	
1 min	Noncardiac origin: anemia	
	acidosis, hypoxia, hypoglycemia,	Acquired
1 h	hypocalcemia, sepsis	
1 d	PDA in premature infants	
1 wk	HPLV	
2 wk	Coarctation	Congenital
1 mo	Ventricular septal defect	
3 mo	Supraventricular tachycardia	
1 y	Myocarditis	
	Cardiomyopathy	Acquired
	Severe anemia	
10 y	Rheumatic fever	

Key: HPLV = hypoplastic left ventricle, PDA = patent ductus arteriosus.

radiogram are an abnormal cardiothoracic index and lack of retrosternal air space due to the direct abutment of the heart against the sternum.

Once CHF is recognized, age-related categories simplify further differential diagnosis (Table 68-2). In contrast to the gradual onset of failure with a ventricular septal defect, coarctation of the aorta can present with abrupt onset of CHF precipitated by a delayed closure of the ductus arteriosus during the second week of life. Onset of CHF after age 3 months usually signifies acquired heart disease. The exception is when pneumonia, endocarditis, or another complication causes a congenital lesion to decompensate.

Myocarditis is often preceded by a viral respiratory illness and needs to be differentiated from pneumonia. As with pneumonia, the infant usually presents in distress with fever, tachypnea, and tachycardia. ECG may show diffuse ST changes, dysrhythmias, or ectopy, signaling increased risk of sudden death. Chest radiogram shows cloudy lung fields from inflammation or pulmonary edema. Cardiomegaly with poor distal pulses and prolonged capillary refill, however, distinguish it from common pneumonia. Once cardiomegaly is discovered, hospital admission and an echocardiogram are indicated.

Usually pericarditis presents as cardiomegaly discovered on a chest radiogram. Clinical signs such as chest pain, muffled heart sounds, and a rub may be present. An echocardiogram is performed urgently to distinguish a pericardial effusion from dilated or hypertrophic cardiomyopathy and to determine the need for pericardiocentesis.

If an infant presents in pure right-side CHF, the primary problem is most likely to be pulmonary, such as cor pulmonale. In early stages, lid edema is often the first noticeable sign. This may progress to hepatomegaly, jugular venous distention, peripheral edema, and anasarca.

Emergency Department Care and Disposition

1. The infant who presents with mild tachypnea, hepatomegaly, and cardiomegaly should be seated upright in a comfortable position, oxygen should be given, and the child should be kept in a neutral thermal envi-

ronment to avoid metabolic stresses imposed by hypothermia or hyperthermia.

2. If the work of breathing is increased or CHF is apparent on chest radiogram, 1 to 2 mg/kg **furosemide** parenterally is indicated.

3. Hypoxemia usually can be corrected by fluid restriction, diuresis, and an increased fraction of inspired oxygen, although continuous positive airway pressure is sometimes necessary.

4. Stabilization and improvement of left ventricular function can often first be accomplished with inotropic agents. **Digoxin** is used in milder forms of CHF. The appropriate first digitalizing dose to be given in the ED would be 0.02 mg/kg.

5. At some point, CHF progresses to cardiogenic shock, in which distal pulses are absent and end-organ perfusion is threatened. In such situations, continuous infusions of inotropic agents, such as **dopamine** or **dobutamine,** are indicated instead of digoxin. The initial starting range is 2 to 10 μg/kg/min.

6. Aggressive management is often necessary for secondary derangements, including respiratory insufficiency, acute renal failure, lactic acidosis, disseminated intravascular coagulation, hypoglycemia, and hypocalcemia.

7. For definitive diagnosis and treatment of congenital lesions presenting in CHF, cardiac catheterization followed by surgical intervention is often necessary. See the previous section for recommendations regarding administration of prostaglandin E_1 as a temporizing measure before surgery.

For further reading in *Emergency Medicine: A Comprehensive Study Guide,* 6th ed., see Chap. 120, "Pediatric Heart Disease," by C. James Corrall.

69 | Otitis Media and Pharyngitis

David M. Cline

OTITIS MEDIA

Otitis media (AOM), an infection of the middle ear, commonly affects infants and young children because of relative immaturity of the upper respiratory tract, especially the eustachian tube. *Streptococcus pneumoniae* is the most prevalent and most virulent cause, accountng for 40% to 50% of infections. *Haemophilus influenzae* nontypeable and β-lactamase–producing *Moraxella catarrhalis* account for another 40%.

Clinical Features

Peak age is 3 to 24 months. Symptoms include fever, poor feeding, irritability, vomiting, ear pulling, and earache. Signs include a dull, bulging, immobile tympanic membrane (TM), loss of visualization of bony landmarks within the middle ear, air-fluid levels or bubbles within the middle ear, and bullae on the TM.

Diagnosis and Differential

Diagnosis is based on presenting symptoms and changes of the TM and middle ear. A red TM alone does not indicate the presence of an ear infection. Fever, prolonged crying, and viral infections can cause hyperemia of the TM. Pneumatic otoscopy can be a helpful diagnostic tool; however, a retracted drum for whatever reason will demonstrate decreased mobility.

Emergency Department Care and Disposition

1. **Amoxicillin** 45 to 60 mg/kg/d orally (PO) divided 2 to 3 times daily remains the first drug of choice despite the increasing incidence of penicillin-resistant *S pneumoniae* and the predominance of β-lactamase–producing *H influenzae* nontypeable and *M catarrhalis*.
2. Risk factors for drug-resistant *S pneumoniae* (DRSP) include age younger than 2 years, day-care attendance, antibiotics in the past 3 months, and immunoincompetence. **High-dose amoxicillin** (80 to 90 mg/kg/d PO divided twice daily) is considered the first-line treatment for those at risk for DRSP.
3. Other antibiotics appropriate for DRSP include **amoxicillin/clavulanate** 45 mg/kg/d PO divided twice daily (high dose can be considered, 80 to 90 mg/kg/d divided twice daily, but do not exceed 10 mg/kg/d of clavulanate component). Other choices include **cefpodoxime** 10 mg/kg/d PO divided twice daily, **cefuroxime axetil** 30 mg/kg/d PO divided twice daily, **cefdinir** 14 mg/kg/d PO divided 1 or 2 times a day, and **ceftriaxone** 50 mg/kg/d intramuscularly (IM) for 3 doses. For patients allergic to the previously mentioned antibiotics, **azithromycin** 10 mg/kg/d PO on the first day followed by 5 mg/kg PO for 4 more days can be used.
4. Infants younger than 30 days with AOM are at risk for infection with group B *Streptococcus, Staphylococcus aureus,* and gram-negative bacilli and should undergo evaluation and treatment for presumed sepsis (see Chap. 66).

5. Recurrent AOM is characterized as 3 or more episodes within 6 months or 4 or more episodes within 12 months.
6. Persistent AOM occurs when the signs and symptoms of AOM do not improve with appropriate antibiotic therapy.
7. High-dose amoxicillin therapy or other antibiotics suitable for DRSP coverage should be considered for recurrent and persistent AOM.
8. In uncomplicated AOM, symptoms resolve within 48 to 72 hours; however, the middle ear effusion may persist as long as 8 to 12 weeks. Routine follow-up is not necessary unless the symptoms persist or worsen.

OTITIS MEDIA WITH EFFUSION

Otitis media with effusion (OME) is fluid within the middle ear without the associated signs and symptoms of an acute infection. Chronic OME (duration >3 months) can result in significant hearing loss and language delay.

Clinical Features

OME is characterized by a middle ear effusion, distortion of bony landmarks, and decreased mobility of the TM. Absent are symptoms of acute infection such as fever, irritability, and otalgia.

Diagnosis and Differential

The diagnosis is based on the appearance of the TM in the absence of systemic symptoms. Audiometry is of limited value for diagnosis but is crucial to the evaluation of hearing deficit.

Emergency Department Care and Disposition

Treatment of OME includes the following:

1. Careful observation for resolution (standard treatment of choice).
2. No indication for antihistamines, decongestants, or steroids.
3. Antibiotics achieve resolution in only 14% of cases.
4. Ear, nose, and throat referral should be sought for hearing evaluation and consideration for myringotomy tubes.

OTITIS EXTERNA

Otitis externa (OE) is an inflammatory process involving the auricle, external auditory canal (EAC), and surface of the TM. It is commonly caused by gram-negative enteric organisms, *Staphylococcus, Pseudomonas,* or fungi.

Clinical Features

Peak seasons for OE are spring and summer, and the peak age is 9 to 19 years. Symptoms include earache, itching, and fever. Signs include erythema, edema of EAC, white exudate on EAC and TM, pain with motion of the tragus or auricle, and periauricular or cervical adenopathy.

Diagnosis and Differential

Diagnosis for OE is based on clinical signs and symptoms. A foreign body within the external canal should be excluded by carefully removing any debris that may be present.

Emergency Department Care and Disposition

1. Cleaning the ear canal with a small tuft of cotton attached to a wire applicator is the first step. The clinician should place a wick in the canal if significant edema obstructs the EAC.

2. Mild OE can be treated with acidifying agents alone, such as Otic Domeboro.

3. Fluoroquinolone otic drops are now considered the preferred agents over neomycin containing drops. **Ciprofloxacin with hydrocortisone,** 0.2% and 1% suspension (Cipro HC), 3 drops twice daily or **ofloxacin** 0.3% solution 10 drops twice daily can be used. Ofloxacin is used when TM rupture is found or suspected.

4. Oral antibiotics are indicated if auricular cellulitis is present.

5. Follow-up should be advised if improvement does not occur within 48 hours; otherwise reevaluation at the end of treatment is sufficient.

6. Cultures of the EAC may identify unusual or resistant organisms. Patients with diabetes or other forms of immunoincompetence can develop malignant otitis externa.

7. Malignant OE is characterized by systemic symptoms and auricular cellulitis. This condition can result in serious complications and requires hospitalization with intravenous antibiotics.

PHARYNGITIS

Etiologies include multiple viruses and bacteria, but only group A β-hemolytic *Streptococcus* (GABHS), Epstein-Barr virus (EBV), and *Neisseria gonorrhea* require accurate diagnosis. The identification and treatment of GABHS pharyngitis is important to prevent the suppurative complications and the sequelae of acute rheumatic fever.

Clinical Features

Peak seasons for GABHS are late winter or early spring, and the peak age is 4 to 11 years. Symptoms (sudden onset) include sore throat, fever, headache, abdominal pain, enlarged anterior cervical nodes, palatal petechiae, and tonsillar hypertrophy. With GABHS there is absence of cough, coryza, laryngitis, stridor, conjunctivitis, and diarrhea. A scarlatina-form rash associated with pharyngitis almost always indicates GABHS and is commonly referred to as *scarlet fever* (see Chap. 82). Diagnosis based on clinical findings alone results in only 50% to 70% accuracy at best.

EBV is a herpes virus and often presents much like streptococcal pharyngitis. Common symptoms are fever, sore throat, and malaise. Cervical adenopathy may be prominent and often is posterior and anterior. Hepatosplenomegaly may be present. EBV should be suspected in the child with pharyngitis nonresponsive to antibiotics in the presence of a negative throat culture.

Gonococcal (CG) pharyngitis in children and nonsexually active adolescents should alert one to the possibility of child abuse. GC pharyngitis tends to have a more benign clinical presentation than GABHS pharyngitis.

Diagnosis and Differential

Definitive diagnosis of GABHS is made with the throat culture; however, this may not always be practical in the emergency department because of the time involved and potential problems with follow-up. Rapid antigen-detection tests, if properly performed, achieve sensitivity and specificity close to those of the throat culture. A negative rapid strep test does not exclude GABHS and should be verified with a throat culture. Other etiologies of pharyngitis to recognize are EBV (infectious mononucleosis) and *N gonorrhea.*

With EBV, the white blood cell count typically will show a lymphocytosis with a preponderance of atypical lymphocytes. Diagnosis is confirmed with a positive heterophil antibody (mono spot). Diagnosis of GC pharyngitis is made by culture on Thayer-Martin medium. Vaginal, cervical, and rectal cultures also should be obtained if GC pharyngitis is suspected.

Emergency Department Care and Disposition

1. Antibiotic choices for GABHS include **Benzathine PCN** 1.2 million U IM (600,000 U IM for patients weighing less than 27 kg), **penicillin V** 1 g PO twice daily for 10 days (500 mg PO twice daily for patients weighing less than 27 kg), **amoxicillin** 60 mg/kg/d PO divided in 3 doses for 10 days, **erythromycin ethylsuccinate** 40 to 50 mg/kg/d PO divided in 3 doses for 10 days, **cefprozil** 30 mg/kg/d PO divided in 2 doses for 10 days, **cefuroxime** 30 mg/kg/d divided in 2 doses for 10 days, and **azithromycin** 12 mg/kg once daily for 5 days.
2. Antibiotic choices GC pharyngitis include **ceftriaxone** 125 mg plus **azithromycin** 12 mg/kg once daily for 5 days or **spectinomycin** 40 mg/kg IM for 7 days plus doxycycline 100 mg twice daily for 7 days.
3. Antipyretics and sometimes analgesics will be necessary during the first 48 to 72 hours of treatment. Appropriate follow-up should be encouraged for treatment failure and symptomatic contacts. Follow-up for suspected GC pharyngitis should include child sexual abuse and social service investigations.
4. An increase in the number of treatment failures with penicillin has been reported. The evidence does not support the abandonment of penicillin as a mainstay of treatment.
5. EBV is usually self-limited and requires only supportive treatment of antipyretics, fluids, and bedrest. Occasionally EBV is complicated by airway obstruction and can be effectively treated with **prednisone** 2.5 mg/kg/d tapered over 5 days or **dexamethasone** 0.5 mg/kg to a maximum of 10 mg daily tapered over 5 days.
6. Steroids also may be helpful in other forms of pharyngitis with moderate to severe swelling.

For further reading in *Emergency Medicine: A Comprehensive Study Guide,* 6th ed., see Chap. 121, "Otitis and Pharyngitis in Children," by Kimberly S. Quayle, Susan Fuchs, and David M. Jaffe.

Skin and Soft Tissue
Infections in Children

David M. Cline

This chapter discusses several common skin and soft tissue infections of childhood. (Impetigo is discussed in Chap. 82.)

CONJUNCTIVITIS

Clinical Features

Older children with conjunctivitis may complain of photophobia, ocular pain, or the sensation of a foreign body in the eye, which is associated with crusting of the eyelids or conjunctival injection. Erythema and increased secretions characterize conjunctivitis, with intense redness and purulence being more common with infectious rather than with allergic causes. Allergic conjunctivitis is typically recurrent, seasonal, and accompanied by pruritus and sneezing. Fever and other systemic manifestations do not occur with isolated conjunctivitis. The duration of symptoms with infectious causes is often 2 to 4 days. Conjunctivitis is the most common ocular infection of childhood and is usually a sporadic illness, but may occur with epidemic periodicity with viral pathogens in summer months. Although *Chlamydia trachomatis* is more common, *Neisseria gonorrhea* poses the greatest threat to the integrity of the eye in the neonate. Later in childhood, the respiratory tract pathogens predominate, particularly nontypeable *Haemophilus* species.

Diagnosis and Differential

The diagnosis of infectious conjunctivitis depends on the clinical examination. A Gram stain should be performed in infants younger than 1 month or in confusing cases. It will show more than 5 white blood cells (WBCs) per field and, in many cases, bacteria. The finding of gram-negative intracellular diplococci identifies *N gonorrhea*. Conjunctival scrapings or cultures may be performed to diagnose *C trachomatis* or other pathogens. Fluorescein staining helps to identify the dendrites of herpes simplex. Conjunctivitis may be a manifestation of a systemic disorder, such as measles or Kawasaki disease. Differential diagnosis of the red eye includes conjunctivitis, orbital and periorbital infections, retained foreign body, corneal abrasion, uveitis, and glaucoma.

Emergency Department Care and Disposition

1. Treatment is directed at the most common causes of conjunctivitis based on the patient's age, examination findings, slit lamp examination, fluorescein staining pattern, and Gram staining, if indicated.
2. Infants younger than 1 month with exceptionally purulent conjunctivitis or gram-stain positive for *N gonorrhoeae* should receive **ceftriaxone** 125 mg intramuscularly. Close follow-up the next day should be arranged. Infants appearing toxic should be admitted.
3. For infants younger than 3 months, treatment with **erythromycin** 50 mg/kg/d divided 4 times a day for 14 days plus erythromycin ointment 0.5% 4 times a day is instituted to treat *C trachomatis* and to prevent later

development of the associated vertically transmitted pneumonia syndrome.

4. Older children require only topical antibiotic instillation into the conjunctival sac such as **tobramycin** or **gentamicin** 1 to 2 drops every 4 hours while awake.

5. For herpes simplex infections, urgent consultation with an ophthalmologist is required. Topical and oral antiviral therapies are indicated. Examples include **trifluridine** 1 drop 9 times daily and **acyclovir** 10 to 20 mg/kg orally (PO) 4 times daily.

6. The administration of **diphenhydramine** (5 mg/kg/d PO divided every 6 hours) or **hydroxyzine** (2 mg/kg/d PO divided every 6 hours) may be useful for allergic conjunctivitis in addition to eradication of exposure to offending agents. In older children, olopatadine 0.1% 1 to 2 drops twice daily can be used.

7. All children with conjunctivitis should have reevaluation within 48 hours of treatment if there is no improvement, and no child should be treated for longer than 5 days with topical therapy without improvement. Failure to improve indicates further investigation and ophthalmologic consultation.

SINUSITIS

Sinusitis is an inflammation of the paranasal sinuses that may be secondary to infection and allergy and may be acute, subacute, or chronic in time course. The major pathogens in childhood are *Streptococcus pneumoniae, Moraxella catarrhalis,* and nontypeable *Haemophilus influenzae.* Other agents have been identified, but their role is unclear.

Clinical Features

Two major types of sinusitis may be differentiated on clinical grounds: acute severe sinusitis and mild subacute sinusitis. Acute severe sinusitis is associated with elevated temperature, headaches, and localized swelling and tenderness or erythema in the facial area corresponding to the sinuses. Such localized findings are seen most often in older adolescents. Mild subacute sinusitis is manifest in childhood as a protracted upper respiratory infection associated with purulent nasal discharge persisting in excess of 2 weeks. Fever is infrequent. This latter type of sinusitis may be confused with congestion of brief duration found with some upper respiratory infections.

Diagnosis and Differential

The diagnosis is made on clinical grounds without laboratory or radiographic studies. Transillumination of the maxillary or frontal sinuses is seldom helpful. Nasal congestion lasting 3 to 7 days often accompanies viral upper respiratory infections and should not be diagnosed as acute sinusitis and does not need treatment with antibiotics. Standard radiographs should be obtained for patients with uncertain clinical diagnosis and in cases of severe sinusitis. The most diagnostic finding is an air-fluid level or complete opacification of the sinus. Computed tomography is a more accurate and expensive tool for cases that fail to respond to standard therapy. Few other conditions masquerade as sinusitis, and the differential is limited, particularly in children.

Emergency Department Care and Disposition

1. For acute severe disease, intravenous therapy is recommended: **ceftriaxone** 75 mg/kg/d or **ampicillin/sulbactam** 200 mg/kg/d of ampicillin divided every 8 hours.
2. Persistent disease demands ear, nose, and throat referral for surgical drainage.
3. Mild subacute disease can be treated with **amoxicillin** 80 mg/kg/d PO divided 3 times a day.
4. Persistent subacute disease can be treated with **cefprozil** 30 mg/kg/d PO divided twice daily or **cefdinir** 14 mg/kg/d PO divided 1 or 2 times daily.
5. Patients failing prior antibiotics can be given **amoxicillin/clavulanate** 40 to 45 mg/kg/d PO divided twice daily or **cefpodoxime** 10 mg/kg/d PO divided twice daily.

CELLULITIS

Cellulitis is an infection of the skin and subcutaneous tissues that extends below the dermis, thus differentiating it from impetigo. It is a frequent infection in warm weather. Under normal circumstances, *Staphylococcus aureus, Streptococcus pyogenes* (group A β-hemolytic streptococcus), and *H influenzae* are the most commonly isolated organisms. Since the advent of effective conjugated vaccines against *H influenzae,* such infections are rare in childhood except in immunocompromised hosts.

Clinical Features

Cellulitis manifests a local inflammatory response at the site of infection with erythema, warmth, and tenderness. Fever is unusual, except in severe cases including those caused by *H influenzae.*

Diagnosis and Differential

The diagnosis of cellulitis is made by inspection. Cellulitis must be differentiated from other causes of erythema and edema including trauma, allergic reaction, and cold-induced lesions. Laboratory studies, including WBC concentration, blood culture, and, rarely, aspirate culture, are obtained in specific circumstances to include immunocompromise, fever, severe local infection, facial involvement, and failure to respond to standard therapy.

Emergency Department Care and Disposition

1. For toxic patients with fever and leukocytosis, intravenous therapy should be used. Antibiotic choices include **nafcillin** 25 to 37 mg/kg given every 6 hours, **oxacillin** 25 to 37 mg/kg given every 6 hours, or **ampicillin/sulbactam** (200 mg/kg/d of ampicillin divided every 8 hours). Alternatives include **cefazolin** 20 mg/kg given every 6 hours plus **gentamicin** 5 to 7.5 mg/kg/d divided every 8 hours.
2. For nontoxic patients, **dicloxacillin** 50 to 100 mg/kg/d divided 4 times daily, **amoxicillin/clavulanate** 45 mg/kg/d PO divided twice daily, or **cephalexin** 50 to 100 mg/kg/d divided 4 times daily can be used.
3. For patients allergic to the previously mentioned antibiotics, **azithromycin** 10 mg/kg/d PO on the first day is followed by 5 mg/kg

PO for 4 more days, or **erythromycin ethylsuccinate** 40 to 50 mg/kg/d PO divided 3 times a day can be used but may be less effective.

4. Patients who fail to respond to reasonable outpatient antibiotic therapy must be further evaluated and considered for admission and intravenous antibiotic therapy. Other underlying conditions, such as diabetes or underlying immune compromise, must be sought.

PERIORBITAL AND ORBITAL CELLULITES

Periorbital cellulitis is an inflammatory process of the tissues anterior to the orbital septum or within the orbit (orbital cellulitis). *Staphylococcus aureus* and *S pneumoniae* are the principal etiologic agents. *Haemophilus influenzae* is declining in frequency. Orbital infections are due most often to *S aureus*, particularly when puncture wounds are involved. Children younger than 3 years are more likely to be bacteremic, so they generally experience highest incidence of periorbital cellulitis. Orbital cellulitis can occur at any age.

Clinical Features

Orbital and periorbital cellulites cause the periorbital area to appear red and swollen. Periorbital edema is usually more pronounced with preseptal infections. Proptosis or limitation of extraocular muscle function indicates orbital involvement. The eye is usually painful to touch but is nonpruritic.

Diagnosis and Differential

Periorbital and orbital cellulites are distinguished from noninfectious disorders on the basis of clinical findings and the WBC concentration. As with cellulitis at other locations, allergic and traumatic causes for edema must be considered. Angioedema typically is nontender and pruritic. Tumors and metabolic disease may cause swelling and discoloration, particularly thyrotoxicosis in adolescents and neuroblastoma in the young child. Leukocytosis occurs frequently with cellulitis and more often with bacteremic preseptal infections. Blood cultures in patients with leukocytosis are often positive. Computed tomography is performed when orbital involvement is likely because it is a very sensitive test.

Emergency Department Care and Disposition

1. Admission and treatment with intravenous antibiotics is the usual course to prevent complications of meningitis and subperiosteal abscess.
2. Antibiotic choices include **nafcillin** 25 to 37 mg/kg intravenously given every 6 hours, **oxacillin** 25 to 37 mg/kg intravenously given every 6 hours, or **ampicillin/sulbactam** (200 mg/kg/d ampicillin divided every 8 hours). Alternatives include **cefazolin** 20 mg/kg given every 6 hours plus **gentamicin** 5 to 7.5 mg/kg/d divided every 8 hours.
3. Surgical drainage may be necessary with abscess formation.

For further reading in *Emergency Medicine: A Comprehensive Study Guide,* 6th ed., see Chap. 122, "Skin and Soft Tissue Infections," by Richard Malley.

71 | Pneumonia

Lance Brown

Most cases of pediatric pneumonia develop from inhalation of infective bacteria or viruses. The clinical presentation, likely etiologic agents, severity of illness, and disposition, are most dependent on the patient's age.

CLINICAL FEATURES

Clinical features of pneumonia are quite variable. In addition to the age of the patient, factors that affect the clinical presentation of pediatric pneumonia include the specific respiratory pathogen, the severity of the disease, and any underlying illnesses. Tachypnea is the most commonly seen physical sign in children with pneumonia. In an otherwise well-appearing child, the absence of tachypnea suggests against the diagnosis of pneumonia. Neonates and young infants with pneumonia typically present with a sepsis syndrome. The signs and symptoms are nonspecific and may include fever or hypothermia, apnea, tachypnea, poor feeding, vomiting, diarrhea, lethargy, grunting, bradycardia, and shock. In older children, signs and symptoms of pneumonia include fever, abnormal lung examination, cough, and pleuritic chest pain. Associated signs and symptoms may include headache, malaise, wheezing, rhinitis, conjunctivitis, pharyngitis, and rash. The clinical manifestations of bacterial and viral pneumonias significantly overlap, thus making the clinical distinction between them problematic. Lower lobe pneumonias may cause significant abdominal pain and distention. This presentation may mislead the unsuspecting physician into pursuing an intraabdominal diagnosis and inappropriately consulting a surgeon.

DIAGNOSIS AND DIFFERENTIAL

Several conditions may present similarly to pneumonia: congestive heart failure, atelectasis, tumors, congenital pulmonary anomalies, aspiration pneumonitis, poor inspiration or technical difficulties with the chest x-ray, allergic alveolitis, and chronic pulmonary diseases. Chest x-rays are commonly used to make the diagnosis of pneumonia. Consolidation on chest x-ray is considered a reliable sign of pneumonia. Viral pneumonias tend to have diffuse interstitial infiltrates with hyperinflation, peribronchial thickening or cuffing, and areas of atelectasis. Bacterial pneumonias tend to have lobar or segmental infiltrates. However, there is overlap in the radiographic appearance of bacterial and viral pneumonias, making this distinction problematic at times. Rapid viral antigen tests are available for respiratory syncytial virus and influenza and may be helpful in identifying a viral etiology in the emergency department. Most children with radiographically evident pneumonia have normal pulse oximetry readings.

EMERGENCY DEPARTMENT CARE AND DISPOSITION

General care of the pediatric patient with pneumonia includes assessing for and treating hypoxia, dehydration, and fever.

1. With significant bronchospasm and wheezing, **albuterol** (by nebulizer or pocket inhaler with a spacer administered 2 puffs every 4 hours) may be helpful.

TABLE 71-1 Empiric Treatment of Pediatric Pneumonias

Patient characteristics	Treatment recommendations
Neonates (<28 d old)	Inpatient treatment with IV Ampicillin 50 mg/kg per dose plus cefotaxime 50 mg/kg per dose or Ampicillin 50 mg/kg per dose plus gentamicin 2.5 mg/kg per dose
1–3 mo old: afebrile, staccato cough, rales, relatively well appearance, 50% have had prior conjunctivitis	Inpatient treatment with IV erythromycin 10 mg/kg per dose
1 mo to 5 y	Inpatient treatment with IV Cefuroxime 50 mg/kg per dose or Ampicillin 50 mg/kg per dose Outpatient treatment with PO Amoxicillin 45 mg/kg per dose bid or Erythromycin 15 mg/kg per dose tid
6–18 y	Inpatient treatment with IV erythromycin 10 mg/kg per dose Outpatient treatment with PO erythromycin 15 mg/kg per dose tid May substitute another macrolide
Critically ill–appearing child and/or resistant *Streptococcus pneumoniae* suspected	To standard therapy add IV vancomycin 20 mg/kg per dose
Technology- or ventilator-dependent child with multiple hospitalizations (suspect *Pseudomonas aeruginosa*)	Inpatient treatment with IV ceftazidime 50 mg/kg per dose

Key: bid = twice daily, IV = intravenous, PO = oral, tid = thrice daily.

2. Empiric antibiotic selection is based on the likely etiologic agents given the patient's age and whether the patient is admitted to the hospital or discharged home (Table 71-1). Most children with pneumonia are treated as outpatients.

3. The exact pulse oximetry threshold at which an otherwise well-appearing young child with pneumonia should be admitted to the hospital is unknown. Indications for admission include age younger than 3 months, a history of apneic episodes or cyanosis, toxic appearance, respiratory distress, oxygen requirement, dehydration, vomiting, failed outpatient therapy, immunocompromised state, associated pleural effusion or pneumatocele, or an unreliable care taker.

4. Pediatric intensive care unit admission should be considered in children with severe respiratory distress or impending respiratory failure.

For further reading in *Emergency Medicine: A Comprehensive Study Guide,* 6th ed., see Chap. 123, "Viral and Bacterial Pneumonia in Children," by Kathleen M. Brown and Willie Gilford Jr.

72 | Asthma and Bronchiolitis

Douglas R. Trocinski

ASTHMA

The incidence of and death from asthma increased significantly in the 1990s. Triggers for an acute asthma exacerbation include allergens, exercise, environmental irritants such as cigarette smoke, and, most commonly, infection. Risk factors that may contribute to asthma deaths include socioeconomic background, limited access to health care, improper medication administration, unrecognized severity or extreme lability of disease, nocturnal asthma, and history of prior respiratory failure and intubation.

Clinical Features

Wheezing is the most common symptom of asthma; however, if there is severe bronchoconstriction one may only hear diminished breath sounds and decreased air movement. Also, persistent nonproductive cough or exercise-induced cough may be the result of bronchospasm. Occasionally, rales or rhonchi may be present in conjunction with wheezing. Tachypnea and tachycardia almost always accompany wheezing. The amount of air movement, retractions, nasal flaring, degree of accessory muscle use, and/or a tripod position usually reflect the severity of the asthma attack. Cyanosis, altered mental status, and somnolence often indicate respiratory failure. Bradycardia and shock herald impending cardiac arrest.

Diagnosis and Differential

The chest x-ray usually shows hyperinflation and flattening of the diaphragm and generally is not useful in the treatment of uncomplicated, chronic asthma. Relative indications for chest x-ray include a first episode of wheezing, asymmetric physical examination, and productive cough or fever. Measurement of peak flow is useful in older children; peak expiratory flow rate of less than 50% of the predicted value indicates severe obstruction. All children should have initial pulse oximetry on room air, with continuous monitoring indicated for oxygen saturation of less than 93%. Arterial blood gases may be indicated in severe exacerbations unresponsive to intensive therapy or with signs of fatigue or impending respiratory failure. Compensatory hyperventilation may cause a fall in Pa_{CO_2} and respiratory alkalosis. Severe obstruction and inadequate alveolar ventilation ultimately result in marked CO_2 retention, respiratory acidosis, and respiratory failure leading to hypercarbia, often the initial sign of respiratory failure. Pseudonormalization of Pa_{CO_2} is therefore ominous.

The most common cause of wheezing in infants and young children is bronchiolitis, especially during fall and winter, when respiratory syncytial virus is prevalent. Infants with bronchopulmonary dysplasia often exhibit wheezing as a manifestation of chronic lung disease or secondary infections. These children also may develop wheezing as a symptom of congestive heart failure, as will children with sickle cell disease or congenital heart disease. Recurrent aspiration resulting from gastroesophageal reflux may cause wheezing in young infants. Structural abnormalities, such as vascular rings, bronchial stenosis, or mediastinal cysts, also may cause wheezing. Often, early cystic fibrosis will present with wheezing and may mimic asthma. Pneumonia in young children also may be accompanied by wheezing. Aspiration of a foreign body may manifest as unilateral wheezing and should be considered in association with sudden onset of respiratory distress preceded by choking.

Emergency Department Care and Disposition

Nebulized β_2-agonist therapy, specifically albuterol, is the mainstay of acute asthma therapy, in addition to the administration of supplemental oxygen and early use of corticosteroids.

1. **Oxygen** should be administered when oxygen saturation is below 94%.
2. **Albuterol** can be administered as episodic treatments at 0.15 mg/kg (2.5-5.0 mg) every 20 minutes. A continuous nebulization of up to 0.5 mg/kg/h (10-15 mg) can be considered for severely ill patients (potassium levels should be monitored).
3. Steroids are indicated for nearly all acute exacerbations to decrease mucosal inflammation, thereby preventing progression of an attack, decreasing the incidence of emergency department visits and hospitalization, and reducing morbidity. **Prednisone or prednisolone** 2 mg/kg/d should be administered early in presentation and can be continued safely for 5 days with no need for a taper. Steroids are contraindicated in varicella-susceptible patients who have known exposure or might have potential exposure to varicella.
4. **Ipratropium** should be considered for most exacerbations in doses of 125 to 250 μg if the patient is younger than 14 years and 500 μg if the patient is 14 years or older and may be mixed with the first 3 doses of albuterol.
5. **Terbutaline,** also a β_2-agonist, may be given as an aerosol and subcutaneously (SC) and intravenously (IV). The nebulized dose is 1 mg of a 0.1% solution in 2 mL saline solution for children younger than 1 year and 2 mg for children older than 1 year every 15 to 20 minutes (maximum, 3 mg). Terbutaline may be given 0.01 mL/kg SC every 15 to 20 minutes (maximum, 0.25 mL). The IV route may be given to refractory patients at a dose of 0.5 to 1.0 μg/kg/min.
6. SC injection of **epinephrine** is rarely used anymore but is an acceptable alternative when nebulized therapy is delayed or unavailable or as initial therapy for the child with severe hypoventilation or apnea. It is given at doses of 0.01 mL/kg SC every 15 to 20 minutes (maximum, 0.3 mL).
7. **Magnesium sulfate** 20 to 50 mg/kg (maximum, 2 g) IV over 20 minutes may benefit a subset of children with severe exacerbation.
8. Helium-oxygen (Heliox) may benefit children with severe exacerbation by decreasing airway resistance and work of breathing.
9. Admission is warranted for children with a persistent oxygen requirement, refractory respiratory distress, or dyspnea on exertion despite intensive therapy over 2 to 4 hours.
10. Children in status asthmaticus may become dehydrated due to decreased oral intake and increased insensible water loss. IV fluids should be administered as maintenance therapy.
11. Treatment of children with respiratory failure includes continuous β_2-agonist nebulization, intravenous β_2-agonist therapy, or mechanical

ventilation. If mechanical ventilation is required, low inflating pressures and long expiratory times may reduce the risk of barotrauma.

12. **Ketamine** 1 to 2 mg/kg IV is a useful induction agent for intubation due to its bronchodilating effects.

13. Children who respond to conventional therapy should be discharged with detailed instructions, β_2-agonist therapy (generally a MDI with spacer), a prescription for oral steroids, and confirmed follow-up with primary care provider.

BRONCHIOLITIS

Bronchiolitis occurs typically during fall to early spring, affects infants younger than 2 years, and is characterized primarily by tachypnea and wheezing. Respiratory syncytial virus accounts for most infections; however, other respiratory viruses have been isolated. Young infants (age <2 months) and those with a history of prematurity, bronchopulmonary dysplasia, congenital heart disease, or immunosuppression are at particular risk for complications.

Clinical Features

Although wheezing is the prominent clinical manifestation, symptoms of upper respiratory infection will precede the respiratory distress. Most infants will exhibit fever, and apnea can occur among those 6 months or younger. Other signs of respiratory distress, such as tachypnea, retractions, nasal flaring, and grunting, may be present. Rales also may be present, alone or in conjunction with wheezing. Decreased breath sounds or absence of breath sounds signifies severe bronchoconstriction. Cyanosis and altered mental status are ominous signs of respiratory failure. Symptoms generally peak in 3 to 5 days and usually resolve within 2 weeks; however, immunity is variable and reinfection may occur.

Diagnosis and Differential

In general, all children should have a chest x-ray with the first episode of wheezing. The chest x-ray in bronchiolitis shows hyperinflation and peribronchial cuffing. Occasionally, small areas of atelectasis may mimic pneumonic infiltrates. True consolidation is indicative of a primary pneumonia or bronchiolitis with superinfection.

Identification of respiratory syncytial virus can be made with fluorescent monoclonal antibody testing of nasal washings. This method may be useful in identifying children at risk for severe disease and as a means to identify admitted children who require respiratory isolation. All children with respiratory distress should have initial pulse oximetry on room air; if the saturated O_2 is less than 93%, pulse oximetry should be continuous. Arterial blood gas analysis indications are similar to those for severe asthma exacerbations. White blood cell count and blood culture are not useful unless a superimposed bacterial infection is suspected.

Emergency Department Care and Disposition

1. Children with bronchiolitis and a history of reactive airway disease may respond to an inhaled β-agonist (albuterol 0.15 mg/kg per dose). If improvement occurs, treatments may be repeated as needed.

2. Nebulized epinephrine (1:1000) 0.5 mL in 2.5 mL normal saline solution

may be beneficial if albuterol fails. It can be administered every 2 hours.

3. **Helium-oxygen** (Heliox) should be considered for children with severe symptoms.

4. Dehydration may complicate bronchiolitis because increased work of breathing prevents adequate oral intake and increases insensible water loss. IV fluids should be administered to children requiring admission, and close attention should be given to the state of hydration of children discharged.

5. Corticosteroids are not indicated in bronchiolitis unless there is a history of underlying reactive airway disease, in which case a dose of 2 mg/kg should be administered.

6. Apnea and respiratory failure mandate endotracheal intubation and mechanical ventilation.

7. Indications for hospitalization include (*a*) apnea, (*b*) respiratory distress, (*c*) hypoxia, (*d*) vomiting and/or dehydration, and (*e*) persistent tachypnea faster than 60 breaths/min.

8. Infants who are not hypoxic, are well hydrated, and have minimal or no respiratory distress may be discharged from the emergency department. Infants who continue to be tachypneic in the absence of wheezing should be observed and considered for admission.

9. Admission also should be considered for children with underlying conditions that predispose to a complicated illness course (bronchopulmonary dysplasia, congenital heart disease, and immunity compromise).

10. All children discharged from the emergency department require confirmed 24-hour follow-up with their primary care provider, and clear instructions should be given to the caregiver regarding signs of worsening respiratory distress and dehydration.

For further reading in *Emergency Medicine: A Comprehensive Study Guide,* 6th ed., see Chap. 124, "Pediatric Asthma and Bronchiolitis," by Maybelle Kou and Thom A. Mayer.

73 | Seizures and Status Epilepticus in Children

Michael C. Plewa

The causes and manifestations of seizure activity are numerous, ranging from benign to life threatening. Idiopathic seizures (eg, epilepsy) comprise the largest category of seizures, and other risk factors are encephalitis, disorders of amino acid metabolism, structural abnormalities (eg, neoplasm, hydrocephalus, shunt malfunction, microcephaly, or arteriovenous malformations), systemic disorders (eg, sickle cell anemia), congenital infections, or neurocutaneous syndromes (eg, tuberous sclerosis, neurofibromatosis, or Sturge-Weber syndrome). Precipitants of seizures can include fever, sepsis, hypoglycemia, hypocalcemia, hypoxemia, hyper- or hyponatremia, hypotension, toxin or medication exposure, and head injury.

CLINICAL FEATURES

Symptoms of seizure may include loss of or alteration in consciousness, including behavioral changes and auditory, sensory or olfactory hallucinations; involuntary motor activity, including vocalizations, tonic or clonic contractions, spasms, automatisms (eg, blinking or lip smacking) or choreoathetoid movements; atony (loss of tone resulting in a fall); and incontinence. Signs may include alteration in consciousness or motor activity; autonomic dysfunction, such as mydriasis, diaphoresis, hypertension, tachypnea or apnea, tachycardia, and salivation; and postictal somnolence.

DIAGNOSIS AND DIFFERENTIAL

The diagnosis of seizure disorder is based primarily on history and physical examination, with laboratory studies (other than a bedside assay for glucose) obtained in a problem-focused manner. Serum drug level determinations are useful for phenobarbital, phenytoin, valproic acid, carbamazepine, and ethosuximide in patients with breakthrough seizures or status epilepticus, whereas levels for patients taking newer seizure medications may not be immediately available or useful in guiding therapy. Serum chemistry studies (ie, electrolytes, magnesium, calcium, creatinine, and serum urea nitrogen levels) usually are not indicated except in neonatal seizures, infantile spasms, febrile seizures that are complex in nature (with duration longer 15 minutes, focal involvement, or several recurrences in 24 hours), status epilepticus, or suspected metabolic or gastrointestinal disorders. Serum ammonia, TORCH (toxoplasmosis, rubella, cytomegalovirus, herpes) titers, and urine and serum amino acid screenings may be useful in neonatal seizures. Blood gas analysis is indicated in neonatal seizures and status epilepticus. Cardiac monitoring is useful to assess the PR and QT intervals and the possibility of cardiac dysrhythmia as the precipitant of seizure. Toxicology screening may be useful if recreational drug use (eg, cocaine) is suspected.

Magnetic resonance imaging is the preferred neuroimaging procedure for most cases of new onset seizures, whereas cerebral ultrasound is useful in neonates and immediate noncontrast computed tomography is indicated in cases of head trauma, nonfebrile status epilepticus, and focal seizures or focal neurologic signs. Lumbar puncture should be performed in patients with neonatal seizure, infantile spasms, complex febrile seizures in those younger than 18 months, meningeal signs, or persistent alteration in consciousness. Emergent electroencephalographic (EEG) monitoring is indicated for neonatal seizures, nonconvulsive status epilepticus, and refractory status epilepticus, especially when a paralytic agent is used.

It is important to differentiate true seizure activity from one of several nonepileptic paroxysmal disorders, such as neonatal jitteriness, shuddering, hyperekplexia (startle disease), near-miss sudden death syndrome, breath-holding spells (of cyanotic or pallid types), hyperventilation, syncope, migraine, pseudo-seizures, narcolepsy, Tourette syndrome, or chorea, which are characterized by normal EEGs and are unresponsive to antiepileptic drugs.

EMERGENCY DEPARTMENT CARE AND DISPOSITION

Essential care for the child with seizures includes:

1. Airway maintenance (supplemental oxygen, suctioning, airway opening, or intubation when necessary).
2. Seizure termination.
3. Correction of reversible causes.
4. Initiation of appropriate diagnostic studies.
5. Arrangement of follow-up or admission, as appropriate.

Termination of seizure activity is important to prevent irreversible pathologic changes and risk of persistent seizure disorder, especially in the setting of status epilepticus, defined as a seizure longer than 30 minutes. For this reason, seizures lasting greater than 10 minutes are treated as status epilepticus. Intravenous (IV) access is essential in cases of neonatal seizures, status epilepticus, and recurrent seizures.

Status Epilepticus

1. Airway maintenance is of primary importance in status epilepticus because all therapeutic agents can result in respiratory depression.
2. With IV access, **lorazepam** 0.1 mg/kg to a total of 8 mg, **diazepam** 0.2 to 0.5 mg/kg to a total of 2.6 mg/kg, or **midazolam** 0.2 mg/kg are the primary agents of choice.
3. Without IV access, alternatives include rectal, nasal, or intramuscular midazolam 0.1 to 0.2 mg/kg; rectal diazepam 0.5 mg/kg; rectal valproic acid 60 mg/kg; or intraosseous (IO) infusion of lorazepam, diazepam, or midazolam (in similar dosages as those of IV dosages).
4. **Fosphenytoin** 20 mg phenytoin equivalent (PE)/kg IV or IO should be started immediately after the primary agent, followed by **phenobarbital** 20 to 30 mg/kg IV or IO repeated 10 mg/kg every 20 minutes to levels of 60 mg/mL or **Depacon** 10 to 30 mg/kg IV (over 15 minutes) if fosphenytoin is ineffective.
5. Hypoglycemia should be treated with **10% dextrose** 5 mL/kg IV or IO.
6. If seizures persist, consider continuous **midazolam** IV infusion 0.04 to 0.05 mg/kg/h, **propofol** 1 mg/kg IV bolus followed by 2 mg/kg/h infusion or general anesthesia (plus continuous EEG monitoring) with pentobarbital 2 mg/kg bolus followed by 1 to 2 mg/kg/h IV infusion or inhalational agents, or IV **lidocaine** 2 mg/kg bolus followed by infusion at 5 to 10 mg/kg/h.

7. Continuous midazolam infusion or oral clonazepam 0.02 to 0.06 mg/kg/d by nasogastric tube can be used for non-continuous status epilepticus.

Treatable causes, such as hyponatremia, toxin exposure (eg, iron, lead, carbon monoxide, salicylates, and stimulants) or infections (eg, meningoencephalitis or brain abscess) should be considered. Specific toxicologic therapy (eg, activated charcoal, hyperbaric oxygen, or chelation therapy) should be used when appropriate for suspected toxin exposure.

First Seizure

1. Only patients with prolonged or repetitive witnessed seizures, especially with concomitant neurologic deficit, are started on antiepileptic drugs. The choice of antiepileptic drug is based on seizure type, side effect profile, and ease of administration and usually should be discussed with the primary physician or neurologist.
2. Generalized tonic-clonic seizures are commonly treated with **valproate** 20 to 60 mg/kg/d, **topiramate** 1 to 10 mg/kg/d, or **lamotrigine** 2 to 15 mg/kg/d (with lower doses when used with valproate). Other drugs are effective.
3. Partial seizures are treated primarily with **carbamazepine** 10 to 40 mg/kg/d. Other first-line agents include **phenytoin** 4 to 8 mg/kg/d, **phenobarbital** 3 to 8 mg/kg/d, and **primidone** 5 to 20 mg/kg/d.
4. Complex partial seizures are commonly treated with **felbamate** 45 mg/kg/d or **gabapentin** 20 to 30 mg/kg/d.
5. Absence seizures are treated primarily (after confirmatory EEG) with **ethosuximide** 20 to 30 mg/kg/d and with valproate, **lamotrigine,** or topiramate, if present with other seizure types.
6. Myoclonic and tonic/atonic seizures are commonly treated with valproate, lamotrigine, topiramate, or felbamate. IV loading can be achieved with the IV form of valproate, **Depacon** 10 to 30 mg/kg over 15 minutes, or **fosphenytoin** 15 to 20 mg PE/kg at 3 PE/kg/min, a phenytoin prodrug without infusion-related complications.
7. Admission should be considered for focal seizure, persistent abnormal neurologic examination, or suspected neurologic or systemic disease. Discharged patients should arrange close follow-ups.

Breakthrough Seizures in the Known Epileptic

Patients with 1 breakthrough seizure should have antiepileptic drug levels measured because low levels (secondary to noncompliance or altered metabolism) or, occasionally, toxic levels may be the cause.

1. Those with recurrent or frequent tonic, tonic-clonic, or clonic seizures and low antiepileptic drug levels should receive rapid loading of antiepileptic drug IV (phenobarbital, fosphenytoin, or Depacon) or rectally (liquid valproate, phenobarbital, phenytoin, primidone, or carbamazepine). Lamotrigine should not be loaded because of risk of rash.
2. A second antiepileptic agent should be considered if levels are in the high therapeutic range, such as phenobarbital, phenytoin, or valproate for focal or partial seizures and lamotrigine, ethosuximide, valproate, clonazepam, or acetazolamide for absence seizures.
3. Admission should be considered for patients with serious medical illness, toxic drug levels, or frequent or recurrent seizures despite therapeutic drug levels.
4. Close outpatient follow-up should be arranged for discharged patients.

Febrile Seizure

Identification and treatment of the cause of fever is the primary goal of therapy for febrile seizures.

1. Fever can be controlled by acetaminophen or ibuprofen and tepid water baths.
2. Antiepileptic drug therapy with oral phenobarbital or valproate are used only in those with an underlying neurologic deficit (eg, cerebral palsy), complex (prolonged or focal) febrile seizure, repeated seizures in the same febrile illness, onset at younger than 6 months, or more than 3 febrile seizures in 6 months. One dose of oral or rectal diazepam 0.2 to 0.5 mg/kg given at the onset of febrile illness also may be effective in these patients.
3. Children with suspected sepsis or meningitis and those with recurrent seizures should be admitted.
4. Antiepileptic drug administration or EEG monitoring and close follow-up should be arranged with the primary care physician for discharged patients.

Neonatal Seizures

The cause of neonatal seizures should be investigated and treated aggressively in an intensive care setting.

1. Seizures of uncertain cause or persistent seizures should be treated with empiric **pyridoxine** 100 mg/d IV; hypoglycemia with **10% dextrose** solution 5 mL/kg IV; hypocalcemia with **calcium gluconate** (10% solution) 200 to 500 mg/kg/d IV (in 4 daily doses) and **magnesium sulfate** 25 to 50 mg/kg IV or intramuscularly; and biotinidase deficiency with **biotin** 10 mg/d.
2. The first-line agent is **phenobarbital** 20 mg/kg IV at 1 mg/kg/min followed by 3 to 4 mg/kg/d.
3. Second-line agents include **fosphenytoin** 20 mg PE/kg IV at 3 mg PE/kg/min and then 4 to 8 mg PE/kg/d, **midazolam** 0.2 mg/kg over 2 minutes, or **lorazepam** 0.1 mg/kg IV over 2 minutes.
4. Refractory seizures are treated with continuous IV infusion of **midazolam** 0.04 to 0.5 mg/kg/h or **pentobarbital** 0.5 to 3.0 mg/kg/h.

Infantile Spasms

Prompt recognition of infantile spasms is essential to optimal outcome. Therapy with adrenocorticotrophic hormone (or with topiramate, clonazepam, vigabatrin, or valproate) is often started in the inpatient setting after specialty consultation. Glucose transporter defect syndrome (diagnosed by lumbar puncture (LP)) is treated with a ketogenic diet.

Head Trauma and Seizures

Immediate seizures after head trauma may require short-term treatment with fosphenytoin, especially after severe head injury. Early and late posttraumatic seizures, if recurrent, may require long-term antiepileptic therapy.

For further reading in *Emergency Medicine: A Comprehensive Study Guide,* 6th ed., see Chap. 125, "Seizures and Status Epilepticus in Children," by Michael A. Nigro.

74 | Vomiting and Diarrhea

Debra G. Perina

Gastroenteritis is a major public health problem, accounting for up to 20% of all acute care outpatient visits to hospitals. Most children who come to the emergency department because of vomiting have a self-limited viral disorder. Likewise, most cases of diarrhea result from self-limited enteric infections. Nevertheless, loss of water and electrolytes can lead to clinical dehydration in 10% of cases and may be life threatening in 1%.

CLINICAL FEATURES

Evaluation of the child's hydration state is most important, regardless of whether the presenting complaint is vomiting or diarrhea. (Guidelines for determining the child's hydration status can be found in Chap. 80.) Viral, bacterial, or other infectious organisms may cause gastroenteritis, and spread occurs by the fecal-to-oral route. Pathogenic agents may be isolated from up to 50% of children with diarrhea. Acute diarrhea is the most prominent symptom in infants and children. Viral etiologies are the most common cause in both groups. Viral pathogens cause disease by tissue invasion and alteration of intestinal absorption of water and electrolytes. Bacterial pathogens cause diarrhea by the production of enterotoxins and cytotoxins and invasion of the mucosal absorptive surface. Dysentery occurs when bacteria invade the mucosa of the terminal ileum and colon, producing diarrhea with blood, mucus, or pus. Table 74-1 lists common causative agents, clinical features, and treatment for diarrhea in children.

DIAGNOSIS AND DIFFERENTIAL

The most important aspect of diagnosis is a thorough history and physical examination, first seeking out life-threatening conditions and rapidly intervening and then determining the degree of dehydration followed by appropriate rehydration. Dehydration caused by diarrhea is usually isotonic, and serum electrolytes determinations are not necessary unless signs of severe dehydration are present. However, one must be alert for the development of hypoglycemia in the setting of protracted vomiting or diarrhea in infants and toddlers. Blood glucose determinations are useful in this setting. Stool cultures should be reserved for cases in which the child is febrile, has numerous episodes of diarrhea, and blood in the stool. The fecal leukocyte test, sometimes used as a screening tool, has poor sensitivity. Likewise, guaiac testing has poor specificity. Positive results should be interpreted in relation to the patient's clinical picture. Vomiting and diarrhea also may be nonspecific presentations for other disease processes, such as otitis media, urinary tract infection, sepsis, malrotation, intussusception, increased intracranial pressure, metabolic acidosis, and drug or toxin ingestion. Particular attention should be paid to infants younger than 1 year because they are at greater risk for rapid dehydration and hypoglycemia. Special attention should be given to those children who have chronically debilitating illnesses, high-risk social situations, or malnutrition because they are at particular risk for rapid decompensation.

TABLE 74-1 Common Agents, Clinical Features, and Treatment of Diarrhea*

Agent	Clinical features	Treatment
Viral		
Rotavirus	Watery diarrhea, winter, most common agent	Rehydration
Enteric adenovirus	Watery diarrhea, concurrent respiratory symptoms	Rehydration
Norwalk	Watery diarrhea, epidemic, fever, headache, myalgias	Rehydration
Bacterial		
Campylobacter jejuni	Fever, abdominal pain, watery or bloody diarrhea, may mimic appendicitis, animal reservoir	Rehydration Erythromycin
Shigella	Fever, abdominal pain, headache, mucoid diarrhea	Rehydration TMP-SMX or **ampicillin**
Salmonella	Fever, bloody diarrhea, animal reservoir, antibiotics prolong the carrier state	Rehydration TMP-SMX if complicated
Escherichia coli		
Enterotoxigenic	Watery diarrhea	Rehydration
Enterohemorrhagic	Dysentery, associated with HUS	TMP-SMX
Enteroinvasive	Dysentery, *Shigella*-like	Rehydration; check CBC, BUN, creatinine; TMP-SMX
Vibrio cholerae	Rice-water diarrhea	Rehydration TMP-SMX
Yersinia enterocolitica	Fever, vomiting, diarrhea, abdominal pain; may mimic appendicitis	Rehydration Ceftriaxone (controversial)
Clostridium difficile	Recent antibiotic use	Rehydration Metronidazole
Staphylococcus aureus	Food poisoning	Rehydration
Parasitic		
Giardia lamblia	Diarrhea, flatulence; exposure to day care centers, mountain streams	Rehydration Metronidazole
Entamoeba histolytica	Bloody, mucoid stools, hepatic abscess	Rehydration Metronidazole

*Doses: ampicillin 50 mg/kg/d divided 4 times daily; ceftriaxone 50 mg/kg/d; erythromycin 40 mg/kg/d divided 4 times daily; metronidazole 30 mg/kg/d divided twice daily; TMP-SMX based on 8 to 12 mg/kg/d of the TMP component divided twice daily.
Key: BUN = serum urea nitrogen, CBC = complete blood count, HUS = hemolytic-uremic syndrome, TMP-SMX = trimethoprim-sulfamethoxazole.

EMERGENCY DEPARTMENT CARE AND DISPOSITION

The following steps should be used if vomiting is the prominent symptom.
1. Because most cases are self-limited, oral rehydration is generally all that is necessary. Vomiting is not a contraindication to oral rehydration with glucose and electrolyte solutions. The key is to give small amounts of the solution frequently.

2. If oral rehydration is not possible or not tolerated by the patient, intravenous rehydration with normal saline may be necessary.

3. Antiemetics are controversial and generally not recommended. If they are used, the physician should be aware of potential adverse side effects associated with these drugs, such as dystonic reactions.

The following steps should be used if diarrhea is the prominent symptom.

1. Children with mild diarrhea who are not dehydrated may continue routine feedings.

2. Children with moderate to severe dehydration should receive adequate rehydration before resuming routine feedings. Food should be reinstated after the rehydration phase is completed and never delayed longer than 24 hours. There is no need to dilute formula because more than 80% of children with acute diarrhea can tolerate full-strength milk safely.

3. Dietary recommendations include a diet high in complex carbohydrates, lean meats, vegetables, fruits, and yogurt. Fatty foods and foods high in simple sugars should be avoided. The BRAT diet is discouraged because it does not provide adequate energy sources.

4. Antimotility drugs are not helpful and should not be used to treat acute diarrhea in children.

5. Antibiotics are considered if the diarrhea has persisted longer than 10 to 14 days or the patient has a significant fever, systemic symptoms, or blood or pus in the stool after a stool culture is sent. Empiric therapy should cover common agents (see Table 74-1), with ampicillin or trimethoprim-sulfamethoxazole being good choices.

6. All infants and children who appear toxic or have high-risk social situations, significant dehydration, intractable vomiting, altered mental status, inability to drink, bloody diarrhea, or laboratory evidence of hemolytic anemia, thrombocytopenia, azotemia, or elevated creatinine should be admitted.

7. Children who respond to oral or intravenous hydration can be discharged. Instructions should be given to return to the emergency department or seek care with the primary physician if the child becomes unable to tolerate oral hydration, develops bilious vomiting, becomes less alert, or exhibits signs of dehydration, such as no longer wetting diapers.

For further reading in *Emergency Medicine: A Comprehensive Study Guide,* 6th ed., see Chap. 126, "Vomiting and Diarrhea in Children," by Christopher M. Holmes and Summer A. Smith.

75 | Pediatric Abdominal Emergencies

Debra G. Perina

Abdominal pain in children is a diagnostic challenge to the emergency department physician. To provide effective treatment, the physician must be able to recognize clinical manifestations of common diseases, develop a differential diagnosis, and know how to approach a child. The child's age will influence the presenting signs and symptoms significantly. Abdominal disease processes can be classified in several ways: with or without fever, abdominal or extraabdominal, obstructive or nonobstructive, or a local or systemic process.

CLINICAL FEATURES

Presenting signs and symptoms differ with the child's age. The key gastrointestinal (GI) signs and symptoms are pain, vomiting, diarrhea, constipation, bleeding, jaundice, and masses. These symptoms can be the result of a benign process or indicate a life-threatening illness. The origin of abdominal pain may be extraabdominal, such as with pneumonia or pharyngitis. Pain in children younger than 2 years usually manifests as fussiness, irritability, or lethargy. Pain may be peritonitic and exacerbated by motion or obstructive, spasmodic, and associated with restlessness. Differentiation between the 2 types can aid in diagnosis. Pain of GI origin is usually referred to the periumbilical area in children 2 to 6 years old. Associated symptoms or the presence of illness in other family members may be useful in arriving at a diagnosis.

Vomiting and diarrhea are common in children. These symptoms may be the result of a benign process or indicate the presence of a life-threatening process (see Chap. 74). Bilious vomiting is always indicative of a serious process. Diarrhea should be evaluated for the presence of blood. Stool cultures should be done in children with bloody stools, toxic appearance, or diarrhea lasting longer than 5 days. Constipation may be functional or pathologic. The shape and girth of the abdomen, presence of bowel sounds or masses, and abnormalities in the anal area should be noted. GI bleeding can be from upper or lower sources. Upper sources are vascular malformation, swallowed maternal blood, bleeding diathesis, foreign body, peptic ulcer disease, and Mallory-Weiss tear. Lower GI bleeding can be from fissures, intussusception, hemolytic uremic syndrome, swallowed maternal blood, vascular malformations, polyps, inflammatory bowel disease, or diverticulum. A small amount of blood in the diaper is most likely related to anal fissure or ingested foodstuffs. The cause of minimal to moderate amounts of blood in the stool is frequently never identified. Jaundice can be an ominous sign, and all icteric patients should be fully evaluated for sepsis, congenital infections, hepatitis, anatomic problems, and enzyme deficiencies.

DIAGNOSIS AND DIFFERENTIAL

Obtaining a thorough history from parent and child (if possible) is essential. The history should include fever, quality and location of pain, chronology of events, feedings, bowel habits, weight changes, quantity of vomiting and bowel losses, and blood in stool. Physical examination should include completely disrobing the patient, inspection and nontouch maneuvers, followed by auscultation and palpation. The rectal examination and guaiac test should never be omitted. Extraabdominal areas, such as the chest, pharynx, testes, scrotum, inguinal area, and neck, should be evaluated. Every child should have a careful abdominal examination. A palpated abdominal mass is worrisome at any age because it may be the first presentation of a tumor or life-threatening pathology, such as neuroblastoma, Wilms tumor, rhabdomyosarcoma, pyloric stenosis, or intussusception. In girls after menarche, ectopic pregnancy should be considered.

The likely etiologies of abdominal pain change with age. Table 75-1 lists common causes of abdominal pain seen in various age groups and identifies

TABLE 75-1 Etiology of Abdominal Pain

Under 2 y	6–11 y
Appendicitis*	Appendicitis*
Colic (first 4 months)	Diabetic ketoacidosis
Congenital abnormalities*	Functional
Gastroenteritis	Gastroenteritis
Incarcerated hernia*	Henoch-Schönlein purpura
Intussusception*	Incarcerated hernia*
Malabsorption	Inflammatory bowel disease
Malrotation	Obstruction
Metabolic acidosis*	Peptic ulcer disease*
Obstruction	Pneumonia*
Sickle cell pain crisis	Renal stones
Toxins*	Sickle cell syndrome
Urinary tract infection	Streptococcal pharyngitis
Volvulus*	Torsion of ovary or testicle
	Toxins*
	Trauma*
	Urinary tract infection
2–5 y	>11 y
Appendicitis*	Appendicitis*
Diabetic ketoacidosis*	Cholecystitis
Gastroenteritis	Diabetic ketoacidosis*
Hemolytic uremic syndrome*	Dysmenorrhea
Henoch-Schonlein purpura	Ectopic pregnancy*
Incarcerated hernia*	Functional
Intussusception*	Gastroenteritis
Malabsorption	Incarcerated hernia*
Metabolic acidosis*	Inflammatory bowel disease
Obstruction	Obstruction
Pneumonia*	Pancreatitis
Sickle cell pain crisis	Peptic ulcer disease*
Toxins*	Pneumonia*
Trauma*	Pregnancy
Urinary tract infection	Renal stones
Volvulus*	Sickle cell syndrome
	Torsion of ovary or testicle
	Toxins*
	Trauma*
	Urinary tract infection

*Life-threatening causes of abdominal pain.

those that are potentially life threatening. It is clinically useful to split the most serious causes of GI emergencies in the first year of life from those seen in older children.

Infants

Common emergencies in the first year of life include malrotation of the gut, incarcerated hernia, intestinal obstruction, pyloric stenosis, and intussusception.

Malrotation of the gut, although rare, can present with a volvulus, which can be life threatening. Presenting symptoms are usually bilious vomiting, abdominal distention, and streaks of blood in the stool. The vast majority of cases presents within the first month of life. Distended loops of bowel overriding the liver on abdominal radiographs are suggestive of this diagnosis.

Incarcerated hernia may present with irritability, poor feeding, vomiting, and an inguinal or scrotal mass. The mass will not be detected unless the infant is totally undressed. The incidence of incarcerated hernia is highest in the first year of life. It is possible to manually reduce the hernia on examination in most cases (see Chap. 43).

Intestinal obstruction may be caused by atresia, stenosis, meconium ileus, malrotation, intussusception, volvulus, incarcerated hernia, imperforate anus, and Hirschsprung disease. Presentation includes irritability, vomiting, and abdominal distention, followed by absence of bowel sounds. Abdominal radiographs show an obstructive pattern with dilated loops of bowel.

Pyloric stenosis usually presents with nonbilious projectile vomiting occurring just after feeding. It is seen most commonly in the second or third week of life. It is familial and male predominant, with first-born males being particularly affected. Palpation of the pyloric mass, or "olive," in the left upper quadrant is diagnostic. Ultrasound may aid in the diagnosis, if clinically suspected but a mass is not palpated.

Intussusception occurs when 1 portion of the gut telescopes into another. GI bleeding and edema give rise to bloody mucus-containing stools, thus producing the classic "currant jelly" stool. The greatest incidence occurs between ages 3 months and 6 years. Presentation is usually sudden epigastric pain with pain-free intervals during which the examination can show the classic sausage-shaped mass in the right side of the abdomen. This mass is present in up to two thirds of cases. A barium enema or insufflation can be diagnostic and therapeutic because the intussusception is reduced while doing this procedure in 80% of cases.

Children 2 Years or Older

Common GI emergencies in children 2 years and older include appendicitis, bleeding, Meckel diverticulum, Henoch-Schönlein purpura, hemolytic uremia syndrome (HUS), colonic polyps, pancreatitis, intraabdominal masses and portal hypertension.

Appendicitis may present with classic symptoms of pain, fever, and anorexia; however, presentation may be extremely varied, making the diagnosis quite challenging. Guarding and rebound may not be found on examination, the temperature may be normal, the white blood cell count may be normal, and the child may be asking for food. Associated gastroenteritis is fairly common. Appendicitis is also seen in children younger than 1 year. The perforation rate is higher in this age group due to the difficulty in making the diagnosis, which is frequently confused with gastroenteritis.

Meckel diverticulum can cause bleeding, volvulus, and intestinal obstruction or act as a nidus for intussusception. Acute inflammation may mimic appendicitis.

Henoch-Schönlein purpura and HUS can cause abdominal pain and bleeding. Associated symptoms in Henoch-Schönlein purpura include joint pain and petechial or purpuric rash on buttocks and lower extremities. Low-grade fever, hematuria, pallor, lethargy, or altered mental status is seen in HUS. A history of gastroenteritis, sometimes with bloody diarrhea, is present up to 2 weeks before the onset of HUS. Hypertension occurs in up to 50% and seizures in up to 40% of cases of HUS.

Colonic polyps can be single or multiple and give rise to painless bright red lower GI bleeding. Multiple polyps may suggest familial polyposis, which is a rare and often premalignant syndrome. A single polyp is most common and frequently palpated by the mother or noticed as a mass protruding from the anus.

Pancreatitis is not common in childhood. The most common cause is abdominal trauma followed by postviral process, drugs and toxin exposure, and idiopathic.

Portal hypertension, although rare, is one of the common causes of major upper GI bleeding. Ascites is the most common presenting sign in infants, whereas massive hematemesis and hematochezia are the usual presenting symptoms in children. Etiologies include congenital liver disease, hepatitis, inborn errors of metabolism, extrahepatic biliary thrombosis, and biliary atresia.

EMERGENCY DEPARTMENT CARE AND DISPOSITION

1. If the child is critically ill, resuscitation efforts should begin immediately while the examination is being done concurrently.
2. All clothing is removed before examination. The examination should always include a rectal examination and testing of stool for occult blood.
3. The most important laboratory studies are complete blood count with differential, urinalysis, and guaiac test for occult blood. Other tests should be guided by how ill the child appears. Determination of electrolyte, hepatic, lipase, and amylase levels and pregnancy test may be indicated.
4. Chest and abdominal radiographs can be useful to diagnose pneumonia, obstruction, or ileus. Abdominal ultrasound is useful in assessment of pyloric stenosis, ectopic pregnancy, or appendicitis. Abdominal computed tomography may be diagnostic with abdominal masses and appendicitis.
5. In some cases, dehydration and electrolyte abnormalities may require correction with oral or intravenous rehydration.

For further reading in *Emergency Medicine, A Comprehensive Study Guide,* 6th ed., see Chap. 127, "Pediatric Abdominal Emergencies," by Robert W. Schafermeyer.

76 | Diabetic Ketoacidosis in Children

David M. Cline

Type 1 or juvenile-onset diabetes (the term preferred to insulin-dependent diabetes mellitus) is clinically detected by the presence of hyperglycemia in association with glucosuria. The diagnosis typically is characterized by polyuria, polydipsia, and polyphagia; however, other common complaints include failure to gain weight, weight loss, enuresis, anorexia, and changes in vision and school performance.

CLINICAL FEATURES

Diabetic ketoacidosis (DKA) is a common complication of type 1 diabetes and is responsible for the majority of deaths in diabetics younger than 24 years. Classic early symptoms include polydipsia, polyuria, and polyphagia. In addition, DKA should be considered in patients who present with hyperventilation, fruity breath odor of ketosis, dehydration, lethargy, vomiting, abdominal pain, and fever. Physical examination may show signs of dehydration (see Chap. 80), mild abdominal tenderness (from vomiting), Kussmaul respirations, decreased level of consciousness, or coma. Cerebral edema is the most dreaded complication and should be suspected in all comatose patients.

DIAGNOSIS AND DIFFERENTIAL

DKA is defined by hyperglycemia (blood glucose >250 mg/dL), ketonemia, and metabolic acidosis (pH <7.2 and plasma bicarbonate level <15 mEq/L) associated with glucosuria and ketonuria. Most such patients are dehydrated and ill in appearance. Laboratory tests required to manage and diagnose DKA include serum electrolytes, urinalysis, blood pH (from an arterial or venous sample), and serum ketones. Children with suspected cerebral edema should have a noncontrast head computed tomography. Sepsis should be considered when the cause of DKA is not apparent, and a complete blood count, a chest radiogram, and appropriate cultures should be obtained. Other causative factors include trauma, vomiting, noncompliance, and overall stress.

EMERGENCY DEPARTMENT CARE AND DISPOSITION

The treatment of DKA consists of volume replacement, insulin therapy, correction of electrolyte abnormalities, and a search for a causative factor. Patients should be placed on a cardiac monitor, noninvasive blood pressure device, and pulse oximetry, and intravenous lines should be established. Initially, hourly monitoring of electrolytes and pH is necessary.

1. In general, to calculate the total fluid deficit, the patient's presenting weight should be compared with a recent weight. If this is not available, assume at least a 10% (100 mL/kg) deficit (see Chap. 80). Volume replacement using a **normal saline** (NS) infusion of 10 to 20 mL/kg over 1 to 2 hours should be given initially to most patients. If evidence of shock is present, a 20-mL/kg bolus of NS is administered. After initial stabilization is complete, the remaining fluid deficit should be replaced over 24 to

48 hours with 0.45% NS. If serum osmolality remains above 320 mosm/L, NS is continued until the osmolality approaches normal. Glucose levels are monitored closely, and 5% dextrose in 0.45% NS is started when blood glucose levels are between 300 and 250 mg/dL.

2. A regular **insulin** infusion of 0.1 U/kg/h should be initiated as soon as a glucose level above 250 mg/dL is obtained. There is no need for an insulin bolus, which may produce unwanted hypoglycemia. If the acidosis has not improved after 2 hours of insulin therapy, the insulin infusion is increased to 0.15 to 0.2 U/kg/h. The insulin infusion and 5% dextrose in 0.45% NS are continued until the acidosis is corrected.

3. Restoration of **sodium** levels is accomplished by administration of NS and 0.45% NS fluid. Patients typically demonstrate sodium deficits of approximately 5 to 10 mEq/kg. Also, the hyperglycemia and hyperlipoidemia associated with DKA cause a falsely low serum sodium level. Serum sodium levels should be monitored closely because a decline of the sodium level is sometimes indicative of developing cerebral edema.

4. Management of **potassium** abnormalities is critical to the care of DKA patients. Because of the shift of potassium to the extracellular space secondary to the acidosis of DKA, one may see falsely elevated serum K^+ levels despite total body depletion. If the pH is 7.10 or lower and the K^+ level is normal or low, replacement therapy is begun immediately by adding 30 to 40 mEq K^+ to each liter of maintenance fluid. Higher doses should be considered if the potassium level is less than 3.0 mEq/L. If the K^+ level is elevated (>6.0 mEq/L), then K^+ therapy should be suspended until urine output is present and K^+ is correcting. Half KCl and half KPO_4 are used in such cases. Calcium levels must be monitored because excess phosphate can cause hypocalcemia.

5. Bicarbonate therapy has not been shown to improve outcome and may lead to cerebral edema, volume overload, hypernatremia, accelerated hypokalemia, and paradoxical central nervous system acidosis. Bicarbonate should be used only in life-threatening situations in which other therapy has failed (including adequate ventilation), such as cardiac dysrhythmias or dysfunction.

6. A potentially fatal complication of DKA in children is development of cerebral edema. This typically occurs 6 to 10 hours after initiating therapy and presents as mental status changes progressing to coma. Although the etiology of this complication is unknown, it is felt that several factors may contribute, including overly aggressive fluid therapy, rapid correction of blood glucose levels, bicarbonate therapy, and failure of the serum sodium level to increase with therapy. Treatment should include **mannitol** 1 to 2 g/kg, intracranial pressure monitoring, possible intubation with hyperventilation, and fluid restriction.

7. Most of these patients will require admission to a high acuity area or pediatric intensive care unit for monitoring and ongoing therapy. Consultation with the patient's primary care physician and possibly a pediatric endocrinologist should be made early in the course of therapy.

For further reading in *Emergency Medicine: A Comprehensive Study Guide*, 6th ed., see Chap 128, "The Diabetic Child and Diabetic Ketoacidosis," by Rick Place and Thom A. Mayer.

77 | Hypoglycemia in Children

Juan A. March

CLINICAL FEATURES

Hypoglycemia occurs as a primary or secondary feature of a large number of clinical conditions (Table 77-1). In children presenting to the emergency department, idiopathic ketotic hypoglycemia is by far the most common cause of hypoglycemia in 58% of cases, whereas 10% are due to insulin-dependent diabetes mellitus. The drugs most commonly associated with clinically significant hypoglycemia in children are insulin, sulfonylurea-type medications, and ethanol. Calcium channel blockers, β-agonists, and anticholinergic drugs can produce hypoglycemia by suppressing the release of glycogen stores.

Hypoglycemic patients typically present with a mixture of neuroglycopenic and adrenergic signs and symptoms. Neurologic symptoms associated with hypoglycemia include confusion, ataxia, depressed consciousness, blurred vision, focal neurologic deficits, and seizures. Adrenergic symptoms associated with hypoglycemia include anxiety, tachycardia, perspiration, tremors, pallor, weakness, abdominal pain, and irritability.

The symptoms of hypoglycemia in neonates and infants are usually less specific and more difficult to classify. These include poor feeding, jitteriness, emesis, ravenous hunger, lethargy, altered personality, repetitive colic-like symptoms, hypotonia, and hypothermia.

Hypoglycemia often accompanies a critical illness (eg, meningococcemia) and the features of that illness may dominate the clinical picture, thereby masking the signs of hypoglycemia. Hypoglycemia should be suspected in all moderately to severely ill children, and bedside glucose testing should be performed immediately for children with unexplained coma, severe hypothermia, and arrest.

TABLE 77-1 Conditions Associated with Hypoglycemia in Infants and Children*

Perinatal period	Infancy and childhood
Infant of a diabetic mother	Idopathic ketotic hypoglycemia/starvation
Congenital heart disease	Diabetes mellitus/endocrine disorder
Infection/sepsis	Infection/sepsis
Adrenal hemorrhage	Inborn errors of metabolism
Hypothermia	Hypothermia
Hypoglycemia-inducing drug use by mother	Drug induced (salicylates, etc)
Maternal eclampsia	Hyperinsulinism
Fetal alcohol syndrome	Idiopathic
Hypopituitarism	

*This is a partial listing; see Chap. 129 in *Emergency Medicine: A Comprehensive Study Guide*, 6th ed., for a complete listing.

DIAGNOSIS AND DIFFERENTIAL

Plasma glucose concentration of less than 60 mg/dL constitutes hypoglycemia in school-age children, adolescents, and adults. Although controversial, in general one should consider hypoglycemia for a plasma glucose of less than 30 mg/dL in the first 24 hours of life and a plasma glucose level of less than 45 mg/dL for the remainder of the neonatal period.

The differential diagnosis of hypoglycemia differs based on age and represents an important clinical finding associated with many disorders, illnesses, and ingestions. A list of common conditions associated with hypoglycemia in infants and children is provided in Table 77-1.

Bedside glucometers have evolved over the years and can produce diagnostic results within 2 minutes. However, one must be cautious because false low readings of bedside glucometers have been associated with abnormal hematocrits, severe dehydration, and hyperosmolar conditions. This is especially true for neonates. Nevertheless, symptomatic patients should be treated based on bedside testing.

EMERGENCY DEPARTMENT CARE AND DISPOSITION

There are 3 important aspects of emergency patient care: (*a*) rapid diagnosis of hypoglycemia, (*b*) acquisition of blood and urine specimens, and (*c*) prompt restoration and maintenance of euglycemia.

1. The Pediatric Advanced Life Support manual recommends that a 5- to 10-mL/kg bolus of **10% dextrose in water** be administered intravenously or intraosseously to hypoglycemic neonates. Older children should receive a bolus of 2 to 4 mL/kg of **25% dextrose in water** ($D_{25}W$). Adolescents typically receive the adult dose of 50 mL of $D_{50}W$. Other sources recommend smaller doses. Administration of $D_{25}W$ and $D_{50}W$ is controversial because both are hyperosmolar, cause pain, and increase the risk in smaller veins for phlebitis, extravasation, and surrounding tissue necrosis. Hyperosmolar loading in premature neonates is associated with increased risk of intracranial germinal matrix hemorrhage and subsequent periventricular leukomalacia. Use of $D_{25}W$ and $D_{50}W$ also may rebound hypoglycemia due to release of endogenous insulin.
2. After the dextrose bolus and return to normal glucose levels, maintenance fluid must be started (see Chap. 80).
3. When intravenous access is unavailable, **glucagon** 0.03 to 0.05 mg/kg intramuscularly can be considered. Glucagon works only in patients with intact glycogen stores, and its use is controversial in the pediatric population. Thus, intraosseous access should be considered when the intravenous route is not possible.
4. When standard therapy fails, **hydrocortisone** 1 to 2 mg/kg intravenouly should be considered for those who cannot achieve euglycemia despite adequate dextrose administration. This is especially true of patients with hypopituitarism and adrenal insufficiency.
5. For idiopathic ketotic hypoglycemia, the best treatment is prevention, which includes avoiding prolonged fasts and providing frequent high carbohydrate, high protein meals. Monitoring these patients by measuring urine for ketones can assist in their management.

For further reading in *Emergency Medicine: A Comprehensive Study Guide*, 6th ed., see Chap. 129, "Hypoglycemia," by Randolph J. Cordle.

| Altered Mental Status and Headache in Children

Debra G. Perina

ALTERED MENTAL STATUS

Altered mental status (AMS) in a child is failure to respond to the external environment after appropriate stimulation in a manner consistent with the child's developmental level. In treating children with AMS, aggressive resuscitation, stabilization, diagnosis, and treatment must occur simultaneously to prevent morbidity and death.

Clinical Features

The spectrum of AMS ranges from confusion to lethargy, stupor, and coma indicative of depression of the cerebral cortex or localized abnormalities of the reticular activating system. Pathologic conditions affecting mental status can be divided into supratentorial lesions, subtentorial lesions, and metabolic encephalopathy. Supratentorial lesions present with focal motor abnormalities, rostral-to-caudal progression of dysfunction, and slow nystagmus toward the lesion with cold calorics. Motor abnormalities generally precede AMS. Subtentorial lesions produce rapid loss of consciousness, cranial nerve abnormalities, abnormal breathing patterns, and asymmetric or fixed pupils. Metabolic encephalopathy produces decreased level of consciousness before exhibiting motor signs, which are symmetrical when present. Pupillary reflexes are intact except with profound anoxia, opiates, barbiturates, and anticholinergics.

Diagnosis and Differential

A thorough history and physical examination are paramount to determining the diagnosis. Key questions must include prodromal events and associated signs and symptoms, such as fever, headache, weakness, vomiting, diarrhea, gait disturbances, head tilt, rash, palpitations, abdominal pain, hematuria, and weight loss. Inquiries also should be made regarding past medical history, family history, and immunization status. The examination should look for signs of occult infection, trauma, toxicity, or metabolic disease. A useful tool for organizing diagnostic possibilities in the mnemonic AEIOU TIPS (Table 78-1).

Diagnostic adjuncts should be guided by the clinical situation but can include analysis of blood, gastric fluid, urine, stool, cerebrospinal fluid, electrocardiography, or selected radiographic studies. Rapid bedside glucose determination is a universally accepted standard. If meningitis or encephalitis is suspected, lumbar puncture and cerebrospinal fluid analysis should be done as rapidly as possible after initial resuscitation and stabilization. A 12-lead electrocardiogram should be obtained in cases in which there are pathologic auscultatory findings or rhythm disturbances.

Emergency Department Care and Disposition

Treatment priorities should concentrate on stabilization and reversal of life-threatening conditions.

359

TABLE 78-1 AEIOU TIPS

A	**Alcohol.** Changes in mental status can occur with serum levels <100 mg/dL. Concurrent hypoglycemia is common. **Acid-base and metabolic.** Hypotonic and hypertonic dehydration. Hepatic dysfunction, inborn errors of metabolism, diabetic ketoacidosis, primary lung disease, and neurologic dysfunction causing hypercapnia. **Dysrhythmia (arrhythmia)/cardiogenic.** Stokes-Adams, supraventricular tachycardia, aortic stenosis, heart block.
E	**Encephalopathy.** Hypertensive encephalopathy can occur with diastolic pressures of 100–110 mm Hg. Reye syndrome. **Endocrinopathy.** AMS is rare as a presentation in this category. Addison disease can present with AMS or psychosis. Thyrotoxicosis can present with ventricular dysrhythmias. Pheochromocytoma can present with hypertensive encephalopathy. **Electrolytes.** Hyponatremia becomes symptomatic around 120 mEq/L. Hypernatremia and disorders of calcium, magnesium, and phosphorus can produce AMS.
I	**Insulin.** AMS from hyperglycemia is rare in children, but diabetic ketoacidosis is the most common cause. Hypoglycemia can be the result of many disorders. Irritability, confusion, seizures, and coma can occur with blood glucose levels <40 mg/dL. **Intussusception.** AMS may be the initial presenting symptom.
O	**Opiates.** Common household exposures are to Lomotil, Imodium, diphenoxylate, and dextromethorphan. Clonidine, an α-agonist, can also produce similar symptoms.
U	**Uremia.** Encephalopathy occurs in over one third of patients with chronic renal failure. Hemolytic uremic syndrome can produce AMS in addition to abdominal pain. Thrombocytopenic purpura and hemolytic anemia also can cause AMS.
T	**Trauma.** Children with blunt trauma are more likely than adults to develop cerebral edema. Remember to look for signs of child abuse, particularly shaken baby syndrome with retinal hemorrhages. **Tumor.** Primary, metastatic, or meningeal leukemic infiltration. **Thermal.** Hypo- or hyperthermia.
I	**Infection.** One of the most common causes of AMS in children. Meningitis should be high on the differential list. **Intracerebral vascular disorders.** Subarachnoid, intracerebral or intraventricular hemorrhages can be seen with trauma, ruptured aneurysm, or arteriovenous malformations. Venous thrombosis can follow severe dehydration or pyogenic infection of the mastoid, orbit, middle ear, or sinuses.
P	**Psychogenic.** Rare in the pediatric age group, characterized by decreased responsiveness with normal neurologic examination incluidng oculovestibular reflexes. **Poisoning.** Drugs or toxins can be ingested by accident, through neglect or abuse, or in a suicide gesture.
S	**Seizure.** Generalized motor seizures are often associated with prolonged unresponsiveness in children. Seizures in a young febrile patient suggests intracranial infection.

Key: AMS = altered mental status.

1. Airway, breathing, and circulation must be ensured.
2. Continuous pulse oximetry and supplemental **oxygen** as needed to correct hypoxia should be provided (bring O_2 saturation up to 90% or above), including bag-valve-mask and intubation when appropriate.
3. Fluid resuscitation with 20-mL/kg fluid boluses of **isotonic crystalloid** is given for hypotension. Fluid boluses may be repeated up to 60 mL/kg, after which the need for pressor agents, such as dopamine, should be considered.
4. Bedside glucose testing and administration of glucose should be performed, if indicated (see Chap. 77).
5. Core body temperature should be controlled to minimize metabolic demands.
6. Seizures, if present, are controlled with benzodiazepines (see Chap. 73).
7. Acid–base balance is restored with hydration and compensatory ventilation. **Bicarbonate** (1 to 2 mEq/kg intravenously, slow infusion) is used sparingly and only if pH is less than 7.0 (see Chap. 4).
8. Patients who appear septic should receive empiric antibiotics as quickly as possible, which may be given before lumbar puncture.
9. Most patients with AMS will require admission and extended observation. Only those with transient, rapidly reversible causes of AMS can be treated and discharged from the emergency department after a period of observation with follow-up scheduled within 24 hours of discharge.

HEADACHE

Up to 2% of emergency department visits are for complaints of headache. The vast majority of headaches in children have a benign etiology. Occipital location of the headache and the inability of the child to describe the quality of the head pain are associated with serious underlying causes.

Clinical Features

Headaches can be classified as primary or secondary. Primary headaches are physiologic (migraine, tension), whereas secondary headaches have an anatomic basis (vascular malformation, tumor, or infection). A careful history and physical examination can greatly aid in differentiating these types. History suggestive of a secondary headache includes acute onset; morning vomiting; behavioral changes; AMS; "worst ever" headache that, awakens the child from sleep; associated with fever, trauma, or toxic exposure, or aggravated by coughing; Valsalva; or lying down. Physical findings suggestive of a secondary headache include blood pressure abnormalities, nuchal rigidity, head tilt, ptosis, retinal hemorrhage or optic nerve distortion, visual field defects, gait disturbances, or focal motor or sensory deficits.

Diagnosis and Differential

There are no evidence-based studies guiding diagnostic workup in children. The selection of studies will depend on findings obtained from the history and physical examination. Blood tests such as complete blood count, blood glucose, basic metabolic panel, or thyroid function tests may be useful. Lumbar puncture is indicated if infection or subarachnoid hemorrhage is suspected. Head computed tomography and magnetic resonance brain imaging may be indicated in trauma or secondary types of headaches (eg, occipital headaches with or without any neurologic symptoms).

Emergency Department Care and Disposition

1. Narcotic or non-narcotic analgesics should be given as appropriate for relief of pain according to the disease process and level of pain. Typically ibuprofen is given, but some patients may require opiates, such as **morphine** 0.1 mg/kg, or **acetaminophen with codeine,** 3 to 6 years old, 5 mL/dose; 7 to 12 years old, 10 mL/dose; older than 12 years, 15 mL/dose.
2. Treatment of the underlying condition identified during diagnostic testing.
3. Any potential precipitating factors should be addressed to avoid reoccurrence of the headache. Addressing these factors may include prophylactic regimens such as β-blockers for migraines.
4. In general, most patients may be discharged after relief of symptoms. Patients with emergent causes of headache such as meningitis, tumor, severe hypertension, or hemorrhage should be admitted for definitive care. Patients with intractable pain also may need admission.

For further reading in *Emergency Medicine: A Comprehensive Study Guide,* 6th ed., see Chap. 130, "Altered Mental Status and Headache in Children," by Nancy Pook, Natalie Cullen, and Jonathan Singer.

79 | Syncope and Sudden Death in Children and Adolescents

Debra G. Perina

Syncope is very common in adolescence. Up to 50% of adolescents experience at least 1 syncopal episode. This condition is transient and usually self-limited, but it may be a symptom of serious cardiac disease.

The rate of sudden, unexpected death in children is 2.3% of all pediatric deaths. Sudden cardiac death makes up about one third of these. Except for trauma, sudden cardiac death is the most common cause of sports-related deaths, particularly with basketball, football, and track. Hypertrophic cardiomyopathy is the most common cause of sudden cardiac death in adolescents without known cardiac disease. Other causes of sudden cardiac death in children are myocarditis, congenital heart disease, and conduction disturbances.

CLINICAL FEATURES

Syncope is sudden onset of falling accompanied by a brief episode of loss of consciousness. Involuntary motor movements may occur with all types of syncopal episodes but are most common with seizures. Two thirds of children experience lightheadedness or dizziness before the episode. There are many causes of syncope in children. Table 79-1 lists the most common causes of syncope by category.

Neurally mediated syncope is the most common cause in children and includes vasovagal, vasodepressor, neurocardiogenic, reflex syncope, and simple fainting. This type of syncope is usually preceded by sensations of nausea, warmth, or lightheadedness with a gradual visual grayout. Cardiac syncope occurs due to an interruption of cardiac output from an intrinsic cardiac problem such as tachydysrhythmia, bradydysrhythmia, outflow obstruction, and myocardial dysfunction. Syncope resulting from cardiac causes usually begins and ends abruptly.

Risk factors associated with serious causes of syncope are presented in Table 79-2. Events easily mistaken for syncope are presented in Table 79-3 in addition to common associated symptoms.

DIAGNOSIS AND DIFFERENTIAL

No specific historical or clinical features reliably distinguish between vasovagal syncope and other causes. However, a thorough history and physical examination can help to arouse suspicion of serious causes. The most important step in evaluation of children with syncope is a detailed history, including medications, drugs, intake, and food. Syncope during exercise suggests a more serious cause. A cardiac dysrhythmia should be suspected if syncope is associated with an intense sympathetic stimulus such as fright, anger, surprise, or exercise. Many of the diseases that cause syncope also cause sudden death in children. Approximately 25% of children who suffer sudden death have a history of syncope. If witnesses note that the patient appeared dead or cardiopulmonary resuscitation was performed, a search for serious pathologic conditions must be undertaken.

363

TABLE 79-1 Causes of Syncope in Children and Adolescents

Neurally mediated: most common cause of syncope in children
  Orthostatic: lightheadedness with standing
  Situational: urination, defecation, coughing, and swallowing may precipitate
  Familial dysautonomia

Cardiac dysrhythmias: events that usually start and end abruptly
  Prolonged Q-T syndrome
  Wolff-Parkinson-White syndrome
  Sick sinus syndrome: assocaited with prior heart surgery
  Supraventricular tachycardia
  Atrioventricular block: most common in children with congenital heart disease
  Pacemaker malfunction

Structural cardiac disease
  Hypertrophic cardiomopathy: exertional syncope most common
  presentation, but infants can present with congestive heart failure and
  cyanosis, echocardiography necessary to confirm
  Dilated cardiomyopathy: may be idiopathic, postmyocarditis, or with
  congenital heart disease
  Congenital heart disease
  Valvular diseases: aortic stenosis usually congenital defect. Ebstein
  malformation, or mitral valve prolapse (which is not associated with
  increased risk of sudden death)
  Dysrhythmogenic right ventricular dysplasia
  Pulmonary hypertension: dyspnea on exertion, exercise intolerance,
  shortness of breath
  Coronary artery abnormalities: aberrant left main artery causing external
  compression during physical exercise

Endocrane abnormalities: hyperthyroid, hyperglycemia, adrenal insufficiency

Medications and drugs: antihypertensives, tricyclic antidepressants, cocaine,
diuretics, antidysrhythmics

Gastrointestinal disorders: reflux

The physical examination should include complete cardiovascular, neurologic, and pulmonary examinations. Particular attention should be paid to the cardiovascular examination. Any abnormalities noted in the cardiovascular examination require an in-depth cardiac workup.

EMERGENCY DEPARTMENT CARE AND DISPOSITION

1. Laboratory assessment is guided by the history, physical examination, and clinical suspicion. Routine laboratory studies are not needed if vasovagal

TABLE 79-2 Risk Factors for Serious Causes of Syncope

Exertion preceding the event

History of cardiac disease in patient

Recurrent episodes

Recumbent episode

Family history of sudden death, cardiac disease, deafness

Chest pain, palpitations

Prolonged loss of consciousness

Medications that affect cardiac conduction

TABLE 79-3 Events Mistaken for Syncope

Basilar migraine: headache, loss of consciousness, neurologic symptoms
Seizure: loss of consciousness, simultaneous motor movements, prolonged recovery
Vertigo: no loss of consciousness, spinning or rotating sensation
Hysteria: no loss of consciousness, indifference to the event
Hypoglycemia: confusion, gradual onset associated with diaphoresis
Breath-holding spell: crying prior to the event, age 6–18 mo
Hyperventilation: severe hypocapnia can cause syncope

syncope is strongly suspected. Those with worrisome associated symptoms should have a chemistry panel and hematocrit, thyroid function, and chest radiograph. A pregnancy test should also be done in females of child-bearing age. Serum drug screening or alcohol level determination also may be useful if ingestion is suspected.

2. An echocardiogram (ECG) should be done on all patients except those with an unquestionable vasovagal episode.

3. An echocardiogram is recommended for patients with known or suspected cardiac disease. If an echocardiogram is not immediately available, the urgency for obtaining the study should be determined in consultation with a cardiologist.

4. If no clear cause if found, the child may be discharged to be further evaluated and followed by the primary care physician unless there are cardiac risk factors or exercise-induced symptoms for which referral to a cardiologist is warranted.

5. Children with documented dysrhythmias should be admitted. Patients with a normal ECG but a history suggesting a dysrhythmic event are candidates for outpatient monitoring and cardiac workup.

6. All children admitted for syncope should undergo cardiac monitoring. Children who are survivors of sudden cardiac arrest should be admitted to a pediatric intensive care unit with emergency department efforts aimed at identifying the probable cause of the arrest to prevent future events.

For further reading in *Emergency Medicine: A Comprehensive Study Guide,* 6th ed., see Chap. 131, "Syncope and Sudden Death," by William E. Hauda II and Thom A. Mayer.

80 | Fluid and Electrolyte Therapy

Lance Brown

The most common cause of fluid and electrolyte disturbances in children is gastroenteritis. Each year in the United States, there are about 3 million physician visits, more than 200,000 hospitalizations, and more than 300 deaths associated with pediatric gastroenteritis.

CLINICAL FEATURES

The clinical appearance of patients with dehydration and fluid and electrolyte disturbances depends on the degree of dehydration, the rate at which the fluid was lost, and the age of the patient. With prolonged diarrhea, older children may tolerate a slow total body water loss as great as 40% of the preillness intracellular volume. Rapid and large volume loss as is seen in some cases of rotavirus diarrhea (or cholera) can cause young infants to rapidly deteriorate to the point of cardiovascular collapse.

Because acute fluid (water) loss can be measured as lost weight (1 L water = 1 kg), the gold standard for assessing dehydration is comparison of a very recent preillness weight with weight at presentation on the same scale. From this comparison, the percentage of dehydration (as represented by percentage of weight loss) can be calculated. Unfortunately, this comparison is almost never available in the emergency department. However, physical examination has been shown to provide a reliable estimation of the degree of dehydration. The dehydration state is classified as mild, moderate, or severe (Table 80-1). An exception to this general pattern occurs in hypernatremic dehydration, when fluid is drawn from the interstitial and intracellular spaces in the face of the increased serum osmolarity. This process protects the circulating blood

TABLE 80-1 Clinical Estimate of Pediatric Dehydration

Clinical characteristic	None to mild dehydration	Moderate dehydration	Severe dehydration
% Dehydrated*	<5	5–10	>10
Overall appearance	Active and playful	Restless and fussy	Limp and sleepy
Eyes	Not sunken	Somewhat sunken	Clearly sunken
Tears	Present when cries	May be absent when cries	Absent when cries
Mouth	Moist mucous membranes	Somewhat dry mucous membranes	Dry mucous membranes
Thirst	Not particularly thirsty	Drinks eagerly	Too sick to drink
Skin pinch	Returns immediately	Returns somewhat slowly	Returns slowly

*The number used to calculate the fluid deficit.

volume. Peripheral perfusion and vital signs may be deceptively normal. The skin may have a characteristic doughy feel.

DIAGNOSIS AND DIFFERENTIAL

In the absence of a reliable preillness comparison weight, the diagnosis of dehydration is based primarily on historical data and physical examination findings. Laboratory values may be helpful in some cases but generally are not needed in mild to moderate cases of dehydration. Laboratory data lend supporting evidence, help classify the type of dehydration (eg, isotonic, hypernatremic, and hyponatremic), and identify related problems (eg, renal failure, ketotic hypoglycemia, and diabetic ketoacidosis). The serum bicarbonate level (or total CO_2) has been inversely related to the degree of dehydration (ie, the lower the serum bicarbonate, the greater the degree of dehydration).

The most common cause of dehydration and fluid and electrolyte imbalances in infants and young children is viral gastroenteritis. The most common enteropathogens identified in the United States are rotavirus and enteric adenoviruses. Other important causes of fluid and electrolyte disturbances in children include burns, diabetic complications, inappropriate formula administration (mixed incorrectly), inappropriate feedings (eg, extensive juice drinking, bottles of water offered to small infants, chicken broth, and boiled milk), diabetes insipidus, adrenal insufficiency, renal tubular acidosis, anorexia due to febrile illnesses, respiratory illnesses interfering with adequate oral intake, and cystic fibrosis. Pyloric stenosis historically has been identified with a hypochloremic metabolic alkalosis. However, with earlier identification of pyloric stenosis, this presentation is becoming increasingly uncommon, and at the time of diagnosis the electrolytes are normal. The differential diagnosis of a metabolic acidosis with an elevated anion gap in infants includes those conditions that are seen in adults (ie, renal failure, lactic acidosis, ketoacidosis, and toxic ingestions) and inborn errors of metabolism. The emergency department presentation of infants with inborn errors of metabolism may include vomiting, abnormal tone, seizures, and coma.

EMERGENCY DEPARTMENT CARE AND DISPOSITION

The management of fluid and electrolyte disturbances in infants and young children revolves around a few basic principles: (*a*) identification and treatment of shock, (*b*) identification and treatment of causes that have a specific treatment (eg, diabetic ketoacidosis, pyloric stenosis, and respiratory distress), and (*c*) administration of appropriate fluids to replace maintenance fluids, fluids already lost, and ongoing fluid losses. The commonly accepted approaches to rehydration involve intravenous therapy or oral rehydration therapy.

1. Hypovolemic shock should be treated with 20-mL/kg boluses of intravenous (or intraosseous) isotonic crystalloid (eg, 0.9% normal saline [NS] or lactated Ringer solution) until improved mental status, vital signs, and peripheral perfusion are noted.
2. Maintenance fluids are calculated as follows: for children weighing 10 kg or less, administer 100 mL/kg/d; for children weighing 11 to 20 kg, administer 1,000 mL plus 50 mL/kg for each additional kg >10 kg over 24 hours; for children weighing more than 20 kg, administer 1,500 mL plus 20 mL/kg for each additional kg >20 kg over 24 hours. Standard solutions

for maintenance fluids are 5% dextrose in 0.2 NS (ie, one fourth NS) for young infants and 5% dextrose in 0.45 NS (ie, one half NS) for older infants and children. After adequate urine output is established, 20 mEq/L potassium chloride is typically added. A rapid means of calculating maintenance fluid rates is as follows: 4 mL/h for every kilogram up to 10, plus 2 mL/h for every kilogram between 10 and 20, plus 1 mL/h for every kilogram over 20.

3. Deficit fluids are determined from the clinical appearance and estimated percentage of dehydration (see Table 80-1). Standard solutions for deficit fluid replacement are the same as those for maintenance fluids. The calculations are performed in the following manner. If the patient weighs 15 kg on presentation and is estimated as 10% dehydrated, then it is estimated that 15 kg × 10% = 1.5 kg of water has been lost: 1.5 kg water equals 1.5 L water. Therefore, 1500 mL is the estimated deficit. Half of this total is given over the first 8 hours and the remaining half is given over the following 16 hours. The hourly intravenous fluid rate is determined by the sum of maintenance and deficit fluid requirements for the patient. To avoid cerebral edema, the fluid deficit is replaced much more slowly in the setting of hypernatremic dehydration. After the fluid deficit calculation, the first half is given over 16 hours instead of 8 hours and the second half is given over 32 hours instead of 16 hours.

4. Oral rehydration has been shown to be as effective as intravenous therapy for rehydrating infants and children and may be administered by having the patient drink or through a nasogastric tube. There is debate as to what the appropriate sodium content of the rehydration solution should be. One frequently used rehydration solution is Rehydralyte (Ross Pharmaceuticals), which has 75 mEq of sodium per liter. The replacement is performed by administering 50 mL/kg orally over 4 hours to mildly dehydrated patients and 100 mL/kg to moderately dehydrated patients. Vomiting is not a contraindication to attempting oral rehydration.

5. Antiemetics are not typically advocated for use in infants and young children with vomiting. As new classes of antiemetics become available, these recommendations may change.

6. Most children with potential fluid and electrolyte disturbances from gastroenteritis can be managed as outpatients without any laboratory evaluation in the emergency department.

7. Admission criteria include young age (typically <3 months), severe dehydration, persistent vomiting with failed attempts at oral rehydration, identified admitting diagnosis (eg, diabetic ketoacidosis), hypernatremic dehydration, suspected inborn error of metabolism, and marked electrolyte abnormalities (eg, serum bicarbonate ≤mEq/L).

For further reading in *Emergency Medicine: A Comprehensive Study Guide*, 6th ed., see Chap. 132, "Fluid and Electrolyte Therapy," by William Ahrens.

81 | Upper Respiratory Emergencies

Juan A. March

Diseases that cause upper respiratory tract (URT) obstruction account for a significant percentage of pediatric emergency department visits. Whereas some diseases of the URT are common and quite benign, others although rare are life threatening. The physical sign common to all causes of URT obstruction is stridor. Laryngomalacia, due to a developmentally weak larynx, accounts for 60% of stridor in the neonatal period, but it is self-limited and rarely requires treatment.

VIRAL CROUP (LARYNGOTRACHEOBRONCHITIS)

Clinical Features

Viral croup is responsible for most cases of stridor after the neonatal period. It is usually a benign, self-limited disease caused by marked edema and inflammation of the subglottic area. Children ages 6 months to 3 years are most commonly affected, with a peak at an age of 12 to 24 months. It occurs mainly in late fall and early winter, with parainfluenza viruses (I, II, and III) being the most common etiology. Typically, there is a 1- to 5-day prodrome of cough and coryza, which is followed by a 3- to 4-day period of classic barking cough. Symptoms peak on days 3 to 4. Physical examination classically shows a biphasic stridor, although the inspiratory component usually is much greater.

Diagnosis and Differential

The differential diagnosis should include epiglottitis, bacterial tracheitis, or foreign body aspiration. Croup usually can be diagnosed on clinical grounds.

X-rays are not necessary, unless other causes are being considered.

A lateral neck and chest x-ray may demonstrate the normally squared shoulders of the subglottic tracheal air shadow as a pencil tip, hourglass, or steeple.

Emergency Department Care and Disposition

1. Patients should be monitored with pulse oximetry and treated with cool mist and oxygen.
2. Administer **dexamethasone** 0.6 mg/kg orally or intramuscularly or an equivalent dose of **prednisone** or **prednisolone** (1 to 2 mg/kg). Nebulized budesonide may be clinically useful in moderate to severe cases.
3. Nebulized **epinephrine,** 0.05 mL/kg/dose up to 0.5 mL of 2.25% solution, should be used to treat moderate to severe cases. Children with stridor only after agitation do not need epinephrine.
4. Although intubation should be performed whenever clinically indicated, if treated aggressively, fewer than 1% of admitted patients require intubation.
5. Helium plus oxygen (Heliox), in a 60:40 mixture, may prevent the need for intubation. However, if the patient requires greater that 40% supplemental oxygen, Heliox should not be given.

6. Discharge criteria include the following: at least 3 hours since the last dose of epinephrine, nontoxic appearance, no clinical signs of dehydration, room air oxygen saturation greater than 90%, parents able to recognize changes in the patient's condition, and no social concerns with access to telephone and relatively short transit time to the hospital.

EPIGLOTTITIS

Clinical Features

Epiglottitis is life threatening and can occur at any age. Since the introduction of the *Haemophilus influenzae* vaccine, the incidence and demographics have changed remarkably, with fewer than 25% of cases caused by *Haemophilus* and a median age of presentation shifting to older children and adults. In immunized children the most cases are due to gram-positive organisms, *Streptococcus pyogenes, Staphylococcus aureus,* and *Streptococcus pneumoniae.* In the immunocompromised child herpes, *Candida* and varicella must be considered. Classically, there is abrupt onset of high fever, sore throat, stridor, dysphagia, and drooling developing over 2 days.

The presentation in older children and adults is much more subtle. The only complaint may be severe sore throat, with or without stridor. The diagnosis is suggested by severe sore throat, with a normal-appearing oropharynx, and a striking tenderness with gentle movement of the hyoid.

Diagnosis and Differential

If the patient is moved to an x-ray suite, a physician trained in airway management should be at the bedside at all times. X-rays are usually unnecessary in patients with a classic presentation. If the diagnosis is uncertain, then lateral neck films must be taken with the neck extended and should be taken during inspiration. The epiglottis is normally tall and thin, but in epiglottitis it is very swollen and appears squat and fat like a thumbprint at the base of the hypopharynx.

False negative radiographic evaluations do occur, and, if suspicion remains, direct visualization of the epiglottis is necessary to exclude the diagnosis. Blood cultures are positive in up to 90% of patients, whereas cultures from the epiglottis are less sensitive.

Emergency Department Care and Disposition

1. If total airway obstruction or apnea does occur, children with epiglottitis sometimes can be effectively ventilated with a bag-valve-mask device.
2. Supportive therapy includes humidified oxygen and nebulized epinephrine. Heliox also can be attempted.
3. The most experienced individual should perform intubation as soon as the diagnosis is made. Use of sedation, paralytics, and vagolytics are used as indicated. Ideally, an otolaryngologist should be present during the intubation to perform a surgical airway if intubation fails. Use of a tube 1 size smaller than usual prevents postextubation stridor.
4. Only after airway management should intravenous (IV) antibiotics be considered. These include use of **cefuroxime** 50 mg/kg IV per dose, **cefotaxime** 50 mg/kg IV per dose, or **ceftriaxone** 80 to 100 mg/kg IV per dose. In regions with increased cephalosporin resistance, vancomycin or nafcillin should be added.

BACTERIAL TRACHEITIS

Clinical Features

Bacterial tracheitis (membranous laryngotracheobronchitis), a more severe form of croup, is usually rare and caused by bacterial superinfection of a preceding viral upper respiratory infection. Bacterial tracheitis is typically seen in children younger than 3 years, but it can be seen in patients between ages 3 months and 13 years. It is usually caused by *S aureus, S pneumoniae,* or β-lactamase–producing gram-negative organisms (*H influenza* and *Moraxella catarrhalis*).

Patients with bacterial tracheobronchitis have more respiratory distress than do patients with croup. Children appear septic and present similarly to those with epiglottitis, with the following exceptions: severe inspiratory and expiratory stridor, occasionally with thick sputum production, and a raspy hoarse voice but no dysphagia.

Diagnosis and Differential

Radiographs of the lateral neck and chest usually demonstrate subglottic narrowing of the trachea, irregular densities maybe seen within the trachea, and its borders may appear ragged and indistinct.

Emergency Department Care and Disposition

1. Management is similar to that for epiglottitis, with more than 85% of these patients requiring intubation. Ideally, these patients should go to the operating room for sedation, paralysis, intubation, and bronchoscopy. Cultures and Gram stain at that time may help guide antibiotic therapy.
2. Empirically, antibiotics therapy includes **vancomycin** 10 mg/kg IV every 6 hours and a third-generation cephalosporin, such as **ceftriaxone** 80 to 100 mg/kg IV per dose.

FOREIGN BODY ASPIRATION

Clinical Features

Foreign body (FB) aspirations cause more than 3,000 deaths each year and have a peak incidence between ages 12 and 36 months, with 90% occurring in children younger than 4 years. In children younger than 6 months, the cause is usually secondary to a feeding by a well-meaning sibling. The most common FB aspirations are peanuts, sunflower seeds, raisins, grapes, hot dogs, and small sausages, but almost any object may be aspirated. Unlike small round metal objects, aspirated vegetable matter commonly causes intense pneumonitis and subsequent pneumonia and suppurative bronchitis.

At presentation many patients will be completely asymptomatic. Patients may have a variety of signs, depending on the location of the FB and the degree of obstruction. Classic teaching is that a FB in the laryngotracheal area causes stridor, whereas a bronchial FB causes wheezing, but there is significant overlap in symptoms. Wheeze is present in 30% of laryngotracheal FB aspirations and stridor is found in up to 10% of bronchial aspirations. Patients with immediate onset of severe stridor and cardiac arrest usually have laryngotracheal aspirations.

A significant percentage of patients present without cough, wheeze, or stridor. Because as many as 33% of the aspirations are not witnessed or remembered by the parent, FB aspirations should be considered in all children with unilateral wheezing.

Diagnosis and Differential

FB aspiration is easily confused with more common causes of URT diseases because 36% of patients have fever, 35% have wheezes, and 38% have rales. In up to one third of cases, plain radiographs are normal; thus, a single negative x-ray does not rule out an FB. In cases of complete obstruction, atelectasis may be found. In partial obstructions, a ball valve effect occurs, with air trapping caused by the FB leading to hyperinflation of the obstructed lung. Thus, in a stable cooperative child, inspiratory and expiratory posteroanterior chest radiographs may be helpful. In a stable but noncooperative child, decubitus films may be used but are less sensitive than fluoroscopy. FB aspiration is definitively diagnosed preoperatively in only one third of cases; thus, if clinically suspected, laryngoscopy is indicated.

Although upper esophageal FB can impinge on the posterior aspect of the trachea and may present with stridor, patients typically have dysphagia and are usually radiopaque. Radiographically, flat FBs such as coins are usually oriented in the sagittal plane when located in the trachea (which appear as a thick line in an anterioposterior chest x-ray) and in the coronal plane when in the esophagus (which appear round on an anterioposterior chest x-ray).

Emergency Department Care and Disposition

1. If FB aspiration or airway obstruction is clearly present, a protocol for obstructed airway should be implemented immediately (see Chap. 1).
2. Use of racemic epinephrine or Heliox may be considered.
3. Ideally, treatment of an airway foreign body is usually with laryngoscopy or rigid bronchoscopy in the operating room under anesthesia.

PERITONSILLAR ABSCESS

Clinical Features

Peritonsillar abscess in children most commonly presents in adolescents with an antecedent sore throat. The patients usually appear acutely ill with fevers, chills, dysphagia, trismus, drooling, and a muffled "hot potato" voice.

The uvula is displaced away from the affected side. As a rule, the affected tonsil is anteriorly and medially displaced.

Diagnosis and Differential

Careful visualization of the oral cavity can reliably rule out peritonsillar abscess in many cases. With uvular deviation, marked soft palate displacement, severe trismus, airway compromise, or localized areas of fluctuance are noted; the diagnosis of peritonsillar abscess can be made with confidence and no imaging studies are required. In cases without these physical findings, differentiation from peritonsillar cellulitis may be difficult. In toxic-appearing patients or those with inconsistent findings, computed tomography (CT) or ultrasound is indicated.

Emergency Department Care and Disposition

1. Most cases of peritonsillar abscess can be safely treated as outpatients with needle aspiration, antibiotics, and pain control.

2. Antibiotic choices include **clindamycin** 25 to 40 mg/kg IV divided every 6 hours or **ampicillin/sulbactam** 200 mg/kg/d divided every 6 hours. Definitive follow-up is essential in all cases.
3. Formal incision and drainage in the operating room are sometimes necessary, especially in young or uncooperative patients.

RETROPHARYNGEAL ABSCESS

Clinical Features

Retropharyngeal abscesses are the second most commonly seen deep neck infections, usually occurring in children ages 6 months to 4 years. Patients classically appear toxic and present with fever, drooling, dysphagia, and inspiratory stridor. Dysphagia and refusal to feed occur before significant respiratory distress. Patients may have rapidly fatal airway obstruction from sudden rupture of the abscess pocket. Aspiration pneumonia, empyema, infection into the mediastinum, and erosion into the jugular vein and carotid artery have been reported.

Diagnosis and Differential

Physical examination of the pharynx may show a retropharyngeal mass. Although palpation commonly will demonstrate fluctuance, this could lead to rupture of the abscess. Lateral neck x-ray performed during inspiration may show a widened retropharyngeal space. CT of the neck is thought to be almost 100% sensitive and very helpful in differentiation between cellulites and abscess.

Emergency Department Care and Disposition

1. Immediate airway stabilization should be the first priority. Unstable patients should be intubated before performing CT.
2. Antibiotic choice is controversial because most retropharyngeal abscesses contain mixed flora. Broad-spectrum coverage can be accomplished with **ampicillin/sulbactam** 200 mg/kg/d divided every 6 hours and/or **clindamycin** 25 to 40 mg/kg IV divided every 6 hours. If there is an allergy to penicillin, clindamycin and a third-generation cephalosporin are recommended.
3. Consultation with an otolaryngologist for operative incision and drainage is indicated. Although cellulitis and some very small abscesses may do well with antibiotics alone, most require surgery.

For further reading in *Emergency Medicine: A Comprehensive Study Guide,* 6th ed., see Chap. 129, "Upper Respiratory Emergencies," by Randolph J. Cordle.

82 | Pediatric Exanthems

Lance Brown

Helpful information to make the diagnosis of rash in a child includes the signs and symptoms that preceded or presented with the exanthem, immunization history, human and animal contacts, and environmental exposures. Pediatric exanthems can be broadly classified by etiologic agent. With few exceptions, outpatient management is appropriate for most of these conditions. Potential bioterrorism agents such as cutaneous anthrax and variola (smallpox) are discussed in Chaps. 94 and 96, respectively.

BACTERIAL INFECTIONS

Bullous Impetigo

Bullous impetigo typically occurs in infants and young children. Lesions are superficial, thin-walled bullae that characteristically occur on the extremities, rupture easily, leave a denuded base, dry to a shiny coating, and contain fluid that harbors staphylococci. The diagnosis usually is made by the appearance of the characteristic bullae (Fig. 82-1 and Color Plate Section between pages 754 and 755). Treatment includes local wound cleaning in addition to oral antistaphylococcal antibiotics such as **cephalexin** (25 mg/kg per dose, 3 times daily) or **dicloxacillin** (5 mg/kg per dose, 4 times daily) and topical **mupirocin.**

Impetigo Contagiosum

This exanthem is a superficial skin infection typically caused by group A β-hemolytic streptococci or *Staphylococcus aureus*. The lesions usually occur in small children, often in areas of insect bites or minor trauma. The lesions start as red macules and papules that then form vesicles and pustules (Fig. 82-2 and

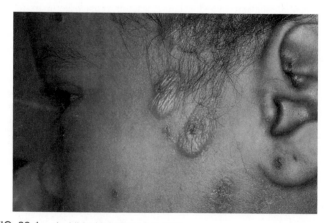

FIG. 82-1.   A child with bullous impetigo.

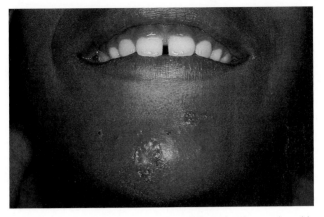

FIG. 82-2.   A young girl with crusting impetiginous lesions on her chin.

Color Plate Section between pages 754 and 755). Rupture of the vesicles results in the formation of a golden crust. The lesions may become confluent. With the exception of lymphadenopathy, fever and systemic signs are rare. Most commonly, affected areas include the face, neck, and extremities. Diagnosis is based on the appearance of the rash. Appropriate antibiotic choices include oral **cephalexin** (25 mg/kg per dose, 3 times daily), **erythromycin** (15 mg/kg per dose, 3 times daily), **clindamycin** (10 mg/kg per dose, 3 times daily), **amoxicillin/clavulanate** (20 mg/kg per dose, twice daily), and **dicloxacillin** (5 mg/kg per dose, 4 times daily). Further treatment includes local wound cleaning and topical **mupirocin.**

Erysipelas

Erysipelas is a cellulitis and lymphangitis of the skin due to group A β-hemolytic streptococci. Fever, chills, malaise, headache, and vomiting are common. The face is the most common site, and the lesion typically forms in the area of a skin wound or pimple. The rash starts as a red plaque that rapidly enlarges. Increased warmth to the touch, swelling, and a raised, sharply demarcated, indurated border are typical. Diagnosis is by history and the appearance of the rash. Initial treatment may be in an inpatient setting and include intravenous **penicillin G** (50,000 U/kg per dose, every 6 hours) or **erythromycin** (10 mg/kg per dose, every 6 hours) in the penicillin-allergic patient. Outpatient treatment may include oral **penicillin V** (15 mg/kg per dose, 3 times daily), **cephalexin** (25 mg/kg per dose, 3 times daily), **erythromycin** (15 mg/kg per dose, 3 times daily), or **clindamycin** (10 mg/kg per dose, 3 times daily). Rapid clinical improvement is expected after treatment has begun.

Mycoplasma Infections

Rashes associated with mycoplasma infections typically occur in the setting of an acute respiratory illness in a school-age child (5-19 years of age). Associated symptoms are typically fever, cough, sore throat, malaise, headache, chills, and rash. Mycoplasma should be suspected in school-age children with pneumonia and a rash. The rash is typically on the trunk and is red and maculopapular. Also seen is erythema multiforme and occasionally Stevens-Johnson syndrome.

The treatment is with an oral macrolide antibiotic such as **erythromycin** (15 mg/kg per dose, 3 times daily) or **azithromycin** (10 mg/kg once on day 1 and 5 mg/kg per dose for days 2–5).

Scarlet Fever

A distinctive rash is seen with scarlet fever. The etiologic agent is typically group A β-hemolytic streptococci (recently group C streptococci also has been implicated). Scarlet fever typically occurs in school-age children and is diagnosed by the presence of exudative pharyngitis, fever, and the characteristic rash (Fig. 82-3 and Color Plate Section between pages 754 and 755). Associated symptoms include sore throat, fever, headache, vomiting, and ab-

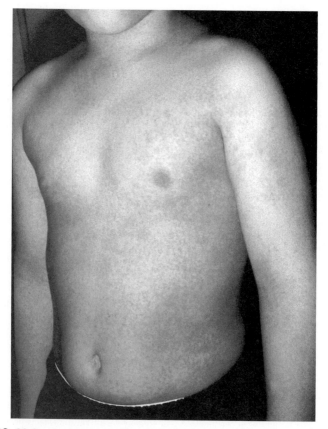

FIG. 82-3. Scarlatiniform rash of scarlet fever.

dominal pain. The rash typically starts in the neck, groin, and axillae, with accentuation at the flexural creases (Pastia lines). The rash is red and punctate, blanches with pressure, and has a rough sandpaper feel. In the early course of the illness, the tongue has a white coating through which hypertrophic, red papillae project (the "white strawberry tongue"). Hemorrhagic spots may be seen on the soft palate. The rash typically develops 1 to 2 days after the illness onset. Facial flushing and circumoral pallor are characteristic. Desquamation occurs with healing approximately 2 weeks after the onset of symptoms.

The diagnosis generally is made on clinical grounds. Throat culture typically shows group A β-hemolytic streptococci or group C streptococci. Treatment is with **penicillin V** (15 mg/kg per dose, 3 times daily) or **erythromycin** (15 mg/kg per dose, 3 times daily) in the penicillin-allergic patient. Antibiotic treatment shortens the course of the illness and reduces the incidence of rheumatic fever.

RICKETTSIAL INFECTIONS

Rocky Mountain Spotted Fever

The etiologic agent is *Rickettsia rickettsii,* which is transmitted by ticks. The major clinical features include headache, fever, toxicity, myalgias, and rash. The rash of Rocky Mountain spotted fever (RMSF) typically appears on the second or third day of illness. The initial lesions typically appear on the ankles and wrists and spread centrally to the trunk. The palms and soles are usually involved. The lesions begin as blanching erythematous macules but rapidly become maculopapular and petechial (See Color Plate in this section). Laboratory confirmation of the diagnosis is challenging. Diagnosis and treatment are usually initiated based on the clinical features. Appropriate antibiotics for the treatment of RMSF include **tetracycline** (10 mg/kg per dose, 4 times daily) in children 8 years and older and **chloramphenicol** (15 mg/kg per dose, 4 times daily), see Chap. 94. The mortality of RMSF is 3% to 6% even if treated.

VIRAL INFECTIONS

Enterovirus

Included in this group are coxsackie viruses and echoviruses that can produce a wide range of clinical presentations. These infections typically occur in the summer and early fall. Also included in this group are polioviruses. Many enteroviral infections lack characteristic features. Clinical presentation of an enteroviral infection may include nonspecific febrile illnesses, upper respiratory tract infections, parotitis, croup, bronchitis, pneumonia, bronchiolitis, vomiting, diarrhea, abdominal pain, hepatitis, pancreatitis, conjunctivitis, pericarditis, myocarditis, orchitis, nephritis, arthritis, meningitis, and encephalitis. The rashes of enteroviral infections also may have a variety of appearances. These include macular eruptions, morbilliform erythema, vesicular lesions, petechial and purpural eruptions, rubelliform rash, roseola-like rash, and scarlatiniform eruptions.

One of the enterovirus infections that is common and has distinctive features is hand-foot-and-mouth disease. At the outset, the patient typically has fever, anorexia, malaise, and a sore mouth. Oral lesions appear on days 2 or 3 of illness followed by skin lesions. The oral lesions start as very painful vesicles on an erythematous base that then ulcerate. The typical location of the oral lesions is on the buccal mucosa, tongue, soft palate, and gingival. The skin lesions start as red papules that change to gray vesicles that ultimately heal in 7 to 10 days. The typical locations of the skin lesions include the palms, soles, and buttocks.

Management of presumed enteroviral infections typically involves symptomatic therapy ensuring adequate hydration, **acetaminophen** (15 mg/kg per dose, every 4 hours as needed for fever), and intraoral analgesics such as **magic mouthwash** (a compounded suspension of 30 mL of 12.5 mg/5 mL diphenhydramine liquid + 60 mL Mylanta + 4 g Carafate) applied in small quantities to the lesions (or swish and spit) 3 times daily and before feeding.

Erythema Infectiosum

Erythema infectiosum (also known as *fifth disease*) is a febrile illness, typically appearing in the spring, most commonly affecting children ages 5 to 15 years. The rash typically starts as an abrupt onset, bright red rash on the cheeks producing the "slapped-cheek appearance" (Fig. 82-4 and Color Plate Section between pages 754 and 755). The lesions are closely grouped, tiny papules on an erythematous base with slightly raised edges. The eyelids and chin are characteristically spared. Circumoral pallor is typical. This rash fades after 4 to 5 days. As the illness progresses, and 1 to 2 days after the facial rash appears, a nonpruritic erythematous macular or maculopapular rash appears on the trunk and limbs. This rash may last for 1 week and is not pruritic. As the rash fades, central clearing of the lesions occurs, leaving a lacy appearance to the rash. Palms and soles are rarely affected.

This rash may recur intermittently in the weeks after the onset of illness. This rash may be exacerbated by sun exposure or hot baths. Associated symptoms include fever, malaise, headache, sore throat, cough, coryza, nausea, vomiting, diarrhea, and myalgias. There is no specific therapy beyond symptomatic therapy.

Measles

Due to immunizations, measles is no longer common. Local epidemics do occur. This myxovirus infection typically occurs in the winter and spring. The incubation period is 10 days. A 3-day prodrome of upper respiratory symptoms followed by malaise, fever, coryza, conjunctivitis, photophobia, and cough is typical. Ill appearance is expected. Just before the development of a rash, Koplik spots, tiny white spots on the buccal mucosa, may be seen. These spots produce a "grains of sand" appearance and are pathognomonic for measles. The rash develops 14 days after exposure. Initially, a red, blanching, maculopapular rash develops. The rash progresses from the head to the feet. The rash rapidly coalesces on the face. The duration of the rash is about 1 week. As the rash resolves, a coppery brown discoloration may be seen and desquamation may occur. Measles is self-limited. Treatment is supportive.

Infectious Mononucleosis

The etiologic agent for infectious mononucleosis is the Epstein-Barr virus, and the disease primarily affects children and young adults. Systemic symptoms include fever, malaise, fatigue, and sore throat. The pharynx is often inflamed with exudate present. Lymphadenopathy typically affects anterior and posterior cervical chains but may be generalized. A generalized erythematous

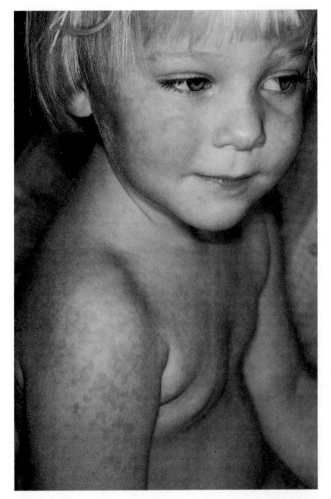

FIG. 82-4. Toddler with the classic slapped cheek appearance of fifth disease.

maculopapular rash with soft palate petechiae is seen in 5% of patients. Nearly all patients who are treated with ampicillin or other related penicillins (eg, amoxicillin) develop an erythematous maculopapular rash. The Monospot test is less reliable in children younger than 5 years. Treatment is supportive. Of note is the splenic enlargement, which occurs with infectious mononucleosis. If a child participates in contact sports or sustains an injury to the left upper quadrant of the abdomen, splenic rupture may occur. Children with mononucleosis must not participate in contact activities until cleared by their primary physician.

Rubella

Now quite rare due to immunizations, rubella (German measles) can be seen in teenagers, typically in the spring. The incubation period is 12 to 25 days. The prodromal symptoms include fever, malaise, headache, sore throat, and upper respiratory tract symptoms. The rash develops as fine, irregular pink macules and papules on the face that then spread to the neck, trunk, and arms in a centrifugal distribution. The rash coalesces on the face as the eruption reaches the lower extremities and then clears in the same order as it appeared. Lymphadenopathy typically involves the suboccipital and posterior auricular nodes. Treatment is supportive.

Varicella (Chicken Pox)

Due to immunizations, the incidence of varicella has declined dramatically. The etiologic agent is the varicella-zoster virus, a herpes virus. It typically occurs in children younger than 10 years but may occur at all ages. Varicella occurs most often in the late winter and early spring. Patients are highly contagious from the prodrome phase of the illness until all lesions are crusted over. The rash starts as faint red macules on the scalp or trunk. Within the first day the lesions begin to vesiculate and develop a red base, thus producing the characteristic appearance (Fig. 82-5 and Color Plate Section between pages 754 and 755). Over the next few days, groups of lesions develop, producing the appearance of simultaneous multiple stages of development. Over the next 1 to 2 weeks, the lesions become dry and crusted. The rash typically spreads centrifugally (outward from the center). The palms and soles are spared. Low-grade fever, malaise, and headache are frequently seen but are typically mild. Treatment is symptomatic and includes **diphenhydramine** (1.25 mg/kg per dose, every 6 hours as needed for itching) and **acetaminophen** (15 mg/kg per dose, every 4 hours as needed for fever). Although not needed in previously healthy children, **varicella-zoster immune globulin** and **acyclovir** (10 mg/kg per dose, 3 times daily) may be needed for immunocompromised children.

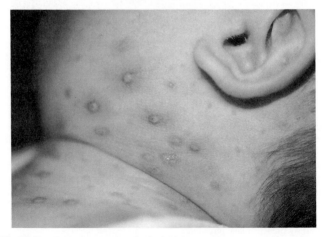

FIG. 82-5.   Typical rash of varicella (chicken pox).

Roseola Infantum (Exanthem Subitum)

Roseola is a common acute febrile illness in children ages 6 months to 3 years and thought to be caused by herpesvirus 6. Roseola initially starts with an abrupt onset, high fever for 3 to 5 days. Associated symptoms are typically mild and may include irritability when the fever is highest, cough, coryza, anorexia, and abdominal discomfort. Febrile seizures may occur. As the fever begins to resolve, blanching macular or maculopapular, rose or pink discrete lesions develop (Fig. 82-6 and Color Plate Section between pages 754 and 755). The areas typically involved with rash include the neck, trunk, and buttocks but may include the face and proximal extremities. Mucous membranes are not involved. The rash lasts 1 to 2 days and rapidly fades. The treatment is symptomatic.

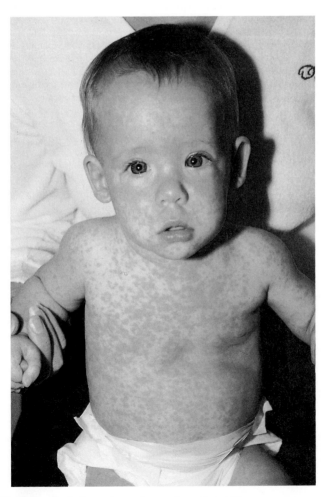

FIG. 82-6. Typical maculopapulur eruptions of roseola.

UNCLEAR ETIOLOGY

Erythema Nodosum

Erythema nodosum is an inflammatory exanthem associated with medications (eg, oral contraceptives), sarcoidosis, *Yersinia* infections, inflammatory bowel disease, leukemia, vasculitis, tuberculosis, fungal diseases, leukemia, and streptococcal infections. The lesions of erythema nodosum are distinctive tender nodules up to 5 cm in size on the shins and extensor prominences. The skin overlying the lesions is red, smooth, and shiny. Ulceration is not seen. Other symptoms include fever, arthralgias, myalgias, and fatigue. The lesions last several weeks. The only known treatment is analgesia.

Kawasaki Disease

Kawasaki disease (mucocutaneous lymph node syndrome) is a generalized vasculitis of unknown cause that typically occurs in children younger than 9 years. Diagnosis depends on the following clinical findings. The patient should have several days of fever and the illness must not be explained by another known disease process. Then, 4 of the following 5 criteria must be met: (*a*) conjunctivitis; (*b*) rash; (*c*) lymphadenopathy; (*d*) oropharyngeal changes, including injection of the pharynx and lips with prominent papillae of the tongue (strawberry tongue); or (*e*) extremity erythema and edema.

Typical rash appearances have been described as erythematous, morbilliform, urticarial, scarlatiniform, or erythema multiforme-like. Perineal rash is not uncommon. Associated findings may include leukocytosis, elevation of acute-phase reactants (eg, erythrocyte sedimentation rate and C-reactive protein), elevated liver function tests, arthritis, arthralgia, and irritability. Later in the illness, findings may include a rise in the platelet count, desquamation of the fingers and toes, and coronary artery aneurysms. One percent to 2% of patients with coronary artery aneurysms develop sudden cardiac death.

Treatment consists of **intravenous γ-globulin** and **aspirin** (25 mg/kg per dose, 4 times daily). The use of steroids is controversial.

Pityriasis Rosea

Pityriasis rosea is seen characteristically in older school-age children and young adults in the spring and fall. Pityriasis rosea does not appear to occur in epidemics and is not contagious. The rash evolves over weeks. The rash begins with a herald patch, ie, 1 red lesion with a raised border on the trunk. One to 2 weeks later, a widespread eruption of pink maculopapular oval patches erupts on the trunk in a pattern following the ribs ("Christmas tree distribution"). There may be mucous membrane involvement. Pityriasis rosea typically lasts 3 to 8 weeks. Testing for secondary syphilis is commonly done because secondary syphilis may appear like pityriasis rosea. Treatment is symptomatic and includes **diphenhydramine** (1.25 mg/kg per dose, every 6 hours as needed for itching).

For further reading in *Emergency Medicine, A Comprehensive Study Guide,* 6th ed., see Chap. 135, "Pediatric Exanthems," by Michael S. Weinstock and Alexander M. Rosenau.

| Musculoskeletal Disorders
in Children

David M. Cline

CHILDHOOD PATTERNS OF INJURY

The growth plate (physis) is the weakest point in children's long bones and the frequent site of fractures. The ligaments and periosteum are stronger than the physis because they tolerate mechanical forces at the expense of physeal injury. The blood supply to the physis arises from the epiphysis, so separation of the physis from the epiphysis may be disastrous for future growth. The Salter-Harris classification is widely used to describe fractures involving the growth plate (Fig. 83-1).

Salter-Harris Type I Fracture

In type I physeal fracture, the epiphysis separates from the metaphysis. The reproductive cells of the physis stay with the epiphysis. There are no bony fragments. Bone growth is undisturbed. Diagnosis is suspected clinically in children with point tenderness over a growth plate. On radiogram, the only abnormality may be an associated joint effusion. There may be epiphyseal displacement from the metaphysis. In the absence of epiphyseal displacement, the diagnosis is clinical and supported by the joint effusion. Treatment consists of splint immobilization, ice, elevation, and referral.

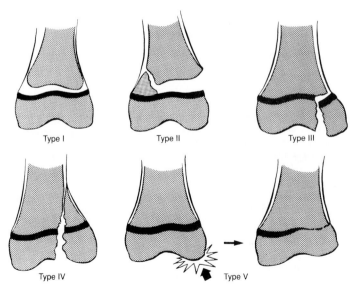

FIG. 83-1. Salter-Harris classification of physeal injuries.

Salter-Harris Type II Fracture

Type II physeal fracture is the most common (75%) physeal fracture. The fracture goes through the physis and out through the metaphysis. The periosteum remains intact over the metaphyseal fragment but is torn on the opposite side. Growth is preserved because the physis remains with the epiphysis. Treatment is closed reduction with analgesia and sedation followed by cast immobilization.

Salter-Harris Type III Fracture

The hallmark of type III physeal fracture is an intraarticular fracture of the epiphysis with the cleavage plane continuing along the physis. The prognosis for bone growth depends on the circulation to the epiphyseal bone fragment and is usually favorable. Reduction of the unstable fragment with anatomic alignment of the articular surface is critical. Open reduction is often required.

Salter-Harris Type IV Fracture

The fracture line of type IV physeal fractures begins at the articular surface and extends through the epiphysis, physis, and metaphysis. Open reduction is required to reduce the risk of premature bone growth arrest.

Salter-Harris Type V Fracture

In type V physeal fracture, the physis is essentially crushed by severe compressive forces. There is no epiphyseal displacement. The diagnosis is often difficult. An initial diagnosis of sprain or type I injury may prove incorrect when later growth arrest occurs. Radiograms may look normal or demonstrate focal narrowing of the epiphyseal plate. There is usually an associated joint effusion. Treatment consists of cast immobilization, non–weight bearing, and close orthopedic follow-up in anticipation of focal bone growth arrest.

Torus Fractures, Greenstick Fractures, and Plastic Deformities

Children's long bones are more compliant than those of adults and tend to bow and bend under forces where an adult's might fracture. Torus (also called *cortical* or *buckle*) fractures involve a bulging or buckling of the bony cortex, usually of the metaphysis. Patients have point tenderness over the fracture site and soft tissue swelling. Radiographs may be subtle but show cortical disruption. Torus fractures are not typically angulated, rotated, or displaced, so reduction is rarely necessary. Splinting or casting in a position of function for 3 to 4 weeks with orthopedic follow-up is recommended.

In greenstick fractures, the cortex and periosteum are disrupted on 1 side of the bone but intact on the other. Treatment is closed reduction and immobilization.

Plastic deformities are seen in the forearm and lower leg in combination with a completed fracture in the companion bone. The diaphyseal cortex is deformed, but the periosteum is intact.

FRACTURES ASSOCIATED WITH CHILD ABUSE

Certain injury patterns are consistently seen in abused children, particularly multiple fractures in various stages of healing. Twisting injuries create spiral fractures in long bones and are highly specific for abuse in nonambulatory children. In ambulatory children, spiral fractures may occur accidentally, the classic example being the spiral fracture of the lower third of the tibia, known as *toddler's fracture,* but they can also be seen with abuse. The injury pattern most closely associated with abuse is the chip fracture of the metaphysis. The tight attachment of the periosteum to the metaphysis will cause avulsion of little chips of the bone with pulling. There is exuberant callus formation and periosteal new bone formation. With direct trauma, subperiosteal hemorrhage characteristically lifts the periosteum off the bone, where it appears as opacified line. Fragmentation of the clavicle and acromion and separation of the costochondral junctions of the ribs are very suggestive of abuse. Bony injuries from shaking are similar to twisting but also include spinal compression fractures and other vertebral injuries. Distraction injuries to the long bones cause hemorrhagic separation of the distal metaphysis, thus creating a lucency proximal to the physis (bucket handle fracture). Squeezing injuries create rib fractures that are highly suggestive of abuse.

SELECTED PEDIATRIC INJURIES

Clavicle Fracture

A clavicle fracture is the most common fracture in children. Fractures may occur in newborns during difficult deliveries. Babies may have nonuse of the arm. If the fracture was not initially appreciated, parents may notice a bony callus at age 2 to 3 weeks. In older infants and children, the usual mechanism is a fall onto the outstretched arm or shoulder. Care of the patient with a clavicle fracture is directed toward pain control. Even displaced fractures usually heal well, although patients may have a residual bump at the fracture site. Figure-of-8 shoulder abduction restraints have been the traditional treatment, but many patients have more pain with this device. A simple sling is equally effective and less painful. Newborns require no specific treatment. Orthopedic follow-up can be arranged in the next week. Orthopedic consultation in the emergency department (ED) is required for an open fracture (which also requires antibiotics), anterior or posterior displacement of the medial clavicle, or a skin-tenting fracture fragment that has the potential to convert to an open fracture.

Supracondylar and Condylar Fractures

The most common elbow fracture in childhood is the supracondylar fracture of the distal humerus. The mechanism occurs when children fall on their outstretched arms. The close proximity of the brachial artery to the fracture predisposes the artery to injury. Subsequent arterial spasm or compression by casts may further compromise distal circulation. A forearm compartment syndrome (ie, Volkmann ischemic contracture) may occur. Symptoms include pain in the proximal forearm on passive finger extension, stocking-glove anesthesia of the hand, and hard forearm swelling. Pulses may remain palpable at the wrist despite serious vascular impairment. Injuries to the ulnar, median, and radial nerves are also common, occurring in 5% to 10% of all supracondylar fractures. Children complain of pain on passive elbow flexion and maintain the forearm pronated. Radiograms show the injury, but the findings may be subtle. A posterior fat pad sign is indicative of intraarticular effusion and thus fracture. Normally, the anterior humeral line, a line drawn along the anterior distal humeral shaft, should bisect the posterior two thirds of the capitellum on the lateral view. In subtle supracondylar fractures, the line often lies more anteriorly.

In cases of neurovascular compromise, immediate fracture reduction is indicated. If an ischemic forearm compartment is suspected after reduction, surgical decompression or arterial exploration may be indicated. Admission is recommended for patients with displaced fractures or significant soft tissue swelling. Open reduction is often required. Outpatient treatment is acceptable for nondisplaced fractures with minimal swelling; however, telephone consultation with an orthopedic surgeon will provide the preferred splinting technique. Such children need orthopedic reassessment within 24 hours.

Lateral and medial condylar fractures and intercondylar and transcondylar fractures carry risks of neurovascular compromise, especially to the ulnar nerve. These patients have soft tissue swelling and tenderness while maintaining the arm in flexion. Most patients require open reduction.

Radial Head Subluxation ("Nursemaid's Elbow")

Radial head subluxation is a very common injury seen most often in children ages 1 to 4 years. The typical history is that the children are lifted up by an adult pulling on the hand or wrist. Sometimes there is a history of trauma and sometimes no event at all but children who refuse to use the arm. The arm is held close to the body, flexed at the elbow, with the forearm pronated. Gentle examination demonstrates no tenderness to direct palpation, but any attempts to supinate the forearm or move the elbow cause pain. If the history and examination is classic, radiographs are not needed, but if the history is atypical or there is a point tenderness or signs of trauma, radiographs should be taken.

There are 2 maneuvers for reduction. The supination technique is performed by holding the patient's elbow at 90° with 1 hand and then firmly supinating the wrist and simultaneously flexing the elbow so that the wrist is directed to the ipsilateral shoulder. There may be a "click" with reduction, and the child may transiently scream and resist. The hyperpronation technique is reported to be more successful, and it can used primarily or as a backup when supination fails. The hyperpronation technique is performed by holding the child's elbow at 90° in 1 hand and then firmly pronating the wrist. Usually the child will resume normal activity in 15 to 30 minutes if reduction is achieved. If the child is not better after a second reduction attempt, alternate diagnoses and radiographs should be considered. No specific therapy is needed after successful reduction. Parents should be reminded to avoid linear traction on the arm because there is an increased risk of recurrence.

Slipped Capital Femoral Epiphysis

Slipped capital femoral epiphysis (SCFE) is more common in boys, with the peak incidence between ages 14 and 16 years and between ages 11 and 13 years in girls. Clinically, the child presents with pain at the hip or referred to the thigh or knee. With a chronic SCFE, children complain of dull pain in the groin, anteromedial thigh, and knee, which becomes worse with activity. With walking, the leg is externally rotated and the gait is antalgic. Hip flexion is restricted and accompanied by external rotation of the thigh. Acute SCFE is due to trauma or may occur in a patient with preexisting chronic SCFE. Patients are in great pain, with marked external rotation of the thigh and leg shortening. The hip should not be forced through the full range of motion because this may displace the epiphysis further.

The differential includes septic arthritis, toxic synovitis, Legg-Calvé-Perthes disease, and other hip fractures. Children with SCFE are not febrile or toxic and have normal white blood cell counts (WBCs) and erythrocyte sedimentation rates (ESRs). On radiogram, medial slips of the femoral epiphysis will be seen on anteroposterior views, whereas frog-leg views detect posterior slips. In the anteroposterior view, a line along the superior femoral neck should transect the lateral quarter of the femoral epiphysis, but not if the epiphysis is slipped.

The management of SCFE is operative. The main long-term complication is avascular necrosis of the femoral head.

SELECTED NONTRAUMATIC MUSCULOSKELETAL DISORDERS OF CHILDHOOD

Kawasaki disease is discussed in Chap. 82.

Acute Suppurative Arthritis

Septic arthritis occurs in all ages, but especially in children younger than 3 years. The hip is most often affected, followed by the knee and elbow. The diagnosis is critical because, if left untreated, purulent joint infection leads to total joint destruction. Bacteria access the joint hematogenously, by direct extension from adjacent osteomyelitis, or from inoculation as in arthrocentesis or femoral venipuncture. The organisms vary with the child's age. In the neonate in which maternal transmission is possible, group B *Streptococcus* and *Neisseria gonorrhoeae* are a concern. In all age groups, *Staphylococcus aureus,* gram-negative bacilli, and *Streptococcus* species should be considered. *Haemophilus influenzae* has diminished due to widespread vaccination. Although systemic symptoms can be subtle in newborns, older children will appear ill, with high fever and irritability. The affected joint is very painful and shows warmth, swelling, and severe tenderness to palpation and movement. Children with hip or knee infection will limp or not walk at all. Children maintain an infected hip in flexion, abduction, and external rotation.

Radiographs show joint effusion, but this is nonspecific. The differential includes osteomyelitis, transient tenosynovitis, cellulitis, septic bursitis, acute pauciarticular juvenile rheumatoid arthritis (JRA), acute rheumatic fever, hemarthrosis, and SCFE. Distinguishing septic arthritis from osteomyelitis may be quite difficult. Osteomyelitis is more tender over the metaphysis, whereas septic arthritis is more tender over the joint line. Joint motion is much more limited in septic arthritis. Prompt arthrocentesis is the key to diagnosis at the bedside or, in the case of the hip, in the operating room or under ultrasound. Synovial fluid shows WBCs and organisms.

Prompt joint drainage is critical in the operating room in the case of the hip or arthroscopically or via arthrocentesis in more superficial joints. In the neonate, **oxacillin** 37 mg/kg intravenously (IV) every 6 hours plus **cefotaxime** 50 mg/kg IV every 8 hours are administered. In the infant older than 3 months or a child, **nafcillin** 37 mg/kg IV every 6 hours plus **cefotaxime** 50 mg/kg IV every 8 hours are administered. If resistant organisms are suspected, **vancomycin** 10 to 15 mg/kg IV every 6 hours is used. The prognosis depends on the duration between symptoms and treatment, which joint is involved (worse for the hip), presence of associated osteomyelitis (worse), and the patient's age (worse for the youngest children).

Henoch-Schönlein Purpura

Henoch-Schönlein purpura (HSP) is a small-vessel vasculitis characterized by purpura, arthritis, abdominal pain, and hematuria. Palpable purpura, the classic vasculitic rash, appears on the trunk, buttocks, and legs. A polymigratory arthritis occurs in two thirds of children, typically of the knees or ankles associated with edema. Involvement of the bowel wall causes colicky abdominal pain and may lead to melena, hematochezia, or intussusception. HSP involves the glomeruli, with resulting hematuria and proteinuria.

HSP is largely a clinical diagnosis; useful laboratory tests include urinalysis, complete blood cell count, tests of renal function, and, sometimes, tests for collagen vascular disease.

Hospital admission is indicated when the diagnosis is in doubt, dehydration occurs, or gastrointestinal or renal complications require close observation. Therapy with IV steroids (1 to 2 mg/kg/d may improve gastrointestinal symptoms but when required is best directed by the admitting pediatrician. Arthritis, when present as an isolated symptom, can be treated with non-steroidal anti-inflammatory drugs.

SELECTED PEDIATRIC RHEUMATOLOGIC DISORDERS

Transient Synovitis of the Hip

Transient synovitis (also called *toxic tenosynovitis*) is the most common cause of hip pain in children younger than 10 years. The peak age is 3 to 6 years, with boys affected more than girls. The cause is unknown. Symptoms may be acute or gradual. Patients have pain in the hip, thigh, and knee and an antalgic gait. Pain limits range of motion of the hip, but in contrast to septic arthritis, passive range of motion remains possible. There may be a low-grade fever, but patients do not appear toxic. The WBC and ESR are usually normal. Radiographs of the hip are normal or show a mild to moderate effusion. The main concern is differentiation from septic arthritis, particularly if the patients are febrile, with elevation of WBC or ESR and effusion. Diagnostic arthrocentesis is required when the diagnosis is in doubt with fluoroscopic or ultrasound guidance at the discretion of the orthopedic surgeon. The fluid in transient tenosynovitis is a sterile clear transudate.

Once septic arthritis and hip fracture have been ruled out, patients can be treated with crutches to avoid weight bearing for 3 to 7 days, no strenuous activity for 1 to 2 weeks, anti-inflammatory agents such as **ibuprofen** 10 mg/kg, and close follow-up.

Legg-Calvé-Perthes Disease

Legg-Calvé-Perthes disease is essentially avascular necrosis of the femoral head with subchondral stress fracture. Collapse and flattening of the femoral head ensues, with a potential for subluxation. The result is a painful hip with limited range of motion, muscle spasm, and soft tissue contractures. Onset of symptoms is between ages 4 and 9 years. The disease is bilateral in 10% of patients. Children have a limp and chronic dull pain in the groin, thigh, and knee, which becomes worse with activity. Systemic symptoms are absent. Hip motion is restricted; there may be a flexion and abduction contracture and thigh muscle atrophy. Initial radiographs (in the first 1 to 3 months) show widening of the cartilage space in the affected hip and diminished ossific nucleus of the femoral head. The second sign is subchondral stress fracture of the femoral head. The third finding is increased femoral head opacification. Deformity of the femoral head then occurs, with subluxation and protrusion of the femoral head from the acetabulum.

Bone scan and magnetic resonance imaging are very helpful in making this diagnosis by showing bone abnormalities well before plain films. The differential diagnosis includes toxic tenosynovitis, tuberculous arthritis, tumors, and bone dyscrasias.

In the ED, the most important thing is to consider this chronic and potentially crippling condition; therefore, orthopedic consultation in the ED is warranted. Nearly all children are hospitalized initially for orthopedic management.

Osgood-Schlatter Disease

Osgood-Schlatter disease is a common syndrome that affects preteen boys more than girls. The cause is repetitive stress on the tibial tuberosity by the quadriceps muscle, which initiates inflammation of the tibial tuberosity without avascular necrosis. Children have pain and tenderness over the anterior knee, which becomes worse with knee bending and better with rest. The patellar tendon is thick and tender, with the tibial tuberosity enlarged and indurated.

Radiographs show soft tissue swelling over the tuberosity and patellar tendon thickening without knee effusion. Normally, the ossification site at the tubercle at this age will be irregular, but the prominence of the tubercle is characteristic of Osgood Schlatter disease.

The disorder is self-limited. Acute symptoms improve after restriction of physical activities involving knee bending for 3 months. Crutches may be necessary, although a knee immobilizer or cylinder cast are only rarely needed. Exercises to stretch taut and hypertrophied quadriceps muscles are also helpful.

Acute Rheumatic Fever

Acute rheumatic fever (ARF) is an acute inflammatory multisystem illness affecting primarily school-age children. It is not common in the United States, but there have been recent epidemics. ARF is preceded by infection with certain strains of group A β-hemolytic *Streptococcus,* which stimulates antibody production to host tissues. Children develop ARF 2 to 6 weeks after symptomatic or asymptomatic streptococcal pharyngitis. Arthritis, which occurs in most initial attacks, is migratory and polyarticular, primarily affecting the large joints. Carditis occurs in 33% of patients and can affect valves, muscle, and pericardium. Sydenham chorea occurs in 10% of patients and may occur months after the initial infection. The rash, erythema marginatum, is fleeting, faint, and serpiginous, usually accompanying carditis. Subcutaneous nodules, found on the extensor surfaces of extremities, are quite rare. Carditis confers greatest mortality and morbidity.

Laboratory tests are used to confirm prior streptococcal infection (throat culture and streptococcal serology) or to assess carditis (electrocardiogram, chest radiograph, and echocardiogram). The differential includes JRA, septic arthritis, Kawasaki disease, leukemia, and other cardiomyopathies and vasculitides. In the ED, carditis is the main management issue. Most patients are admitted.

Significant carditis is managed initially with **prednisone** 1 to 2 mg/kg/d. Arthritis is treated with high-dose aspirin (75 to 100 mg/kg/d to start. All children with ARF are treated with **penicillin** (or **erythromycin,** if allergic): **benzathine penicillin** 1.2 million U intramuscularly, **procaine penicillin G** 600,000 U intramuscularly daily for 10 days, or oral **penicillin VK** 25 to 50 mg/kg/d divided 4 times a day for 10 days. Long-term prophylaxis is indicated for patients with ARF, and lifelong prophylaxis is recommended for patients with carditis.

Poststreptococcal Reactive Arthritis

Because of increased group A β-hemolytic streptococcal infections, post-streptococcal reactive arthritis (PSRA) is also increasing. PSRA is a sterile, inflammatory, nonmigratory mono- or oligoarthritis occurring with infection at a distant site with β-hemolytic *Streptococcus* and with *Staphylococcus* and *Salmonella.* Unlike ARF, PSRA is not associated with carditis and in general is a milder illness. However, the arthritis in PSRA is more severe and prolonged as compared with ARF and may be resistant to salicylates.

To establish the diagnosis of PSRA, antecedent infection with group A *Streptococcus* must be established with throat culture or 4-fold rise in ASO or anti-DNase B titer.

PSRA is responsive to nonsteroidal anti-inflammatory drugs. The issue of penicillin prophylaxis, a mainstay of therapy in ARF, is controversial in PSRA. However, if group A *Streptococcus* is recovered from the throat, treatment with penicillin or erythromycin should be instituted.

Juvenile Rheumatoid Arthritis

The group of diseases comprising JRA share the findings of chronic noninfectious synovitis and arthritis, with systemic manifestations. Pauciarticular disease is the most common form, usually involving a single large joint such as the knee. Permanent joint damage occurs infrequently. Polyarticular disease occurs in one third of cases. Large and small joints are affected, and there may be progressive joint damage. Systemic JRA occurs in 20% of patients. This form is associated with high fevers and chills. Extraarticular manifestations are common, including a red macular coalescent rash, hepatosplenomegaly, and serositis. The arthritis in this form may progress to permanent joint damage.

In the ED, laboratory tests focus mostly on excluding other diagnoses. Complete blood count, ESR, and C-reactive protein may be normal. Arthrocentesis may be necessary to exclude septic arthritis, particularly in pauciarticular disease. Radiographs initially show joint effusions but are nonspecific. The diagnosis of JRA likely will not be made in the ED.

Initial therapy for patients with an established diagnosis includes aspirin or nonsteroidal anti-inflammatory drugs. Glucocorticoids are occasionally used, for example, for unresponsive uveitis or decompensated pericarditis or myocarditis.

For further reading in *Emergency Medicine: A Comprehensive Study Guide,* 6th ed., see Chap. 136, "Musculoskeletal Disorders in Children," by Courney Hopkins Mann, David Leader, Donna Sutherland, and Richard Christoph.

84 | Sickle Cell Anemia in Children

Douglas R. Trocinski

Sickle cell emergencies in children include vasoocclusive crises, hematologic crises, and infections. Children with sickle cell disease (SCD) can present great diagnostic and therapeutic challenges for emergency department (ED) physicians. All children with SCD presenting with fever, pain, respiratory distress, or a change in neurologic function require a rapid and thorough ED evaluation.

VASOOCCLUSIVE CRISES

Vasoocclusive sickle episodes are due to intravascular sickling, which leads to tissue ischemia and infarction. Bones, soft tissue, viscera, and the central nervous system (CNS) may be affected. Pain may be the only symptom; however, children also may have symptoms related to the affected organ system.

PAIN CRISES

Clinical Features

The classic sickle cell pain crisis is usually typical in location, character, and severity of pain. These symptoms may be triggered by stress, extremes of cold, dehydration, hypoxia, or infection but most often occur without a specific cause. Although typically there are no physical findings, pain, local tenderness, swelling, and warmth may occur. Infants, rarely younger than 5 or 6 months, initially may present with dactylitis, a swelling of hands or feet, and low-grade temperature caused by ischemia and infarction of the bone marrow. As children age, the array of presentations may expand from the extremities to the abdomen, chest, and lumbosacral area.

Diagnosis and Differential

Infections can cause vasoocclusive pain crises; therefore, determining the presence of an infectious process is critical. Painful crises can be associated with low-grade fever and leukocytosis, but temperatures higher than 38.3°C (101.0°F) are more likely to be due to an infectious cause than to tissue ischemia. Vasoocclusive pain crises usually present in a stereotypical fashion. Atypical pain or new sites of pain warrant further investigation for infection or complications of SCD. Osteomyelitis or septic arthritis should be considered in the differential diagnosis.

Abdominal pain crises are common and are characterized by abrupt onset, lack of localization, and recurrent nature. It is important to determine whether the abdominal pain in SCD patients has substantially changed in character, quality, duration, severity, and associated symptoms. If such changes are present, infection or other related diagnoses (eg, cholecystitis, appendicitis, pancreatitis, hepatitis, perforated viscous, pelvic inflammatory disease, or other gynecologic pathology) should be considered and explored. Ultrasound examination or computed tomography of the abdomen or pelvis may be useful in determining the diagnosis. If the diagnosis cannot be readily clarified and

391

the cause of the abdominal pain is not clear, then prompt surgical consultation should be initiated.

Emergency Department Care and Disposition

Treatment objectives for painful crises consist of thorough evaluation for etiology of the crisis and treatment of discomfort. Pain management must be individualized, with previous effective regimens as a guide.

1. Aggressive hydration should be attempted with oral fluids as tolerated or age-appropriate intravenous (IV) maintenance fluids, 5% dextrose (D_5) in 0.25 normal saline solution (NS), or D_5 0.45 NS at 1.5 the maintenance rate. Lactated Ringer solution or NS is indicated in the hypotensive patient, with careful attention to avoid fluid overload.
2. Mild to moderate pain often can be managed with oral hydration and analgesics, such as narcotic and acetaminophen combinations and nonsteroidal anti-inflammatory drugs.
3. Parenteral, long-acting narcotics, **morphine** 0.1 to 0.15 mg/kg IV or **hydromorphone** 0.015 mg/kg IV, are indicated for failure of oral regimens.

Admission is warranted for poor pain control or inadequate oral fluid intake. Children who have presented repeatedly for the same pain crisis also should be considered for admission. It is essential for any child discharged from the ED for a pain crisis to be reevaluated within 24 hours by the child's pediatrician or hematologist.

ACUTE CHEST SYNDROME

Acute chest syndrome is believed to be attributable to a combination of pneumonia, pulmonary infarction, and pulmonary emboli from necrotic bone marrow. It is a major cause of death in all patients with SCD, but especially in those older than 10 years.

Clinical Features

Acute chest syndrome should be considered in all patients with SCD who present with complaints of chest pain, especially when associated with tachypnea, dyspnea, cough, or other symptoms of respiratory distress. Significant hypoxia and rapid deterioration to respiratory failure can occur.

Diagnosis and Differential

Chest x-rays should be obtained but may be normal during the first hours to days. There are no specific laboratory abnormalities typical of acute chest syndrome; however, a complete blood count (CBC), reticulocyte count, and blood culture should be obtained. Sputum Gram stain and culture should be obtained, when possible. Noninvasive pulse oximetry should be instituted, and arterial blood gas analysis should be obtained in the presence of significant oxygen desaturation or respiratory distress.

Emergency Department Care and Disposition

All children in whom the diagnosis of acute chest syndrome is being considered should be monitored closely for changes in work of breathing and oxygenation because deterioration can be rapid.

1. Supplemental oxygen should be provided if respiratory distress is present or if oxygen saturation is persistently less than or equal to 94%.

2. Adequate analgesia for chest pain should be provided (see above) in addition to age-appropriate IV fluid hydration at 1 to 1.5 maintenance.
3. Treat potential underlying bacterial pneumonia with empiric antibiotic therapy such as **ceftriaxone** 75 mg/kg/d or **cefotaxime** 50 to 75 mg/kg/d divided every 8 hours.
4. Simple **red blood cell transfusion** (10-15 mL red blood cells per kilogram) or exchange transfusion should be considered in children with severe anemia (hemoglobin level <5 g/dL) or rapidly worsening hypoxia. Transfusion decisions should be made early and in consultation with a pediatric hematologist.

All children with suspected acute chest syndrome should be admitted to the hospital for further care.

ACUTE CENTRAL NERVOUS SYSTEM EVENTS

Clinical Features

Acute CNS crisis should be considered in any patient with SCD who presents with sudden onset headache or neurologic changes, including hemiparesis, seizures, speech defects, sensory hearing loss, visual disturbances, transient ischemic attacks, dizziness, vertigo, cranial nerve palsies, paresthesias, or inexplicable coma.

Diagnosis and Differential

When CNS vasoocclusion is suspected, computed tomography or magnetic resonance imaging of the brain should be obtained. A lumbar puncture may be necessary to exclude subarachnoid hemorrhage. No specific hematologic changes are associated with CNS vasoocclusion; however, a CBC and reticulocyte count should be obtained, and blood typing and screening should be ordered in case an exchange transfusion is necessary.

Emergency Department Care and Disposition

Suspected CNS vasoocclusion necessitates immediate stabilization and careful monitoring. Once intracranial hemorrhage or infarction is confirmed, a 1.5- to 2-vol exchange transfusion should be begun as soon as possible in consultation with a pediatric hematologist. A pediatric neurosurgeon should be consulted once intracranial bleeding has been confirmed. All children with diagnosed or suspected CNS vasoocclusion should be admitted to the pediatric intensive care unit for close monitoring and further care.

PRIAPISM

Clinical Features and Diagnosis

Priapism, a painful sustained erection in the absence of sexual stimulation, occurs when sickled cells accumulate in the corpora cavernosa. It can affect any male with SCD regardless of age, and severe prolonged attacks can cause impotence.

Emergency Department Care and Disposition

Patients with priapism should receive IV hydration with D_5 0.45 NS at 1.5 to 2 times maintenance, appropriate analgesia, and bladder catheterization if the patient is unable to void spontaneously. Treatment options include an oral α-adrenergic agonist (eg, terbutaline or pseudoephedrine), intrapenile injection of vasodilators (eg, hydralazine) or dilute epinephrine, or needle aspiration of the corpora cavernosa. Management and admission decisions should be made promptly in consultation with a urologist and pediatric hematologist.

HEMATOLOGICAL CRISES

ACUTE SEQUESTRATION CRISES

Clinical Features and Diagnosis

Sequestration crises are the second most common cause of death in children with SCD younger than 5 years. The spleen of a young child with SCD can massively enlarge, trapping a considerable portion of the circulating blood volume. This condition can quickly progress to hypotension, shock, and death. Such crises are often preceded by a viral infection.

Classically, children present with sudden onset left upper quadrant pain; pallor and lethargy; a markedly enlarged, tender, and firm spleen on abdominal examination; and signs of cardiovascular collapse, including hypotension and tachycardia. A CBC shows a profound anemia (hemoglobin drops to <6 g/dL, or 3 g/dL lower than the patient's baseline level). Minor episodes can occur with insidious onset of abdominal pain, slowly progressive splenomegaly, and a more minor fall in hemoglobin level (generally the hemoglobin level remains >6 g/dL).

Splenic sequestration crises may be characterized by thrombocytopenia and higher than normal reticulocyte counts. Less commonly, sequestration can occur in the liver. Clinical features include an enlarged and tender liver with associated hyperbilirubinemia, severe anemia, and elevated reticulocyte count. Cardiovascular collapse is rare in this condition.

Emergency Department Care and Disposition

Early recognition and prompt initiation of treatment are the keys to successful management. The goal of treatment is to quickly expand the intravascular volume with the rapid infusion of resuscitative crystalloid or colloid fluids. Transfusion with packed red blood cell or exchange transfusion are often required and should be instituted immediately. Even children with minor episodes should be admitted to the hospital.

APLASTIC EPISODES

Potentially life-threatening aplastic episodes are precipitated primarily by viral infections (typically parvovirus B19) but also can be caused by bacterial infections, folic acid deficiency, or bone-marrow–suppressive or toxic drugs.

Patients usually present with gradual onset of pallor, dyspnea, fatigue, and jaundice. CBC shows an unusually low hematocrit ($\leq10\%$) with decreased to absent reticulocytosis. White blood cell and platelet counts remain stable. Pain is not a hallmark of this crisis unless there is an associated vasoocclusive crisis. Cultures should be obtained if the source of infection is not apparent.

If anemia is severe, the patient should be admitted for red blood cell transfusion to avoid secondary cardiopulmonary complications.

HEMOLYTIC CRISES

Bacterial and viral infections in children with SCD also can precipitate an increasing degree of active hemolysis.

Onset is usually sudden. A CBC shows hemoglobin level decreased from baseline, with markedly increased reticulocytosis. Increased jaundice and pallor may be noticed on physical examination, in addition to other signs and symptoms of the precipitating infection.

Specific therapy is rarely required. Hematologic values return to normal as the infectious process resolves. Care should be directed toward treating the underlying infection. Close follow-up to monitor hemoglobin level and reticulocyte count should be arranged at discharge.

INFECTIONS

Clinical Features

Children with SCD are functionally asplenic and have deficient antibody production and impaired phagocytosis. Therefore, bacterial infections, especially with encapsulated organisms, pose a serious and potentially fatal threat to young children with SCD.

Because sepsis can be rapid, overwhelming, and fatal, particularly in children younger than 5 years, all children with SCD and fever should be quickly and carefully examined and managed aggressively.

Diagnosis and Differential

CBC, reticulocyte count, and blood cultures should be obtained for all children with SCD and fever or history of fever. Cultures (urine, throat, and sputum) should be obtained as indicated by physical examination. Pulse oximetry should be evaluated and a chest x-ray obtained if the patient is hypoxic or presenting with signs of respiratory distress. A lumbar puncture is indicated if clinical signs or symptoms of meningitis are present. Knowledge regarding a child's immunization status (particularly whether that child has been immunized against *Haemophilus influenzae* B or pneumococcus) and compliance with the home penicillin prophylaxis is helpful.

Emergency Department Care and Disposition

Children who appear ill on presentation should be treated parenterally with an antibiotic with activity against *Streptococcus pneumoniae* and *H influenzae* (eg, ceftriaxone 50 mg/kg IV or intramuscularly) before evaluation is complete and test results are available. Vancomycin should be added if the patient is at high risk for penicillin-resistant pneumococcal infection. Septic shock must be managed aggressively with IV fluids, vasoactive medications, and possible transfusion as indicated, with admission to the appropriate level of care for the severity of presentation. Fever without a source must be treated aggressively in SCD in consultation with a pediatric hematologist.

DISPOSITION GUIDELINES

Hospital admission is warranted for the following conditions:

1. Temperature higher than 38.4°C with a white blood cell count higher than 30,000, left shift, or hematologic parameters markedly altered from patient baseline
2. Any signs of respiratory distress, hypoxia, or lobar infiltrate on chest x-ray.
3. Splenic or liver sequestration or aplastic crisis.
4. Any new CNS findings or presentations.

5. Evidence of acute abdomen.
6. Prolonged priapism.
7. Any vasoocclusive crises not responsive to analgesia and hydration.
8. Inability to maintain adequate hydration.
9. Uncertain diagnosis.
10. Inadequate follow-up assurance.
11. Blood transfusions are often necessary in children undergoing splenic sequestration crisis and severe aplastic crisis. Transfusions may be required for management of cerebrovascular accident, priapism, or perioperative management before surgery. Transfusion should be considered when hemoglobin is below 6 g/dL; reticulocyte count is less than 20%; and there is evidence of heart failure, hypotension resistant to fluids and oxygen therapy, or marked fatigue. In cases of acute deterioration, packed red blood cell transfusion is indicated while arranging for an exchange transfusion.

VARIANTS OF SICKLE CELL DISEASE

Sickle cell trait is the carrier state of SCD and the most common variant. These patients are asymptomatic and hematologically normal. They will have sickling and concomitant vasoocclusive complications only in the presence of extreme hypoxia or high altitude. They have minimal complications, the most common being hematuria (1%), most likely due to papillary necrosis in the renal medullary tissue.

Sickle cell hemoglobin C disease is a heterozygous condition characterized by mild to moderate anemia and mild reticulocytosis. A smear shows abundant target cells and few sickled cells. Many adults have splenomegaly, and these patients are at risk for pain crisis and organ infarcts. Most patients, however, have few clinical complications.

Sickle cell β-thalassemia disease is a heterozygous condition with different degrees of severity of symptoms depending on the amount of normal β-hemoglobin chains that is produced. The severity can range from mild symptoms to a syndrome similar to SCD.

For further reading in *Emergency Medicine: A Comprehensive Study Guide,* 6th ed., see Chap. 137, "Sickle Cell Disease," by Peter J. Paganussi, Thom Mayer, and Maybelle Kou.

85 | Pediatric Urinary Tract Infections

Lance Brown

Urinary tract infections (UTIs) are relatively common from infancy through adolescence. The incidence and clinical presentation of pediatric UTIs change with age and sex.

CLINICAL FEATURES

There are 3 age-based clinical presentations for pediatric UTIs. Neonates present with a clinical presentation indistinguishable from that of sepsis, and they may have symptoms that include fever, jaundice, poor feeding, irritability, and lethargy. Older infants and young children typically present with gastrointestinal complaints that may include fever, abdominal pain, vomiting, and a change in appetite. School-age children and adolescents typically present with adult-type complaints such as dysuria, urinary frequency, urgency, and hesitancy. Although making the clinical distinction between infantile cystitis with fever and pyelonephritis is unlikely in the emergency department, older children typically will have fever, flank pain, and flank tenderness on percussion when they have pyelonephritis but not when they have simple cystitis.

DIAGNOSIS AND DIFFERENTIAL

The gold standard for confirming the diagnosis of pediatric UTI is the growth of a single urinary pathogen from a culture of properly obtained urine. For infants and young children in diapers, urine is properly obtained by catheterization or, rarely, suprapubic aspiration. For children who are toilet trained, urine is properly collected as a supervised clean catch specimen. Because urine culture takes much longer than an emergency department visit, emergency physicians typically rely on urinary test strips ("urine dip") and microscopic urinalysis to assist in making the diagnosis of pediatric UTI.

Urinary test strips positive for leukocyte esterase or nitrite poorly correlate with positive urine cultures, with a sensitivity of less than 50%. Microscopic urinalysis is typically considered positive for infection if more than 5 white blood cells per high power field and bacteria are seen. A positive microscopic urinalysis has a sensitivity of 65% for identifying culture-proven UTI. Neither urinary test strips nor microscopic urinalysis can be used to definitively rule out pediatric UTI. The clinical context must be taken into account. Because of the reliance on culture results for definitive diagnosis and frequent specimen contamination from the perineum, bagged urine specimens have essentially no role in diagnosis of pediatric UTI in a child who can be catheterized or produce a clean catch specimen.

Adolescents may have urinary symptoms as their manifestation of a sexually transmitted disease such as *Chlamydia trachomatis*. An appropriate sexual history and pelvic examination may be indicated and helpful in making this diagnosis (for a discussion of sexually transmitted diseases, see Chap. 86).

EMERGENCY DEPARTMENT CARE AND DISPOSITION

The treatment and disposition of infants and children with UTI depend on age and are based on the severity of concurrent symptoms.

1. Neonates are treated as if they have sepsis. Neonates with UTI are admitted to the hospital for intravenous antibiotics. Appropriate antibiotic selections include **ampicillin** (50 mg/kg per dose) plus **cefotaxime** (50 mg/kg per dose) or **ampicillin** (50 mg/kg per dose) plus **gentamicin** (2.5 mg/kg per dose).

2. Infants from 1 to 3 months of age and children older than 3 months who are dehydrated, have persistent vomiting, appear ill or septic, or are medically complicated typically are admitted to the hospital for intravenous treatment with **cefotaxime, ceftriaxone,** or **cefepime** (all are dosed at 50 mg/kg per dose).

3. Children older than 3 months who are otherwise doing well and tolerating oral fluids are treated as outpatients with a single parenteral dose of **ceftriaxone** (50 mg/kg) in the emergency department and then oral antibiotics for at least 7 days with close follow-up with their primary doctors because many of these children will undergo renal imaging studies. Emergency physicians should be familiar with the antibiotic-resistance patterns in their geographic area. Appropriate oral antibiotic choices to treat pediatric UTIs include **amoxicillin** (15 mg/kg per dose, given 3 times a day), **amoxicillin/clavulanate** (20 mg/kg per dose, given twice daily), **trimethoprim/sulfamethoxazole** (5 mg/kg per dose of the trimethoprim component, given twice daily), **cephalexin** (25 mg/kg per dose, given 3 times a day), or **cefixime** (4 mg/kg per dose, given twice daily).

4. Adolescent females with cystitis or acute pyelonephritis are treated similarly to adults (see Chap. 53).

For further reading in *Emergency Medicine: A Comprehensive Study Guide,* 6th ed., see Chap. 140, "Pediatric Urinary Tract Infections," by Michael F. Altieri, Mary Camarca, and Thom A. Mayer.

11 | INFECTIOUS DISEASES

Gregory S. Hall

This chapter covers the major sexually transmitted diseases (STDs) in the United States, with the exception of human immunodeficiency virus, which is discussed in Chap. 89. Vaginitis and pelvic inflammatory disease (PID) are covered separately in Chaps. 62 and 63, respectively.

GENERAL RECOMMENDATIONS

When treating STDs in the emergency department, one must remember that multiple infections frequently occur concurrently, that compliance and follow-up are often limited or unreliable, and that infertility and other long-term morbidities may result from lack of treatment. For these reasons, STDs should be treated in the following ways.

1. Even when an STD is only suspected, it should be treated with an emphasis on single-dose "observed" therapy, if feasible.
2. Serologic testing should be done for syphilis in patients with other STDs and always when treating any ulcerative STDs.
3. Pregnancy tests should be performed in all female patients with STDs.
4. Patients should be counseled about STD prevention.
5. Patients should be counseled or referred for human immunodeficiency virus testing.
6. Patients should be advised that partners must be treated to prevent reinfection. If partners are present during the emergency department visit, they are evaluated and treated at that time.
7. Many states have laws requiring the reporting of cases of STDs to the local health department for follow-up. Physicians should be aware of local state laws regarding the reporting of STDs (the new federal Health Information Privacy Protection Act [HIPPA] regulations do not prohibit such reporting if required by state health laws).

CHLAMYDIAL INFECTIONS

Clinical Features

Chlamydia trachomatis is an obligate intracellular bacterium that causes urethritis, epididymitis, orchitis, proctitis, or Reiter syndrome (nongonococcal urethritis, conjunctivitis, and rash) in men and urethritis, cervicitis, PID, and infertility in women. In both sexes, asymptomatic infection is common. There is a high incidence of coinfection with *Neisseria gonorrhoeae*. The incubation period varies from 1 to 3 weeks, with symptoms ranging from mild dysuria with purulent or mucoid urethral discharge to sterile pyuria and frequency (urethritis). Women may present with mild or even asymptomatic cervicitis or with abdominal pain, findings of PID, and possibly even peritonitis. Men may present with a tender swollen epididymis or testicle.

401

Diagnosis and Differential

Diagnosis is best made with indirect detection methods—such as enzyme-linked immunosorbent assay or DNA probes, which have a sensitivity of 75% to 90%. The Centers for Disease Control and Prevention (CDC) recommends a nucleic acid amplification test such as Amplicor, Abbott LCx, BD Probe TEC, or Gen-Probe APTIMA to be used as screening tests for *Chlamydia*. Culture is possible but difficult and produces a low yield.

Emergency Department Care and Disposition

1. **Doxycycline** 100 mg orally (PO) twice daily for 7 days or **azithromycin** 1 g PO as a single dose is the treatment of choice for uncomplicated urethritis or cervicitis.
2. Alternatives include 7-day treatment with **erythromycin** 500 mg PO 4 times a day, **ofloxacin** 300 mg twice daily, or **levofloxacin** 500 mg PO daily.

GONOCOCCAL INFECTIONS

Clinical Features

Neisseria gonorrhoeae (GC) is a gram-negative diplococcus that causes urethritis, epididymitis, orchitis, and prostatitis in men and urethritis, cervicitis, PID, and infertility in women. Rectal infection and proctitis with mucopurulent anal discharge and pain can occur in both sexes. Asymptomatic or subclinical infection, particularly in women, is possible. The incubation period ranges from 3 to 14 days. Women tend to present with nonspecific lower abdominal pain and mucopurulent vaginal discharge with findings of cervicitis and possibly PID. Eighty percent to 90% of men develop symptoms of urethritis: dysuria and purulent penile discharge within 2 weeks. Men also may present with acute epididymitis and orchitis or prostatitis. Occasionally, GC can be isolated from the throat, but it rarely causes symptomatic pharyngitis. Disseminated GC is a systemic infection that occurs in 2% of untreated patients with GC, most often women, and is the most common cause of infectious arthritis in young adults. Although there is overlap, disseminated GC tends to be biphasic. An initial febrile bacteremic stage includes skin lesions (tender pustules on a red base, usually on the extremities, and may include palms and soles), tenosynovitis, and myalgias. Over the next week, these symptoms subside, followed by mono- or oligoarticular arthritis with purulent joint fluid.

Diagnosis and Differential

For uncomplicated GC, urethral or cervical cultures are the standard diagnostic tests. A Gram stain of urethral discharge showing intracellular gram-negative diplococci is very useful in men; cervical smears are unreliable in women. Diagnosis of disseminated GC is often clinical because results of culture of blood, skin lesions, and joint fluid are positive in only 20% to 50% of patients. Culturing the cervix, rectum, and pharynx may improve the yield. A positive GC culture result from a partner may be very helpful.

Emergency Department Care and Disposition

1. Effective therapy for uncomplicated gonorrhea (not PID) includes single-dose regimens of **cefixime** 400 mg PO, **ceftriaxone** 125 mg intramuscularly (IM), **ciprofloxacin** 500 mg PO, or **ofloxacin** 400 mg PO.
2. Alternatives include single-dose regimens of **spectinomycin** 2 g IM, **norfloxacin** 800 mg PO, or **gatifloxacin** 400 mg PO.
3. Disseminated gonorrhea is treated initially with parenteral **ceftriaxone** 1 g/d IM for 7 to 10 days.
4. Treatment for possible coinfection with *Chlamydia* also should be given.

TRICHOMONAS INFECTIONS

Clinical Features

Trichomonas vaginalis is a flagellated protozoan that causes vaginitis with malodorous yellow-green discharge and urethritis. Abdominal pain also may be present. Trichomoniasis in pregnancy has been associated with premature rupture of membranes, preterm delivery, and low birthweight. In men, infection is often asymptomatic (90% to 95%), but urethritis may be present. The incubation period varies from 3 to 28 days.

Diagnosis and Differential

Diagnosis is based on finding the motile, flagellated organism on a saline wet preparation of vaginal discharge or in a spun urine specimen.

Emergency Department Care and Disposition

1. **Metronidazole** 2 g PO in a single dose is the treatment of choice (alternatively, 500 mg PO twice daily for 7 days).
2. Metronidazole gel is much less effective, achieving cure in fewer than 50% of patients.
3. Oral metronidazole is still considered to be a class C agent in pregnancy by many authorities, and many clinicians avoid treatment during the first trimester. However, the CDC points out that multiple studies of metronidazole use in pregnancy have not demonstrated a consistent association with teratogenic or mutagenic effects. The CDC guidelines state that pregnant women may be treated with a single 2-g PO dose of metronidazole.

SYPHILIS

Clinical Features

Treponema pallidum, a spirochete, causes syphilis. It enters the body through mucous membranes and nonintact skin. The incidence of syphilis in the United States has risen remarkably over the past decade and is thought to be related to the epidemic use of "crack" cocaine and other street drugs. Syphilis occurs in 3 stages. The primary stage is characterized by the chancre, a single painless ulcer with indurated borders that develops after an incubation period of 21 days on the penis, vulva, or other areas of sexual contact (including the vagina or cervix). The primary chancre heals and disappears after 3 to 6 weeks. The secondary stage occurs several weeks after the chancre disappears. Rash and lymphadenopathy are the most common symptoms. The rash starts on the trunk, spreads to the palms and soles, and is polymorphous, most often dull red and papular (similar to that of *Pityriasis rosacea*), but it may also take on other forms such as psoriatic or pustular lesions. The rash is not pruritic. Constitutional symptoms are common, including fever, malaise, headache, and sore throat. Mucous membrane involvement ("mucous patches") includes oral or vaginal lesions, and condyloma lata, which are flat, moist, wartlike growths, may occur at the perineum, anogenital region, or adjacent areas (thighs). This stage also resolves spontaneously. *Latency* refers to the period between stages during which a patient is asymptomatic. Any patient with secondary or latent syphilis who presents with neurologic symptoms or findings should have a lumbar puncture and cerebrospinal fluid testing for neurosyphilis. Late stage or tertiary syphilis, which is much less common (classically found in 33% of untreated patients), occurs years after the initial infection and affects primarily the cardiovascular and neurologic systems. Specific manifestations include neuropathy (tabes dorsalis), meningitis, dementia, and aortitis with aortic insufficiency and thoracic aneurysm formation.

Diagnosis and Differential

Syphilis may be diagnosed in the early stages with dark-field microscopic identification of the treponemes from the primary chancre or secondary condyloma or oral lesions. Serologic tests include nontreponemal (VDRL and rapid plasma reagin) and treponemal (fluorescent treponemal antibody absorption test). Nontreponemal test results are positive about 14 days after the appearance of the chancre. There is a false positive rate of approximately 1% to 2% of the population. Treponemal tests are more sensitive and specific but harder to perform.

Emergency Department Care and Disposition

1. Syphilis in all stages remains sensitive to penicillin, which is the drug of choice: **benzathine penicillin G** 2.4 million U IM as a single dose. Latent or tertiary syphilis is treated as above with 3 weekly IM injections.
2. Intravenous high-dose penicillin is the only treatment with proven benefit for neurosyphilis.

HERPES SIMPLEX INFECTIONS

Clinical Features

Herpes simplex virus type 2 and, less often, type 1 cause genital herpes by invading mucosal surfaces or nonintact skin. In primary infections, clusters of painful pustules or vesicles on an erythematous base occur 7 to 10 days after contact with an infected person. These lesions ulcerate and may coalesce over the next 3 to 5 days, and in women a profuse watery vaginal discharge may develop. Tender inguinal adenopathy is usually present. Dysuria is common and may lead to frank urinary retention due to severe pain. Systemic symptoms are common in first infections and include fever, chills, headache, and myalgias. The untreated illness lasts 2 to 3 weeks and then heals without scarring. The virus remains latent in the body, however, and continues to be shed in urogenital secretions of asymptomatic patients, making transmission to partners possible. Recurrences occur in most patients (60% to 90%) but are usually briefer and milder without systemic symptoms.

Diagnosis and Differential

The diagnosis is usually clinical, based on the characteristic appearance. Viral cultures for herpes simplex virus taken from vesicles or early ulcers are more reliable than the Tzanck smear for intranuclear inclusions.

Emergency Department Care and Disposition

1. Treatment of choice for primary genital herpes is a 7- to 10-day course of **acyclovir** 400 mg PO 3 times daily, **valacyclovir** 1 g PO twice daily, or **famciclovir** 250 mg PO 3 times daily.
2. In those cases severe enough to require hospitalization, treatment with intravenous **acyclovir** 5 to 10 mg/kg body weight every 8 hours may be given.
3. Treatment for episodes of recurrent genital herpes consist of a 5-day course of **acyclovir** 400 mg PO 3 times daily, **valacyclovir** 500 mg PO twice daily, or **famciclovir** 125 mg PO 3 times daily. If started at the onset of symptoms, antiviral therapy may reduce the severity and duration of the episode.

CHANCROID

Clinical Features

Caused by *Haemophilus ducreyi,* a pleomorphic gram-negative bacillus, chancroid is more common in the tropics, but in recent years there has been a rise in cases in the United States, with epidemic outbreaks. After an incubation period of 4 to 10 days, a tender papule on an erythematous base appears on the external genitalia and then over 1 to 2 days erodes to become a painful purulent or pustular ulcer with irregular edges. Multiple ulcers may be present. The ulcers are usually 1 to 2 cm in diameter with sharp, undermined margins and are very painful. "Kissing lesions" may occur due to autoinoculation of adjacent skin. Tender inguinal adenopathy, usually unilateral, follows in 50% of untreated patients within 1 to 2 weeks, and these nodes may mat together to form a mass (bubo) that becomes necrotic, suppurates, and drains. Constitutional symptoms are rare.

Diagnosis and Differential

Diagnosis is usually clinical, with care to exclude syphilis. Sometimes the organism may be cultured from a swab of the ulcer or pus from a bubo, but special media are required.

Emergency Department Care and Disposition

1. Treatment regimens include **azithromycin** 1 g PO as a single dose, **ceftriaxone** 250 mg IM as a single dose, **erythromycin** 500 mg PO 4 times a day for 7 days, or **ciprofloxacin** 500 mg PO twice daily for 3 days. Symptoms usually improve within 3 days, but large ulcers may require 2 to 3 weeks to heal.
2. Buboes may be aspirated to relieve pain from swelling but should not be excised.

LYMPHOGRANULOMA VENEREUM

Clinical Features

Three serotypes of *C trachomatis* are associated with lymphogranuloma venereum (LGV), which is endemic in other parts of the world but uncommon in the United States. The primary lesion, usually occurring 5 to 21 days after exposure, is a painless, small papule or vesicle that may go unnoticed and heals spontaneously in a 2 to 3 days. After anal intercourse, primary LGV may present as painful mucopurulent or bloody proctitis. Several weeks to months after the primary lesion, painful inguinal adenopathy (unilateral in 60%) occurs. The nodes mat together to form a bubo (often with a purplish hue to the overlying skin) and often suppurate and form fistulae. "Groove sign," an indentation across the bubo that parallels the inguinal ligament, may be seen. Systemic symptoms may include fever, chills, arthralgias, erythema nodosum, and, rarely, meningoencephalitis. Late sequelae include scarring; urethral, vaginal, and anal strictures; and occasionally lymphatic obstruction.

Diagnosis and Differential

Diagnosis is through serologic testing and culture of LGV from a lesion. A complement fixation titer for LGV greater than 1:64 is consistent with infection.

Emergency Department Care and Disposition

1. Doxycycline 100 mg PO twice daily for 21 days is the treatment of choice.
2. An alternative is erythromycin 500 mg PO 4 times daily for 21 days.

For further reading in *Emergency Medicine: A Comprehensive Study Guide,* 6th ed., see Chap. 141, "Sexually Transmitted Diseases," by Joel Kravitz and Susan B. Promes.

87 | Toxic Shock

Kevin J. Corcoran

TOXIC SHOCK SYNDROME

Toxic shock syndrome (TSS) is a severe, life-threatening syndrome that initially was associated with the use of tampons by menstruating women. The overall incidence of menstrual-related TSS and the number of cases associated with the use of tampons have decreased dramatically over the past 20 years. Most TSS cases have been directly associated with colonization or infection with *Staphylococcus aureus*. Currently 41% of TSS cases are non–menstrual-related TSS and include nasal packing, contraceptive sponges, diaphragms, body art and piercing as a few of the pathways for illness.

Clinical Features

TSS is characterized by high fever, profound hypotension, diffuse erythro-dermatous rash, mucus membrane hyperemia, diffuse myalgias, headache, vomiting, diarrhea, and constitutional symptoms that rapidly progress to multisystem dysfunction. When associated with menstruation, women typically present between the third and fifth day of menses. The rash associated with TSS is described as "painless sunburn" that typically fades within 3 days and is followed by full-thickness desquamation. Adult respiratory distress syndrome with refractory hypotension represents the ultimate end-organ damage secondary to TSS.

Diagnosis and Differential

TSS must be considered in any acute febrile illness associated with erythro-derma, hypotension, and multiorgan involvement. Diagnostic criteria are listed in Table 87-1. Other syndromes to consider in the differential diagnosis of TSS include streptococcal TSS (STSS), Kawasaki disease, staphylococcal scalded skin syndrome, Rocky Mountain spotted fever, and septic shock. When considering TSS, the evaluation should include arterial blood gas analysis; a complete blood count with a differential count; electrolyte determinations, including magnesium, calcium, and coagulation panel; urinalysis; electrocardiogram; and a chest x-ray.

Emergency Department Care and Disposition

The treatment of TSS consists of airway management, aggressive management of circulatory shock, continuous monitoring of vital signs and urinary output, use of antistaphylococcal antimicrobial agents with β-lactamase-stability, and the search for a focus of infection.

1. Crystalloid intravenous (IV) fluids should be used initially for hypotension and fluid resuscitation. A central venous pressure catheter or Swan-Ganz catheter may be necessary if there is no response to an initial fluid bolus of 1 to 2 L normal saline. Large volumes of fluid may be required (up to 20 L) over the first 24 hours.
2. A **dopamine** infusion may be necessary to augment fluid resuscitation for refractory hypotension to maintain a systolic blood pressure of 90 mm Hg.

407

TABLE 87-1 Diagnostic Criteria for Toxic Shock Syndrome

Fever: temperature ≥38.9°C (≥102.0°F)
Rash: diffuse macular erythroderma
Desquamation: 1–2 wk after onset of illness
Hypotension
Multisystem involvement (≥3 of the following)

1. Gastrointestinal: vomiting or diarrhea at onset of illness
2. Muscular: severe myalgias or creatine kinase elevation twice the normal level
3. Mucous membrane: vaginal, oropharyngeal, or conjunctival hyperemia
4. Renal: serum urea nitrogen or creatinine at least twice the upper limit of normal for laboratory or urinary sediment with pyuria (≥5 leukocytes/high power field) in the absence of urinary tract infection
5. Hepatic: total bilirubin, alanine aminotransferase enzyme, or aspartate aminotransferase enzyme levels at least twice the upper limit of normal for the laboratory
6. Hematologic: platelets <100,000/mL
7. Central nervous system: disorientation or alterations in consciousness

3. Fresh-frozen plasma, packed red blood cells, or platelets may be given to correct any coagulation abnormalities (see Chap. 138).
4. All potentially infected sites, including blood, should be cultured before initiating antibiotic therapy.
5. Tampons or nasal packing should be removed.
6. Antistaphylococcal antimicrobial therapy with β-lactamase stability should be initiated. Antistaphylococcal penicillin, such as **nafcillin or oxacillin** 1 to 2 g IV every 4 hours, or a cephalosporin with β-lactamase stability, such as **cefazolin** 2 g every 6 hours. In penicillin-allergic patients, clindamycin, vancomycin, or, potentially, cephalosporins may be used.
7. Other considerations include the use of methylprednisolone and IV immunoglobulin.
8. Patients are typically admitted to the intensive care unit.

STREPTOCOCCAL TOXIC SHOCK SYNDROME

STSS is defined as any group A streptococcal infection associated with invasive soft tissue infection, early onset of shock, and organ failure. STSS is very similar to TSS but is associated with soft tissue infection that is culture positive for *Streptococcus pyogenes*. Labeled the "flesh-eating bacteria" by the news media, group A streptococcal infections cause streptococcal necrotizing fasciitis, with mortality rates of 30% to 80%.

Clinical Features

Pain is the most common presenting symptom, whereas fever is the most common presenting sign followed closely by shock. STSS typically presents with the abrupt onset of severe pain that precedes physical findings. Eight percent of patients have signs of soft tissue infection, most commonly affecting the extremities. The development of vesicles and bullae at the site of soft tissue infection that progresses to violaceous or blue discoloration is an ominous sign of necrotizing fasciitis or myositis. Necrotizing fasciitis may

TABLE 87-2 Diagnostic Criteria for Streptococcal Toxic Shock Syndrome

Hypotension

Multiorgan involvement (characterized by ≥2 of the following)
1. Renal impairment: creatinine level twice normal
2. Coagulopathy
3. Liver involvement: enzyme or bilirubin level twice normal
4. Acute respiratory distress syndrome
5. Generalized erythematous macular rash that may desquamate
6. Soft tissue necrosis, including necrotizing fascitis or myositis or gangrene

develop rapidly and carries a poor prognosis. Adult respiratory distress syndrome develops in 55% of patients, usually after the onset of hypotension. Patients are usually febrile, hypotensive, and confused and develop multisystem organ dysfunction.

Diagnosis and Differential

Diagnostic criteria are listed in Table 87-2. The differential diagnosis should include TSS in addition to other infections caused by group A streptococcus, *Clostridium perfringens,* and other bacteria; Kawasaki disease; Rocky Mountain spotted fever; and septic shock. When considering STSS, signs of soft tissue infection should be sought and the suspected site should be cultured. Laboratory evaluation includes a complete blood count with a differential count; arterial blood gas analysis; liver function tests; serum electrolyte, magnesium, and calcium determinations; a coagulation profile; blood cultures; electrocardiogram; chest x-ray; and urinalysis.

Emergency Department Care and Disposition

1. Treatment is similar to that for TSS, with airway management and aggressive fluid resuscitation with vasopressors, as needed.
2. Antistreptococcal antimicrobial therapy is started with IV **penicillin** G 24 million U/d in divided doses and IV **clindamycin** 900 mg every 8 hours. **Erythromycin** 1.0 g IV every 6 hours can be substituted in penicillin-allergic patients, or **ceftriaxone** 2 g IV every 24 hours and clindamycin 900 mg IV every 8 hours can be used.
3. Immediate surgical consultation should be obtained because 70% of patients with STSS require debridement, fasciotomy, or amputation.
4. IV immunoglobulin may be considered.
5. Patients require admission to the intensive care unit.

For further reading in *Emergency Medicine: A Comprehensive Study Guide,* 6th ed., see Chap. 142, "Toxic Shock Syndrome and Streptococcal Toxic Shock Syndrome," by Shawna J. Perry and Ashley E. Booth.

88 | Common Viral Infections

Matthew J. Scholer

Viral illnesses are among the most common reasons that people come to an emergency department. This chapter focuses on the viral illness for which antiviral therapy has been developed. Treatment of primary herpes zoster and mononucleosis is discussed in Chap. 82, and genital herpes is discussed in Chap. 86. Treatment of the human immunodeficiency virus is covered in Chap. 89, and treatment of cytomegalovirus is discussed in Chap. 97.

INFLUENZAE A AND B

Flu occurs worldwide, in the winter months, and sporadically year round in the tropics. Influenza is spread by droplets generated by coughing. After exposure, the incubation period is usually about 2 days.

Clinical Features

Classic flu symptoms include fever of 38.6°C to 39.8°C (101°F to 103°F) with chills or rigor, headache, myalgia, and generalized malaise. Respiratory symptoms include dry cough, rhinorrhea, and sore throat, frequently with bilateral tender, enlarged cervical lymph nodes. The elderly usually do not have classic symptoms and may present with only fever, malaise, confusion, and nasal congestion. Almost 50% of affected children have gastrointestinal symptoms, but these are unusual in adults.

The fever generally lasts 2 to 4 days, followed by rapid recovery from most of the systemic symptoms. Cough and fatigue may persist for several weeks.

Common complications of acute influenza infection include primary influenza pneumonitis, secondary bacterial pneumonia, croup, exacerbation of chronic obstructive pulmonary disease, and Reye syndrome. The presence of dyspnea and hypoxia should raise the suspicion for pulmonary involvement. Aspirin therapy should not be used for fevers caused by influenza or varicella due to the association with Reye syndrome.

Diagnosis and Differential

A clinical diagnosis of flu during a known outbreak has an accuracy of approximately 85%, but bacteremia also should be considered in patients with rigor and myalgia.

Newer rapid antigen tests are available that may change the approach to flulike illnesses and decrease the empirical use of antibiotics. Commercially available tests take less than 30 minutes to perform and have sensitivities of 57% to 81% and specificities of 93% to 100%.

Emergency Department Care and Disposition

1. Amantadine and rimantadine are antiviral drugs approved for the treatment of influenza A. Neither has activity against influenza B. Oseltamivir and zanamivir are neuraminidase inhibitors that are active against influenzae A and B. For maximal effectiveness, these medications need to be started within 48 hours of onset of symptoms and can reduce the duration of systemic symptoms by 1 to 2 days.

2. The dose for **amantadine** and **rimantadine** is 100 mg twice daily for 5 days. Amantadine causes an increase in seizure activity in patients with a preexisting seizure disorder. Rimantadine has a significantly lower incidence of central nervous system side effects than does amantadine but is more expensive.
3. **Zanamivir** is an inhaled medicine, 2 5 mg inhalations per dose, dosed twice a day for 5 days. It may cause bronchospasm and should not be given to patients with underlying pulmonary disease.
4. **Oseltamivir** is dosed at 75 mg twice a day orally for 5 days. Nausea is reported frequently with oseltamivir and can be decreased by taking the drug with food.
5. All four anti-influenza medicines are effective in preventing flu, with efficacy rates of 70% to 90% when used at treatment doses (as above) for a prolonged duration (zanamivir is not approved by the US Food and Drug Administration for this indication).

HERPES SIMPLEX VIRUS 1

Transmission of herpes simplex virus (HSV) occurs by contact of infected secretions (saliva or genital) with mucous membranes or open skin.

Clinical Features

HSV-1 primarily causes oral lesions but may cause genital infection. The primary infection of HSV-1 is often mild or asymptomatic. The lesions are distributed throughout the mouth and consist of small, thin-walled vesicles on an erythematous base, although they do not always become vesicular. The primary lesions generally last 1 to 2 weeks. In children younger than 5 years, it may present as a pharyngitis or gingivostomatitis associated with fever and cervical lymphadenopathy. The diagnosis is largely clinical because viral cultures take days to weeks to be performed and thus are of little use in an emergency department setting. HSV-2 is spread primarily sexually. It causes identical lesions, primarily genital, but may cause oral lesions.

Recurrent oral lesions occur in 60% to 90% of infected individuals and are usually milder and generally occur on the lower lip at the outer vermilion border. The recurrences often are triggered by local trauma, sunburn, or stress. Patients may have pain or tingling before developing lesions. The lesions may begin as erythematous papules and then become vesicular.

Emergency Department Care and Disposition

1. Oral acyclovir has been shown to shorten the duration of symptoms in children if begun within the first 72 hours of symptoms.
2. Treatment of recurrent oral herpes labialis with oral **acyclovir** 400 mg 5 times per day or topical **penciclovir** applied every 2 hours for 4 days shortens duration of symptoms in adults.

HERPES ZOSTER

Herpes zoster (shingles) is the reactivation of latent herpes zoster virus infection. There is a lifetime incidence of almost 20%, with most cases being among the elderly.

Clinical Features

The lesions of shingles are identical to those of chickenpox but are limited to a single dermatome in distribution. Thoracic and lumber dermatomes are most common. The disease begins with a prodrome of pain in the affected area for 1 to 3 days, followed by the outbreak of a maculopapular rash that quickly progresses to a vesicular rash. The course of the disease is usually approximately 2 weeks but may persist for a full month. Rash involving more than 1 dermatome or crossing the midline should raise the suspicion of disseminated disease.

The cranial nerves (CNs) also may be affected, with the potential complications of herpes zoster ophthalmicus (HZO) and Ramsay-Hunt syndrome. HZO is due to involvement of the ocular branch of CN V and is a vision-threatening condition. Ocular involvement can be seen in the presence of only a slight rash on the forehead. The Hutchinson sign (lesions on the tip of the nose) may be seen before ocular involvement is recognized, but its absence does not rule out HZO. Occasionally, a red eye may precede the appearance of the rash. HZO induces keratitis and may be followed by involvement of deeper structures. A dendriform corneal ulcer often can be identified with fluorescein staining. Involvement of CN VII may result in Ramsay-Hunt syndrome, which presents clinically as a facial nerve palsy resembling Bell palsy and is treated in the same fashion.

The most common complication of shingles is postherpetic neuralgia (PHN). PHN occurs in 10% to 20% of all patients after an episode of acute zoster, but in up to 70% of patients 70 years or older. It generally resolves in 1 to 2 months but may last longer than 1 year in some patients.

Emergency Department Care and Disposition

The treatment of herpes zoster in the normal host is aimed at decreasing the risk of PHN because the antivirals have a clinically small, but statistically significant, effect on the duration of the acute disease.

1. Treatment should begin as soon as possible and within 72 hours of disease onset for maximal benefit. There is a suggestion that **famciclovir** (500 mg 3 times a day for 7 days) and **valacyclovir** (1,000 mg 3 times a day for 7 days) may be more effective than **acyclovir** (800 mg 5 times a day for 7 days), but this has not been shown to be clinically significant.
2. Patients with evidence of disseminated disease should be admitted for intravenous acyclovir.
3. Treatment with antiherpes agents has been shown to decrease the duration of PHN but not reduce its incidence.
4. Initial treatment of patient with PHN is typically systemic analgesia, often narcotics. Patients should be referred back to their primary care provider because first-line agents often fail, and a trial of oral **gabapentin** 300 mg to 600 mg 3 times daily or carbamazepine may be tried as second-line therapy.
5. HZO or suspected HZO mandates an ophthalmologic consultation due to the threat to vision.

For further reading in *Emergency Medicine: A Comprehensive Study Guide,* 6th ed., see Chap. 143, "Common Viral Infections: Influenzaviruses and Herpesviruses," by Robert A. Brownstein.

89 | HIV Infections and AIDS

David M. Cline

Risk factors commonly associated with the human immunodeficiency virus (HIV) include homosexuality or bisexuality, injected drug use, heterosexual exposure, receipt of a blood transfusion before 1985, and vertical and horizontal maternal-to-neonatal transmission.

CLINICAL FEATURES

Acute HIV infection, essentially indistinguishable from a "flulike" illness, usually goes unrecognized but is reported to occur in 50% to 90% of patients. The time from exposure to onset of symptoms is usually 2 to 4 weeks, and the most common symptoms include fever (>90%), fatigue (70–90%), sore throat (>70%), rash (40-80%), headache (30-80%), and lymphadenopathy (40-70%). Other reported symptoms include myalgias, diarrhea, and weight loss. Seroconversion, reflecting detectable antibody response to HIV, usually occurs 3 to 8 weeks after infection. This is followed by a long period of asymptomatic infection during which patients generally have no findings on physical examination except for possible persistent generalized lymphadenopathy. The mean incubation times from exposure to the development of acquired immunodeficiency syndrome (AIDS) is estimated at 8.23 years for adults and 1.97 years for children younger than 5 years. Early symptomatic infection is characterized by conditions that are more common and more severe in the presence of HIV infection but, by definition, are not AIDS indicator conditions. Examples include thrush, persistent vulvovaginal candidiasis, peripheral neuropathy, cervical dysplasia, recurrent herpes zoster infection, and idiopathic thrombocytopenic purpura. At this time CD4 counts are 200 to 500/μL. As the CD4 count drops below 200 cells/μL, the frequency of opportunistic infections dramatically increases. AIDS is defined by the appearance of any indicator condition (Table 89-1) including a CD4 count smaller than 200 cells/μL. Median survival time after the CD4 count has fallen to below 200 cells/μL is 3.7 years. Late symptomatic or advanced HIV infection exists in patients with a CD4 count smaller than 50 cells/μL or clinical evidence of end-stage disease, including disseminated *Mycobacterium avium* complex or disseminated cytomegalovirus (CMV).

Constitutional Symptoms and Febrile Illnesses

Systemic symptoms, such as fever, weight loss, and malaise, are common in HIV-infected patients and account for most HIV-related ED presentations. Appropriate laboratory investigation includes electrolytes, complete blood count, blood cultures, urinalysis and culture, liver function tests, chest radiographs, and serologic testing for syphilis, cryptococcosis, toxoplasmosis, CMV, and coccidioidomycosis. Lumbar puncture should be considered if there are neurologic signs or symptoms or unexplained fever.

In HIV patients without obvious focalizing signs or symptoms, sources of fever vary by stage of disease. Patients with CD4 counts larger than 500 cells/μL generally have sources of fever similar to those in nonimmunocompromised patients. Those with CD4 counts between 200 and 500 cells/μL are most likely to have early bacterial respiratory infections. For patients with

TABLE 89-1 Indicator Conditions for Acquired Immunodeficiency Syndrome

CD4 count <200 cell/μL
Cervical cancer (invasive)
Cryptococcosis
Cryptosporidiosis
Cytomegalovirus retinitis
Esophageal candidiasis
Herpes simplex virus
Histoplasmosis, disseminated
HIV encephalopathy
HIV wasting syndrome
Isosporiasis
Kaposi sarcoma
Lymphoma (brain)
Mycobacterium avium complex
Mycobacterium tuberculosis disease
Pneumocystis carinii pneumonia
Progressive multifocal leukoencephalopathy
Recurrent bacterial pneumonia
Salmonella septicemia (recurrent)
Toxoplasmosis (brain)
Tuberculosis (pulmonary)

Key: HIV = human immunodeficiency virus.

CD4 counts smaller than 200 cells/μL, likely infections include *Pneumocystis carinii* pneumonia (PCP), central line infection, *M avium* complex (MAC), *Mycobacterium tuberculosis*, CMV, drug fever, and sinusitis. Disseminated MAC occurs predominately in patients with CD4 counts below 100 cells/μL. Persistent fever and night sweats are typical. Associated symptoms include weight loss, diarrhea, malaise, and anorexia. Diagnosis is made with acid-fast stain of stool or other body fluids or culture. A more focal and invasive form of MAC has emerged, called *immune reconstitution illness to MAC*, which presents with lymphadenitis and follows weeks to months after starting highly active antiretroviral therapy.

CMV is the most common cause of serious opportunistic viral disease in HIV-infected patients. Disseminated disease commonly involves the gastrointestinal or pulmonary system. The most important manifestation is retinitis.

Infective endocarditis is a concern especially in intravenous (IV) drug users (see Chap. 90). Non-Hodgkin lymphoma is the most commonly occurring neoplasm in HIV patients and typically presents as a high-grade, rapidly growing mass lesion.

Pulmonary Complications

Pulmonary presentations are among the most common reasons for ED visits by HIV-infected patients. Presenting complaints frequently are nonspecific and include cough, hemoptysis, shortness of breath, and chest pain. The most common causes of pulmonary abnormalities in HIV-infected patients include community-acquired bacterial pneumonia, PCP, *Mycobacterium tuberculosis,* CMV, *Cryptococcus neoformans, Histoplasma capsulatum,* and neoplasms. Evaluation should include pulse oximetry, arterial blood gas analysis, sputum culture and Gram stain, acid-fast stain, blood cultures, and chest radiograph.

The classic presenting symptoms of PCP are fever, cough (typically nonproductive), and shortness of breath (progressing from being present only with exertion to being present at rest). Negative radiographs are reported in 15% to 20% of patients. Hypoxia or increased alveolar-arterial gradient identify patients at risk.

Classic pulmonary manifestations of tuberculosis (TB) include cough with hemoptysis, night sweats, prolonged fevers, weight loss, and anorexia. TB is common in patients with CD4 counts between 200 and 500 cells/μL. Classic upper lobe involvement and cavitary lesions are less common, particularly among late-stage AIDS patients. False negative purified protein derivative TB test results are frequent among AIDS patients due to immunosuppression.

Nonopportunistic bacterial pneumonias are the most common pulmonary infections in HIV-infected patients. Common pathogens include *Streptococcus pneumoniae, Haemophilus influenzae,* and *Staphylococcus aureus.* Productive cough, leukocytosis, and the presence of a focal infiltrate suggest bacterial pneumonia, especially in those with earlier-stage disease.

Neurologic Complications

Central nervous system (CNS) disease occurs in 90% of patients with AIDS, and 10% to 20% of HIV-infected patients initially present with CNS symptoms. ED evaluation includes computed tomography and lumbar puncture. Cerebrospinal fluid studies should include blood pressures; complete cell count; glucose; protein; Gram stain; India ink stain; bacterial, viral, and fungal cultures; toxoplasmosis; and *Cryptococcosis* antigen and coccidioidomycosis titer.

The most common causes of neurologic symptoms include AIDS dementia, *Toxoplasma gondii,* and *Cryptococcus neoformans.* Symptoms may include headache, fever, focal neurologic deficits, altered mental status, or seizures.

AIDS dementia complex (also referred to as HIV encephalopathy or subacute encephalitis) is a progressive process commonly heralded by subtle impairment of recent memory and other cognitive deficits caused by direct HIV infection.

Other, less common CNS infections that should be considered in the presence of neurologic symptoms include bacterial meningitis, histoplasmosis (usually disseminated), CMV, progressive multifocal leukoencephalopathy, herpes simplex virus, neurosyphilis, and TB.

Fifty percent of HIV patients will experience HIV neuropathy characterized by painful sensory symptoms of the feet.

Gastrointestinal Complications

Approximately 50% of AIDS patients will present with gastrointestinal complaints at some time during their illness. The most frequent presenting symptoms include odynophagia, abdominal pain, bleeding, and diarrhea. ED evaluation includes stool for leukocytes, ova, parasites, acid-fast staining, and culture.

Diarrhea is the most frequent gastrointestinal complaint and is estimated to occur in 50% to 90% of AIDS patients. Common causes include bacterial organisms, such as *Shigella, Salmonella,* enteroadherent *Escherichia coli,* and *Campylobacter;* parasitic organisms, such as *Giardia, Cryptosporidium, Entamoeba histolytica,* and *Isospora belli;* CMV; *M avium intracellulare;* and antibiotic therapy.

Oral candidiasis, or thrush, affects more than 80% of AIDS patients. The tongue and buccal mucosa are commonly involved, and the plaques characteristically can be easily scraped from an erythematous base.

Esophageal involvement may occur with *Candida,* herpes simplex, and CMV. Complaints of odynophagia or dysphagia are usually indicative of esophagitis and may be extremely debilitating.

Hepatomegaly occurs in approximately 50% of AIDS patients. Elevation of alkaline phosphatase levels are frequently seen. Jaundice is rare. Coinfection with hepatitis B and hepatitis C is common, especially among IV drug users.

Anorectal disease is common in AIDS patients. Proctitis is characterized by painful defecation, rectal discharge, and tenesmus. Common causative organisms include *Neisseria gonorrhoeae, Chlamydia trachomatis,* syphilis, and herpes simplex.

Cutaneous Manifestations

Kaposi sarcoma appears more often in homosexual men than in other risk groups. Clinically, it consists of painless, raised brown-black or purple papules and nodules that do not blanch. Common sites are the face, chest, genitals, and oral cavity; however, widespread dissemination involving internal organs may occur.

Reactivation of varicella zoster virus is more common in patients with HIV infection and AIDS than in the general population. Herpes simplex virus infections are common. HIV patients may develop bullous impetigo and *Pseudomonas* associated chronic ulcerations.

Ophthalmologic Manifestations

Seventy-five percent of patients with AIDS develop ocular complications.

CMV retinitis is the most frequent and serious ocular opportunistic infection and the leading cause of blindness in AIDS patients. The prevalence is estimated to be up to 40%. The presentation of CMV retinitis is variable. It may be asymptomatic early on but later causes changes in visual acuity, visual field cuts, photophobia, scotoma, or eye redness or pain. Herpes zoster ophthalmicus is another diagnosis to consider and is recognized by the typical zoster rash.

DIAGNOSIS AND DIFFERENTIAL

The most common assay used to detect viral antibody is an enzyme-linked immunoassay (EIA) and a confirming western blot test on EIA-positive specimens. EIA is approximately 99% specific and 98.5% sensitive; the western blot test is nearly 100% sensitive and specific if performed under ideal laboratory circumstances. Diagnosis of acute-stage HIV infection is not possible with standard serologic tests because seroconversion has not yet occurred. Methods for earlier detection of HIV-1 include techniques to detect DNA, RNA, or HIV antigens. The single-use diagnostic system is used to screen rapidly for antibodies to HIV-1 in serum or plasma. OraSure manufactures saliva-based and fingerstick blood assays for rapid HIV testing.

Knowledge of current or recent CD4 counts and a HIV viremia load will help in the management of HIV patients. CD4 counts below 200 cells/μL and viral load greater than 50 000 is associated with increased risk of progression to AIDS-defining illness.

EMERGENCY DEPARTMENT CARE AND DISPOSITION

1. The initial evaluation of HIV-infected and AIDS patients begins with a heightened awareness of the need for universal precautions. All blood and body fluid exposures should be considered infective. Respiratory isolation should be instituted for patients with suspected TB.
2. All unstable patients should have airway management as indicated, oxygen, pulse oximetry, cardiac monitoring, and IV access. Shock, with its myriad causes, should be managed in standard fashion.
3. Seizures, altered mental status, gastrointestinal bleeding, and coma should be managed with standard protocols.
4. Suspected bacterial sepsis and focal bacterial infections should be treated with standard antibiotics.
5. Systemic *M avium* should be treated with **clarithromycin** 500 mg orally (PO) twice daily plus **ethambutol** 15 mg/kg/d PO plus **rifabutin** 300 mg daily. Treatment of immune reconstitution illness to MAC should be continuation of highly active antiretroviral therapy, antimicrobials as above, and possibly steroids.
6. Systemic CMV should be treated with **ganciclovir** 2.5 mg/kg IV every 8 hours or **foscarnet** 90 mg/kg IV every 12 hours.
7. Ophthalmologic CMV is treated with a ganciclovir implant plus **ganciclovir** 1.0 to 1.5 g PO twice daily or 5 mg/kg IV twice daily for 14 to 21 days.
8. Pulmonary PCP should be treated with **trimethoprim-sulfamethoxazole** (TMP-SMX), with TMP 15 to 20 mg/kg/d and SMX 75 to 100 mg/kg/d PO, for 3 weeks. The typical oral dose is 2 tablets of TMP-SMX double strength 3 times daily. An alternative is **pentamidine** 4 mg/kg/d IV or intramuscularly for 3 weeks. Oral steroids should be given if hypoxic: prednisone 40 mg twice daily for 5 days, then 40 mg daily for 5 days, and then 20 mg daily for 11 more days.
9. Pulmonary TB may be treated with **INH** 5 mg/kg/d PO plus **rifabutin** 10 mg/kg/d PO plus **pyrazinamide** 15 to 30 mg/kg/d PO plus **streptomycin** 15 mg/kg/d intramuscularly.
10. CNS toxoplasmosis can be treated with **pyrimethamine** 50 to 100 mg/d PO plus **sulfadiazine** 4.8 mg/kg/d PO plus folinic acid 10 mg/d PO.
11. CNS cryptococcosis can be treated with **amphotericin** B 0.7 mg/kg/d IV. When improved, **fluconazole** 400 mg daily for 8 to 10 weeks can be used.
12. Candidiasis (thrush) can be treated with **clotrimazole** 10 mg troches 5 times per day or **nystatin** 500,000 U gargle 5 times per day.
13. Esophagitis can be treated with **fluconazole** 100 to 400 mg daily PO.
14. Salmonellosis can be treated with **ciprofloxacin** 500 mg twice daily for 2 to 4 weeks.
15. Cutaneous herpes simplex can be treated with **acyclovir** 1000 mg/d or **famciclovir** 250 mg PO 3 times a day for 14 to 21 days.

16. Cutaneous herpes zoster can be treated with **acyclovir** 4000 mg/d PO, **valacyclovir** 1 g PO twice daily, or **famciclovir** 500 mg PO 3 times daily.
17. Herpes zoster ophthalmicus should be treated with **acyclovir** 30 to 36 mg/kg/d IV for at least 7 days and then with oral therapy.
18. Although rarely started in the ED, antiretroviral therapy is started for CD4 counts below 350 cells/μL or for a HIV viral load greater than 55,000 copies/mL. Initial treatment includes 2 nucleoside reverse transcriptase inhibitors plus 1 or 2 protease inhibitors or 1 non-nucleoside reverse transcriptase inhibitor drug. An updated guide for their use can be found on the Web site of the Centers for Disease Control and Prevention: www.cdc.gov/hiv/pubs/mmwr.
19. The decision to admit an AIDS patient should be based on severity of illness, with attention to new presentation of fever of unknown origin, hypoxia worse than baseline or Pao_2 below 60, suspected PCP, suspected TB, new CNS symptoms, intractable diarrhea, suspected CMV retinitis, herpes zoster ophthalmicus, or a patient unable to perform self-care.

For further reading in *Emergency Medicine: A Comprehensive Study Guide,* 6th ed., see Chap. 144, "HIV Infection and AIDS," by Richard E. Rothman, Catherine Marco, and Gabor D. Kelen.

90 | Infective Endocarditis

Chadwick D. Miller

Infective endocarditis (IE) has 3 main classifications determined by the patient population in which it occurs. The classifications describe likely causative organisms and guide treatment. Native valve endocarditis, representing 59% to 70% of IE, most commonly involves the aortic valve. Patients often have predisposing factors such as congenital heart defects, valve pathology, indwelling lines, poor dentition, or human immunodeficiency virus. Common organisms include streptococci (>50%), staphylococci, and enterococci. Intravenous drug users have a 2% to 5% annual risk of endocarditis. The tricuspid valve is most commonly involved and *Staphylococcus aureus* represents more than 50% of causative organisms. Prosthetic valve endocarditis is divided by proximity to surgery into early (<6 months from surgery) and late IE. Early disease is associated with *Staphylococcus epidermidis* and has a higher mortality. Late disease has similar bacteriology to native valve endocarditis.

CLINICAL FEATURES

IE presents along a continuum from a subacute to acute illness. Acute IE is associated with highly virulent organisms *(S aureus)* and presents with abrupt onset of high fever, hemodynamic deterioration, and may lead to death. Subacute IE is classically associated with less virulent organisms *(Streptococcus viridians)* and progresses along a more indolent course, with complications taking weeks or months to develop.

Signs and symptoms are divided into those caused by bacteremia, cardiac findings, embolic sequelae, and circulating immune complexes. Bacteremia presents with constitutional symptoms of fever (>38°C present in more than 90%), chills, nausea, and fatigue. Cardiac murmurs are detectable in up to 85% of patients with IE and represent destruction of valvular or supporting tissue. Congestive heart failure, the most common complication, is the leading cause of death in IE and is detectable in up to 70% of patients as dyspnea, frothy sputum, or chest pain. Arterial embolization of valve vegetation fragments is the second most common complication and may affect many systems including the central nervous system (20% to 40%) as an embolic stroke, pulmonary system (infarction and pneumonia), and kidneys (hematuria and flank pain). Circulating immune complexes cause skin findings in 18% to 50% of patients (Table 90-1).

DIAGNOSIS AND DIFFERENTIAL

Definitive diagnosis of IE relies on blood culture results and echocardiographic findings of valvular injury or vegetations. Blood cultures should be obtained from 3 different sites before the initiation of antibiotic therapy. Echocardiography should not delay appropriate treatment and antibiotics. Nonspecific laboratory findings that support the diagnosis include leukocytosis, elevated C-reactive protein, normocytic anemia, hematuria, and pyuria.

Due to the high incidence of disease, the following patient populations should be routinely admitted for a complete evaluation for IE: (*a*) all febrile

TABLE 90-1 Findings from Circulating Immune Complexes in Infective Endocarditis

Finding	Location	Description	Frequency
Petechiae	Buccal mucosa, conjunctiva, extremities	Nonblanching erythematous pinpoint macules	20–40%
Osler nodes	Pads of fingers and toes	Small tender subcutaneous nodules	25%
Splinter hemorrhages	Under fingernails or toenails	Linear dark streaks	15%
Janeway lesions	Palms and soles	Small painless hemorrhagic plaques	<10%
Roth spots	Retina	Oval retinal hemorrhages with pale centers near optic disc	

intravenous drug-using patients, (*b*) patients with a cardiac prosthesis and fever, and (*c*) patients with a new or changed murmur and evidence of vascular complications.

EMERGENCY DEPARTMENT CARE AND DISPOSITION

The first priority in the care of patients with IE is stabilization of respiratory and cardiac symptoms.

1. For patients with mental status changes and hypoxia or a compromised airway, control of the airway with oral intubation may be required. Cardiac decompensation is usually due to left-side valvular incompetence or rupture.
2. Acute rupture of the mitral or aortic valve should be stabilized with afterload reducers, such as sodium nitroprusside, and insertion of a Swan-Ganz catheter for monitoring therapy as soon as possible (see Chap. 24). Preparation for emergency surgery should be made for patients with suspected acute valvular rupture or those who may be surgical candidates. Aortic balloon counterpulsation may be helpful for mitral valve rupture but is contraindicated for wide-open aortic valve rupture.
3. The second priority is drawing 3 blood cultures from different sites and then starting empiric antibiotic therapy.
4. Table 90-2 lists current empiric antibiotic treatment guidelines and dosages.
5. Prophylaxis against endocarditis should be performed before invasive procedures for patients with risk factors for endocarditis, such as prosthetic valves, history of endocarditis, congenital cardiac abnormalities, acquired valvular dysfunction, and mitral valve prolapse with documented regurgitation. Acceptable regimens for dental procedures known to cause bleeding include **amoxicillin** 2 g orally (PO) 1 hour before intervention or **ampicillin** 2 g intravenously (IV) or intramuscularly (IM) 30 minutes before intervention or **clindamycin** 600 mg PO or IV. For genitourinary in-

TABLE 90-2 Empiric Therapy of Suspected Bacterial Endocarditis*

Patient Characteristics	Recommended Agents	Initial Dose
Uncomplicated history	Ceftriaxone	1–2 g IV
	or nafcillin	2 g IV
	plus gentamycin	1–3 mg/kg IV
Injection drug use, congenital heart disease, hospital-acquired, suspected MRSA, or already on oral antibiotics	Nafcillin	2 g IV
	plus gentamycin	1–3 mg/kg IV
	plus vancomycin	15 mg/kg IV
Prosthetic heart valve	Vancomycin	15 mg/kg IV
	plus gentamycin	1–3 mg/kg IV
	plus rifampin	300 mg PO

*Because of controversy in the literature regarding the optimal regimen for empiric treatment, antibiotic selection should be based on patient characteristics, local resistance patterns, and current authoritative recommendations.

terventions, add **gentamicin** 1.5 mg/kg IV or IM to the regimen above. For incision and drainage of infected tissue, administer **cefazolin** 1.0 g IV or IM 30 minutes before the procedure or **cephalexin** 2 g PO 1 hour before the procedure.

For further reading in *Emergency Medicine: A Comprehensive Study Guide,* 6th ed., see Chap. 145, "Infective Endocarditis," by R. E. Rothman, S. Yang, and C. Marco.

C. James Corrall

TETANUS

Tetanus is an acute, frequently fatal spasmodic disease that results from a wound infected with the organism *Clostridium tetani*. The clinical manifestations of tetanus are secondary to an exotoxin elaborated within the wound site.

Clinical Features

Tetanus occurs most frequently after an acute unreported injury, most commonly a puncture wound, but it can also develop after minor trauma, surgical procedures, abortions, or in neonates because of inadequate umbilical cord care. The incubation period of tetanus can range from shorter than 24 hours to longer than 30 days. Clinically, tetanus can be categorized into 4 forms based on site of inoculation and the incubation period: local, generalized, cephalic, and neonatal.

Local tetanus is manifested by persistent rigidity of muscles in close proximity to the injury site and usually resolves without sequelae. Generalized tetanus is the most common form of the disease and most frequently presents with pain and stiffness in the jaw and trunk muscles. Later, the rigidity leads to the development of trismus and the characteristic facial expression, *risus sardonicus* (devil's smile). Reflex spasms and tonic contractions of all muscle groups are responsible for the other symptoms of the disease, which include dysphagia, opisthotonos, flexing of the arms, fist clenching, and extension of the lower extremities. Patients are conscious and alert throughout these spasms unless laryngospasm and tetanic contraction of respiratory muscles causes respiratory compromise.

Autonomic nervous system dysfunction resulting in a hypersympathetic state occurs in the second week of the illness and is manifested as tachycardia, labile hypertension, profuse sweating, and hyperpyrexia. Such autonomic dysfunction contributes to morbidity and mortality and is difficult to manage.

Cephalic tetanus follows injuries to the head and neck area and occasionally results in dysfunction of cranial nerves, most often the seventh nerve. This form of tetanus has a particularly poor prognosis.

Neonatal tetanus carries an extremely high mortality rate and is uniformly associated with inadequate maternal immunization and poor umbilical cord care.

Diagnosis and Differential

Tetanus is diagnosed solely on the basis of the clinical examination. A history of active immunization with a booster within the previous 10 years eliminates tetanus as a diagnostic possibility. There are no confirmatory laboratory or microbiological tests. The differential diagnosis includes strychnine poisoning, dystonic reactions to phenothiazine, hypocalcemic tetany, rabies, and temporomandibular joint disease.

Emergency Department Care and Disposition

Patients with tetanus should be managed in an intensive care unit due to the potential for respiratory compromise. Environmental stimuli must be minimized to prevent precipitation of reflex convulsive spasms. Identification and debridement of the inciting wound, if present, is necessary to minimize further toxin production.

1. **Tetanus immune globulin** 3,000 to 6,000 U intramuscularly in a single injection should be given. It should be given before any wound debridement because more exotoxin may be released during wound manipulation.
2. Antibiotics are of questionable value in the treatment of tetanus. If warranted, parenteral **metronidazole** (500 mg intravenously [IV] every 6 hours) is the antibiotic of choice. Penicillin is contraindicated because it may potentiate the effects of tetanospasmin.
3. **Midazolam** (5 to 15 mg IV as a continuous drip to effect) has been used extensively and results in sedation and amnesia, but **lorazepam** (2 mg IV to effect), because of its long duration of action, may be superior and the drug of choice.
4. Neuromuscular blockade may be required to control ventilation and muscular spasm and to prevent fractures and rhabdomyolysis. In such cases, **vecuronium** (6 to 8 mg/h IV) is the agent of choice because of its minimal cardiovascular side effects. Sedation during neuromuscular blockade is mandatory.
5. The combined α- and β-adrenergic blocking agent, **labetalol** (0.25 to 1 mg/min continuous IV infusion), has been used to treat the manifestation of sympathetic hyperactivity, but it may precipitate myocardial depression. **Magnesium sulfate** (70 mg/kg loading, then 1 to 4 g/h IV) has been advocated as a treatment for this condition. **Morphine sulfate** (0.5 to 1 mg/kg/h is also useful and provides sympathetic control without compromising cardiac output. **Clonidine** (300 μg every 8 hours nasogastrically), an α-receptor agonist, may be helpful in the management of cardiovascular instability.
6. Patients who recover from clinical tetanus *must* undergo active immunization (see Chap. 12 for treatment schedule).

RABIES

Rabies is most commonly fatal and is transmitted by inoculation with infectious saliva or by salivary contact with a break in the skin or mucous membranes.

In the United States, dog and cat bites are the most common reason for implementation of postexposure prophylaxis, but the most important source of active rabies is wildlife transmission. Animal bites contracted outside the United States in an undeveloped country should be considered at high risk for rabies transmission.

Rabid wildlife species include skunks, bats, raccoons, cows, dogs, foxes, and cats. Rodents (squirrels, chipmunks, rats, mice, etc) and lagomorphs (rabbits, hares, and gophers) may be infected by rabies, but no transmission to humans has been documented from these animals. Most rabid animals are agitated and labile, may indiscriminately attack anything that moves, and may wander aimlessly. Feeble bark, drooling, stupor, and convulsions mark more advanced disease preceding death of the animal.

As human rabies has decreased in the United States, the proportion of rabies patients without animal-bite exposure has increased. In 60% of the cases in the 1980s, a source of infection was not identified. Incubation periods average 35 to 64 days; periods as short as 12 days or as long as 700 days have been reported. Most of these cases of cryptic rabies virus exposure are associated with insectivorous bats.

Clinical Features

The initial symptoms of human rabies are nonspecific and last 1 to 4 days: fever, malaise, headache, anorexia, nausea, sore throat, cough, and pain, or paresthesia at the bite site (80%). Subsequently, central nervous system involvement becomes apparent with restlessness and agitation, altered mental status, painful bulbar and peripheral muscular spasms, opisthotonos, and bulbar or focal motor paresis. Alternatively, in 20%, an ascending, symmetric, flaccid, and areflexic paralysis, comparable to the Landry-Guillain-Barré syndrome, may be seen. Hypersensitivity to sensory stimuli and hydrophobia may occur at this stage, with the latter resulting from the sight, sound, swallowing, or even mention of water. Progressively lucid and confused intervals may become interspersed, cholinergic nervous abnormalities may manifest (hyperpyrexia, mydriasis, and increased lacrimation and salivation), and brainstem dysfunction (dysphagia, optic neuritis, and facial palsies) with hyperreflexia may occur. Extensor plantar responses may be positive and may mimic toxidromes and botulism. Common complications include adult respiratory distress syndrome, diabetes insipidus, syndrome of inappropriate secretion of antidiuretic hormone, hypovolemia, electrolyte abnormalities, pneumonia, and cardiogenic shock with hypotension and dysrhythmia from rabies myocarditis. Coma, convulsions, and apnea are the final manifestations of rabid death.

Diagnosis and Differential

The diagnosis of rabies in the emergency department is clinical. A final diagnosis is made by postmortem analysis of brain tissue. Cerebrospinal fluid and serum antibody titers should be sent to a laboratory skilled in rabies antibody analysis. Elevated cerebrospinal fluid protein and a mononuclear pleocytosis are also seen.

The differential diagnosis includes viral or other infectious encephalitis, polio, tetanus, viral process, meningitis, brain abscess, septic cavernous sinus thrombosis, cholinergic poisoning, and the Landry-Guillain-Barré syndrome. The diagnosis is especially difficult without history of exposure but should be considered for patients with a picture of progressive and unexplained encephalitis.

Emergency Department Care and Disposition

The treatment of rabies exposure consists of assessment of risk of rabies, public health and animal control notification, and, if warranted, the administration of specific immunobiological products to protect against rabies.

1. Debridement of devitalized tissue, if any, is important in reducing the viral inoculum. Wounds of special concern should not be sutured because this promotes rabies virus replication.
2. Tetanus should always be considered and primary or reimmunization prophylaxis should be administered (see Chap. 12).
3. **Human rabies immune globulin** is administered only once at the outset of therapy. The dose is 20 IU/kg, with half of the dose (based on tissue vol-

ume constraints) infiltrated locally at the exposure site and the remainder administered intramuscularly.

4. **Human diploid cell vaccine** (HDCV), for active immunization, is available in 2 formulations of the same vaccine. The HDCV can be administered intramuscularly or intradermally in 5 1-mL doses on days 0, 3, 7, 14, and 28. The World Health Organization recommends a sixth dose on day 90, but this is not universally accepted.

5. Human rabies immune globulin and HDCV should be administered in the deltoid muscle rather than in the gluteal area or anterolateral area of the thigh in children due to vaccine failures at the gluteal site, unless the vaccine requires intradermal administration.

6. Ordinarily, domestic dogs and cats with normal behavior are quarantined for 10 days, which is sufficient for the disease to manifest if the animal is infected. If no signs become apparent, the animal can be considered nonrabid. The principal indication for the initiation of prophylaxis is a bite wound by an un-captured dog or cat in an endemic area or a bite wound by an un-captured bat or appropriate species of carnivore in an unprovoked attack.

7. State or local officials should be consulted regarding the possibility of rabies in local animal populations before decisions on initiating rabies prophylaxis are made. This action may not be possible before the first treatment but may affect subsequent treatments. Animal bites should be reported to the local animal control unit or police department so that appropriate animals can be captured or quarantined for observation in a timely fashion.

8. The Centers for Disease Control and state or county health departments can provide assistance in the management of complications. The most current information available on the rabies home page is produced and updated regularly by the Centers for Disease Control at www.cdc.gov/ncidod/dvrd/rabies.

For further reading in *Emergency Medicine: A Comprehensive Study Guide,* 6th ed., see Chap. 146, "Tetanus," by Donna L. Carden; and Chap. 147, "Rabies," by David J. Weber, David Wohl, and William A. Rutala.

92 | Malaria

Gregory S. Hall

Malaria must be considered in any person who has traveled to the tropics and presents with an unexplained febrile illness. Four species of the protozoa *Plasmodium* infect humans: *P vivax, P ovale, P malariae,* and *P falciparum.* The organism is transmitted by the anopheline mosquito bite and travels hematogenously first to the liver, where asexual reproduction occurs (exo-erythrocytic stage). The liver cell ruptures, releasing merozoites that invade erythrocytes, multiply, and cause hemolysis (erythrocytic stage). Malaria also may be transmitted by blood transfusion or passed transplacentally from mother to fetus.

Malaria transmission occurs in large areas of Central and South America, the Caribbean, sub-Saharan Africa, the Indian subcontinent, Southeast Asia, the Middle East, and Oceania (New Guinea, Solomon Islands, etc). More than 50% of all US cases of malaria, including most cases due to *P falciparum,* arise from travel to sub-Saharan Africa. Resistance of *P falciparum* to chloroquine and other drugs including Fansidar (pyrimethamine-sulfadoxine) continues to spread. Strains of *P vivax* with chloroquine resistance recently have been identified. The Centers for Disease Control and Prevention (CDC) has a 24-hour hotline and fax-back service (888-232-3228), which can provide the most recent information on resistance patterns. Alternatively, the CDC Internet site can be accessed at http://www.cdc.gov/travel for information on resistance patterns in various countries and information on malaria prophylaxis and treatment. When in doubt, chloroquine resistance for initial treatment should be assumed.

CLINICAL FEATURES

The incubation period ranges from 1 to 3 weeks. Partial chemoprophylaxis or incomplete immunity can prolong the incubation period to months or even years. The hallmark of malaria is the cyclical recurring febrile paroxysm, with each episode corresponding to hemolysis of infected erythrocytes. With *P falciparum,* hemolysis can be severe because red cells of all ages are affected. Infected red blood cells also lose flexibility and further obstruct the microcirculation, causing tissue anoxia of the lungs, kidneys, brain, and other vital organs. Patients commonly have a prodrome of malaise, myalgias, headache, and low-grade fever and chills. The early manifestations are nonspecific and may resemble viral illness, influenza, or hepatitis. Febrile episodes progress to high fever, severe chills, orthostatic dizziness, and extreme weakness with spontaneous resolution after several hours. The malarial paroxysm—rigor and fever followed by profuse diaphoresis and exhaustion—occurs at regular intervals. The paroxysms may not be present in *P falciparum* malaria.

Physical examination findings are also nonspecific. During a febrile paroxysm, most patients appear acutely ill, with high fever, tachycardia, and tachypnea. Splenomegaly is common. In *P falciparum* infections, hepatomegaly, edema, and icterus often occur. Laboratory features include normocytic normochromic anemia with evidence of hemolysis and thrombocytopenia. The white blood cell count is normal or low.

Complications of malaria can occur rapidly, particularly with *P falciparum.* All forms cause hemolysis and splenomegaly, and splenic rupture may occur.

Hypersplenism with subsequent pancytopenia may be seen in advanced cases. Glomerulonephritis, most often in *P malariae* infections, and nephrotic syndrome may occur. *Plasmodium falciparum* infections are especially virulent and can be rapidly fatal. Cerebral malaria, characterized by somnolence, coma, delirium, and seizures, has a mortality rate greater than 20%. Other life-threatening complications associated with *P falciparum* include noncardiogenic pulmonary edema and metabolic abnormalities, including lactic acidosis and profound hypoglycemia. Blackwater fever is a severe complication seen almost exclusively in *P falciparum* infections, with massive intravascular hemolysis, jaundice, hemoglobinuria (dark urine), and acute renal failure.

DIAGNOSIS AND DIFFERENTIAL

The definitive diagnosis is established by identification of the parasite on Giemsa-stained thin and thick smears of peripheral blood. In early infection, especially *with P falciparum,* parasitemia may be undetectable initially due to intraorgan sequestration. Parasite load in the peripheral circulation fluctuates over time and is highest during an acute rising fever with chills. Therapy should *not* be withheld if malaria is suspected, even though the parasite is not detected on initial blood smears. If plasmodia are not visualized, repeated smears should be taken at least twice daily (preferably during febrile episodes) for 3 days to fully exclude malaria.

Once plasmodia are identified, the smear is also evaluated for the degree of parasitemia (percentage of red blood cells infected), which correlates with prognosis, and which species (in particular *P falciparum*) is present.

EMERGENCY DEPARTMENT CARE AND DISPOSITION

1. If *P falciparum* can be excluded, most patients with adequate home care and oral hydration can be treated as outpatients with close follow-up, including repeated blood smears to assess treatment response. The drug of choice for treatment of infection due to *P vivax, P ovale,* and *P malariae* is chloroquine. Table 92-1 summarizes recommended treatment regimens.
2. Newer agents including mefloquine with or without doxycycline and atovaquone-proguanil are highly effective against chloroquine-resistant plasmodia.
3. Chloroquine has no effect on the exoerythrocytic forms of *P vivax* and *P ovale,* which remain dormant in the liver. Unless treated with primaquine, relapse will occur. Primaquine should be avoided in patients with glucose-6-phosphate dehydrogenase deficiency because of hemolysis.
4. Unless it is certain that a patient could *not* have a chloroquine-resistant case, based on history of geographic exposure, the infection must be assumed to be resistant and treated with 1 of the chloroquine-resistant regimens listed in Table 92-1.
5. Patients with significant hemolysis or with comorbid conditions that can be aggravated by high fevers or hemolysis are best hospitalized, as are infants and pregnant women. *Plasmodium falciparum* infections are best managed in the hospital, as are patients with more than 3% parasitemia.
6. Patients with complications due to *P falciparum* or with high parasitemia but unable to tolerate oral medication should receive intravenous treatment.

TABLE 92-1 Treatment Regimens for Malaria

Clinical setting	Drug	Dosage guidelines Adults	Children
Uncomplicated infection with *P. vivax*, *P. ovale*, *P. malariae*, and chloroquine-sensitive *P. falciparum*	Chloroquine phosphate	1-g load (600-mg base), then 500 mg (300-mg base) in 6 h, then 500 mg (300-mg base) per day for 2 d (total dose 2.5 g)	10-mg/kg base to maximum of 600 mg load, then 5-mg/kg base in 6 h and 5-mg/kg base per day for 2 d
	plus		
	Primaquine phosphate*	26.3-mg load (15-mg base) per day for 14 d on completion of chloroquine therapy	0.3-mg/kg base for 14 d on completion of chloroquine therapy
Uncomplicated infection with chloroquine-resistant *P. falciparum*	Quinine sulfate	650 mg PO tid for 3–7 d	8.3 mg/kg PO tid for 3–7 d
	plus		
	Doxycycline†	100 mg PO bid for 7 d	Contraindicated in children <8 y of age†
	Plus or minus		
	Pyrimethamine-sulfadoxine (fansidar)‡	3 tablets (75 mg/1500 mg) PO × 1 dose	Over 2 months old >50 kg 3 tabs 30–50 kg 2 tabs 15–29 kg 1 tab 10–14 kg $\frac{1}{2}$ tab 4–9 kg $\frac{1}{4}$ tab
	or		
	Mefloquine	750 mg PO initially followed by 500 mg in 6–8 h	10–15 mg/kg base followed by 5–10 mg/kg base in 6–8 h
	plus		
	doxycycline§	See above	See above
	or		

Atovaquone-proguanil (Malarone)	4 tablets adult strength (250/100) daily × 3 d	>40 kg, adult dose 31–40 kg, 3 adult tablets × 3 d 21–30 kg, 2 adult tablets × 3 d 11–20 kg, 1 adult tablet × 3 d
Complicated infection with chloroquine-resistant *Plasmodium falciparum*	Quinidine gluconate	10-mg/kg load over 2 h (maximum, 600 mg), then 0.02 mg/kg/min continuous infusion until patient is stabilized and able to tolerate PO therapy (see above)	Same as adults§
	plus Doxycycline†	100 mg IV q12h until tolerating PO therapy (see above)	Contraindicated in children <8 y of age†

*Terminal treatment for *Plasmodium vivax* and *P. ovale* only

†Clindamycin is an alternate to doxycycline at dose of 10 mg/kg (maximum 900 mg) every 8 hours for 3 to 7 days.

‡Optional; of unlikely value if acquisition occurs with Fansidar resistance.

#Optional; many experts feel comfortable with mefloquine alone.

§Consult an expert in pediatric infectious disease immediately for guidance.

Key: IV = intravenously, PO = oral.

7. Quinidine is the intravenous drug of choice. Parenteral quinidine and quinine can cause severe hypoglycemia. They are also myocardial depressants and are contraindicated in patients with heart disease. Cardiac monitoring is required during administration.
8. Aggressive supportive care should be provided to all hospitalized ill patients, including judicious fluid replacement, correction of metabolic derangements, and advanced support (dialysis, mechanical ventilation, etc).
9. A recently published meta-analysis reported no survival benefit for exchange transfusion as compared with antimalarial chemotherapy.

For further reading in *Emergency Medicine: A Comprehensive Study Guide,* 6th ed., see Chap. 148, "Malaria," by Jeffrey D. Band.

93 | Infections from Helminths

Phillip A. Clement

Parasitic infections are increasingly common in the United States. This is due to immigration from Asia, Africa, and Latin America; to increased travel by US citizens to the developing world; and to the rise of parasitic infections among immunosuppressed individuals. Parasitic diseases are a significant cause of morbidity and mortality worldwide and may be acquired through the consumption of infected food or water, walking barefoot on contaminated soil, and from insect bites. The agents that cause parasitic diseases belong to 3 major groups: helminths (worms), protozoa, and arthropods. This chapter reviews infections from helminths. For more information concerning the treatment of parasitic disease, see the Web site of the Centers for Disease Control and Prevention: www.cdc.gov/ncidod/diseases/list_parasites.

CLINICAL FEATURES

Parasitic diseases present with a wide variety of symptoms (Table 93-1) and may be acute or chronic. Presentations range from common complaints, such as headache, fever, cough, and malaise, to life-threatening complications, such as seizures, hemoptysis, melena, and intestinal obstruction.

DIAGNOSIS AND DIFFERENTIAL

Parasites flourish in warm, moist climates with poor sanitation and nutrition. Information about travel to or immigration from high-risk areas should be sought. Children are more often infected than adults because of their poor hygiene, oral behavior, and inability to ward off arthropod vectors. The diagnosis is complicated by the fact that the latent period between exposure and symptoms may be months to years. Parasitic disease should be considered in any patient with fever, abdominal pain, persistent or bloody diarrhea, skin rash, ulcers, or eosinophilia. Most helminth infections can be diagnosed by testing the stool for ova and parasites. *Ascaris lumbricoides, Necator americanus, Ancylostoma duodenale,* and *Strongyloides stercoralis* larvae may be found in the sputum. For pinworms, a cellophane tape anal swab is the most useful test. The larvae of *Strongyloides* may be detected via duodenal aspirate. Eosinophilia is present in most helminth infections. The enzyme-linked immunosorbent assay (ELISA) technique can be used to make a serologic diagnosis of many parasitic infections.

EMERGENCY DEPARTMENT CARE AND DISPOSITION

1. Patients who are dehydrated from gastrointestinal losses or fever should receive intravenous hydration.
2. Those patients who appear severely ill or toxic, those who cannot tolerate anything by mouth, those with significant dehydration, and those with multiple organ system involvement (eg, lung, blood, or central nervous system [CNS]) should be admitted for intravenous hydration, further diagnostic evaluation, and antiparasitic drug treatment, as indicated.
3. For treatment of specific helminths, see below.

TABLE 93-1 Common Symptoms of Helminth Infections*

Symptom	Possible cause
Abdominal pain	*Ascaris*, hookworm, *Trichuris*, *Schistosoma*, *Clonorchis*, *Fasciola*, *Taenia*, *Hymenolepis*, *Diphyllobothrium*
Anemia	*Diphyllobothrium*, hookworm, *Trichuris*
CNS symptoms	*Hymenolepis*, *Trichinella*, *Paragonimus*, *Echinococcus*, *Tanenia solium*, *Toxocara*, *Strongyloides*
Diarrhea	Hookworms, *Strongloides*, *Trichuris*, *Trichinella*, *Schistosoma*, *Fasciola*, *Fasciolopsis*, *Taenia*, *Hymenolepis*
Eosinophilia	*Strongyloides*, hookworms, *Trichuris*, *Drancunculus*, *Fasciola*, *Toxocara*, *Ascaris*, *Trichinella*, filariae, *(Wuchereria bancrofti, Brugia malayi) Hymenolepis*, *Schistosoma*, fluke, *Paragonimus westermani*, *C sinensis, Fasciolopsis buski), Taenia*
Fever	*Ascaris*, *Toxocara*, hookworms, *Trichuris*, *Trichinella*, filariae *(W bancrofti)*, *Schistosoma*, fluke *(C sinensis)*, *Fasciola*
Hepatomegaly	*Toxocara*, *Schistosoma*, fluke *(C sinensis, Opisthorchis viverrini, Fasciola)*, tapeworm *(Echinococcus)*
Intestinal obstruction	*Ascaris*, *Strongyloides*, fluke *(F buski)*, *Taenia*, *Diphyllobothrium*
Jaundice	Fluke *(C sinensis, O viverrini)*, *Fasciola*
Cardiac symptoms	*Taenia*, *Trichinella*
Nausea and vomiting	*Ascaris*, *Trichuris*, *Trichinella*, *Taenia*
Ocular disease	Filariae *(Onchocerca volvulus)*, *Taenia*, *Trichinella*, *Toxocara canis*, *Ascaris*, hookworm, *Echinococcus*
Pruritus	*Enterobius*, *Trichuris*, filariae *(O volvulus)*
Pulmonary symptoms	*Ascaris*, filariae *(W bancrofti, B malayi)*, fluke *(P westermani)*, hookworms, *Strongyloides*, *Trichinella*, *Paragonimus*, *Echinococcus*, *Toxocara*
Dermatological symptoms	*Dracunculus*, hookworm *(Ancylostoma duodenale)*, *Toxocara*, *Schistosoma*, *Ascaris*, *Strongyloides*, *Trichinella*, *Fasciola*, *Trichinella*

*For more information, see the Web site of the Centers for Disease Control and Prevention: www.cdc.gov/ncidod/diseases/list_parasites.
Key: CNS = central nervous system.

HELMINTHS

Helminths are multicellular worms and include nematodes (roundworms), trematodes (flukes), and cestodes (flatworms).

Nematodes (Roundworms)

Nematodes are cylindrical, unsegmented, elongated white worms. Humans are infected by egg ingestion, penetration through the skin, or inoculation by insect bite. The intestinal nematodes include hookworm, roundworm, and whipworm, in which a soil phase is needed for fecally passed eggs to develop.

These infections occur in areas of poor sanitation. Pinworm eggs are infectious when excreted, thus facilitating person-to-person spread. The tissue nematodes include filariae, arthropod-borne worms that induce lymphatic, ocular, and skin diseases.

Ascaris lumbricoides

Ascaris has a worldwide distribution. Infection is by the ingestion of eggs. Larvae migrate through the lungs and mature in the small intestines. Adult worms are 25 to 35 cm in length. Eggs are passed via feces. Clinical disease is due to pulmonary hypersensitivity or intestinal complications. During the lung phase, patients may develop pulmonary infiltrates, fever, cough, dyspnea, hemoptysis, and eosinophilia. Adult worms in the gut may be asymptomatic or may cause abdominal pain and lead to intestinal obstruction in heavy infections. This is especially true in children. Worm migration into the biliary tract may cause biliary obstruction and pancreatitis. The diagnosis is made by finding eggs or an adult worm in the stool. Chest radiograph may show eosinophilic pneumonitis (Loeffler syndrome). Serologic tests may be helpful. Treatment is with oral (PO) **mebendazole** 100 mg twice a day for 3 days, **albendazole** 400 mg PO once, or **pyrantel pamoate** 11 mg/kg PO once up to 1 g. Intestinal obstruction may necessitate surgery.

Enterobius vermicularis (Pinworm)

Enterobius infection is most prevalent in temperate climates during the winter and fall and most often affects children. Infection is by the ingestion of eggs.

Adult pinworms are small (2-5 mm) and reside in the cecum, appendix, ileum, and ascending colon. The gravid female migrates to the anus, especially at night, depositing eggs and causing intense pruritus. Autoinfection with hand-to-mouth transmission occurs after scratching. Organisms often can be seen by direct examination of the anus. The diagnosis is confirmed by finding eggs on a cellophane tape swab of the anus. Eosinophilia is usually absent. All close household contacts should be examined and treated. Treatment consists of **pyrantel pamoate** 11 mg/kg PO once up to 1 g, **mebendazole** 100 mg PO once, or **albendazole** 400 mg PO once. Treatment must be repeated in 2 weeks.

Strongyloides stercoralis (Threadworm)

Infection is through skin penetration by filariform larvae. Adult threadworms reside in the small intestine but migrate through the lungs. Entry of the parasite through the skin can lead to allergic manifestations causing pruritus and an erythematous rash. Cough, dyspnea, and pneumonitis may occur from migration through lung parenchyma. The intestinal phase may produce abdominal pain, diarrhea with mucus and blood, and eosinophilia. Diagnosis is made by finding larvae in the stool, duodenal contents, or sputum. An ELISA test is also available. An upper gastrointestinal series may show a deformed duodenal bulb and *may* be confused with ulcer disease. Treatment consists of **ivermectin** 200 μg/kg/d PO for 1 to 2 days or **thiabendazole** 50 mg/kg/d in 2 doses (maximum, 3 g/d) for 2 days.

Necator americanus, Ancylostoma duodenale (Hookworm)

Hookworms prevail in the southern United States and are often seen in immigrants from warmer climates. Infection is by filariform larval migration through the skin and is associated with the use of human feces as fertilizer, the lack of shoes, and the lack of latrines. Obligate larval lung migration occurs before the organism matures in the intestinal mucosa. Infection through the skin may induce rash. There may be pulmonary and gastrointestinal symptoms as the worms migrate. Patients may have cough, low-grade fever, abdominal pain, diarrhea, weakness, weight loss, heme-positive stools, and eosinophilia. This worm also ingests blood, leading to iron-deficiency anemia. Pica and geophagy are often seen in infected children. The diagnosis is made by finding ova in the stool. Cutaneous larva migrans is a related infection due to the larvae of *Ancylostoma braziliense* (dog or cat hookworm). Larval migration through the skin causes pruritus and a rash described as the "creeping eruption." Treatment is the same as for *Ascaris* (above).

Trichuris trichiura (Whipworm)

Trichuris trichiura is most common in the rural south of the United States and occurs most often in children who play in the soil. Infection is by the ingestion of eggs. Adult worms reside in the cecum and reach 3 to 5 cm in length. Symptoms are usually gastrointestinal. Patients may complain of anorexia, insomnia, abdominal pain, fever, flatulence, bloody diarrhea, weight loss, and pruritus. There may be an associated eosinophilia and microcytic hypochromic anemia. Large infections can cause tenesmus, colitis, or rectal prolapse in children. The diagnosis is made by finding ova in the stool. Treatment is as for *Ascaris* (above).

Trichinella spiralis

Trichinosis occurs in Mexico and the United States and results from the ingestion of pork, bear, or walrus meat containing encysted larvae. Symptoms depend on the parasite load and on the site of invasion and may include nausea, vomiting, diarrhea, urticaria, headache, muscle weakness, fever, stiff neck, CNS manifestations, and psychiatric disturbances. Patients may present with acute myocarditis, nonsuppurative meningitis, bronchopneumonia, or catarrhal enteritis. The triad of periorbital edema, diffuse myalgias, and eosinophilia strongly suggests trichinosis. Pathognomonic splinter hemorrhages and subconjunctival hemorrhages also may occur. The diagnosis may be confirmed serologically. Stool specimens are helpful only early in the infection course, ie, during the gastrointestinal stage. Laboratory manifestations of trichinosis include leukocytosis, eosinophilia, elevated creatine phosphokinase, and electrocardiographic changes. Most cases are mild and resolve with only symptomatic treatment. **Mebendazole** 200 to 400 mg PO 3 times a day for 3 days and then 400 to 500 mg PO 3 times a day for 10 days is indicated for the intestinal phase but may not be effective after encystment. Steroids are indicated for severe infections, such as CNS disease and myocarditis, but are not advocated routinely because their use can increase the number of circulating larvae.

Blood and Tissue Nematodes (Filariae)

Transmission is by an arthropod vector (usually fly or mosquito). The larval stages are microscopic and are found in the cutaneous tissues or the blood.

Treatment is with diethylcarbamazine or ivermectin.

Trematodes (Flukes)

Trematodes are leaflike, symmetrical flatworms possessing a ventral sucker to hold their position. They are found in the tropics and require intermediate hosts such as snails, crabs, or fish. Trematodes shed their eggs from the human host in the feces, urine, or sputum.

Schistosomiasis

Schistosomiasis is the most common fluke-borne illness. *Schistosoma mansoni, Schistosoma japonicum,* and *Schistosoma haematobium* have freshwater snails as intermediate hosts. Cercariae, the larval form, live freely in freshwater and directly penetrate the skin, thereby inducing dermatitis. Pathology is caused by inflammation induced by the eggs. Acute disease may include fever, diarrhea, abdominal pain, melena, cough, hematemesis, lymphadenopathy, hepatosplenomegaly, urticaria, and eosinophilia. Chronic disease occurs from egg deposition in the bladder, intestines, and liver, leading to portal hypertension, ascites, liver failure, and obstructive hydroureter. Adults of *S mansoni* and *S japonicum* reside in mesenteric veins. Eggs are usually passed in the stool. Adults of *S haematobium* reside in vesical, prostatic, and uterine plexuses. Eggs may be found in urine. The diagnosis is suggested by a positive immunofluorescent antibody test and confirmed by finding eggs in the feces or urine or on rectal biopsy. Treatment consists of **praziquantel** 40 to 60 mg/kg/d PO in 2 to 3 doses for 1 day.

Cestodes (Flatworms)

The cestodes are flatworms commonly referred to as *tapeworms.* They have a scolex, or head, equipped with suckers, or hooks. Cestodes grow by segmentation, extending proglottids from the neck.

Hymenolepis nana (Dwarf Tapeworm)

Hymenolepis nana is the most common tapeworm in the United States and occurs most often in children and institutionalized patients. Transmission is by the ingestion of eggs. Symptoms are mild and may include diarrhea and abdominal discomfort. Treatment is with **praziquantel** 25 mg/kg PO once.

Taenia saginata (Beef Tapeworm)

Infection is by the consumption of raw beef containing cysticercus larvae. Adult worms live in the small intestine and may reach 9 m in length. Infections may be asymptomatic or may cause gastrointestinal distress, abdominal pain, and weight loss. Diagnosis is by stool examination for proglottids. Treatment is with **praziquantel** 10 mg/kg PO once.

Taenia solium (Pork Tapeworm)

Taenia solium is encountered primarily in immigrants or visitors from Central America or the Middle East. Infection is by the ingestion of raw or undercooked pork containing cysticercus larvae or by the ingestion of food or water containing eggs. Infected patients may be asymptomatic or may present with nausea and vomiting, headache, abdominal pain, pruritus, constipation, diarrhea, and intestinal obstruction. The larval stage produces the clinical disease cysticercosis and may lead to seizures and hydrocephalus. Cysticercosis should be considered in patients from endemic areas with new onset seizures or other neurologic symptoms. Radiographs of the soft tissues may show curvilinear calcifications indicative of cysts. Cysts also may be seen in the meninges and brain parenchyma on computed tomography. The diagnosis is made by finding gravid proglottids in the stool. An ELISA or hemagglutination reaction may be helpful, but results of both can be falsely negative if the cysts are calcified. Treatment of the adult (intestinal) stage is with **praziquantel** 10 mg/kg PO once. The larval (tissue) stage is treated with **albendazole.** For cysticercosis, **albendazole** 15 mg/kg/d PO in 2 to 3 doses for 8 to 30 days or **praziquantel** 50 mg/kg/d PO in 3 doses for 15 days is recommended. Adjunctive surgery also may be necessary to remove cysts.

Diphyllobothrium

This fish tapeworm, *Diphyllobothrium latum,* occurs in people who eat raw, larvae-encysted fish (eg, sushi, sashimi, and gefilte fish). Patients may be asymptomatic or exhibit mild gastrointestinal symptoms. Pernicious anemia may occur, presumably by competition by the worm with the host for vitamin B_{12}.

Treatment is the same as for *Taenia saginata.*

For further reading in *Emergency Medicine: A Comprehensive Study Guide,* 6th ed., see Chap. 149, "Common Parasitic Infections," by Harold H. Osborn.

94 | Zoonotic Infections

Gregory S. Hall

Zoonoses are those diseases and infections that are naturally transmitted between vertebrate animals and humans by direct contact with an infected animal or animal product, by ingestion of contaminated water or food products, by inhalation, or through arthropod vectors. Pets, farm animals, and common wildlife are the primary reservoirs, and arthropods, in particular ticks, are the primary vectors. These diseases may be caused by a myriad of organisms including bacteria, viruses, *Rickettsia,* and parasites. The high morbidity and mortality rates often associated with these illnesses mandate their careful consideration in patients who present with fever, chills, myalgias, rash, and other nonspecific symptoms. In such cases, specific risk factors for zoonotic infection should always be sought, namely exposure to household pets; domesticated and nondomesticated animals; recent travel or residence in rural areas or underdeveloped countries; dressing, skinning, or handling animal skins or raw flesh; animal bites or scratches; or ingestion of animal or dairy products. In the United States, where most zoonoses have a higher incidence in spring and summer, ticks are the most prolific agents of disease transmission. Unfortunately, many patients with tick-acquired infections do not give a history of recent tick bite; hence, clinical suspicion should remain high for patients in endemic areas.

LYME DISEASE

Lyme disease remains the most common vector-borne zoonotic infection in the United States, with approximately 15,000 cases reported annually. Cases have been reported in all 48 continental states, but the highest prevalence remains the northeastern region of the United States. The spirochete *Borrelia burgdorferi* is responsible for this disease via transmission by bite of the *Ixode*s species ticks. Small mammals (eg, rabbits and rodents) and deer serve as host reservoirs in the wild. Fewer than 33% of patients can recall a tick bite.

Clinical Features

Lyme disease is a multiorgan infection that is typically divided into 3 distinct stages. Not all patients progress through all 3 stages, stages may overlap, and there are often remissions between stages. The hallmark of stage I is erythema migrans (EM), an annular erythematous skin rash with central clearing, which forms at the site of the tick bite, usually 2 to 20 days after the bite. It is the most common manifestation of Lyme disease, occurring in 60% to 80% of cases and results from local vasculitis. Untreated, the EM lesion may persist for 3 to 4 weeks, resolve spontaneously, but then may recur in the secondary stage.

Stage II corresponds to dissemination of the spirochete within a few days to 6 months after initial infection, and results in multiple secondary annular red skin lesions (EM), fever, lymphadenopathy, arthralgias, splenomegaly, cardiac abnormalities, and flulike symptoms. Approximately 15% of untreated stage II patients develop neurologic disease, including headache, meningoencephalitis, and, most commonly, cranial neuritis, ie, often a

437

uni- or bilateral facial nerve palsy. In addition, other peripheral neuropathies can develop, in addition to asymmetric oligoarticular arthritis, usually of the large joints. Cardiac disease is seen in 8% of patients: they may develop first-, second-, or third-degree atrioventricular nodal block or myopericarditis.

Stage III represents chronic persistent infection, occurs years after initial infection, and includes chronic arthritis, myocarditis, subacute encephalopathy, axonal polyneuropathy, and leukoencephalopathy. Chronic arthritis usually takes the form of brief, recurrent episodes of migratory oligoarthritis, most commonly affecting (in declining order of frequency) the knee, shoulder, temporomandibular joint, ankle, wrist, hip, and small joints of the hands and feet.

Diagnosis and Differential

Diagnosis initially must rely on clinical features. Confirmation may be obtained via polymerase chain reaction testing, polyvalent fluorescence immunoassay, or western immunoblot testing.

Emergency Department Care and Disposition

Lyme disease generally responds well to antimicrobial therapy, if begun early in the course.

1. For early Lyme disease (stage I or II), antimicrobials should be given for 10 to 21 days. Treatment regimens may include **doxycycline** 100 mg orally (PO) twice daily, **amoxicillin** 500 mg PO 3 times daily, **cefuroxime** 500 mg PO twice daily, **clarithromycin** 500 mg PO twice daily, **azithromycin** 250 mg PO daily, or parenteral daily **ceftriaxone** 1 g.
2. Bell palsy, mild arthritis, or mild cardiac manifestations may be managed similarly to EM rash by using oral doxycycline or amoxicillin (preferred in children).
3. Serious central nervous system disease (eg, meningitis, encephalitis, encephalopathy, or neuropathy), serious cardiac manifestations, or severe arthritis is probably best managed by hospital admission for supportive care and a 14- to 21-day course of intravenous (IV) ceftriaxone or penicillin G and possibly further continuation of oral therapy to complete 28 to 60 days of treatment.
4. Late stage III disease may not respond to even aggressive IV antimicrobial therapy.
5. A recombinant vaccine is commercially available with an efficacy of 76% and is given at 0, 1, and 12 months, with subsequent booster immunization every 1 to 3 years. It is recommended for high-risk individuals between ages 15 and 70 years who live in, work in, or repeatedly visit very high-risk areas and have frequent or prolonged exposure to *Ixodes scapularis* ticks.
6. Timely consultation with an infectious disease expert and the patient's primary physician are strongly recommended for any patient with suspected Lyme disease. Close follow-up is crucial for any patient who will be treated as an outpatient.

ROCKY MOUNTAIN SPOTTED FEVER

Rocky Mountain spotted fever (RMSF), the most frequently reported rickettsial zoonosis in the United States, is caused by *Rickettsia rickettsii,* a pleomorphic obligate intracellular coccobacillus. *Dermacentor* species ticks serve as the primary vector, with deer, rodents, horses, cattle, cats, and dogs as the usual animal hosts. Ninety-five percent of cases reported occur between April 1 and September 30, with two thirds of cases reported in children younger than 15 years. The highest incidence of RMSF appears to occur in the mid-Atlantic states, but cases have been reported in the majority of continental states.

Clinical Features

RSMF affects multiple organ systems, and most patients develop moderate to severe symptoms unless treated early. A triad of fever, rash, and history of tick exposure have classically defined RMSF. Unfortunately, only about 50% of infected patients can recall a tick bite. The incubation period is usually 4 to 10 days, followed by abrupt or insidious onset of symptoms. Initial findings that are nonspecific, can lead to misdiagnosis, and include fever, malaise, severe headache, myalgias, nausea, vomiting, diarrhea, anorexia, abdominal pain, and photophobia. Other signs or symptoms that may develop are lymphadenopathy, hepatosplenomegaly, conjunctivitis, confusion, meningismus, renal and respiratory failure, and myocarditis.

Rash, the hallmark feature of RMSF, usually develops within the first 2 weeks of illness, often between the third and fifth days. Initially the rash is maculopapular and typically begins on the extremities on the hands, feet, wrists, and ankles (and may involve palms or soles) and spreads centripetally up the trunk, usually sparing the face. Rash may be absent in about 20% of patients with "spotless RMSF"; most often this occurs in African Americans, the elderly, and severe fatal cases. Gastrointestinal symptoms are often prominent features and may precede the onset of rash, leading to misdiagnosis of gastroenteritis or even acute abdomen. Pneumonitis, a common and potentially fatal complication, typically presents with cough, dyspnea, pulmonary edema, and systemic hypoxia. Serious neurologic involvement may occur in 23% to 28% of cases, with symptoms including confusion, stupor, ataxia, coma, and seizures. The pathophysiology of RMSF is a vasculitis; as a consequence, the initial maculopapular rash often evolves into a petechial or purpuric rash. Late sequelae can include disseminated intravascular coagulopathy and the loss of circulation to extremities requiring amputation, similar to the sequelae seen with meningococcemia.

Diagnosis and Differential

Early recognition of RMSF is crucial because mortality rates are nearly 0 for patients treated before the sixth day of illness, whereas untreated patients may have up to 25% mortality. Thus, a high index of clinical suspicion must be maintained, especially because the early symptoms are often nonspecific and the characteristic rash, which aids in the diagnosis, may be absent. Laboratory abnormalities are nonspecific and may include a normal or elevated white blood cell count, thrombocytopenia, elevated liver function tests, hyponatremia, and cerebrospinal fluid (CSF) pleocytosis with elevated protein levels. Chest radiograph may be normal or may show diffuse interstitial infiltrates and pleural effusions. Serologic tests may help confirm RMSF; however, because results do not reliably become positive until 6 to 10 days *after* the onset of symptoms, the diagnosis must be made on clinical grounds to ensure correct early therapy. RMSF can be confirmed with a rise in antibody titer between acute and convalescent sera or via skin biopsy of the rash with immunofluorescence antibody testing (however, negative skin biopsy results do not exclude RMSF). The differential diagnosis includes viral illnesses (eg, measles, rubella, hepatitis, mononucleosis, encephalitis, or enteroviral exanthem), gastroenteritis, acute abdomen, disseminated gonorrhea, meningitis (meningococcus), secondary syphilis, leptospirosis, pneumonia, typhoid fever, and streptococcal infection (pharyngitis with rash).

Emergency Department Care and Disposition

1. Early therapy with appropriate antimicrobials produces a dramatic reduction in mortality rates from RMSF.

2. Appropriate therapy for adults includes **doxycycline** 100 mg PO twice daily, **tetracycline** 500 mg PO 4 times daily, or **chloramphenicol** 50 to 75 mg/kg/d IV in 4 divided doses.

3. Appropriate therapy for children weighing less than 45 kg, or 100 lb, includes **doxycycline** 4.4 mg/kg/d PO in 2 divided doses on day 1 and then 2.2 mg/kg/d in 2 divided doses thereafter. Alternatives include **tetracycline** 30 to 40 mg/kg/d PO in 4 divided doses for children older than 8 years and **chloramphenicol** 100 mg/kg/d (3 g maximum) IV in 4 divided doses. Doxycycline has been used for short courses in children without significant staining of the teeth, but these cosmetic risks must be balanced against the potentially serious adverse effects of chloramphenicol (myelosuppression). It would be prudent to discuss these risks with the parents and primary care physicians at the onset of therapy to reach a consensus on treatment.

4. Antimicrobial therapy is generally recommended for 7 to 14 days and continued until the patient is afebrile and clinically improving for at least 2 days.

5. Hospital admission for IV doxycycline, tetracycline, or chloramphenicol is strongly recommended for any patient with nausea, vomiting, or significant systemic disease. Seriously ill patients often require aggressive supportive care and careful attention to fluid and electrolyte imbalances. Those discharged home should have close follow-up to ensure their clinical improvement.

WEST NILE VIRUS ENCEPHALITIS

Clinical Features

The West Nile virus (WNV) was first seen in the western hemisphere in 1999. The mode of transmission involves mosquitoes of the *Culex* species, with infected birds such as crows, raven, and jays serving as the natural animal reservoirs. Transmission to humans and other vertebrates occurs when carrier mosquitoes bite and take a blood meal. The incubation period varies from 3 to 15 days. Approximately 20% of patients bitten develop fever and a flulike illness, ie, "West Nile fever." The classic presentation is a mild dengue-like illness of sudden onset with fever, lymphadenopathy, headache, abdominal pain, vomiting, rash, conjunctivitis, eye pain, and anorexia. Duration is typically from 3 to 6 days. Meningoencephalitis occurs in about 1 in 150 patients and is more common than viral meningitis. Immunocompromised patients (those with human immunodeficiency virus, tuberculosis, malaria, etc) and those of advanced age are at greatest risk for meningoencephalitis. Complaints of weakness out of proportion to physical examiantion findings are common, and myoclonus is a nearly universal finding. Complete flaccid paralysis may occur and can be easily confused with Guillain-Barré syndrome. Other neurologic findings include parkinsonian-like signs, ataxia, extrapyramidal signs, cranial nerve abnormalities, myelitis, optic neuritis, and seizures.

Diagnosis and Differential

Laboratory findings may include a normal or slightly elevated white blood cell count during the complete blood count, hyponatremia (especially with encephalitis), CSF protein elevation with normal glucose, and CSF lymphocytosis. Brain computed tomography is often normal, although progression to meningoencephalitis cerebral edema may be seen. Diagnosis is made by identifying WNV-specific immunoglobulin (Ig) M antibody in the serum or CSF. IgM-specific antibody is an acute phase identifier that can persist in the serum for up to 12 months postinfection. IgG WNV-specific antibody is found in the convalescent phase in serum and CSF. Polymerase chain reaction testing is still in an experimental stage.

Emergency Department Care and Disposition

1. Treatment is entirely supportive, and the decision to admit rests entirely on the severity of clinical symptoms and the age and overall condition of the patient.
2. Close follow-up should be arranged for any patient discharged from the emergency department with suspected WNV infection.

TICK PARALYSIS

Clinical Features

Tick paralysis, a relatively uncommon disease, is important to recognize because it is potentially fatal yet easily cured. It is thought to be caused by a neurotoxic venom secreted from female tick salivary glands, which produce a conduction block at the motor end plate of peripheral nerves. *Dermacentor* species ticks have been the usual vector. Incidence is highest in spring to late summer, with children most commonly affected. Symptoms usually begin within 4 to 7 days after attachment by the female tick. An initial prodrome of malaise, irritability, restlessness, and paresthesias of the hand or foot is followed by a symmetrical, ascending, flaccid paralysis similar to that of Guillain-Barré syndrome. Fever is generally absent. Loss of deep tendon reflexes, difficulty swallowing, and involuntary eye movements also may occur, but sensation remains intact. Poor coordination and ataxia may indicate cerebellar involvement. In severe untreated cases, respiratory paralysis may lead to death.

Diagnosis and Differential

Diagnosis requires recognition of the clinical features and the discovery of an attached tick.

Emergency Department Care and Disposition

1. Patients should be searched carefully for ticks, including the entire scalp. Prompt and careful removal of the tick leads to cure, with most patients experiencing complete recovery within 48 to 72 hours.

2. Aggressive supportive care, especially ventilatory support, is indicated for patients with respiratory compromise before tick removal.

TULAREMIA

Clinical Features

Tularemia (rabbit skinner's disease) is caused by *Francisella tularensis,* a small, gram-negative coccobacillus. Principal zoonotic vectors are ticks of the *Dermacentor* and *Amblyomma* species and the deerfly. Natural animal reservoirs include rabbits and hares, deer, muskrats, beavers, and some domestic animals. Although widely reported throughout the continental United States, the highest incidence of tularemia occurs in Arkansas, Missouri, and Oklahoma. Cases can occur year round but may be more common in early winter in adults and early summer in children. Methods of transmission include tick or deerfly bites; animal bites; inoculation of broken skin, conjunctiva, or oral mucosa by blood or tissue from an infected host; and handling or ingestion of contaminated meat, soil, grain, hay, or water.

The average incubation period is 3 to 5 days, followed by sudden onset of fever, chills, headache, anorexia, malaise, and fatigue. Myalgias, cough, vomiting, pharyngitis, abdominal pain, and diarrhea also may develop. Fever often persists for several days, remits briefly, and then recurs. Clinical features at presentation depend on the route of inoculation. Ulceroglandular fever, the most common syndrome, follows tick bites or animal contact and is characterized by a papule at the bite site, which evolves into a tender, necrotic ulcer with painful regional adenopathy. Glandular tularemia consists of tender regional adenopathy without a skin lesion. Oculoglandular tularemia results in a painful conjunctivitis and in periauricular, submandibular, and cervical adenopathy. Pharyngeal tularemia, acquired from ingestion of contaminated food or water, presents with exudative pharyngitis or tonsillitis. Typhoidal tularemia may occur with any form of transmission and includes diarrhea, myalgias, hepatosplenomegaly, cough, and pneumonitis. Tularemic pneumonitis can occur via inhalation of the organism, with no signs or symptoms or a productive cough, pleuritic chest pain, rales, consolidation, and pleural rub.

Laboratory findings are nonspecific for all forms of tularemia, and the key to diagnosis rests on the clinical features coupled with a history of potential exposure. Serologic studies (enzyme-linked immunosorbent assay) to determine acute and convalescent titers or culture from blood, wounds, lymph nodes, or sputum may confirm the diagnosis. The multiple clinical variations of tularemia lead to a broad differential diagnosis that must include pyogenic bacterial infection, syphilis, anthrax, plague, Q fever, psittacosis, typhoid, brucellosis, and rickettsial infection. Tularemia has the potential to be used as a biologic "weapon of mass destruction" through contamination of water supplies or food sources.

Emergency Department Care and Disposition

1. Preferred therapy includes **streptomycin** 7.5 to 10 mg/kg every 12 hours intramuscularly (IM) or IV for 7 to 14 days. The pediatric dose is 30 to 40 mg/kg IM or IV in 2 divided doses for 7 days.
2. Alternatives include **gentamicin** 3 to 5 mg/kg/d IV divided every 8 hours for 7 to 14 days. Chloramphenicol may be added if meningitis is

suspected. Other potentially effective agents include tobramycin, doxycycline, ciprofloxacin, and azithromycin.

3. A live, attenuated vaccine is available for research workers and laboratory personnel. Patients with isolated skin lesions who are not systemically ill may be treated as outpatients with oral antimicrobials but must have very close follow-up to ensure recovery.

4. Any patient with systemic illness, and particularly if the diagnosis is uncertain, is probably best admitted to the hospital for antimicrobial therapy, supportive care, and consultation with an infectious disease specialist.

EHRLICHIOSIS

Clinical Features

Ehrlichia are small, gram-negative coccobacilli that infect circulating leukocytes. Animal reservoirs include deer, dogs, and other mammals, with *Ixodes* and *Amblyomma* species ticks serving as vectors. Approximately 90% of patients report a tick bite within the 3 weeks before symptom onset, and the incubation period varies from 1 to 21 days (median, 7 days). Characteristic clinical features are consistent with a nonspecific febrile illness, including high fever, headache, nausea, vomiting, malaise, abdominal pain, anorexia, and myalgias. In 20% of cases, a maculopapular or petechial rash develops which only infrequently involves the palms or soles and occurs in the initial stage of illness. A minority of patients progress to serious complications that may include renal failure, respiratory failure, disseminated intravascular coagulopathy, cardiomegaly, encephalitis, and seizures.

Diagnosis and Differential

Laboratory findings are most prominent after 5 to 7 days of illness and may include leukocytopenia, thrombocytopenia, and liver dysfunction. Rarely, CSF pleocytosis is seen. Diagnosis initially must be made on clinical grounds but may be confirmed with an indirect immunofluorescent antibody test on serum. A 4-fold rise or an increase in antibody titer between acute and convalescent phases of the illness suggests the diagnosis. The differential diagnosis includes the other rickettsial diseases and bacterial meningitis.

Emergency Department Care and Disposition

1. Treatment consists of **doxycycline** 100 mg PO or IV twice daily for 7 to 14 days. Tetracycline is an acceptable alternative.

2. There is no current alternative recommendation for children or in pregnancy.

COLORADO TICK FEVER

Clinical Features

Colorado tick fever is an acute viral illness caused by an RNA virus of the *Coltivirus* species, with *Dermacentor* species ticks serving as the vector. Most cases occur between late May and early July in the mountainous western regions of the United States. Symptoms begin suddenly 3 to 6 days after a tick bite and include fever, chills, severe headache, photophobia, and myalgias. Symptoms usually persist for 5 to 8 days and then spontaneously remit. Fifty percent of patients experience a secondary phase, with return of symptoms, usually 3 days after initial remission. The secondary phase lasts 2 to 4 days and may be accompanied by transient, generalized maculopapular, or petechial rash.

Diagnosis and Differential

Diagnosis must be suspected by clinical features but may be confirmed with serologic studies or isolation of the virus from blood or CSF that is inoculated into suckling mice. Laboratory abnormalities may include leukocytosis and thrombocytopenia. The differential diagnosis includes meningitis and rickettsial infections.

Emergency Department Care and Disposition

1. No specific therapy exists, and supportive care usually is sufficient. Recovery is spontaneous, typically within 3 weeks.
2. Empiric antimicrobial therapy to cover other potential diagnoses (especially *Rickettsia* and bacterial meningitis) pending serologic confirmation is prudent.

ANTHRAX

Clinical Features

Anthrax, although extremely rare in North America, remains a significant threat, in part because of its potential as an agent of biological warfare. Anthrax is an acute bacterial infection caused by *Bacillus anthracis,* an aerobic gram-positive rod that forms central oval spores. (Oxygen is required for sporulation but not for germination of the spores.) In nature, the disease is seen most commonly in domestic herbivores (cattle, sheep, horses, and goats) and wild herbivores. Human infection can result from inhalation of spores, inoculation of broken skin, arthropod bite (fleas), or ingestion of inadequately cooked, infected meat.

Inhaled or pulmonic anthrax usually results from handling unsterilized, imported animal hides or imported raw wool. It results in a mediastinitis, rather than in true pneumonia, and is universally fatal. Initial presentation consists of flulike symptoms, which progress over 3 to 4 days to include marked mediastinal and hilar edema and respiratory failure. Cutaneous anthrax (woolsorter's disease) accounts for 95% of infections seen in United States. It begins with a small red macule at the site of inoculation, which progresses over 1 week's time through papular, vesicular, or pustular forms to result in an ulcer with a black eschar and adjacent brawny edema. Once fully developed, it may be painless and it typically sloughs off spontaneously in about 2 weeks and spontaneously heals in most cases. A small minority of untreated patients develops rapidly fatal bacteremia. Gastrointestinal anthrax exhibits various symptoms such as fever, nausea, vomiting, abdominal pain, bloody diarrhea, ascites, pharyngitis, and tonsillitis.

Diagnosis and Differential

Gram stain, direct fluorescent antibody stain, or culture of skin lesions or fluid from vesicle may establish the diagnosis. Blood cultures may also be positive. Laboratory abnormalities may include normal leukocyte counts in mild cases or leukocytosis. Sera also may be tested for antibody to *B anthracis.*

Emergency Department Care and Disposition

1. Treatment consists of **ciprofloxacin** 750 mg PO twice daily, 400 mg IV for 7 to 10 days, or **doxycycline** 100 mg PO or IV twice daily. Penicillin G and erythromycin are alternatives.
2. A vaccine is available and is currently being given to active-duty US military personnel.
3. Although there is great concern for the potential use of anthrax as a terrorist warfare agent, the delivery system required to generate and distribute large volumes of cultured spores would not be easy to use in a large population center.

PLAGUE

Clinical Features

Plague *(Yersinia pestis)* is a gram-negative aerobic bacillus of the Enterobacteriaceae family endemic to the United States. It is found most often in rock squirrels and ground rodents of the southwest but also may be carried by cats or dogs. The rodent flea serves as the primary vector. Transmission to humans occurs through the bite of a flea from an infected animal host or through ingestion of infected rodents. Plague may take 3 forms: bubonic or suppurative (most common), pneumonic, or septicemic. The incubation period ranges from 2 to 7 days after the flea bite, which some patients may not recall. Frequently, an eschar develops at the initial bite wound, which is followed by the development of a painful, sometimes suppurative, bubo (enlarged regional lymph nodes), often in the groin. Associated symptoms may include fever, headache, malaise, abdominal pain, nausea, vomiting, and bloody diarrhea. After the lymphatic system, the lung is the organ most commonly affected, with 10% to 20% of patients progressing to secondary pneumonia. This may include multilobar infiltrates, bloody sputum, and respiratory failure. The pneumonic form is highly contagious and can be transmitted from person to person via aerosolized respiratory secretions. Subclinical disseminated intravascular coagulation also may occur in a large number of patients. Untreated bubonic plague may proceed (without other organ systems involved) to generalized sepsis, hypotension, and death.

Diagnosis and Differential

Diagnosis must be made on clinical findings in a patient with possible contact with a vector or animal host. Needle aspiration of a bubo with direct staining of the aspirate using Wayson or Giemsa stain reveals bipolar, safety pin-shaped organisms. Fluorescent antibody staining of a biopsy or antibody titers of acute and convalescent sera also may confirm the diagnosis. Laboratory findings are nonspecific and may include leukocytosis, modest elevations of serum hepatic transaminases, and evidence of disseminated intravascular coagulation (eg, thrombocytopenia, prolonged partial thromboplastin time, and fibrin degradation products). Chest radiography may show infiltrates, frequently with pleural effusion. The differential diagnosis includes lymphogranuloma venereum, syphilis, staphylococcal or streptococcal lymphadenitis, or tularemia. Because plague is a rapidly progressive infection, therapy should begin immediately for any suspected case.

Emergency Department Care and Disposition

1. Recommended antimicrobials are **gentamicin** 2 mg/kg IV loading dose followed by 1.7 mg/kg IV every 8 hours and **streptomycin** 1 g IV or IM every 12 hours.
2. Alternatives include doxycycline plus an aminoglycoside or chloramphenicol.
3. Hospital admission is recommended, and patients with suspected pneumonic plague should be under strict respiratory isolation.

For further reading in *Emergency Medicine: A Comprehensive Study Guide,* 6th ed., see Chap. 151, "Zoonotic Infections" by John T. Meredith.

95 | Soft Tissue Infections

Chris Melton

Patients with soft tissue infections present frequently to the emergency department (ED). The management of these infections involves an understanding of appropriate antibiotic treatment, outpatient or inpatient, and an understanding of when surgical intervention is necessary.

GAS GANGRENE

Clinical Features

Gas gangrene, or clostridial myonecrosis, is a rapidly progressive life- and limb-threatening disease. Patients present with pain out of proportion to physical findings and a sense of heaviness in the affected part. Physical findings typically include a combination of edema, brownish skin discoloration, bullae, malodorous serosanguineous discharge, and crepitance. The patient frequently has a low-grade fever and tachycardia out of proportion to the fever. Mental status changes, including delirium and irritability, may accompany gas gangrene.

Diagnosis and Differential

Familiarity with the disease and an appreciation of the subtle physical findings are the most important factors in making the diagnosis of gas gangrene. Additional findings that may confirm the clinical suspicion include gas within soft tissue on plain radiographs, metabolic acidosis, leukocytosis, anemia, thrombocytopenia, myoglobinuria, and renal or hepatic dysfunction.

The differential diagnosis includes other gas-forming infections, such as necrotizing fasciitis, streptococcal myositis, acute streptococcal hemolytic gangrene, and crepitant cellulitis. When crepitance is present, it should be differentiated from that caused by laryngeal or tracheal fracture, pneumothorax, and pneumomediastinum.

Emergency Department Care and Disposition

1. The patient with gas gangrene should be adequately resuscitated with crystalloid intravenous (IV) fluids and packed red blood cells if there is significant hemolysis with anemia.
2. Urine output and central venous pressure readings should be used to assess volume status. Vasoconstrictors should be avoided in these patients because of compromised perfusion in the affected extremity.
3. Antibiotic therapy should be administered **penicillin G** 24 million U/d in divided doses. Because mixed infections are common, the addition of an aminoglycoside, such as **gentamicin** 1 to 1.5 mg/kg every 8 hours, plus a penicillinase-resistant penicillin, such as **nafcillin** 2 g IV every 4 hours, or **vancomycin** 1 g IV every 12 hours, is recommended.
4. In the penicillin-allergic patient, **clindamycin** 600 to 900 mg IV every 8 hours, **metronidazole** 15 mg/kg loading dose and then 7.5 mg/kg IV every 6 hours, or chloramphenicol may be used.
5. Tetanus prophylaxis should be administered as indicated.

6. Surgical consultation for debridement should be obtained immediately and may include fasciotomy or amputation. Hyperbaric oxygen therapy should be initiated as soon as possible after surgery.

GAS GANGRENE (NONCLOSTRIDIAL MYONECROSIS)

The clinical presentation and management are similar to those of clostridial myonecrosis. The pain associated with the onset of infection is typically not as pronounced as clostridial myonecrosis. This may explain the significant mortality rate, 43% in 1 study, in nonclostridial myonecrosis. This infection typically involves 2 to 10 bacterial species and requires broad-spectrum antibiotic therapy. Current recommendations include **penicillin G** 24 million U/d in divided doses plus an aminoglycoside, such as **gentamicin** 1 to 1.5 mg/kg every 8 hours, plus **metronidazole** 15 mg/kg loading dose and then 7.5 mg/kg IV every 6 hours or **clindamycin** 600 to 900 mg IV every 8 hours.

NECROTIZING FASCIITIS

Clinical Features

The most common type is polymicrobial, followed by the single-organism form typically caused by group A *Streptococcus*. Both forms are characterized by necrosis of subcutaneous tissue and fascia, but not by extending through the fascia into the muscle layers. Whereas the polymicrobial form may form gas in the tissues, group A *Streptococcus* infection does not. The primary complaint is pain out of proportion to physical examination. Initially the skin appears erythematous and edematous and then develops discoloration, vesicles, and crepitus. Tachycardia and low-grade fever are common.

Diagnosis and Differential

Diagnosis is based primarily on clinical suspicion; however, definitive diagnosis can be made by bedside soft tissue biopsy. Early surgical consultation is necessary in all suspected cases.

Emergency Department Care and Disposition

The treatment consists of 4 phases.

1. Aggressive fluid and blood resuscitation and avoidance of vasopressors.
2. Antibiotic therapy is the same as that with nonclostridial myonecrosis. If group A *Streptococcus* is identified, **penicillin G** 24 million U/d plus **clindamycin** 600 to 900 mg IV every 8 hours is adequate coverage.
3. Surgical debridement should be accomplished.
4. Hyperbaric oxygen therapy is effective for polymicrobial infections. Group A *Streptococcus* does not respond to hyperbaric oxygen therapy.

CELLULITIS

Cellulitis is a local soft tissue inflammatory response secondary to bacterial invasion of the skin. It is more common in the elderly, immunocompromised patients, and patients with peripheral vascular disease.

Clinical Features

Cellulitis presents as localized tenderness, erythema, and induration. Lymphangitis and lymphadenitis may accompany cellulitis and indicate a more severe infection. Patients may become bacteremic and have fever and chills.

Diagnosis and Differential

The clinical presentation is usually sufficient for diagnosis. In patients with underlying disease or signs of bacteremia, blood cultures and leukocyte counts are indicated. Otherwise, no further investigation is necessary. The differential diagnosis includes any erythematous skin condition. Cellulitis is sometimes complicated by deep venous thrombosis and may require venogram or Doppler studies for a complete evaluation.

Emergency Department Care and Disposition

1. Simple cellulitis can be treated in an outpatient setting using oral (PO) **dicloxacillin** 500 mg every 6 hours, **amoxicillin/clavulanate** 875 mg/125 mg PO every 12 hours, or a macrolide such as **clarithromycin** 500 mg PO every 12 hours, for 10 days.
2. All patients discharged should have close follow-up to evaluate the cellulitis and response to therapy.
3. Patients with diabetes mellitus, alcoholism, evidence of bacteremia, or other immunosuppressive disorders and all patients with significant cellulitis involving the head or neck should be admitted for IV antibiotics.
4. IV antibiotics, such as a first-generation cephalosporin (**cefazolin** 1 g IV every 6 hours) or a penicillinase-resistant penicillin (**nafcillin** 2 g IV every 4 hours), may be used unless the patient has diabetes.
5. In patients with diabetes, **ceftriaxone** 1 to 2 g IV can be used; in severe cases, **imipenem** 500 mg IV every 6 hours is indicated.

ERYSIPELAS

Erysipelas is a superficial cellulitis with lymphatic involvement caused primarily by group A *Streptococcus*. Infection is usually through a portal of entry in the skin.

Clinical Features

Onset is acute, with sudden high fever, chills, malaise, and nausea. Over the next 1 to 2 days, a small area of erythema with a burning sensation develops. The erythema is sharply demarcated from the surrounding skin and is tense and painful. Lymphangitis and lymphadenitis are common. Purpura, bullae, and necrosis may accompany the erythema. It is primarily an infection of the lower extremities.

Diagnosis and Differential

The diagnosis is based primarily on physical findings. Leukocytosis is common. Cultures, ASO titers, and anti-DNAase B titers are of little use in the ED. Differential diagnosis includes other forms of local cellulitis. Some believe necrotizing fasciitis is a complication of erysipelas and should be considered in all cases.

Emergency Department Care and Disposition

1. **Penicillin G** 1 to 2 million U IV every 6 hours may be used in nondiabetic patients.
2. Penicillinase-resistant penicillins, such as **nafcillin** 2 g IV every 4 hours, or parental second- or third-generation cephalosporins, such as **ceftriaxone** 1 to 2 g/d, should be used in diabetic patients and in those with facial involvement.
3. **Imipenem** 500 mg IV every 6 hours is indicated in severe cases.
4. In patients allergic to penicillin, a macrolide may be used, such as **azithromycin** 500 mg/d IV for 2 days and then PO.
5. Most patients are admitted for IV antibiotics.

CUTANEOUS ABSCESSES

Cutaneous abscesses are the result of a breakdown in the cutaneous barrier, with subsequent contamination with resident bacterial flora. Incision and drainage (I&D) is usually the only necessary treatment.

Clinical Features and Diagnosis

Patients present with an area of swelling, tenderness, and erythema. The area of swelling is frequently fluctuant. Cutaneous abscesses are usually localized, although they may cause systemic toxicity in the immunosuppressed. Cutaneous abscesses should be inspected closely for predisposing injury and foreign bodies. Radiography may be indicated if foreign body is suspected.

Emergency Department Care and Disposition

1. See Chap. 10 for information on conscious sedation.
2. *Bartholin gland abscess* presents as unilateral painful swelling of the labia with a fluctuant 1- to 2-cm mass. *Neisseria gonorrhoeae* and *Chlamydia trachomatis* are commonly found in these abscesses. Cervical cultures should be done in all women with a Bartholin abscess. Routine antimicrobial treatment is not necessary unless there is a suspicion of sexually transmitted disease. Treatment involves I&D along the vaginal mucosal surface of the abscess, followed by the insertion of a Word catheter.
3. *Hidradenitis suppurativa* is a recurrent chronic infection involving the apocrine sweat glands. These abscesses tend to occur in the axilla and in the groin. The causative organism is usually *Staphylococcus*, although *Streptococcus* also may be present. The abscesses are typically multiple and in different stages of progression. ED treatment involves the I&D of any acute abscess, treating with antibiotics for any cellulitis that may be present, and referral to a surgeon for definitive treatment.
4. *Infected sebaceous cysts* may develop in the sebaceous glands, which occur diffusely throughout the skin. Cysts present with an erythematous, tender, cutaneous mass that is often fluctuant. I&D is the appropriate ED treatment, with wound rechecks in 2 to 3 days in the ED or surgeon's office.
5. *Pilonidal abscess* presents as a tender, swollen, and fluctuant mass along the superior gluteal fold. Treatment includes I&D and subsequent iodoform gauze packing. The patient should be rechecked in 2 to 3 days, and the wound should be repacked. Surgical referral is usually necessary for definitive treatment. Antibiotics are not necessary unless there is an accompanying cellulitis.

6. *Staphylococcal soft tissue abscess* causes folliculitis, the inflammation of a hair follicle caused by bacterial invasion, and is usually treated with warm compresses. When deeper invasion occurs, the soft tissue surrounding the hair follicle becomes infected, and a furuncle (boil) is formed. Warm compresses are usually adequate to promote spontaneous drainage. If several furuncles coalesce, they may form a large area of interconnected sinus tracts and abscesses called a *carbuncle.* Carbuncles usually require surgical referral for wide excision.

7. In the healthy, immunocompetent patient, routine use of antibiotics is not indicated unless there is a secondary infection.

8. In the potentially immunocompromised patient, the threshold for antibiotic use should be lowered. Patients presenting with secondary cellulitis or systemic symptoms should be considered for antibiotic therapy. Abscesses involving the hands and face also should be treated more aggressively with antibiotics. Appropriate choices if antibiotics are used include a first-generation cephalosporin such as **cephalexin** 500 mg PO every 6 hours, **clindamycin** 300 mg PO every 6 hours, or **amoxicillin/clavulanate** 875 mg/125 mg PO every 12 hours.

9. Prophylaxis for endocarditis in patients with structural cardiac abnormalities should be considered (see Chap. 90 for information on those at risk).

SPOROTRICHOSIS

Sporotrichosis is caused by traumatic inoculation of the fungus *Sporothrix schenckii,* which is found on plants and in the soil.

Clinical Features

After a 3-week incubation period, 3 types of infection may occur. The fixed cutaneous type is at the site of inoculation and looks like a crusted ulcer or verrucous plaque. The local cutaneous type also remains at the site of inoculation but presents as a subcutaneous nodule or pustule. The surrounding skin may become erythematous. The lymphocutaneous type is the most common of the 3. It presents as a painless nodule at the site of inoculation that develops subcutaneous nodules that migrate along lymphatic channels.

Diagnosis and Differential

The diagnosis is based on the history and physical examination. Tissue biopsy cultures are often diagnostic but of limited use in the ED. The differential diagnosis includes tuberculosis, tularemia, cat-scratch disease, leishmaniasis, nocardiosis, and staphylococcal lymphangitis.

Emergency Department Care and Disposition

1. **Itraconazole** 100 to 200 mg/d PO for 3 to 6 months is highly effective when treating sporotrichosis.

2. If disseminated, sporotrichosis may be treated with IV **amphotericin B** 0.5 mg/kg/d.

3. Most cases of cutaneous sporotrichosis can be treated on an outpatient basis. Those patients who have systemic symptoms or who are acutely ill should be admitted for possible treatment with amphotericin B.

For further reading in *Emergency Medicine: A Comprehensive Study Guide,* 6th ed., see Chap. 152, "Soft Tissue Infections," by Steven G. Folstad.

96 | Bioterrorism

Roy Alson

Because of similar presentations between biological weapons (BWs) and endemic diseases, detection can be difficult. Challenges faced by the clinician include detecting an attack, identification of the agent, lack of familiarity with the diseases, initiating treatment or prophylaxis, and dealing with the psychosocial implications of such an attack.

RESPONSE PLANNING

Local resources for sheltering, decontamination, and treatment of multiple patients must be identified before the event. Planning should include how to notify state and federal agencies, how to integrate outside assets such as the National Pharmaceutical Stockpile into the operation, and dealing with the potential for large numbers of fatalities. Bioterrorist events are also crime scenes, and personnel will have to assist the Federal Bureau of Investigation and other law enforcement agencies. Preplanning should involve emergency management, emergency medical services, fire departments, law enforcement, and the medical community.

DETECTION OF AN ATTACK

A BW attack may be difficult to recognize. The signs and symptoms of the agent may be similar to more common or even endemic illnesses in the area. Complicating the issue is a lack of rapid and reliable tests for most of BW agents. Many tests require specimens to be sent to state or federal laboratories, which can be overwhelmed during a suspected attack (as was seen during the anthrax attack in the United States in the fall of 2001).

Clinicians must be aware of the common presenting signs and symptoms of BWs. When confronted with a cluster of patients who fit the pattern of signs and symptoms, or even a single patient with appropriate findings and history, the clinician should initiate notification of public health authorities and begin appropriate testing and treatment.

Real-time testing of suspect specimens and specific diagnostic tests for most BWs are still under development. Thus emergency physicians must combine knowledge of specific disease processes with information regarding the characteristics of the (possible) exposure to stratify the risk to the patient and the community. These same factors will determine the initiation of therapy and activation of local responses.

RESPONSE ACTIONS

All emergency departments should have in place a plan to deal with contaminated and BW victims. Once identified as possibly exposed or infected, the patient should be placed into the appropriate area, based on the suspected agent and mode of transmission. All staff should wear appropriate personal protective equipment. At a minimum this equipment should consist of gowns, gloves, eye protection, and a HEPA mask.

Information collected from patients should include occupation, travel history, social events, recent close contacts, and what steps, if any, have been taken for treatment or decontamination. The local health department, hospital epidemiologist, and the hospital media relation's representative must be notified. Accurate information, distributed appropriately to the public, will decrease the number of "worried well" who would seek care and effectively "clog up" the system. To be effective, the BW response plan must be integrated into the hospital and community disaster response plans.

SPECIFIC AGENTS

The Centers for Disease Control and Prevention (CDC) has divided BW agents into 3 classes based on their ability to affect a community, the ease of dissemination, and requirements for management. Class A agents are easily disseminated and cause widespread disease or death (Table 96-1). Class B agents have less of a threat because of the disease caused or difficulties in dissemination. Class C agents are those that can be a threat in the future. (Anthrax, plague, and tularemia are discussed in Chap. 92 of this manual. Class B and C agents are discussed in Chap. 7 of *Emergency Medicine: A Comprehensive Study Guide,* 6th ed.)

BW agents may be live, infectious agents or toxins produced by organisms. After entering the body, toxins behave like chemical agents, whereas infectious organisms induce specific diseases. Infectious agents can be classified as contagious or not. Contagious BW agents are smallpox, plague, and viral hemorrhagic fevers (eg, Ebola). Many infectious BW agents are zoonoses, and veterinarians may be an additional information resource.

Smallpox

Having been eradicated in the wild due to vaccination, it presents a high risk due to suspension of vaccination programs and because prior vaccination does not convey lifelong immunity. The virus is transmitted by droplet nuclei, with an incubation of 10 to 14 days. A prodrome of "flulike" symptoms, with headache, myalgias, and fevers, is followed 2 to 4 days later by a macular rash. The rash can involve the palms and soles and, unlike chicken pox, all of the lesions appear to be of the same age. The rash progresses to vesicles and then pustules that scab over. The patient is contagious until the scabs slough (17-21 days). Vaccine (vaccina) given within 3 days of exposure is protective. Exposed persons should be quarantined for 18 days. Care of infected patient is supportive. Mortality of unvaccinated persons is about 30%, with flat and hemorrhagic forms having higher mortality.

Botulism

Botulinum toxin is produced by *Clostridia botulinum,* a spore-forming obligate anaerobe, found throughout the world. The toxin (it has 7 different antigenic types) blocks acetylcholine release at the synapse, causing a flaccid paralysis. Natural cases are food borne (consumption of toxin) or wound or intestinal infection. Inhalation of toxin can occur and is felt to be the best route for "weaponization." Symptoms begin 12 to 72 hours post inhalation and from 1 to 4 days after oral intake. The patient, who remains alert, is afebrile and develops multiple cranial nerve palsies. Care is symptomatic because death usually results from respiratory failure. Antitoxin should be given. Avoid aminoglycosides, which can worsen paralysis.

TABLE 96-1 "Class A" Biological Agents

Agent	Disease	Signs and symptoms	Prophylaxis	Treatment
Variola major	Smallpox	10–14 d incubation, prodrome of flulike symptoms: fever, myalgias; rash: face to trunk: vesicles to pustules, all with the same age Contagious until scabs fall off	Vaccine within 3 d is protective Mortality 30% in unvaccinated	Supportive
Bacillus anthracis	Cutaneous anthrax	1–14 d. macule to papule developing eschar	Vaccine available to military	Respiratory support for inhalational form
	Inhalational	<1 wk (up to 6 wk): flulike symptoms, cough, and dyspnea Wide mediastinum on x-ray after CV collapse and death (see text for GI symptoms)	Ciprofloxacin for up to 2 mo Doxycycline also effective	Ciprofloxacin or doxycycline plus 2 others: clindamycin, aminoglycoside, vancomycin, or streptomycin
Yersinia pestis	Bubonic plague	2–8 d: fever, chills, suppurative nodes, buboes	Ciprofloxacin or doxycycline for 7–10 d	Treat sepsis and pulmonary failure: streptomycin or gentamicin; ciprofloxacin also useful
	Pneumonic plague	2–3 d: fever, chills, cough SOB, becomes septic; contagious.		
	Septicemic plague	2–8 d: fever, chills, suppurative nodes, buboes then become septic		
Clostridium botulinum	Food-borne botulism	1–5 d: GI symptoms: nausea, vomiting, followed by progressive bulbar palsies, descending paralysis	Not applicable	Support ventilations; need may be prolonged; administer antitoxin from CDC
	Inhalational botulism	May not have GI symptoms, will have descending paralysis		
Francisella tularensis	Tularemia	2–5 d followed by febrile illness that can progress to pneumonitis: may have ulcerative skin lesions	Investigational vaccine Ciprofloxacin or doxycycline for 14 d	Streptomycin, ciprofloxacin, or doxycycline
Filovirus and arenavirus	Viral hemorrhagic fevers	2 d to 3 wk: flulike illness with fever, progresses to GI bleeding, shock, and death; contagious	None	Supportive: 90% mortality; ribavirin may be helpful

Key: CDC = Centers for Disease Control and Prevention, CV = cardiovascular, GI = gastrointestinal.

Ricin

Ricin is a byproduct of the extraction of castor oil from the castor bean *(Ricinus communis)*. It can be inhaled or ingested and has been used as an injected assassination weapon. It causes cell destruction by interfering with protein synthesis. Symptom onset varies with route of exposure. Inhalation (the most likely weapons route) causes fever, cough, chest tightness, and weakness, leading to pulmonary edema and cardiovascular collapse. With ingestion, gastrointestinal symptoms predominate. Death follows in 36 to 48 hours. No known antidote exists. Treatment is supportive.

Ebola and Marburg

Viral hemorrhagic fevers (filovirus and arenavirus) such as Ebola and Marburg are highly contagious between persons. After a 3- to 21-day incubation, prodrome of high fever and myalgias is followed by gastrointestinal and other mucosal bleeding, petechiae, edema, hypotension, and cardiovascular collapse. Mortality approaches 90%. Strict isolation in a negative pressure room plus the use of HEPA masks and gowns are key to limiting spread. Ribavirin may be effective post exposure (Argentine hemorrhagic fever).

MANAGEMENT ISSUES

Decontamination of exposed persons who may have agents on them is important to limit spread. Removal of contaminated clothing followed by shower with soap and water are effective. The clothing should be kept in a bag as evidence. Use of dilute hypochlorite bleach should be limited to decontaminating surfaces and equipment. Staff will need to wear appropriate protective equipment. Be aware that prolonged wearing of such gear can cause physical and psychological stressors on staff.

As this field is evolving rapidly, additional information can be found at the following Web sites: http://www.bt.cdc.gov (CDC), http://pubs. ama-assn.org/bioterror.html *(Journal of the American Medical Association),* and http://www.usamriid.army.mil (US Army Research Institute for Infectious Diseases).

For further reading in *Emergency Medicine: A Comprehensive Study Guide,* 6th ed., see Chap. 7, "Bioterrorism Response" by Anthony Macintyre and Joseph Barberra.

97 | Management of the Transplant Patient

David M. Cline

Management of the transplant patient in the emergency department can be divided into 2 general areas: disorders specific to the transplanted organ and disorders common to all transplant patients due to their immunosuppressed state or antirejection medication. Disorders specific to the transplanted organ are manifestations of acute rejection, surgical complications specific to the procedure performed, and altered physiology (most important in cardiac transplantation). In addition, the management of routine injuries or illnesses may be complicated by the patient's immunosuppressed state or medication. Before prescribing any new drug for a transplant recipient, the treatment plan should be discussed with a representative from the transplant team.

POSTTRANSPLANT INFECTIOUS COMPLICATIONS

Infections after transplantation are a common and feared complication. Predisposing factors include ongoing immunosuppression in all patients and the presence of diabetes mellitus, advanced age, obesity, and other host factors in some. Table 97-1 lists the broad array of potential infections and the time after transplant they are most apt to occur.

The most common infection in recipients of solid organs, especially in bone marrow graft recipients, is cytomegalovirus (CMV). This infection may manifest with daily fever and malaise in its mildest form. Progressively more serious disease manifestations include leukopenia, hepatopathy (elevated transaminase enzymes), enteropathy (epigastric pain and diarrhea), and pneumonitis. Mortality associated with CMV pneumonitis exceeds 50%. A patient presenting with a febrile illness should have as part of the assessment a complete blood count, chest radiograph, and measurement of liver function. During active CMV infection, immunosuppression is maintained at the minimum possible level and, if liver, gut, or pulmonary involvement is documented, intravenous ganciclovir therapy, often in conjunction with immune globulin, is prescribed.

The initial presentation of a potentially life-threatening infectious illness may be quite subtle in transplant recipients. The transplant recipient receiving glucocorticoids may not mount an impressive febrile response. A nonproductive cough with little or no findings on physical examination may be the only clue to emerging *Pneumocystis carinii* pneumonia or CMV pneumonia. The threshold for obtaining chest radiographs for these patients should be low. Central nervous system infections are more common in transplant recipients than in other patients. Common etiologies include *Listeria monocytogenes* and cryptococci. Complaints of recurrent headaches, therefore, with or without fever, should be investigated vigorously, first with a structural study to exclude a mass lesion (central nervous system lymphomas occur with increased frequency, too) and then with a lumbar puncture. Moreover, a significant subset of renal transplant recipients has undergone intentional splenectomy to improve allograft survival. Although this procedure is no longer routinely practiced, these patients, as in other postsplenectomy patients, are at

TABLE 97-1 Infectious Complications of Whole-Organ Transplantation

First month posttransplant
Bacterial
Wound infection (*Staphylococcus aureus, Staphylococcus epidermidis* gram-negative bacilli)
Pneumonia (gram-negative bacilli)
Urinary tract infection (gram-negative bacilli, enterococcus)
Line-related sepsis (*S aureus, S epidermidis,* gram-negative bacilli)
Intraabdominal infections (liver transplant)
Viral
HSV
Fungal
Candidal pharyngitis, esophagitis, cystitis
Second to sixth months posttransplant
Bacterial
Pneumonia: pneumococcal and other community acquired
Meningitis *(Listeria monocytogenes)*
Urinary tract infection
Nocardial infection
Listeriosis
Viral
Cytomegalovirus, EBV, HSV, varicella zoster
Adenovirus
Hepatitis A, B, C
Fungal
Aspergillosis
Candidal pharyngitis, esophagitis, cystitis
Other opportunistic infection
Pneumocystis carinii pneumonia, tuberculosis, toxoplasmosis
Beyond sixth months posttransplant
Bacterial
Pneumonia: pneumococcal and other community acquired
Urinary tract infection
Listeriosis
Viral
Cytomegalovirus chorioretinitis
Varicella zoster
Hepatitis C, B
Fungal
Cryptococcal
Other opportunistic infection
P carinii pneumonia

Key: EBV = Epstein-Barr virus, HSV = herpes simplex virus.

particularly high risk for overwhelming sepsis caused by encapsulated bacteria such as pneumococci or meningococci.

Liver transplant patients are especially susceptible to intraabdominal infections during the first postoperative month. Lung transplant patients are especially prone to pneumonia during the first 3 postoperative months. Cardiac transplant patients may develop mediastinitis during the first postoperative month.

Emergency Department Care and Disposition

1. Drug choice, dose, and ultimate management should be accomplished in consultation with the transplant team.

2. For skin and superficial wounds, probable offending organisms are gram-positive cocci, especially *Staphylococcus aureus,* and treatment should be with a penicillinase-resistant penicillin such as **nafcillin** or **oxacillin** 1 to 2 g intravenously (IV) every 4 hours or a first-generation cephalosporin, such as **cefazolin** 2 g IV every 8 hours.

3. If there is a suspicion for methicillin-resistant organisms or sensitivity to β-lactams, **vancomycin** 1 g IV every 12 hours should be used.

4. Nosocomial pneumonia is likely due to gram-negative organisms such as *Escherichia coli, Enterobacter,* or *Pseudomonas.* Treatment options include **imipenem** 500 mg IV every 6 hours, **meropenem** 1 g IV every 8 hours, **cefotaxime** 1 to 2 g IV every 6 to 8 hours plus **gentamicin** 1 to 2 mg/kg IV every 8 hours, or **piperacillin/tazobactam** 3.375 g IV every 6 hours. Community-acquired pneumonia should be treated as such with a fluoroquinolone such as **levofloxacin** 500 mg IV every day, with the proviso that opportunistic infection may also be present.

5. Intraabdominal infection may be due to enterococci, gram-negative bacilli, or anaerobes and sometimes *S aureus.* Triple coverage may be necessary empirically, with **ampicillin** 500 mg IV every 6 hours or vancomycin plus an aminoglycoside such as gentamicin to treat enterococci; a broad-spectrum penicillin or second- or third-generation cephalosporin may be used to treat gram-negative organisms such as piperacillin or cefotaxime, and **clindamycin** 900 mg IV every 8 hours or metronidazole 500 mg IV every 12 hours may be used to treat anaerobes. Penicillins with β-lactamase inhibitors (eg, sulbactam and clavulanic acid) such as **ticarcillin/sulbactam** 3.1 g IV every 6 hours or **ampicillin/sulbactam** 3 g IV every 6 hours have broad coverage against gram-positive cocci, gram-negative bacilli, and anaerobes.

6. Meningitis is frequently due to *L monocytogenes,* and patients with suspected meningitis should be treated with **ampicillin** 2 g IV every 4 hours plus **cefotaxime** 2 g IV every 6 hours. The addition of vancomycin should be considered.

7. The mainstay of fungal treatment has been **amphotericin B** 0.7 mg/kg/d IV, but **fluconazole** 400 mg daily IV is an alternative. *Candida albicans* can be treated first with fluconazole 100 mg/d orally (PO).

8. Viral therapy depends on the disease syndrome and the offending agent. CMV disease is treated with **ganciclovir,** with a dose of 5 mg/kg IV twice daily.

9. Varicella and herpes simplex virus are typically treated with **acyclovir** 800 mg IV 5 times a day for dissemination or ocular involvement. Acyclovir has renal excretion, and the dose must be adjusted for renal insufficiency. Epstein-Barr virus is typically treated with a reduction in the immunosuppression regimen.

10. Treatment of choice for *P carinii* pneumonia is with **trimethoprim/ sulfamethoxazole** (TMP-SMX), TMP 15 mg/kg/d IV divided every 8 hours while critically ill. Prednisone should be given before TMP-SMX. Oral therapy is TMP-SMX double strength (DS) 2 tablets PO every 8 hours for 3 weeks of total therapy. **Pentamidine** 4 mg/kg/d IV or in-tramuscularly for 3 weeks is reserved as an alternative therapy if TMP-SMX is not tolerated.

11. Toxoplasmosis can be treated initially with **pyrimethamine** 50 to 100 mg PO plus **sulfadiazine** 1 to 1.5 g PO plus folinic acid 10 mg PO.

12. Urinary tract infections, invasive gastroenteritis (due to *Salmonella, Campylobacter,* and *Listeria*), and diverticulitis can be treated with the usual antimicrobial agents.

COMPLICATIONS OF IMMUNOSUPPRESSIVE AGENTS

Therapeutic immunosuppression is accompanied by a number of side effects and complications (Table 97-2). Combined toxicities can produce or worsen preexisting renal insufficiency, hypertension, and hyperglycemia. Elevated

TABLE 97-2 Antirejection Medication Side Effects

Medication	Side Effects
Cyclosporine	Nephrotoxicity
	Neurotoxicity
	Hyperkalemia
	Hypomagnesemia
	Hyperuricemia
	Hypertension
	Anorexia
	Hyperbilirubinemia
	Cholestasis
	Gastric dysmotility
	Hirsutism
	Hypercholesterolemia
Tacrolimus	Nephrotoxicity
	Neurotoxicity
	Hyperkalemia
	Hypomagnesemia
	Hyperglycemia
	Anemia
	Headache
	Diarrhea
	Hypertension
	Nausea
Azathioprine	Leukopenia
	Thrombocytopenia
	Cholestatic jaundice
	Alopecia
Mycophenolate mofetil	Diarrhea
	Abdominal pain
	Vomiting
	Leukopenia
	Anemia
	Peripheral edema
Prednisone	Cushing syndrome
	Osteoporosis
	Adrenal suppression
	Hypertension
	Hyperglycemia
	Peptic ulcer disease
	Myopathy
	Cataracts
	Poor wound healing

cyclosporine levels cause renal arteriolar constriction, which reduces glomerular blood flow, stimulates the renin-angiotensin system, and elevates blood pressure. Glucocorticoids promote renal salt and water retention, which further aggravate hypertension. A headache syndrome often indistinguishable from migraine is common in transplant recipients and usually develops within the first 2 months of immunosuppression. An important differential must include infectious causes and malignancy when headache first presents and usually requires computed tomography of the head with subsequent biochemical analysis of cerebrospinal fluid.

Any illness that prevents transplant patients from taking or retaining their immunosuppressive therapy warrants hospital admission for IV therapy, preferably at a transplant center. Starting even simple medications can precipitate complications. For example, nonsteroidal anti-inflammatory drugs may increase nephrotoxicity. In general, any new medications should be discussed with a representative of the patient's transplant team.

CARDIAC TRANSPLANTATION

Transplantation results in a denervated heart that does not respond with centrally medicated tachycardia in response to stress or exercise but does respond to circulating catecholamines and increased preload. Patients may complain of fatigue or shortness of breath with the onset of exercise, which resolves with continued exertion as an appropriate tachycardia develops.

The donor heart is implanted with its sinus node intact to preserve normal atrioventricular conduction. The normal heart rate for a transplanted heart is 90 to 100 beats/min. The technique of cardiac transplantation also results in the preservation of the recipient's sinus node at the superior cavoatrial junction. The atrial suture line renders the 2 sinus nodes electrically isolated from each other. Thus, electrocardiograms frequently will have 2 distinct P waves. The sinus node of the donor heart is easily identified by its constant 1:1 relation to the QRS complex, whereas the native P wave marches independently through the donor heart rhythm.

Clinical Features

Because the heart is denervated, myocardial ischemia does not present with angina. Instead, recipients present with heart failure secondary to silent myocardial infarctions or with sudden death. Transplant recipients who have new onset shortness of breath, chest fullness, or symptoms of congestive heart failure should be evaluated, in routine fashion with an electrocardiogram and serial cardiac enzymes levels, for the presence of myocardial ischemia or infarction.

Although most episodes of acute rejection are asymptomatic, symptoms can occur. The most common presenting symptoms are dysrhythmias and generalized fatigue. The development of atrial or ventricular dysrhythmia in a cardiac transplant recipient (or congestive heart failure) must be assumed to be due to acute rejection until proven otherwise. In children, rejection may present with low-grade fever, fussiness, and poor feeding.

Emergency Department Care

1. Consultation: Differentiating rejection from other acute illnesses in the transplant patient can be difficult. Treatment for rejection without biopsy

confirmation is contraindicated except when patients are hemodynamically unstable.

2. Rejection: Management of acute rejection is **methylprednisolone** 1 g IV after consultation with a representative from the transplant center.

3. Dysrhythmias: If patients are hemodynamically compromised by dysrhythmias, empiric therapy for rejection with methylprednisolone 1 g IV may be given after consultation. Atropine has no effect on the denervated heart; isoproterenol is the drug of choice for bradydysrhythmia in these patients. Patients who present in extremis should be treated with standard cardiopulmonary resuscitation measures.

4. Hypotension: Low-output syndrome, or hypotension, should be treated with inotropic agents such as dopamine or dobutamine when specific treatment for rejection is instituted.

5. Hospitalization: Transplant patients suspected of having rejection or acute illness should be hospitalized, preferably at the transplant center, if stable for transfer.

LUNG TRANSPLANTATION

Clinical Features

Clinically, the patient suffering rejection may have a cough, chest tightness, fatigue, and fever (>0.5°C above baseline). Acute rejection may be manifest with frightening rapidity, causing a severe decline in patient status in only 1 day. Isolated fever may be the only finding. Spirometry may show a 15% drop in forced expiratory volume in 1 second, the patient may be newly hypoxic, and examination may show rales and adventitious sounds. Chest radiograph may demonstrate bilateral interstitial infiltrates or effusions but may be normal when rejection occurs late in the course. The longer a patient is from transplant, the less classic a chest radiograph may appear for acute rejection. Infection, such as interstitial pneumonia, may present with a clinical picture similar to acute rejection. Diagnostically, bronchoscopy with transbronchial biopsy is usually needed not only to confirm rejection but also to exclude infection.

Two late complications of lung transplant are obliterative bronchiolitis and posttransplant lymphoproliferative disease (PTLD). Obliterative bronchiolitis presents with episodes of recurrent bronchitis, small airway obliteration, wheezing, and eventually respiratory failure. PTLD is associated with Epstein-Barr virus and presents with painful lymphadenopathy and otitis media (due to tonsillar involvement) or may present with malaise, fever, and myalgia.

Diagnosis and Differential

Evaluation of the lung transplant patient should include chest radiograph, arterial blood gas analysis, spirometry, complete blood cell count, serum electrolytes, creatinine and magnesium levels, and appropriate drug levels.

Emergency Department Care and Disposition

1. Consultation: Communication should be made directly with the transplant center (often a nurse coordinator). Coordinators should have patients' current medication doses, recent infection history, and knowledge of complications for which patients may be at risk.

2. Rejection: If clinically indicated (ie, infection is excluded), **methylpred-nisolone** 500 to 1,000 mg IV should be given. Patients who have a history of seizures associated with the administration of high-dose glucocorticoids also will need concurrent benzodiazepines to prevent further seizure episodes.

3. Late complications: Obliterative bronchiolitis is treated with increased immunosuppression including high-dose steroids, whereas PTLD is treated with reduced immunosuppression and the addition of high-dose acyclovir. These decisions should be made in consultation with specialists from the transplant center.

RENAL TRANSPLANT

Clinical Features

Diagnosis and treatment of acute rejection is most critical. Without timely recognition and intervention, allograft function may deteriorate irreversibly in a few days.

Renal transplant recipients, when symptomatic from acute rejection, complain of vague tenderness over the allograft (in the left or right iliac fossa). Patients also may describe decreased urine output, rapid weight gain (from fluid retention), low-grade fever, and generalized malaise. Physical examination may disclose worsening hypertension, allograft tenderness, and peripheral edema. The absence of these symptoms and signs, however, does not exclude the possibility of acute rejection. With improved methods of maintenance immunosuppression, the only clue may be an asymptomatic decline in renal function. Even a change in creatinine levels from 1.0 mg/dL to 1.2 or 1.3 mg/dL may be important. When such changes in creatinine levels are reproducible, a careful workup consists of complete urinalysis, renal ultrasonography, and a trough level of cyclosporine, in addition to a careful history and examination. It is critical to interpret changes in renal function in the context of prior data (eg, trends of recent serum creatinine levels, recent history of rejection, or other causes of allograft dysfunction). Evaluation should consider the multiple etiologies of decreased renal function in the renal transplant recipient. The 2 most common causes, apart from acute rejection causing an increase in creatinine, are volume contraction and cyclosporine-induced nephrotoxicity.

Emergency Department Care and Disposition

1. Consultation: Communication should be made directly with the transplant center (often a nurse coordinator). Coordinators should have patients' current medication doses, recent infection history, and a knowledge of complications for which patients may be at risk.

2. Rejection: Treatment of allograft rejection consists of high-dose glucocorticoids, typically **methylprednisolone** 500 mg IV.

LIVER TRANSPLANT

Clinical Features

Although frequently subtle in presentation, a syndrome of acute rejection includes fever, liver tenderness, lymphocytosis, eosinophilia, liver enzyme elevation, and a change in bile color or production. In the perioperative period, the differential diagnosis must include infection, acute biliary obstruction, or vascular insufficiency. Diagnosis can be made with certainty only by hepatic ultrasound and biopsy, which usually requires referral back to the transplant center for management and follow up.

Two possible surgical complications in liver transplant patients are biliary obstruction or leakage and hepatic artery thrombosis. Biliary obstruction follows 3 typical presentations. The most common is intermittent episodes of fever and fluctuating liver function tests. The second is a gradual worsening of liver function tests without symptoms. Third, obstruction may present as acute bacterial cholangitis with fever, chills, abdominal pain, jaundice, and bacteremia. It can be difficult to distinguish clinically from rejection, hepatic artery thrombosis, CMV infection, or a recurrence of a preexisting disease, especially hepatitis.

If a biliary complication is suspected, all patients should have a complete blood count; serum chemistry levels; liver function tests; basic coagulation studies; amylase and lipase levels; cultures of blood, urine, bile, and ascites, if present; chest radiograph; and abdominal ultrasound. Ultrasound rules out the presence of fluid collections, screens for the presence of thrombosis of the hepatic artery or portal vein, and identifies any dilatation of the biliary tree. Alternatively, abdominal computed tomography can be used.

Biliary leakage is associated with 50% mortality. It occurs most frequently in the third or fourth postoperative week. The high mortality may be related to a high incidence of concomitant hepatic artery thrombosis, infection of leaked bile, or difficult bile repair when the tissue is inflamed. Patients most often have peritoneal signs and fever, but these signs may be masked by concomitant use of steroids and immunosuppressive agents. Presentation is signaled by elevated prothrombin time and transaminase levels and little or no bile production, but this complication also may present as acute graft failure, liver abscess, unexplained sepsis, or a biliary tract problem (leak, obstruction, abscess, or breakdown of the anastomosis).

Emergency Department Care and Disposition

1. Consultation: Communication should be made directly with the transplant center (often a nurse coordinator). Coordinators should have patients' current medication doses, recent infection history, and a knowledge of complications for which patients may be at risk.
2. Rejection: Acute rejection is managed with a high-dose glucocorticoid bolus of **methylprednisolone** 500 to 1,000 mg IV.
3. Surgical complications are best managed at the transplant center. Biliary obstruction is managed with balloon dilatation, and all patients should receive broad-spectrum antibiotics against gram-negative and gram-positive enteric organisms. Biliary leakage is treated with reoperation, and hepatic artery thrombosis is treated with retransplantation.

For further reading in *Emergency Medicine: A Comprehensive Study Guide,* 6th ed., see Chap. 60, "Cardiac Transplantation," by Michael R. Mill and Michelle S. Mill; Chap. 70, "The Lung Transplant Patient," by Thomas P. Noeller; Chap. 90, "The Liver Transplant Patient," by Steven Kronick; and Chap. 99, "The Renal Transplant Patient," by Richard Sinert and Mert Erogul.

12 | TOXICOLOGY AND PHARMACOLOGY

98 | General Management of the Poisoned Patient

Sandra L. Najarian

It is estimated that more than 2 million poisonings occur annually in the United States. The poisoned patient requires a thorough, systematic evaluation. Poison centers are an invaluable resource. Prompt consultation can aid in diagnosis and help ensure efficient and cost-effective management of the poisoned patient.

CLINICAL FEATURES

A detailed history of the poisoning is essential. Every attempt should be made to ascertain the number of persons exposed and the timing, type, amount, and route of exposure. Family members, witnesses, prehospital care providers, and the patient's primary physician are important sources of information. They should be used to corroborate the patient's entire history. Details about the environment in which the patient was found (eg, presence of pill bottles or empty containers, drug paraphernalia, unusual odors or smells, or presence of a suicide note) should be gathered because these may provide clues to identifying the poison.

A thorough physical examination on a fully disrobed patient is necessary. Caution should be used when searching the patient's clothing for substances. Attention to vital signs, general appearance, skin, pupils, mucous membranes, heart, lung, gastrointestinal, and neurologic examinations is important because exposure to certain substances results in specific clinical signs and symptoms called *toxidromes* (Table 98-1). If the poisoning is unknown, recognition of these toxidromes can assist the physician in narrowing the differential diagnosis (Table 98-2).

DIAGNOSIS AND DIFFERENTIAL

Diagnosis is based on history and clinical presentation. If there is a question of a toxic ingestion, having the actual container, pill remnants, or liquids is very important. Family, friends, or emergency personnel should be dispatched to retrieve these items. Laboratory studies may be useful but often serve only to confirm the diagnosis. Toxicologic drug screens also may be useful for certain ingestions but rarely alter management. Acetaminophen and aspirin are common coingestants in suicide attempts, so consideration should be given to perform routine testing for these medications. Other tests that may be useful include electrocardiogram, arterial blood gas analysis, urine pregnancy test, and electrolyte and glucose levels.

EMERGENCY DEPARTMENT CARE AND DISPOSITION

1. Attention to airway, breathing, and circulation (ABCs) always take precedence in managing the poisoned patient. Patients require **oxygen** administration, cardiac monitoring, and intravenous (IV) access. Once the ABCs are secured, decontamination, elimination of the toxin, and administration of the antidote should take place (Table 98-3).

467

TABLE 98-1 Toxidromes

Toxidrome	Representative agents(s)	Most common findings	Additional signs and symptoms	Potential interventions
Opioid	Heroin Morphine	CNS depression, miosis, respiratory depression	Hypothermia, bradycardia. Death may result from respiratory arrest, pulmonary edema	Ventilation or naloxone
Sympathomimetic	Cocaine Amphetamine	Psychomotor agitation, mydriasis, diaphoresis, tachycardia, hypertension, hyperthermia	Seizures, rhabdomyolysis, myocardial infarction Death may result from seizures, cardiac arrest, hyperthermia	Cooling, sedation with benzodiazepines, hydration
Cholinergic	Organophosphate insecticides Carbamate insecticides	Salivation, lacrimation, diaphoresis, nausea, vomiting, urination, defecation, muscle fasciculations, weakness, bronchorrhea	Bradycardia, miosis/mydriasis, seizures, respiratory failure, paralysis Death may result from respiratory arrest 2° to paralysis and/or bronchorrhea, seizures	Airway protection and ventilation, atropine, pralidoxime
Anticholinergic	Scopolamine Atropine	Altered mental status, mydriasis, dry/flushed skin, urinary retention, decreased bowel sounds, hyperthermia, dry mucous membranes	Seizures, dysrhythmias, rhabdomyolysis Death may result from hyperthermia and dysrhythmias	Physostigmine (if appropriate), sedation with benzodiazepines, cooling, supportive management

Salicylates	Aspirin Oil of wintergreen	Altered mental status, respiratory alkalosis, metabolic acidosis, tinnitus, hyperpnea, tachycardia, diaphoresis, nausea, vomiting	Low-grade fever, ketonuria Death may result from pulmonary edema, cardiorespiratory arrest	MDAC, alkalinization of the urine with potassium repletion, hemodialysis, hydration
Hypoglycemia	Sulfonylureas Insulin	Altered mental status, diaphoresis, tachycardia, hypertension	Paralysis, slurring of speech, bizarre behavior, seizures Death may result from seizures, altered behavior	Glucose containing solution intravenously, and oral feedings if able, frequent capillary blood for glucose measurement
Serotonin syndrome	Meperidine/dextromethorphan + MAOI; SSRI + TCA, SSRI/TCA/MAOI + amphetamines, SSRI overdose	Altered mental status, increased muscle tone, hyperreflexia, hyperthermia	"Wet dog shakes" (intermittent whole body tremor) Death may result from hyperthermia	Cooling, sedation with benzodiazepines, supportive management, theoretical benefit—cyproheptadine

Key: CNS = central nervous system, MDAC = multidose activated charcoal, MAOI = monoamine oxidase inhibitor, SSRI = selective serotonin reuptake inhibitor, TCA = tricyclic antidepressant.

TABLE 98-2 Agents that May Alter Presenting Signs or Symptoms*

Drugs	Seizures	Change in blood pressure	Change in ventilation	Change in heart rate	Temperature change
Alcohol withdrawal	✓	↑		↑	↑
Amphetamines	✓	↑	↑	↑	↑
Anticholinergic	✓	↑	↑	↑	↑
Baclofen	✓	↓	↓	↓	↓
Caffeine	✓	↑	↑	↑	
Camphor	✓				
Cocaine	✓	↑	↑	↑	↑
Gyrometria esculenta (mushroom)	✓				
Isoniazid	✓				
Lithium	✓				
Methaqualone	✓	↓	↓	↓	
Serotonin syndrome	✓	↑	↑	↑	↑
Theophylline	✓	↓	↑	↑	
Tricyclic antidepressants	✓	↑	↓	↓	
β-Adrenergic antagonists		↓		↓	
Calcium channel blockers		↓		↓	
Clonidine		↓	↓	↓	↓

This page presents a rotated table of toxicologic agents with associated vital-sign changes (indicated by ↑/↓ arrows) and an additional marked column (↘). The row labels, in order, are:

- Ethanol
- Phenothiazines
- Opioids
- Organophosphates ↘
- Meprobamate
- Monoamine oxidase inhibitor overdose ↘
- Phencyclidine ↘
- Sedative hypnotic withdrawal
- Phenylpropanolamine
- Barbiturates
- Ethchlorvynol
- Glutethamide
- Salicylates
- Nicotine ↘
- Hydrocarbons ↘
- Toxic alcohols ↘
- Iron ↘

Agent	Col 1	Col 2	Col 3	Col 4
Ethanol	→		→	→
Phenothiazines	→	←	→	→
Opioids		←	→	→
Organophosphates		→	→	→
Meprobamate	→	→	→	→
Monoamine oxidase inhibitor overdose	←		→	←
Phencyclidine	←	←	←	←
Sedative hypnotic withdrawal		←	→	←
Phenylpropanolamine	→		←	←
Barbiturates		←	←	→
Ethchlorvynol		→	→	→
Glutethamide		→	→	→
Salicylates	←		→	←
Nicotine		←	←	→
Hydrocarbons		←	←	→
Toxic alcohols		←	←	→
Iron		←	←	→

*Listed are the most common or most classically seen with the agent.

471

TABLE 98-3 Poison Antidotes

Antidote	Dose		Poison
	Child	Adult	
N-acetylcysteine	140 mg/kg PO load, followed by 70 mg/kg PO q4h for 18 total doses		Acetaminophen
Activated charcoal	1 g/kg PO		Most ingested poisons
Antivenom Fab	4–6 vials IV initially over 1 h may be repeated; 2 vials every 6 h for 18 h		Envenomation by *Crotalidae*
Calcium gluconate 10% (9 mg/mL elemental calcium)	0.6–0.8 mL/kg IV	30 mL IV	Hypermagnesemia, hypocalcemia (ethylene glycol, hydrofluoric acid), calcium channel antagonists, black widow spider
Calcium chloride 10% (27.2 mg/mL elemental calcium)	0.2–0.25 mL/kg IV	10 mL IV	
Cyanide antidote kit Amyl nitrate	Not typically used	1 ampule in oxygen chamber of ambu-bag 30 s on/30 s off	Cyanide poisoning
Sodium nitrite	Sodium nitrite 0.33 mL/kg IV (3% solution)	Sodium nitrite 10 mL (3% solution)	Hydrogen sulfide (use only sodium nitrate)
Thiosulfate	Thiosulfate 1.65 mL/kg IV	Thiosulfate 12.5 g IV	
Deferoxamine	90 mg/kg IM (1 g max) or 15 mg//kg/h IV (1 g max)	2 g IM or 15 mg//kg/h (6–8 g/d max)	Iron
Dextrose	1–1.5 g/kg IV		Hypoglycemia

Digoxin Fab
  Acute
  Chronic
	10–20 vials IV
	1–2 vials IV
		
		3–6 vials IV
			Digoxin and cardiac glycosides

Ethanol 10% for IV	0.8 g/kg = 8-mL/kg load then 1/10 qh		Ethylene glycol, methanol
20% PO	0.8 g/kg = 4 mL/kg, then 1/10 qh		
Folic acid/ Leucovorin	1–2 mg/kg q4–6 h IV		Methanol, methotrexate (only Leucovorin)
Fomepizole	15 mg/kg IV, then 10 mg/kg q12h		Methanol, ethylene glycol, disulfiram

(continued)

TABLE 98-3 Poison Antidotes *(continued)*

Antidote	Dose — Child	Dose — Adult	Poison
Glucagon	50 µg/kg	1–10 mg IV	Calcium channel blocker, β-blocker
Methylene blue	1–2 mg/kg Neonates: 0.3–1 mg/kg	1–2 mg/kg	Oxidizing chemicals (eg, nitrites, benzocaine, sulfonamides)
Octreatide	1 µg/kg q6h SC	50 µg SC q6h	Refractory hypoglycemia after oral hypoglycemic agent ingestion
Naloxone	As much as is needed. Typical starting dose 0.4 mg– 10 mg IV		Opioid, clonidine
Physostigmine	0.02 mg/kg IV	1–2 mg IV	Anticholinergic substances (not TCAs)
Pralidoxime (2-PAM)	20–40 mg/kg IV	1–2 g IV	Cholinergic substances
Protamine	1 mg neutralizes 100 U administered heparin; 0.6 mg/kg administered over 15 min	25–50 mg IV, empiric	Heparin
Pyridoxine	Gram-for-gram ingestion if amount of INH is known 70 mg/kg IV	5 g IV	INH, *Gyromitra esculenta*, rocket fuel
Sodium bicarbonate	1–2-mEq/kg IV bolus followed by 1-2 mEq/kg/h		Sodium channel blockers, alkalinization of urine or serum
Thiamine	10–100 mg IV	100 mg IV	Ethylene glycol, Wernicke syndrome, "wet" beri-beri
Vitamin K$_1$	2–5 mg/d PO	25–50 mg TID	Anticoagulants
Whole bowel irrigation	0.5 L/h PO	1.5–2 L/h PO	Multiple indications (eg, sustained-release products, body packers)

Key: IM = intramuscularly, INH = isoniazid, IV = intravenously, max = maximum, PO = orally, q = every, SC = subcutaneously, TCA = tricyclic antidepressant, TID = 3 times a day.

2. Primary evaluation includes assessment of airway patency and quality of respirations. Early **endotracheal intubation** should be considered, especially if gastric lavage is indicated in a patient with a depressed level of consciousness. Respiratory status should be monitored continuously. Abnormalities in breathing are not usually the direct effect of a toxin, but rather a result of the patient's altered level of consciousness.

3. Hypotension should be corrected with IV fluids; pressors are rarely required. Ventricular dysrhythmias should be treated according to standard ACLS protocol unless treatment of a particular toxin dictates an alternative treatment. Atropine should be used for bradyarrhythmias; cardiac pacing may be necessary.

4. For those patients found unresponsive or with altered mental status, administration of **naloxone** (0.2–2.0 mg IV in adults), **glucose** (50 mL 50% dextrose IV), and **thiamine** (100 mg IV) should be considered after taking into account the history, vital signs, and immediate laboratory data. Routine use of flumazenil, a benzodiazepine antagonist, is not recommended. A Foley catheter should be placed in unconscious patients. Administration of naloxone, a competitive opioid antagonist, may precipitate acute withdrawal syndrome, especially if large doses are given.

5. Seizures should be treated with benzodiazepines (**lorazepam** 2 mg IV) initially, followed by phenobarbital if necessary. (Phenytoin is less useful for the poisoned patient.)

6. Physical and chemical restraints should be considered in the agitated patient. Short-acting benzodiazepines or **haloperidol** may be useful.

7. Decontamination of the poisoned patient is the mainstay of therapy. **Gross (surface) decontamination** is the initial step. If patients are being contaminated by a toxin through dermal contact, they should be removed from the toxic substance; this includes undressing patients completely and washing their skin with copious amounts of water. Properly gowned staff should assist the patient in an isolated area to avoid contamination of other patients and staff. With ocular exposure, the eyes must be flushed immediately with irrigation solution until the pH of the eyes returns to a physiologic range.

8. Gastric decontamination includes gastric emptying, adsorption of the toxin in the gut, and irrigation of the bowel. Selecting the appropriate method is dependent on the toxin, timing of exposure, and clinical status of the patient. **Gastric lavage** is the preferred method of gastric emptying. Ipecac is contraindicated. Gastric lavage should be reserved for patients with a recent ingestion (usually within 60 minutes) of a potentially life-threatening toxin. When performed, a large-bore orogastric tube with connections for infusion and drainage should be used. The patient should be placed in the left lateral decubitus position, with the head lower than the feet. Roughly 250-mL aliquots of tap water should be infused until the return is clear. Before removing the tube, **activated charcoal** (1 g/kg) should be administered to help bind any remaining toxin. Activated charcoal may be given orally or per nasogastric tube when gastric lavage is not indicated. Osmotic cathartics (1 g/kg 70% sorbitol or 4 mg/kg 10% magnesium citrate) may be given with activated charcoal to reduce transit time through the gastrointestinal tract. Multiple-dose activated charcoal is an option usually reserved for very large ingestions, life-threatening toxins known to slow gut motility, or slow-release toxins. **Whole bowel irrigation** may be useful in eliminating sustained-release preparations, toxins not known to be adsorbed by activated charcoal, or packages of toxic drugs (body packers). **Polyethylene glycol** 2 L/h should be administered in adults (50-250 mL/kg/h in pediatric patients) until rectal effluent is clear.

9. Once decontamination is underway, specific antidotes or other special treatment may be given. Enhancing elimination of certain toxins may be

indicated; these methods include urinary **alkalization, hemoperfusion,** or **hemodialysis** for specific toxins.

10. Disposition of patients depends on the nature of the exposure and underlying conditions. Consideration should be given to delayed effects and absorption of toxins. Psychiatric consultation should be obtained for all intentional overdoses. Poisonings in children older than 5 years should be considered suspicious and warrant social work consultation or law enforcement involvement. Patients and families should be given instructions on prevention of poisonings.

For further reading in *Emergency Medicine: A Comprehensive Study Guide,* 6th ed., see Chap. 156, "General Management of Poisoned Patients," by Jason B. Hack and Robert S. Hoffman.

O. John Ma

Anticholinergic toxicity is commonly seen in the emergency department. Table 99-1 lists the important anticholinergic agents and the classes to which they belong.

CLINICAL FEATURES

Clinical findings include mydriasis, hypo- or hypertension, hypoactive or absent bowel sounds, tachycardia, flushed skin, disorientation, urinary retention, hyperthermia, dry skin and mucus membranes, confusion, agitation, and auditory and visual hallucinations.

DIAGNOSIS AND DIFFERENTIAL

Diagnosis is primarily clinical. In isolated anticholinergic toxicity, routine laboratory studies should be normal, and toxicology screening is of little value. Nonetheless, electrolytes, glucose, and pulse-oximetry should be obtained in the presence of altered mental status. The differential diagnosis includes viral encephalitis, Reye syndrome, head trauma, other intoxications, neuroleptic malignant syndrome, delirium tremens, acute psychiatric disorders, and sympathomimetic toxicity.

EMERGENCY DEPARTMENT CARE AND DISPOSITION

Treatment is primarily supportive.

1. The patient should be placed on a cardiac monitor and intravenous access secured.
2. Gastric lavage may be useful within 1 hour of ingestion. **Activated charcoal** may decrease drug absorption.
3. Temperature monitoring is essential. Hyperthermia is treated conventionally.
4. Hypertension usually does not require intervention but may be treated conventionally, as necessary.
5. Standard antiarrhythmics are usually effective, but class Ia medications should be avoided. Dysrhythmias, widened QRS complexes, and hypotension from sodium blocking agents (eg, cyclic antidepressants) can be treated with intravenous sodium bicarbonate.
6. Seizures should be treated with benzodiazepines (lorazepam 2 mg intravenously).
7. Agitation should be treated with benzodiazepines (**lorazepam** 2–4 mg intravenously). Phenothiazine should be avoided.
8. **Physostigmine** treatment is controversial. It is indicated only if conventional therapy fails to control seizures, agitation, unstable dysrhythmias, coma with respiratory depression, malignant hypertension, or hypotension. The initial dose is 0.5 to 2 mg intravenously, slowly administered over 5 minutes. When effective, a significant decrease in agitation may be apparent within 15 to 20 minutes. Physostigmine may worsen cyclic antidepressant toxicity and lead to bradycardia and asystole. It is contraindicated in patients with cardiovascular or peripheral vascular disease,

TABLE 99-1 Anticholinergic Substances

Antihistamines
  Ethanolamines
    Dimenhydrinate (Dramamine)
    Diphenhydramine (Benadryl)
  Ethylenediamines
    Tripelennamine (Pyribenzamine)
  Alkylamines
    Chlorpheniramine (Teldrin)
  Piperazines
    Astemizole (Hismanal)
    Terfenadine (Seldane)
    Loratadine (Claritin)
    Cyclizine (Marezine)
    Meclizine (Antivert)
  Phenothiazines
    Prochlorperazine (Compazine)
    Promethazine (Phenergan)
Antiparkinsonian drugs
  Benztropine mesylate (Cogentin)
  Biperiden (Akineton)
  Ethopropazine (Parsidol)
  Trihexyphenidyl (Artane)
  Procyclidine (Kemadrin)
Antipsychotics
  Phenothiazines
    Chlorpromazine (Thorazine)
    Thioridazine (Mellaril)
    Perphenazine (Trilafon)
  Nonphenothiazines
    Clozaril (Clozapine)
    Molindone (Moban)
    Loxapine (Loxitane)
Antispasmodics
  Clidinium bromide (Quarzan,
    Librax)
  Dicyclomine (Bentyl)
  Methantheline bromide (Banthine)
  Propantheline bromide
    (Pro-Banthine)
  Tridihexethyl chloride (Pathilon)
Plants
  Deadly nightshade
  Mandrake
  Jimsonweed

Belladonna alkaloids, synthetic cogeners
  Atropine (Hyoscyamine)
  Belladonna alkaloid mixtures
  Glycopyrrolate (Robinul)
  Homatropine (Dia-Quel, Malcotran)
  Methscopolamine bromide (Pamine)
  Scopolamine hydrobromide (Hyoscine)
Cyclic antidepressants
  Amitryptyline hydrochloride (Elavil,
    Amitril, Endep)
  Desipramine hydrochloride (Norpramin,
    Pertofrane)
  Doxepin hydrochloride (Sinequan,
    Adapin)
  Imipramine hydrochloride (Tofranil,
    Pramine)
  Nortriptyline hydrochloride (Aventyl,
    Pamelor)
  Protriptyline hydrochloride (Vivactil)
  Trimipramine (Surmontil)
  Maprotiline hydrochloride (Ludiomil)
  Zimelidine hydrochloride
  Fluoxetine (Prozac)
  Amoxapine (Asendin)
Ophthalmic products
  Atropine and scopolamine solutions
  Cyclopentolate hydrochloride (Cyclogyl)
  Tropicamide (Mydriacyl)
OTC medications (including
  antihistamines and belladonna alkaloids)
  Analgesics: Excedrin PM, Percogesic
  Cold remedies: Actifed, Allerest,
    Coricidin, Dristan, Flavihist, Romex,
    Sine-Off
  Hypnotics: Compoz, Sleep-Eze,
    Sominex
  Menstrual products: Pamprin, Premesyn
    PMS
Skeletal muscle relaxants
  Orphenadrine citrate (Norflex)
  Cyclobenzaprine hydrochloride (Flexeril)
Mushrooms
  Amanita muscaria
  Amanita pantherina
Other
  Diphenidol (Cephadol, Vontrol)

Key: OTC = over the counter.
Source: Adapted from Goldfrank et al, Goldfrank's Toxicologic Emergencies,
7th ed. McGraw-Hill, New York, 2002. With permission.

bronchospasm, intestinal obstruction, heart block, or bladder obstruction. The patient should be observed for cholinergic excess.

9. Patients with mild anticholinergic toxicity can be discharged after 6 hours of observation if their symptoms are improving. More symptomatic patients should be admitted for 24 hours of observation. Patients receiving physostigmine usually require at least a 24-hour admission.

For further reading in *Emergency Medicine: A Comprehensive Study Guide,* 6th ed., see Chap. 183, "Anticholinergic Toxicity," by Paul M. Wax.

100 | Psychopharmacologic Agents

C. Crawford Mechem

SEROTONIN SYNDROME

Serotonin syndrome is a rare, idiosyncratic complication of antidepressant therapy characterized by cognitive impairment and autonomic and neuromuscular dysfunctions. It may be caused by any drug or combination of drugs that increases central serotonin transmission. Most cases occur at therapeutic drug levels.

Clinical Features

The diagnosis is made on clinical grounds. Cognitive and behavioral findings include confusion, agitation, coma, anxiety, hypomania, lethargy, seizures, insomnia, hallucinations, and dizziness. Autonomic signs include hyperthermia, diaphoresis, sinus tachycardia, hypertension, tachypnea, dilated or unreactive pupils, flushed skin, hypotension, diarrhea, abdominal cramps, and salivation. Neuromuscular findings include myoclonus, hyperreflexia, muscle rigidity, tremor, hyperactivity, ataxia, shivering, Babinski sign, nystagmus, teeth chattering, opisthotonus, and trismus.

Emergency Department Care and Disposition

Therapy involves discontinuing all serotoninergic agents and providing supportive care.

1. Antiserotoninergic agents may have a role. Most experience has been with **cyproheptadine** 4 to 8 mg orally (PO) and repeated in 2 hours if no response is noted. Additional dosing should be discontinued if the patient fails to respond to 16 mg. Patients who do respond are then given 4 mg PO every 6 hours for 48 hours.
2. **Benzodiazepines** may be used to relieve muscle rigidity and discomfort.
3. Patients with muscle rigidity, seizures, or hyperthermia should be monitored for development of rhabdomyolysis and/or metabolic acidosis. All patients require admission.

TRICYCLIC ANTIDEPRESSANTS

Although their popularity is decreasing, tricyclic antidepressants (TCAs) continue to be used for a variety of conditions including depression, obsessive-compulsive disorder, and chronic pain. They are associated with significant toxicity and cause more drug-related deaths than do any other class of prescription medication.

Clinical Features

Mild to moderate TCA toxicity may present as drowsiness, confusion, slurred speech, ataxia, dry mucous membranes, sinus tachycardia, urinary retention, myoclonus, hyperreflexia, decreased bowel sounds, and ileus. Serious toxicity almost always manifests within 6 hours of major ingestion and consists of cardiac conduction delays, supraventricular tachycardia, premature ventricular contractions, ventricular tachycardia, hypotension, coma, respiratory

479

depression, and seizures. Secondary complications include aspiration pneumonia, anoxic encephalopathy, hyperthermia, rhabdomyolysis, and pulmonary edema.

Diagnosis and Differential

Diagnosis is made on clinical grounds. Most cases of serious toxicity are associated with elevated TCA plasma levels, but the results are rarely available to the emergency physician. Electrocardiographic (ECG) abnormalities are common and may be useful in identifying patients at risk for seizures and ventricular dysrhythmias. Classic ECG findings in TCA toxicity include sinus tachycardia, right axis deviation of the terminal for 40 milliseconds (a positive terminal R wave in lead aVR and a negative S wave in lead I), and prolongation of PR, QRS, and QT_c intervals. Life-threatening complications are more likely when the QRS interval is longer than 100 milliseconds or right axis deviation of the terminal is 40 milliseconds. However, complications can occur in the absence of significant ECG abnormalities.

Appropriate laboratory studies may include serum electrolytes, creatinine, glucose, arterial blood gas, and acetaminophen and aspirin levels. A baseline ECG should be obtained.

The differential diagnosis includes toxicity due to carbamazepine, cyclobenzaprine, diphenhydramine, phenothiazine, class Ia and Ic antiarrhythmics, propranolol, propoxyphene, cocaine, lithium, and hyperkalemia.

Emergency Department Care and Disposition

1. All patients should be promptly evaluated for altered mental status, hemodynamic instability, and respiratory impairment. Intravenous (IV) access and cardiac monitoring should be initiated.
2. All patients should receive **activated charcoal** 1 g/kg PO or per nasogastric tube. Gastric lavage is indicated early (<2 hours) after ingestion.
3. **Sodium bicarbonate** 1 to 2 mEq/kg IV bolus is given for a QRS interval longer than 100 milliseconds, hypotension refractory to hydration, terminal rightward axis in the aVR lead, or ventricular dysrhythmias. It may be repeated until the patient improves or until the serum pH is 7.50 to 7.55. As an alternative to repeat boluses, an IV infusion may be mixed by adding 3 ampules to 1 L 5% dextrose in water and run at 2 to 3 mL/kg/h. Serum potassium should be closely monitored.
4. Ventricular dysrhythmias refractory to sodium bicarbonate should be treated with **lidocaine.** Synchronized cardioversion is indicated for unstable patients. Torsade de pointes should be treated initially with **magnesium sulfate** 2 g IV.
5. **Thiamine** and **naloxone** are warranted for altered mental status, and a fingerstick serum glucose level should be obtained.
6. Seizures should be controlled with IV **lorazepam** or **diazepam**. Refractory cases are treated with **phenobarbital** at an initial loading dose of 15 mg/kg IV. Hypotension and respiratory depression should be anticipated. If neuromuscular blockade and endotracheal intubation prove necessary, electroencephalographic monitoring and continued anticonvulsant therapy are required.
7. **Crystalloid IV fluids** should be administered in increments of 10 mL/kg for hypotension, and the patient should be watched closely for signs of

pulmonary edema. **Norepinephrine** is the vasopressor of choice in cases refractory to IV fluids and sodium bicarbonate.
8. Patients who remain asymptomatic 6 hours after ingestion may be medically cleared. Psychiatric consultation should be considered, based on the circumstances. All symptomatic patients require admission to a monitored setting.

NEWER ANTIDEPRESSANTS

The newer antidepressants are the most popular psychopharmacologic agents used for the treatment of depression. They are more selective in their activity and have a toxicologic behavior very different from those of the TCAs and monoamine oxidase inhibitors (MAOIs). However, like the TCAs and MAOIs, they can cause the serotonin syndrome.

TRAZODONE AND NEFAZODONE

Clinical Features

Adverse effects due to trazodone include orthostatic hypotension, drowsiness, dizziness, dry mouth, nausea, vomiting, liver toxicity, and priapism. Cardiac dysrhythmias may include sinus bradycardia, atrial fibrillation, sinus arrest, atrioventricular blocks, premature ventricular contractions, and torsade de pointes. Nefazodone produces headache, dizziness, drowsiness, asthenia, tremor, dry mouth, nausea, constipation, and blurred vision. It can inhibit metabolism of terfenadine, astemizole, cisapride, and pimozide, resulting in QT_c interval prolongation and torsades de pointes. It also potentiates central nervous system (CNS) depression caused by benzodiazepines. Its use is less commonly associated with orthostatic hypotension and priapism than is the case with trazodone.

In acute trazodone overdose, serious toxicity is rare at doses smaller than 2 g. Manifestations include CNS depression, orthostatic hypotension, nausea, vomiting, abdominal pain, muscle weakness, priapism, ataxia, dizziness, seizures, and coma. Respiratory depression is rarely seen. On ECG, QT_c interval prolongation may be seen, rarely leading to torsades de pointes. In acute nefazodone overdose, nausea, vomiting, and somnolence have been reported.

Emergency Department Care and Disposition

In most trazodone or nefazodone overdoses, supportive care is sufficient. The patient should be assessed for respiratory or hemodynamic compromise from a coingestion and an acetaminophen level obtained.

1. An IV line should be started, and cardiac monitoring should be initiated for all patients.
2. **Activated charcoal** 1 g/kg should be administered. Gastric lavage is unnecessary unless there is a clear history of life-threatening coingestion.
3. Hypotension is best treated initially with **crystalloid IV fluids.** In refractory cases, **norepinephrine** is the vasopressor of choice.
4. Patients who remain asymptomatic 6 hours after ingestion can be medically cleared. Symptomatic patients should be admitted to a monitored setting.

BUPROPION

Clinical Features

Adverse effects include dry mouth, dizziness, agitation, nausea, headache, constipation, tremor, anxiety, confusion, blurred vision, and increased motor activity. It rarely causes catatonia, hallucinations, psychosis, and paranoia.

Bupropion has a low toxic-to-therapeutic ratio. Toxicity may be seen at doses at, or just above, the maximum therapeutic dose of 450 mg/d. Findings include sinus tachycardia, lethargy, tremor, seizures, confusion, vomiting, and mild hyperthermia. The hallmark of overdose is seizures, which usually develop within the first 4 hours, often without associated signs of toxicity. Sustained-release preparations may causes seizures up to 14 hours postingestion.

Emergency Department Care and Disposition

Seizures should be anticipated in all patients. Significant cardiotoxicity is unlikely except in mixed overdoses.

1. IV access should be established, and the patient should be placed on a cardiac monitor.
2. Gastric lavage for acute ingestions (<1 hour) and **activated charcoal** 1 g/kg are recommended.
3. Seizures should be controlled with **benzodiazepines** and **phenobarbital.**
4. Admission to a monitored setting is indicated for patients with sinus tachycardia, lethargy, or seizures. Patients who remain asymptomatic 8 hours after ingestion of regular-release bupropion may be medically cleared. Ingestion of more than 450 mg of a sustained-release preparation warrants admission for further monitoring.

MIRTAZAPINE

Clinical Features

Adverse effects include weight gain and somnolence. Mirtazapine has limited toxicity in acute overdose. The patient may present with sedation, confusion, sinus tachycardia, and mild hypertension. Respiratory depression or coma may be seen at higher doses or when combined with another CNS depressant.

Emergency Department Care and Disposition

Experience with mirtazapine overdose is limited, so early consultation with a poison control center is recommended. Supportive care is usually sufficient.

1. **Activated charcoal** 1 g/kg should be administered. Gastric lavage may be indicated early after large overdoses or with significant coingestants.
2. Symptomatic patients should be admitted to a monitored bed. Asymptomatic patients may be medically cleared after 8 hours of observation.

SELECTIVE SEROTONIN REUPTAKE INHIBITORS

Clinical Features

The selective serotonin reuptake inhibitors (SSRIs) have a high therapeutic-to-toxic ratio. The most serious adverse effect is development of serotonin syndrome. Other effects include headache, sedation, insomnia, dizziness, fatigue, tremor, and nervousness. Seizures occur rarely. Dystonic reactions, akathisia, dyskinesia, hypokinesia, and parkinsonism have been reported. Other adverse effects include nausea, vomiting, diarrhea, constipation, anorexia, dry mouth, increased sweating, blurred vision, priapism, hyponatremia, and hypoglycemia.

In acute overdose, patients may present with nausea, vomiting, sedation, tremor, and sinus tachycardia. Less commonly, mydriasis, seizures, diarrhea, agitation, hallucinations, hypertension, and hypotension may be noted. Although cardiotoxicity is uncommon, sinus bradycardia may be observed in fluvoxamine overdoses, and citalopram may cause QRS interval widening and QT_c interval prolongation.

Emergency Department Care and Disposition

Pure SSRI overdoses are rarely associated with serious toxicity. However, the patient should be carefully observed for the development of seizures or serotonin syndrome.

1. All patients should have IV access and cardiac monitoring.
2. **Activated charcoal** 1 g/kg should be administered. Gastric lavage is indicated only in the setting of very large overdoses or mixed ingestions.
3. **Sodium bicarbonate** should be used to treat QRS interval prolongation.
4. **Benzodiazepines** are recommended as initial anticonvulsant therapy.
5. All patients should be observed for 6 hours postingestion. Patients who continue to manifest toxicity, such as tachycardia or lethargy, should be admitted for further monitoring.

VENLAFAXINE

Clinical Features

Adverse effects are similar to those with SSRIs, including development of serotonin syndrome. It also produces hypertension in doses exceeding 225 mg/d.

In acute overdose, signs and symptoms include tachycardia, hypertension, diaphoresis, tremor, and mydriasis. CNS depression and generalized seizures are common. Severe hypotension requiring vasopressors has been reported. ECG findings include sinus tachycardia, QRS interval widening, and QT_c interval prolongation.

Emergency Department Care and Disposition

Venlafaxine has greater toxicity in overdose than do SSRIs, and onset of symptoms may be precipitous.

1. All patients should have IV access and be placed on a cardiac monitor.
2. Early gastric lavage should be strongly considered.
3. **Activated charcoal** 1 g/kg should be administered to all patients.
4. **Benzodiazepines** are the anticonvulsants of choice.
5. Hypertension and tachycardia may require pharmacologic management. Administration of a **β-blocker** should be considered.
6. **IV sodium bicarbonate** should be considered for QRS interval longer than 100 milliseconds.
7. Patients should be observed for 6 hours postingestion. Symptomatic patients should be admitted to a monitored bed.

MONOAMINE OXIDASE INHIBITORS

Because of their inherent toxicity, MAOIs have for the most part been replaced by safer antidepressants. However, they are still used for refractory cases. MAOIs cause accumulation of neurotransmitters in presynaptic nerve terminals and decrease clearance of dietary biogenic amines such as tyramine. They have a low therapeutic index, lead to potentially fatal food and drug interactions, and cause severe toxicity in overdose.

Tyramine is a dietary amine found in aged meats, cheeses, and red wine. Coingestion with MAOIs results in release of norepinephrine, epinephrine, serotonin, and dopamine.

Clinical Features

Within 90 minutes of ingestion of tyramine, patients taking MAOIs may develop hypertension, diaphoresis, headache, mydriasis, neck stiffness, neuromuscular excitation, palpitations, and chest pain. Symptoms generally resolve within 6 hours, but deaths, usually due to intracranial hemorrhage or myocardial infarction, have been reported.

When MAOIs are combined with certain other medications (Table 100-1), several potentially serious types of drug interactions may develop. These include a hyperadrenergic state similar to the tyramine reaction when taken with sympathomimetics. MAOIs inhibit the clearance of other drugs, including opiates and sedative-hypnotics. Tranylcypromine and phenelzine stimulate insulin secretion leading to hypoglycemia in patients on sulfonylureas. Serotonin syndrome has been reported, especially when combined with other serotonergic agents such meperidine, dextromethorphan, or tramadol.

In acute overdose, toxicity may develop at doses smaller than 2 mg/kg. A dose of 4 to 6 mg/kg may be fatal. Signs and symptoms usually develop 6 to 12 hours postingestion but may be delayed up to 24 hours. Symptoms include headache, agitation, irritability, nausea, palpitations, and tremor. Signs include sinus tachycardia, hyperreflexia, hyperactivity, fasciculations, mydriasis, hyperventilation, nystagmus, and generalized flushing. Opisthotonus, muscle rigidity, diaphoresis, chest pain, hypertension, diarrhea, hallucinations, combativeness, confusion, marked hyperthermia, and trismus may develop. "Ping-pong" gaze, or bilateral wandering horizontal eye movements, may be noted. Severe toxicity presents with bradycardia, worsening hyperthermia, papilledema, seizures, coma, and cardiac arrest. Hypotension is associated with a poor prognosis.

Diagnosis and Differential

The diagnosis is a clinical one. Laboratory tests are used to detect complications such as hypoxia, rhabdomyolysis, renal failure, hyperkalemia, metabolic acidosis, hemolysis, and disseminated intravascular coagulation.

The differential diagnosis for MAOI toxicity includes all causes of a hyperadrenergic state, altered mental status, and/or muscle rigidity (Table 100-2).

Emergency Department Care and Disposition

Emergency department management involves supportive care and early recognition and treatment of complications.

1. All patients require IV access, cardiac monitoring, and supplemental **oxygen.**

TABLE 100-1 Drugs Contraindicated with Monoamine Oxidase Inhibitors

Indirect sympathomimetics	Miscellaneous drugs
Benzphetamine	Beta blockers
Bretylium	Bupropion
Cocaine	Buspirone
Dexfenfluramine	Caffeine
Diethylpropion	Carbamazepine
Dopamine	Cyclobenzaprine
Ephedrine	Dextromethorphan
Fenfluramine	Disulfiram
Guanethidine	Ergot alkaloids
Isometheptene	Fentanyl
Mephentermine	Furazolidone
Metaraminol	Ketamine
Methamphetamine	Levodopa (L-dopa)
3,4-Methylenedioxymethamphetamine	Lithium
Methyldopa	Meperidine
Methylphenidate	Mirtazapine
Pemoline	Oral hypoglycemic agents
Phentermine	Phenothiazines
Phencyclidine	Procarbazine
Phenylpropanolamine	St. John's wort
Propylhexedrine	Sumatriptan
Pseudoephedrine	Theophylline
Reserpine	Tramadol
Ritodrine	Tricyclic antidepressants
Tyramine	

2. Gastric lavage within 2 hours of significant overdose is recommended.
3. A single dose of **activated charcoal** 1 g/kg should be administered.
4. **Phentolamine** 2.5 to 5 mg IV every 10 to 15 minutes is used to treat hypertension. An infusion of 0.2 to 5.0 mg/min may be used for maintenance therapy. **Sodium nitroprusside,** starting at 0.5 to 1.0 μg/kg/min, is an effective alternative, as is **fenoldopam,** administered as a titratable infusion starting at 0.05 to 0.1 μg/kg/min.
5. Hypotension is treated with **crystalloid IV fluid** boluses of 10 to 20 mL/kg.
6. **Norepinephrine** is the preferred vasopressor in refractory hypotension.
7. **Lidocaine, procainamide,** and **phenytoin** are used to treat dysrhythmias. Bradycardia is treated with **atropine, isoproterenol,** and **dobutamine.**
8. **Benzodiazepines** are the agents of choice for seizure control. Barbiturates are alternatives but may precipitate hypotension and respiratory depression.
9. Hyperthermia is managed with cool mist sprays, fans, or ice baths. Benzodiazepines may be given to minimize muscle hyperactivity and associated heat production. **Nondepolarizing neuromuscular blockers** or

TABLE 100-2 Differential Diagnosis of Monoamine Oxidase
Inhibitor Overdose

Intoxications
Amphetamines
Antimuscarinics
Cathinone
Clonidine (early)
Cocaine
Lysergic acid diethylamide
Methylphenidate
MDMA
Nicotine (early)
Phencyclidine
Phenylpropanolamine
Strychnine
Theophylline
Tricyclic antidepressants (early)
Withdrawal states
Ethanol (delirium tremens)
Sedative-hypnotics
Clonidine
β-Blockers
Medical conditions
Heat stroke
Hypoglycemia
Hyperthyroidism
Pheochromocytoma
Infectious diseases
Encephalitis
Meningitis
Rabies
Sepsis
Tetanus
Adverse drug reactions
Dystonic reactions
Malignant hyperthermia
Serotonin syndrome
Tyramine reaction
Spontaneous hypertensive crisis
Neuroleptic malignant syndrome
Psychaitric
Lethal catatonia

Key: MDMA = 3,4-methylenedioxymethamphetamine.

    dantrolene 0.5 to 2.5 mg IV every 6 hours may be required for muscle relaxation in refractory cases.
10. With few exceptions, all patients with MAOI exposures should be monitored for at least 24 hours. All intentional overdoses and accidental exposures of greater than 1 mg/kg should be admitted to an intensive care unit; others usually can be admitted to a monitored floor.

ANTIPSYCHOTICS

Antipsychotics are used to manage schizophrenia and other psychoses; for chemical restraint; as antiemetics; and to control hiccups, various headache syndromes, and certain involuntary motor disorders, such as Tourette syndrome. Older agents, referred to as *typical* antipsychotics, have numerous adverse effects. A new generation of *atypical* antipsychotics has a greater safety profile.

Clinical Features

Antipsychotics have a high therapeutic index. However, they have adverse effects related to their anticholinergic, antihistaminic, and antiadrenergic properties. They also can cause dystonic reactions, akathisia, bradykinesia, tardive dyskinesia, and neuroleptic malignant syndrome.

In acute overdose, patients present with CNS depression, seizures, tachycardia, hypotension, and impaired thermoregulation. Cardiac conduction disturbances may develop, ranging from asymptomatic QT_c interval prolongation to ventricular dysrhythmias, including torsades de pointes. Fatalities in acute overdose are rare.

Emergency Department Care and Disposition

Management is supportive. All patients require an ECG and continuous cardiac monitoring.

1. Patients with altered mental status should receive **oxygen** and **naloxone,** and their blood sugar should be determined at bedside.
2. Hypotension is treated with **crystalloid IV fluids.** If vasopressors are required, those with β-adrenergic properties (epinephrine, dopamine, and isoproterenol) should be avoided. **Norepinephrine** is the vasopressor of choice.
3. **Activated charcoal** 1 g/kg should be administered. Gastric lavage may be appropriate early after a large overdose.
4. Ventricular dysrhythmias are treated with class Ib antidysrhythmics (eg, **lidocaine**); the Ia agents (quinidine, procainamide, and disopyramide) should be avoided. Wide complex tachycardias should be treated with **sodium bicarbonate** 1 to 2 mEq/kg IV bolus followed by an infusion of 100 to 150 mEq in 1 L 5% dextrose in water titrated over 4 to 6 hours, with a target arterial pH of 7.5. Torsade de pointes is treated with **magnesium sulfate** 2 to 4 g IV or overdrive pacing.
5. Seizures may be controlled with **benzodiazepines, phenobarbital,** or **phenytoin.**
6. Patients with altered mental status or cardiotoxicity should be admitted to an intensive care unit. All patients who have ingested thioridazine or mesoridazine should be monitored for at least 24 hours. Other patients may be medically cleared if asymptomatic 6 hours postingestion, their physical examination is normal, and there is no QTc interval widening on ECG.

LITHIUM

Lithium is used to treat bipolar disorder and other medical and psychiatric conditions. Most patients on chronic lithium therapy will develop some form of toxicity.

Clinical Features

The most common adverse effects are hand tremor, polyuria, and rash. Nephrogenic diabetes insipidus and incomplete distal renal tubular acidosis have been reported. Neurologic effects include memory loss, decreased concentration, fatigue, ataxia, and dysarthria.

Toxicity results from acute or chronic exposure or decreased drug clearance. Patients with renal insufficiency or volume depletion are at increased risk. After an acute overdose, patients with mild toxicity may present with nausea, vomiting, tremor, hyperreflexia, ataxia, agitation, and muscle weakness. With increasing toxicity, patients may manifest depressed mental status, rigidity, and hypotension. Severe toxicity may present with coma, seizures, myoclonus, and cardiovascular collapse. Serum lithium levels correlate poorly with toxicity in the acute setting. Cardiac abnormalities include the presence of U waves, T-wave changes, ST-segment depression, QT_c interval prolongation, bundle branch block, junctional rhythms, and bradycardia. Patients with chronic toxicity tend to show a preponderance of neurologic symptoms. Serum lithium levels correlate better with toxicity than in the acute setting.

Emergency Department Care and Disposition

Initial treatment includes cardiovascular and respiratory stabilization, continuous cardiac monitoring, baseline laboratory studies, and ECG.

1. **Activated charcoal** does not bind lithium but may be indicated for coingestions. Early gastric lavage or whole bowel irrigation also should be considered.
2. Seizures may be controlled with **benzodiazepines** or **phenobarbital.**
3. Aggressive hydration with **IV normal saline** enhances lithium elimination.
4. **Hemodialysis** is used in severe cases to reduce the serum lithium level to below 1 mEq/L. Indications include a level higher than 3.5 mEq/L (4.0 mEq/L in acute overdose), little change in a level of 1.5 to 3.5 mEq/L after 6 hours of hydration, an increasing level, renal failure, or ingestion of sustained-release preparations.
5. **Sodium polystyrene sulfonate** 15 g PO 4 times a day or 30 g rectally may be useful in clearing lithium in mild to moderate toxicity.
6. Although serum levels do not correlate well with symptoms, it is recommended that patients with levels above 1.5 mEq/L be admitted, as should patients who have ingested sustained-release preparations.
7. In acute overdose, patients who remain asymptomatic after 6 hours may be medically cleared.
8. In chronic toxicity, patients with mild symptoms and no other risk factors may be hydrated for 4 to 6 hours and discharged if their levels drop below 1.5 mEq/L and there is clinical improvement. Patients with more severe manifestations should be admitted.

For further reading in *Emergency Medicine: A Comprehensive Study Guide,* 6th ed., see Chap. 158, "Tricyclic Antidepressants," Chap. 159, "Newer Antidepressants and Serotonin Syndrome," and Chap. 160, "Monoamine Oxidase Inhibitors," by Kirk C. Mills; Chap. 161, "Antipsychotics," by Richard A. Harrigan and William J. Brady; and Chap. 162, "Lithium," by Sandra M. Schneider and Daniel S. Cobaugh.

101 | Sedatives and Hypnotics

Keith L. Mausner

Sedative and hypnotic agents include barbiturates, benzodiazepines, and non-benzodiazepine drugs such as chloral hydrate, ethchlorvynol, glutethimide, meprobamate, methaqualone, buspirone, zolpidem, zaleplon, and γ-hydroxy-butyrate (GHB).

BARBITURATES

Clinical Features

Barbiturates depress activity in nerve and muscle cells. Mild to moderate intoxication resembles alcohol intoxication; drowsiness, disinhibition, ataxia, slurred speech, and confusion worsen with increasing dose. Stupor, coma, or complete neurologic unresponsiveness occurs with severe intoxication and with respiratory depression, hypotension, and hypothermia. Pulse rate is not diagnostic, and pupil size and reactivity, nystagmus, and deep tendon reflexes are variable. Gastrointestinal (GI) motility is slowed, thus delaying gastric emptying. Hypoglycemia may be seen.

Early death from barbiturate overdose usually results from cardiovascular collapse and respiratory arrest. Complications include aspiration pneumonia, noncardiogenic pulmonary edema, and adult respiratory distress syndrome. Severe poisoning can be assumed if greater than 10 times the hypnotic dose is ingested at one time.

Diagnosis and Differential

Barbiturate serum levels may establish the diagnosis and are useful to distinguish long- from short-acting barbiturates; this distinction is important because the treatment approach is different. Long-acting agents include barbital and phenobarbital (duration of action, >6 hours). Amobarbital is an intermediate acting agent (3- to 6-hour duration). Pentobarbital and secobarbital are short-acting agents (duration of action, <3 hours), and thiopental and methohexital are ultra short-acting (duration of action, 0.3 hour). The differential diagnosis of barbiturate poisoning includes intoxication with other sedative-hypnotics or alcohol and with environmental hypothermia and other causes of coma. Barbiturates are more likely than benzodiazepines to produce coma and myocardial depression. Chloral hydrate is associated with cardiac arrhythmias. Ethchlorvynol may produce a vinyl-like odor and prolonged coma. Glutethimide may cause fluctuating central nervous system (CNS) impairment and anticholinergic signs.

Bedside glucose determination is indicated for all patients with altered levels of consciousness, as is consideration of naloxone and thiamine administration. Laboratory studies should include electrolytes, blood urea nitrogen, creatinine, and glucose levels; complete blood count; toxicology screen, including acetaminophen to exclude coingestion; electrocardiogram; and chest radiograph. An arterial blood gas analysis may be useful.

Emergency Department Care and Disposition

1. Emergent priorities remain airway, breathing, and circulation. **Endotracheal intubation** is often necessary in severe sedative-hypnotic overdose.

Cardiac monitoring and an intravenous (IV) line should be instituted. Volume expansion with **isotonic saline** is the primary treatment for shock and hypotension. In elderly patients or those with a history of heart failure or renal failure, 250-mL boluses may be prudent. **Dopamine** or **norepinephrine** may be necessary if volume resuscitation is ineffective.

2. **Activated charcoal** 1 to 2 g/kg should be administered because it decreases absorption; the addition of a cathartic such as sorbitol has no proven benefit. The airway should be secured first if there is significant risk of aspiration. Multiple-dose activated charcoal 25 to 50 g every 4 hours may decrease barbiturate serum levels. There is no evidence of any benefit of gastric lavage over activated charcoal. Ipecac has no role in management because of CNS depression and risk of aspiration.

3. Forced diuresis with saline and furosemide, titrating urine output to 4 to 6 mL/kg/h, is beneficial in phenobarbital poisoning.

4. **Urinary alkalinization** promotes the excretion of long-acting barbiturates. **Sodium bicarbonate** 1 to 2 mEq/kg IV bolus should be administered. Then, 50 to 100 mEq bicarbonate should be added to 500 mL of 5% dextrose in water, and the drip rate should be adjusted to maintain an arterial pH of 7.45 to 7.50, urinary pH of 8.0, and urine output of 2 mL/kg/h. The serum potassium level must remain at a minimum of 4.0 mEq/L for alkalinization to be effective. Electrolytes and effectiveness of therapy should be monitored every 2 to 4 hours.

5. **Hemodialysis** and **hemoperfusion** are indicated for patients who deteriorate despite aggressive supportive care.

6. Close monitoring over 6 to 8 hours and documentation of improvement in neurologic and vital signs may allow patients with mild to moderate toxicity to be discharged to psychiatric care or home, if appropriate. Severe toxicity requires admission, and toxicology consultation is recommended.

Barbiturate abstinence syndrome occurs with abrupt withdrawal in chronic users and produces minor withdrawal findings within 24 hours and major life-threatening manifestations in 2 to 8 days. Short-acting agents produce more severe withdrawal than do long-acting agents. Clinical manifestations are similar to alcohol withdrawal. Minor findings include anxiety, depression, insomnia, anorexia, nausea, vomiting, muscle twitching, abdominal cramping, and sweating. Severe manifestations include psychosis, hallucinations, delirium, seizures, hyperthermia, and cardiovascular collapse. Treatment consists of aggressive supportive care and IV benzodiazepines or barbiturates, with subsequent tapering of dose.

BENZODIAZEPINES

Clinical Features

Isolated benzodiazepine overdose has a relatively low morbidity and mortality; serious toxicity usually occurs with coingestion of other agents or with parenteral administration. Fatal isolated benzodiazepine overdose is more likely with short-acting agents such as triazolam, alprazolam, or temazepam.

The most significant effects of benzodiazepines are on the CNS, which include drowsiness, dizziness, slurred speech, confusion, and cognitive impairment. Other reported effects are headache, nausea, vomiting, chest pain, arthralgias, diarrhea, and incontinence. Rare paradoxical reactions include rage and delirium. Respiratory depression and hypotension are more likely to occur with parenteral administration or with coingestants. The elderly are more susceptible to the adverse effects of benzodiazepines.

Diagnosis and Differential

Toxicology screening may be useful in establishing the diagnosis, but the laboratory may not routinely screen for all available benzodiazepines. Therefore, it is essential to know the laboratory's limitations. Serum benzodiazepine levels are not clinically useful in overdoses. The findings of benzodiazepine toxicity are nonspecific.

Emergency Department Care and Disposition

1. Emergent priorities remain airway, breathing, and circulation (see the preceding section on barbiturate toxicity for initial guidelines on monitoring, resuscitation, and laboratory evaluation).
2. **Activated charcoal** 1 to 2 g/kg should be administered; there is no role for multiple-dose activated charcoal.
3. Flumazenil, a benzodiazepine antagonist, is not indicated for empiric administration in poisoned patients. Seizures may occur in mixed ingestions, especially those involving tricyclic antidepressants, and in patients chronically dependent on benzodiazepines or with underlying seizure disorders. Flumazenil also is contraindicated in suspected elevated intracranial pressure or head injury. Its primary use is in reversing the effects of benzodiazepines administered acutely for sedation. Due to its short half-life (approximately 1 hour), it is mainly effective with short-acting agents such as midazolam. Flumazenil is administered 0.2 mg IV every minute to response or a total dose of 3 mg.
4. Forced diuresis, urinary alkalinization, hemodialysis, and hemoperfusion are not effective in enhancing benzodiazepine elimination.
5. Care for benzodiazepine ingestions is primarily supportive. Hospital admission is indicated for significant alterations in mental status, respiratory depression, and hypotension. Psychiatric consultation is indicated for intentional overdoses.

Chronic benzodiazepine users may experience a withdrawal syndrome similar to alcohol or barbiturate withdrawal (see the preceding section on barbiturate abstinence syndrome).

NONBENZODIAZEPINE SEDATIVE-HYPNOTICS

Clinical Features

γ-Hydroxybutyrate

GHB is used abroad as an anesthetic and in the treatment of narcolepsy and substance withdrawal. In the United States, only sodium oxybate (Xyrem), a form of GHB, is approved for the treatment of cataplexy associated with narcolepsy. γ-Hydroxybutrolactone and 1,4-butanediol are metabolized after ingestion of GHB. These drugs are increasingly abused and implicated in overdose and drug-facilitated sexual assault. Effects are dose-dependent. Abrupt onset of aggressive behavior followed by drowsiness, dizziness, euphoria, or coma with rapid awakening and amnesia may be seen. Other findings may include nystagmus, ataxia, apnea, seizure-like activity, and bradycardia. Marked agitation on stimulation such as a sternal rub or intubation is common. Improperly synthesized GHB may contain sodium hydroxide, which may cause esophageal burns or pulmonary injury in the event of aspiration. Chronic GHB users may be at risk for an abstinence syndrome similar to alcohol withdrawal, which may be severe and last from 5 to 15 days.

Buspirone

Buspirone is unrelated to the other sedative-hypnotics and does not appear to be addictive. Overdoses of up to 3 g (150 times the average anxiolytic dose) have produced no lasting ill effects. Symptoms of overdose include drowsiness and dysphoria. Rare findings include hypotension, bradycardia, seizures, GI upset, dystonia, and priapism. Hypertensive reactions may occur with coadministration of monoamine oxidase inhibitors.

Chloral Hydrate

Toxic doses produce severe CNS, respiratory, and cardiovascular depressions and resistant ventricular arrhythmias, which are the leading cause of mortality in overdose. Clues to ingestion include a combination of a pearlike breath odor, hypotension, and dysrhythmias. It is also a GI irritant, and overdose may be associated with GI bleeding or intestinal perforation. Chloral hydrate is radiopaque, and abdominal radiographs may be useful in diagnosis and to exclude perforation.

Ethchlorvynol

CNS effects of overdose include nystagmus, lethargy, and prolonged coma. Hypothermia, hypotension, bradycardia, and noncardiogenic pulmonary edema may occur. A distinct vinyl-like breath odor may be a clue to diagnosis.

Glutethimide

The manifestations of glutethimide overdose are similar to those of barbiturate toxicity except for the presence of prominent anticholinergic findings and a fluctuating, prolonged coma.

Meprobamate

The CNS manifestations of meprobamate toxicity are similar to those of other sedative-hypnotics. Hypotension is a common feature of serious overdose. Seizures, cardiac arrhythmias, and pulmonary edema also have been reported. Prolonged fluctuating coma may occur secondary to continued absorption from GI concretions of the drug. Meprobamate is the active metabolite of carisoprodol (Soma), a commonly prescribed, noncontrolled muscle relaxant.

Methaqualone

Methaqualone has CNS, respiratory, and cardiovascular effects similar to those of the other sedative hypnotics. Unlike the others, it also causes hypertonicity, clonus, hyperreflexia, and muscle twitching. It often impairs judgment and impulse control, thereby increasing risk of morbidity and mortality from trauma.

Zaleplon and Zolpidem

Zaleplon and zolpidem are used for the treatment of insomnia. Zaleplon was only recently released, and there have been no case reports of fatalities in single-agent ingestions. Findings in zolpidem overdose include drowsiness, vomiting, and, rarely, coma and respiratory depression. Flumazenil may reverse some of the effects of zolpidem, but its use is not recommended in most overdose situations for the reasons outlined in the section on benzodiazepines.

Emergency Department Care and Disposition

1. Emergent priorities remain airway, breathing, and circulation (see the preceding section on barbiturate toxicity for initial guidelines for monitoring and laboratory evaluation). Specific serum levels are not particularly useful except in helping establish the diagnosis. Serum levels also may guide the decision to treat patients not responding to standard supportive therapy with **hemoperfusion,** which is more effective than hemodialysis.
2. Treatment for nonbenzodiazepine sedative-hypnotic toxicity is primarily supportive. Because these agents may cause pulmonary edema, judicious administration of IV fluids plus early vasopressors is indicated to treat hypotension.
3. **Activated charcoal** 1 to 2 g/kg should be administered. Because of the tendency of meprobamate to form GI concretions, **whole bowel irrigation** using 2 L/h polyethylene glycol (40 mL/kg/h in children) until rectal effluent is clear may be of benefit once GI perforation is excluded. Forced diuresis is not effective with the nonbenzodiazepine agents due to limited renal excretion.
4. Chloral hydrate–induced arrhythmias may respond to β**-blockers.** Overdrive pacing may be necessary for ventricular tachycardia. β-Adrenergic agents (epinephrine, isoproterenol, and dopamine) may worsen chloral hydrate–induced arrhythmias; if a pressor is needed for hypotension, an α-acting agent such as **norepinephrine** should be used.
5. There should be a low threshold for hospital admission of these patients, especially with any significant CNS or respiratory depression, hypotension, or arrhythmias. Glutethimide and meprobamate are of special concern because of the potential for fluctuating or delayed manifestations.

For further reading in *Emergency Medicine: A Comprehensive Study Guide,* 6th ed., see Chap. 163, "Barbiturates," by R. M. Schears; Chap. 164, "Benzodiazepines," by G. M. Bosse; and Chap. 165, "Nonbenzodiazepine Hypnosedatives," by R. M. Schears.

102 | Alcohols

Michael P. Kefer

In discussing the toxicity of common alcohols, an understanding of the osmolal gap is important. The presence of an elevated osmolal gap suggests the presence of a low-molecular-weight substance such as ethanol, isopropanol, methanol, or ethylene glycol.

$$\text{osmolal gap} = \text{osmoles measured} - \text{osmoles calculated}$$
$$\text{normal osmolal gap} < 10 \text{ mOsm/L}$$
$$\text{osmoles measured} = \text{laboratory determination by freezing point depression}$$
$$\text{osmoles calculated} = 2(\text{Na}) + (\text{blood urea nitrogen}/2.8) + (\text{glucose}/18)$$

ETHANOL

Although acute ethanol intoxication may cause death directly from respiratory depression, morbidity and mortality are usually related to accidental injury from impaired cognitive function. Ethanol intoxication predisposes patients to trauma and complicates evaluation of the injured patient. On average, nondrinkers eliminate ethanol from the bloodstream at a rate of 15 to 20 mg/dL/h and chronic drinkers do so at 25 to 35 mg/dL/h.

Clinical Features

Signs and symptoms of ethanol intoxication include slurred speech, disinhibited behavior, central nervous system (CNS) depression, and altered coordination. Manifestations of serious head injury may be identical to, or clouded by, ethanol intoxication. Ethanol use is associated with abuse of other illicit drugs.

Emergency Department Care and Disposition

The mainstay of treatment is observation of the patient until clinically sober. A careful physical examination should be performed to evaluate for complicating injury or illness.

1. Hypoglycemia should be excluded by measuring fingerstick glucose. **Thiamine** 100 mg intravenously (IV) or intramuscularly should be administered. If required, IV fluids should contain 5% dextrose because these patients are often glycogen depleted.
2. Any deterioration or lack of improvement during observation should be considered secondary to causes other than ethanol and managed accordingly. The patient can be discharged once intoxication has resolved to the extent that the patient does not pose a threat to self or others. Those who plan to operate a motor vehicle should have nearly undetectable serum ethanol levels.

ISOPROPANOL

Isopropanol is commonly found in rubbing alcohol, solvents, skin and hair products, paint thinners, and antifreeze. Its CNS depressant effects are twice as potent and last twice as long as those of ethanol. Acetone is the principal metabolite.

Clinical Features

Clinically, isopropanol intoxication manifests similarly to ethanol intoxication except the duration is longer and the CNS depressant effects are more profound. The smell of rubbing alcohol or the fruity odor of ketones may be noted on the patient's breath. Severe poisoning is marked by early onset coma, respiratory depression, and hypotension. Hemorrhagic gastritis is a characteristic finding that causes nausea, vomiting, and abdominal pain. Upper gastrointestinal bleeding may be severe. Other less common complications include hepatic dysfunction, acute tubular necrosis, and rhabdomyolysis.

Diagnosis and Differential

Calculation of the osmolal gap is useful if isopropanol testing is not immediately available. In addition to an elevated isopropanol level, laboratory investigation may show ketonemia and ketonuria, from accumulation of acetone, without hyperglycemia or glycosuria, and the presence of an osmolal gap. Mild acidosis may be present from acetone metabolism to acetate and formate or hypotension with resultant lactic acidosis.

Isopropanol intoxication is characteristically distinguished from that of other common alcohols by the significant osmolal gap without a significant anion gap metabolic acidosis and a negative ethanol level.

Emergency Department Care and Disposition

1. General supportive measures are indicated. As with any patient who presents with altered mental status, administration of glucose, thiamine, and naloxone should be considered.
2. Charcoal does not bind alcohols, so it is useful only if there is co-ingestion of an absorbable substance.
3. Hypotension usually responds to IV fluids, but vasopressors may be necessary. Severe hemorrhagic gastritis may require transfusion.
4. Hemodialysis is indicated for refractory hypotension or when the predicted peak level of isopropanol is higher than 400 mg/dL. Hemodialysis removes isopropanol and acetone.
5. Patients with prolonged CNS depression require admission. Those who are asymptomatic after 6 to 8 hours of observation can be discharged or referred for psychiatric evaluation, if indicated.

METHANOL AND ETHYLENE GLYCOL

Methanol (wood alcohol) is commonly found as a solvent in paint products, windshield washing fluids, and antifreeze. Ethylene glycol is commonly used as a coolant and preservative and is found in polishes and detergents. Toxicity from these alcohols is due to formation of their toxic metabolites, which result in a high anion-gap metabolic acidosis ($Na^+ - [Cl^- + HCO3^-]$ $>12 + 4$ mEq/L). Prognosis is related to the severity of the acidosis.

Clinical Features of Methanol

Methanol metabolism results in formation of formaldehyde and formic acid. Symptoms may not appear for 12 to 18 hours after ingestion because these toxic metabolites must accumulate. Time to symptom onset may be longer if ethanol is consumed because ethanol inhibits methanol metabolism.

Symptoms include CNS depression, visual disturbances (classically, a complaint of looking at a snowstorm), abdominal pain, nausea, and vomiting. The gastrointestinal symptoms may be due to mucosal irritation or pancreatitis. On examination, CNS signs can vary from lethargy to coma. Funduscopic examination may show retinal edema or hyperemia of the optic disk caused by formaldehyde.

Clinical Features of Ethylene Glycol

Ethylene glycol poisoning often exhibits 3 distinct clinical phases after ingestion due to the toxic metabolites. First, within 12 hours, CNS effects predominate. The patient appears intoxicated without the odor of ethanol on the breath. Second, 12 to 24 hours after ingestion, cardiopulmonary effects predominate. Elevated heart and respiratory rate and blood pressure are common. Congestive heart failure, respiratory distress syndrome, and circulatory collapse are also noted. Third, 24 to 72 hours after ingestion, renal effects predominate. Flank pain with costovertebral angle tenderness is noted. Acute tubular necrosis with acute renal failure occurs if appropriate treatment is not received.

Hypocalcemia may result from precipitation of calcium oxalate into tissues and may be severe enough to cause tetany and typical electrocardiogram changes. Calcium oxalate crystals are noted on urinalysis. Elevated creatine kinase levels may be seen.

Diagnosis and Differential

The diagnosis is based on clinical presentation and laboratory findings of a high anion-gap metabolic acidosis with elevated levels of methanol or ethylene glycol. An elevated osmolal gap is present, and calculation of this is useful if methanol or ethylene glycol testing is not immediately available. Basic laboratory investigation should include a complete blood count, electrolytes, blood urea nitrogen, creatinine, glucose, arterial blood gas, urinalysis, and methanol or ethylene glycol level.

The differential diagnosis includes other causes of an anion-gap metabolic acidosis and is recalled by the acronym MUDPILES (Table 102-1). Ethylene glycol poisoning differs from methanol poisoning in that visual disturbances and funduscopic abnormalities are absent and calcium oxalate crystals are present in the urine.

TABLE 102-1 Differential Diagnosis of an Anion-Gap Metabolic Acidosis Is Recalled by the Acronym MUDPILES

Methanol
Uremia
Diabetic ketoacidosis
Paraldehyde
Iron, isoniazid, inhalants
Lactic acidosis
Ethanol, ethylene glycol
Salicylates

Emergency Department Care and Disposition

Treatment is based on preventing formation of the toxic metabolites and removing them from the body.

1. General supportive measures are indicated, including the administration of glucose, thiamine, and naloxone in the patient with altered mental status.
2. Sodium bicarbonate may be required to correct acidosis.
3. **Fomepizole** as a 15 mg/kg IV load followed by 10 mg/kg every 12 hours for 4 doses is now favored over ethanol infusion as the treatment of choice for methanol and ethylene glycol toxicities. Fomepizole is a potent inhibitor of alcohol dehydrogenase, with 8,000 times greater affinity than ethanol and with fewer side effects. Indications for fomepizole administration include (*a*) suspected methanol or ethylene glycol poisoning, (*b*) the presence of an anion-gap metabolic acidosis, (*c*) a methanol or ethylene glycol level above 20 mg/dL, and (*d*) any patient requiring hemodialysis.
4. If fomepizole is not available, ethanol infusion should be administered. **Ethanol** 0.6 gm/kg IV is administered as a loading dose, followed by a continuous infusion of 0.11 g/kg/h in the average drinker and 0.15 g/kg/h in the heavy drinker. The continuous infusion is adjusted accordingly to keep the blood ethanol level between 100 and 150 mg/dL. Ethanol inhibits formation of toxic metabolites because it has 10 to 20 times greater affinity for alcohol dehydrogenase than for methanol and 100 times that of ethylene glycol. Indications for ethanol treatment are the same as those for fomepizole. Additional indications are allergy to or unavailability of fomepizole.
5. If necessary, oral therapy with commercial alcoholic beverages can be initiated. The amount of ethanol contained in these is calculated by:

$$\text{ethanol (g)} = \text{beverage (mL)} \times 0.9 \times (\text{proof}/200)$$

6. Serum glucose should be monitored during treatment with ethanol because hypoglycemia may be induced, especially in children.
7. **Dialysis** eliminates methanol and ethylene glycol and their toxic metabolites. Indications for dialysis are (*a*) signs or symptoms of significant toxicity, (*b*) the presence of an anion-gap metabolic acidosis, (*c*) a methanol or ethylene glycol level above 20 mg/dL, and (*d*) signs of ocular toxicity from methanol or nephrotoxicity from ethylene glycol. Peritoneal dialysis is considered only when hemodialysis is not available.
8. Use of fomepizole or ethanol does not affect indications for dialysis. Fomepizole and ethanol are dialyzable. Therefore, during dialysis, the dosing interval of fomepizole is increased to every 4 hours. The continuous infusion rate of ethanol is doubled initially and readjusted accordingly to maintain the level between 100 and 150 mg/dL.
9. Treatment with dialysis, fomepizole, or ethanol is continued until the methanol or ethylene glycol level is 0 and acidosis has resolved.
10. Vitamin therapy also is important. In methanol poisoning, **folate** 50 mg IV every 4 hours should be administered as a cofactor for the conversion of formic acid to carbon dioxide. In ethylene glycol poisoning, **pyridoxine** 100 mg and **thiamine** 100 mg IV or intramuscularly every day should be administered as cofactors for the conversion of toxic metabolites to nontoxic compounds.

11. Calcium replacement may be necessary from ethylene glycol toxicity.
12. Any patient with serious signs or symptoms of toxicity should be admitted to a facility capable of intensive care and hemodialysis. Asymptomatic individuals should be admitted for observation because of possible delayed onset of toxic symptoms.

For further reading in *Emergency Medicine: A Comprehensive Study Guide,* 6th ed., see Chap. 166, "Alcohols," by William A. Burke and Wilma V. Henderson.

103 | Drugs of Abuse

Jeffrey N. Glaspy

OPIOIDS

Clinical Features

Opioid overdose and withdrawal are frequently encountered in the emergency department (ED). Opioids cause different degrees of respiratory depression, altered mental status, miosis, orthostatic hypotension, nausea, vomiting, histamine release (resulting in urticaria and bronchospasm), decreased gastrointestinal motility, and urinary retention. Although the classic triad of opioid overdose is coma, miosis, and respiratory depression, miosis is not universally present. Normal pupillary size or mydriasis has been reported with the use of meperidine, morphine, propoxyphene, pentazocine, and diphenoxylate. Mydriasis also may result from coingestants or with severe cerebral hypoxia.

Opioid withdrawal usually manifests in feelings of anxiety, insomnia, yawning, lacrimation, diaphoresis, rhinorrhea, diffuse myalgias, piloerection, mydriasis, nausea, vomiting, diarrhea, and abdominal cramping. Opioid withdrawal is rarely life threatening.

Diagnosis and Differential

Opioid overdose or withdrawal is a clinical diagnosis. The classic triad of coma, miosis, and respiratory depression strongly suggests acute or chronic opioid intoxication. Detection of opioids in the urine may aid in diagnosis of opioid overdose; however, there is a high false negative rate and the results of the urine test are not immediately available to the clinician. An acetaminophen level should be obtained in cases of propoxyphene, oxycodone, hydrocodone, tramadol, and codeine overdose and in any intentional suicidal ingestion.

The differential diagnosis of opioid overdose includes ingestion of clonidine, organophosphates, carbamates, phenothiazine, sedative-hypnotic agents, or γ-hydroxybutyrate; carbon monoxide poisoning; hypoglycemia; central nervous system (CNS) infection; postictal state; and pontine hemorrhage.

The diagnosis of opioid withdrawal is established when a constellation of withdrawal symptoms is temporally related to the abrupt cessation of an opioid agent. The differential diagnosis of opioid withdrawal includes drugs and toxins that promote an adrenergic state, other drug withdrawal, and hyperthyroidism.

Emergency Department Care and Disposition

1. Airway management is the most crucial aspect in the initial treatment of opioid overdose. Bag-valve-mask support may be needed to maintain oxygenation while naloxone and/or endotracheal intubation are being prepared.
2. **Naloxone** is a pure competitive antagonist at all opioid receptors. It can be given intravenously (IV), intratracheally, intramuscularly, subcutaneously, and intralingually. Onset after IV administration is 1 to 2 minutes; it has a 20- to 60-minute duration of action. For patients presenting with significant respiratory depression, a 2-mg IV dose should be given. Repeated doses of

499

2 mg IV every 3 minutes are then administered until respiratory depression is reversed or until a maximum dose of 10 mg has been reached. Propoxyphene, fentanyl, pentazocine, dextromethorphan, and sustained preparations of oxycodone may require administration of serial 2-mg doses.

3. For opioid-dependent individuals without respiratory depression, smaller doses of naloxone (eg, 0.05 mg IV) may be used to prevent opioid withdrawal. For non–opioid-dependent individuals without respiratory depression, an initial dose of 0.4 mg IV may be given.

4. A **continuous naloxone infusion** should be administered only if the patient has required multiple boluses of naloxone. The IV infusion dosage is two thirds of the total reversal dose per hour. Patients on naloxone infusions may require additional bolus doses and/or upward (for respiratory depression) or downward (for opioid withdrawal) adjustments in the infusion rate and should be admitted to an intensive care unit or monitored setting.

5. **Activated charcoal** should be administered if large amounts of opioid have been ingested or if coingestion is a possibility. Multiple-dose–activated charcoal administration is indicated in diphenoxylate hydrochloride-atropine sulfate (Lomotil) ingestion and in cases of large ingestions of sustained-release preparations.

6. An ED observation period of 4 to 6 hours is recommended for most cases of opioid intoxication. For longer-acting opioids (propoxyphene or methadone) or for sustained-release preparations, a 24- to 48-hour hospital admission is indicated.

7. Opioid withdrawal is rarely life threatening. Supportive care with **clonidine** 0.1 to 0.2 mg orally, antiemetics, and antidiarrheals may alleviate discomfort.

COCAINE, AMPHETAMINES, AND OTHER STIMULANTS

Clinical Features

Cocaine is a water-soluble, hydrochloride salt that is rapidly absorbed across all mucous membranes. Ether extraction yields crack cocaine, which is heat stable and commonly smoked. Intranasal use of cocaine causes a peak effect in 30 minutes and a duration of effect of 1 to 3 hours. Inhalational (smoked) and IV use of cocaine produce a rapid (1 to 2 minutes) effect and a short (15 to 30 minutes) duration. Cocaine has quinidine-like effects on cardiac conduction, which may cause a wide QRS interval complex and QT interval prolongation. In large doses, myocardial toxicity may result in negative inotropy, wide complex dysrhythmia, bradycardia, and hypotension. Central effects are mediated through activation of the sympathetic nervous system, which produce characteristic effects of mydriasis, tachycardia, hypertension, and diaphoresis. These effects predispose the user to dysrhythmias, seizures, and hyperthermia.

Cocaine induces dysrhythmias, myocarditis, cardiomyopathy, myocardial ischemia and infarction, aortic rupture, and aortic and coronary artery dissection. Even at low doses, it can produce coronary artery vasoconstriction. Animal data have demonstrated increased platelet aggregation, thrombogenesis, accelerated atherosclerosis, myocardial toxicity, and increased myocardial oxygen demand. Any route of cocaine administration may induce Q-wave and non–Q-wave myocardial infarction in patients, even those without coronary artery disease. Cocaine abuse during pregnancy increases risk for spontaneous abortion, abruptio placentae, fetal prematurity, and intrauterine growth retardation.

Crack cocaine use has been associated with pulmonary hemorrhage, pneumonitis, asthma, pulmonary edema, pneumomediastinum, pneumothorax, and pneumopericardium. "Body stuffers" (ingestion of small, poorly wrapped bags) and "body packers" (ingestion of large amounts of well-packaged bags) may die or demonstrate signs of severe cocaine toxicity if even a single bag ruptures. Intestinal ischemia, bowel necrosis, ischemic colitis, gastrointestinal bleeding, bowel perforation, and splenic infarction may be induced by cocaine.

Methamphetamine is abused by ingestion, IV injection, inhalation, or insufflation. Mortality from amphetamine toxicity is most commonly the result of hyperthermia, dysrhythmias, seizures, hypertension that results in intracranial infarction or hemorrhage, and encephalopathy. Methamphetamine abuse during pregnancy also has detrimental effects on fetal growth.

Stimulants, such as ephedrine and phenylpropanolamine, produce toxic effects similar to those of cocaine and amphetamines. Ephedrine has been linked to significant cardiovascular and neurologic toxicities, psychosis, severe hypertension, and death. Rhabdomyolysis also may occur with cocaine or amphetamine use.

The cocaine- or amphetamine-intoxicated patient may demonstrate tachycardia, tachypnea, hypertension, hyperthermia, and any degree of altered mental status. Common symptoms include chest pain, palpitations, dyspnea, headache, focal neurologic complaints, and seizure.

Diagnosis and Differential

Diagnosis of cocaine, amphetamine, or stimulant intoxication is usually made clinically. Urine drug screening for the cocaine metabolite benzoylecgonine will be positive in most cases if cocaine use has occurred within the past 72 hours. This test is fairly specific and exhibits little crossreactivity. Urine drug screens for amphetamines, however, are not specific and have high false negative and false positive results.

Patients with hyperthermia and agitation should have a chemistry panel, blood urea nitrogen, creatinine, and creatine kinase (CK) screen for metabolic acidosis, renal failure, and rhabdomyolysis. If altered mental status does not respond to standard therapy, a head computed tomographic should be obtained. Electrocardiogram, chest radiograph, and cardiac enzymes should be considered in cocaine- or amphetamine-intoxicated patients presenting with chest pain. Traumatic injury and hypoglycemia should be included in the differential diagnosis. Concomitant use of substances such as alcohol or opioids may significantly alter the presentation.

Emergency Department Care and Disposition

1. Treatment of cocaine and amphetamine toxicities involves adequate sedation and assessment of vital signs. Benzodiazepines, such as **lorazepam** 2 mg IV or **diazepam** 5 mg IV, often will improve tachycardia and hypertension. **Active cooling,** with mist spray and fanning, is used to treat moderate or severe hyperthermia.
2. Seizures also should be treated with **benzodiazepines;** however, phenobarbital loading or neuromuscular blockade may be necessary for status epilepticus.

3. Cardiac ischemia or infarction should be treated with **aspirin, nitrates, morphine,** and **benzodiazepines.** β-blockers are contraindicated due to unopposed α-receptor stimulation. Fibrinolytic therapy should be used with great caution because cocaine-associated intracranial hemorrhage and aortic or coronary artery dissection are contraindications to thrombolysis.

4. Cocaine-induced wide complex tachydysrhythmia and QRS interval prolongation should be treated by alkalinizing the serum to a pH of 7.45 to 7.5 with **sodium bicarbonate.** Acidification of the urine for amphetamine intoxication is not recommended.

5. Hypertensive emergencies should be treated with **nitroprusside** or **phentolamine.**

6. Asymptomatic "body packers" should be given 1 dose of **activated charcoal,** followed by polyethylene glycol electrolyte solution (GoLYTELY). If symptomatic, these patients should be given benzodiazepines and have immediate surgical consultation for laparotomy and packet removal.

7. Patient disposition depends on initial presentation, response to treatment, stimulant involved, and expected duration of effect. Amphetamines have a longer duration of effect than does cocaine; therefore, intoxication may require longer periods of observation or hospital admission.

8. Patients with significantly increased CK levels, hyperthermia, myoglobinuria, or electrocardiogram changes consistent with myocardial ischemia should be hospitalized in an intensive care unit setting.

HALLUCINOGENS

Clinical Features

Table 103-1 summarizes the classification, mechanism, typical dose, duration of action, features, complications, and specific treatments of commonly abused hallucinogens.

Diagnosis and Differential

Diagnosis of lysergic acid diethylamide abuse is based on history of use and the presence of sympathomimetic signs. Routine drug screens will not detect psilocybin or mescaline. Urine tests for phencyclidine (PCP) may be falsely negative in acute intoxication or falsely positive weeks after use in chronic abusers. Traumatic injuries, hypoglycemia, elevated CK level, and rhabdomyolysis should be ruled out in suspected cases of PCP intoxication. Urine tests for marijuana are unreliable indicators of acute use because patients may be positive for days to weeks after their last use.

The differential diagnosis of hallucinogen intoxication includes alcohol and benzodiazepine withdrawals, hypoglycemia, anticholinergic poisoning, thyrotoxicosis, CNS infections, structural CNS lesions, and acute psychosis.

Emergency Department Care and Disposition

1. Initial management of patients with hallucinogen intoxication is support of airway, breathing, and circulation. Hypoxia and hypoglycemia must be diagnosed and treated immediately.

2. Supportive care is usually all that is needed to manage a patient with lysergic acid diethylamide intoxication. IV **benzodiazepines** may be given for extremely agitated patients. Haloperidol should be considered as a second-line therapy because it may lower the seizure threshold. Most patients may

TABLE 103-1 Characteristics of Hallucinogens

Drug	Chemical classification	Mechanism of action	Typical dose	Duration of action	Clinical features	Complications	Specific treatment
LSD	Indole alkylamine	5-HT$_2$ agonist	50–300 μg	8–12 h	Mydriasis, sympathomimetic symptoms, nausea, muscle tension	Persistent psychosis, hallucinogen persisting perception disorder	Supportive benzodiazepines
Psilocybin	Indole alkylamine	5-HT$_2$ agonist	5–100 mushrooms, 4–6 mg psilocybin	4–6 h	Mydriasis, sympathomimetic symptoms, nausea	Seizures (rare), hyperthermia (rare)	Supportive benzodiazepines
Mescaline	Phenylethylamine	5-HT$_2$ agonist	3–12 "buttons" 200–500 mg mescaline	6–12 h	Mydriasis, abdominal pain, vomiting, dizziness, sympathomimetic symptoms	Rare	Supportive benzodiazepines
MDMA	Phenylethylamine	5-HT release	50–200 mg	4–6 h	Mydriasis, sympathomimetic symptoms, bruxism, jaw tension, ataxia	Arrhythmias, hypertension, seizures, hyperthermia, rhabdomyolysis, DIC, chronic neuropsychiatric problems	Benzodiazepines, hydration, active cooling
Phencyclidine (PCP)	Piperadine derivative	Glutamate agonist at NMDA receptor	1–9 mg	4–6 h	Miosis or midsized pupils; nystagmus; hypertension; sympathomimetic, anticholinergic, and cholinergic symptoms	Coma, seizures, hyperthermia rhabdomyolysis, hypertension, hypoglycemia	Benzodiazepines, hydration, active cooling, multiple doses of activated charcoal, alkalinize urine (for rhabdomyolysis)
Marijuana	Cannabinoid	Binds cannabinoid receptor	5–15 mg THC	2–4 h	Tachycardia, conjunctival injection	Rare	Supportive benzodiazepines

Key: DIC = disseminated intravascular coagulation; LSD = lysergic acid diethylamide; MDMA = 3,4-methylenedioxymethamphetamine; NMDA = N-methyl-D-aspartic acid; THC = tetrahydrocannabinol.

be safely discharged after a period of observation, although patients with symptoms lasting longer than 8 to 12 hours may require hospital admission.

3. Management of patients with psilocybin intoxication and mescaline ingestion is supportive. Coingestion of abused substances should be considered.

4. Treatment of 3,4-methylenedioxymethamphetamine (Ecstasy) use includes **activated charcoal** if ingestion is recent and standard treatment of arrhythmias. Benzodiazepines may alleviate hypertension and tachycardia, although **nitroprusside** or **phentolamine** should be used for severe cases.

5. Management of the PCP-intoxicated patient is generally supportive. If possible, **activated charcoal** should be given to patients with large or recent use. Sedation with benzodiazepines is preferred over physical restraint of PCP-intoxicated patients. Seizures should be controlled with **benzodiazepines** but may require additional therapy. Hypertension may require use of **nitroprusside.** Rhabdomyolysis should be treated in the typical fashion. Patients with significant medical complications should be admitted to the hospital.

6. Most patients with hallucinogen intoxication can be safely discharged from the ED after a period of observation. Patients with serious medical complications, such as severe hyperthermia or hypertension, seizure, or rhabdomyolysis, should be admitted to the hospital.

For further reading in *Emergency Medicine: A Comprehensive Study Guide,* 6th ed., see Chap. 167, "Opioids," by Suzanne Doyon; Chap. 168, "Cocaine, Amphetamines, and Other Stimulants," by Jeanmarie Perrone and Robert S. Hoffman; and Chap. 169, "Hallucinogens," by Karen N. Hansen and Katherine M. Prybys.

104 Analgesics

Keith L. Mausner

Salicylate and acetaminophen overdoses are potentially life threatening and must be rapidly identified and treated. Nonsteroidal anti-inflammatory drug (NSAID) overdoses are rarely fatal and usually require only supportive care.

SALICYLATES

Clinical Features

In addition to aspirin, salicylate containing products such as Pepto-Bismol, oil of wintergreen (methyl salicylate), and vaporizer liniments with methyl salicylate have significant potential to produce severe or fatal toxicity. The clinical manifestations of salicylate toxicity depend on the dose, whether exposure is acute or chronic, and the patient's age. Acute ingestion of less than 150 mg/kg usually produces mild toxicity with nausea, vomiting, and gastrointestinal (GI) irritation. Acute ingestion of 150 to 300 mg/kg usually results in moderate toxicity with vomiting, hyperventilation, sweating, and tinnitus. In adults, these findings often coincide with salicylate levels above 30 mg/dL.

The pathognomonic acid-base disturbance of salicylate toxicity is (*a*) increased anion-gap acidosis, (*b*) metabolic alkalosis (due to volume contraction), and (*c*) respiratory alkalosis. However, the most common clinical picture is combined respiratory alkalosis and increased anion-gap metabolic acidosis. In addition, coingestion of sedative drugs may impair the respiratory drive and result in respiratory acidosis.

Toxicity from ingestion of more than 300 mg/kg is usually severe. Uncommon manifestations of severe acute salicylate toxicity include fever, neurologic dysfunction, renal failure, pulmonary edema, and adult respiratory distress syndrome. Rarely, rhabdomyolysis, gastric perforation, and GI hemorrhage occur. Fatality is more likely with advanced age. Unconsciousness, fever, severe acidosis, seizures, and dysrhythmias are also associated with increased mortality risk.

In children, acute salicylate overdoses generally present within a few hours of ingestion. Children younger than 4 years tend to develop metabolic acidosis (pH <7.38), whereas children older than 4 years usually have mixed acid-base disturbance as in adults.

Chronic salicylate toxicity (associated with long-term therapeutic use) is usually seen in elderly patients with underlying medical problems. It may present with hyperventilation, tremor, papilledema, agitation, paranoia, bizarre behavior, memory loss, confusion, and stupor. Chronic salicylism should be considered in any patient with unexplained nonfocal neurologic and behavioral abnormalities, especially with coexisting acid-base disturbance, tachypnea, dyspnea, or noncardiogenic pulmonary edema. Patients taking carbonic anhydrase inhibitors to treat glaucoma are at increased risk for chronic salicylism. The carbonic anhydrase inhibitor produces a metabolic acidosis, which increases the volume of distribution of salicylates, leading to increased central nervous system (CNS) salicylate levels and possible toxicity despite a "therapeutic" serum salicylate level.

In children, chronic (repeated dose) salicylate toxicity is usually more serious than acute toxicity and more likely to be lethal. It may take several days for symptoms to appear, and there may be an underlying illness that triggered the salicylate administration. Chronic salicylism may be mistaken for an infectious process. The child presents with hyperventilation, volume depletion, acidosis, marked hypokalemia, and CNS disturbances. Fever indicates a worse prognosis. Renal failure is a severe complication. Pulmonary edema is rare in pediatric patients.

Diagnosis and Differential

Clinical status is the key to diagnosis and treatment. Salicylate levels should be interpreted cautiously because severe toxicity may be present despite a "therapeutic" or declining level. The use of the Done nomogram, which was developed to predict toxicity after acute ingestion within a known time frame, may be misleading and is *not* recommended.

Bedside glucose determination is indicated for altered level of consciousness or seizures. Laboratory studies should include electrolytes, glucose, blood urea nitrogen (BUN), creatinine, complete blood count (CBC), prothrombin time (PT), salicylate level, acetaminophen level (to exclude coingestion), and an arterial blood gas to determine acid-base status. Hypo- or hyperglycemia may be seen with severe or chronic toxicity. Elevated PT due to hypoprothrombinemia may occur in severe chronic toxicity.

The differential diagnosis of salicylate toxicity includes theophylline toxicity, caffeine overdose, acute iron poisoning, Reye syndrome, diabetic ketoacidosis, sepsis, and meningitis.

Emergency Department Care and Disposition

1. Emergent priorities remain airway, breathing, and circulation. Cardiac monitoring and an intravenous (IV) line should be instituted.
2. **Activated charcoal** 1 g/kg should be administered to minimize absorption and hasten elimination. Multiple doses probably are not beneficial. **Whole bowel irrigation** may be effective when toxicity is due to sustained-release or enteric-coated aspirin.
3. **IV normal saline** should be administered to patients with evidence of volume depletion. Except for the initial saline resuscitation, all subsequent fluids should contain at least 5% dextrose; if hypoglycemia or neurologic symptoms are present, then administration of IV fluids with 10% dextrose should be considered. After adequate urine output (1–2 mL/kg/h) is established and, if not contraindicated by initial electrolyte and renal function test results, potassium 40 mEq/L should be added to the patient's IV fluids.
4. **Alkalinization of the serum and urine** enhances salicylate protein binding and urinary elimination. This may be accomplished with a second IV concurrent with volume resuscitation. A bolus of 1 to 2 mEq/kg of sodium bicarbonate should be administered. Then, 150 mEq (3 ampules) of sodium bicarbonate should be added to 1 L 5% dextrose in water and infused at 1.5 to 2.0 times the patient's maintenance rate; the infusion should be adjusted to maintain urine pH above 7.5.
5. Severe salicylate toxicity may result in significant volume depletion and metabolic abnormalities; during resuscitation, frequent clinical evaluation and at least hourly monitoring of urine pH, salicylate level, electrolytes,

glucose, and acid-base status are indicated. Bicarbonate administration will further exacerbate hypokalemia; potassium levels should be closely followed. A sudden drop in serum pH due to respiratory failure may acutely worsen salicylate toxicity; early intubation and controlled ventilation are indicated in the event of impending respiratory failure.

6. **Hemodialysis** is indicated for clinical deterioration despite supportive care and alkalinization, renal insufficiency or failure, severe acid–base disturbance, altered mental status, or adult respiratory distress syndrome.

7. Hemorrhage due to elevated PT in chronic salicylism is rarely seen but may be treated with **fresh-frozen plasma.**

8. Dysrhythmias should be treated by correcting metabolic abnormalities and with standard antiarrhythmics.

In significant ingestions, patients should undergo serial examinations, and the salicylate levels should be checked every 2 hours until the peak occurs and then every 4 to 6 hours until the level is nontoxic. In severe ingestions, hourly levels correlated with clinical status are indicated. Except with ingestion of enteric-coated or sustained-release formulations, a patient may be discharged from the emergency department (ED) if there is progressive clinical improvement, no significant acid-base abnormality, and a decline in serial salicylate levels toward the therapeutic range. In deliberate overdoses, a psychiatric consultation should be obtained before discharge.

With enteric-coated and sustained-release salicylates, peak serum levels may not occur until 10 to 60 hours after ingestion. In potentially large ingestions, the patient should be admitted and observed for at least 24 hours to ensure declining serial salicylate levels and improving clinical status. Enteric-coated aspirin may be visible on plain radiographs; however, a negative radiograph does not exclude the ingestion.

ACETAMINOPHEN

Clinical Features

Acute acetaminophen toxicity presents in 4 stages. (*a*) During the first 24 hours, the patient may be asymptomatic or have nonspecific symptoms such as anorexia, nausea, vomiting, and malaise. (*b*) On days 2 to 3, nausea and vomiting may improve, but evidence of hepatotoxicity, such as right upper quadrant abdominal pain and tenderness with elevated transaminases and bilirubin, may be present. (*c*) On days 3 to 4, there may be progression to fulminant hepatic failure with lactic acidosis, coagulopathy, renal failure, and encephalopathy, in addition to recurrent nausea and vomiting. (*d*) Those who survive hepatic failure will begin to recover over the next weeks with complete resolution of hepatic dysfunction. Massive acetaminophen ingestion (4-hour acetaminophen level >800 μg/mL) may be associated with acute onset of coma or agitation and lactic acidosis.

Diagnosis and Differential

Acetaminophen toxicity may occur with acute ingestion of more than 140 mg/kg or when more than 7.5 g is ingested by an adult in a 24-hour period. The diagnosis of a significant ingestion depends on laboratory testing because symptoms initially may be absent or nonspecific. An acetaminophen level should be measured in all patients presenting with any drug overdose because acetaminophen is a common coingestant.

An acetaminophen level, drawn as soon as possible within 4 to 24 hours of ingestion, will guide subsequent ED management. In a single large overdose, the Rumack-Matthew nomogram (Fig. 104-1) accurately predicts acetaminophen toxicity based on the serum acetaminophen level measured 4 to 24 hours after the estimated time of ingestion. The nomogram is not useful outside of this 4- to 24-hour window. A 4-hour level greater than 150 μg/dL is usually toxic. After 24 hours, a detectable acetaminophen level or the presence or elevated transaminases may predict toxicity.

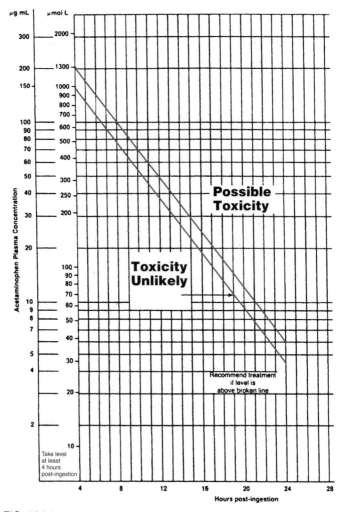

FIG. 104-1. Rumack-Matthew nomogram.

When multiple ingestions have occurred over a specific period, assessment is problematic. One approach is to assume a single ingestion at the earliest possible point in time and use the Rumack-Matthew nomogram accordingly.

Clinical experience with Tylenol Arthritis Pain Extended Relief ingestion is limited. If a 4- to 8-hour level is in the toxic range, then therapy should be initiated. If the 4- to 8-hour level is elevated but below the toxicity cutoff value on the nomogram, then a second level 4 to 6 hours later should be obtained and therapy initiated if the second level is in the toxic range.

The differential diagnosis of acetaminophen toxicity includes viral and alcoholic hepatitis, other drug- or toxin-induced hepatitides, and hepatobiliary disease. Acute acetaminophen poisoning often can be distinguished from other forms of hepatitis by its acute onset, rapid progression, and markedly elevated transaminase levels.

Other laboratory studies, including electrolytes, glucose, BUN, creatinine, transaminases, CBC, and PT, should be drawn if clinically indicated or if the acetaminophen level falls in the toxic range on the Rumack-Matthew nomogram.

Emergency Department Care and Disposition

1. Emergent priorities remain airway, breathing, and circulation. Cardiac monitoring and an IV line should be instituted.
2. **Activated charcoal** 1 g/kg is indicated for GI decontamination and in case of coingestion of other drugs.
3. *N*-acetylcysteine (NAC) is the specific antidote. It effectively prevents toxicity if administered within 8 hours of ingestion, significantly reduces hepatotoxicity if administered within 24 hours of ingestion, and may be of value even after 24 hours. If the acetaminophen level will not be available within 8 hours of ingestion, then NAC therapy should be initiated and continued, if indicated, based on the subsequent acetaminophen level.
4. NAC is administered orally or by nasogastric tube as a 140-mg/kg loading dose, followed by 70 mg/kg every 4 hours for 17 additional doses. NAC may be administered immediately after activated charcoal; there is no evidence that activated charcoal decreases the effectiveness of NAC. NAC is safe in pregnancy.
5. Nausea and vomiting during NAC therapy may be reduced by diluting NAC in a beverage and by administration of antiemetics such as metoclopramide or ondansetron.
6. Intravenous NAC therapy is not approved in the United States but may be used in consultation with a toxicologist for patients unable to tolerate or receive oral therapy.
7. Treatment of fulminant hepatic failure includes NAC therapy, correction of coagulopathy and acidosis, treatment of cerebral edema, supportive measures for multiorgan system failure, and early referral to a liver transplant center.
8. Patients with nontoxic acetaminophen levels based on the Rumack-Matthew nomogram may be discharged from the ED if there is no evidence of other drug ingestion. In deliberate overdoses, a psychiatric evaluation should be obtained before discharge. All patients receiving NAC therapy should be admitted.

NONSTEROIDAL ANTI-INFLAMMATORY DRUGS

Clinical Features

Toxicity associated with therapeutic use of NSAIDs is more common than with acute overdose. The most frequent problems are GI bleeding and renal insufficiency. CNS effects such as headache, mental status changes, and aseptic meningitis may be seen. Seizures have been seen with large ingestions, especially of mefenamic acid. Pulmonary manifestations such as bronchospasm and hypersensitivity pneumonitis have been reported. Hepatic dysfunction may occur, especially in the elderly and in patients with autoimmune disease. Inhibition of platelet aggregation may lead to bleeding. The cyclooxygenase-2 (COX-2) inhibitors (eg, rofecoxib and celecoxib) have less antiplatelet effect than do conventional NSAIDs; the lack of platelet inhibition with COX-2 inhibitors may increase the risk of acute coronary syndrome or thromboembolic stroke in at-risk patients who were previously on conventional NSAIDs. Bone marrow suppression, including aplastic anemia, has been reported. In addition, NSAIDs account for approximately 10% of cutaneous drug reactions, ranging from benign rashes and phototoxic reactions to severe Stevens-Johnson syndrome and toxic epidermal necrolysis. Fetal NSAID exposure may lead to premature closure of the ductus arteriosus, oligohydramnios, renal dysfunction, necrotizing enterocolitis, and CNS hemorrhage.

The NSAIDs have a number of clinically significant drug interactions. Phenylbutazone and naproxen may displace warfarin from plasma proteins, resulting in elevated PTs. Phenylbutazone also decreases the elimination of warfarin. The selective COX-2 inhibitors have been reported to slightly elevate the PT at therapeutic doses. Other NSAIDs do not interact in these ways with warfarin, but nonselective NSAID use is contraindicated with warfarin because NSAID platelet aggregation inhibition may significantly increase the risk of bleeding. NSAIDs may decrease the effectiveness of antihypertensives, including diuretics, α-adrenergic blockers, angiotensin-converting enzyme inhibitors, and β-adrenergic blockers. NSAIDs inhibit the renal clearance of lithium and methotrexate and may cause toxicity from these drugs.

Acute NSAID overdose generally has low morbidity and usually becomes clinically apparent within 4 hours of ingestion. Abdominal pain, nausea, and vomiting may occur. CNS manifestations include altered mental status, diplopia, nystagmus, headache, and, rarely, seizures. Hypotension and bradydysrhythmia have been reported. Renal failure may occur and be associated with serum electrolyte abnormalities and volume overload.

Diagnosis and Differential

The manifestations of NSAID toxicity are nonspecific. NSAID levels are not readily available and are not clinically useful in assessing toxicity. Acetaminophen and salicylate levels will exclude coingestion of these agents. Laboratory evaluation should include electrolytes, glucose, renal and hepatic function tests, acetaminophen level, salicylate level, and CBC. Bedside glucose determination is indicated for altered mental status or seizures.

Emergency Department Care and Disposition

1. Emergent priorities remain airway, breathing, and circulation. Cardiac monitoring and an IV line should be instituted.

2. **Activated charcoal** 1 g/kg is indicated for GI decontamination.
3. **Volume resuscitation,** correction of acid–base and electrolyte disorders, and standard treatment of other complications such as seizures, dysrhythmias, and renal failure are performed as indicated.
4. Patients with asymptomatic NSAID ingestions may be safely discharged from the ED after screening for coingestants and a 4- to 6-hour observation period. In deliberate overdoses, a psychiatric consultation should be obtained before discharge.

For further reading in *Emergency Medicine: A Comprehensive Study Guide,* 6th ed., see Chap. 170, "Salicylates," by L. Yip; Chap. 171, "Acetaminophen," by O. Hung and L. Nelson; and Chap. 172, "Nonsteroidal Anti-inflammatory Drugs," by G. R. Bruno and W. A. Carter.

105 | Theophylline

Mark B. Rogers

The role of theophylline in the management of acute asthma and chronic obstructive pulmonary disease remains controversial due to efficacy and toxicity issues. Theophylline has a narrow therapeutic window and a metabolism dependent on comorbid conditions and other medications taken. Because most bronchodilation effects occur with serum levels of 15 μg/mL, toxicity can be avoided by decreasing target levels from the traditional 20 μg/mL.

CLINICAL FEATURES

Theophylline toxicity can cause life-threatening cardiac, neurologic, and metabolic abnormalities. Even therapeutic levels of theophylline can cause significant side effects. Elderly patients with concomitant medical problems are more susceptible to life-threatening toxicity after chronic overmedication than are younger patients after an acute overdose.

Cardiac side effects include sinus tachycardia, premature atrial contractions, atrial flutter, and atrial fibrillation. Premature ventricular contractions and ventricular tachycardia are seen, particularly in the elderly with chronic overdoses and levels between 40 and 60 μg/mL. Younger patients with acute ingestions may tolerate levels above 100 μg/mL. Hypotension may occur.

Neurologic side effects include agitation, headache, irritability, sleeplessness, tremors, and seizures. Seizures are seen in patients with high serum levels or with a history of epilepsy. Hallucinations and psychosis may be seen.

Metabolic side effects include an increase in catecholamine, glucose, free fatty acid, and insulin levels. Hypokalemia may occur and be worsened by β-agonist therapy. Gastrointestinal effects commonly include nausea and vomiting. Gastrointestinal bleeding and epigastric pain may occur.

DIAGNOSIS AND DIFFERENTIAL

Therapeutic serum theophylline levels of 10 to 20 μg/mL may produce toxic effects. It is a common misnomer that the severity of symptoms is dependent on the serum level. Life-threatening effects may occur with little warning and before minor symptoms are evident. Smoking cessation, disease states such as congestive heart failure and chronic obstructive pulmonary disease, and numerous medications, such as cimetidine and erythromycin, increase the half-life of theophylline. In addition to obtaining a serum theophylline level, clinicians should order an electrolyte panel and an electrocardiogram.

EMERGENCY DEPARTMENT CARE AND DISPOSITION

Treatment of theophylline toxicity consists of initial stabilization, gastric decontamination and elimination, treatment of life-threatening toxic effects, and, in severe cases, hemoperfusion or dialysis. Patients should be placed on a cardiac monitor, noninvasive blood pressure device, and pulse oximeter. An intravenous (IV) line should be inserted.

1. **Gastric lavage** should be considered for acute ingestions of toxic doses within 2 to 4 hours. Ipecac should not be used.

TABLE 105-1 Indications for Hemoperfusion and Hemodialysis

Clinical conditions	Recommendation
Life-threatening toxicity (ie, seizures, tachydysrhythmia) not responsive to other therapy	Indicated
Acute overdose with level ≥100 μg/mL	Possibly indicated
Chronic overdose with level ≥60 μg/mL	Possibly indicated
Elderly patient with prolonged half-life, severe liver or severe cardiac disease, or level ≥40 μg/mL	Controversial
Theophylline level ≤30 μg/mL	Not indicated

2. Multiple doses of oral **activated charcoal** (1 g/kg), mixed with a cathartic such as sorbitol, should be administered every 2 to 4 hours in the first 24 hours due to hepatobiliary enteric circulation.
3. **Ranitidine** 50 mg IV is useful for the nausea and vomiting associated with toxicity.
4. Seizure activity may be treated with diazepam, phenobarbital, or phenytoin.
5. Hypotension initially should be treated with IV isotonic crystalloid. In patients unresponsive to IV fluids or conventional vasopressors, an α-adrenergic agent such as phenylephrine should be considered.
6. Cardiac arrhythmias may be treated cautiously with β-blockers such as metoprolol and esmolol or a calcium channel blocker such as diltiazem. Ventricular dysrhythmias have been treated with lidocaine, phenytoin, and digoxin. Adenosine for supraventricular tachycardia may induce bronchospasm. Hypokalemia should be considered in recurrent dysrhythmias and treated.
7. Indications for **hemoperfusion or hemodialysis** remain controversial and are listed in Table 105-1.
8. Patients with seizures or ventricular dysrhythmias should be monitored until their levels normalize. Patients with mild symptoms or levels below 25 μg/mL do not require specific treatment or admission, but their medication dosing should be decreased or discontinued. Patients with levels above 30 μg/mL should be treated with oral activated charcoal and monitored for toxic side effects.

For further reading in *Emergency Medicine: A Comprehensive Study Guide,* 6th ed., see Chap. 173, "Theophylline," by Heather Marshall and Charles L. Emerman.

106 | Cardiac Medications
C. Crawford Mechem

DIGITALIS GLYCOSIDES

Digitalis glycosides, found in medications and plants such as foxglove and oleander, are used to treat supraventricular tachydysrhythmia and congestive heart failure.

Clinical Features

Toxicity results from accidental ingestion, intentional overdose, or chronic therapy. At increased risk are the elderly and patients with underlying conditions such as chronic obstructive pulmonary disease, cardiac or hepatic disease, or hypokalemia. Drug interactions, such as those involving class Ia antidysrhythmics, may potentiate toxicity. *Acute overdose* presents with cardiac dysrhythmias, such as supraventricular tachycardia with atrioventricular block, bradycardia, and ventricular dysrhythmias. Patients may develop nausea, vomiting, and mental status changes. *Chronic toxicity* is more common in elderly patients with renal insufficiency or taking diuretics and presents with gastrointestinal symptoms, weakness, altered mental status, seizures, and cardiac dysrhythmias.

Diagnosis and Differential

Diagnosis requires a careful history, physical examination, and laboratory studies. Hyperkalemia is often seen in acute poisoning but may be absent in chronic toxicity. Serum digoxin levels are neither sensitive nor specific for toxicity. However, the higher the serum level, the more likely the patient will experience toxicity.

The differential diagnosis includes sinus node disease or toxicity from calcium channel blockers, β-blockers, class Ia antidysrhythmics (quinidine or procainamide), clonidine, organophosphates, or cardiotoxic plants such as rhododendron or yew berry.

Emergency Department Care and Disposition

Management includes supportive care, prevention of further absorption, treatment of complications, and antidote administration. All patients require continuous cardiac monitoring, intravenous (IV) access, and frequent reevaluation.

1. **Activated charcoal,** 1 g/kg initially followed by 0.5 g/kg every 4 to 6 hours, should be administered.
2. **Atropine** 0.5 to 2.0 mg IV and cardiac pacing may be used to treat bradydysrhythmia.
3. Ventricular dysrhythmias are treated with **phenytoin** 15 mg/kg infused no faster than 25 mg/min; **lidocaine** 1 mg/kg; or **magnesium sulfate** 2 to 4 g IV. Electro-cardioversion may induce refractory ventricular dysrhythmias and should be considered only as a last resort. The initial setting should be 10 to 25 J.
4. Hyperkalemia is treated with glucose followed by insulin; other options are sodium bicarbonate, potassium-binding resin, or hemodialysis. Calcium chloride should be avoided.

5. **Digoxin-specific Fab** is indicated for ventricular dysrhythmias, hemodynamically significant bradydysrhythmia unresponsive to standard therapy, and hyperkalemia greater than 5.5 mEq/L. Dosage is based on the estimated total body load of digoxin. If this is unknown, 5 to 10 vials is recommended as the initial dose in severe cases.

6. Patients with signs of toxicity or with a history of a large overdose should be admitted to a monitored setting. Patients receiving Fab fragments should be admitted to an intensive care unit (ICU). Patients who are asymptomatic after 12 hours of observation may be medically cleared.

β-BLOCKERS

β-blockers have many uses, including the management of acute myocardial infarction, angina, dysrhythmias, hypertension, thyrotoxicosis, migraines, and glaucoma. In overdose, their negative inotropic and chronotropic effects may cause cardiac decompensation and death.

Clinical Features

Toxicity usually develops within 2 to 4 hours of acute ingestion. In the case of sustained-release preparations, toxicity has not been reported more than 6 hours postingestion. Cardiac manifestations include hypotension, bradycardia, conduction abnormalities, cardiogenic shock, and asystole. Sotalol, unlike other β-blockers, is a class III antidysrhythmic. As such, it may cause QT-interval prolongation and ventricular tachycardia, torsade de pointes, and ventricular fibrillation. Noncardiac manifestations of toxicity include altered mental status, psychosis, seizures, hypoglycemia, bronchospasm, and respiratory depression.

Diagnosis and Differential

The diagnosis is made on clinical grounds. Drug levels correlate poorly with clinical effects. A 12-lead electrocardiogram should be obtained in all cases. Laboratory studies are directed at identifying underlying medical conditions or complications. The differential diagnosis includes overdose of calcium channel blockers, centrally acting α-agonists, digoxin, organophosphates, cyanide, hydrogen sulfide, plants such as oleander and rhododendron, and Chinese herbal preparations containing cardiac glycosides.

Emergency Department Care and Disposition

The goal of specific cardiovascular drug therapy is restoration of perfusion to critical organs by increasing heart rate and myocardial contractility.

1. All patients require supportive care, continuous cardiac monitoring, and IV access. Oxygen should be administered to correct hypoxia. IV crystalloid boluses are appropriate to treat hypotension.

2. Bedside serum glucose determination is warranted in the setting of altered mental status.

3. **Activated charcoal** 1 g/kg should be administered. Gastric lavage before administration of charcoal may be beneficial if performed within 1 to 2 hours of ingestion.

4. **Glucagon** has positive inotropic and chronotropic effects and is a first-line agent. It is administered as an IV bolus of 0.05 to 0.15 mg/kg. This is followed by a continuous infusion of 1 to 10 mg/h.

5. **Amrinone,** given as a 10 mg/kg bolus over 2 minutes followed by a continuous infusion of 5 to 20 μg/kg/min, may be used if glucagon is unavailable. Atropine is unlikely to treat β-blocker–induced bradycardia or hypotension.

6. **Epinephrine** is used for refractory hypotension.

7. Cardiac pacing may be used to treat bradycardia refractory to other measures but is not always successful and may not reverse hypotension.

8. **Lidocaine, magnesium sulfate, isoproterenol,** and **overdrive pacing** are used to treat sotalol-induced ventricular dysrhythmias.

9. Patients who develop bradycardia, hypotension, conduction disturbances, or altered mental status should be managed in an ICU. Patients who have ingested multiple cardioactive agents or a sustained-release preparation should be admitted to a monitored setting due to concern for delayed toxicity.

10. Those patients who remain asymptomatic 6 hours after ingestion in most cases can be medically cleared. However, this period may need to be extended in cases of sotalol ingestion.

CALCIUM CHANNEL BLOCKERS

Clinical applications of calcium channel blockers include the treatment of hypertension and angina, rate control of supraventricular tachydysrhythmia, and management of esophageal and arterial spasms. Three widely used classes of calcium channel blockers are the phenyl alkylamines (verapamil), benzodiazepines (diltiazem), and dihydropyridines (nifedipine and most newer agents).

Clinical Features

Cardiac manifestations of toxicity consist of sinus bradycardia, atrioventricular block, and hypotension. In dihydropyridine overdose, reflex tachycardia is common. In severe cases, all classes of calcium channel blockers can cause complete heart block, depressed myocardial contractility, and vasodilatation, ultimately resulting in cardiovascular collapse. Noncardiac consequences include hyperglycemia, lactic acidosis, hypokalemia, noncardiogenic pulmonary edema, seizures, delirium, and coma. Altered mental status is usually due to hypoperfusion. If noted in the setting of a normal blood pressure, other causes should be sought.

Diagnosis and Differential

A careful history should be obtained in all cases, including the agent taken, whether it is a sustained-release preparation, any coingestants, and time of ingestion. The physical examination is often unremarkable except for a slow pulse relative to the blood pressure. In the setting of dihydropyridine overdose, vasodilatation may result in flushed skin, hypotension, and tachycardia. Laboratory studies help to identify complications. Lactic acidosis manifesting with an elevated anion gap and low serum bicarbonate may be noted. Hyperglycemia is common and helps to distinguish calcium channel blocker from β-blocker toxicity, which is often associated with hypoglycemia. Hypokalemia may be seen in severe overdoses. Serum acetaminophen and aspirin levels should be obtained in all patients after a suicide attempt by overdose.

The differential diagnosis for bradycardia and hypotension includes hypothermia, acute coronary syndrome, hyperkalemia, and toxicity due to cardiac glycosides, β-blockers, class Ia and Ic antidysrhythmics, and central α-adrenergic agonists (clonidine).

Emergency Department Care and Disposition

Treatment is supportive, with an emphasis on decontamination and cardiovascular stabilization.

1. All patients require supplemental oxygen, cardiac monitoring, and IV access. Patients with altered mental status should receive an opiate antagonist and have a bedside serum glucose determination.
2. The endpoint of treatment of bradycardia and hypotension is adequate end-organ perfusion.
3. **Gastric lavage** is indicated for all patients presenting within 60 minutes of a potentially life-threatening calcium channel blocker overdose and for those patients requiring endotracheal intubation. Because of the associated risk of aspiration with gastric lavage, definitive airway management is often required.
4. **Activated charcoal** 1 g/kg is indicated for all patients. **Whole bowel irrigation** has been advocated for sustained-release preparations.
5. **Crystalloid IV fluids** should be administered for hypotension, with care to avoid fluid overload.
6. Hypotension refractory to IV fluids is treated with a 1- to 3-g IV bolus of **calcium chloride,** repeated as needed or administered as an infusion of 2 to 6 g/h. Care should be exercised in avoiding extravasation, which may result in tissue necrosis. **Calcium gluconate** is an alternative therapy but provides one third the amount of calcium on a weight-to-weight basis.
7. **Glucagon** is a first-line agent for moderate to severe calcium channel blocker toxicity. It is administered as a 0.05-mg/kg bolus, which may be repeated every 10 minutes to a total dose of 0.15 mg/kg. Patients who respond should be started on an infusion of 0.075 to 0.15 mg/kg/h. Because glucagon may cause vomiting, prophylactic endotracheal intubation should be considered.
8. Dopamine, epinephrine, norepinephrine, amrinone, or milrinone may be used to treat refractory hypotension.
9. Anecdotal evidence supports the **coadministration of regular insulin and dextrose** to patients with a severe overdose who fail to respond to other measures. After checking the serum glucose level, regular insulin is administered as a 1.0-U/kg IV bolus followed by an infusion of 0.5 U/kg/h. A 10% dextrose infusion is run at 200 to 300 mL/h (15–20 mL/kg/h in children), and blood sugar and potassium levels are monitored every 20 minutes. The target blood sugar range is 150 to 300 mg/dL.
10. Symptomatic patients should be admitted to a monitored setting or ICU. Patients who have taken a sustained-release preparation should be admitted to a monitored setting for 24 hours.
11. Patients who are asymptomatic, have received charcoal decontamination, and have normal vital signs after a 6-hour observation period after ingestion of a non–sustained-release product may be medically cleared.

ANTIHYPERTENSIVES

In addition to β-blockers and calcium channel blockers, other antihypertensives include diuretics, clonidine and other centrally acting agents, peripheral α_1-adrenergic receptor antagonists, direct vasodilators, dopamine agonists, angiotensin converting enzyme inhibitors, and angiotensin II receptor antagonists. Because they are widely prescribed, the potential for intentional or accidental overdose is high.

DIURETICS

Diuretics include *thiazides* (hydrochlorothiazide), *loop diuretics* (furosemide, bumetanide, ethacrynic acid, and torsemide), *potassium-sparing diuretics* (spironolactone, triamterene, and amiloride), *carbonic anhydrase inhibitors* (acetazolamide), and *osmotic agents* (mannitol).

Clinical Features

Thiazides and loop diuretics   Patients present with hypotension, tachycardia, altered mental status, hyponatremia, hypokalemia, hypocalcemia (loop diuretics), hypomagnesemia, hyperuricemia (thiazides), and hypochloremic metabolic alkalosis. Patients also may develop rash, pruritus, hearing loss, leukopenia, and thrombocytopenia.

Potassium-sparing diuretics   Toxicity manifests with volume depletion, hyperkalemia, hyponatremia, and hypochloremia.

Carbonic anhydrase inhibitors   Overdose results in volume depletion, electrolyte disturbances, and non–anion-gap metabolic acidosis.

Osmotic agents   Signs of toxicity include volume depletion and electrolyte imbalances. Pulmonary edema, anaphylaxis, and acute renal failure have also been reported.

Emergency Department Care and Disposition

Management is supportive and includes fluid resuscitation and correction of electrolyte and pH abnormalities. All patients require continuous cardiac monitoring and IV access.

1. **IV normal saline** is used to correct hypovolemia, hyponatremia, and alkalosis.
2. **Dopamine** is used for hypotension refractory to volume resuscitation.
3. Potassium abnormalities should be aggressively corrected using standard measures. Patients with severe hyperkalemia from potassium-sparing diuretics may require dialysis.
4. Most asymptomatic patients can be medically cleared after therapy and observation. Patients with electrolyte abnormalities may require admission.

CLONIDINE AND OTHER CENTRALLY ACTING AGENTS

Clonidine, guanabenz, guanfacine, and methyldopa are used for the management of hypertension. Clonidine is also used to mitigate opiate and ethanol withdrawal symptoms.

Clinical Features

Clonidine toxicity causes hypotension and bradycardia, leading to myocardial ischemia and congestive heart failure. Other findings include respiratory depression, hypothermia, mental status changes, miosis, and seizures. *Guanabenz, guanfacine, methyldopa,* and *reserpine* can cause hypotension, symptomatic bradycardia, dry mouth, and mental status changes.

Emergency Department Care and Disposition

Management is supportive, with special attention to correcting hypotension.

1. Recurrent apnea from clonidine, most commonly seen in children, may warrant endotracheal intubation. All patients require continuous cardiac monitoring and IV access.
2. **IV crystalloid** should be administered for hypotension.
3. **Dopamine** or **norepinephrine** is used for hypotension refractory to fluid resuscitation.
4. **Atropine** is indicated for management of symptomatic bradycardia.
5. **Naloxone** may be effective for cases of refractory hypotension or altered mental status.
6. **Tolazoline,** 10 mg IV titrated every 15 minutes to a total of 40 mg, is recommended for treatment of clonidine-induced cardiovascular effects that fail to respond to fluids, dopamine, atropine, and naloxone.
7. Seizures are controlled with standard anticonvulsants.
8. Dialysis may be warranted in severe cases of methyldopa toxicity.
9. Symptoms of clonidine toxicity can persist for up to 72 hours, so admission should be considered for any patient suspected of clonidine overdose.

PERIPHERAL α₁-ADRENERGIC RECEPTOR ANTAGONISTS

Agents include *doxazosin, prazosin, terazosin,* and *phenoxybenzamine.* Toxicity is uncommon but may include hypotension and tachycardia. Syncope, headache, paresthesias, vertigo, gastrointestinal discomfort, and weakness have also been reported. Treatment is supportive and includes IV fluid administration, vasopressors, if needed, and inpatient cardiac monitoring.

DIRECT VASODILATORS

Agents include hydralazine, minoxidil, and sodium nitroprusside.

Clinical Features

Toxicity from *hydralazine* is uncommon. Hypotension is the most common presentation. Symptomatic tachycardia also may be noted. *Minoxidil* causes hypotension and tachycardia. Toxicity from *sodium nitroprusside* includes hypotension, altered mental status, and dysrhythmias and is more common after prolonged infusion and in patients with hepatic or renal failure. Less commonly, thiocyanate toxicity with tinnitus, altered mental status, nausea, and abdominal pain may develop. Rarely, cyanide toxicity presents with acidosis, coma, and respiratory arrest. In very rare cases, methemoglobinemia and cellular hypoxia develop.

Emergency Department Care and Disposition

1. **IV fluids** are used to treat hypotension. Hypotension from sodium nitroprusside infusion is best avoided by careful monitoring and titration of dosage.
2. **Vasopressors** can induce dysrhythmias in cases of hydralazine-induced hypotension, so it should be used with caution. **Dopamine** is the preferred

agent. For minoxidil-induced hypotension, dopamine or **phenylephrine** should be considered because vasopressors such as epinephrine that have β-adrenergic activity can result in excessive cardiac stimulation.

3. **β-blockers** can be used to treat symptomatic tachycardias.
4. Thiocyanate toxicity may be avoided by limiting the duration of infusion and restricting the use of nitroprusside in patients with renal insufficiency. In severe cases, thiocyanate may be removed by dialysis.
5. Cyanide toxicity is avoided by coadministration of sodium thiosulfate or by limiting the duration of infusion.

DOPAMINE AGONISTS

Fenoldopam is used to treat acute, severe hypertension and is an alternative to sodium nitroprusside in patients with renal insufficiency. Experience with this agent is limited, but toxicity theoretically may result in hypotension. Care is supportive. Hypotension is best treated with IV fluids and vasopressors such as dopamine or norepinephrine.

ANGIOTENSIN-CONVERTING ENZYME INHIBITORS

Agents include *captopril, enalapril,* and *enalaprilat.* Hypotension is the most common concern in overdose. Care is supportive. Hypotension may be treated with IV normal saline, followed by vasopressors such as dopamine. Naloxone has been reported to reverse captopril-induced hypotension, but its mechanism of action is unknown.

ANGIOTENSIN II RECEPTOR ANTAGONISTS

Agents include *losartan, valsartan,* and *candesartan.* Experience with toxicity is limited, but hypotension and tachycardia are the most common toxic effects. Vagally mediated bradycardia may occur. Hyperkalemia also has been reported. Therapy is supportive and includes IV fluid administration, correction of electrolyte disturbances, and cardiac monitoring for at least 6 hours.

For further reading in *Emergency Medicine: A Comprehensive Study Guide,* 6th ed., see Chap. 174, "Digitalis Glycosides," by William Dribben and Mark Kirk; Chap. 175, "Beta-Blocker Toxicity," by Teresa Carlin; Chap. 176, "Calcium Channel Blockers," by Kennon Heard and Jeffrey A. Kline; and Chap. 177, "Antihypertensives," by Arjun Chanmugam and Keith Thomasset.

107 | Phenytoin and Fosphenytoin Toxicity

Mark B. Rogers

Intentional phenytoin overdose rarely leads to death, provided adequate supportive care is administered. Most phenytoin-related deaths have been caused by rapid intravenous (IV) administration and hypersensitivity reactions.

CLINICAL FEATURES

Phenytoin toxicity depends on the duration of exposure, dosage taken, and, most importantly, route of administration. An acute oral overdose is typically dose related and usually presents with nystagmus, nausea, vomiting, ataxia, dysarthria, choreoathetosis, opisthotonos, and central nervous system (CNS) depression or excitation. Death from oral overdose alone is extremely rare. Life-threatening effects such as hypotension, bradycardia, and asystole can be seen with IV administration and are secondary to the diluent of the IV preparation, propylene glycol. This morbidity can be avoided by slowing the rate of administration.

Fosphenytoin, a prodrug of phenytoin, is more soluble and less irritating to tissues. IV fosphenytoin can cause pruritus and hypotension. Blood pressure and cardiac monitoring are recommended when loading fosphenytoin intravenously but not intramuscularly. The adverse and toxic effects of fosphenytoin are the same as those of phenytoin, except the toxic effects of propylene glycol are not present.

CNS toxicity begins with horizontal nystagmus; however, vertical, bidirectional, or alternating nystagmus may occur with severe intoxication. A depressed level of consciousness is common, with sedation, lethargy, ataxic gait, and dysarthria progressing to confusion, seizures, coma, and apnea in a large overdose. Depressed or hyperactive deep tendon reflexes, clonus, and extensor toe responses may be noted. Acute dystonia and movement disorders, such as opisthotonos and choreoathetosis, may occur. Peripheral neuropathy and ataxia may persist for months.

Cardiovascular toxicity is usually associated with IV administration only. In an otherwise healthy patient, cardiac toxicity has never been reported after an oral overdose of phenytoin; when observed, this requires assessment for other causes. Cardiovascular toxicity includes hypotension, bradycardia, conduction delays (which may progress to complete atrioventricular nodal block), ventricular tachycardia, ventricular fibrillation, and asystole. Electrocardiographic changes include increased PR interval, widened QRS interval, and altered ST-wave and T-wave segments. Bradycardia, hypotension, and syncope in healthy volunteers have been reported after small IV doses. Most of these side effects are due to the propylene glycol.

Phenytoin causes significant soft tissue toxicity. Intramuscular injection can result in localized crystallization of the drug, hematoma, sterile abscess, and myonecrosis. Reported complications of extravasation after IV infusion have included skin and soft tissue necrosis, compartment syndrome, gangrene, and death. Fosphenytoin is well tolerated intramuscularly or intravenously.

Hypersensitivity reactions usually occur within 1 to 6 weeks of initiation of phenytoin therapy. Reactions can include systemic lupus erythematosus, erythema multiforme, toxic epidermal necrosis, Stevens-Johnson syndrome, hepatitis, rhabdomyolysis, acute interstitial pneumonitis, lymphadenopathy, leukopenia, disseminated intravascular coagulation, and renal failure. Gingival hyperplasia is a common side effect of phenytoin, and its absence may suggest poor compliance.

Phenytoin is teratogenic and should never be initiated in a pregnant patient without consulting a neurologist and obstetrician.

DIAGNOSIS AND DIFFERENTIAL

Therapeutic levels are between 10 and 20 μg/mL (40–80 μmol/L). Some patients require levels above 20 μg/mL for adequate seizure control. Individual variation in toxicity depends on baseline neurologic status, response to the drug, and free drug fraction. Patients with underlying brain disease are predisposed to toxicity and may become toxic at low levels. Toxicity generally correlates with increasing plasma levels (Table 107-1). Due to erratic absorption, serial phenytoin levels should be obtained to ensure the level has peaked.

Almost any CNS-active drug, such as ethanol, carbamazepine, benzodiazepines, barbiturates, and lithium, can mimic phenytoin toxicity. Disease states that resemble phenytoin toxicity include hypoglycemia, Wernicke encephalopathy, and posterior fossa hemorrhage or tumor. Seizures caused by phenytoin toxicity are uncommon, and other causes such as trauma or alcohol withdrawal should be investigated.

EMERGENCY DEPARTMENT CARE AND DISPOSITION

The treatment of phenytoin toxicity consists of initial stabilization, activated charcoal, and observation. Patients should be placed on a cardiac monitor, noninvasive blood pressure device, and pulse oximeter. An IV line should be established.

1. Supplemental oxygen should be administered to maintain an adequate pulse oximetry reading. Respiratory acidosis should be avoided.
2. Hypotension from IV administration of phenytoin should be treated with IV isotonic crystalloid and the discontinuation of the infusion.
3. For an acute oral overdose, multiple doses of oral **activated charcoal** (1 g/kg), mixed with a cathartic such as sorbitol, should be given every 2 to 4 hours in the first 24 hours due to the extended absorptive phase.
4. Bradydysrhythmia may require atropine or cardiac pacing.
5. Seizures may be treated with a benzodiazepine or phenobarbital.

TABLE 107-1 Correlation of Plasma Phenytoin Level and Side Effects

Plasma level (μ/mL)	Side effects
<10	Usually none
10–20	Occasional mild nystagmus
20–30	Nystagmus
30–40	Ataxia, slurred speech, nausea and vomiting
40–50	Lethargy, confusion
>50	Coma, seizures

Hemodialysis and hemoperfusion are of no benefit. Appropriate orthopedic or plastic surgery consultation should be obtained for any signs of local soft tissue toxicity.

After an oral ingestion, patients with serious complications (eg, seizures, coma, altered mental status, and ataxia) should be admitted. With mild symptoms, the patient may be treated with activated charcoal in the emergency department and discharged home if repeat serum levels return to normal and the patient is not actively suicidal. Patients with symptomatic chronic intoxication should be admitted for observation unless the toxic effects are minimal, adequate care can be obtained at home, and they are 8 to 12 hours from their last dose. Phenytoin should be stopped and levels rechecked in 2 to 3 days.

After IV administration of phenytoin, patients with significant or persistent complications should be admitted for observation on a telemetry unit. Those with transient effects can be discharged.

For further reading in *Emergency Medicine: A Comprehensive Study Guide,* 6th ed., see Chap. 178, "Phenytoin and Fosphenytoin Toxicity," by Harold H. Osborn.

108 | Iron

O. John Ma

Iron toxicity from an intentional or accidental ingestion is a common poisoning. When determining a patient's potential for experiencing toxicity, elemental iron must be used in calculations. Ferrous sulfate contains 20% elemental iron, and pediatric multivitamins typically contain 10 to 18 mg of elemental iron per tablet.

CLINICAL FEATURES

Based on clinical findings, iron poisoning can be divided into 5 stages. Patients can die in any stage of iron poisoning.

The first stage develops within the first few hours after the ingestion. The direct irritative effects of iron on the gastrointestinal (GI) tract produce abdominal pain, vomiting, and diarrhea. Hematemesis is not unusual. Vomiting is the clinical sign most consistently associated with acute iron toxicity. The absence of these symptoms within 6 hours of ingestion essentially excludes a diagnosis of significant iron toxicity.

During the second stage, which may continue for up to 24 hours after ingestion, the patient's GI symptoms may resolve, thereby producing a false sense of security despite toxic amounts of iron being absorbed into the body. Patients may not be symptomatic but still appear ill and may have abnormal vital signs and evidence of poor tissue perfusion because of ongoing volume loss and worsening metabolic acidosis.

The third stage may appear early or develop hours after the second stage. Shock and a metabolic acidosis develop. Iron-induced coagulopathy may worsen bleeding and hypovolemia. Hepatic dysfunction, cardiomyopathy, and renal failure also may occur.

The fourth stage develops 2 to 5 days after ingestion. It manifests as elevation of aminotransferase and may progress to hepatic failure.

The fifth stage, which occurs 4 to 6 weeks after ingestion, involves gastric outlet obstruction secondary to the corrosive effects of iron on the pyloric mucosa.

DIAGNOSIS AND DIFFERENTIAL

The diagnosis of iron poisoning is based on the clinical picture and the history provided by the patient, significant others, or out-of-hospital care providers. Toxic effects have been reported after oral doses as low as 10 to 20 mg/kg elemental iron. Moderate toxicity occurs at doses of 20 to 60 mg/kg elemental iron, and severe toxicity can be expected after doses larger than 60 mg/kg elemental iron.

Laboratory work should be sent for serum electrolytes, blood urea nitrogen, serum glucose, coagulation studies, complete blood count, hepatic enzymes, and serum iron level. It is crucial to note that the determination of a single serum iron level does not reflect what iron levels have been previously, what direction they are going, or the degree of iron toxicity in the tissues. A single low serum level does not exclude the diagnosis of iron toxicity because there are variable times to peak level after ingestion of different iron preparations. Serum iron levels have limited use in directing management because excess iron is toxic intracellularly and not in the blood. In general, serum iron levels between 300 and 500 μg/dL correlate with mild systemic toxicity and iron levels between 500 and 1,000 μg/dL correlate with moderate systemic toxicity. Levels higher than 1,000 μg/dL are associated with significant morbidity. The total iron-binding capacity (TIBC) is currently thought to have little value in the assessment of iron-poisoned patients because it becomes falsely elevated in the presence of elevated serum iron levels or deferoxamine.

A plain radiograph of the kidneys, ureters, and bladder may show iron in the GI tract; however, many iron preparations are not routinely detected, so negative radiographs do not exclude iron ingestion.

EMERGENCY DEPARTMENT CARE AND DISPOSITION

Patients who have remained asymptomatic for 6 hours after ingestion of iron and who have a normal physical examination do not require medical treatment for iron toxicity. Patients whose symptoms resolve after a short period and who have normal vital signs usually have mild toxicity and require only supportive care. This subset of patients still requires an observation period.

Patients who are symptomatic or demonstrate signs of hemodynamic instability after iron ingestion should be managed aggressively in the emergency department.

1. Patients should receive supplemental oxygen, be placed on a cardiac monitor, and have 2 large-bore intravenous (IV) lines established.
2. Patients should receive vigorous IV **crystalloid infusion** to help correct hypovolemia and tissue hypoperfusion.
3. Patients who present within 2 hours of ingestion should undergo **gastric lavage.** Activated charcoal does not bind iron, and its use is not recommended.
4. Whole bowel irrigation with **polyethylene glycol** solution has been demonstrated to be efficacious. Administration of 250 to 500 mL/h in children and 2 L/h in adults via nasogastric tube may clear the GI tract of iron pills before absorption occurs.
5. Antiemetics such as **promethazine** (25 mg intramuscularly [IM] in adults; 0.25-0.5 mg/kg IM in pediatric patients) or **ondansetron** (4 mg IV in adults; 0.1 mg/kg to a maximum dose of 4 mg in pediatric patients) should be administered.
6. Coagulopathy should be corrected with **vitamin K_1** (5-25 mg subcutaneously (SQ) and **fresh-frozen plasma** (10-25 mL/kg in adults; 10 mL/kg in pediatric patients). Blood should be typed and screened or crossmatched, as necessary.
7. **Deferoxamine** is a chelating agent that can remove iron from tissues and free iron from plasma. Deferoxamine combines with iron to form water-soluble ferrioxamine, which is excreted in the urine. Deferoxamine is safe to administer to children and pregnant women.
8. Patients with mild iron toxicity may be treated with **deferoxamine** 90 mg/kg IM, up to 1 g in children and 2 g in adults. The dose may be repeated every 4 to 6 hours, as clinically indicated.
9. For patients with more severe iron toxicity, the preferred route of deferoxamine administration is as an IV infusion. Because hypotension is the rate-limiting factor for IV infusion, it is recommended to begin with a slow IV infusion at 5 mg/kg/h. The deferoxamine infusion rate can be increased to 15 mg/kg/h, as tolerated, within the first

hour of treatment. It is recommended not to exceed a total daily dose of 6 to 8 g. In a clinically ill patient with a known acute ingestion of iron, deferoxamine therapy should be initiated without waiting for the serum iron level result.

10. Determination for the efficacy of deferoxamine involves evaluating serial urine samples. As ferrioxamine is excreted, the urine changes to the classic *vin rose* appearance. Clinical recovery of the patient is probably the most important factor in terminating deferoxamine therapy.

11. Patients who remain asymptomatic after 6 hours of observation and have a reliable history of an insignificant ingestion may be considered for discharge. Patients initially symptomatic who become asymptomatic nevertheless should be admitted because this may represent the second stage. Patients who receive deferoxamine therapy should be admitted to an intensive care setting. All patients should be assessed for suicide risk. Child abuse or neglect should be considered in pediatric cases.

For further reading in *Emergency Medicine: A Comprehensive Study Guide,* 6th edition, see chapter 179, "Iron," by Joseph G. Rella and Lewis S. Nelson.

109 | Hydrocarbons and Volatile Substances

J. Christian Fox

Products containing hydrocarbons are found in many household and workplace settings; these include fuels, lighter fluids, paint removers, pesticides, polishers, degreasers, and lubricants. Volatile substances containing hydrocarbons such as glue, propellants, and gasoline are occasionally used for abuse. Exposure to hydrocarbons and volatile substances may cause life-threatening toxicity and even sudden death.

CLINICAL FEATURES

Toxicity depends on route of exposure (ingestion, inhalation, or dermal), physical characteristics (volatility, viscosity, and surface tension), chemical characteristics (aliphatic, aromatic, or hydrogenated), and the presence of toxic additives (eg, lead or pesticides). Pulmonary and cardiac toxicities are the most common. Toxicity is reviewed by chemical composition in Table 109-1.

Chemical pneumonitis, the most common pulmonary complication, results from aspiration of the highly volatile aliphatic substances such as gasoline,

TABLE 109-1 Chemical Toxicity

Chemical composition	Example	Commercial use	Toxicity
Aliphatic (open chain)	Short chain		Pulmonary
	Methane	Fuel	Negligible GI
	Butane		absorption
	Propane		
	Intermediate chain		Hemolysis
	Gasoline	Motor fuel	
	Kerosene	Stove fuel	
	Mineral seal oil	Furniture polish	
	Long chain		Polyneuropathy
	N-hexane	Tar	
	Ketone	Rubber cement	
Aromatic (benzene ring)	Benzene	Gasoline	Dysrhythmias
	Toluene	Airplane glue	Aplastic anemia
	Xylene	Cleaning agent Degreaser	CML
Halogenated (substituted halogen group)	Carbon-tetrachloride	Refrigerant	Dysrhythmias
	Chloroform	Propellant	Hepatic toxicity
	Trichloroethylene	Solvent	Acute renal failure
	Trichloroethane	Spot remover Degreaser	Hemolysis

Key: CML = chronic myelogenous leukemia, GI = gastrointestinal.

kerosene, methane, or butane. Additional complications include pneumomediastinum, pneumothorax, and pneumatocele. Patients present with coughing, dyspnea, choking, and gasping. Physical examination findings include tachypnea, wheezing, grunting, and decreased breath sounds. Radiographic findings lag behind the clinical picture by 4 to 6 hours.

Toxicity of the central nervous system is most common with the volatile petroleum distillates such as toluene and trichloroethane. Symptoms range from giddiness, slurred speech, ataxia, and hallucinations to seizures, lethargy, obtundation, and coma. Chronic exposure may cause cerebellar ataxia and mood lability.

Cardiac toxicity from aromatic and halogenated hydrocarbons is due to the sensitization of the myocardium to catecholamines. This may cause serious dysrhythmias (ventricular tachycardia or fibrillation), decreased contractility, bradycardia, and heart blocks.

Hepatic toxicity from halogenated hydrocarbons such as carbon tetrachloride and chloroform cause hepatocellular injury. Liver enzymes may be elevated within 24 hours, and right upper quadrant abdominal pain and jaundice develop within 48 to 96 hours. Chronic exposure causes cirrhosis and hepatoma.

Hematologic toxicity due to gasoline, kerosene, and trichloroethane can cause hemolysis. Chronic benzene abuse can cause aplastic anemia and hematologic malignancies.

Dermal toxicity includes rashes (erythema, papules, vesicles, or scarlatiniform rash), eczematous dermatitis, and burns.

DIAGNOSIS AND DIFFERENTIAL

Diagnosis is made by the history and accompanying physical examination findings. Laboratory tests that should be ordered include arterial blood gas, liver function panel, blood urea nitrogen, creatinine, hematocrit, and carboxyhemoglobin level (in methylene chloride exposure). A chest radiograph to evaluate for pneumonitis and a kidney-ureter-bladder radiograph to investigate for radiopaque substances (eg, chlorinated hydrocarbons) should be ordered.

EMERGENCY DEPARTMENT CARE AND DISPOSITION

1. All symptomatic patients should be administered supplemental **oxygen** and placed on a cardiac monitor. Strong consideration for **endotracheal intubation** should be given to patients having respiratory distress. Positive end-expiratory pressure may be added, if necessary, but pneumothorax or pneumatocele are potential complications. In severe pulmonary aspiration resulting in refractory hypoxemia, treatment with extracorporeal membrane oxygenation and high-frequency jet ventilation has proved to be successful.
2. Decontamination of the patient should follow standard hazardous material measures, which preferably should occur in the out-of-hospital setting.
3. Hypotension should be treated with intravenous **crystalloid** infusion. Catecholamines may precipitate life-threatening dysrhythmias and should be avoided except in cases of cardiac arrest. Tachydysrhythmia may be treated with **propranolol** (1 mg intravenously; may repeat if blood pressure is stable). Seizures should be managed using standard regimens.

4. Because some hydrocarbons, such as the CHAMP (camphor, halogenated, aromatic, metals, pesticides) agents and wood distillates (turpentine or pine oil), get absorbed through the gastrointestinal (GI) tract, patients with these ingestions should undergo **GI decontamination.** Most hydrocarbon ingestions, which consist of aliphatic mixtures, do not require GI decontamination. Aliphatic hydrocarbons are poorly absorbed from the GI tract and carry a risk of aspiration during GI decontamination measures. Activated charcoal and cathartics are of no benefit with any hydrocarbon ingestion.

5. **Hyperbaric oxygen** therapy may be indicated for patients who develop significant carbon monoxide toxicity after exposure to methylene chloride.

6. Because most fatalities occur in the first 24 to 48 hours, all patients who are symptomatic at the time of evaluation should be admitted. Patients exposed to significant amounts of methemoglobinemia-producing hydrocarbons also should be admitted. Asymptomatic patients with a normal chest radiograph who remain free of symptoms after 6 hours of observation may be discharged. All discharged patients should receive close follow-up because delayed toxicity (>18 hours) has been reported.

For further reading in *Emergency Medicine: A Comprehensive Study Guide,* 6th ed., see Chap. 180, "Hydrocarbons and Volatile Substances," by Paul M. Wax.

110 | Caustics

Christian A. Tomaszewski

Most exposures to caustic agents are unintentional in children, whereas most serious sequelae result from intentional suicide attempts in adults. The variety of caustics includes alkalis, such as sodium hydroxide in drain cleaners and sodium hypochlorite in household bleach, and acids, such as hydrochloric and sulfuric acids in cleaners and hydrofluoric acid in rust removers. Typically, these caustic agents cause local tissue inflammation and eventually necrosis on any exposed dermal surface (eg, skin, mucous membranes, or eye) depending on the strength and concentration of the agent and duration of exposure.

CLINICAL FEATURES

Alkali injuries cause deep liquefaction necrosis, typically in the esophagus, which can lead to perforation or delayed stricture. Strong acids produce coagulation necrosis, which limits the extent of deep tissue injury. Although acids can cause damage to the esophagus, they also tend to pool in the stomach, leading to gastric hemorrhage, necrosis, and even perforation. In addition, acids that are absorbed by the patient can cause metabolic acidosis, hemolysis, and renal failure.

Caustic ingestions can cause distal gastrointestinal (GI) injury without necessarily causing oral or facial burns. More distal injury may lead to vomiting, dysphagia, odynophagia, and epigastric pain. Laryngotracheal injury is usually marked by dysphonia, drooling, stridor, and respiratory distress.

Dermal exposures to caustics usually produce only local pain and irritation. However, sodium hydrofluoric acid differs in its ability to cause deep, often delayed, tissue necrosis accompanied by hypocalcemia and hypomagnesemia, which may lead to death from ventricular dysrhythmias. Caustic exposures to the cornea are particularly serious if they involve alkalis. Acid exposures tend to be superficial and usually do not lead to perforation or scarring as can be seen with alkali exposure.

DIAGNOSIS AND DIFFERENTIAL

Clinically, it is difficult to exclude esophageal or gastric injury and therefore the need for endoscopy. The absence of burns to the mouth or oropharynx does not necessarily exclude significant esophageal or gastric injury.

Laboratory tests are not generally useful in caustic ingestions. In serious cases (particularly after acid ingestion) in which the patient is symptomatic, arterial blood gas and electrolytes may be useful. In hydrofluoric acid exposures, calcium and magnesium levels, and an electrocardiogram may be useful. An upright chest radiograph will evaluate for aspiration, pneumomediastinum, or pneumoperitoneum from gastric perforation.

Endoscopy is the diagnostic test of choice in evaluating for serious esophageal or gastric injury. It is indicated in all patients with signs or symptoms of serious injury (eg, vomiting, drooling, dyspnea, or stridor) or severe oropharyngeal burns. Asymptomatic patients who intentionally ingest strong acids also may benefit from endoscopy to exclude occult gastric injury. Early endoscopy, within several hours of ingestion, can be safe and useful in determining the extent of injury and the need for admission.

Computed tomography may be a useful screen in patients with symptoms referable to the GI tract distal to the stomach. Ultrasonography can be used to follow up gastric injury after caustic ingestion.

EMERGENCY DEPARTMENT CARE AND DISPOSITION

1. **One hundred percent oxygen** should be administered to any patient with respiratory symptoms, followed by endotracheal intubation under direct visualization for any patient with respiratory distress. Cardiac monitor and pulse oximetry should be applied.
2. Gastric decontamination in the form of activated charcoal, ipecac, or gastric lavage is contraindicated. Only in cases of strong acid ingestions may a nasogastric tube be inserted for removal of excessive acid in the stomach. This is especially true for hydrofluoric acid, for which fluoride binding can be effected with **milk** (8 oz) orally or **magnesium citrate** 300 mL by nasogastric tube.
3. Dilution is indicated only for solid alkali ingestions; particles should be washed away with water or milk. For other caustic ingestions, dilution is contraindicated because it can precipitate vomiting. Neutralization cannot be routinely recommended.
4. Steroids are controversial in alkali ingestions. They may be indicated within the first 6 hours of ingestion for patients at risk of esophageal strictures, in particular those with deep, discrete, or circumferential ulcerations, but without evidence of necrosis. **Dexamethasone** 0.1 mg/kg or **methylprednisolone** 2 mg/kg intravenous (IV) bolus are recommended. **Antibiotics** (eg, **ampicillin** 500 mg IV every 6 hours) are reserved for patients placed on IV steroids or who have suspected esophageal or gastric perforation.
5. Emergent GI consultation should be obtained for any caustic ingestion other than an unintentional, benign ingestion. Patients who experienced unintentional ingestions usually can be discharged home after a few hours of observation if they remain asymptomatic and tolerate liquids well. Intentional ingestion warrants endoscopy and admission regardless of symptoms. Psychiatric consultation also should be initiated.
6. Ocular exposures should be treated with **copious irrigation** for at least 20 to 30 minutes with 1 to 2 L normal saline. Alkali exposures usually require more prolonged irrigation. The final pH of the conjunctivae should be below 8.0 before ceasing irrigation.
7. Dermal exposures to caustics usually only require copious irrigation with water. Hydrofluoric acid dermal exposures require additional treatment. Small areas of skin initially can be treated with a topical application of **calcium gluconate gel** (3.5 g mixed with 5 oz water-soluble surgical lubricant) every 4 to 8 hours, as dictated by pain relief. In nondigital areas, if no relief is obtained or an extensive area is involved, then 10% **intradermal calcium gluconate** (0.5 mL/cm^2) should be administered. In digits, **intraarterial calcium gluconate** (10 mL of 10% in 50 mL 5% dextrose in water over 4 hours) should be administered into the radial artery of the affected extremity.
8. Oral ingestions of hydrofluoric acid and ammonium bifluoride and severe dermal exposures (>20% concentration) usually require systemic treatment. Known or suspected hypocalcemia can be treated with 10% **calcium chloride** 0.02 to 0.04 mL/kg in adults (0.1–0.3 mL/kg in children). Alternatively, 10% **calcium gluconate** can be used at 3 times the dose with less

concern for local tissue necrosis if infiltrated. Prolonged QT-interval or ventricular dysrhythmias also can be treated with **magnesium sulfate** 2 to 4 g IV (25–50 mg/kg in children).
9. Suspected disc battery ingestions require a chest radiograph to exclude esophageal lodgment. If it is discovered in the esophagus, then immediate endoscopic removal is indicated to help prevent esophageal perforation.

For further reading in *Emergency Medicine: A Comprehensive Study Guide,* 6th ed., see Chap. 181, "Caustics," by G. Richard Bruno and Wallace A. Carter.

111 | Insecticides, Herbicides, and Rodenticides

Christian A. Tomaszewski

Pesticides are divided into the target-based groupings of insecticides, herbicides, and rodenticides. They are responsible for a large number of accidental, occupational, and intentional exposures each year. Mass poisoning may be seen with organophosphates in the setting of terrorist activity or chemical warfare. Pesticide toxicity can come from all exposure routes, with the notable attribute of systemic toxicity from dermal exposure. Acute exposure may result in a class-specific toxidrome within 12 to 24 hours; however, early presentation, high lipid solubility, the presence of other "inert" ingredients, and chronic low-grade poisoning may contribute to less than clear clinical features in individual cases. Poison center consultation is recommended for management strategies.

CLINICAL FEATURES

Among all pesticides, organophosphorus insecticides are the most common cause of major toxicity. Patients usually become symptomatic within 8 hours of dermal exposure; nerve gas agents (eg, VX gas) can cause immediate effects via dermal or inhalation routes. The main exceptions are the fat-soluble agents (eg, fenthion), which can cause delayed or persistent symptoms. The effects of organophosphates, which inhibit cholinesterase, are manifested in muscarinic, nicotinic, and central nervous system (CNS) effects. Muscarinic over-stimulation results in the *SLUDGE syndrome* (salivation, lacrimation, urination, defecation, gastrointestinal, emesis) and the *Killer Bees* (bradycardia, bronchospasm, and bronchorrhea). In addition, especially with nerve gas agents, the patient may have blurred vision associated with miosis. Nicotinic stimulation leads to fasciculations and muscle weakness, which is most pronounced in the ventilatory system already compromised by muscarinic effects. Nicotinic effects also can lead to paradoxical tachycardia and mydriasis. CNS effects, which often predominate in children, include tremor, restlessness, confusion, seizures, and coma.

A variety of nonacute effects are associated with organophosphorus insecticide poisoning. An intermediate syndrome, which occurs 1 to 4 days after acute poisoning, may present with paralysis or weakness of neck, facial, and respiratory muscles. This can result in respiratory arrest if not treated. Organophosphate-induced delayed neuropathy occurs 1 to 3 weeks after acute poisoning. By inhibiting neuronal esterase, the patient develops a distal motor-sensory polyneuropathy. Carbamates produce a cholinergic toxidrome similar to that of organophosphates, but of shorter duration and with less CNS symptomatology.

Several other classes of pesticides, such as organophosphates, can cause seizures. Organic chlorines (eg, dichlorodiphenyltrichloroethane) are represented by methoxychlor, endosulfan, toxaphene, and the therapeutic agent lindane. Acute poisoning with organic chlorines primarily produces CNS stimulation, with headache, excitability, myoclonus, and seizures. This may be associated with hyperpyrexia. Pyrethroids, synthetic derivatives of pyrethrins, are probably the safest insecticides. In massive ingestion, however, they may cause gastrointestinal (GI) distress and, rarely, seizures. The main issue with pyrethrins and pyrethroids is the occasional allergic response, which can include contact dermatitis, rhinitis, and refractory asthma. N,N-diethyl-3-methylbenzamide (DEET), the extensively used insect repellent, can lead to neuronal toxicity after ingestion or multiple applications, particularly in small children. These patients may present with restlessness, confusion, ataxia, lethargy, seizures, or coma.

Herbicide toxicity leads to a wide variety of symptoms based on which organ system has been exposed. Topical exposure causes local irritation, and ingestion may result in vomiting, diarrhea, and pulmonary edema. Chlorophenoxy compounds (eg, 2,4-diclorophenoxyactic acid) may cause tachycardia, dysrhythmias, and hypotension in addition to muscle toxicity manifested by muscle pain, fasciculations, and rhabdomyolysis. Paraquat is especially toxic, with caustic effects resulting in severe dermal, corneal, and mucus membrane burns, including burns of the respiratory and GI epithelia. Cardiovascular collapse may occur early, especially in the case of large ingestions. If patients survive the initial insult, they can develop liver and renal necrosis, followed by irreversible pulmonary fibrosis weeks later. Diquat is very similar in toxicity to paraquat, although it lacks the pulmonary toxicity, but is more prone to produce brainstem hemorrhage. A cross between organophosphates and herbicides is glyphosate, which generally causes only mild dermatitis and mucosal irritation on contact. Massive ingestions of concentrated solution have caused widespread organ dysfunction, including pulmonary edema, acidosis, and hyperkalemia.

The clinical signs of rodenticide poisoning vary widely, and specific features are associated with individual agents. Sodium mono fluoroacetate and related compounds typically demonstrate delayed toxicity until metabolites block aerobic metabolic pathways, which lead to lactic acidosis. Patients exhibit nausea and anxiety followed by respiratory depression, pulmonary edema, cardiovascular collapse, coma, and seizures. Strychnine toxicity blocks the spinal cord inhibitor glycine and results in "awake seizures," which are characterized by facial grimacing, muscle twitching, severe extensor spasms, and opisthotonos. This can lead to rhabdomyolysis, hyperthermia, and lactic acidosis. Exposure to thallium sulfate initially causes GI hemorrhage and vomiting, which are followed days later by neurologic sequelae. Patients can develop painful paresthesias, weakness, tremors, ataxia, seizures, and coma. Death is typically due to respiratory failure and dysrhythmias. Zinc phosphide ingestion results in the liberation of phosphine gas that subsequently causes GI irritation, hepatocellular toxicity, pulmonary edema, altered mental status, seizures, and cardiovascular collapse; hypomagnesemia and hypocalcemia also can result. Yellow phosphorous causes severe topical burns and also may cause jaundice, seizures, and cardiovascular collapse. Within hours of ingestion, barium carbonate can cause GI distress with dysrhythmias, respiratory failure, weakness, and paralysis. This is often accompanied by hypokalemia. N-3-pyridylmethly-N-*p*-nitrophylurea (Vacor) has the unique ability to induce insulin deficiency and peripheral neuropathy. Death is due to GI perforation, diabetic ketoacidosis, or cardiac dysrhythmias. Arsenic may present initially with nausea and vomiting, hypotension, bloody diarrhea, altered mental status, and seizures. If the patient survives, peripheral neuropathies ensue with weakness and muscle wasting.

As for the moderately toxic rodenticides, α-naphthyl-thiourea exhibits primarily pulmonary effects with dyspnea, pleuritic chest pain, and noncardiogenic pulmonary edema. Cholecalciferol causes the typical symptoms of vitamin D excess. Red Squill poisoning is a mildly toxic rodenticide that can present with severe GI distress and cardiac dysrhythmias due to digitalis effect. After large deliberate ingestions, bromethalin can cause headache, confusion, tremors, seizures, and coma. Norbormide causes dermatitis from chronic handling.

The most common rodenticide exposures are due to superwarfarins (eg, brodifacoum), which are present in a variety of grain-based rodent baits. Because of their extraordinary half-lives, exposures may come to attention months later with symptoms of unexplained coagulopathy. This coagulopathy may manifest itself when the patient experiences hematuria, epistaxis, GI hemorrhage, spontaneous hemoperitoneum, or fatal intracranial hemorrhage.

DIAGNOSIS AND DIFFERENTIAL

The diagnosis of pesticide poisoning is made clinically in the overwhelming majority of cases. In the case of organophosphate poisoning, clues at the bedside include the odor of garlic or hydrocarbons. A positive response to atropine and pralidoxime usually will confirm the diagnosis of organophosphate poisoning.

Laboratory confirmation of pesticide exposure is usually unavailable in the emergency department. For delayed confirmation of organophosphate poisoning, an assay of plasma (easier to obtain) or red blood cell (more accurate) cholinesterase activity can be obtained for diagnosis and treatment guidance. Qualitative and quantitative assays of blood and urine for paraquat at times may be clinically useful in confirming exposure and prognostication. In deliberate or massive ingestions of superwarfarins, a 48-hour postingestion prothrombin time is needed. Other routine laboratory testing is nondiagnostic but may show hyperglycemia, electrolyte abnormalities, metabolic acidosis, leukocytosis, hyperamylasemia, or liver enzyme abnormalities. In cases involving severe respiratory distress, a chest radiograph may show signs of pulmonary edema. Electrocardiographic findings are variable and may include tachydysrhythmia, ventricular blocks, bradydysrhythmia, or QT interval prolongation with ensuing torsades de pointes.

Pesticide poisoning can easily be mistaken for routine illnesses. Bronchospasm and pulmonary edema may be attributed to asthma or congestive heart failure exacerbations. Vomiting and diarrhea could be mistaken for gastroenteritis. The differential diagnosis for organophosphate poisoning includes these illnesses and a variety of cardiopulmonary and neurologic emergencies. In addition, other toxic agents may mimic the same effects of organophosphates: muscarinic effects may arise from bethanecol or the mushrooms *Clitocybe* and *Inocybe;* agitation and diaphoresis may arise from sympathomimetics like cocaine; nicotinic effects may arise from tobacco toxicity; and seizures may be due to a variety of toxins.

EMERGENCY DEPARTMENT CARE AND DISPOSITION

1. Before encountering the pesticide-poisoned patient (especially when involving organophosphates), health care workers should wear at least gown and glove (neoprene or nitrile) to prevent secondary contamination.

2. Symptomatic patients require emergent attention to airway protection and ventilation. Supplemental **oxygen** should be administered to maintain oxygen saturation greater than 95%. **Endotracheal intubation** and mechanical ventilation may be necessary in severe poisoning; the effects of succinylcholine may exacerbate certain conditions, and its use should be carefully considered during rapid sequence intubation.

3. **Decontamination** in dermal exposures can be performed with soap and water or with dilute bleach. In recent significant ingestions, aspiration of gastric contents with a nasogastric tube and administration of activated charcoal may be helpful, especially if a coingestion may be involved.

4. The mainstay of treatment for pesticide exposure is identification of the specific agent involved, supportive monitoring, and treatment. Continuous cardiac, blood pressure, and pulse oximetry monitoring are essential; intravenous (IV) access should be secured. Maintenance of intravascular volume and urine output should be ensured. Cardiac dysrhythmias should be treated in standard fashion.

5. Benzodiazepines (eg, **lorazepam** 2 mg IV) remain the initial therapy for seizures.

6. If the prothrombin time or international normalized ratio is elevated after superwarfarin ingestion, **vitamin K$_1$** 10 to 20 mg subcutaneously or IV

TABLE 111-1 Pesticides and Specific Antidotes

Pesticide	Antidote	Dosing
Organophosphates	Atropine	0.05 mg/kg up to 1–2 mg IV initially q5–15 min; consider IV infusion and titrate to effect (drying secretions)
	2-PAM	20–40 mg/kg up to 1 g IV; may repeat in 1–2 h, then every 6–8 h for 48 h
Carbamates	Atropine	Same as for organophosphates
	2-PAM	Use is controversial
Zinc phosphide	NaHCO$_3$	50–100 mEq (1 ampule) for intragastric alkalinization
	Calcium gluconate	10 mL of 10% IV (for hypocalcemia)
Yellow phosphorous	K permanganate or H$_2$O$_2$	1:5000 dilution used for gastric lavage
Sodium mono fluoroacetate	Ethanol	10 mL/kg 10% IV bolus, then 1.5 mL/(kg · h)
PNU (Vacor)	Niacinamide	500 mg IV
Arsenic	BAL	3–5 mg/kg IM q4h
	DMSA	10 mg/kg PO q8h
Red Squill	Fab fragments	May start with 5 vials in severe toxicity
Superwarfarins	Vitamin K$_1$	Up to 20 mg IV, repeated and titrated to effect

Key: 2-PAM = pralidoxime; BAL = dimercaprol (British Anti-Lewisite); DMSA = succimer (dimercaptosuccinic acid); H$_2$O$_2$ = hydrogen peroxide; IM = intramuscularly; IV = intravenously; NaHCO$_3$ = sodium bicarbonate; PNU = N-3-pyridylmethyl-N-p-nitrophenyl urea; PO = orally; q = every.

can be administered; if serious bleeding is present; **fresh-frozen plasma** also may be required.

7. Administration of a **specific antidote** may be appropriate for selected agents (Table 111-1).

8. Disposition depends on the pesticide involved in the exposure. Asymptomatic patients with a history of contact with a pesticide may require decontamination and a 4- to 6-hour observation period. Close follow-up should be arranged for exposures to rodenticides that produce delayed symptoms. A low threshold for admission should be maintained for patients with intentional ingestions or symptoms. Any patient with a history of paraquat or diquat exposure should be admitted because of the extreme lethality of these compounds.

For further reading in *Emergency Medicine: A Comprehensive Study Guide,* 6th ed., see Chap. 182, "Insecticides, Herbicides, and Rodenticides," by Walter C. Robey III and William J. Meggs.

112 | Metals and Metalloids

Lance H. Hoffman

Even though patients rarely present to the emergency department for acute metal or metalloid poisoning, this diagnosis should be considered when more common disease entities have been excluded as the etiology for the patient's symptoms. In general, metal and metalloid poisonings result in a combination of neurologic, gastrointestinal, hematologic, and renal symptoms secondary to enzymatic dysfunction caused by the metal combining with sulfhydryl groups of enzymatic systems.

LEAD POISONING

Clinical Features

Lead poisoning is the most common cause of chronic metal poisoning, with an estimated 890,000 children between the ages of 1 and 5 years having a serum lead level higher than 10 μg/dL. Lead poisoning manifests as signs and symptoms affecting a variety of organ systems (Table 112-1).

Diagnosis and Differential

Lead poisoning should be suspected in any individual, especially a child, demonstrating central or peripheral neurologic dysfunction and anemia while complaining of abdominal pain, nausea, and vomiting. Even though the differential diagnosis is broad for neurologic dysfunction, anemia, and abdominal pain, this combination of signs and symptoms should prompt an investigation into the possibility of lead poisoning. Lead exposure may occur through occupational, recreational, or environmental exposure. An elevated serum lead level confirms the diagnosis, but the results of this test are often delayed in the emergency department. Other findings suggestive of lead poisoning include basophilic stippling of erythrocytes, metaphyseal long bone lead bands on radiographs, and radiopaque material in the alimentary tract or retained bullet fragments on radiographs.

Emergency Department Care and Disposition

1. Life-threatening ventilatory and circulatory problems should be addressed through airway management and fluid resuscitation.
2. Gastrointestinal decontamination with **whole bowel irrigation** using polyethylene glycol solution is indicated for lead ingestion. The adult rate of instillation is 500 to 2,000 mL/h, and the pediatric rate of instillation is 100 to 500 mL/h.
3. Chelation therapy is the mainstay of treatment. Symptomatic individuals should receive **dimercaprol (British Anti-Lewisite [BAL])** 50 to 75 mg/m^2 intramuscularly (IM) followed in 4 hours with a continuous intravenous infusion of **CaNa$_2$ ethylene-diamine-tetraacetic acid** 1,500 mg/m^2/d, with higher dosing being reserved for patients with encephalopathy. Adults with a serum lead level of 70 to 100 μg/dL or children with a serum lead level of 45 to 69 μg/dL and with little or no symptoms should receive **succimer (dimercaptosuccinic acid)** 350 mg/m^2 orally 3 times daily for 5 days and then twice daily for 14 days. Chelation

TABLE 112-1 Common Signs and Symptoms of Lead Poisoning

System	Clinical manifestations
Central nervous system	**Acute:** encephalopathy, seizures, altered mental status, papilledema, optic neuritis, ataxia **Chronic:** headache, irritability, depression, fatigue, mood and behavioral changes, memory deficit, sleep disturbance
Peripheral nervous system	Paresthesias, motor weakness (classic wrist drop) depressed/absent DTRs, sensory function intact
Gastrointestinal	Abdominal pain (mostly with acute poisoning), constipation, diarrhea
Renal	**Acute:** Fanconi syndrome (aminoaciduria, glucosuria, phosphaturia), renal tubular acidosis **Chronic:** interstitial nephritis, renal insufficiency, hypertension, gout
Hematologic	Hypoproliferative and/or hemolytic anemia; basophilic stippling (rare and nonspecific)
Reproductive	Decreased libido, impotence, sterility, abortions, premature births, decreased or abnormal sperm production

Key: DTR = deep tendon reflexes.

therapy is not indicated for asymptomatic adults with a serum lead level below 70 μg/dL or children with a serum lead level below 45 μg/dL. Only removal from the exposure is needed in these cases.

4. Patients requiring parenteral chelation therapy or whose only option is to return to the environment producing the lead exposure should be admitted to the hospital.

ARSENIC POISONING

Clinical Features

Arsenic poisoning is the most common cause of acute metal poisoning and the second most common cause of chronic metal poisoning. Arsenic is used in a variety of insecticides and herbicides and in mining and smelting processes. Acute ingestion results in a profound gastroenteritis within hours of exposure. Hypotension and tachycardia may be present secondary to intravascular volume depletion and direct myocardial dysfunction. Encephalopathy, pulmonary edema, acute renal failure, and rhabdomyolysis also have been described. Chronic poisoning causes stocking glove peripheral neuropathies, morbilliform skin rash, malaise, myalgia, abdominal pain, memory loss, and personality changes. Transverse white lines of the nails (Mees lines) may be evident 4 to 6 weeks postingestion.

Diagnosis and Differential

An exposure history is most useful in identifying arsenic poisoning. However, the diagnosis should be considered in patients with hypotension preceded by a profound gastroenteritis and a variety of neurologic and gastrointestinal complaints. Radiopaque alimentary foreign bodies may be seen on abdominal radiographs in arsenic ingestion. An electrocardiogram may show QT-interval prolongation. The diagnosis is confirmed by demonstrating an elevated 24-hour urine arsenic level. Other diagnoses to consider include septic shock, encephalopathy, peripheral neuropathy, Addison disease, hypo- and hyperthyroidism, porphyria, and other metal poisonings.

Emergency Department Care and Disposition

1. Ventilatory and cardiovascular abnormalities require immediate treatment. Tracheal intubation may be required to protect the airway in obtunded patients. Hypotension should be treated with volume resuscitation and vasopressors. Dysrhythmias are managed by the ACLS protocol, with the need to avoid antiarrhythmia agents that prolong the QT interval (class Ia, Ic, and III agents).
2. **Whole bowel irrigation** with polyethylene glycol solution is indicated for patients with an arsenic ingestion and an abdominal radiograph demonstrating radiopaque foreign bodies in the alimentary tract.
3. Chelation therapy is the definitive treatment. **Dimercaprol (BAL)** 3 to 5 mg/kg IM every 4 hours should be administered initially. **Succimer** (350 mg/m^2 orally 3 times daily for 5 days and then twice daily for 14 days) is the preferred chelating agent for patients who can tolerate oral intake, are hemodynamically stable, and can be treated as an outpatient without risk of repeated exposure to arsenic.

MERCURY POISONING

Clinical Features

Short-chain alkyl mercury (methyl, dimethyl, and ethyl) and elemental mercury produce a constellation of neurologic abnormalities collectively referred to as *erethism*. This constellation includes mood alterations, anxiety, sleep disturbances, memory loss, paresthesias, ataxia, muscle rigidity and spasticity, visual and hearing impairment, and tremors. Inhalation of elemental mercury can result in pneumonitis, acute respiratory distress syndrome, and pulmonary fibrosis. Ingestion of mercury salts results in a severe gastroenteritis and acute tubular necrosis but does not affect the central nervous system. *Acrodynia* describes an immune-mediated condition that affects children exposed to mercury. Features include a generalized rash, fever, irritability, splenomegaly, and hypotonia.

Diagnosis and Differential

The key to diagnosing mercury poisoning is obtaining a history of exposure to mercury. An elevated 24-hour urine mercury level confirms the diagnosis for all forms of mercury except the short-chain alkyl mercury compounds, which are excreted in the bile, undergo extensive enterohepatic recirculation, and accumulate in erythrocytes. An elevated whole blood mercury level must be used to confirm poisoning from these types of mercury compounds. The differential diagnosis of symptoms caused by mercury poisoning is extensive and includes all causes of encephalopathy or tremor. Alternative causes of corrosive gastroenteritis (ingestion of iron, arsenic, phosphorus, acids, and alkalis) should be considered if mercury salt ingestion is suspected.

Emergency Department Care and Disposition

1. Aggressive management of ventilatory and cardiovascular abnormalities is of primary importance.
2. Gastric lavage and **activated charcoal** should be considered. A cathartic is not indicated if profuse diarrhea is present.
3. Chelation therapy should begin prior to confirming the diagnosis. **Dimercaprol (BAL)** 5 mg/kg IM is the preferred chelating agent for mercury poisonings not involving methyl mercury because central neurologic symptoms are exacerbated with this combination. **Succimer (dimercaptosuccinic acid)** 10 mg/kg orally every 8 hours may be the agent of choice in short-chain alkyl mercury poisonings.

For further reading in *Emergency Medicine: A Comprehensive Study Guide,* 6th ed., see Chap. 184, "Metals and Metalloids," by Heather Long and Lewis S. Nelson.

113 | Hazardous Materials

Christian A. Tomaszewski

A hazardous material is any substance (chemical, biological, or nuclear) that poses a risk to health, safety, property, or the environment. Well over a half million, potentially toxic compounds have been produced, ranging from industrial chemicals to hazardous nuclear, biological, and chemical agents, known as *weapons of mass destruction*. Exposure to hazardous materials results in direct toxicity and is frequently associated with trauma, burns, and respiratory compromise.

Hazardous materials incidents, although rare, can quickly overwhelm a medical facility, especially when mass casualties are involved. Prior planning is essential to coordinate resources, minimize loss of life, and prevent secondary contamination of health care workers. Data about involved chemicals are essential. Sources include regional poison centers, material safety data sheets, transportation specific markings (Department of Transportation placards, shipping papers, bills of lading), private agencies (Chemtrec), government agencies (Nuclear Regulatory Commission, Environmental Protection Agency, Centers for Disease Control and Prevention, Agency for Toxic Substance and Disease Registry, and Radiation Emergency Assistance Center/Training Site), and computerized databases (Micromedex and ToxNet).

DECONTAMINATION

The goal of decontamination is to decrease further exposure to victims and to prevent secondary contamination of health care workers. Decontamination is performed in 3 "zones." The *hot zone* is the area at the scene or outside the hospital, where contaminated patients are held and where only immediate life-threatening conditions are addressed. The *warm zone* is the area outside (or physically isolated from) the hospital, where decontamination and further stabilization of the patient occur. The *cold zone* is where fully decontaminated victims are transferred. There should be no movement of health care personnel between zones.

Because of the risk of contamination, access to the hot and warm zones is restricted to personnel with suitable protective clothing. The minimum personal protection available for hospital personnel caring for contaminated patients is level C: splash protection with chemical-resistant clothing (eg, Tyvec or Saranex) and a full-face, air-purifying, canister-equipped respirator. Higher levels of protection are available but are not generally practical for hospital personnel.

Triage should occur outside the hospital, where urgency of care and adequacy of decontamination are assessed. First, contaminated patients should not be allowed to enter the hospital premises. Second, personnel without appropriate personal protective gear should not be allowed into the decontamination or triage area. Medical stabilization before decontamination is limited to opening the airway, cervical spine stabilization, oxygen administration, ventilatory support, and application of direct pressure to arterial bleeding.

As patients are triaged, decontamination commences in the warm zone by removing all the victims' clothing and brushing away gross particulate matter. Ocular and wound decontaminations are initiated by focused irrigation of those sites. Whole body irrigation is performed by using copious amounts of water and mild soap or detergent, beginning at the hands and head; this is followed by showering for 3 to 5 minutes.

Many chemicals require special irrigation. Dilute household bleach (1 part to 9 parts water) will inactivate organophosphate pesticides, nerve agents, and most biological agents. Phenol burns may benefit from polyethylene glycol. Water-reactive metals such as sodium, lithium, and potassium initially should be covered with mineral or vegetable oil, removed or brushed off, and then irrigated with water. Other water-reactive substances include acetic anhydride, chlorosulfonic acid, dry lime (calcium oxide), hydrides (bornanes and silanes), titanium tetrachloride, and organometallics (alkylaluminums and zinc phosphide). In the absence of proper decontamination solutions for these agents, especially in critically ill patients, large volumes of water may be considered once the agents are mechanically removed as much as possible. In contrast to these agents, white phosphorus ignites in air, and burns from it should be kept continuously moist with water or saline dressings. Tar burns cannot be readily débrided and usually will benefit from repeated application of Neosporin cream, petroleum jelly, or mayonnaise.

Vomiting by the contaminated patient also may be a source of secondary contamination. This is especially true for organophosphates. In addition, some materials, such as sodium azide, react to produce toxic gases, namely hydrogen cyanide, when combined with stomach acid. Gastric emptying or activated charcoal should be considered early in such ingestions.

After decontamination, patients can be wrapped in clean blankets and transferred to the cold zone, where medical assessment and treatment can be completed. Until definitive identification of the chemical and its risk is made, emergency department personnel should maintain protective gear. After performing the primary survey, the secondary survey can be carried out with the goal of identifying the specific hazardous material toxidrome, which may require a specific antidote.

EMERGENCY DEPARTMENT CARE AND DISPOSITION

Inhaled Toxins

Inhaled toxins include gases, dusts, fumes, and aerosols and generally result in upper airway damage or pulmonary toxicity. Agents larger than 10 μm in particle size or highly water-soluble agents are deposited primarily in the upper airway. Water-soluble gases include ammonia, sulfur dioxide, and various acids such as hydrochloric acid. These patients rapidly develop symptoms and complain of mucous membrane irritation accompanied by coughing and wheezing. Smaller particles or non–water-soluble agents, such as phosgene, ozone, or nitrogen oxides, reach deeper into the pulmonary system and tend to inflict delayed effects. A gas of intermediate solubility, such as chlorine gas, can cause early upper irritant symptoms followed by delayed pulmonary edema. Many of these irritant chemicals are carried in smoke and are responsible for the ensuing respiratory distress. Systemic toxicity from carbon monoxide and cyanide toxicity should be considered if a history of combustion is present. The mainstay of treatment in inhaled toxins is to administer 100% oxygen, consider bronchodilators, and examine the upper airway for signs of compromise. Patients should be intubated early if they develop respiratory distress or airway edema.

Neurotoxins

Hydrocarbon inhalation victims may present with headache, dizziness, confusion, lethargy, and coma. Central nervous system stimulants (eg, organophosphates or nitrophenol) can cause agitation, seizures, and hyperthermia. Some inhaled agents, such as carbon monoxide, hydrogen sulfide, methanol, certain metals, and pesticides, can cause serious delayed neurotoxic effects. Simple asphyxiants (eg, nitrogen, carbon dioxide, or natural gas) can cause dramatic loss of consciousness in an enclosed space. Before loss of consciousness, patients may experience headache, dizziness, nausea, or confusion. Treatment for neurotoxins is 100% oxygen after removal from the environment.

Dermal Toxins

Solvents and heat exposure may increase the dermal absorption of toxins, in particular organophosphate or organic chlorine pesticides. In addition, systemic toxicity can result from any of the following agents that can also be readily absorbed through intact skin: acrylamide, acetonitrile, aniline, chlordane, dinitrophenol, hydrogen cyanide, hydrofluoric acid, organic mercury, methyl bromide, nerve agents, nitrobenzene, and phenol.

Corrosive effects from hazardous materials may be immediately obvious in the case of mineral acids or delayed after alkaline corrosives or hydrofluoric acid. Alkaline burns can be particularly problematic because of the deeper penetration associated with liquefaction necrosis, as opposed to the coagulation necrosis seen with acids. Another dermal effect from hazardous materials is frostbite from liquid phosphine, phosgene, ammonia, chlorine, hydrogen sulfide, or propane. Hydrocarbons further promote the absorption of hazardous material because of their ability to defat in addition to burning. Treatment consists of copious irrigation with pH monitoring of the skin.

Phenol can cause skin destruction, thus facilitating its absorption into the circulation. This may lead to central nervous system depression, intravascular hemolysis, pulmonary edema, and hepatorenal dysfunction. Phenol absorption is enhanced by water; however, copious irrigation should obviate this problem. Alternatively, the burn area may be soaked with gauze impregnated with polyethylene glycol. Hydrofluoric acid burns also require special therapy with topical, systemic, and intradermal calcium salts.

Ocular Exposures

Ocular chemical burns are marked by conjunctival injection, blepharospasm, and clouding of the cornea. The main threat is ulceration and globe perforation. Ocular exposures demand emergent irrigation with large volumes of water. In stable patients, immediate prehospital irrigation for up to 20 minutes before transport is recommended. Gross particulate matter should be brushed away from the eye, and contact lenses should be removed. Absence of pain may not indicate cessation of ocular damage; irrigation should continue until ocular pH returns to 7.4.

Metabolic Toxins

Hydrogen sulfide is a colorless gas used in industry and encountered in sewage treatment or manure collections. Although it has a distinct "rotten egg" odor, this olfactory warning is lost with extended exposure or high concentrations. It causes cellular asphyxia with production of lactate and ensuing metabolic acidosis. In high concentrations, rapid loss of consciousness, seizures, and death may occur after a few breaths. Survivors may develop pulmonary edema and corneal damage from irritant effects. Other similar metabolic poisons are carbon monoxide and hydrogen cyanide. After decontamination, the patient may benefit from sodium nitrite administration.

Myocardial Toxins

Certain solvents, such as freon and halogenated and aromatic hydrocarbons, can sensitize the myocardium to dysrhythmic effects of catecholamines. Refraining from the use of sympathomimetic drugs may decrease the chance of inducing fatal ventricular tachydysrhythmia. In cases of hydrocarbon exposure, if the patient is soaked, countershocking may need to be avoided because of flammability issues. Cases of hydrofluoric acid exposure can present with dysrhythmias from hypocalcemia and hypomagnesemia. Intravenous calcium therapy may be life saving.

POST-INCIDENT RESPONSE

Prolonged observation in the emergency department or hospital admission should be considered for exposures to certain hazardous materials. For example, the nitriles can form cyanide; methylene chloride can be metabolized to carbon monoxide; aniline can cause hemolysis; and delayed pulmonary edema can result from cadmium, chlorine, halogenated solvents, methyl bromide, nitrogen oxides, ozone, paraquat, phosgene, phosphine, and zinc phosphide. In addition, ethylene oxide and metals can cause hepatorenal toxicity. In many cases, patients require follow-up for symptomatic care and counseling for posttraumatic stress and fears of carcinogenic or harmful reproductive side effects. Hepatic and renal tests may indicate delayed toxicity.

For further reading in *Emergency Medicine: A Comprehensive Study Guide,* 6th ed., see Chap. 185, "Hazardous Materials Exposure," by Suzanne R. White and Col Edward M. Eitzen Jr.

114 | Herbals and Vitamins

Christian A. Tomaszewski

Sales of over-the-counter herbal preparations exceeded $1.5 billion in 1997, all without US Food and Drug Administration control except for label wording. Other dietary supplements that are considered innocuous by most of the public are vitamins. Many of these herbal and vitamin products have the capability to induce significant toxicity, especially if used in excess.

CLINICAL FEATURES

The daily recommended doses of vitamin A for adult men and women are 5000 IU and 4000 IU, respectively. Hypervitaminosis A usually occurs when children are given excessive amounts of high-potency supplements. Dialysis patients are also at risk for bone resorption with resulting hypercalcemia. Symptoms and signs of vitamin A toxicity are related primarily to the skin, central nervous system, and hepatic function. Patients may have dry or abnormally pigmented skin, pruritus, and loss of hair. Central nervous system complaints can include blurred vision and headache; pseudotumor cerebri may develop. Because of storage of vitamin A in the liver, patients may develop hepatomegaly. Hypercalcemia from toxicity can cause ectopic calcifications and bone pain.

Vitamin D is also associated with hypercalcemia at doses larger than 1,000 IU/kg, although infants may experience toxic effects at 2000 IU. Patients may present with anorexia, nausea, abdominal pain, lethargy, weight loss, polyuria, constipation, and confusion. Eventually, high calcium levels can lead to ectopic bone formation and renal failure.

Although nontoxic at daily doses up to 600 IU, vitamin E at higher doses can antagonize vitamin K production. This can be important as a potential cause of bleeding, particularly for patients on anticoagulants. Chronic use of large doses can lead to nausea, fatigue, headache, weakness, and blurred vision.

Vitamin K, despite being fat soluble, does not tend to accumulate in the body and is readily excreted in the urine. At low doses, it is required for maintenance of clotting function; at higher doses, vitamin K_3 (menadione) can cause hemolytic anemia, kernicterus, and hemoglobinuria in infants. Of note, there are rare reports of cardiovascular collapse with rapid intravenous (IV) injection of vitamin K_1 (phytonadione).

Vitamin B_3 (niacin) consists of water-soluble nicotinic acid and its active metabolite nicotinamide. Acute ingestion of as little as 100 mg of nicotinic acid can cause "niacin flush," which is characterized by burning, itching, and redness of the face, neck, and chest due to histamine release. Higher doses can cause nausea, abdominal cramps, diarrhea, and headache. Chronic toxicity from high doses (>2,000 mg/d) can cause elevated liver enzymes, impaired glucose tolerance, hyperuricemia, and skin dryness and discoloration.

Vitamin B_6 (pyridoxine) in chronic high doses can cause a sensory axonal neuropathy. Typically, more than 5 g/d must be taken over several weeks. Patients may present with unstable gait and numbness of the feet. This can progress to similar symptoms in the upper extremities accompanied by loss of position and vibratory senses. A unique interaction of vitamin B_6 is the inactivation of levodopa, which may pose problems for patients with Parkinson disease.

Excessive doses of the water-soluble vitamins B_1 (thiamine), B_2 (riboflavin), B_{12}, biotin, and folic acid do not cause medical problems. High doses of vitamin C can precipitate gout and nephrolithiasis in susceptible patients; diarrhea and abdominal cramps also may ensue.

Among dietary supplements, herbal medicines present a larger threat than vitamins. Because the US Food and Drug Administration allows them to be marketed for their intended, but not proven, effects, there are presently no regulations on the safety and composition of such products. Many of these preparations can lead to toxicity, often because of contaminants or deliberate adulterants.

There are several popular herbal preparations that have potential for serious toxicity. Chaparral, derived from the creosote bush and used for cancer and pain relief, can be hepatotoxic. By adding in 2 to 4 teaspoons of nutmeg, enterprising individuals may experience hallucinations. High doses also can cause gastrointestinal upset, agitation, miosis, coma, and hypertension. Ephedra, used for weight loss, contains ephedrine and can cause sympathomimetic toxicity, particularly in large doses. It has been associated with deaths from stroke, seizures, and cardiac toxicity. Yohimbine, an α_2-adrenergic receptor antagonist, also can cause sympathomimetic excess, especially when taken with a decongestant such as phenylpropanolamine. Toxic effects include hallucinations, weakness, hypertension, and paralysis.

There are some less common herbal preparations that are equally unsafe. Distributed as a European liquor, absinthe (wormwood) contains volatile oils that can cause psychosis, intellectual deterioration, ataxia, headache, and vomiting. Black (or blue) cohosh, used to treat menopause, can induce nausea, vomiting, dizziness, and weakness. Juniper, used as a diuretic, can cause renal toxicity, nausea, and vomiting. Lobelia, used for asthma, can produce anticholinergic syndrome.

Even purportedly safer herbal agents can cause adverse effects. Chamomile and echinacea have been associated with anaphylaxis. Garlic, ginkgo, and ginseng have antithrombotic activity, which may precipitate bleeding in patients on warfarin. St John's wort, in conjunction with other antidepressants, may precipitate serotonin syndrome.

DIAGNOSIS AND DIFFERENTIAL

Diagnosis is usually made clinically. If patients are unable to recall the precise herbal or vitamin compounds they are taking, then arrangements should be made for someone to retrieve the substances from the patients' homes. Under the appropriate clinical setting, laboratory studies that should be obtained may include a chemistry panel, blood urea nitrogen, creatinine, calcium level, hepatic enzymes, coagulation studies, bleeding time, toxicology screen, and urine pregnancy test. An electrocardiogram may be indicated.

EMERGENCY DEPARTMENT CARE AND DISPOSITION

1. Discontinuation of the vitamin, particularly water-soluble ones, or herbal preparation is usually all that is needed if a patient presents with mild toxicity.
2. In vitamin A overdoses, gastric decontamination with **activated charcoal** 1 g/kg orally (PO) is indicated for acute ingestions of more than 300,000 IU in children or 1,000,000 IU in adults. Only deliberate massive overdoses

of vitamin D, such as 100 or more multivitamin tablets, should be considered for decontamination.

3. Hypercalcemia, from vitamin A or D ingestion, can be treated with IV fluids, prednisone, and furosemide. In addition, lumbar puncture may be useful in pseudotumor cerebri from massive vitamin A ingestion.

4. **Diphenhydramine** 25 to 50 mg IV or PO can be given to patients with "niacin flush" symptoms.

5. Administration of **N-acetylcysteine** 140 mg/kg PO or IV should be considered for treating severe hepatotoxicity from herbal preparations such as chaparral or pennyroyal oil.

For further reading in *Emergency Medicine: A Comprehensive Study Guide,* 6th ed., see Chap. 186, "Herbals and Vitamins," by G. Richard Braen.

115 | Antimicrobials

Christian A. Tomaszewski

Although antimicrobial overdoses are frequently reported, they seldom result in death. Observation is usually all that is required, except for agents such as isoniazid, chloroquine, and quinine.

ISONIAZID

Clinical Features

Patients taking isoniazid as prophylaxis or treatment for *Mycobacterium tuberculosis* are increasingly commonplace in most emergency departments. The initial features of overdose include nausea, vomiting, and altered mental status. Severe signs include seizures, coma, and lactate acidosis. Seizures are usually seen within 1 hour of acute ingestions larger than 30 mg/kg.

Diagnosis and Differential

In general, the diagnosis of isoniazid overdose is made clinically and should be considered in any patient with refractory seizures. A serum isoniazid level can be used for confirmation. Acute isoniazid overdose usually presents with an anion-gap metabolic acidosis (see Table 102-1). In severe cases with prolonged seizure activity, serial arterial blood gas analysis to follow lactic acidosis and serial creatine kinase levels to exclude rhabdomyolysis may be helpful. A fingerstick serum glucose level is essential for patients experiencing altered mental status or seizures. Hepatic profile may be useful in cases of chronic use.

Emergency Department Care and Disposition

1. In addition to managing seizure activity or coma in the standard approach, the emergency physician should treat the patient with **pyridoxine** (vitamin B_6) at a dose of 1 g for every gram of isoniazid ingested. If the amount is unknown, then administer 5 g (70 mg/kg in children) intravenously (IV) over 30 minutes. Additional doses of 1 g every 2 to 3 minutes can be administered until seizures resolve.
2. Most patients will manifest serious symptoms within 2 hours and can be discharged after 6 hours if they remain asymptomatic.

ANTIMALARIAL DRUGS

Clinical Features

Although not commonly used, antimalarials have the most potential among antimicrobials for toxic effects. Common agents are quinine, chloroquine, mefloquine, and primaquine. Quinine and chloroquine can cause headache, altered mental status, and seizures. Both can cause prolonged intervals on electrocardiogram and hypotension. Quinine has the unique property to cause blindness.

Diagnosis and Differential

Quinine also should be considered in the differential diagnosis of hypoglycemia. Chloroquine can lead to hypokalemia. Electrolytes and an electrocardiogram

549

should be obtained. Patients who have overdosed on dapsone, chloroquine, or primaquine may benefit from a methemoglobinemia determination if they are cyanotic or dyspneic.

Emergency Department Care and Disposition

1. Attention to early **intubation, gastric decontamination,** and sedation with **benzodiazepines** may decrease mortality in serious overdoses.
2. The pressor of choice for hypotension is **epinephrine** starting at 0.25 μg/kg/min IV.
3. **Sodium bicarbonate** 50 mEq IV (1 mEq/kg in children) push can be used for prolonged QRS interval, particularly in the face of hypotension.
4. Any ingestion of more than a daily therapeutic dose, especially in children, warrants at least 6 hours of observation on a cardiac monitor.

PENICILLINS AND THE β-LACTAM AGENTS

Clinical Features

Most overdoses of penicillins and β-lactams are relatively benign. However, high-dose penicillin G, cephalosporins, and imipenem have caused confusion, agitation, myoclonic jerking, and seizures. Amoxicillin has been associated with renal failure.

Diagnosis and Differential

Central nervous system toxicity from β-lactams usually occurs only in renal failure patients receiving high doses who have underlying central nervous system abnormalities. Renal function tests and electrolytes may be indicated in large symptomatic overdoses.

Emergency Department Care and Disposition

Seizures should be treated in the standard fashion, starting with **lorazepam** 2 mg IV or intramuscularly (0.05 mg/kg in children).

AMINOGLYCOSIDES

Clinical Features

Most toxic exposures to aminoglycosides involve iatrogenic administration. These usually result in ototoxity and nephrotoxicity.

Diagnosis and Differential

The potential for hearing loss is associated with prolonged or high-dose therapy, with neomycin being the worst offender. The risk for nephrotoxicity is due to a combination of factors: dose, duration, hydration, and extremes of age.

Emergency Department Care and Disposition

1. **Intravenous hydration** (3–6 mL/kg/h) with monitoring of renal and hearing functions is the main approach to most acute toxic exposures.
2. **Hemodialysis** should be considered only in patients with renal failure.

For further reading in *Emergency Medicine: A Comprehensive Study Guide,* 6th ed., see Chap. 187, "Antimicrobials," by G. Richard Bruno and Wallace A. Carter.

116 | Cyanide

Mark E. Hoffmann

Cyanide is a chemical present in many industrial products and is a naturally occurring potent cellular toxin. Poisoning may occur from accidental or intentional exposures (cyanide gas; cyanide salts; nitriles; burning plastics, wool, silk, polyurethane, or vinyl), ingestion of plants or foods containing cyanogenic glycosides (apricot pits, cassava, or bitter almonds), or iatrogenic toxicity from the use of nitroprusside.

CLINICAL FEATURES

An occupational history, particularly in a suicidal patient, may provide a clue to the possibility of cyanide poisoning. Symptoms begin immediately after inhalation of cyanide gas. Ingestion of cyanide salts may cause toxicity within minutes. Ingestion of cyanogenic compounds (eg, acetonitrile in nail removal solvents, or amygdaline in apricot pits) may take hours to cause symptoms.

Patients with cyanide toxicity may complain of mucous membrane irritation, anxiety, headache, dyspnea, confusion, seizures, and coma. Early tachycardia, hypertension, and tachypnea are replaced by bradycardia, hypotension, apnea, and asystole. Mydriasis, cherry red retinal vessels, oral burns, the smell of bitter almonds, and dyspnea with high venous oxygen saturations are clues to the diagnosis. A metabolic acidosis with high lactate levels and a wide anion gap is commonly encountered. The hallmark of cyanide poisoning is apparent hypoxia without cyanosis.

DIAGNOSIS AND DIFFERENTIAL

The diagnosis of cyanide toxicity should be considered in patients with profound high anion-gap metabolic acidosis with a normal Pao_2. Laboratory tests that may be helpful include arterial blood gas analysis, chemistry panel, serum lactate level, and serum cyanide level, if available.

The differential diagnosis includes poisonings that accumulate lactate (iron, methemoglobin inducers, methanol, biguanides, or strychnine), other cellular toxins or asphyxiants (salicylates, carbon monoxide, hydrogen sulfide, azides, arsine, phosphine, nerve agents, or organophosphates), and seizure-inducing agents (cocaine and other stimulants, theophylline, camphor, or cicutoxin).

EMERGENCY DEPARTMENT CARE AND DISPOSITION

1. All patients with suspected cyanide toxicity should be placed on continuous cardiac monitoring with frequent blood pressure monitoring and **100% oxygen** and have adequate intravenous (IV) access. Those with altered mental status must be considered for IV glucose, thiamine, and naloxone administration. Airway management and resuscitation should always take priority over decontamination.
2. Decontamination should include copious irrigation of dermal exposures and gastric lavage followed by **activated charcoal** for acute ingestions.
3. Specific antidote therapy with **nitrite-thiosulfate** in the form of a kit from Taylor Pharmaceuticals should be considered in symptomatic patients (Table 116-1).

551

TABLE 116-1 Treatment of Cyanide Poisoning

Adults
1. 100% oxygen
2. Amyl nitrite; crack vial and inhale for 30 s*
3. Sodium nitrite (3% $NaNO_2$): 10 mL IV (10-mL ampule 3% solution = 300 mg)†
4. Sodium thiosulfate (25% $Na_2S_2O_3$): 50 mL IV (50-mL ampule 25% solution = 12.5 g)
5. May repeat at half dose if symptoms persist

Children
1. 100% oxygen
2. Administration of IV sodium nitrite and sodium thiosulfate

Hb (g/100 mL)	3% $NaNO_2$ (mL/kg)	25% $Na_2S_2O_3$ (mL/kg)
7	0.19	1.65
8	0.22	1.65
9	0.25	1.65
10	0.27	1.65
11	0.30	1.65
12	0.33	1.65
13	0.36	1.65
14	0.39	1.65

3. May repeat once at half dose if symptoms persist
4. Monitor methemoglobin to keep level <30%

*Not necessary if IV *line* is in place.

†Avoid nitrites in the presence of severe hypotension if diagnosis is unclear.

Key: Hb = hemoglobin, IV = intravenously.

4. Due to the potential side effects of hypotension and induction of methemoglobinemia, patients who are hypotensive and acidotic and without a clear history of cyanide toxicity or smoke inhalation should receive IV **sodium thiosulfate** only. **Hydroxocobalamin,** which has orphan drug status in the United States, will be an ideal agent in this setting.
5. All patients who receive antidotal therapy or patients who have ingested a substance that may result in delayed toxicity should be admitted to a monitored bed.

For further reading in *Emergency Medicine: A Comprehensive Study Guide,* 6th ed., see Chap. 188, "Cyanide," by Larissa Velez and Kathleen Delaney.

117 | Dyshemoglobinemias

Howard E. Jarvis III

The dyshemoglobinemias are a group of disorders in which the hemoglobin molecule is structurally altered and prevented from carrying oxygen. The most relevant of these are carboxyhemoglobinemia, methemoglobinemia, and sulfhemoglobinemia. Carboxyhemoglobinemia follows carbon monoxide exposure (see Chap. 128). Acquired methemoglobinemia and sulfhemoglobinemia are typically caused by exposures to various drugs and chemicals that cause an oxidant stress. Hereditary methemoglobinemia also occurs but is typically a chronic, stable disorder.

CLINICAL FEATURES

The clinical suspicion of methemoglobinemia should be raised when the pulse oximetry approaches 80% to 85% and there is no response to supplemental oxygen. The patient may display a brownish-blue skin. "Chocolate-brown" blood discoloration typically is noted on venipuncture. Exposure to known causes, such as nitrates (in well water and vegetables) and certain medications, also should raise concern. Medications that may precipitate this condition include phenazopyridine (Pyridium), benzocaine (a topical anesthetic), and dapsone (an antibiotic often used in therapy related to the human immunodeficiency virus). There may be significant time delays from exposure to symptoms with some agents.

Patients with normal hemoglobin concentrations do not develop clinically significant effects until methemoglobin levels rise above 20% of the total hemoglobin. They may seek evaluation for cyanosis that occurs when the methemoglobin level approaches 1.5 g/dL, which is approximately 10% of the total hemoglobin in normal individuals. Patients with anemia require a higher percentage because it is an absolute concentration (1.5 g/dL) that determines cyanosis. When levels reach 20% to 30%, symptoms may include anxiety, headache, weakness, and lightheadedness. Tachypnea and sinus tachycardia may occur. Methemoglobin concentrations of 50% to 60% impair oxygen delivery to vital tissues, causing myocardial ischemia, dysrhythmias, depressed mental status (including coma), seizures, and lactic acidosis. Levels above 70% are largely incompatible with life. Patients with anemia and those with preexisting diseases that impair oxygen delivery (eg, emphysema and congestive heart failure) may be symptomatic at lower concentrations of methemoglobin. Neonates and infants are more susceptible. Gastroenteritis may precipitate methemoglobinemia in infants.

Sulfhemoglobinemia is caused by many of the same agents that cause methemoglobinemia, although it is clinically less concerning. Cyanosis may occur at levels of 0.5 g/dL due to increased pigmentation.

DIAGNOSIS AND DIFFERENTIAL

The diagnosis of methemoglobinemia must be considered in any cyanotic patient, especially if the cyanosis is unresponsive to oxygen. The blood has a "chocolate-brown" color, and comparison of color with that of normal blood is useful. Pulse oximetry must be interpreted with caution because it cannot properly differentiate oxyhemoglobin from methemoglobin. Pulse oximetry

553

trends toward 80% to 85% in those with methemoglobinemia, and it will suggest a falsely high oxygen saturation in those with methemoglobin levels above 20%. The oxygen saturation obtained from an arterial blood gas analysis also will be falsely normal because it is calculated from dissolved oxygen tension, which is appropriately normal.

Definitive identification of methemoglobin relies on cooximetry, which is a widely available test and requires only venous blood (although arterial blood can be used). It can differentiate oxyhemoglobin, deoxyhemoglobin, carboxyhemoglobin, and methemoglobin species.

Sulfhemoglobin is differentiated from methemoglobin by the addition of cyanide to the laboratory cooximetry sample. Failure to eliminate the methemoglobin peak with the addition of cyanide confirms the diagnosis of sulfhemoglobinemia.

EMERGENCY DEPARTMENT CARE AND DISPOSITION

Patients with methemoglobinemia require optimal supportive measures to ensure oxygen delivery.

1. The effectiveness of gastric decontamination is limited because there is often a substantial time from exposure to development of methemoglobin. If an ongoing source of exposure exists, a single dose of oral **activated charcoal** 1 g/kg is indicated.
2. Antidotal therapy with **methylene blue** is reserved for those with documented methemoglobinemia or a high clinical suspicion of disease. Unstable patients should receive methylene blue but may require blood transfusion or exchange transfusion for immediate enhancement of oxygen delivery. The initial dose of methylene blue is 1 to 2 mg/kg intravenously, and its effect should be seen within 20 minutes. Repeat dosing of methylene blue is acceptable, but high doses (>7 mg/kg) actually may induce methemoglobin formation.
3. Treatment failures occur in some patients, including those with glucose-6-phosphate dehydrogenase deficiency and other enzyme deficiencies, and may occur in the presence of hemolysis. Hemolysis is seen with some inducers of methemoglobinemia, such as chlorates. Agents with long half-lives, such as dapsone, may require repetitive dosing of methylene blue.
4. Patients with the clinically indistinguishable sulfhemoglobinemia do not respond to methylene blue and should be treated supportively. They may require blood transfusions in cases of severe toxicity. Likewise, those with methemoglobinemia unresponsive to methylene blue should be treated supportively. If clinically unstable, the use of blood transfusions or exchange transfusions is indicated. If newly transfused red blood cell hemoglobin undergoes oxidation, it likely will respond to methylene blue therapy.

For further reading in *Emergency Medicine: A Comprehensive Study Guide*, 6th ed., see Chap. 189, "Dyshemoglobinemias," by Sean M. Rees and Lewis S. Nelson.

118 | Hypoglycemic Agents

Christian A. Tomaszewski

Patients commonly experience intentional and unintentional poisonings from hypoglycemic agents. In 2002, there were more than 6,000 symptomatic cases that resulted in several deaths.

CLINICAL FEATURES

The body's autonomic response to hypoglycemia, defined as a serum glucose level below 60 mg/dL, consists of diaphoresis, anxiety, nausea, tremors, and palpitations. Ultimately, the organ most dependent on a constant supply of glucose is the brain. Neurologic symptoms and signs of hypoglycemia include dizziness, confusion, headache, diplopia, dysarthria, lethargy, coma, and seizures. Patients also may present with focal neurologic deficits as profound as hemiparesis. Chronic ethanol abuse, extremes of age, and medications that blunt counter regulatory mechanisms (eg, β-adrenergic antagonists) may impair the ability of patients to avoid hypoglycemic spells.

The only parenteral hypoglycemic agent, and the most commonly involved with severe symptomatic hypoglycemia, is insulin. This is especially true in patients with tight glycemic control. The duration of action of insulin usually is based on the form taken; however, a large subcutaneous injection of regular insulin may behave like a long-acting formulation, thus resulting in delayed or prolonged hypoglycemia.

The most common oral agents for diabetes are the sulfonylureas; as a result, they are implicated most often in hypoglycemia cases. These agents cause the release of insulin from the pancreas, reduce hepatic glucose production, and increase peripheral insulin sensitivity. Second-generation sulfonylureas have supplanted the first-generation agents primarily because they are not solely dependent on renal elimination. Nonetheless, they have a long duration of action, particularly after overdose, which can lead to delayed hypoglycemia as late as 16 hours after ingestion.

More popular agents for the initial control of diabetes are the biguanides, represented by metformin. It suppresses glucose output by the liver and stimulates its uptake by muscle. Although metformin does not specifically cause hypoglycemia, it can increase this risk in patients on concomitant sulfonylureas or insulin. The more serious adverse effect of metformin is lactic acidosis, which is due in part to inhibition of gluconeogenesis. It can occur after overdose but more commonly is associated with renal insufficiency or the administration of intravascular iodinated contrast media.

Thiazolidinediones are becoming as popular as sulfonylureas because of their ability to ameliorate hyperglycemia without increasing insulin secretion. In addition to increasing insulin sensitivity, these agents decrease hepatic glucose output and increase muscle glucose uptake. Hepatically metabolized, there have been rare cases of liver failure associated with these agents.

The benzoic acid derivative, repaglinide, increases insulin secretion. Like sulfonylureas, the risk of developing hypoglycemia exists, even though overdose experience is lacking.

Another group of diabetic agents that has not been associated with hypoglycemia is the α-glucosidase inhibitor agent. Acarbose, miglitol, and voglibose decrease gastrointestinal absorption of carbohydrates. Adverse effects include flatulence, bloating, and malabsorption; rare cases of hepatic toxicity have occurred with acarbose.

DIAGNOSIS AND DIFFERENTIAL

Hypoglycemia should be considered in all patients with altered mental status. In addition, all patients with stroke-like symptoms, seizures, or hypothermia should be screened. Rapid glucose determination can be done with a reagent strip or glucometer at the bedside, with confirmation by formal laboratory testing if hypoglycemia is still suspected. Patients who have been involved in a single-vehicle crash also may warrant screening for hypoglycemia.

There are many pharmaceutical agents and medical conditions that can precipitate hypoglycemia. Angiotensin-converting enzyme inhibitors, chloramphenicol, disopyramide, pentamidine, salicylates, quinidine, and streptozocin have been implicated in patients experiencing hypoglycemic episodes. Ethanol, especially in the presence of malnutrition, can induce hypoglycemia. The unripe, fresh ackee fruit from Jamaica can cause hypoglycemia, which is usually associated with severe vomiting. Medical causes of hypoglycemia include insulinoma, endocrine insufficiency, hepatic disease, sepsis, and autoimmune disease.

EMERGENCY DEPARTMENT CARE AND DISPOSITION

1. Once hypoglycemia is suspected or determined, a 50-mL intravenous (IV) bolus of **50% dextrose solution** should be given. Children may receive 25% dextrose at 2 mL/kg, and neonates can tolerate 10% dextrose at 2 mL/kg.
2. A repeat glucose determination should be performed every 30 to 60 minutes after the initial dextrose administration. If hypoglycemia recurs or is expected to recur, then the patient can receive another bolus of 50% dextrose solution 50 mL IV or start a continuous infusion of 10% dextrose in water at 1 to 2 mL/kg/h.
3. If IV access cannot be established, **glucagon** 1 to 2 mg intramuscularly or subcutaneously (0.1 mg/kg in children, up to 2 mg) can be administered. Glucagon will not work well in patients with depleted glycogen stores or after sulfonylurea toxicity.
4. **Diazoxide** 300 mg IV has been used successfully in sulfonylurea overdose. Because it can cause hypotension and does not work well in insulin overdoses, its use is limited.
5. In cases of sulfonylurea overdose with extreme glucose requirements, **octreotide** 50 μg subcutaneously every 6 hours can be used.
6. Gastric decontamination with **activated charcoal** 1 g/kg orally may be indicated early after oral overdoses of hypoglycemic agents. In addition, whole bowel irrigation with polyethylene glycol–based electrolyte solutions may benefit massive overdoses of sustained-release preparations.
7. **Urine alkalinization** will increase the clearance of chlorpropamide.
8. **Thiamine** 100 mg IV may be warranted when administering glucose to patients who are hypoglycemic secondary to ethanol abuse or malnutrition.
9. Metformin overdoses should be monitored for lactic acidosis. Aggressive treatment of acidosis should be instituted with **sodium bicarbonate** therapy; **hemodialysis** should be reserved for refractory cases.

10. Disposition of certain patients may be problematic. Patients with unintentional hypoglycemia from a short- or intermediate-acting insulin can be discharged after several hours of observation, particularly if they have eaten, have not had a recurrence of hypoglycemia, and have a reliable individual who lives with them. Because of the long duration of action of sulfonylureas, patients with symptomatic overdoses of sulfonylureas should be admitted for regular glucose monitoring. Such patients include those with an episode of hypoglycemia from a therapeutic dose of the sulfonylurea agent. Asymptomatic patients should be observed for at least 12 to 16 hours after an overdose, depending on the particular sulfonylurea taken, because of the danger of delayed hypoglycemia.

For further reading in *Emergency Medicine: A Comprehensive Study Guide,* 6th ed., see Chap. 190, "Hypoglycemic Agents," by Joseph G. Rella and Lewis S. Nelson.

13 | ENVIRONMENTAL INJURIES

119 | Frostbite and Hypothermia

Mark E. Hoffmann

Hypothermia results from heat loss by conduction, convection, radiation, or evaporation. Local cold injuries and frostbite occur when hypothermia causes increased blood viscosity and intracellular injury.

CLINICAL FEATURES

Frostnip is a less severe form of frostbite that resolves with rewarming and involves no tissue loss. Trench foot results from cooling of tissue in a wet environment at above-freezing temperatures over several hours to days. Long-term hyperhidrosis and cold insensitivity are common. Chilblains (pernio) presents with painful and inflamed skin lesions caused by chronic, intermittent exposure to damp, nonfreezing ambient temperatures. Once affected by chilblains, frostnip, or frostbite, the involved body part becomes more susceptible to reinjury.

First- and second-degree frostbites are superficial injuries that present with edema, burning, erythema, and blistering (second-degree). Third-degree frostbite is a deeper injury involving the full-thickness skin and the subdermal tissue. Fourth-degree injury includes subcutaneous tissue, muscle, tendon, and bone. Patients present with cyanotic and insensate tissue that may have hemorrhagic blisters and skin necrosis. Subsequently, this tissue appears mummified (Table 119-1).

Mild hypothermia, 32°C (89.6°F) to 35°C (95°F), presents with shivering, tachycardia, and elevated blood pressure. Shivering ceases as heart rate and blood pressure fall when core temperatures drop below 32°C (89.6°F). Mentation slows and there is a loss of cough and gag reflexes. Aspiration is a common complication. Impaired renal concentrating ability leads to a "cold diuresis" with resulting dehydration.

With progressively lower core temperatures, patients become lethargic and comatose. Prolonged immobility increases the risk of rhabdomyolysis and acute renal failure. Hemoconcentration and volume depletion may lead to intravascular thrombosis and disseminated intravascular coagulation. Hyperglycemia is common; however, up to 40% of patients are hypoglycemic. Acid-base disturbances are usually present but do not follow a uniform pattern.

The electrocardiogram may show PR-, QRS-, and QT-interval prolongations and Osborn J waves. The cardiac rhythm progresses from tachycardia to bradycardia to atrial fibrillation, with a slow ventricular rate to ventricular fibrillation, to asystole as the core temperature falls.

DIAGNOSIS AND DIFFERENTIAL

Hypothermia is diagnosed when the core body temperature is below 35°C (95°F).

Underlying disease states that may result in hypothermia, such as thyroid deficiency, adrenal insufficiency, central nervous system dysfunction, infection, sepsis, dermal disease, drug intoxication, and metabolic derangement, need to be considered and evaluated. Localized cold-related injuries are diagnosed by history and physical examination.

TABLE 119-1 Classification of Cold Injury According to Severity

Classification	Symptoms
Superficial	
First-degree: partial skin freezing	Transient stinging and burning
Erythema, edema, hyperemia	Throbbing and aching possible
No blisters or necrosis	May have hyperhidrosis
Occasional skin desquamation (5–10 d later)	
Second-degree: full-thickness injury	Numbness
Erythema, substantial edema, vesicles with clear fluid	Vasomotor disturbances in severe cases
Blisters that desquamate and form blackened eschar	
Deep	
Third-degree: full-thickness skin and subcutaneous freezing	Initially, no sensation
Violaceous or hemorrhagic blisters	Tissue feels like "block of wood"
Blue-gray discoloration	Later, shooting pains, burning, throbbing, aching
Fourth-degree: full-thickness skin subcutaneous tissue, muscle, tendon, and bone freezing	Possible joint discomfort
Little edema	
Initially mottled, deep red, or cyanotic	
Eventually dry, black, mummified	

Source: Britt LD, Dascombe W, Rodriquez A. New horizons in management of hypothermia and frostbite injury. *Surg Clin North Am.* 1991;71:359.

EMERGENCY DEPARTMENT CARE AND DISPOSITION

1. Chilblains and trench foot should be managed with elevation, warming, and bandaging of the affected tissues. **Nifedipine** 20 mg orally 3 times daily, **topical corticosteroids, prednisone,** and prostaglandin E_1 (**Limaprost** 20 μg orally 3 times daily) may be helpful.
2. Rapid rewarming with **circulating water at 42°C (107°F)** for 10 to 30 minutes results in thawing of frostbitten extremities. Dry air rewarming may cause further tissue injury and should be avoided. Patients should receive narcotics, ibuprofen, and aloe vera. **Penicillin G** 500,000 U every 6 hours for 48 to 72 hours has been shown to be beneficial.
3. Clear blisters rich in prostaglandins and thromboxane should be débrided or aspirated. Hemorrhagic blisters should be left intact.
4. **Rewarming techniques** include passive rewarming, active external rewarming, and active core rewarming (Table 119-2).
5. Patients with mild hypothermia may be warmed passively by removal from the cold environment and with the use of insulating blankets.
6. Patients with more severe hypothermia should be placed on pulse oximetry, cardiac monitor, and continued core temperature monitoring (rectal or esophageal probe).
7. Attention should be placed on the ABCs and initial resuscitation. If the is no cardiovascular instability, active external warming may be applied (radiant heat, warmed blankets, warm water immersion, and heated objects)

TABLE 119-2 Frostbite Treatment Summary

Thaw
  Thaw in warm water bath (40°C to 42°C) for 10–30 min until extremity is
  pliable and erythematous
  Parenteral opioid analgesics (eg, morphine 0.1 mg/kg intravenously)
Postthaw
  Débride clear blisters
  Leave hemorrhagic blisters intact
  Dress injured area and blisters with aloe vera cream
  Tetanus immunization prophylaxis
  Ibuprofen 12 mg/kg/d in divided doses
  Consider limaprost 20 μg orally 3 times daily
  Begin daily hydrotherapy

in conjunction with warmed intravenous (IV) fluids and warmed humidified oxygen.

8. If cardiovascular instability is present, more aggressive active core rewarming is required **(gastric, bladder, peritoneal, and pleural lavage).**
These lavage fluids should be heated to 42°C (107°F).

9. Patients with suspected thiamine depletion and alcoholism should receive
thiamine 100 mg IV or intramuscularly and **50% glucose** 50 to 100 mL
IV if rapid glucose testing is not available or is low.

10. Patients with suspected hypothyroidism or adrenal insufficiency may require IV **thyroxine** and **hydrocortisone** (100 mg).

11. Ventricular fibrillation is usually refractory to defibrillation until a temperature of 30°C (86°F) is obtained, although 3 countershocks should be
attempted.

12. Rewarming through an **extracorporeal circuit** is the method of choice in
the severely hypothermic patient in cardiac arrest. If this equipment is not
available, resuscitative thoracotomy with internal cardiac message and
mediastinal lavage is an acceptable alternative.

13. All patients with more than isolated superficial frostbite or mild hypothermia should be admitted to the hospital. Patients should not be discharged unless they can return to a warm environment.

For further reading in *Emergency Medicine: A Comprehensive Study Guide,* 6th ed., see
Chap. 191, "Frostbite and Other Localized Cold-Related Injuries," by Mark B.
Rabold; and Chap. 192, "Hypothermia," by Howard A. Bessen.

120 | Heat Emergencies

T. Paul Tran

Heat-related illnesses comprise a spectrum of disorders, ranging from minor heat disorders such as prickly heat, heat cramps, and heat exhaustion to the life-threatening condition known as *heat stroke*. Mostly preventable, these illnesses tend to occur in patients whose cooling and adaptive mechanisms are impaired in an environment of elevated heat stress. Heat stroke occurs in classic (nonexertional) form when it results from exposure to a hot environment and exertional form when it results from physical activity.

HEAT STROKE

Clinical Features

Patients with heat stroke have an alteration in mental status and an elevated body temperature. A history of environmental or occupational heat exposure usually can be discerned. Core temperature ranges from 40°C to 47°C. Neurologic abnormalities include ataxia, confusion, bizarre behavior, agitation, seizures, obtundation, and coma. Anhidrosis is not invariably present.

Risk factors for heat related injuries include extremes of age (<4 years and >75 years), predisposing conditions (heart failure, psychiatric illnesses, alcohol abuse, dehydration, poverty, or social isolation), certain medications (anticholinergics, β-blocker, or calcium channel blocker), and persons who lack access to air conditioning, have poor physical conditioning, and are poorly acclimatized to hot weather.

Diagnosis and Differential

Heat stroke is a true time-dependent medical emergency and should be considered in the clinical context of environmental heat stress, hyperthermia, and altered mental status. Patients are tachycardic, hyperventilating, and have respiratory alkalosis. About 20% of heat stroke patients are hypotensive. In contrast to classic heat stroke, patients with exertional heat stroke may have respiratory alkalosis and lactic acidosis. Exertional heat stroke patients may present with rhabdomyolysis, hyperkalemia, hyperphosphatemia, and hypocalcemia.

Initial diagnostic studies should include a complete blood count, electrolyte panel, creatinine kinase, hepatic panel, serum alcohol level, toxicology screen, coagulation studies, urinalysis, urine myoglobin, urine pregnancy, arterial blood gas, chest radiograph, and electrocardiogram. Neuroimaging studies and other evaluations (eg, septic workup) can be individualized as clinically indicated. The differential diagnosis includes infection (sepsis, meningitis, encephalitis, malaria, or typhoid fever), toxins (serotonin syndrome, anticholinergics, phenothiazine, salicylate, phencyclidine (PCP), sympathomimetics abuse, or alcohol withdrawal), metabolic and endocrinologic emergencies (thyrotoxicosis or diabetic ketoacidosis), central nervous system disorders (status epilepticus or stroke syndrome), neuroleptic malignant syndrome, and malignant hyperthermia.

Emergency Department Care and Disposition

1. Emergent priorities remain airway, breathing, and circulation. Cardiac monitoring and an intravenous (IV) line should be established. High-flow

supplemental oxygen should be administered. Patients with significant altered mental status, diminished gag reflex, or hypoxia should undergo **endotracheal intubation.**

2. Core temperature should be obtained immediately with a rectal (or bladder) probe and continuously monitored.

3. Volume-depleted patients should be rehydrated with IV normal saline or lactated Ringer solution to maintain mean arterial pressure above 60 mm Hg. Care should be used to avoid volume overloading the patient. A central venous catheter line or pulmonary artery catheter may be required to guide fluid therapy. Inotropic support and pressors may be required.

4. **Evaporative cooling** is the most efficient and practical means of cooling hyperthermic patients in the emergency department. Fans are positioned near the completely disrobed patient who is then sprayed with tepid water. Spraying with ice water should be avoided because this may cause shivering, which induces thermogenesis. Excessive shivering can be treated with benzodiazepines (midazolam 2 mg IV). The goal is to bring the core temperature below 40°C.

5. Other methods of cooling such as immersion cooling, cold water gastric and urinary bladder lavage, thoracostomy lavage, and cardiopulmonary bypass may be considered as clinically indicated and logistically feasible.

6. Seizures can be treated with **benzodiazepines.** Rhabdomyolysis can be treated with IV hydration, diuretics (furosemide 40 mg IV), sodium bicarbonate (3 ampules in 1 L 5% dextrose in water at 250 mL/h). Hyperkalemia should be treated with standard regimens. The patient's electrolytes should be monitored every hour initially.

7. Heat stroke patients need to be admitted to an intensive care unit for further observation and monitoring.

OTHER MINOR HEAT ILLNESSES

Heat exhaustion is a clinical syndrome that results from heat exposure. It is characterized by nonspecific signs and symptoms, including malaise, fatigue, weakness, dizziness, syncope, headache, nausea, vomiting, myalgias, diaphoresis, tachypnea, tachycardia, and orthostatic hypotension. Core body temperature is frequently elevated but may be normal. Although a patient may complain of neurologic symptoms, the patient's sensorium and neurologic examination should be normal. Laboratory examination usually demonstrates hemoconcentration. A creatinine kinase level should be checked to exclude rhabdomyolysis. Treatment consists of rest, evaporative cooling, and administration of IV normal saline or oral electrolyte solution, depending on clinical situation. Because heat exhaustion has the potential to evolve into heat stroke, patients should be treated aggressively and observed until symptoms resolve. Most patients can be discharged home. Those patients with significant comorbid conditions (heart failure or poor social support) or severe electrolyte abnormality may require hospitalization.

Heat syncope results from volume depletion, peripheral vasodilation, and decreased vasomotor tone. It occurs most commonly in the elderly and poorly acclimatized individuals. Postural vital signs may or may not be demonstrable on presentation to the emergency department. Patients should be evaluated for any trauma resulting from a fall. Potentially serious causes of syncope (eg, cardiovascular, neurologic, infectious, endocrine, and electrolyte abnormalities) should be investigated, especially in the elderly. Treatment for heat syncope consists of rest and oral or IV rehydration.

Heat cramps are characterized by painful muscle spasms, especially in the calves, thighs, and shoulders. Common during athletic events, they are thought to result from dilutional hyponatremia as individuals replace evaporative losses with free water but not with salt. Core body temperature may be normal or elevated. Treatment consists of rest and administration of oral electrolyte solution or IV normal saline. Patients should be instructed to replace future fluid losses with a balanced electrolyte solution.

Heat tetany is due to the effects of respiratory alkalosis that results when an individual hyperventilates in response to an intense heat stress. Patients may complain of paresthesia of the extremities, circumoral paresthesia, and carpopedal spasm. Muscle cramps are minimal or nonexistent. Treatment consists of removal from the heat stress and self-rebreathing through a paper bag.

Heat edema is a self-limited, mild swelling of dependent extremities (hands and feet) that occurs in the first few days of exposure to a new hot environment. It is due to cutaneous vasodilation and pooling of interstitial fluid in dependent extremities. Treatment consists of elevation of the extremities and, in severe cases, application of compressive stockings. Administration of diuretics may exacerbate volume depletion and should be avoided.

Heat rash (prickly heat) is a maculopapular eruption that is found most commonly over clothed areas of the body. It results from inflammation and obstruction of sweat ducts. Early stages present with a pruritic, erythematous rash best treated with antihistamines and chlorhexidine cream or lotion. Continued blockage of pores results in a nonpruritic, nonerythematous, whitish papular rash known as the *profunda stage* of prickly heat. This is best treated with anti-staphylococcal antibiotics and application of 1% salicylic acid to affected areas 3 times daily.

For further reading in *Emergency Medicine: A Comprehensive Study Guide,* 6th ed., see Chap. 193, "Heat Emergencies," by James S. Walker and David E. Hogan.

121 | Bites and Stings

Burton Bentley II

HYMENOPTERA (WASPS, BEES, AND STINGING ANTS)

Wasps, bees, and stinging ants are members of the order Hymenoptera. Local and generalized reactions may occur in response to an encounter.

Clinical Features

Local reactions consist of edema at the sting site. Although it may involve neighboring joints, local reactions cause no systemic symptoms. Severe local reactions increase the likelihood of serious systemic reactions if the patient is exposed again at a later time. *Toxic reactions* are a nonantigenic response to multiple stings. They have many of the same features that are seen in true systemic (allergic) reactions, but there is a greater frequency of gastrointestinal disturbance, whereas bronchospasm and urticaria do not occur. *Systemic* or *anaphylactic reactions* are true allergic reactions that range from mild to fatal. In general, the shorter the interval between the sting and the onset of symptoms, the more severe the reaction. Initial symptoms usually consist of itchy eyes, urticaria, and cough. As the reaction progresses, patients may experience respiratory failure and cardiovascular collapse. *Delayed reactions* may appear 10 to 14 days after a sting. Symptoms of delayed reactions resemble serum sickness and include fever, malaise, headache, urticaria, lymphadenopathy, and polyarthritis.

Emergency Department Care and Disposition

1. The treatment for all Hymenoptera encounters is the same. First, **any bee stinger remaining in the patient should be removed immediately,** and the wound should be cleaned. Ice packs and elevation may reduce the degree of swelling.
2. Erythema and swelling seen in local reactions may be difficult to distinguish from cellulitis. As a general rule, infection is present in a minority of cases. For minor local reactions, oral antihistamines and analgesics may be the only treatment needed.
3. More severe reactions, such as chest constriction, nausea, presyncope, or a change in mental status, require treatment with **1:1,000 epinephrine subcutaneously,** 0.3 to 0.5 mL for an adult and 0.01 mL/kg for a child (0.3 mL maximum). Some patients may require a second epinephrine injection in 10 to 15 minutes.
4. Parenteral **H_1- and H_2-receptor antagonists** (eg, diphenhydramine and ranitidine) and **steroids** (eg, methylprednisolone) should be rapidly administered. Bronchospasm responds to courses of **inhaled β-agonists** (eg, albuterol). Hypotension should be treated aggressively with crystalloid, although **dopamine** and **epinephrine** infusions may be required.
5. Patients with minor symptoms who respond well to conservative measures may be discharged after monitoring for several hours. Severe reactions require admission to the hospital. All patients with Hymenoptera reactions should be referred to an allergist for further evaluation and prescribed a pre-measured epinephrine injector (EpiPen).

ANTS (FORMICOIDEA)

There are several species of fire ants *(Solenopsis)* in the United States, and their venom may crossreact in individuals sensitized to other Hymenoptera stings. Fire ants swarm during an attack, and each sting results in a papule that evolves to a sterile pustule over 6 to 24 hours. Local necrosis and scarring in addition to systemic reactions can occur. Treatment is the same as for other Hymenoptera stings, and appropriate referral should be made for desensitization therapy.

ARACHNIDA (SPIDERS, SCABIES, CHIGGERS, AND SCORPIONS)

BROWN RECLUSE SPIDER *(LOXOSCELES RECLUSA)*

Clinical Features

The *L reclusa* bite causes a mild, erythematous lesion that may become firm and heal over several days to weeks. Occasionally, a severe reaction with immediate pain, blister formation, and bluish discoloration may occur. These lesions often become necrotic over the next 3 to 4 days and form an eschar 1 to 30 cm in diameter. *Loxoscelism* is a systemic reaction that may occur 1 to 2 days after envenomation. Signs and symptoms may include fever, chills, vomiting, arthralgias, myalgias, petechiae, and hemolysis; severe cases progress to seizure, renal failure, disseminated intravascular coagulation, and death. The diagnosis of *L reclusa* envenomation may need to be made on clinical grounds because the bite often is not witnessed. There is no laboratory test that specifically confirms *L reclusa* poisoning, but all patients with suspected envenomation should have the following tests performed: complete blood count, blood urea nitrogen, creatinine, electrolytes, coagulation profile, and urinalysis for hemoglobinuria.

Emergency Department Care and Disposition

1. Treatment of the brown recluse spider bite includes the usual supportive measures. Currently, there is no commercially available antivenom. Tetanus prophylaxis, analgesics, and antibiotics may be offered when appropriate.
2. Surgery is reserved for lesions larger than 2 cm and is deferred for 2 to 3 weeks after the bite.
3. The roles of **dapsone** (50–200 mg/d) and **hyperbaric oxygen** recently have been challenged but may prevent some ongoing local necrosis. Patients with systemic reactions and hemolysis must be hospitalized for consideration of blood transfusion and hemodialysis.

HOBO SPIDER *(TEGENARIA AGRESTIS)*

Clinical Features

The hobo spider, also known as the Northwestern brown spider, causes clinical signs and symptoms that are quite similar to those of the brown recluse spider bite. The skin site is initially painless before developing induration, erythema, blistering, and necrosis. Victims also may experience headache, vomiting, and fatigue.

Emergency Department Care and Disposition

There is no specific diagnostic test or therapeutic intervention for hobo spider bites. Surgical repair may be required, although it must be delayed until the necrotizing process is complete.

BLACK WIDOW SPIDER *(LATRODECTUS MACTANS)*

Clinical Features

Black widow spider bites induce an immediate pinprick sensation that often allows the victim to identify the offending spider. Within 1 hour, the patient may experience erythematous skin lesions (often "target" shaped), swelling, and diffuse muscle cramps. Large muscle groups are involved, resulting in painful cramping of the abdominal wall musculature that may mimic peritonitis. Severe pain may wax and wane for several days. Serious acute complications include hypertension, respiratory failure, shock, and coma.

Emergency Department Care and Disposition

1. Initial therapy includes local wound treatment and supportive care. **Analgesics** and **benzodiazepines** will relieve pain and cramping.
2. For severe envenomation, hospitalization is required for parenteral pain medication and antivenin therapy. The **antivenin,** derived from horse serum, is rapidly effective for severe envenomation. If the patient tolerates placement of a standard cutaneous test dose, the usual intravenous (IV) dose is 1 to 2 diluted vials delivered over 30 minutes. Anaphylaxis has rarely been reported with this therapy.
3. Patients receiving antivenin may be discharged from the emergency department if the treatment is successful in reversing the symptoms of envenomation.

TARANTULAS

Clinical Features

When threatened, tarantulas may flick some of their barbed hairs into their victim. Although North American tarantula hairs rarely penetrate human skin, they can embed deeply into the conjunctiva and cornea. This may result in a local or generalized ocular inflammatory response. Tarantulas also may render a painful bite resulting in erythema, swelling, and local joint stiffness.

Emergency Department Care and Disposition

Any patient complaining of ocular symptoms after exposure to a tarantula should undergo a thorough slit lamp examination. Treatment includes **topical steroids** and consultation with an ophthalmologist for surgical removal of the hairs. The bite of a tarantula requires only local wound care and appropriate analgesia.

SCORPION (SCORPIONIDA)

Clinical Features

Of all North American scorpions, only the bark scorpion *(Centruroides exilicauda)* of the western United States is capable of producing systemic toxicity. Venom from *C exilicauda* causes immediate burning and stinging, although no local injury is visible. Systemic effects are infrequent and occur mainly at the extremes of patient age. Findings may include tachycardia, excessive secretions, roving eye movements, opisthotonos, and fasciculations. The diagnosis may be elusive if the scorpion is not seen, although roving eye movements are pathognomonic. A positive "tap test" (ie, exquisite local tenderness when the area is lightly tapped) is also suggestive.

Emergency Department Care and Disposition

1. Treatment is supportive, including local wound care. Reassurance is also important because many patients harbor misconceptions about the lethality of scorpion stings. Patients with pain in the absence of other toxic symptoms may be observed briefly before they are discharged with analgesics.
2. The application of ice often provides immediate relief of local pain. Muscle spasm and fasciculations respond promptly to **benzodiazepines.**
3. Severe toxicity may warrant **scorpion antivenin,** a product in dwindling supply that is currently available only in Arizona. One to two vials of this goat-derived product affords immediate symptomatic resolution.

SCABIES *(SARCOPTES SCABIEI)*

Clinical Features

Scabies bites are concentrated in the web spaces between fingers and toes. Other common areas include the penis, children's faces and scalps, and the female nipple. Transmission is typically by direct contact. The distinctive feature of scabies infestation is intense pruritus with "burrows." These white, threadlike channels form zigzag patterns with small gray spots at the closed end where the parasite rests. Undisturbed burrows can be traced with a hand lens, and the female mite is easily scraped out with a blade edge. Associated vesicles, papules, crusts, and eczematization may obscure the diagnosis.

Emergency Department Care and Disposition

Adult treatment of scabies infestation consists of a thorough application of **permethrin** (Elimite) from the neck down; infants may require additional application to the scalp, temple, and forehead. The patient should first bathe in warm soapy water, apply the medication, and then bathe again in 12 hours. Reapplication is necessary only if mites are found 2 weeks after treatment, although the pruritus may last for several weeks after successful therapy.

CHIGGERS (TROMBICULIDAE)

Clinical Features

Chiggers are tiny mite larvae that cause intense pruritus when they feed on host epidermal cells. Itchiness begins within a few hours, followed by a papule that enlarges to a nodule over the next 1 to 2 days. Single bites also can cause soft tissue edema, whereas infestation has been associated with fever and erythema multiforme. Children who have been sitting on lawns are prone to chigger lesions in the genital area. The diagnosis of chigger bites is based on typical skin lesions in the context of known outdoor exposure.

Emergency Department Care and Disposition

Treatment consists of symptomatic relief with oral or topical antihistamines, although oral steroids may be required in more severe cases. Annihilation of the mites requires topical application of **lindane** (Kwell), **permethrin** (Elimite), or **crotamiton** (Eurax). The package insert provides techniques for proper use.

FLEAS (SIPHONAPTERA)

Flea bites are frequently found in zigzag lines, especially on the legs and waist. They are intensely pruritic lesions with hemorrhagic puncta, surrounding erythema, and urticaria. Discomfort is relieved with **starch baths** (1 kg starch in a tub of water), **calamine lotion,** and oral **antihistamines.** Severe irritation may require topical steroid creams. Patients may develop impetigo and other local infections from scratching. Fingernails should be cut short, and infections should be treated in the standard manner.

LICE (ANOPLURA)

Body lice concentrate on the waist, shoulders, axillae, and neck. Their bites produce red spots that progress to papules and wheals. They are so intensely pruritic that linear scratch marks are suggestive of infestation. The white ova of *head lice* are adherent to the hair shaft and therefore can be distinguished from dandruff. *Pubic lice* are spread by sexual contact. They cause intense pruritus, and their small white eggs (nits) are visible on hair shafts. Reactions to lice saliva and feces may cause fever, malaise, and lymphadenopathy. As with scabies, **permethrin** is the primary treatment for body lice infestation. Treatment of any hair-borne infestation requires a thorough application of **pyrethrin with piperonyl butoxide** (RID Lice Killing Shampoo) with mandatory reapplication in 10 days. A fine-tooth comb will aid in removal of dead lice and nits. Clothing, bedding, and personal articles must be sterilized in hot (>52°C) water to prevent reinfestation.

KISSING BUG, PUSS CATERPILLAR, AND BLISTER BEETLE

Kissing Bugs and Bed Bugs (Hemiptera)

Kissing bugs (also known as conenose beetles) and bed bugs feed on blood as they attack the exposed surface of a sleeping victim. The initial bite is painless, and the victim may be unaware of the attack. Proper identification is difficult if the insect is not recovered. Bites are often multiple and result in wheals or hemorrhagic papules and bullae. Anaphylaxis commonly occurs in the sensitized individual. Treatment consists of local wound care and analgesics. Allergic reactions must be treated as previously outlined for Hymenoptera envenomation. Hypersensitive individuals should be referred to an allergist for possible immunotherapy.

Puss Caterpillar *(Megalopyge opercularis)*

The puss caterpillar has stinging spines on its body that provoke immediate, intense, and rhythmic pain. Local edema is often followed by pruritic vesicles and hemorrhagic papules. Infrequently, fever, muscle cramps, anxiety, and shocklike symptoms may occur. Lymphadenopathy with local desquamation may develop in a few days. Treatment consists of **immediate spine removal with cellophane tape.** Antihistamines and steroids may help to reduce pruritus. Intravenous **calcium gluconate,** 10 mL of a 10% solution, may be effective in relieving severe pain. Intravenous fluids and subcutaneous epinephrine will be required for the rare case of hypotension.

Blister Beetle (Coleoptera)

Blister beetles produce local irritation and blistering within hours of contact, although they provoke intense gastrointestinal disturbances if ingested. Treatment consists of an occlusive dressing to protect the bullae from trauma. Large bullae should be drained and covered with a topical antibiotic ointment. Application of steroid creams also may speed recovery.

CROTALINAE (PIT VIPER) BITES

There are approximately 8,000 venomous snakebites each year in the United States, but only about 10 deaths result. In fact, 25% of bites are "dry strikes," with no effect from the venom. Except for imported species and coral snakes, the only venomous North American snakes are the crotaline snakes (eg, rattlesnakes, copperhead, water moccasin, and massasauga). Crotaline snakes, commonly known as pit vipers, are identified by their 2 retractable fangs and by the heat-sensitive depressions ("pits") located bilaterally between each eye and nostril.

Clinical Features

The effects of crotaline envenomation depend on the size and species of snake, the age and size of the victim, the time elapsed since the bite, and the characteristics of the bite itself. The hallmark of pit viper envenomation is fang marks with local pain and swelling, but there are 3 classes of criteria that determine the severity of a rattlesnake bite: (*a*) degree of local injury (swelling, pain, and ecchymosis), (*b*) degree of systemic involvement (hypotension, tachycardia, and paresthesia), and (*c*) evolving coagulopathy (thrombocytopenia, elevated prothrombin time, and hypofibrinogenemia). Abnormalities in any of these 3 areas indicate that envenomation has occurred. Conversely, the absence of any clinical findings after 8 to 12 hours effectively rules out venom injection. Because the degree of poisoning after an encounter is variable, it is crucial to remember that initially benign-appearing bites may still evolve with devastating complications.

Diagnosis and Differential

The diagnosis of crotaline envenomation is based on the clinical findings and corroborating laboratory data. In general, all envenomated patients will have swelling within 30 minutes, although some may take up to 12 hours. The degree of envenomation is graded on a progressive continuum. *Minimal* envenomation describes cases with local swelling, no systemic signs, and no laboratory abnormalities. *Moderate* envenomation causes increased swelling that spreads from the site. These patients also may have systemic signs such as nausea, paresthesia, hypotension, and tachycardia. Coagulation parameters may be abnormal, but there is no significant bleeding. *Severe* envenomation causes extensive swelling, potentially life-threatening systemic signs (eg, hypotension, altered mental status, and respiratory distress), and markedly abnormal coagulation parameters that may result in hemorrhage. Laboratory studies that should be obtained include complete blood count, coagulation tests, urinalysis, and blood typing.

Emergency Department Care and Disposition

1. All patients bitten by a pit viper must be evaluated at a medical facility; first aid measures must not delay definitive care. Consultation with a specialist familiar with snakebite is recommended for all but the simplest cases; one resource is the Arizona Poison Control Center (520-626-6016). The patient should minimize physical activity, remain calm, and immobilize any bitten extremity in a neutral position below the level of the heart.

2. Cardiac monitoring and IV access should be established. The patient should be aggressively resuscitated according to ACLS protocols.

3. Local wound care and tetanus immunization should be given, but prophylactic antibiotics and steroids have no proven benefit. Limb circumference at several sites above and below the wound should be checked every 30 minutes, and the border of advancing edema should be marked.

4. Any patient with progressive local swelling, systemic effects, or coagulopathy should immediately receive antivenin therapy. **Polyvalent Crotalidae Immune Fab** (CroFab), a new sheep-derived antivenin, has generally replaced Antivenin (Crotalidae) Polyvalent, an equine-derived product. Polyvalent Crotalidae Immune Fab is administered as an initial dose of 4 to 6 vials IV; there is no need for a prior intradermal skin test. The initial dose of Polyvalent Crotalidae Immune Fab is diluted in 250 mL normal saline and infused IV over 60 minutes. Because allergic reactions may occur, the infusion should proceed at a slow rate of 25 to 50 mL/h for the first 10 minutes. If the patient remains stable, the infusion rate may be increased to the full 250-mL/h rate. Because the goal of therapy is to neutralize the existing venom, dosing regimens are exactly the same for children and adults (although the amount of diluent will need proper adjustment).

5. One hour after the initial dose has been administered, the patient must be reexamined to determine whether local swelling has been arrested, coagulation tests have normalized, and systemic symptoms have abated. If the initial dose was ineffective in any of these 3 areas, then a repeat dose of 4 to 6 vials should be administered.

6. Laboratory determinations are repeated every 4 hours or after each course of antivenin, whichever is more frequent.

7. Because the endpoint of antivenin therapy is the arrest of progressive symptoms and coagulopathy, the administration of antivenin must continue until complete control of the envenomation is achieved. Once initial control has been achieved, the protocol is completed by administering additional 2-vial doses every 6 hours for an additional 18 hours (ie, 3 more doses). The antivenin package insert will guide in administration, and the physician must be prepared to treat severe allergic and anaphylactic reactions.

Compartment syndrome may occur secondary to envenomation. If suspected, the compartment pressure must be determined. Pressures above 30 mm Hg require limb elevation and **repeat dosing of antivenin.** Persistently elevated pressures may require **mannitol** (1-2 g/kg IV over 30 minutes) and surgical consultation for emergent **fasciotomy.** Active bleeding due to severe coagulopathy may require the transfusion of blood products, although the mainstay of uncomplicated coagulopathy remains antivenin therapy.

All patients with a pit viper bite must be observed for at least 8 hours. Patients with severe bites and those receiving antivenin must be admitted to the intensive care unit. Patients with mild envenomation who have completed antivenin therapy may be admitted to the general ward. Patients with no evidence of envenomation after 8 to 12 hours may be discharged. All patients who receive Polyvalent Crotalidae Immune Fab antivenin should be counseled about serum sickness because this occurs in 16% of patients at 7 to 14 days after therapy. Oral **prednisone,** 60 mg/d tapering over 1 to 2 weeks, is the standard treatment for serum sickness.

CORAL SNAKE BITE

Clinical Features

Coral snakes are brightly colored with a pattern of black, red, and yellow bands. All true coral snakes have their yellow bands directly touching the red bands; nonpoisonous impostors have an intervening black band. This consistent and distinctive pattern establishes the familiar mnemonic for North American snakes: "Red on yellow, kill a fellow; red on black, venom lack." Only the bite of the eastern coral snake *(Micrurus fulvius fulvius)* requires significant treatment; the bite of the Sonoran (Arizona) coral snake is mild and needs only local care. Eastern coral snake venom is a potent neurotoxin capable of causing tremor, salivation, respiratory paralysis, seizures, and bulbar palsies (eg, dysarthria, diplopia, and dysphagia).

Emergency Department Care and Disposition

Patients with possible envenomation must be admitted to the hospital for 24 to 48 hours of observation. The toxic effects of coral snake venom may be preventable, but they are not easily reversed. Therefore, all patients who have potential envenomation should receive 3 vials of **antivenin** *(M fulvius)*. Additional doses are required if symptoms appear, and these patients must be admitted to an intensive care unit.

GILA MONSTER BITE

Gila monster bites result in pain and swelling. Systemic toxicity is rare but may consist of diaphoresis, paresthesia, weakness, and hypertension. The bite may be tenacious, and the reptile should be removed as soon as possible. If the reptile is still attached, it may loosen its bite when placed on a solid surface where it is not suspended in midair. Other techniques include submersion of the animal in water, use of a cast spreader, or local application of an irritating flame. Once removed, standard wound care should be performed, including a search for implanted teeth. No further treatment is required.

For further reading in *Emergency Medicine: A Comprehensive Study Guide,* 6th ed., see Chap. 194, "Arthropod Bites and Stings," by Richard F. Clark and Aaron B. Schneir; and Chap. 195, "Reptile Bites," by Richard C. Dart and Frank F. S. Daly.

| Trauma and Envenomation from Marine Fauna

Christian A. Tomaszewski

The population growth along coastal areas of the United States has made exposure to hazardous marine fauna an increasingly common event. The popularity of home aquariums has generated additional exposure to these unique problems across the entire country. Marine fauna can inflict injury through direct bite or envenomation, usually via a stinging apparatus or cells.

CLINICAL FEATURES

Marine animals reported in attacks include sharks, great barracudas, moray eels, giant groupers, sea lions, seals, crocodiles, alligators, needlefish, wahoos, piranhas, and trigger fish. They have inflicted abrasions, puncture wounds, lacerations, and crush injuries. With shark bites, there is the added issue of substantial tissue loss associated with hemorrhagic shock, hypothermia, and near-drowning.

Coral cuts and scrapes are the most common underwater injury and cause local stinging pain, erythema, urticaria, and pruritus. This may progress to cellulitis with lymphangitis and, in worse cases, ulceration and wound necrosis.

Ocean water contains many potentially pathogenic bacteria, including *Aeromonas hydrophila, Bacteroides fragilis, Chromobacterium violaceum, Clostridium perfringens, Escherichia coli, Salmonella enteritidis, Staphylococcus aureus,* and *Streptococcus* species. But among the most serious infections are those due to the species from the genera Vibrio and Aeromonas (both gram-negative rods). Vibrio infections are some of the most virulent, causing rapid infections marked by pain, swelling, hemorrhagic bullae, vasculitis, and even necrotizing fascitis and sepsis. Immunosuppressed patients, particularly those with chronic liver disease, are especially susceptible to sepsis and death (up to 60%) with *Vibrio vulnificus* infections. *Erysipelothrix rhusiopathiae,* the bacterium implicated in fish handler's disease, causes painful, marginating plaques on the hand after a cutaneous puncture wound. Another unique marine bacterium is *Mycobacterium marinum,* an acid-fast bacillus that can cause a chronic cutaneous granuloma 3 to 4 weeks after exposure.

Numerous invertebrate and vertebrate marine species are venomous. These venoms can be cytotoxic, hematoxic, myotoxic, and neurotoxic. Most are heat labile. The invertebrates consist of five phyla: Cnidaria, Porifera, Echinodermata, Annelida, and Mollusca.

Cnidaria include true jellyfish (Scyphozoa), box jellyfish (Cubozoa), anemones (Anthozoa), fire corals, and Portuguese man-of-war (Hydrozoa). Most of these organisms have tentacles with nematocysts or stinging cells that release venom upon contact. Most reactions are localized, with resulting pain, erythema, and urticaria. *Physalia* (the Portuguese man-of-war) also causes severe pain, respiratory distress, and even death (possibly due to anaphylaxis). The deadliest Cnidarians are the box jellyfish, in particular *Chironex fleckeri* in Australia and *Chiropsalmus,* which even exists in the Gulf of Mexico. Death is rapid by cardiovascular demise. Another Australian box jellyfish, *Carukia barnesi,* can cause the Irukandji syndrome, which is characterized by diffuse pain, hypertension, tachycardia, diaphoresis, and pulmonary edema (rarely).

575

Porifera are sponges that produce a stinging dermatitis. In addition, spicules of silica or calcium carbonate carried by the sponge become embedded in the skin. In severe cases, chronic inflammatory changes may develop and result in a papulovesicular rash and erythema multiforme.

Echinodermata include sea urchins, sea stars, and sea cucumbers. Sea urchin spines produce immediate pain followed by erythema, myalgia, and local swelling. Delayed effects consist of granulomas from retained spines. Systemic envenomation rarely occurs and is manifested by nausea, paresthesia, paralysis, abdominal pain, syncope, respiratory distress, and hypotension. The most notorious sea star, *Acanthaster planci,* has sharp rigid spines that cause burning pain and local inflammation. Although uncommon, severe envenomation can cause nausea, vomiting, paresthesia, and paralysis.

Annelida include bristle worms, which embed bristles in the skin, causing pain and erythema. Mollusca include gastropods and octopuses. The Indo-Pacific cone shell, *Conus,* has a poison dart whose envenomation is similar to that of bee stings; however, it may induce muscle paralysis and respiratory failure within 30 minutes. The blue-ringed octopus, *Hapalochalena,* can inject tetrodotoxin and cause paresthesias, flaccid paralysis, and respiratory failure.

Vertebrate envenomations are primarily due to stingrays (order Rajiformes), with an occasional sting from venomous spined fish and bites from sea snakes. The stingray has a venomous spine, which punctures or lacerates the skin and causes an intense painful local reaction. The spine sheath and even the spine itself may break off as a retained body. Systemic manifestations may include weakness, nausea, vomiting, diarrhea, syncope, seizures, paralysis, hypotension, and dysrhythmias. There are many spined venomous fish, including scorpion fish (popular in aquariums), rockfish, catfish, weever fish, toadfish, rat fish, rabbit fish, stargazers, and scats. All have spines associated with venom glands but cause only severe local pain, erythema, and edema, with an occasional retained spine. The most venomous is the Indo-Pacific stone fish *(Synaceja),* which, in addition to severe local effects, can cause diaphoresis, nausea, and hypotension.

Sea snakes, which live in tropical Indo-Pacific oceans, have venom that contains a paralyzing neurotoxin and myotoxin. Symptoms, occurring 30 minutes to 4 hours after the bite, include myalgia, ophthalmoplegia, ascending paralysis, and respiratory failure; myoglobinuria and elevated liver enzymes may be found. If death occurs, it is usually due to ventilatory failure that occurs within 6 hours.

EMERGENCY DEPARTMENT CARE AND DISPOSITION

1. Attention should be focused on airway, breathing, circulation, treatment of life-threatening injuries, and correction of hypothermia.
2. Lacerations should be **copiously irrigated,** explored for foreign matter, and débrided of devitalized tissue. Soft tissue radiographs may help locate foreign bodies. Most wounds should undergo delayed primary closure. Tetanus prophylaxis should be updated as appropriate.
3. Empiric antibiotic therapy is not indicated for routine minor wounds in healthy patients. Patients who are immunocompromised and have liver disease or have grossly contaminated or extensive lacerations require antibiotics; in high-risk patients, the initial dose should be parenteral. Aerobic and anaerobic cultures should be ordered, and the laboratory should be

alerted because special media may be needed. Antibiotic therapy should cover *Staphylococcus* and *Streptococcus* species; in ocean-related infections, *Vibrio* species should be covered with a **third-generation cephalosporin** or **quinolone.** Granulomas from *Mycobacterium marinum* require several months of treatment with **clarithromycin** or **rifampin plus ethambutol** for deep-seated infections.

4. For Cnidaria envenomation, the wound should be **rinsed with saline;** fresh water should be avoided because it may cause further envenomation. To deactivate attached nematocysts, particularly from the deadly box jellyfish and Portuguese man-of-war, **5% acetic acid** (vinegar) should be applied for 30 minutes or until pain is resolved. Of note, greater clinical success is achieved by immersing the wound of a Hawaiian box jellyfish *(Carybdea alata)* in **hot water** (>40°C); wounds of some other species of true jellyfish should be immersed in a slurry of **sodium bicarbonate.** Subsequently, retained tentacles and nematocysts can be picked off with gloved hands or scraped off. Chronic inflammatory problems can be treated with **topical steroids.** Corneal envenomation should be irrigated copiously; persistent symptoms may require topical steroids. Patients with systemic symptoms should be observed for at least 8 hours. There is an **antivenin** for systemic symptoms from the box jellyfish *Chironex* venom.

5. Sponge-induced dermatitis should be treated with gentle drying of the skin and removal of spicules with **adhesive tape.** Antihistamines and topical steroids may be beneficial in chronic inflammatory reactions.

6. Echinodermata envenomation should be treated by removing gross spines and with **hot water immersion** (45° C) for 30 to 90 minutes. In Annelida envenomation, bristles should be removed with adhesive tape or forceps.

7. With stingray, scorpion fish, and other vertebrate envenomations, the affected area should be immersed in **hot water,** spines should be removed, and the wound should be explored and débrided as necessary. The patient should be observed for 4 hours to exclude systemic toxicity.

8. With sea snake bites, the injured area should be kept immobilized and dependent; the application of local pressure such as with an elastic bandage may help sequester the venom. **Sea snake antivenin,** monovalent (for the beaked sea snake in southeast Asia) or polyvalent, is indicated for any systemic symptoms and may be beneficial up to 36 hours after envenomation. If no symptoms develop after 8 hours, then envenomation can be excluded.

For further reading in *Emergency Medicine: A Comprehensive Study Guide,* 6th ed., see Chap. 196, "Trauma and Envenomation from Marine Fauna," by Geoffrey K. Isbister and David G. Caldicott.

High-Altitude Medical Problems

Keith L. Mausner

High-altitude syndromes are due primarily to hypoxia; the rapidity and height of ascent influence the risk of occurrence.

CLINICAL FEATURES

Acute mountain sickness (AMS) is usually seen in non-acclimated people making a rapid ascent higher than 2,000 m (6,600 ft) above sea level. The earliest symptoms are lightheadedness and mild breathlessness. Symptoms similar to a hangover may develop within 6 hours after arrival at altitude but may be delayed as long as 1 day. These symptoms include bifrontal headache, anorexia, nausea, weakness, and fatigue. Worsening headache, vomiting, oliguria, dyspnea, and weakness indicate progression of AMS. There are few specific physical examination findings. Postural hypotension and peripheral and facial edemas may occur. Localized rales are noted in 20% of cases. Funduscopy shows tortuous and dilated veins; retinal hemorrhages are common at altitudes higher than 5,000 m.

High-altitude cerebral edema (HACE) is an extreme progression of AMS and usually is associated with pulmonary edema. It presents with altered mental status, ataxia, stupor, and progression to coma. Focal neurologic signs such as third and sixth cranial nerve palsies may be present.

High-altitude pulmonary edema (HAPE) is the most lethal of the high-altitude syndromes. Risk factors include heavy exertion, rapid ascent, cold exposure, excessive salt intake, use of sleeping medications, and previous history of HAPE. Individuals with pulmonary hypertension and children with acute respiratory infections may be more susceptible to HAPE.

Early findings of HAPE include a dry cough, impaired exercise capacity, and localized rales, usually in the right midlung field. Progression of the disease leads to tachycardia, tachypnea, resting dyspnea, severe weakness, productive cough, cyanosis, and generalized rales. Low-grade fever is common. As hypoxemia worsens, consciousness is impaired, and, without treatment, coma and death usually follow. Other findings may include signs of pulmonary hypertension such as a prominent P_2, right ventricular heave on cardiac examination, and right axis deviation and a right ventricular strain pattern on electrocardiogram. Early recognition of HAPE, descent, and treatment is essential to prevent progression.

High altitude may adversely affect patients with chronic obstructive pulmonary disease, heart disease, sickle cell disease, and pregnancy. Patients with chronic obstructive pulmonary disease may require supplemental O_2 or an increase in their usual O_2 flow rate. Patients with atherosclerotic heart disease do surprisingly well at high altitude, but there may be a risk of earlier onset of angina and worsening of heart failure. Ascent to 1,500 to 2,000 m may cause a vasoocclusive crisis in individuals with sickle cell disease or sickle thalassemia. Individuals with sickle trait usually do well at high altitude, but splenic infarction has been reported during heavy exercise. Pregnant long-term high-altitude residents have an increased risk of hypertension, low-birthweight infants, and neonatal jaundice, but no increase in pregnancy complications has been reported in pregnant visitors to high altitude who engage in reasonable activities. However, it is reasonable to advise pregnant women to avoid altitudes above which oxygen saturation falls below 85%; this level corresponds to a sleeping altitude of approximately 10,000 ft.

DIAGNOSIS AND DIFFERENTIAL

The differential diagnosis of the high-altitude syndromes includes hypothermia, carbon monoxide poisoning, pulmonary or central nervous system infections, dehydration, and exhaustion. HACE may be difficult to distinguish in the field from other high-altitude neurologic syndromes. Strokes due to arterial or venous thrombosis or arterial hemorrhage have been reported at high altitude in individuals without classic risk factors. Reversible focal neurologic signs or symptoms may occur and may be due to vasospasm, migraine headache, or transient ischemic attack. These syndromes typically have more focal findings than does HACE. Previously asymptomatic brain tumors may be unmasked by ascent to high altitude. Underlying epilepsy may be worsened by hyperventilation, which is part of the normal acclimatization response. HAPE must be distinguished from pulmonary embolus, cardiogenic pulmonary edema, and pneumonia. A key to diagnosis is the clinical response to treatment.

CARE AND DISPOSITION IN THE FIELD AND EMERGENCY DEPARTMENT

1. Mild AMS usually improves or resolves in 12 to 36 hours if farther ascent is delayed and acclimatization is allowed. A decrease in altitude of 500 to 1,000 m may provide prompt relief of symptoms. **Oxygen** relieves symptoms, and nocturnal low-flow O_2 (0.5 to 1 L/min) is helpful. Patients with mild AMS should not ascend to a higher sleeping elevation. Descent is indicated if symptoms persist or worsen. Immediate descent and treatment are indicated if there is a change in the level of consciousness, ataxia, or pulmonary edema. Gradual ascent is effective at preventing AMS. A reasonable recommendation for sea-level dwellers is to spend a night at 1,500 to 2,000 m before sleeping at altitudes above 2,500 m. High-altitude trekkers should allow 2 nights for each 1,000-m gain in sleeping altitude, starting at 3,000 m. Eating a high carbohydrate diet and avoiding overexertion, alcohol, and respiratory depressants also may help prevent AMS.

2. **Acetazolamide** causes a bicarbonate diuresis, leading to a mild metabolic acidosis. This acidosis stimulates ventilation and pharmacologically produces an acclimatization response. Acetazolamide is effective in prophylaxis and treatment. Specific indications for acetazolamide are (*a*) prior history of altitude illness, (*b*) abrupt ascent higher than 3,000 m (10,000 ft), (*c*) treatment of AMS, and (*d*) symptomatic periodic breathing during sleep at high altitude. The adult dose is 125 mg orally (PO) twice daily or 5 mg/kg/d in 2 or 3 divided doses; it is continued until symptoms resolve or is started 24 hours before ascent and continued for 2 days at high altitude as a prophylaxis. It should be restarted if symptoms recur. Acetazolamide is contraindicated in sulfa-allergic patients.

3. **Dexamethasone** (4 mg PO, intramuscularly [IM], or intravenously [IV] every 6 hours) is effective in moderate to severe AMS. Tapering of the dose over several days may be necessary to prevent rebound.

4. **Aspirin** or **acetaminophen** may improve headache in AMS. **Prochlor-perazine** (5-10 mg IM, IV, or PO) may help with nausea and vomiting. Diuretics may be useful for treating fluid retention but should be used with caution to avoid intravascular volume depletion.

5. HACE mandates **immediate descent or evacuation. Oxygen** and **dexamethasone** (8 mg PO, IM, or IV and then 4 mg every 6 hours) should be administered. **Furosemide** (40-80 mg) may help reduce brain edema. **Intubation** and **hyperventilation** are necessary in severe cases. Careful monitoring of arterial blood gases are needed to prevent excessive lowering of P_{CO_2} (<30 mm Hg), which may cause cerebral ischemia. **Mannitol** should be considered in severe cases not responding to treatment.

6. HAPE also should be treated with **immediate descent. Oxygen** may be lifesaving if descent is delayed. The patient should be kept warm and exertion should be minimized. Drugs are second-line treatment after descent and oxygen. **Nifedipine** (10 mg PO every 4-6 hours, or 30 mg extended release every 12 hours), morphine, and furosemide may be effective. These patients are usually volume depleted, and care should be taken to avoid precipitating drug-induced hypotension. An expiratory positive airway pressure mask may be useful in the field and, without supplemental O_2, can increase oxygen saturation by 10% to 20%. Portable fabric inflatable hyperbaric chambers may be effective in the field when immediate descent is not possible.

7. In individuals with prior episodes of HAPE, **nifedipine** 20 mg (slow-release preparation) every 8 hours during ascent may be effective as prophylaxis. **Inhaled salmeterol** twice daily also may help prevent recurrent HAPE.

For further reading in *Emergency Medicine: A Comprehensive Study Guide,* 6th ed., see Chap. 207, "High Altitude Medical Problems," by Peter H. Hackett.

124 | Dysbarism and Complications of Diving

Christian A. Tomaszewski

Dysbarism is commonly encountered in scuba divers and refers to complications associated with changes in environmental ambient pressure and with breathing compressed gases. These effects are governed by the gas laws: the Boyle law states that, at a constant temperature, the pressure and volume of a gas are inversely related; the Henry law states that, at equilibrium, the quantity of gas in solution is proportional to the partial pressure of the gas.

CLINICAL FEATURES

Barotrauma is the most common diving-related affliction and is caused by the direct mechanical effects of pressure, as gas-filled cavities in the body contract with pressure. Middle ear squeeze, or barotitis media, is the most frequently seen form of barotrauma. It occurs secondary to eustachian tube dysfunction during descent. If the dive is not aborted or pressure is not equalized, the eardrum may rupture, and the diver may have a sensation of escaping air bubbles from the ear, with nausea and vertigo. The patient may complain of ear pain or fullness on presentation. On physical examination, there may be blood behind the tympanic membrane or within the canal, mild conductive hearing loss, and tympanic membrane perforation.

If the sinus ostia are occluded on descent, an impending squeeze can cause bleeding from the maxillary or frontal sinuses, with subsequent pain and epistaxis. Squeeze also may manifest as subconjunctival hemorrhage if a diver does not exhale into the mask and equalize pressure during descent.

A rare but serious condition is inner ear barotrauma. This typically occurs during rapid descent, when the diver does an overly forceful Valsalva maneuver. Instead of clearing the ears or rupturing the tympanic membrane, pressure is transmitted through vestibular and cochlear structures. This may lead to serious inner ear damage, including rupture of the oval or round window, fistula formation, or rupture of Reissner membrane. Inner ear barotrauma may present with roaring tinnitus, vertigo, sensorineural hearing loss, a feeling of ear fullness, nausea, and vomiting. Insufflation of the tympanic membrane on the affected side may cause contralateral eye deviation, known as a positive fistula test.

Barotrauma during ascent is due to expansion of gas in body cavities. Although rare, "reverse squeeze" may affect the ear or sinuses during ascent with rupture. Alternobaric vertigo can temporarily occur during ascent due to unbalanced vestibular stimulation from unequal middle ear pressures. Although rare, tooth squeeze may be noted during ascent from air-filled dental cavities. Gastrointestinal barotrauma presents with abdominal fullness, colicky abdominal pain, belching, and flatulence. Severe cases of air swallowing have resulted in stomach rupture on ascent.

Pulmonary over-pressurization syndrome (POPS) may occur during ascent, resulting in mediastinal and subcutaneous emphysema. Although rapid ascents without exhalation are the usual cause of POPS, patients with obstructive lung disease and congenital cysts also may have air trapping. After the dive, these patients may experience gradual onset of increasing hoarseness, neck fullness, substernal chest pain, dyspnea, and dysphagia; in severe cases, syncope and pneumothorax may occur.

Air embolism is the most severe form of pulmonary barotrauma. Gas bubbles may enter the pulmonary venous circulation and embolize to the brain, causing cerebral arterial gas embolism. This can result from as shallow a dive as 4 ft: a full breath of compressed air taken at the bottom of a swimming pool and the diver ascends in a panic without exhaling. This condition typically presents acutely in a diver surfacing after a rapid ascent. This also can occur in patients with central venous catheters or on cardiac bypass, when an inadvertent air embolus enters the right side of the heart and crosses over into the left atrium via a patent foramen ovale. Returning venous air in a severe decompression sickness (DCS) case can produce the same condition. Regardless of the source, cerebral arterial gas embolism can result in immediate apnea and death, as seen in 4% of dive-related cases. If patients survive the acute insult, they usually present within 1 hour of the dive with syncope, seizure, disorientation, or hemiplegia. Milder cases may present with sensory disturbances, confusion, or vertigo.

DCS is not a form of barotrauma. It is due to gas bubble formation as inert gas comes out of solution in blood and tissues, if ascent is too rapid, without adequate time for decompression. Although usually seen in scuba divers who have violated the limits of safe diving as defined by the US Navy or have flown within 12 to 24 hours of diving, it also can occur in high-altitude pilots and caisson workers. In conventional compressed air diving, the culprit is nitrogen. DCS is a multiorgan system disorder due to the direct effects of nitrogen bubbles on circulation and cells and to secondary inflammatory responses and activation of clotting mechanisms. Type I DCS (pain only) typically involves the joints, extremities, and at times the skin, which is manifested by purple mottling. Type II DCS is more serious and involves the central nervous system, typically the spine, and occasionally the vestibular ("staggers") and cardiopulmonary ("chokes") systems. The symptoms of DCS often cannot be distinguished from barotrauma and are lumped together as *decompression illness.*

The most common initial symptoms of DCS may be nonspecific; they include fatigue, headache, nausea, and dizziness. Divers with type I DCS typically have deep pain in the knee or shoulder that is relieved with movement. Type II DCS may present with vague patchy paresthesias. On physical examination, the patient may have ataxia, bladder dysfunction, and partial paralysis. In pulmonary DCS, the patient may present with cough, hemoptysis, dyspnea, and substernal chest pain. Vestibular DCS, which may be mistaken for inner ear barotrauma, can present with vertigo, hearing loss, tinnitus, and dysequilibrium.

DIAGNOSIS AND DIFFERENTIAL

The time of symptom onset in relation to the dive profile, ie, depth, duration, and repetitiveness, and in relation to descent or ascent are the most useful historical factors in distinguishing decompression illness from other disorders. During descent, the most common maladies are the squeeze syndromes. During the ascent phase, barotrauma or alternobaric vertigo is most likely to occur. DCS, if severe, may become symptomatic during ascent.

Onset of severe symptoms within 10 minutes of surfacing is an air embolism until proven otherwise. POPS and other forms of barotrauma also usually present shortly after ascent. DCS tends to be less catastrophic initially, more severe symptoms develop 1 to 6 hours after surfacing but may be delayed for up to 48 hours.

The differential diagnosis for DCS is broad. Musculoskeletal complaints could be due to joint strain or a newly symptomatic herniated cervical disk. Chest pain may be due to cardiac ischemia from overexertion. Acute pulmonary edema from cardiogenic causes has occurred in young people during strenuous dives, particularly in cold water. Sudden loss of consciousness or seizure may be idiopathic or from subarachnoid hemorrhage. Paresthesias, in particular hot-and-cold sensation reversal, may occur within a day of eating a ciguatera-contaminated predatory fish. In challenging cases, patients with these diverse symptoms may benefit from a trial of pressure within a hyperbaric chamber, which would result in dramatic clinical improvement if symptoms are related to DCS.

EMERGENCY DEPARTMENT CARE AND DISPOSITION

1. Attention should be focused on airway, breathing, circulation, treatment of life-threatening injuries, and correction of hypothermia. **High-flow oxygen** should be administered.
2. If air embolism is suspected, the **patient should be placed in a supine position;** left lateral decubitus may be used if vomiting occurs, but the Trendelenburg position is no longer recommended. **Lidocaine** as a 1-mg/kg bolus may be given, followed by a continuous infusion at 1 mg/min. There is no support for the use of heparin, aspirin, or corticosteroids at this time.
3. If air embolism or DCS is suspected, **recompression chamber therapy** should be initiated as quickly as possible. Aeromedical transport should be at an altitude of less than 1000 ft or in an aircraft that can be pressurized to 1 atmosphere absolute. Most DCS patients are volume depleted; **intravenous fluids** should be administered if not otherwise contraindicated.
4. Patients with middle ear and other squeeze syndromes should stop diving until symptoms resolve. **Decongestants** and **analgesics** may be helpful. **Antibiotics,** such as amoxicillin, are indicated if the tympanic membrane is ruptured; diving is contraindicated until it has healed. Sinus squeeze is treated similarly to middle ear squeeze; antibiotics are optional. Inner ear barotrauma usually mandates ear, nose, and throat consultation because surgical repair may be indicated. These patients should avoid straining, be prescribed medications for nausea and vertigo, and be placed on bedrest with the head elevated.
5. POPS may require **needle decompression** or **tube thoracostomy** if a pneumothorax develops. POPS usually resolves with rest and supplemental oxygen and rarely requires recompression therapy.
6. For assistance in treating dive-related conditions and for the location of the nearest recompression unit, call the National Diving Alert Network at Duke University, 24 hours a day, at (919) 684-8111.

For further reading in *Emergency Medicine: A Comprehensive Study Guide,* 6th ed., see Chap. 197, "Dysbarism and Complications of Diving," by Brain Snyder and Tom Neuman.

125 | Near Drowning

Richard A. Walker

Near drowning is defined as survival longer than 24 hours after a submersion event and tends to occur in otherwise healthy, young individuals. The prognosis depends on the degree of pulmonary and central nervous system injury and therefore is highly dependent on early rescue and resuscitation. Prevention is the most important means to reduce associated morbidly and mortality.

CLINICAL FEATURES

Dry drowning results from laryngospasm causing hypoxemia and different degrees of neurologic insult and represents up to 20% of submersion injuries. *Wet drowning* consists of aspiration of water into the lungs causing washout of surfactant, which results in diminished alveolar gas transfer, atelectasis, and ventilation perfusion mismatch. Noncardiogenic pulmonary edema results from moderate to severe aspiration. Physical examination may show clear lungs, rales, rhonchi, or wheezes. Mental status may range from normal to comatose. Patients are at risk for hypothermia even in "warm water" submersions.

DIAGNOSIS AND DIFFERENTIAL

The diagnosis of near drowning is usually not problematic, but associated injuries and underlying precipitating disorders should be sought. Spinal cord injuries may occur in association with diving or surfing injuries or in boating accidents. Syncope, seizures, hypoglycemia, and underlying heart disease, including acute myocardial infarction and dysrhythmias, have been associated with near drowning. Laboratory findings may include metabolic acidosis and electrolyte abnormalities if there is associated renal injury from hypoxemia, hemoglobinuria, or myoglobinuria. Massive hemolysis may occur with very large volumes of aspirated fresh water. Disseminated intravascular coagulation is rare. Essential diagnostic tests include a chest radiograph and arterial blood gas analysis. The chest radiograph may show generalized pulmonary edema or perihilar infiltrates or be normal. Because the chest radiograph may not correlate with the arterial Po_2, an arterial blood gas to assess oxygen saturation and metabolic acidosis is important.

EMERGENCY DEPARTMENT CARE AND DISPOSITION

1. All patients should have their airway, ventilation, and oxygenation status assessed, and the cervical spine should be stabilized and evaluated in cases of diving accidents, multiple trauma, or if the circumstances are unknown.
2. **Warmed intravenous normal saline** and **warming adjuncts** (overhead warmer, bear hugger, etc) should be used if the patient is hypothermic. The patient's core temperature should be monitored.
3. Near drowning victims can be divided into 2 groups based on the Glasgow Coma Scale (GCS). Patients with a GCS score of at least 14 should receive supplemental **oxygen** to maintain oxygen saturation (Sao_2) above 95%. They may be discharged home after a 4- to 6-hour observation period as long as their pulmonary and neurologic examinations and Sao_2 remain

normal. The patient with an oxygen requirement or abnormal examination after 4 to 6 hours should be admitted.

4. Patients with a GCS score lower than 14 should be administered supplemental **oxygen. Intubation and mechanical ventilation** are indicated if the Pao_2 cannot be maintained above 60 mm Hg in adults or above 80 mm Hg in children despite high-flow oxygen (40% to 60%).

5. Pediatric victims of fresh-water near drowning rarely develop dilutional hyponatremia and seizures, which are usually easily controlled by correction of the electrolyte abnormality.

6. Prophylactic antibiotics are not indicated because the development of bacterial pneumonia is rare.

7. Efforts at "brain resuscitation," including the use of mannitol, loop diuretics, hypertonic saline, fluid restriction, mechanical hyperventilation, controlled hypothermia, barbiturate coma, and intracranial pressure monitoring, have not shown benefit.

8. Asystole outside the hospital arena or in the emergency department is a poor prognostic sign in pediatric warm-water submersion injuries, but there are anecdotal reports of neurologic recovery. Patients with short warm-water submersion time and short transport time should undergo vigorous resuscitation attempts. Continuous infusion of vasopressors may be required in the postresuscitation phase. Consideration should be given to withholding resuscitation in patients with prolonged submersion and transport.

9. Reports of complete and near complete neurologic recovery after asystole in adults and children have been reported in prolonged icy-water submersion. Hypothermic victims of cold-water submersion in cardiac arrest should undergo prolonged and aggressive resuscitation maneuvers until they are normothermic or considered not viable.

For further reading in *Emergency Medicine: A Comprehensive Study Guide,* 6th ed., see Chap. 198, "Near Drowning," by Alan L. Causey and Mark A. Nichter.

126 | Thermal and Chemical Burns

Robert J. French

THERMAL BURNS

Approximately 1 million burn injuries occur each year, resulting in 700,000 emergency department visits, 45,000 hospitalizations, and 4,500 deaths. Nearly 70% of pediatric burn injuries are due to scalds. Up to 20% of pediatric burn injuries result from child abuse. The risk of death from a major burn is associated with increased burn size, advanced age, concomitant inhalation injury, and female sex. Improved survival and long-term outcomes are largely due to medical advances in burn management, development of specialized burn centers, and emergence of burn care as a surgical subspecialty.

Clinical Features

Burns are categorized by their size and depth. Burn size is calculated as the percentage of body surface area (BSA) involved. The most common method to estimate the percentage of BSA is the "rule of 9s" (Fig. 126-1). A more accurate tool to determine the percentage of BSA, especially in infants and children, is the Lund and Browder burn diagram (Fig. 126-2). For smaller burns,

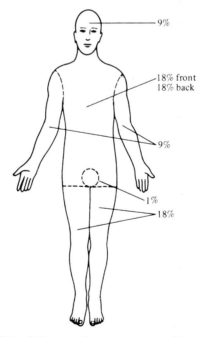

FIG. 126-1. Rule of Nines to estimate percentage of burn.

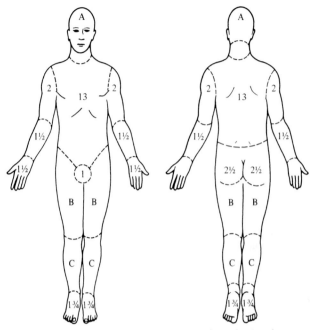

Relative Percentages of Areas Affected by Growth (Age in Years)

	0	1	5	10	15	Adult
A: half of head	9½	8½	6½	5½	4½	3½
B: half of thigh	2¾	3¼	4	4¼	4½	4¾
C: half of leg	2½	2½	2¾	3	3¼	3½

Second-degree _____ and

Third-degree _____ =

Total percent burned ____

FIG. 126-2.   Lund and Browder diagram to estimate percentage of pediatric burn.

the patient's hand can be used as a "ruler" to estimate the percentage of BSA. This area represents approximately 1% of the patient's BSA.

Burn depth historically has been described in degrees: first, second, third, and fourth. A more clinically relevant classification scheme, used to determine the need for surgical intervention, categorizes burns as superficial partial thickness, deep partial thickness, and full thickness. A first-degree burn (eg, sunburn) involves only the epidermal layer. The burned skin is red, painful, dry, and tender without blister formation. This usually heals within 7 days without scarring. Second-degree burns extend into the dermis and are classified as superficial partial-thickness and deep partial-thickness burns. Superficial partial-thickness burns blister and are very painful. The exposed dermis is red and moist, with intact capillary refill. Healing occurs in 14 to 21 days with little to no scar formation. Deep partial-thickness burns are white to yellow in color. Pressure applied to the skin can be felt, but 2-point discrimination is diminished. Capillary refill and pain sensation are absent. These are difficult to differentiate from full-thickness burns. Healing occurs in 3 weeks to 3 months and scarring is common. Third-degree or full-thickness burns are charred, pale, leathery, and painless. These injuries do not heal spontaneously because all dermal elements are destroyed. Surgical repair and skin grafting are needed. Fourth-degree burns are those that extend through the subcutaneous fat, muscle, and bone. Amputation or extensive reconstruction is required.

Inhalation injury occurs most frequently in closed-space fires and in patients with decreased cognition (alcohol intoxication, drug abuse, head injury, or dementia). Injury can occur to the upper and lower airways due to exposure from heat, particulate matter, and toxic gases. Upper airway edema, secondary to thermal injury, can result in acute airway compromise. Smoke contains particulate material generated from incomplete combustion of organic material, which can reach the terminal bronchioles and lead to bronchospasm and edema. Clinical indicators of smoke inhalation injury include facial burns, singed nasal hair, soot in the nose or mouth, hoarseness, carbonaceous sputum, and wheezing. Carbon monoxide poisoning should be suspected in all patients with smoke inhalation injury. Clinical signs include headache, vomiting, confusion, lethargy, and coma. Hydrogen cyanide poisoning should be suspected in fires involving nitrogen-containing polymer products such as wool, silk, polyurethane, and vinyl.

Diagnosis and Differential

The American Burn Association classifies burns into major, moderate, and minor. Examples of major burns include (a) partial-thickness burns greater than 20% of BSA in adults or greater than 10% in children (<10 years) or older adults (>50 years); (b) full-thickness burns greater than 5% of BSA; (c) significant burns to face, eyes, ears, genitalia, hands, feet, or major joints; and (d) concomitant smoke inhalation or major trauma. Examples of minor burns are (a) partial-thickness burns of less than 10% of BSA in adults or less than 5% in children or older adults and (b) full-thickness burns of less than 2%. Moderate burns are those not meeting criteria for major or minor burns. The BSA, depth, and location affect treatment and disposition decisions. Estimation of burn depth is often difficult in the first few hours post-burn and requires serial examinations to improve accuracy. Medical conditions such as heart disease, chronic pulmonary disease, and diabetes increase morbidity and mortality. The diagnosis of inhalation injury is made primarily by history and physical examination findings. Chest radiograph may be normal initially. Flexible fiberoptic bronchoscopy can confirm the diagnosis. Carboxyhemoglobin levels should be obtained if carbon monoxide poisoning is suspected.

Emergency Department Care and Disposition

Care begins in the prehospital setting and continues in the emergency department. Attention to airway, breathing, hemodynamic status; appropriate fluid resuscitation; and accurate burn assessment are critical elements in caring for burn patients.

1. Administration of **100% oxygen** is performed initially. If there are signs of airway compromise or an airway burn, then the patient should undergo **endotracheal intubation** for airway protection. An arterial blood gas, carboxyhemoglobin level, and chest radiograph should be obtained.

2. At least 2 intravenous (IV) lines should be established over unburned areas. Initial **fluid resuscitation,** which should be guided by the Parkland formula, is 2 to 4 mL/kg per BSA percentage per 24 hours. Half the calculated amount is given in the first 8 hours, and the remainder is given over the next 16 hours. **Lactated Ringer** solution is recommended. The 24-hour interval begins from the time the patient sustained the burn injuries, not from the time of resuscitation onset. The BSA percentage used in this calculation should include only second- and third-degree burns.

3. A Foley catheter should be placed and urine output maintained at 0.5 to 1 mL/kg/h. Other physiologic resuscitative guides include mental status, capillary refill, blood pressure, pulse rate, and base deficit.

4. A seriously burned individual should be evaluated and treated as a multiple trauma patient. There is significant morbidity due to missed injuries. Liberal use of computed tomography of the head and abdomen is justified.

5. Burns should be cooled immediately by immersion in cold water or application of a cool compress. Immediate cooling of small wounds helps limit burn depth and decrease release of damaging inflammatory mediators. Prolonged cooling of larger BSAs for longer than 30 minutes can result in severe hypothermia. Ice should not be applied directly to the wound because it can cause tissue injury from frostbite.

6. Intravenous **narcotic analgesia** should be administered early and titrated to the patient's pain. Anxiolytic agents should be used as an adjuvant in pain management.

7. Minor burns can be treated on an outpatient basis. The burn wound should be cleaned with mild soap and water or a dilute antiseptic solution. Large blisters (>2 cm) or those involving mobile joints should be drained or débrided. Small blisters on nonmobile areas should be left intact. Topical antibiotics should be used to prevent wound infection and sepsis. The most common agent is **1% silver sulfadiazine.** This agent has low systemic toxicity and a broad antibiotic spectrum and can be applied without causing pain. Silver sulfadiazine should not be applied to patients with sulfa allergy or on the face because of potential staining. Alternate topical agents such as **bacitracin or triple-antibiotic (neomycin, polymyxin B, and bacitracin zinc)** ointment can be used. Honey appears to be an effective topical alternative for minor burn wound care. Synthetic occlusive dressings, instead of topical agents, are another method of managing partial-thickness wounds on an outpatient basis.

8. Moderate and major burns require inpatient admission. These patients generally should be referred to a hospital with a burn center. The American Burn Association's burn unit referral criteria are listed in Table 126-1. After evaluation and resuscitation, sterile drapes should be placed over the burns. Topical antibiotic agents should not be used until the admitting service evaluates the burn wound. Empiric IV antibiotics are not recommended.

9. Patients with circumferential burns of the limbs may develop compromise of the distal circulation. Circumferential burns of the chest and neck

TABLE 126-1 American Burn Association Burn Unit Referral Criteria

Partial-thickness burns >10% of total body surface area

Burns that involve the face, hand, feet, genitalia, perineum, or major burns

Third-degree burns in any age group

Electrical burns, including lightning injury

Chemical burns

Inhalation injury

Burn injury in patients with preexisting medical disorders that could complicate management, prolong recovery, or affect mortality

Any patients with burns and concomitant trauma (eg, fractures) in which the burn injury poses the greatest risk of morbidity or mortality

Burned children in hospitals without qualified personnel or equipment for the care of children

Burn injury in patients who will require special social, emotional, or long-term rehabilitative intervention

Source: American Burn Association. Available at: www.ameriburn.org.

    may cause mechanical ventilatory restriction. Escharotomy may be needed in these cases.
10. Treatment of inhalation injury may include humidified oxygen, endotracheal intubation and mechanical ventilation, bronchodilators, and pulmonary toilet. **Hyperbaric oxygen therapy** is used for severe carbon monoxide poisoning.
11. Routine **tetanus toxoid** prophylaxis should be administered based on the patient's immunization history. **Tetanus immune globulin** should be given in patients without primary immunization.

CHEMICAL BURNS

More than 25,000 products are capable of producing chemical burns. Chemical burn injuries account for 5% to 10% of burn center admissions.

Clinical Features

Clinical features of chemical burns depend on the type of agent, concentration, volume, and duration of exposure. Most acids produce a coagulation necrosis due to desiccating action on the superficial tissue proteins. Superficial and full-thickness burns may result. Hydrofluoric (HF) acid rapidly penetrates intact skin and can cause progressive pain and deep tissue destruction. The onset of pain can be delayed up to 12 hours postexposure. The presenting complaint of acute topical HF acid exposure is pain, often in the absence of any physical evidence of burn. As tissue injury progresses, the involved skin may develop a blue-gray appearance with surrounding erythema.

    Alkalis cause a liquefaction necrosis that permits the passage of hydroxyl ions into deep tissues. Soft, gelatinous, friable, brownish eschars are produced. Airbags deploy by ignition of a solid propellant (sodium azide) that creates an exothermic reaction and certain corrosive byproducts (sodium hydroxide, nitric oxide, and ammonia). Airbag deployment may cause a combination of friction, thermal, and chemical burns.

Chemical burns of the eye are true ocular emergencies that cause redness, pain, and tearing. Acid ocular burns quickly precipitate proteins in the superficial eye structures resulting in the typical "ground glass" appearance. Alkali ocular burns are more severe due to deeper penetration secondary to liquefaction necrosis. Severe chemosis, blanched conjunctiva, and opacified cornea obscuring the view of the iris and lens can occur. Lacrimators (tear gas) such as chloroacetophenone, chlorobenzylidenemalonitrile, dibenzoxazepine, and trichloronitromethane (pepper mace) can cause ocular, mucous membrane, and pulmonary irritation.

Systemic toxicity can result from topical exposure of certain chemical agents such as (*a*) acids (acidosis, hypotension, and shock); (*b*) oxalic and HF acid (hypocalcemia, hypomagnesemia, hyperkalemia, cardiac arrhythmias, and sudden death); (*c*) tannic, formic, and chromic acid (hepatic necrosis and nephrotoxicity); and (*d*) phenol and creosol (methemoglobinemia, massive hemolysis, and multisystem organ failure).

Diagnosis and Differential

The diagnosis of chemical burn usually is made by history of exposure to a chemical agent. Sensitive questions regarding possible exposure are needed in certain scenarios. Chemical topical exposures should be considered in all cases of skin irritation and/or pain. For ocular exposures, pH paper can help distinguish alkali from acid exposure.

Emergency Department Care and Disposition

1. The first priority in the treatment of chemical burns is to terminate the burning process. This is accomplished by removal of garments and **copious irrigation** of the skin. Dry chemical particles should be removed manually before irrigation. Elemental metals (sodium, lithium, calcium, and magnesium) can ignite spontaneously when exposed to air. Water should not be used to extinguish burning particles because of the explosive exothermic reaction that results. These burning elemental metal particles should be covered with **mineral oil** or extinguished with a class D fire extinguisher.
2. In cases of ocular exposure to alkalis, acids, or lacrimators, eye irrigation with 2 L normal saline for a minimum of 1 hour is needed. With alkali or acid ocular exposure, return of the pH to neutral is a measurable endpoint for irrigation. Visual acuity check and pH testing should follow, not precede, ocular irrigation.
3. Phenol and phenolic compounds should be irrigated immediately with water. Water lavage may be ineffective because the phenol compound may become entrapped beneath the water-impermeable necrotic eschar. In these cases, phenol should be decontaminated with a **polyethylene glycol solution (PEG 300 or PEG 400), glycerol, or isopropyl alcohol.**
4. In addition to copious irrigation, HF acid burns often require **calcium gluconate** to bind fluoride and neutralize its toxic effects. Calcium gluconate can be administered as (*a*) calcium gluconate gel applied **topically** (mixed with Surgilube or dimethyl sulfoxide to a concentration of 2.5% to 10%), (*b*) **subcutaneous and intradermal injections** of 5% solution of calcium gluconate via 30-gauge needle with a maximum dose of 1 mL for each square centimeter of burned tissue, or (*c*) **intraarterial** infusion of calcium gluconate.

5. After initial measures, treatment for systemic toxicity is similar to that for thermal burns, with IV fluid resuscitation, analgesia, and tetanus immunoprophylaxis.

For further reading in *Emergency Medicine: A Comprehensive Study Guide,* 6th ed., see Chap. 199, "Thermal Burns," by Lawrence R. Schwartz and Chenicheri Balakrishnan; and Chapter 200, "Chemical Burns," by Fred P. Harchelroad Jr and David M. Rottinghaus.

127 Electrical and Lightning Injuries

Howard E. Jarvis III

ELECTRICAL INJURIES

Electrical injuries present with a wide spectrum of damage, from superficial skin burn to multisystem injury and death. It is important to suspect occult injury to tissue and organs in the path of the current. Most electrical injuries occur in young children, adolescents, and workers exposed to electrical hazards.

Clinical Features

Electricity causes damage by direct effects of current on cells and by thermal damage from the heat generated by the resistance of tissues. Energy is greatest at the contact point; thus the skin often has the greatest observable damage. The exit wound is often larger than the entrance site. As current flows through the body, the greatest damage is sustained by nerves, blood vessels, and muscles. This may result in coagulation necrosis, neuronal death, and damage to blood vessels. As a result, the overall picture often resembles a crush more than a thermal burn. Because the size of the skin injury does not correlate well with the underlying damage, a careful search for deeper injuries is necessary. Traumatic injuries frequently accompany electrical injuries. Specific complications are summarized in Table 127-1.

Diagnosis and Differential

Diagnosis of electrical injury is usually based on history. The type of current (high-tension wires produce the greatest injury) and surrounding circumstances, such as falls or intoxication, should be noted. In unclear cases, characteristic skin lesions or oral lesions in children may be helpful. A thorough examination to exclude occult injuries is essential. An investigation for fractures and dislocations should be made, even without a history of trauma. The absence of findings on initial examination does not exclude serious injury. Laboratory studies should include a complete blood count, electrolytes, calcium, blood urea nitrogen, creatinine, coagulation studies, arterial blood gas analysis, myoglobin (MB), creatinine kinase (CK), and CK-MB. The CK-MB may be elevated without myocardial damage due to extensive muscle injury. Urinalysis should include an MB screen. Liver function studies and amylase are indicated for suspected abdominal injury. Blood should be typed and crossmatched for those with severe injuries. An electrocardiogram (ECG) should be performed in addition to radiographic studies of sites with suspected injuries. Computed tomography of the head is indicated for those with severe head injury, coma, or unresolved mental status changes.

Emergency Department Care and Disposition

1. The airway, breathing, and circulation should be stabilized. Spinal immobilization should be instituted for any non-witnessed events or when there is a potential for spine injury.

TABLE 127-1 Complications of Electrical Injuries

Cardiovascular	Sudden death (ventricular fibrillation, asystole), chest pain, dysrhythmias, ST-T–segment abnormalities, bundle branch block, myocardial damage, ventricular dysfunction, myocardial infarction (rare), hypotension (volume depletion), hypertension (catecholamine release)
Neurologic	Altered mental status, agitation, coma, seizures, cerebral edema, hypoxic encephalopathy, headache, aphasia, weakness, paraplegia, quadriplegia, spinal cord dysfunction (may be delayed), peripheral neuropathy, cognitive impairment, insomnia, emotional lability
Cutaneous	Electrothermal contact injuries, noncontact arc and "flash" burns, secondary thermal burns (clothing ignition, heating of metal)
Vascular	Thrombosis, coagulation necrosis, disseminated intravascular coagulation, delayed vessel rupture, aneurysm, compartment syndrome
Pulmonary	Respiratory arrest (central or peripheral, eg, muscular tetany), aspiration pneumonia, pulmonary edema, pulmonary contusion, inhalation injury
Renal/metabolic	Acute renal failure (due to heme pigment deposition and hypovolemia), myoglobinuria, metabolic (lactic) acidosis, hypokalemia, hypocalcemia, hyperglycemia
Gastrointestinal	Perforation, stress ulcer (Curling ulcer), GI bleeding, GI tract dysfunction various reports of lethal injuries at autopsy
Muscular	Myonecrosis, compartment syndrome
Skeletal	Vertebral compression fractures, long bone fractures, shoulder dislocations (anterior and posterior), scapular fractures
Ophthalmologic	Corneal burns, delayed cataracts, intraocular hemorrhage or thrombosis, uveitis, retinal detachment, orbital fracture
Auditory	Hearing loss, tinnitus, tympanic membrane perforation (rare), delayed mastoiditis or meningitis
Oral burns	Delayed labial artery hemorrhage, scarring and facial deformity, delayed speech development, impaired mandibular/dentition development
Obstetric	Spontaneous abortion, fetal death

Key: GI = gastrointestinal.

2. High-flow oxygen should be administered by face mask.
3. Patients should have continuous cardiac monitoring, pulse oximetry, non-invasive blood pressure monitoring, and preferably 2 large-bore intravenous (IV) lines.
4. Ventricular fibrillation, asystole, or ventricular tachycardia should be treated by standard ACLS protocols. Other dysrhythmias are usually transient and do not need immediate therapy.
5. IV crystalloid fluid should be given with an initial bolus of 20 to 40 mL/kg over the first hour. Fluid requirements are generally higher than those of thermal burn patients. A Foley catheter for urine output measurement is useful in severely injured patients.

6. If evidence of rhabdomyolysis is present, then fluid loading is desirable to prevent renal failure.
7. **Tetanus** prophylaxis should be given.
8. Prophylactic antibiotics are not necessary initially unless large open wounds are present.
9. Seizures are treated with standard therapy.
10. Fractures should be reduced and splinted as appropriate.
11. Skin burns can be treated with silver sulfadiazine after cleaning.
12. It is appropriate to consult a general surgeon if there is evidence of systemic or deep tissue injury. These patients may require formal wound exploration, debridement, fasciotomy, and long-term care. Children with oral injuries should be evaluated by an ENT specialist or plastic surgeon. All pregnant patients should undergo obstetric consultation for admission and fetal monitoring. Patients with severe electrical injuries should be admitted to a regional burn or trauma center.
13. Table 127-2 summarizes admission criteria. Patients with an unclear history of exposure or degree of injury should be admitted.
14. Children with isolated oral injuries or isolated hand wounds usually can be discharged. Parents should be given instructions for controlling delayed labial artery bleeding.
15. Asymptomatic patients with household voltage exposure (110 to 220 V), a normal ECG, and a normal examination may be discharged.

LIGHTNING INJURIES

There are approximately 300 lightning injuries reported each year in the United States, with approximately 100 deaths. Unlike electrical injuries, extensive tissue damage and renal failure are rare, although as many as 75% of survivors sustain significant morbidity and permanent sequelae.

Clinical Features

Lightning injuries can vary in severity depending on the circumstances of the strike and range from minor injuries to cardiac arrest. Minor injuries produce a stunned patient. These people appear well. Their vital signs will be normal

---

TABLE 127-2 Indications for Admission for Patients with Electrical Injuries

High voltage >600 V

Symptoms suggestive of systemic injury
  Cardiovascular: chest pain, palpitations
  Neurologic: loss of consciousness, confusion, weakness, headache, paresthesias
  Respiratory: dyspnea
  Gastrointestinal: abdominal pain, vomiting

Evidence of neurologic or vascular injury to a digit or extremity

Burns with evidence of subcutaneous tissue damage

Dysrhythmia or abnormal electrocardiogram

Suspected foul play, abuse, suicidal intent, or unreliable social situation

High-risk exposures

Associated injuries requiring admission

Comorbid diseases (cardiac, renal, neurologic)

or they will exhibit a mild tachycardia or hypertension. They may have signs of confusion, amnesia, and short-term memory problems. Other symptoms include headache, muscle pain, paresthesias, and temporary visual or auditory problems. Most patients with minor lightning injuries have a gradual improvement and little long-term sequelae. Complications associated with lightning injuries are summarized in Table 127-3.

Diagnosis and Differential

The diagnosis of lightning injury is based on history and should be considered in a patient found unconscious or in arrest who was outside during appropriate weather conditions. Pupillary dilatation or anisocoria may occur and has no prognostic value. Ruptured tympanic membranes or fernlike erythematous skin markings should alert the physician to potential lightning injury. A careful examination should assess neurologic status, otologic and ophthalmologic injuries, and blunt trauma. Diagnostic tests should include an ECG, complete blood count, electrolytes, blood urea nitrogen, creatinine, urinalysis with myoglobin, and a CK-MB level. For patients with more severe injuries, head computed tomography, chest radiograph, and cervical spine films should be considered. Misdiagnoses include stroke or intracranial hemorrhage, seizure disorder, and cerebral, spinal cord, or other neurologic trauma.

Emergency Department Care and Disposition

Unlike other trauma, priority is given to people who appear dead when there are multiple victims. Aggressive resuscitation measures are indicated because

TABLE 127-3 Complications Associated with Lightning Injuries

System	Injury
Cardiovascular	Dysrhythmias (asystole, ventricular fibrillation/tachycardia, premature ventricular contractions), electrocardiographic changes, myocardial infarction (unusual)
Neurologic	(Immediate or delayed, permanent or transient); loss of consciousness, confusion, amnesia, intracranial hemorrhage, hemiplegia, amnesia, respiratory center paralysis, cerebral edema, neuritis, seizures, parkinsonian syndromes, cerebral infarction, myelopathy, progressive muscular atrophy, progressive cerebellar syndrome, transient paralysis, paresthesias, myelopathy, autonomic dysfunction
Cutaneous	Burns (first to third degree), scars, contractures
Ophthalmologic	Cataracts (often delayed), corneal lesions, uveitis, iridocyclitis, vitreous hemorrhage, macular degeneration, optic atrophy, diplopia, chorioretinitis, retinal detachment, hyphema
Otologic	Tympanic membrane rupture, temporary or permanent deafness, tinnitus, ataxia, vertigo, nystagmus
Renal	Myoglobinuria, hemoglobinuria, renal failure (rare)
Obstetric	Fetal death, placental abruption
Miscellaneous	Secondary blunt trauma, compartment syndrome, disseminated intravascular coagulation

survival has been reported after prolonged respiratory arrest. Spinal immobilization should be used in non-witnessed events or when there is potential spine injury. Continuous cardiac monitoring, pulse oximetry, noninvasive blood pressure monitoring, and at least 1 large-bore IV should be used. Hypotension is unexpected and should prompt investigation for hemorrhage. Treatment, particularly in moderate to severe cases, should include the following steps.

1. High-flow oxygen should be administered by face mask
2. Ventricular tachycardia or fibrillation and asystole should be treated with standard ACLS protocols.
3. Fluid resuscitation is usually unnecessary.
4. **Tetanus** prophylaxis should be given.
5. Seizures may be treated with standard therapy.
6. Fractures and dislocations should be reduced and splinted as appropriate. Extensive wound debridement is rarely necessary.
7. Those with moderate or severe injuries should be admitted to a critical care unit with appropriate consultation. Most patients with minor injuries should be admitted for close monitoring of cardiac and neurologic status. All pregnant patients should be admitted and undergo fetal monitoring.

For further reading in *Emergency Medicine: A Comprehensive Study Guide*, 6th ed., see Chap. 201, "Electrical Injuries," and Chap. 202, "Lightning Injuries," by Raymond M. Fish.

128 | Carbon Monoxide

Christian A. Tomaszewski

Carbon monoxide is a colorless, odorless, nonirritating gas that displaces oxygen from hemoglobin, resulting in early tissue hypoxia and delayed neurologic damage. Sources of exposure to carbon monoxide include the incomplete combustion of carbonaceous fuel (eg, gasoline, kerosene, natural gas, and charcoal) and the metabolism of methylene chloride (paint stripper). Background carboxyhemoglobin (COHb) levels in tobacco smokers can range as high as 10%.

Carbon monoxide causes symptoms acutely from a combination of poor oxygen delivery (carbon monoxide has more than 200 times greater affinity for hemoglobin than for oxygen) and binding to cytochrome Aa3, which impedes oxygen use at the cellular level within mitochondria. During resuscitation, ischemic tissue is reperfused, producing free radicals from leukocytes adherent to the brain microvasculature. The subsequent lipid peroxidation and release of excitatory neurotransmitters causes neuronal death.

CLINICAL FEATURES

Clinical symptoms and signs of carbon monoxide poisoning primarily relate to the cardiovascular and neurologic systems. Patients initially present with flulike symptoms: headache, dizziness, nausea, and vomiting. With increasing exposure, the patient may develop dyspnea, altered mental status, coma, seizures, and respiratory arrest. Cardiovascular signs and symptoms include chest pain from myocardial ischemia, palpitations from dysrhythmias, hypotension, and, ultimately, cardiac arrest. Patients occasionally may develop rhabdomyolysis and subsequent renal failure if unconscious for a prolonged period.

If patients survive the acute insult from carbon monoxide poisoning, they are still susceptible to secondary problems, primarily from the ischemic reperfusion injury. They may develop persistent or delayed neurologic sequelae resulting in deficiencies in learning and memory, chronic headaches, and, rarely, parkinsonism. Early predictors of such sequelae are alterations in mental status or cerebellar dysfunction (abnormal past-pointing or ataxia).

DIAGNOSIS AND DIFFERENTIAL

Any patient with flulike illness, particularly in winter with any carbonaceous heating source, should be considered for COHb determination. This can be done by co-oximeter on venous blood, even hours old, provided it has been drawn in a closed heparinized tube. Breath analysis also can be used for screening, although false positives may occur from ethanol. Although COHb levels confirm exposure, they do not correlate with symptoms or prognosis, in part because of variability in initial treatment with oxygen and delay to testing. In general, a level greater than 10% confirms poisoning in smokers, and a level greater than 5% confirms poisoning in a nonsmoker. Adjunctive testing may include other toxicologic assays and assessment of acid-base status by evaluating for lactic acidosis. It is important to note that pulse oximetry may be minimally depressed in patients with severely elevated COHb levels. Pulse oximetry, although useful if abnormal, overestimates the oxygen saturation of hemoglobin. It confuses COHb for oxyhemoglobin, thus providing false reassurance

In seriously ill patients, arterial blood gas analysis may be useful to determine base deficit. In susceptible patients complaining of chest pain or who may be unconscious, electrocardiogram and cardiac enzyme determinations are recommended. Chest radiographs are generally obtained for smoke inhalation victims. In comatose patients with poor prognosis, computed tomography or magnetic resonance imaging of the brain may identify generalized cerebral edema or specific lesions, particularly infarcts of the globus pallidus.

Although COHb may help confirm exposure, careful neurologic examination will help determine the seriousness of poisoning and the potential need for hyperbaric oxygen therapy. A bedside Mini-Mental Status Examination may demonstrate memory and learning deficits. In addition, patients may have cerebellar dysfunction manifested by abnormal past-pointing or ataxia.

The differential diagnosis for carbon monoxide poisoning is extremely broad because of the wide spectrum of disease entities associated with dizziness, headache, or nausea. The differential most commonly includes flulike illness or gastroenteritis. A variety of toxins, infectious agents, and cardiac diseases may account for the signs and symptoms of carbon monoxide poisoning. Smoke inhalation victims, particularly if enclosed during exposure, should be evaluated specifically for carbon monoxide poisoning.

EMERGENCY DEPARTMENT CARE AND DISPOSITION

1. Initially, patients must be removed from the source of exposure, and immediate attention should focus on the airway, breathing, and circulation. **High-flow 100% oxygen** should be administered with a tightly fitting mask and reservoir; cardiac monitoring and intravenous access should be established. Oxygen therapy should be continued until the patient becomes asymptomatic.
2. **Hyperbaric oxygen therapy** is indicated for severe poisoning based on clinical findings and the COHb level (Table 128-1). The best predictors of delayed or persistent neurologic sequelae and, therefore, the need for hyperbaric oxygen therapy are loss of consciousness and cerebellar dysfunction. COHb levels over 25% and a base deficit greater than 2 mmol/L are also worrisome. The goals of treatment are amelioration of the acute event

TABLE 128-1 Indications for Hyperbaric Oxygen Treatment Within 24 Hours of Acute Carbon Monoxide Poisoning

Definite indication	Relative indication
Abnormal neurologic examination (eg, altered mental status, coma)	Persistent neurologic symptoms (eg, headache or dizziness) after 4 h of 100% normobaric oxygen
Syncope	Carboxyhemoglobin level >25%
Seizure	Persistent metabolic acidosis (base deficit >2 mmol/L)
Cerebellar dysfunction (eg, abnormal past-pointing, ataxia)	Pregnancy (particularly if symptomatic with level elevated >10% or fetal distress)
	Myocardial ischemia

and, more importantly, prevention of delayed neuropsychiatric sequelae. Hyperbaric oxygen therapy should be carefully considered, especially for patients at the extremes of age and in pregnancy, which is not a contraindication to treatment.

For further reading in *Emergency Medicine: A Comprehensive Study Guide,* 6th ed., see Chap. 203, "Carbon Monoxide Poisoning," by Keith W. Van Meter.

Poisonous Plants and Mushrooms

Sandra L. Najarian

Plants and mushrooms have evolved a diverse array of metabolites that are harmful to humans. Chemicals applied to cultivated plants also may cause toxicity. Mushroom ingestion can lead to morbidity and even mortality among amateur foragers and recreational drug users, with *Amanita* and *Gyromitra* species responsible for most fatalities.

CLINICAL FEATURES

Signs and symptoms of plant toxicity are highly variable, often depending on which part of the plant is ingested or contacted. In most cases, patients are asymptomatic or have mild gastrointestinal (GI) symptoms. Nausea, vomiting, hematemesis, abdominal pain, and diarrhea (at times bloody) may follow ingestion of *Acted* (baneberry), *Abrus*, aloe, *Cicuta macualta* (water hemlock), *Conium* (poison hemlock), *Convallaria* (lily of the valley), daphne, *Euphorbia* (poinsettia), *Ilex* (holly), *Phytolacca* (pokeweed), rhododendron, *Ricinus*, *Solanum* (nightshades), and *Taxus* (yews). Fatalities occur from electrolyte abnormalities.

Direct irritation and chemical burns to the oropharynx have been reported after ingestion of *Actaea*, *Abrus* (rosary pea), *Capsicum* (ornamental peppers), daphne, *Dieffenbachia*, and rhododendron. *Capsicum*, *Laportea*, toxidendron, and *Urtica* also can cause a contact dermatitis. Cardiovascular symptoms, including hypotension, dysrhythmias, and conduction defects, have been reported after ingestion of *Convallaria*, *Taxus*, rhododendron, and oleander and may be life threatening.

Ingestion of *Datura* (jimson weed) seeds or smoking its leaves may cause hallucinations. These can be attributed to the plant's anticholinergic properties. Hallucinations have been reported with *Actaea* ingestion. Seizures may be seen after ingestion of *Conium*, *Actaea*, and *Ricinus*. Amygdalin, found in the pits of peaches, apricots, pear, crab apple and hydrangea, is metabolized to hydrocyanic acid and can lead to acute cyanide poisoning if ingested in sufficient quantities.

Mushroom poisoning can be classified according to clinical toxicity and onset of symptoms. Early toxicity (within 1 hour of ingestion) generally indicates a benign course. Delayed toxicity (longer than 6 hours) suggests a more toxic ingestion, which can lead to hepatic failure, renal failure, and even death (Table 129-1).

DIAGNOSIS AND DIFFERENTIAL

Diagnosis of plant and mushroom poisoning is mainly clinical. Most patients are asymptomatic or have mild GI symptoms that might be attributed to gastroenteritis. Patients at risk should be routinely asked about plant or mushroom ingestion. The type and quantity consumed should be ascertained. The time between ingestion and onset of symptoms should be determined. This is most important in mushroom poisoning.

TABLE 129-1 Mushrooms: Symptoms, Toxicity, and Treatment

Symptoms	Mushrooms	Toxicity	Treatment
Gastrointestinal symptoms Onset <2 h	Chlorophyllum molybdites Omphalotus illudens Cantharellus cibarius Amanita caesarea	Nausea, vomiting, diarrhea (occasional bloody) Initial: nausea, vomiting, diarrhea	IV hydration Antiemetics IV hydration, glucose, monitor, AST, ALT, PT, ALT, PT, PTT, bilirubin, BUN, creatinine
Onset 6–24 h	Gyromitra esculenta: fall season Amanita phalloides, Amanita verna, and Amanita virosa: spring season	Day 2: rise in AST, ALT Day 3: hepatic failure	For Amanita: activated charcoal Penicillin G 300,000–1,000 000 U/(kg · d) Silymarin 20–40 mg/(kg · d) Consider cimetidine 4–10 g/d Hyperbaric oxygen
Muscarinic (SLUDGE) syndrome Onset <30 min	Inocybe Clitocybe	Salivation, lacrimation, diarrhea, gastrointestinal distress, emesis	Supportive atropine 0.01 mg/kg repeated as needed for severe secretions
CNS excitement Onset <30 min	Amanita muscaria Amanita pantherina	Intoxication, dizziness, ataxia, visual disturbances, seizures, tachycardia, hypertension, warm dry skin, dry mouth, mydriasis (anticholinergic effects)	Supportive sedation with phenobarbital 30 mg IV or diazepam 2–5 mg IV as needed for adults
Hallucinations Onset <30 min	Psilocybe Gymnopilus	Visual hallucinations, ataxia	Supportive sedation with phenobarbital 0.5 mg/kg or, for adults, 30–60 mg IV, or diazepam 0.1 mg/kg or 5 mg IV for adults
Disulfiram 2–72 h after mushroom, and <30 min after alcohol	Coprinus	Headache, flushing, tachycardia, hyperventilation, shortness of breath, palpitations	Supportive IV hydration Propranolol for supraventricular tachycardia Norepinephrine for refractory hypotension

Key: ALT = alanine aminotransferase, AST = aspartate aminotransferase, BUN = blood urea nitrogen, CNS = central nervous system, IV = intravenous, PT = prothrombin time, PTT = partial thromboplastin time, SLUDGE syndrome = salivation, lacrimation, urination, defecation, gastrointestinal hypermotility, and emesis.

Physical examination should include mental status assessment and hydration status. It is important to search for evidence of cholinergic, anticholinergic, or sympathetic nervous system stimulation. The patient's pharynx and skin should be examined for signs of irritation. Any jaundice should be noted. A complete cardiopulmonary examination is important, especially in those individuals at risk for arrhythmias or cardiac conduction defects.

Laboratory studies are rarely helpful in identifying the type of plant ingested and should be used only if clinically indicated. With mushroom poisonings, however, laboratory studies may have a higher yield and should include a complete blood count, electrolytes, blood urea nitrogen, creatinine, glucose level, and urinalysis. If symptoms are suggestive of ingestion of a cytotoxic mushroom, serum amylase, liver function tests, and coagulation panel should be obtained. An electrocardiogram is appropriate for patients with hemodynamic compromise. If available, a sample of the mushroom or plant should be sent to a botanist or mycologist for identification.

EMERGENCY DEPARTMENT CARE AND DISPOSITION

1. Initial treatment is mainly supportive. Airway management, ventilation, and fluid resuscitation with isotonic saline take priority. A fingerstick glucose level should be obtained in any patient with altered mental status. Standard cooling measures for hyperthermia should be used.
2. **Benzodiazepines** (lorazepam 2 mg intravenously) should be administered to control seizures and agitation.
3. Any acid-base and electrolyte abnormalities should be corrected.
4. The GI tract should be decontaminated. **Activated charcoal** (1 g/kg orally or per nasogastric tube) should be administered with a cathartic such as sorbitol. Consideration should be given to **whole bowel irrigation** (0.5 to 2 L/h of GoLYTELY orally or per nasogastric tube) in a patient suspected of ingesting a cytotoxic mushroom and presenting within 24 hours. Table 129-1 reviews treatment principles for mushroom toxicity.
5. Those patients with early onset of GI, neurologic, or muscarinic symptoms are treated with supportive therapy.
6. Those patients with delayed onset of symptoms or with refractory symptoms should be admitted and monitored for at least 48 hours for the development of hepatic or renal failure. The use of hemodialysis and charcoal hemoperfusion in treating amatoxin poisoning has questionable benefit. **Pyridoxine** (25 mg/kg intravenously over 15 to 30 minutes) may reverse the neurologic toxicity in gyromitrin poisoning but generally has no effect on the development or course of hepatic failure.
7. Patients may be discharged if free of symptoms after 4 to 6 hours of observation or treatment. They should be instructed to return at once if they develop vomiting, abdominal pain, diarrhea, or hallucinations.

For further reading in *Emergency Medicine: A Comprehensive Study Guide,* 6th ed., see Chap. 204, "Mushroom Poisoning," by Sandra M. Schneider and Anne Brayer; and Chap. 205, "Poisonous Plants," by Mark A Hostetler and Sandra M. Schneider.

14 | ENDOCRINE EMERGENCIES

130 | Diabetic Emergencies
Michael P. Kefer

HYPOGLYCEMIA

Glucose is the main energy source of the brain. Severe hypoglycemia can cause brain damage or death. Diabetics on insulin or oral hypoglycemic therapy are especially at risk. Also at risk are patients with alcoholism, sepsis, adrenal insufficiency, hypothyroidism, or malnutrition.

Hypoglycemic agents are the mainstays of treatment for diabetics. Overdose of these agents, intentional or accidental, is a common cause of hypoglycemia. Long-acting forms of insulin and the sulfonylureas have long half-lives that can lead to recurrent episodes of hypoglycemia.

Many medications have been recently introduced for managing diabetic patients. Repaglinide and nateglinide are non-sulfonylurea secretagogs that can cause hypoglycemia. Metformin (a biguanide), rosiglitazone and pioglitazone (thiazolidinediones), and acarbose and miglitol (α-glucosidase inhibitors) are not associated with hypoglycemia.

Clinical Features

Typical symptoms of hypoglycemia include sweating, shakiness, anxiety, nausea, dizziness, confusion, slurred speech, blurred vision, headache, lethargy, and coma. Neurologic manifestations are cranial nerve palsies, hemiplegia, seizure, and decerebrate posturing.

Diagnosis and Differential

The actual blood glucose level that defines hypoglycemia is arbitrary. Some people with low glucose levels are asymptomatic, and some with normal levels are symptomatic. Therefore, the diagnosis is based on the glucose level in conjunction with the clinical presentation. The history usually gives important clues to the cause of hypoglycemia. For example, consider the patient who presents with hypoglycemia and depression that is, or has a family member, being treated with an oral hypoglycemic agent. Unsuspected hypoglycemia easily can be misdiagnosed as a primary neurologic, psychiatric, or cardiovascular condition.

Emergency Department Care and Disposition

1. Treatment is glucose administration, orally or intravenously (IV), as the patient's condition warrants. Initially, **dextrose** 1 g/kg IV as a 50% dextrose solution is administered. A continuous infusion of a 10% dextrose solution may be required to maintain the blood glucose above 100 mg/dL.
2. If there is any concern of malnutrition, **thiamine** 100 mg IV should be administered before giving glucose to prevent precipitation of Wernicke encephalopathy.
3. If there is not a prompt response to glucose infusion, or if adrenal insufficiency is suspected, **hydrocortisone** 100 to 200 mg IV should be administered. If there is difficulty gaining IV access, **glucagon** 1 mg can be administered intramuscularly (IM) or subcutaneously (SC).
4. Refractory hypoglycemia secondary to the sulfonylureas may respond to the somatostatin analog **octreotide** 50 to 125 μg SC.

5. Factors considered in determining disposition include the patient's response to treatment, cause of hypoglycemia, comorbid conditions, and social situation. Most diabetics with uncomplicated insulin reactions respond rapidly. They can be discharged with instructions to continue oral intake of carbohydrates and closely monitor their finger stick glucose. All patients with sulfonylurea-induced hypoglycemia should be admitted due to the prolonged half-life and, hence, risk of recurrence from these agents.

DIABETIC KETOACIDOSIS

Diabetic ketoacidosis (DKA) results from a relative insulin deficiency and counterregulatory hormone excess causing hyperglycemia and ketonemia. DKA is precipitated by noncompliance with insulin therapy, infection, stroke, myocardial infarction, trauma, pregnancy, and many other physiologic stresses. DKA occurs in type 1 and type 2 diabetics.

Clinical Features

Clinical manifestations are directly related to metabolic derangements. Hyperglycemia causes an osmotic diuresis with dehydration, hypotension, and tachycardia. Ketonemia causes an acidosis with myocardial depression, vasodilation, and compensatory Kussmaul respiration. Nausea, vomiting, and abdominal pain are also common. Inappropriate normothermia is seen clinically so infection must be considered even in the absence of fever.

Diagnosis and Differential

Laboratory investigation shows decreased levels of sodium, chloride, calcium, phosphorus, and magnesium from osmotic diuresis. Serum and urine glucose and ketones are elevated. Pseudohyponatremia is common; for each 100 mg/dL increase in blood glucose, the sodium decreases by 1.6 mEq/L. Serum potassium may be low, from osmotic diuresis and vomiting, normal, or high, from acidosis. In acidosis, potassium is driven extracellularly. Therefore, the acidotic patient with normal or low potassium has marked depletion of total body potassium.

An anion-gap metabolic acidosis results from formation of ketone bodies. Acetone, formed from oxidation of ketone bodies, causes the characteristic fruity odor of the patient's breath.

Diagnosis of DKA is based on clinical presentation and laboratory values of a glucose above 250 mg/dL, bicarbonate below 15 mEq/L, pH below 7.3, and a moderate ketonemia.

The differential diagnosis includes other causes of an anion-gap metabolic acidosis, recalled by the acronym MUDPILES (see Table 102-1). Hypoglycemia and hyperosmolar hyperglycemic state also should be considered.

In DKA, formation of β-hydroxybutyrate from acetoacetate is favored. Therefore, the patient may have low levels of acetoacetate and high levels of β-hydroxybutyrate. If the nitroprusside test is used to detect serum or urine ketones, it may be falsely low or negative because it only detects acetoacetate, not β-hydroxybutyrate.

Basic laboratory investigation consists of serum glucose, electrolytes, blood urea nitrogen, creatinine, phosphorus, magnesium, complete blood count, urinalysis (and pregnancy, if indicated), electrocardiogram, and chest radiograph to assess the severity of DKA and search for the underlying cause.

Emergency Department Care and Disposition

The goal of treatment is to correct the volume deficit, acid-base imbalance, and electrolyte abnormalities, administer insulin, and treat the underlying cause.

1. **Isotonic fluid resuscitation** is the most important initial step to restore intravascular volume and tissue perfusion. The average patient in DKA has a body water deficit of 5 to 10 L. The first liter is administered over 30 to 60 minutes. Once intravascular volume is restored, or if the serum sodium is above 155 mEq/L, hypotonic solution is infused to provide free water for intracellular volume replacement. Patients with heart disease may need invasive monitoring to avoid congestive heart failure.

2. **Insulin** is required to shut off ketosis and resume glucose utilization. Insulin should be administered by continuous infusion. This allows close control of effect, as compared with IM or SC administration, in which absorption may be erratic or delayed in an unstable patient. The half-life of regular insulin is 5 minutes when administered IV and 2 hours when administered IM or SC. Initiating a **continuous infusion of insulin** at 0.1 U/kg/h is recommended. A loading dose of 0.1 U/kg IV is optional. If there is no response within the first hour of treatment, insulin resistance is suggested, and the infusion rate is doubled each hour until a response is obtained. Hyperglycemia is controlled much more rapidly with insulin than is ketoacidosis. To reverse ketoacidosis, insulin treatment must continue despite decreasing serum glucose. Therefore, to prevent hypoglycemia, glucose infusion will be necessary when the serum glucose falls below 300 mg/dL.

3. **Potassium** is administered to maintain normal serum levels. Upon initiating treatment for DKA, potassium levels will fall due to dilution from volume replacement, correction of acidosis, renal excretion, and the insulin effect of driving potassium intracellularly. To avoid the dangerous effects of hypokalemia, if the potassium level is below 3.3 mEq/L, potassium replacement should begin 30 minutes before insulin is administered and immediately if the level is between 3.3 and 5 mEq/L and urine output is adequate. To avoid the dangerous effects of hyperkalemia, potassium should not be administered until the level is below 5 mEq/L. Potassium chloride 10 to 20 mEq may be added to each liter of IV fluid, as required, by close monitoring of serum potassium. Potassium phosphate 10 to 20 mEq may be used if phosphorus supplementation is also required.

4. **Phosphorus** has an important role in energy production (adenosine triphosphate), oxygen delivery (2,3–diphosphoglycerate [DPG]), and enzymatic reactions. Acute deficiency has been associated with all types of muscle dysfunction. Phosphorus replacement is recommended if the serum level is below 1 mg/dL.

5. **Magnesium** is administered if levels are low or the patient has symptoms of hypomagnesemia.

6. Bicarbonate therapy remains controversial as to when the benefits of correcting the effects of acidosis (vasodilation, depression of cardiac contractility and respiration, and central nervous system depression) outweigh the risk of bicarbonate treatment (paradoxical cerebrospinal fluid acidosis, hypokalemia, impaired oxyhemoglobin dissociation, rebound alkalosis, and sodium overload). This therapy is recommended as a last resort in the face of severe acidosis.

7. The blood glucose, anion gap, potassium, and bicarbonate should be monitored hourly until recovery is well established.

All patients on an insulin infusion will require close monitoring to avoid complications of treatment. Cerebral edema occurs predominately in children. It has been associated with rehydration rates exceeding 50 mL/kg in the first 4 hours of treatment, so this rate serves as a guideline. It tends to develop 4 to 12 hours into treatment and typically manifests as deterioration in neurologic status. Treatment with mannitol 1 g/kg should be initiated before the diagnosis is confirmed by computed tomography.

HYPEROSMOLAR HYPERGLYCEMIC STATE

Hyperosmolar hyperglycemic state (HHS) is preferred terminology over non-ketotic hyperosmolar coma. HHS is distinguished from DKA by the absence of significant ketosis. It is a relatively common presentation of new onset diabetes. Similar to DKA, precipitating factors include noncompliance, myocardial infarction, stroke, infection, pregnancy, and trauma. Drugs such as thiazide diuretics, β-blockers, and steroids also predispose to this condition.

Clinical Features

The typical patient is elderly with type 2 diabetes, presents with complaints of weakness or mental status changes, and has preexisting renal or heart disease. Because metabolic changes progress slowly, symptoms often signal advanced HHS.

Physical examination shows signs of dehydration with orthostasis, dry skin and mucous membranes, and altered mental status. Kussmaul respiration and the smell of acetone on the breath are not present. Mental status changes range from confusion to coma. Focal deficits and focal or generalized seizures also occur.

Diagnosis and Differential

Diagnosis is based on clinical and laboratory findings. HHS is distinguished from DKA by laboratory investigation. Typically, ketones are absent, the degree of acidosis is less, and the degree of hyperglycemia is marked.

Defining laboratory parameters are a serum glucose above 600 mg/dL, serum osmolality above 315 mOsm/kg, pH above 7.3, and negative or mildly elevated ketones. Pseudohyponatremia is more prominent than in DKA. Hypovolemia from osmotic diuresis initially causes a contraction metabolic alkalosis. With continued volume loss, a metabolic acidosis develops from azotemia and lactic acidosis. Osmotic diuresis also causes low levels of sodium, potassium, chloride, calcium, phosphorus, and magnesium.

Emergency Department Care and Disposition

Therapy consists of correcting the volume deficit, electrolyte imbalance, and hyperosmolality and treating the underlying cause.

1. **Isotonic 0.9 normal saline** is used initially to restore intravascular volume. This is followed by hypotonic 0.45 normal saline to provide free water to restore intracellular volume. The average fluid deficit is 8 to 12 L. One half the deficit is replaced over 12 hours, and the other one half over the next 24 hours. Particularly in children, a rehydration rate slower than 50 mL/kg in the first 4 hours is suggested to avoid cerebral edema.
2. Potassium, magnesium, and phosphorus replacement principles are identical to those of DKA discussed previously.

3. An **insulin drip** 0.1 U/kg/h can be initiated. In less severe cases, the patient will correct with fluids alone or may require only 1 to 2 bolus doses of regular insulin 0.1 U/kg in conjunction with fluid therapy.

For further reading in *Emergency Medicine: A Comprehensive Study Guide*, 6th ed., see Chap. 210, "Hypoglycemia," by William Brady and Richard A. Harrigan; Chap. 211, "Diabetic Ketoacidosis," by Michael E. Chansky and Cary Lubilin; and Chap. 214, "Hyperosmolar Hyperglycemic State," by Charles S. Graffeo.

| Alcoholic Ketoacidosis

Michael P. Kefer

Alcoholic ketoacidosis results from heavy alcohol intake, either acute or chronic, and minimal or no food intake. Alcohol and body fat metabolism generate ketoacids, with a resultant anion-gap metabolic acidosis.

CLINICAL FEATURES

The patient with alcoholic ketoacidosis typically presents with complaints of nausea, vomiting, orthostasis, and abdominal pain 24 to 72 hours after the last alcohol intake. Physical examination shows the patient to be acutely ill and dehydrated with a tender abdomen. Abdominal tenderness is typically diffuse and nonspecific or is a result of other causes associated with the use of alcohol, such as gastritis, hepatitis, or pancreatitis. The presentation may be confounded by other complications of alcoholism, such as infection or alcohol withdrawal.

DIAGNOSIS AND DIFFERENTIAL

Laboratory investigation shows an anion-gap ($Na^+ - [Cl^- + HCO3^-]$ $>12 \pm 4$ mEq/L) metabolic acidosis. However, the serum pH may be low, normal, or high, because these patients often have mixed acid–base disorders, such as a metabolic acidosis from alcoholic ketoacidosis and a metabolic alkalosis from vomiting and volume depletion. Blood glucose ranges from low to mildly elevated. The alcohol level is usually low or 0 because vomiting and abdominal pain limit intake. Serum ketones, acetoacetate and β-hydroxybutyrate, are elevated. Serum and urine ketones are semiquantitatively measured by the nitroprusside test that detects acetoacetate but not β-hydroxybutyrate. Although ketones are usually detected in significant amounts, the redox state may be such that most or all acetoacetate is reduced to β-hydroxybutyrate resulting in a false negative or falsely low estimate of the severity of ketoacidosis. If the diagnosis is unclear, serum levels of acetoacetate and β-hydroxybutyrate can be measured directly.

The diagnosis of alcoholic ketoacidosis is established in the patient with a history of recent heavy alcohol consumption, decreased food intake, vomiting, abdominal pain, and laboratory findings of an anion-gap metabolic acidosis, a positive nitroprusside test for ketones, and a low to mildly elevated glucose.

The differential diagnosis includes other causes of an anion-gap metabolic acidosis, commonly recalled by the acronym MUDPILES (see Table 102-1). These can be excluded by clinical and laboratory data.

EMERGENCY DEPARTMENT CARE AND DISPOSITION

1. Treatment of alcoholic ketoacidosis consists of intravenous infusion of **5% dextrose in normal saline.** The crystalloid solution restores intravascular volume. Glucose administration stimulates insulin release, which inhibits ketosis. Unlike treatment for diabetic ketoacidosis, insulin administration is not necessary because endogenous insulin secretion occurs normally with restoration of volume and glucose administration.

2. Administration of **thiamine** 50 to 100 mg intravenously is recommended before glucose administration to prevent precipitation of Wernicke disease.
3. Other electrolytes and vitamins should be supplemented as the condition warrants.
4. Treatment should be continued until the acidosis is reversed, which is usually within 12 to 18 hours, and the patient is tolerating oral intake.

For further reading in *Emergency Medicine: A Comprehensive Study Guide,* 6th ed., see Chap. 213, "Alcoholic Ketoacidosis," by William A. Woods and Debra G. Perina.

132 | Thyroid Disease Emergencies

Matthew A. Bridges

THYROID STORM

Thyroid storm is a rare, life-threatening condition due to hyperthyroidism. It is seen most often in patients with antecedent Graves disease and is usually precipitated by infection or some other stressful event.

Clinical Features

The signs and symptoms associated with thyroid storm are related to enhanced sympathetic nervous system activity. The most common signs are fever, tachycardia, altered mental status, and diaphoresis. Clues to the diagnosis include a history of hyperthyroidism, exophthalmos, a widened pulse pressure, and a palpable goiter. Central nervous system disturbances are common and include confusion, delirium, seizure, and coma. Cardiovascular abnormalities are often present, with sinus tachycardia being the most common; other dysrhythmias include atrial fibrillation and premature ventricular contractions. Patients may present with signs and symptoms of congestive heart failure. Gastrointestinal symptoms, such as diarrhea and hyper-defecation, occur in most patients. Apathetic thyrotoxicosis is a distinct presentation seen in elderly patients, in which the characteristic symptoms are absent, and lethargy, slowed mentation, and apathetic facies are seen. Goiter, weight loss, and proximal muscle weakness are present. Atrial fibrillation and congestive heart failure may occur.

Diagnosis and Differential

Thyroid storm is a clinical diagnosis because laboratory tests do not help to distinguish it from thyrotoxicosis. Diagnostic criteria include fever; tachycardia out of proportion to fever; dysfunction of the central nervous system, cardiovascular, and/or gastrointestinal systems; and exaggerated peripheral manifestations of thyrotoxicosis. In this clinical setting, an elevated L-thyroxine level (T_4) and a suppressed thyroid-stimulating hormone (TSH) level confirm the diagnosis. The differential diagnosis includes sepsis, other causes of congestive heart failure, stroke, complications of diabetes (eg, diabetic ketoacidosis or hypoglycemia), heat stroke, delirium tremens, malignant hyperthermia, neuroleptic malignant syndrome, pheochromocytoma, medication withdrawal, and sympathomimetic drug overdose. Many of these entities may coincide with or precipitate thyroid storm, thus complicating the diagnosis.

Emergency Department Care and Disposition

The importance of early treatment of thyroid storm based on clinical suspicion must be emphasized. Treatment can be divided into 5 areas: general supportive care, inhibition of thyroid hormone synthesis, retardation of thyroid hormone release, blockade of peripheral thyroid hormone effects, and identification and treatment of precipitating events.

1. Airway stabilization, supplemental oxygen, intravenous fluids, and cardiac monitoring are indicated.

TABLE 132-1 Drug Treatment of Thyroid Storm

Decrease de nova synthesis	
Propylthiouracil	600–1,000 mg PO initially, followed by 200–250 mg q4 h
Methimazole	40 mg PO initial dose, then 25 mg PO q6 h
Prevent release of hormone (after synthesis blockade has been initiated)	
Iodine	Iapanoic acid (Telepaque) 1 g IV q8 h for the first 24 h, then 500 mg IV bid
	Potassium iodide 5 drops PO q6 h
	Lugol solution 8–10 drops PO q6 h
Lithium carbonate	800–1200 mg PO daily
Prevent peripheral effects	
β-blockade	Propranolol (IV) titrate 1–2 mg q5 min PRN (may need 240–480 mg PO daily)
	Esmolol (IV) 500 μg/kg bolus, then 50–200 μg/kg/min maintenance
Guanethidine	30–40 mg PO q6 h
Reserpine	2.5–5 mg IM q4–6 h
Other considerations	
Corticosteroids	Hydrocortisone 100 mg IV q8 h
	Dexamethasone 2 mg IV q6 h
Antipyretics	Cooling blanket
	Acetaminophen 650 mg PO q4 h

Key: bid = twice daily, IM = intramuscularly, IV = intravenously, PO = orally.

2. The pharmacologic treatment of thyroid storm is summarized in Table 132-1.
3. Appropriate cultures and antibiotics may be indicated.
4. All patients should be monitored closely and admitted to the intensive care unit.

HYPOTHYROIDISM AND MYXEDEMA COMA

Myxedema coma is a rare, life-threatening expression of severe hypothyroidism. It is seen most often during the winter months in elderly women with undiagnosed or under-treated hypothyroidism. Precipitating events include infection, congestive heart failure, drugs, trauma, and exposure to a cold environment.

Clinical Features

The typical symptoms of hypothyroidism include fatigue, weakness, cold intolerance, constipation, weight gain, and deepening of the voice. Cutaneous signs include dry, scaly, yellow skin; nonpitting, waxy edema of the face and extremities (myxedema); and thinning eyebrows. Cardiac findings include bradycardia, enlarged heart, and low-voltage electrocardiogram. Paresthesia, ataxia, and prolongation of the deep tendon reflexes are characteristic neurologic findings. A thyroidectomy scar may be present, but a goiter is uncommon. The patient with myxedema coma will present with several additional findings: hypothermia, altered mental status, hyponatremia, hypoglycemia, hypotension, and bradycardia. Respiratory failure with hypoventilation, hypercapnia, and hypoxia is common. Delusions and psychosis (myxedema madness) may occur.

Diagnosis and Differential

The diagnosis of myxedema coma must be suspected based on the clinical presentation and characteristic laboratory abnormalities previously mentioned. Confirmatory thyroid tests typically will demonstrate a low free T_4 level and elevated TSH level. Arterial blood gases, chest radiograph, electrocardiogram, and serum electrolytes may prove useful. The patient's core temperature will be low. The differential diagnosis includes coma secondary to respiratory failure, hyponatremia, hypothermia, congestive heart failure, stroke, and drug overdose.

Emergency Department Care and Disposition

1. Airway stabilization and establishment of adequate oxygenation and ventilation are vital. Cardiovascular status should be supported and monitored.
2. Hypothermic patients should be rewarmed gradually. Hyponatremia typically responds to fluid restriction but may require **hypertonic saline solution** and furosemide in severe cases. Vasopressors are usually ineffective in this setting and should be used only for severe hypotension. Sedating drugs, such as phenothiazine, generally should be avoided.
3. Precipitating causes should be sought and treated. Antibiotics are indicated for underlying infection. In addition, **hydrocortisone** 100 mg intravenously (IV) every 8 hours should be administered.
4. Thyroid hormone is the most specific therapy for myxedema coma. Intravenous levothyroxine in an initial dose of 300 to 500 μg should be given by slow IV infusion; this is followed by 50 to 100 μg IV daily. Alternative treatment consists of **L-triiodothyronine** 25 μg IV or orally every 8 hours. L-triiodothyronine dosage should be halved in patients with cardiovascular disease.
5. Patients should be admitted to a monitored setting. Overall clinical improvement should be seen in 24 to 36 hours with either regimen.

For further reading in *Emergency Medicine: A Comprehensive Study Guide*, 6th ed., see Chap. 215, "Hyperthyroidism and Thyroid Storm," and Chap. 216, "Hypothyroidism and Myxedema Coma," by Horace K. Liang.

133 | Adrenal Insufficiency and Adrenal Crisis

Michael P. Kefer

Adrenal insufficiency may be acute or chronic, and results when the physiologic demand for glucocorticoids and mineralocorticoids exceeds the supply from the adrenal cortex. The hypothalamus secretes corticotropin-releasing factor, which stimulates the pituitary to secrete adrenocorticotrophin hormone (ACTH) and associated melanocyte-stimulating hormone (MSH). ACTH stimulates the adrenal cortex to secrete cortisol (and aldosterone to a minor degree). Cortisol has negative feedback on the pituitary to inhibit secretion of ACTH and MSH. Adrenal insufficiency is described as primary, secondary, or tertiary based on whether the insufficiency occurs at the level of the adrenal glands, pituitary, or hypothalamus, respectively. The adrenal cortex as a source of androgens is much more important in women than in men.

CLINICAL FEATURES

Clinical features of adrenal insufficiency vary in number and severity depending on the etiology and duration of onset. Manifestations of primary adrenal insufficiency are due to cortisol and aldosterone deficiencies and include weakness, dehydration, hypotension, anorexia, nausea, vomiting, weight loss, and abdominal pain. Hyperpigmentation of exposed and unexposed skin and mucous membrane occurs as a result of uninhibited MSH secretion in conjunction with ACTH. Androgen deficiency in women manifests as thinning of pubic and axillary hair.

Secondary and tertiary adrenal insufficiencies result from inadequate secretion of ACTH and corticotropin-releasing factor, respectively, with resultant cortisol deficiency. Aldosterone levels are not significantly affected because of regulation through the renin–angiotensin system. Therefore, hyperpigmentation and hyperkalemia are not seen.

Adrenal crisis is the acute, life-threatening form of adrenal insufficiency. Clinical features are as described above, but to the extreme and accompanied by shock and altered mental status.

DIAGNOSIS AND DIFFERENTIAL

The diagnosis of adrenal insufficiency may be difficult because the clinical features are nonspecific. The diagnosis can be made in the emergency department based on the presence of the clinical features and performing a cosyntropin (synthetic ACTH) stimulation test. This test is performed by drawing a baseline cortisol level and then administering cosyntropin 0.25 mg intramuscularly or intravenously (IV). After 60 minutes, a repeat cortisol level is drawn and should be double the baseline level. In primary adrenal insufficiency, the diseased adrenal cortex does not respond to ACTH and will not increase the cortisol level. In secondary and tertiary adrenal insufficiencies, the adrenal cortex does respond to ACTH and will increase the cortisol level.

For primary adrenal insufficiency, laboratory investigation shows different degrees of hyponatremia, hyperkalemia, hypoglycemia, anemia, metabolic

617

acidosis, and prerenal azotemia. All patients with adrenal insufficiency have low plasma cortisol levels.

The most common cause of adrenal insufficiency and adrenal crisis is adrenal suppression from prolonged steroid use with abrupt steroid withdrawal or exposure to increased physiologic stress such as injury, illness, or surgery. Adrenal suppression can occur with steroids given by any route (oral, topical, intrathecal, or inhaled). In general, there is no adrenal suppression regardless of the daily dose of steroids if the duration of use is shorter than 3 weeks and regardless of duration of use if the daily dose does not exceed 5 mg. It may take up to 1 year for the hypothalamic-pituitary-adrenal axis to recover after prolonged suppression with steroid treatment.

Other causes of adrenal insufficiency include autoimmune, idiopathic, metastatic cancer, sarcoidosis, infection (most commonly with tuberculosis or the human immunodeficiency virus), ketoconazole use, bilateral adrenal hemorrhage associated with meningococcemia (Waterhouse-Friderichsen syndrome) or heparin therapy, and pituitary hemorrhage from head trauma or postpartum necrosis (Sheehan syndrome).

EMERGENCY DEPARTMENT CARE AND DISPOSITION

1. Outpatient management of stable patients with known or suspected adrenal insufficiency consists of steroid replacement therapy and is best managed by the consultant.
2. Treatment of adrenal crisis includes resuscitation with crystalloid fluids, glucocorticoids, and mineralocorticoids to correct volume, glucose, and sodium deficits. **5% dextrose in normal saline** is the initial fluid of choice. **Hydrocortisone** 100 to 300 mg IV every 6 to 8 hours provides adequate glucocorticoid and mineralocorticoid activities. If a cosyntropin stimulation test is being performed, then dexamethasone 4 mg IV should be substituted for hydrocortisone to avoid a false positive test. In refractory cases, additional hydrocortisone or vasopressors may be necessary.

For further reading in *Emergency Medicine: A Comprehensive Study Guide,* 6th ed., see Chap. 217, "Adrenal Insufficiency," by C. N. Shoenfeld.

15 | HEMATOLOGIC AND ONCOLOGIC EMERGENCIES

134 | Evaluation of Anemia and the Bleeding Patient

Sandra L. Najarian

Anemia may be chronic and unrelated to the chief complaint, or it may result from acute blood loss as seen in trauma, gastrointestinal bleeding, or other acute hemorrhage. Underlying bleeding disorders must be suspected in patients presenting with spontaneous bleeding from multiple sites, bleeding from nontraumatized sites, delayed bleeding several hours after injury, or bleeding into deep tissues or joints.

CLINICAL FEATURES

The rate of the development of the anemia, the extent of the anemia, and the ability of the cardiovascular system to compensate for the decreased oxygen-carrying capacity determine the severity of the patient's symptoms and clinical presentation. Patients may complain of palpitations, dizziness, postural faintness, easy fatigability, exertional intolerance, and tinnitus. On physical examination, patients may have pale conjunctiva, skin, and nail beds. Tachycardia, hyperdynamic precordium, and systolic murmurs may be present. Tachypnea at rest and hypotension are late signs. Use of ethanol, prescription drugs, and recreational drugs may alter the patient's ability to compensate for the anemia.

Patients with bleeding may or may not have an obvious site of hemorrhage. When suspecting an underlying bleeding disorder, the presence of excessive or abnormal bleeding in the patient and other family members should be investigated. Historical data about liver disease and drug use, such as use of ethanol, aspirin, nonsteroidal anti-inflammatory drugs, coumadin, antibiotics, and other aspirin-containing products, should be gathered. Mucocutaneous bleeding (including petechiae, ecchymoses, purpura, and epistaxis), gastrointestinal, genitourinary, or heavy menstrual bleeding are features of those patients with qualitative or quantitative platelet disorders. Patients with deficiencies of coagulation factor often present with delayed bleeding, hemarthroses, or bleeding into potential spaces such as between fascial planes and into the retroperitoneum. Patients with combination abnormalities of platelets and coagulation factor, such as disseminated intravascular coagulation, present with both mucocutaneous and deep space bleeding.

DIAGNOSIS AND DIFFERENTIAL

Presence of decreased red blood cell (RBC) count, hemoglobin, and hematocrit is diagnostic for anemia. Determining the exact etiology of the anemia is not essential in the emergency department, except in the face of acute hemorrhage. The initial evaluation of newly diagnosed anemia should include a complete blood count, review of RBC indices, reticulocyte count, stool hemoccult examination, urine pregnancy test, and examination of the peripheral blood smear (Table 134-1). The mean cellular volume and reticulocyte count can assist in classifying the anemia and can aid in differential diagnosis (Figure 134-1).

TABLE 134-1 Tests in the Evaluation of Anemia

Test	Interpretation	Clinical correlation
MCV	Measure of the average red blood cell size	Decreased MCV (microcytosis) is seen in chronic iron deficiency, thalassemia, anemia of chronic disease Increased MCV (macrocytosis) is seen in B_{12} or folate deficiency, alcohol abuse, liver disease, phenytoin, some HIV drugs
Mean cellular hemoglobin	Reflects the weight of hemoglobin in average red blood cells	
Mean cellular hemoglobin concentration	Reflects concentration of hemoglobin in average red blood cell	
Reticulocyte count	These red blood cells of intermediate maturity are a marker of production by the bone marrow	Decreased reticulocytes count reflects impaired red blood cell production Increased counts are a marker of accelerated red cell production
Peripheral blood smear	Allows visualization of the red blood cell morphology Allows evaluation for abnormal cell shapes Allows examination of the white blood cells and platelets	
Direct and indirect Coombs test	Direct Coombs is used to detect antibodies on red blood cells Indirect Coombs is used to detect antibodies in the sera	Direct Coombs is positive in hemolytic disease, transfusion reactions, autoimmune hemolytic anemias induced by drugs Indirect Coombs is used routinely in compatibility testing before transfusion

Key: HIV = human immunodeficiency virus, MCV = mean cellular volume.

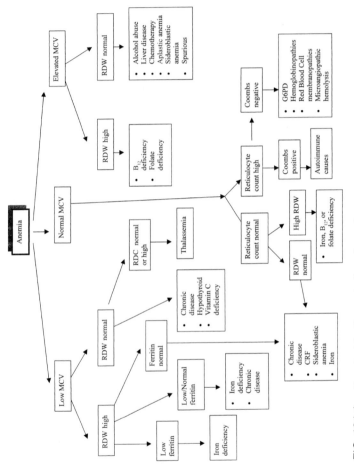

FIG. 134-1. Flowchart for the evaluation of anemia.

TABLE 134-2 Tests of Hemostasis

Screening tests	Normal value	Measures	Clinical correlations
Primary hemostasis			
Platelet count	150,000–300,000/µL	Number of platelets per µL	Decreased platelet count (thrombocytopenia)
			Bleeding usually not a problem until platelet count <50,000/µL; high risk of spontaneous bleeding including CNS with count <10,000/µL.
			Causes
			Decreased production—viral infections (measles); marrow infiltration; drugs (thiazides, ethanol, estrogens, interferon-α)
			Increased destruction—viral infections (mumps, varicella, EBV, HIV); ITP, TTP, DIC, HUS; drugs (heparin, protamine)
			Splenic sequestration (hypersplenism, hypothermia)
			Loss of platelets (hemorrhage, hemodialysis, extracorporeal circulation)
			Pseudothrombocytopenia—platelets are clumped but not truly decreased in number; examine blood smear to recognize this
			Elevated platelet count (thrombocytosis)—commonly reactive to inflammation or malignancy, or in polycythemia vera; can be associated with hemorrhage or thrombosis
Bleeding time (BT)	2.5–10 min (template BT)	Interaction between platelets and the subendothelium	Prolonged BT caused by
			Thrombocytopenia (platelet count <50,000/µL)
			Abnormal platelet function (vWD, ASA, NSAIDs, uremia, liver disease)
			Collagen abnormalities (congenital abnormality or prolonged use of steroids)

Secondary hemostasis			
Prothrombin time (PT)	10–12 s, but laboratory variation	Extrinsic system and common pathway—factors VII, X, V, prothrombin, and fibrinogen	*Prolonged PT* most commonly caused by: Use of warfarin (inhibits vitamin K–dependent factors II, VII, IX, and X) Liver disease with decreased factor synthesis Antibiotics, some cephalosporins, (moxalactam, cefamandole, cefotaxime, cefoperazone) that inhibit vitamin K–dependent factors
Activated partial thromboplastin time (aPTT)	Depends on type of thromboplastin used; "activated" with Kaolin	Intrinsic system and common pathway including factors XII, XI, IX, VIII, X, V, prothrombin, and fibrinogen	*Prolongation of aPTT* most commonly caused by Heparin therapy Factor deficiencies; factor levels have to be <30% of normal to cause prolongation Note: high doses of heparin or warfarin can cause prolongation of both the PT and aPTT due to their activity in the common pathway.
Thrombin clotting time (TCT)	10–12 s	Conversion of fibrinogen to fibrin monomer	*Prolonged TCT* caused by: Low fibrinogen level (DIC) Abnormal fibrinogen molecule (liver disease) Presence of heparin, FDPs or a paraprotein (multiple myeloma); these interfere with the conversion Very high fibrinogen level (acute phase reactant)
"Mixes"	Variable	Performed when ≥1 of the above screening tests is prolonged; the patients plasma ("abnormal") is mixed with "normal" plasma and the screening test is repeated	*If the "mix" corrects the screening test*, one or more factor deficiencies are present. *If the "mix" does not correct the screening test*, an inhibitor is present.

(continued)

TABLE 134-2 Tests of Hemostasis (continued)

Screening tests	Normal value	Measures	Clinical correlations
Other hemostatic tests			
Fibrin degradation products and D-dimer (evaluate fibrinolysis)	Variable	*FDPs* measure breakdown products from fibrinogen and fibrin monomer; *D-Dimer* measures breakdown products of crosslinked fibrin	Levels of these are elevated in DIC, thrombosis, pulmonary embolus, liver disease.
Factor level assays	60–130% (0.60–1.30 U/mL	Measures the percent activity of a specified factor compared to normal	Used to identify specific factor deficiencies and in therapeutic management of patients with deficiencies
Inhibitor screens	Variable	Verifies the presence or absence of antibodies directed against one or more of the coagulation factors	*Specific inhibitors* directed against one coagulation factor, most commonly against factor VIII; can be in patients with congenital or acquired deficiency. *Nonspecific inhibitors* directed against more than one of the coagulation factors; example is lupus-type anticoagulant

Key: ASA = aspirin, CNS = central nervous system, DIC = disseminated intravascular coagulation, EBV = Epstein-Barr virus, FDPs = fibrin degradation products, HIV = human immunodeficiency virus, HUS = hemolytic uremic syndrome, ITP = idiopathic thrombocytopenic purpura, NSAIDs = nonsteroidal anti-inflammatory drugs, TTP = thrombotic thrombocytopenic purpura, vWD = von Willebrand disease.

Laboratory studies used to diagnose bleeding disorders can be divided into the following 3 categories: (*a*) those that test the initial formation of a platelet plug (primary hemostasis); (*b*) those that assess the formation of crosslinked fibrin (secondary hemostasis); and (*c*) those that test the fibrinolytic system, which is responsible for limiting the size of the fibrin clots formed (Table 134-2). A complete blood count with platelet count, prothrombin time, and partial thromboplastin time are the initial studies needed in patients with suspected bleeding disorders. The clinical situation can guide any further laboratory testing.

EMERGENCY DEPARTMENT CARE AND DISPOSITION

Management of anemia depends on the etiology of the anemia and clinical status of the patient.

1. Stabilizing the airway, assisting ventilation, providing circulatory support, and controlling direct hemorrhage are the priorities.
2. Blood should be typed and crossmatched in those patients with anemia and ongoing blood loss so that it is available for transfusion, if necessary.
3. Immediate transfusion of **packed RBCs** should be considered in symptomatic patients who are hemodynamically unstable and have evidence of tissue hypoxia or have limited cardiopulmonary reserve.
4. Patients with anemia and ongoing blood loss should be admitted to the hospital for further evaluation and treatment. Patients with chronic anemia or newly diagnosed anemia with unclear etiology require admission if they are hemodynamically unstable, hypoxic, acidotic, or demonstrating cardiac ischemia.
5. **Hematology consultation** should be considered to assist in evaluation of those patients with anemia of unclear etiology, anemic patients with concomitant abnormalities of platelets and white blood cell counts, and patients with suspected bleeding disorders.

For further reading in *Emergency Medicine: A Comprehensive Study Guide*, 6th ed., see Chap. 218, "Evaluation of Anemia and the Bleeding Patient," by Robin R. Hemphill.

135 | Acquired Bleeding Disorders

Matthew A. Bridges

Acquired bleeding disorders can be caused by platelet abnormalities, coagulation factor deficiencies, drugs, systemic illness, and endogenous anticoagulants. Early recognition of these disorders is required for prompt, etiology-specific treatment.

BLEEDING DUE TO PLATELET ABNORMALITIES

Acquired platelet abnormalities include qualitative and quantitative platelet defects. Quantitative platelet disorders include those caused by decreased platelet production (eg, marrow infiltration, aplastic anemia, viral infections, and drugs), increased platelet destruction (eg, idiopathic thrombocytopenic purpura, thrombotic thrombocytopenic purpura, hemolytic uremic syndrome, disseminated intravascular coagulation [DIC], and viral infection), increased platelet loss (eg, hemorrhage and hemodialysis), and splenic sequestration. Qualitative platelet disorders are the result of abnormal platelet function and result in excess bleeding regardless of the platelet count. Common causes of qualitative platelet disorders include uremia, liver disease, DIC, drugs, and antiplatelet antibodies.

Emergency Department Care and Disposition

1. **Platelet transfusion** is warranted in all patients with a platelet count lower than 10,000/μL, regardless of etiology or symptomatology.
2. Most patients with a platelet count lower than 50,000/μL and active bleeding should receive platelet transfusion. However, hematologic consultation should be obtained because some conditions, such as DIC and thrombotic thrombocytopenic purpura, may be worsened by platelet transfusion.
3. The patient with idiopathic thrombocytopenic purpura should be started on **prednisone** at 60 to 100 mg/d.

BLEEDING DUE TO WARFARIN USE OR VITAMIN K DEFICIENCY

Vitamin K is a necessary cofactor in the production of coagulation factors II, VII, IX, and X and the anticoagulant proteins C and S. Warfarin is the most commonly used vitamin K antagonist in the United States. Patients with liver disease, those with vitamin K deficiency due to poor nutrition or malabsorption, and patients taking warfarin are at increased risk of bleeding.

Emergency Department Care and Disposition

Guidelines for treatment of warfarin-related bleeding are summarized in Table 135-1.

BLEEDING IN LIVER DISEASE

Patients with liver disease have an increased risk of bleeding for multiple reasons including decreased synthesis of coagulation factors due to hepatocyte destruction or vitamin K deficiency, thrombocytopenia, and increased fibrinolysis.

TABLE 135-1 Warfarin Reversal Guidelines

INR value	Bleeding	Recommendations
Any elevation	Major to life threatening	Withhold warfarin Replace coagulation factors with FFP or factor complex concentrates Vitamin K 5–10 mg IV (dose dependent on INR)
Any elevation	Mild to moderate	Withhold warfarin Vitamin K 2–4 mg PO (dose dependent on INR)
<5	None	Withhold warfarin until INR is therapeutic and then restart at same or lower dose
5–9	None	Withhold warfarin Vitamin K 1–2 mg PO
>9	None	Withhold warfarin Vitamin K 2–4 mg PO

Key: FFP = fresh-frozen plasma, INR = international normalized ratio, IV = intravenously, PO = orally.

Emergency Department Care and Disposition

1. All patients with liver disease and active bleeding should receive **vitamin K** (10 mg subcutaneously [SC] or intramuscularly).
2. Patients with severe bleeding should receive **fresh-frozen plasma** (FFP) to rapidly replace coagulation factors.
3. Platelet transfusion can be used in severe bleeding with associated thrombocytopenia.
4. **Desmopressin** (0.3 μg/kg SC or IV) may shorten bleeding times in some patients.
5. **Cryoprecipitate** may be beneficial in patients with active bleeding and fibrinogen levels below 100 mg/dL.

BLEEDING IN RENAL DISEASE

The bleeding tendency exhibited by patients with renal disease is related to the degree and duration of uremia. Bleeding is a result of platelet dysfunction, deficiency of coagulation factors, and thrombocytopenia.

Emergency Department Care and Disposition

1. Transfusion of packed red blood cells to maintain a hematocrit between 26 and 30 optimizes platelet function.
2. **Hemodialysis** improves platelet function transiently for 1 to 2 days.
3. **Desmopressin** (0.3 μg/kg SC or IV) shortens bleeding time in most patients.
4. **Conjugated estrogens** improve bleeding time in most patients.
5. **Platelet transfusions** and **cryoprecipitate** are indicated for life-threatening bleeding only and are to be used in conjunction with the previously listed therapies.

BLEEDING DUE TO HEPARIN USE OR FIBRINOLYTIC THERAPY

Bleeding is the most common side effect of the use of heparin (low-molecular-weight or unfractionated) or fibrinolytic therapy. All fibrinolytic agents have similar rates of major and minor bleeding complications, including a 1% to 2% risk of intracranial hemorrhage.

Emergency Department Care and Disposition

1. Heparin or fibrinolytic therapy should be discontinued if bleeding cannot be controlled by local measures.
2. **Protamine** can be used to neutralize heparin at a dose of 1 mg intravenously (IV) per 100 U of infused heparin in the previous 4 hours. Protamine is partly effective in reversing the effects of low-molecular-weight heparin.
3. Bleeding or thrombosis associated with heparin-induced thrombocytopenia should be treated with discontinuation of heparin and anticoagulation with a different agent (eg, danaparoid, ancrod, or hirudin). Low-molecular-weight heparins should not be used. Platelet counts recover 4 to 6 days after cessation of heparin.
4. Massive bleeding associated with fibrinolytic therapy should be treated with **cryoprecipitate** (10 U IV). If bleeding persists, treatment with **FFP** (2 U IV) should be initiated. Further treatment should be in conjunction with a hematologist but may include platelet transfusion or aminocaproic acid administration.

BLEEDING IN DISSEMINATED INTRAVASCULAR COAGULATION

DIC results from the activation of the coagulation and fibrinolytic systems and is triggered by the activation of tissue factor. The most common conditions associated with DIC are listed in Table 135-2.

Clinical Features

The complications of DIC are related to bleeding and thrombosis, although one or the other usually predominates in an individual patient. Bleeding typically occurs in the skin and mucous membranes. The skin may show signs of petechiae or ecchymoses. Bleeding from several sites, including venipuncture sites and surgical wounds, is common. Gastrointestinal, urinary tract, and central nervous system bleeding also may occur. Other patients show primarily thrombotic symptoms. Depending on the site of the thrombosis, patients may exhibit focal ischemia of the extremities, mental status changes, oliguria, or symptoms of adult respiratory distress syndrome. Purpura fulminans develops when there is widespread thrombosis resulting in gangrene of the extremities and hemorrhagic infarction of the skin.

Diagnosis and Differential

The diagnosis of DIC is based on the clinical setting and characteristic laboratory abnormalities listed in Table 135-3.

Emergency Department Care and Disposition

1. Hemodynamic stabilization should be provided through intravenous fluids or packed red blood cell transfusion.

TABLE 135-2 Conditions Associated with DIC

Clinical setting	Comments
Infection	
Bacterial	Probably the most common cause of DIC; 10–20% of patients with gram-negative sepsis have DIC; endotoxins stimulate monocytes and endothelial cells to express tissue factor; Rocky Mountain spotted fever causes direct endothelial damage; DIC more likely to develop in asplenic patients or those with cirrhosis; septic patients are more likely to have thrombosis than bleeding
Viral	
Fungal	
Carcinoma	Malignant cells may cause endothelial damage and allow the expression of tissue factor as well as other procoagulant materials; most adenocarcinomas tend to have thrombosis (Trousseau syndrome), except prostate cancer tends to have more bleeding; DIC is often chronic and compensated
Adenocarcinoma	
Lymphoma	
Acute leukemia	DIC most common with promyelocytic leukemia (M_3); blast cells release procoagulation enzymes; there is excessive release at time of cell lysis (chemotherapy); more likely to have bleeding than thrombosis
Trauma	DIC especially with brain injury, crush injury, burns, hypothermia, hyperthermia, rhabdomyolysis, fat embolism, hypoxia
Shock	
Liver disease	May have chronic compensated DIC; have acute DIC in the setting of acute hepatic failure, tissue factor is released from the injured hepatocytes
Pregnancy	Placental abruption, amniotic fluid embolus, septic abortion, intrauterine fetal death (can be chronic DIC); can get DIC in HELLP syndrome
Vascular disease	Large aortic aneurysms (chronic DIC can become acute at time of surgery); giant hemangiomas, vasculitis, multiple telangiectasias
Envenomation	DIC can develop with bites of rattlesnakes and other vipers; the venom damages the endothelial cells; bleeding is not as bad as expected from laboratory values
ARDS	Microthrombi are deposited in the small pulmonary vessels, the pulmonary capillary endothelium is damaged; 20% of patients with ARDS develop DIC and 20% of patients with DIC develop ARDS
Transfusion reactions	DIC with severe bleeding, shock, and acute renal failure
Acute hemolytic reaction	
Massive transfusion	
Surgical procedures	
Liver transplantation	
Vascular surgery	

Key: ARDS = adult respiratory distress syndrome, DIC = disseminated intravascular coagulation, HELLP syndrome = hemolysis, elevated liver enzymes, low platelets.

TABLE 135-3 Laboratory Abnormalities Characteristic of Disseminated Intravascular Coagulation

Studies	Result
	Most useful
Prothrombin time	Prolonged
Platelet count*	Usually low
Fibrinogen level†	Low
	Helpful
Activated partial thromboplastin time	Usually prolonged
Thrombin clot time‡	Prolonged
Fragmented red blood cells#	Should be present
FDPs and D-dimers§	Elevated
*Specific factor assays***	
Factor II	Low
Factor V	Low
Factor VII††	Low
Factor VIII‡‡	Low, normal, high
Factor IX	Low (decreases later than other factors)
Factor X	Low

*Platelet count usually low; most important that it is falling if it started at an elevated level.

†Fibrinogen level correlates best with bleeding complications; it is an acute phase reactant so it may actually start out at an elevated level; fibrinogen level below 100 mg/dL correlates with severe DIC.

‡Not a sensitive test; prolonged by many abnormalities.

#Fragmented red blood cells and schistocytes are not specific for DIC.

§Levels may be chronically elevated in patients with liver or renal disease.

**The factors in the extrinsic pathway are most affected (VII, X, V, and II).

††Factor VII is usually low early because it has the shortest half-life.

‡‡Factor VIII is an acute phase reactant so its level may be normal, low, or elevated in DIC.

Key: DIC = disseminated intravascular coagulation, FDPs = fibrin degradation products.

2. The underlying medical or surgical illness should be treated.
3. If bleeding predominates and the prothrombin time (PT) is elevated longer than 2 seconds, replacement of coagulation factors is indicated. **FFP** is infused 2 U at a time. **Cryoprecipitate** is used to replace fibrinogen; it is typically infused 10 bags at a time. If the platelet count is lower than 50,000/μL with active bleeding or lower than 10,000/μL regardless of bleeding, **platelet transfusion** should be initiated. All patients with bleeding due to DIC also should receive **vitamin K** (10 mg SC or intramuscularly) and **folate** (1 mg IV).
4. If thrombosis predominates, heparinization should be considered, although this is controversial. Heparin is most likely to be beneficial if the underlying medical condition is carcinoma, acute promyelocytic leukemia, or retained uterine products, or if the patient exhibits signs of purpura fulminans.

BLEEDING DUE TO CIRCULATING ANTICOAGULANTS

Circulating anticoagulants are antibodies directed against 1 or more of the coagulation factors. The 2 most common circulating anticoagulants are factor VIII inhibitor (a specific inhibitor directed against only factor VIII) and antiphospholipid antibodies, including lupus anticoagulant and anticardiolipin antibody (nonspecific inhibitors directed against several coagulation factors).

Clinical Features

Patients with factor VIII inhibitor have massive spontaneous bruises, ecchymoses, and hematomas. Patients with antiphospholipid antibodies may have thromboses or recurrent fetal loss. Bleeding abnormalities are rare in patients with antiphospholipid antibodies.

Diagnosis and Differential

Laboratory studies in patients with factor VIII inhibitor show a normal PT, normal thrombin clot time, and a greatly prolonged activated partial thromboplastin time that does not correct with mixing. A factor VIII-specific assay will show low or absent factor VIII activity. Patients with antiphospholipid antibodies will have a normal or slightly prolonged PT, a normal thrombin clot time, and a moderately prolonged activated partial thromboplastin time that also does not correct with mixing. Factor specific assays will show a decrease in all factor levels.

Emergency Department Care and Disposition

1. Patients with factor VIII inhibitor and active bleeding should be managed in conjunction with a hematologist. Treatment options include concentrates of factor VIIa, factor VIII, factor IX, prothrombin complex, and plasmapheresis.
2. Patients with antiphospholipid antibodies and arterial or venous thrombosis should be treated with long-term warfarin anticoagulation.

BLEEDING DUE TO INFECTION WITH HUMAN IMMUNODEFICIENCY VIRUS

Infection with the human immunodeficiency virus (HIV) is associated with several abnormalities of hemostasis. Most common are thrombocytopenia and circulating anticoagulants. The most common symptoms are easy bruising, petechiae, and mucosal bleeding. Clinically significant bleeding is rare. HIV-positive patients with antiphospholipid antibodies have a lower risk of thrombosis than do HIV-negative patients.

Emergency Department Care and Disposition

The treatment of the HIV infected patient with bleeding associated with thrombocytopenia or circulating anticoagulants is identical to the treatment of those conditions in the non–HIV-infected patient discussed previously.

For further reading in *Emergency Medicine: A Comprehensive Study Guide,* 6th ed., see Chap. 219, "Acquired Bleeding Disorders," by Mary A. Wittler and Rubin R. Hemphill.

136 | Hemophilias and von Willebrand Disease

Jeffrey N. Glaspy

HEMOPHILIAS

Clinical Features

Hemophilia is a genetic deficiency or defect in one of the circulating coagulation proteins. The most common hemophilias are due to deficiencies of factor VIII (hemophilia A) or factor IX (hemophilia B). Hemophilias A and B are recessive X-linked disorders. Patients with hemophilia are classified as having severe disease if the factor VIII or factor IX deficiency is less than 1% of normal controls. Moderate disease (1%-5% of normal factor activity) and mild disease (5%-25% of normal factor activity) make up the rest of the classification system. Bleeding complications depend on severity of the disease. Easy bruising, hemarthrosis, and hematoma are the most common bleeding complications. These conditions may occur spontaneously or with any degree of trauma. Life-threatening bleeding may occur if patients bleed into the central nervous system, neck, pharynx, abdomen, or the retroperitoneum. Compartment syndromes may occur if hematoma occurs in the extremities. Unless there is another underlying disease, most patients with hemophilia do not have problems with minor cuts or abrasions.

Diagnosis and Differential

Clinically, it is impossible to differentiate between hemophilias A and B. Laboratory testing in patients with hemophilia most often shows a normal prothrombin time (PT), prolonged partial thromboplastin time (PTT), and a normal bleeding time. However, if greater than 30% of factor activity is present, the PTT may be normal. Specific factor assays may be used to differentiate between the types of hemophilia. Approximately 10% to 25% of patients with hemophilia A and 1% to 2% of patients with hemophilia B will develop an inhibitor, which is an antibody against the deficient factor. An inhibitor is diagnosed by mixing the patient's plasma 50-50 with plasma of a normal control and finding that the mixture still has a prolonged PTT. The quantity of inhibitor is measured by the Bethesda inhibitor assay (BIA) and is reported in BIA units. The presence of an inhibitor makes treatment more difficult.

Emergency Department Care and Disposition

The mainstay of therapy for bleeding episodes is early and complete factor replacement; however, the site and severity of bleeding, severity of hemophilia, and presence or absence of an inhibitor affect the specific treatment. Early consultation with a hematologist or transfer to a center with a hematology specialist is recommended. The approach to a bleeding emergency in a patient with hemophilia is outlined below.

1. **Determine the type of hemophilia and the presence or absence of inhibitor.** Most patients with hemophilia and their families are very knowledgeable about this disease. Further, many hospitals keep detailed records

of the diagnosis and treatment strategies for patients with bleeding disorders. Old medical records and medic-alert bracelets also may provide necessary information. If it is a new diagnosis, or if the type of hemophilia is unknown, then fresh-frozen plasma (FFP) is the best initial treatment. If an inhibitor is present, then see item 5.

2. **Determine the site and severity of bleeding.** The site and severity of bleeding determine the potential life or limb threat and dictate the initial factor replacement guidelines (Table 136-1). Factor replacement may need to be instituted before definitive imaging in cases of potentially severe trauma. For example, in a patient with hemophilia who has sustained head trauma, factor replacement should be given before obtaining computed tomography of the head.

3. **Determine the desired factor activity level.** Factor activity level determines how much factor replacement is required. Calculation of the amount of factor needed can be done by using the patient's weight and the desired increase in factor:

units of factor VIII required = weight (kg) $\times$ 0.5
$$\times \, (\% \text{ activity desired} - \% \text{ intrinsic activity})$$
units of factor IX required = weight (kg) $\times$ 1.0
$$\times \, (\% \text{ activity desired} - \% \text{ intrinsic activity})$$

For severe hemophilia, assume 0% intrinsic activity.

4. **Determine the best product for replacement.** Specific factor replacement (factor VIII or factor IX) is the most effective treatment for bleeding episodes in patients with hemophilia. Table 136-2 lists the products available for treatment of hemophilia. The 2 main categories are purified, plasma-derived factors and recombinant factors. Advantages of the purified, plasma-derived factors are lower cost and greater availability. Advantages of the recombinant factors are greater purity and decreased risk of viral transmission. Porcine factor VIII products are also available and have no reported viral transmission to humans. The duration of factor replacement depends on the condition being treated (see Table 136-1). If specific factor replacement is not available, FFP should be used.

5. **Determine the presence of an inhibitor.** The use of factor replacement in patients with an inhibitor is guided by the concentration of the inhibitor (measured in BIA units) and the type of response these patients have to factor concentrates (Table 136-3). In patients with inhibitor titers of less than 5 BIA and who are not vigorous antibody responders, an increased dose of factor can be given in an attempt to overwhelm the existing antibody. Alternative therapies include porcine factor VIII, prothrombin complex concentrates, activated prothrombin complex concentrates, and recombinant activated factor VII. Early consultation with a hematologist is recommended for patients with an inhibitor.

6. If a patient presents with an undiagnosed bleeding disorder, then **FFP** is the treatment of choice. FFP contains all the plasma clotting factors, with an average factor VIII concentration of 1 U/mL. However, 1 unit of FFP will raise the factor IX level by only 3%, so volume overload may limit the effectiveness of FFP in patients with hemophilia B. **Specific factor assays** should be sent to guide further therapy. **Cryoprecipitate,** which contains factor VIII and von Willebrand factor (vWF), may be used if hemophilia B is not suspected. Each bag of cryoprecipitate contains about 100 U factor VIII.

TABLE 136-1 Initial Factor Replacement Guidelines

Site	Minimum initial factor level	Hemophilia A initial dose	Hemophilia B initial dose	Details
Deep muscle	40–50%	20–40 U/kg	40–60 U/kg	Admit, monitor total blood loss, watch for compartment syndrome; duration of replacement 1–3 d
Joint	30–50%	20–40 U/kg	30–40 U/kg	Orthopedic consult for splinting, physical therapy, and follow-up; duration of replacement: 1–3 d
Epistaxis	80–100%	40–50 U/kg	80–100 U/kg	Local measures should be used; replacement is given until bleeding resolves
Oral mucosa	50%	25 U/kg	50 U/kg	Local measures and antifibrinolytic therapy will decrease the need for additional factor replacement; duration of replacement: 1–2 d
Gastrointestinal bleeding	100%	40–50 U/kg	80–100 U/kg	Consultation with gastrointestinal specialist is appropriate to identify a lesion; duration of replacement: 7–10 d
Central nervous system	100%	50 U/kg	100 U/kg	Neurosurgical consultation should be early; lumbar puncture requires factor replacement

TABLE 136-2 Available Products for Hemophilia Treatment

Hemophilia type	Available products	Comments
Hemophilia A	Human plasma-derived factor VIII products Koate-HP (gel chromatography, solvent, detergent purified) Humate-P (heat treated) Alphanate (solvent and detergent purified)	All have a low risk of HIV and hepatitis transmission
	Human plasma-derived factor VII with immunoaffinity purification Hemofil-M (monoclonal, solvent, detergent purification) Monoclate-P (monoclonal and heat treated)	Both have reduced amounts of vWF; Monoclate-P is highly purified source of factor VIII
	Recombinate factor VIII products Recombinate (recombinant DNA product) Gelixate (recombinant DNA product) Bioclate (recombinant DNA product) Kogenate (recombinant DNA product)	Low to no risk of hepatitis and HIV
	Porcine factor VIII products Antihemophilic factor (cryoprecipitate fractionation, screened for porcine viruses) Hyate-C (cryoprecipitate fractionation, screened for porcine viruses)	No evidence that human viral infection occurs
Hemophilia B	Factor IX complex products Koyne-80 factor IX complex (heat treated) Proplex T factor IX complex (heat treated) Profilnine SD (solvent and detergent) Bebulin VH (2-step vapor heat treatment)	Propex-T: HIV seroconversion has occurred Other products have low risk of HIV and hepatitis transmission
	Activated factor IX complex products Autoplex T (heat treated) Feiba VH (2-step vapor heat treatment)	Low risk of HIV and hepatitis transmission
	Purified factor IX products Alpha Nine SD (solvent, detergent, polysorbate) Mononine (monoclonal antibody purification, ultrafiltration)	Low risk of HIV and hepatitis
	Recombinant factor IX BeneFIX (recombinant DNA product)	No known risk of transmission

Key: HIV = human immunodeficiency virus, vWF = von Willebrand factor.

TABLE 136-3 Replacement Therapy for Hemophilias A and B in Patients with Inhibitors

Type of product	Hemophilia A dose	Hemophilia B dose	Comments
Factor VII concentrates	5000–10,000 U bolus followed by a continuous infusion	Not applicable	
Prothrombin complex concentrates Contain factors II, VII, IX, X	75–100 U/kg	75–100 U/kg	Risk of DIC, thromboembolic disease, and low risk of hepatitis transmission
Activated prothrombin complex concentrates Contain factors II, VII, IX, X, with variable amounts of activated factors VIIa, IXa, Xa	75–100 U/kg	~75 U/kg	Similar risks as with the prothrombin complex concentrates
Recombinant factor VIIa (NovoSeven)	Variable	Variable	No risk of viral transmission
Porcine factor VIII (Hyate-C)	Variable	Not applicable	Patients may develop inhibitors
Highly purified factor IX concentrates	Not applicable	Variable	

Key: DIC = disseminated intravascular coagulation.

7. For patients with mild hemophilia A who have mild bleeding, **desmopressin** (DDAVP) may be given. The dose is 0.3 μg/kg intravenously over 30 minutes or subcutaneously. For children older than 5 years, intranasal DDAVP may be given as a single spray in 1 nostril (150 μg). For adolescents and adults, the intranasal dose of DDAVP is a single spray in both nostrils (300 μg). For very mild mucosal bleeding antifibrinolytic agents, such as **ε-aminocaproic acid** (EACA) or **tranexamic acid,** may be used. The dose of EACA is 75 to 100 mg/kg every 6 hours for children and 6 g every 6 hours for adults.

8. Indications for admission include (*a*) bleeding involving the central nervous system, neck, pharynx, retropharynx, abdomen or retroperitoneum; (*b*) potential compartment syndrome; (*c*) inability to control pain; (*d*) inability to administer or lack of access for factor replacement; and (*e*) treatment requiring more than 3 doses (relative indication).

VON WILLEBRAND DISEASE

Clinical Features

Von Willebrand disease (vWD) is a group of disorders caused by a defect or deficiency of vWF. vWF is a cofactor for platelet adhesion and a carrier protein for factor VIII in the plasma. There are 3 main types of vWD. Type I (80% of patients with vWD) is a mild form, with bleeding episodes usually manifesting as epistaxis, easy bruising, menorrhagia, or dental bleeding. Type II is a qualitative disorder accounting for about 10% of patients with vWD. Type III is a severe form accounting for fewer than 10% of cases. These patients manifest with severe bleeding episodes that may resemble the hemophilias (hemarthrosis and hematomas). In mild cases of vWD, the patient may not be aware of the disease until a traumatic episode or surgical procedure.

Diagnosis and Differential

In patients with vWD, the PT and PTT are usually normal. The bleeding time is prolonged and vWF activity is low. Occasionally, the PT and factor VIII level may be abnormal, making it difficult to distinguish vWD from hemophilia A.

Emergency Department Care and Disposition

The treatment of vWD depends on the type of disease and the severity of bleeding.

1. For most patients with vWD, **DDAVP** is the mainstay of treatment. DDAVP works by stimulating endothelial cells to secrete stored vWF and possibly by promoting hemostasis via additional endothelial effects. The dose of DDAVP is 0.3 μg/kg subcutaneously or intravenously over 30 minutes every 12 hours. Three or 4 doses are the maximum because further administration may induce tachyphylaxis. The dose of the concentrated intranasal form of DDAVP is 1 spray in 1 nostril (150 μg) for children older than 5 years and 1 spray in each nostril (300 μg) for adolescents and adults.

2. For patients who do not respond to DDAVP or for patients with type II or III disease, factor VIII concentrate that has significant amounts of vWF is required. The most commonly used factor VIII concentrates are **Humate-P** and **Koate-HP** (see Table 136-2).

3. **Cryoprecipitate** also contains high concentrations of vWF and may be used to treat patients with vWD. There is, however, a greater risk of viral transmission; therefore, the purified products such as Humate are recommended. If used, 10 bags of cryoprecipitate every 12 to 24 hours usually will control bleeding.

4. **Platelet transfusions** may benefit patients with certain types of vWD (type III) who do not respond to factor VIII concentrates.

5. For women with vWD and menorrhagia, birth control pills may help increase the vWF levels and limit the menstrual bleeding. For dental injuries or for planned dental procedures, EACA or tranexamic acid should be used for 5 to 10 days after the injury or procedure.

For further reading in *Emergency Medicine: A Comprehensive Study Guide,* 6th ed., see Chapter 220, "Hemophilias and Von Willebrand's Disease," by Robin R. Hemphill.

137 | Hemolytic Anemias

Sandra L. Najarian

Hemolytic anemias are divided into hereditary and acquired types. Hereditary anemias include sickle cell anemia and its variants, glucose-6-phosphate de-hydrogenase (G-6-PD) deficiency, and hereditary spherocytosis. Acquired anemias may be mediated by an antibody or result from fragmentation, direct toxicity, mechanical injury, or hypersplenism.

HEREDITARY HEMOLYTIC ANEMIAS

SICKLE CELL DISEASE

Clinical Features

Patients with sickle cell disease present with a wide variety of symptoms that can involve nearly every organ system. As a result of this chronic hemolytic anemia, patients may have flow murmurs, congestive heart failure (CHF), cardiomegaly, cor pulmonale, lower extremity ulcerations, icterus, and hep-atomegaly. Patients with acute chest syndrome will have pulmonary manifes-tations such as pleuritic chest pain, fever, sudden decrease in pulmonary func-tion, and hypoxia. Neurologic manifestations include cerebral infarction in children, cerebral hemorrhage in adults, transient ischemic attack, headache, seizure, and coma.

Painful vasoocclusive crises are the most common reason for emergency department (ED) visits. Common precipitants include cold exposure, dehy-dration, high altitude, and infections, particularly with encapsulated organ-isms such as *Haemophilus influenza* or *Pneumococcus*. Patients may present with joint, muscle, or bone pain or diffuse abdominal pain.

Hematologic crises present with weakness, dyspnea, fatigue, worsening CHF, or shock in the setting of a precipitous drop in hemoglobin. Acute splenic sequestration of blood and bone marrow suppression (aplastic crisis) are 2 types of hematologic crisis.

Other clinical presentations of sickle cell disease include priapism, swelling of hands or feet due to vaso-occlusion (dactylitis), and infarction of the renal medulla, associated with flank pain and hematuria.

Diagnosis and Differential

The clinical presentation guides the ED evaluation. For patients suffering an acute crisis, a drop in hemoglobin by 2 g/dL from the patient's baseline sug-gests hematologic crisis or blood loss. A reticulocyte count is necessary in these patients; a count lower than the baseline of 5% to 15% may reflect aplastic crisis. Leukocytosis and a left shift should raise the suspicion of in-fection. Electrolytes should be checked in patients with evidence of dehydra-tion. A urinalysis should be obtained in patients with urinary symptoms. Liver enzymes are indicated in patients with abdominal pain. Arterial blood gas analysis is warranted in patients with respiratory complaints and evidence of hypoxia on pulse oximetry. Patients with sickle cell disease may have a mild to moderate hypoxia; however, a Pao_2 below 60 mm Hg suggests an acute problem. Radiographic studies may include chest radiograph for patients with pulmonary symptoms, abdominal computed tomography or ultrasound for abdominal pain, computed tomography of the head for neurologic complaints, and plain radiographs for patients with focal bone pain.

Differential diagnosis for complaints related to sickle cell disease is extensive and includes osteomyelitis, acute arthritides, pancreatitis, hepatitis, pelvic inflammatory disease, pyelonephritis, pneumonia, pulmonary embolus, and meningitis.

Emergency Department Care and Disposition

Management is primarily supportive, with close attention to possible precipitants of acute crises.

1. Patients with evidence of dehydration or acute pain should be rehydrated orally if they can tolerate fluids or with intravenous fluids, such as 0.45 normal saline or normal saline at 1.5 times maintenance.
2. **Narcotics** should be administered promptly for severe pain. Patients who present to the ED frequently will benefit from a protocol treatment plan.
3. Supplemental **oxygen** is necessary only when the patient is hypoxic. Cardiac monitoring is appropriate for patients with cardiopulmonary symptoms.
4. Patients with symptoms of acute infection or with a temperature higher than 38°C should have the appropriate cultures drawn. Broad-spectrum antibiotics, such as **cefuroxime** or **ceftriaxone,** should be administered.
5. Patients with significant cardiopulmonary decompensation, an acute central nervous system event, or priapism should receive **exchange transfusions.**
6. Patients with priapism require hydration, analgesia, and immediate urologic consultation.
7. Patients with acute bone pain suggestive of osteomyelitis should have cultures drawn and receive intravenous antibiotic therapy to cover *Staphylococcus aureus* and *Salmonella typhimurium.*
8. Admission criteria include pulmonary, neurologic, aplastic, or infectious crises; splenic sequestration; intractable pain; persistent nausea and vomiting; or an uncertain diagnosis. Discharged patients should receive oral analgesics, close follow-up, and instructions to return immediately for temperature above 38°C or worsening symptoms.

VARIANTS OF SICKLE CELL DISEASE

The most common variant of sickle cell disease is sickle cell trait. These carriers have minimal complications, and sickling is not seen except in conditions of extreme hypoxia. These patients are generally asymptomatic and have normal life expectancy. Mild to moderate hemolytic anemia, mild reticulocytosis, and splenomegaly may be seen in patients with sickle cell hemoglobin C disease. Most patients usually present with mild complications, whereas others can present with painful crises and complications similar to those patients with sickle cell disease. Presentation and complications from sickle cell β-thalassemia disease depends on the type of β-thalassemia gene that is inherited. Presentations can range from mild to severe hemolytic anemia and vasoocclusive crises.

GLUCOSE-6-PHOSPHATE DEHYDROGENASE DEFICIENCY

African-American males are most commonly affected by G-6-PD deficiency and may present with acute hemolytic crises, hemoglobinuria, and vascular collapse due to infections, exposure to oxidant drugs, metabolic acidosis, and ingestion of fava beans. The diagnosis is made by decreased G-6-PD activity on quantitative assay. There is no specific treatment; prevention involves early treatment of infection and avoidance of oxidant stress.

HEREDITARY SPHEROCYTOSIS

Hereditary spherocytosis is seen in people of northern European descent and is characterized by mild hemolytic anemia, splenomegaly, and intermittent jaundice. Laboratory features include mild anemia, spherocytes on peripheral smear, a normal mean cell volume, and an increased mean cellular hemoglobin concentration ($>36\%$). Splenectomy is the treatment of choice.

ACQUIRED HEMOLYTIC ANEMIAS

Clinical Features

Antibody-mediated hemolytic anemias include warm and cold antibody types. The warm type is more common in elderly female patients with underlying medical conditions, such as lymphoproliferative disorders and systemic autoimmune diseases. In children, it may develop after acute infections or immunizations. Patients may present with mild anemia and splenomegaly to life-threatening anemia, splenomegaly, pulmonary edema, mental status changes, and venous thrombosis.

Cold antibody hemolytic anemia presents in 2 forms. Cold agglutinin syndrome may present as an acute disease in younger people after infections such as *Mycoplasma pneumonia.* The anemia is usually mild. The chronic form is seen in elderly patients with underlying lymphoproliferative disorders and involves hemolysis in parts of the body exposed to cold. Paroxysmal cold hemoglobinemia is another acute form found in patients with untreated syphilis or viral illnesses and presents with fever, chills, hemoglobinuria, and pain involving the back, legs, and abdomen.

Autoimmune hemolytic anemia also can be induced by drugs, specifically α-methyldopa, penicillin, sulfa drugs, and quinidine. Hemolysis ceases after discontinuation of the drug. Alloimmune hemolytic anemia includes hemolytic disease of the newborn and hemolytic transfusion reactions. In hemolytic disease of the newborn, maternal alloantibodies form after rhesus D–negative maternal red blood cells (RBCs) are exposed to rhesus D–positive fetal blood. These alloantibodies cross the placenta and destroy fetal RBCs, which can lead to mild anemia, fetal hydrops, and intrauterine fetal demise. Patients with hemolytic transfusion reactions often have a history of previous transfusion in which sensitization to allogenic RBC antigens occurs. With subsequent transfusions, patients may develop fever, chest and flank pain, tachypnea, tachycardia, hypotension, hemoglobinuria, and oliguria.

Microangiopathic hemolytic anemia (MAHA) results from fragmentation hemolysis. This includes damage to RBCs from passage through artificial heart valves, calcified aortic valves, or arterioles and microcirculation damaged by thrombotic thrombocytopenia purpura (TTP), hemolytic uremic syndrome (HUS), pregnancy, vasculitis, malignant hypertension, and certain malignancies.

TTP more commonly affects women and presents with fever, neurologic changes, hemorrhage, and renal insufficiency. HUS is a disease of early childhood and presents with fever, acute renal failure, and neurologic deficits after a prodromal infection. Fragmentation hemolysis in pregnancy is seen in preeclampsia, eclampsia, and abruption.

Direct toxic effects causing hemolysis may result from infection (malaria being the most common) and from the venom of bees, wasps, certain spiders, and cobras. Oxidative hemolysis of RBCs results from methemoglobin-producing drugs, such as lidocaine and sulfonamides.

Mechanical damage to RBCs can result in hemolysis and hemoglobinuria. Etiologies include extensive burns and strenuous physical activity. Patients who have been on cardiopulmonary bypass can develop hemolysis, fever, and leukopenia, known as *postperfusion syndrome.* The passage of blood through the oxygenator activates complement, leading to acute intravascular hemolysis.

Hemolysis as a result of sequestration and destruction of RBCs in the spleen, or hypersplenism, is seen most commonly in portal hypertension, infiltrative disease, and infections.

Diagnosis and Differential

Diagnosis is based on recognition of clinical signs and symptoms and obtaining appropriate laboratory studies. Complete blood cell count will show anemia. Review of the peripheral blood smear is vital and often will give keys to the diagnosis. Schistocytes (fragmented RBCs) are seen in MAHA and are the result of direct trauma. Spherocytes are evidence of warm antibody immune hemolysis and hereditary spherocytosis. Other laboratory abnormalities include elevations in lactic acid dehydrogenase and indirect bilirubin. A decrease in haptoglobin level is another indicator of intravascular hemolysis. Patients with evidence of MAHA and thrombocytopenia must be assumed to have TTP until proven otherwise. In TTP, the platelet count is often lower than 20,000/μL. Patients with HUS will have thrombocytopenia, although not to the degree of those with TTP. An elevated serum urea nitrogen and creatinine levels are seen in HUS and TTP. An elevated reticulocyte count is the best indicator of a normal bone marrow in the setting of hemolysis and may be as high as 30% to 40%. The direct Coombs test is positive in those patients with immune-mediated hemolysis. Patients with HELLP syndrome demonstrate hemolysis, elevated liver function enzymes, and low platelets in the setting of preeclampsia.

Emergency Department Care and Disposition

Treatment is directed at stabilization of vital signs and correction of the underlying disease process.

1. **Prednisone** 1.0 mg/kg/d is the initial treatment for warm antibody hemolytic anemia and TTP. **Azathioprine** and **cyclophosphamide** are used occasionally, and splenectomy may be required for those who fail or cannot tolerate steroids.
2. **Plasma exchange transfusion** is the foundation of therapy for TTP. If unavailable, **fresh-frozen plasma** should be infused while arranging transfer to a tertiary care center. Except in cases of life-threatening bleeding or intracranial hemorrhage, platelet transfusions should be avoided because they can aggravate the thrombotic process. Aspirin should be avoided because it may worsen hemorrhagic complications in the face of severe thrombocytopenia. **Immunotherapy** also may be initiated for patients who are refractory to treatment.
3. **Transfusion of packed RBCs** is indicated for angina, CHF, mental status changes, or hypoxia.

4. Patients with cold antibody hemolytic anemia should be kept in a warm environment.
5. Early **dialysis** should be considered in the management of HUS. Otherwise, supportive therapy is indicated for mild HUS.
6. Prompt delivery of the infant followed by supportive care is mandatory for patients with HELLP syndrome.
7. **Iron** and **folate** should be given to patients with traumatic hemolysis due to artificial heart valves. If hemolysis is severe, the defective valve may need replacement.

For further reading in *Emergency Medicine: A Comprehensive Study Guide,* 6th ed., see Chap. 221, "Hereditary Hemolytic Anemias," by Robin R. Hemphill; and Chap. 222, "Acquired Hemolytic Anemias," by Patty Chu.

138 | Transfusion Therapy
Walter N. Simmons

An understanding of available blood products, their indications, and potential complications of transfusions is increasingly important for those caring for patients in the emergency department. The decision to transfuse depends on the underlying cause and rate of blood loss, the patient's health status, and cardiopulmonary reserve. Acute blood loss, circulatory shock, and even chronic symptomatic anemia may necessitate the transfusion. This chapter reviews available blood products, their indications, and associated complications of transfusion.

WHOLE BLOOD

The total blood volume of a 70-kg adult is approximately 75 mL/kg, or 5 L. Whole blood has limited usefulness as a transfusion therapy. Although it can provide volume and oxygen-carrying capacity, this is often better achieved by using the individual blood components. Disadvantages of whole blood, in part because of degradation during storage, include low levels of clotting factors; frequently elevated levels of potassium, hydrogen ion, and ammonia; and the presence of a large number of antigens. A unit of whole blood contains about 500 mL of blood plus a preservative anticoagulant, usually citrate phosphate dextrose adenine type 1.

PACKED RED BLOOD CELLS

Red blood cell (RBC) replacement is usually done with packed RBCs (PRBCs). One unit of PRBCs, about 250 mL in volume, raises an adult's hemoglobin by 1 g/dL or the hematocrit by 3% and is usually transfused over 1 to 2 hours unless there is hemodynamic instability. The major indications for PRBC transfusion include: (*a*) acute hemorrhage is defined as blood loss greater than 25% to 30% of blood volume (1500 mL) in otherwise healthy adults and usually requires transfusion of PRBCs to replace oxygen-carrying capacity and crystalloid infusion to replace volume; (*b*) surgical blood loss greater than 2 L usually requires transfusion of PRBCs and crystalloid; and (*c*) in chronic anemia, transfusion may be indicated for symptomatic patients, those with underlying cardiopulmonary disease, and those with hemoglobin levels less than 7 g/dL. Patients with hemoglobin levels greater than 10 g/dL rarely will benefit from transfusion.

Most patients can be typed (ABO and RhD blood group type) in about 15 minutes. A type and crossmatch against blood intended for transfusion takes approximately 1 hour. RBCs are available as leukocyte poor, frozen, or washed. Leukocyte-poor RBCs have up to 85% of the leukocytes removed and are indicated for transplant recipients or candidates and for patients with a history of febrile nonhemolytic transfusion reactions. Frozen RBCs are a source of rare blood types and provide reduced antigen exposure. Washed RBCs are for patients who have hypersensitive reactions to plasma, for neonatal transfusions, and for those with paroxysmal nocturnal hemoglobinuria.

PLATELETS

Platelet transfusions may be used in thrombocytopenic patients to prevent bleeding or to help stop active bleeding. One unit contains 3 to 6×10^{11} platelets in a volume of 250 to 350 mL and is transfused using ABO compatibility. Dosing is usually 1 U per 10 kg (approximately 6 to 8 U for an adult), which raises the platelet count about 50,000/μL. ABO- and Rh-compatible platelets are preferable. The platelet count should be checked 1 and 24 hours after infusion. Transfused platelets survive 3 to 5 days unless there is platelet consumption.

If the platelet count is above 50,000/μL, bleeding from thrombocytopenia is unlikely unless there is platelet dysfunction. Principles for platelet transfusions in adults include: (*a*) maintaining the platelet count greater than 50,000/μL in patients undergoing major surgery or with significant bleeding; (*b*) a platelet count between 10,000 and 50,000/μL increases the risk of bleeding with trauma or invasive procedures, and patients with platelet dysfunction (eg, renal or liver disease) may have spontaneous hemorrhage with these counts; and (c) a platelet count below 10,000/μL presents a high risk for spontaneous bleeding, and prophylactic transfusion is indicated. In thrombocytopenia due to platelet destruction, however, platelet transfusion may have little effect.

FRESH-FROZEN PLASMA

Fresh-frozen plasma (FFP) is indicated for: (*a*) acquired coagulopathy with active bleeding or before invasive procedures when there is greater than 1.5 times prolongation of the prothrombin time or partial thromboplastin time, or a coagulation factor assay less than 25% of normal; (*b*) congenital isolated factor deficiencies when specific, virally safe products are not available; (*c*) thrombotic thrombocytopenic purpura patients undergoing plasma exchange; (*d*) patients receiving massive transfusion who develop coagulopathy and active bleeding, and (*e*) antithrombin III (ATIII) deficiency when ATIII concentrate is not available. One bag of FFP contains 200 to 250 mL, 1 U/mL of each coagulation factor, and 1 to 2 mg/mL fibrinogen. FFP should be ABO compatible, with a typical starting dose of 8 to 10 mL/kg, or 2 to 4 bags. One unit of FFP will increase most coagulation factors by 3% to 5%.

CRYOPRECIPITATE

Cryoprecipitate is derived from FFP; 1 bag contains 80 to 100 U factor VIIIC, 80 U von Willebrand factor, 200 to 300 mg fibrinogen, 40 to 60 U factor XIII, and variable amounts of fibronectin. The usual dose is 2 to 4 bags per 10 kg of body weight (10 to 20 bags); ABO-compatible bags are preferable. Indications for cryoprecipitate therapy are: (*a*) fibrinogen level below 100 mg/dL associated with disseminated intravascular coagulation or congenital fibrinogen deficiency; (*b*) von Willebrand disease with active bleeding when desmopressin is not effective and factor VIII concentrate containing von Willebrand factor is not available; (*c*) hemophilia A when virally inactivated factor VIII concentrates are not available; (*d*) use as fibrin glue surgical adhesives; and (*e*) fibronectin replacement.

INTRAVENOUS IMMUNOGLOBULINS

Indications for intravenous immunoglobulins include the treatment of primary and secondary immunodeficiencies and treatment of immune or inflammatory disorders, such as immune thrombocytopenia and Kawasaki syndrome. Adverse reactions include anaphylaxis, febrile reactions, headache, and renal failure. There have been some documented cases of patients developing a positive serology to hepatitis C after intravenous immunoglobulin therapy.

ANTITHROMBIN III

ATIII is a serum protein that inhibits coagulation factors, thrombin, and activated factors IX, X, XI, and XII. Deficiency can be congenital or acquired. ATIII is used mainly for prophylaxis of thrombosis or to treat thromboembolism in patients with hereditary ATIII deficiency.

ALBUMIN

Albumin is available for patients with decreased intravascular oncotic pressure; however, due to cost and lack of proven efficacy, its use is controversial and is currently used infrequently.

SPECIFIC FACTOR REPLACEMENT THERAPY

Table 138-1 outlines therapy for congenital coagulation factor deficiencies.

COMPLICATIONS OF TRANSFUSIONS

Adverse reactions occur in up to 20% of transfusions and are usually mild. Transfusion reactions can be immediate or delayed. Table 138-2 summarizes the types of immediate reactions and their recognition, management, and evaluation.

DELAYED TRANSFUSION REACTIONS

1. Delayed hemolytic reactions can occur 7 to 10 days after transfusion.
2. Infection may result from transfusion. There is a small risk of transmission of the human immunodeficiency virus, hepatitis B and C, cytomegalovirus, parvovirus, and human T-cell lymphotropic viruses I and II. Other rare but reported pathogens include Epstein-Barr virus, syphilis, malaria, babesiosis, toxoplasmosis, and trypanosomiasis.
3. Hypothermia may occur from rapid transfusions of refrigerated blood.
4. Noncardiogenic pulmonary edema may be caused by incompatible, passively transferred leukocyte antibodies and usually occurs within 4 hours of transfusion. Clinical findings are respiratory distress, fever, chills, tachycardia, and patchy infiltrates on chest radiograph without cardiomegaly. There is no evidence of fluid overload. Most cases resolve with supportive care.
5. Electrolyte imbalance may occur. Citrate is part of the preservative solution and chelates calcium. Significant hypocalcemia even with massive transfusion is rare because patients with normal hepatic function readily metabolize citrate into bicarbonate. Hypokalemia can occur with large transfusions due to the metabolism of citrate to bicarbonate, leading to alkalosis, which drives potassium ions to the intracellular space. Hyperkalemia can occur in patients with renal failure or in neonates.

TABLE 138-1 Replacement Therapy for Congenital Factor Deficiencies

Coagulation factor	Incidence*	Replacement therapy
Factor I (fibrinogen)	150 cases	Cryoprecipitate
Factor II (prothrombin)	>30 cases	FFP for minor bleeding episodes Prothrombin complex concentrate for major bleeding
Factor V	150 cases	FFP
Factor VII	150 cases	FFP for minor bleeding episodes Prothrombin complex concentrates for major bleeding Recombinant factor VII (experimental)
Factor VIII	1 in 10,000 males	Factor VIII concentrates (cryoprecipitate or FFP if not available) Desmopressin for those with mild hemophilia
von Willebrand disease	up to 1 in 100 persons	Desmopressin (or some factor VIII concentrates or cryoprecipitate)
Factor IX	1 in 30,000 males	Factor IX concentrates
Factor X	1 in 500,000	FFP for minor bleeding episodes Prothrombin complex concentrates for major bleeding
Factor XI#	3 in 10,000 Ashkenazi Jews 1 in 1 000,000 in general	FFP
Factor XII	Several hundred cases	Replacement not required
Factor XIII	>100 cases	FFP or cryoprecipitate

*Incidence as of 1998.

#Factor XI levels correlate poorly with bleeding complications; many patients have low levels, but not bleeding complications.

Key: FFP = fresh-frozen plasma.

6. Graft-versus-host disease, fatal in more than 90% of cases, occurs when nonirradiated lymphocytes are inadvertently transfused into an immunocompromised patient.

EMERGENCY TRANSFUSIONS

Use of type O or type-specific, incompletely crossmatched blood may be life-saving but carries the risk of life-threatening transfusion reactions. Its use should be limited to the early resuscitation of patients with severe hemorrhage without adequate response to crystalloid infusion. Before transfusing, blood for baseline laboratory tests and type and crossmatching should be obtained. Rh-negative blood is preferable when it is not fully crossmatched.

TABLE 138-2 Acute Transfusion Reactions: Recognition, Management, Evaluation

Reaction type	Signs and symptoms	Management	Evaluation
Acute intravascular hemolytic reaction	Fever, chills, low back pain, flushing dyspnea, tachycardia, shock, hemoglobinuria	Immediately stop transfusion IV hydration to maintain diuresis; diuretics may be necessary Cardiorespiratory support as indicated Can be life threatening	Retype and crossmatch Direct and indirect Coombs tests CBC, creatinine, PT, aPTT Haptoglobin, indirect bilirubin, LDH, plasma free hemoglobin Urine for hemoglobin
Acute extravascular hemolytic reaction	Often have low-grade fever but may be entirely asymptomatic	Stop transfusion Rarely causes clinical instability	Hemolytic workup as above to rule out the possibility of intravascular hemolysis
Febrile nonhemolytic transfusion reaction	Fever, chills	Stop transfusion Manage as in intravascular hemolytic reaction (above) because cannot initially distinguish between the 2 Can treat fever and chills with acetaminophen and meperidine Usually mild but can be life threatening in patients with tenuous cardiopulmonary status Consider infectious workup	Hemolytic workup as above because initially cannot distinguish the etiology

Allergic reaction	If mild, urticaria, pruritus If severe, dyspnea, bronchospasm, hypotension, tachycardia, shock	Stop transfusion If mild, reaction can treat with diphenhydramine; if symptoms resolve, can restart transfusion If severe, may require cardiopulmonary support; do not restart transfusion	For mild symptoms that resolve with diphenhydramine, no further workup is necessary, although blood bank should be notified For severe reaction, do hemolytic workup as above because initially will be indistinguishable from a hemolytic reaction
Hypervolemic	Dyspnea, tachycardia, hypertension, headache, jugular venous distention, pulmonary rales, hypoxia	Stop transfusion or decrease rate to 1 mL/kg/h Diuresis Can be difficult to distinguish from a hemolytic reaction; if cannot distinguish, stop transfusion and treat as if intravascular hemolytic reaction	If clearly hypervolemic, no further evaluation is needed; CXR may be helpful If hemolytic reaction is a possibility, do hemolytic workup as above

Key: aPTT = activated partial thromboplastin time, CBC = complete blood count, CXR = chest radiograph, IV = intravenous, LDH = lactate dehydrogenase, PT = prothrombin time.

MASSIVE TRANSFUSION

Massive transfusion is the approximate replacement of a patient's total blood volume within a 24-hour period. Complications include bleeding, citrate toxicity, and hypothermia. Bleeding may result from thrombocytopenia, platelet dysfunction, disseminated intravascular coagulation, or coagulation factor deficiencies. Platelet transfusions are indicated only if there is thrombocytopenia with bleeding, and FFP is indicated only if there are documented coagulopathy and bleeding. Patients receiving more than 5 U of whole blood, those with liver disease, and neonates are at risk for hypocalcemia from citrate toxicity. The QT interval is not a reliable indicator in this setting; an ionized calcium level is necessary. Hypocalcemia should be treated with 5 to 10 mL of intravenous calcium gluconate slowly. Physicians should be wary of hypothermia when administering 3 U or more of blood rapidly.

BLOOD ADMINISTRATION

The correct identification of the patient and the unit to be transfused should always be ensured. A 16-gauge or larger intravenous catheter is preferred to prevent hemolysis and to permit rapid infusion; micropore filters should be used to filter out microaggregates of platelets, fibrin, and leukocytes. Normal saline solution is the only crystalloid compatible with PRBCs. Warmed saline solution (39°C to 43°C or 102.2°F to 109.4°F) may be given concurrently, or a blood warmer can be used to prevent hypothermia; the blood itself will hemolyze if warmed to greater than 40°C (104°F). Rapid transfusion may be facilitated by the use of pressure infusion devices. Patients at risk of hypervolemia should receive each unit over 3 to 4 hours.

For further reading in *Emergency Medicine: A Comprehensive Study Guide,* 6th ed., see Chap. 223, "Transfusion Therapy," by Sally A Santen.

Exogenous Anticoagulants and Antiplatelet Agents

Robert A. Schwab

This chapter reviews the major antithrombotic agents, their indications, contraindications, and complications of therapy.

ANTITHROMBOTIC AGENTS

Oral Anticoagulants

Oral anticoagulants inhibit thrombus formation or propagation and reduce the risk of embolization in patients with existing thrombosis. Sodium warfarin inhibits synthesis of vitamin K-dependent clotting factors and antithrombotic proteins C and S; dosing is guided by the international normalized ratio (INR), which is derived from the prothrombin time. The desired INR is between 2.0 and 2.5. Drug interactions and certain disease states can interfere with warfarin absorption or metabolism; these interactions may be clinically significant. Warfarin is contraindicated in pregnancy.

Full anticoagulation occurs 3 to 4 days after initiating therapy. During the first 24 to 36 hours, a hypercoagulable state occurs due to variable half-lives of clotting factors and antithrombotic proteins; the effects of this can be minimized by beginning with a warfarin dose of 5 mg/d. In situations where immediate anticoagulation is critical, a heparin product should be used until an adequate INR is achieved.

Parenteral Anticoagulants

Unfractionated heparin (UFH) is a heterogenous mixture of polysaccharides that binds antithrombin III; this complex inhibits multiple steps in the coagulation cascade. It is administered subcutaneously (SC) or intravenously (IV). The SC route is adequate only for prophylaxis. A bolus of 70 to 80 U/kg IV is followed by IV infusion at 15 to 18 U/kg/h. Therapy is monitored by the activated partial thromboplastin time; the therapeutic range is 1.5 to 2.5 times the normal value.

Low-molecular-weight heparin (LMWH) fractions (enoxaparin, dalteparin, and ardeparin) are derived from UFH; advantages of LMWH over UFH include longer half-life and decreased binding to plasma proteins, endothelial cells, and macrophages. LMWH is a much more predictable anticoagulant, with fixed dose-response relationships, and can be given once or twice daily SC. Enoxaparin is given in doses of 1 mg/kg SC twice daily; dalteparin is given in doses of 100 IU/kg SC twice daily. All are safe in pregnancy. Caution should be used in patients with renal disease.

UFH and LMWH are indicated for deep venous thrombosis (DVT) prophylaxis and treatment, pulmonary embolism (PE), unstable angina, and acute myocardial infarction. Only enoxaparin is approved for outpatient management of DVT. Laboratory monitoring is not necessary, except in patients with renal disease.

Direct Thrombin Inhibitors

Hirudin is a protein derived from leeches that is now prepared by using recombinant technology. Hirudin and its analogs inhibit circulating and clot-bound thrombin.

They are currently approved for use in patients with heparin-induced thrombocytopenia and as an anticoagulant during percutaneous coronary intervention.

Inhibitors of Platelet Activation

Aspirin is an irreversible inhibitor of cyclooxygenase, an enzyme that produces competing effects on platelet aggregation. At low doses, inhibitory effects predominate; the recommended antiplatelet dose is usually 81 to 162 mg/d. Side effects are usually related to the gastrointestinal tract; active gastrointestinal bleeding is a contraindication. Patients with guaiac-positive stool and no active bleeding can be treated with careful monitoring.

Nonsteroidal anti-inflammatory drugs reversibly inhibit cyclooxygenase; platelet inhibition usually lasts less than 24 hours.

Inhibitors of Platelet Aggregation

Platelet aggregation involves binding of fibrinogen to the platelet glycoprotein IIb and IIIa receptors. Platelet-membrane–altering agents ticlopidine 250 mg twice daily and clopidogrel 75 mg/d inhibit binding of adenosine diphosphate to the receptor, rendering it ineffective. These agents should be used in patients with acute coronary syndromes who cannot take aspirin. Glycoprotein IIb and IIIa inhibitors (abciximab, eptifibatide, and tirofiban) inhibit aggregation, prevent thrombosis, and may augment fibrinolysis. These agents can improve outcomes in selected patients with unstable angina and non-ST elevation myocardial infarction; they should be used in consultation with interventional cardiologists.

Fibrinolytic Agents

Fibrinolytic agents convert plasminogen to plasmin, which dissolves clots. Streptokinase and anistreplase (APSAC) are antigenic; retreatment should not occur within 6 months of the initial therapy. Tissue plasminogen activator is theoretically more "clot specific" than streptokinase or APSAC. Reteplase and tenecteplase are modified versions of tissue plasminogen activator, designed to improve efficacy and safety. Although the side effect profile of these agents is similar, bolus-dose fibrinolytics (APSAC, reteplase, and tenecteplase) result in significantly fewer medication errors.

INDICATIONS FOR ANTITHROMBOTIC THERAPY

Acute Myocardial Infarction

Fibrinolytic therapy should be initiated within 30 minutes or angioplasty within 90 minutes of arrival at the emergency department. Criteria include presentation within 12 hours of symptom onset, ST-segment elevation in 2 or more contiguous leads, or new onset left bundle branch block, and absence of contraindications (Table 139-1). Angioplasty is preferred in patients with cardiogenic shock. Timely initiation of therapy is more important than the spe-

TABLE 139-1 Contraindications to Fibrinolytic Therapy*

Absolute
  Active or recent internal bleeding (≤14 d)
  CVA <2–6 mo or hemorrhagic CVA†
  Intracranial or intraspinal surgery or trauma ≤2 mo
  Intracranial or intraspinal neoplasm, aneurysm, or arteriovenous
  malformation
  Known severe bleeding diathesis
  On anticoagulants (warfarin, PT >15 s, heparin, increased aPTT)
  Uncontrolled hypertension (ie, blood pressure >185/100 mm Hg)
  Suspected aortic dissection or pericarditis
  Pregnancy
Relative
  Active peptic ulcer disease
  Cardiopulmonary resuscitation >10 min
  Hemorrhagic opthalmic conditions
  Puncture of noncompressible vessel <10 d
  Advanced age >75 y
  Significant trauma or major surgery >2 wk and <2 mo
  Advanced kidney or liver disease

*Concurrent menses is *not* a contraindication.
†In ischemic CVA, symptoms longer than 3 hours, severe hemispheric stroke, plate-lets below 100/mL, and glucose below 50 or above 400 mg/dL are additional contraindications.
Key: aPTT = activated partial thromplastic time, CVA = cardiovascular accident, PT = prothrombin time.

cific agent used; fibrinolytics can be initiated in the prehospital setting. Aspirin or other platelet aggregation inhibitors should be given immediately.

Deep Venous Thrombosis or Pulmonary Embolism

Treatment of DVT or PE can be initiated with UFH or LMWH. LMWH is as effective as UFH, with fewer side effects, and allows for outpatient management of selected patients. Evidence for the role of fibrinolytic therapy in the management of PE is inconclusive.

Ischemic Stroke

The role of fibrinolytic therapy in acute stroke is controversial. Some benefit has been shown in patients treated within 3 hours of symptom onset, but overall mortality is not improved. The risk of cerebral hemorrhage is increased substantially; treatment policies should be developed in conjunction with radiologists and neurologists (see Chap. 142).

COMPLICATIONS OF ANTICOAGULATION AND ANTITHROMBOTIC THERAPY

Treatment for the complications of warfarin, heparin, and fibrinolytic therapy are discussed in Chap. 135.

For further reading in *Emergency Medicine: A Comprehensive Study Guide*, 6th ed., see Chap. 224, "Exogenous Anticoagulants and Antiplatelet Agents," by James Edward Weber, F. Michael Jaggi, and Charles V. Pollack Jr.

140 | Emergency Complications of Malignancy

T. Paul Tran

The emergency physician is frequently required to identify and manage a wide range of emergency complications related to malignancy. These oncologic emergencies arise from the underlying malignancy, complications of radiation or chemotherapy, or both.

BONE EMERGENCIES

Carcinomas of the breast, lung, prostate, kidney, bladder, and thyroid in addition to multiple myeloma and Hodgkin disease frequently metastasize to the proximal aspects of the limbs, pelvis, ribs, sternum, skull, and vertebrae. This metastasization may produce pain at the site, pathologic fracture, and, rarely, nerve root and spinal cord compressions. Primary bone tumors are rare, accounting for fewer than 1% of malignant bone lesions. Whereas certain cancers may cause osteolysis (eg, renal) and osteogenesis (eg, prostate), most cancers may produce simultaneous osteolytic and osteoblastic lesions.

Clinical Features

Patients with a known history of primary cancer may present with bone pain. The pain may be vague and insidious in onset, developing over days or weeks, and may even be the first sign of metastatic disease.

Diagnosis and Differential

The emergency physician should keep a high index of suspicion in patients who are at risk for metastatic disease. Clinical examination and plain radiographs are usually sufficient for the initial screening. Computed tomography (CT) can be used to evaluate bone integrity and soft tissue extension. Older women may suffer from osteoporosis in which cortical bone is preserved. In contrast, cortical bone is destroyed in metastatic bone cancer.

Emergency Department Care and Disposition

Patients with metastatic bone pain without fractures should be administered **narcotic analgesics** and have the plan of care discussed with an oncologist. Patients with pathologic fracture should be administered intravenous (IV) narcotics and have the fracture sites immobilized. Most pathologic fractures benefit from surgical intervention. Nondisplaced fractures involving non–weight-bearing bones can be treated conservatively. Indications for hospitalization include hemodynamic instability, irreducible fractures, neurovascular compromise, disabling fractures (eg, fractures of hip or femur), intractable pain, and inadequate home care.

ACUTE SPINAL CORD COMPRESSION

Clinical Features

Patients with epidural spinal cord compression may present with back pain (locally or with radiculopathy), bilateral motor weakness, sensory changes (hyperesthesia or anesthesia), and bladder or bowel retention or incontinence. Back pain is progressive, unrelenting, and worsened by recumbency. The thoracic spine is most commonly involved (70%), followed by the lumbar (20%) and cervical (10%) spine.

Diagnosis and Differential

Acute spinal cord compression can be misdiagnosed in patients with altered mentation and diabetic neuropathy. Intramedullary primary or metastatic disease may present similarly, but the extremity weakness is usually unilateral. The neurologic examination may show vertebral percussion tenderness, motor weakness, diminished or absent rectal tone and anal "wink," extremity areflexia, saddle anesthesia, and extremity sensory deficit. Postvoid bladder residual should be checked to determine whether more than 150 mL of urine is retained. Plain radiographs (or bone scan) can be ordered to identify the level of vertebral involvement, but gadolinium-enhanced magnetic resonance imaging of the entire spine is required to ascertain the diagnosis.

Emergency Department Care and Disposition

If epidural spinal cord compromise is clinically suspected, patients initially should be administered **dexamethasone** 24 mg IV every 6 hours. Adequate parenteral narcotic analgesics also should be given for pain control. Emergent consultation with specialists in radiation oncology and neurosurgery should be initiated for acute **radiation therapy** and/or **surgical decompression.**

UPPER AIRWAY OBSTRUCTION

Clinical Features

Tumors in the oropharynx, larynx, trachea, thyroid, and lung can cause upper airway obstruction. Acute airway obstruction occurs when a vulnerable upper airway is further compromised by a foreign body, airway edema, new bleeding, secretions, or infection. Patients may complain of dyspnea on exertion, wheezing, and orthopnea. Physical examination signs may include tachycardia, tachypnea, wheezing, stridor, intercostal retraction, and accessory muscle use. Stridor is an ominous sign. Bradycardia, cyanosis, or obtundation may be the harbingers of cardiac arrest.

Diagnosis and Differential

Metastatic disease, tracheomalacia, oropharyngeal infections (Ludwig angina and epiglottitis), and lower airway tumors also can produce the clinical syndrome of airway obstruction.

Emergency Department Care and Disposition

Measures should be taken immediately to ensure a patent airway. In consultation with an otolaryngologist or anesthesiologist, emergent **orotracheal intubation** using fiberoptic laryngoscopy or bronchoscopy should be performed. Newer modalities such as laryngeal airway masks may be used. Surgical **cricothyrotomy** and **tracheostomy** should be considered strongly if these methods fail or the site of obstruction is high (upper one third of the trachea). Percutaneous jet ventilation is contraindicated in upper airway obstruction.

MALIGNANT PERICARDIAL EFFUSION WITH TAMPONADE

Clinical Features

Symptomatic pericardial effusion is an uncommon but important entity to recognize because it can develop into cardiac tamponade. The rate of accumulation and distensibility of the pericardial sac determine the degree of hemodynamic instability. Patients may present with fatigue, chest heaviness, dyspnea, palpitations, cough, and syncope. Physical examination findings of tamponade include tachycardia, narrowed pulse pressure, hypotension, distended neck vein, muffled heart tone, and pulsus paradoxus. Common malignancies related to malignant pericardial effusions are breast carcinoma, lung carcinoma, and malignant melanoma.

Diagnosis and Differential

Chest radiograph may demonstrate an enlarged cardiac silhouette and pleural effusion. Electrocardiogram (ECG) may show sinus tachycardia, low QRS amplitude, and pulsus alternans. Transthoracic echocardiogram is diagnostic. Chemotherapy-induced cardiomyopathy and radiation-induced cardiac disease should be considered in the differential diagnosis.

Emergency Department Care and Disposition

Echocardiography-guided **percutaneous pericardiocentesis** under local anesthesia (general anesthesia is contraindicated) is the treatment of choice for cardiac tamponade. Oxygen, volume expansion with crystalloid, and dopamine, up to 20 μg/kg/min IV, can be initiated as temporizing measures before pericardiocentesis. Care of patients with malignant pericardial effusion without tamponade should be discussed with the oncologist.

SUPERIOR VENA CAVA SYNDROME

Clinical Features

Once considered a medical emergency, superior vena cava syndrome is currently recognized as a clinical entity that requires urgent diagnosis and treatment but rarely causes life-threatening complications. Patients may present with an insidious onset of dyspnea, chest pain, cough, and facial and arm swelling. Physical examination signs include distended neck and chest veins, nonpitting edema of the neck, distended arm veins and arm swelling, tongue and facial swelling, and cyanosis.

Diagnosis and Differential

Superior vena cava syndrome usually can be diagnosed based on characteristic history and physical examination findings. Chest radiograph may show a widened mediastinum. Contrast-enhanced CT of the chest is diagnostic.

Emergency Department Care and Disposition

Emergency therapy includes supplemental oxygen, sedation, bedrest, and elevation of the head and upper body. Increases in intracranial pressure can be treated with **methylprednisolone** 125 to 250 mg IV or **dexamethasone** 20 mg IV. Airway compromise should be managed with orotracheal intubation. Furosemide has been suggested as a temporizing measure, but its efficacy and safety are controversial. Diuresis can further exacerbate the already reduced cardiac output, leading to more hemodynamic instability. Intravascular stenting, chemotherapy, and radiotherapy are effective therapeutic measures after the specific tumor type is determined.

THROMBOEMBOLISM

Several factors place cancer patients at high risk for thromboembolic disease. Malignancy is often associated with a hypercoagulable state. Neoplastic cells and chemotherapy can cause intimal injury. Obstructive tumors often cause venous stasis, which is exacerbated by decreased mobility. Approximately 90% of pulmonary embolisms result from emboli originating in the deep veins of the pelvis and legs.

Clinical Features

Patients may present with dyspnea, fever, cough, dyspnea on exertion, pleuritic chest pain, leg pain or swelling, and, rarely, hemoptysis. Low-grade fever, tachypnea, tachycardia, pleural rub, and unilateral lower extremity swelling are some of the nonspecific findings that may be present on physical examination.

Diagnosis and Differential

Nonspecific T-wave inversion on ECG is a common abnormal finding. Alveolar arterial oxygen tension was abnormal in more than 60% of patients in the PIOPED study. The chest radiograph may demonstrate local infiltrates, ipsilateral diaphragm elevation, and Westermark (decreased lung markings from oligemia) or Hampton signs (wedge infiltrate). The D-dimer assay is sensitive but not specific for pulmonary embolism. Ventilation-perfusion scan and spiral CT are often diagnostic, but a pulmonary angiogram occasionally may be necessary to diagnose pulmonary embolism.

Emergency Department Care and Disposition

Resuscitative measures should be initiated on hemodynamically unstable patients, in addition to low-molecular-weight heparin (**enoxaparin** 1 mg/kg subcutaneously [SC]) or heparin therapy. Thrombolytic therapy should be considered in very selected cases. Admission into the hospital should be made in consultation with the patient's oncologist.

HYPERCALCEMIA OF MALIGNANCY

Clinical Features

Hypercalcemia associated with malignancy is caused most often by a parathyroid hormone-related peptide secreted by the cancer cells. This hormone activates the parathyroid hormone receptor, thereby stimulating osteoclastic activity and promoting renal reabsorption of calcium. Mild hypercalcemia (<12 mg/dL) usually is asymptomatic. More severe hypercalcemia may cause polydipsia, polyuria, generalized weakness, lethargy, anorexia, nausea, vomiting, constipation, abdominal pain, volume depletion, altered mentation, and frank psychosis. Malignancies known to cause hypercalcemia include multiple myeloma, carcinoma of the breast, squamous cell carcinoma of the lung, lymphoma, and renal cell carcinoma.

Diagnosis and Differential

ECG may demonstrate shortened QT interval, ST depression, and atrioventricular blocks. Total serum calcium level should be corrected for protein binding. Measurement of ionized calcium is confirmatory. Medications (diuretics), granulomatous disorders, primary hyperparathyroidism, and other endocrine disorders also can cause hypercalcemia.

Emergency Department Care and Disposition

Volume depletion should be corrected with IV crystalloid infusion. **Furosemide** 40 to 80 mg IV every 2 hours can then be added. Bisphosphonates such as **zoledronic acid** 4 mg IV over 15 minutes or **pamidronate** 60 to 90 mg IV over 4 to 24 hours can be initiated in the emergency department. Second-line drugs include **calcitonin** 4 IU/kg SC every 12 hours. **Hemodialysis** provides definitive treatment. Hypercalcemia of malignancy is a marker of advanced carcinomatosis, with median survival ranging from 1 month for patients without an effective anticancer option to 3 months for patients with treatment options. Withdrawal of treatment for hypercalcemia has been argued as a humane option for those with the 1-month median survival rate.

TUMOR LYSIS SYNDROME

Tumor lysis syndrome (TLS) usually occurs 1 to 3 days after the last radiochemotherapy of hematologic malignancies, especially Burkitt lymphoma. TLS refers to a constellation of metabolic abnormalities ignited by the death of neoplastic cells, which releases large quantities of intracellular contents and uric acid into the blood stream. TLS is characterized metabolically by hyperkalemia, hyperphosphatemia, hyperuricemia, secondary hypocalcemia, renal insufficiency, and renal failure. Acute renal failure exacerbates the hyperkalemia, which, with hypocalcemia, contributes to the development of potentially fatal cardiac arrhythmias.

Clinical Features

Patients may present with fatigue, lethargy, nausea, vomiting, and cloudy urine. Hypocalcemia may cause neuromuscular irritability, muscular spasm, seizure, and altered mentation.

Diagnosis and Differential

An electrolyte panel, including renal function, calcium, phosphate, and uric acid, in the proper clinical context is diagnostic. An ECG may show the peaked T waves of hyperkalemia.

Emergency Department Care and Disposition

Preventive measures by oncologists have reduced the incidence of TLS. Hyperkalemia should be treated in the usual fashion with **IV calcium, insulin, and bicarbonate and oral Kayexalate.** Hyperuricemia is treated by alkalinizing the urine with 2 ampules of sodium bicarbonate in 1 L 5% dextrose in water infused to maintain urine pH between 7.1 and 7.5. **Emergency hemodialysis** should be considered in the setting of serum potassium levels above 6.0 mEq/L, uric acid levels above 10.0 mg/dL, phosphate levels above

10 mg/dL, creatinine levels above 10 mg/dL, symptomatic hypocalcemia, or volume overload.

ADRENAL CRISIS

Clinical Features

Infiltration of adrenal tissue with cancer cells, additional physiologic stress of disease or procedure, and steroid withdrawal can precipitate an acute adrenal crisis (see Chap. 133). Patients may complain of fatigue, weakness, nausea, vomiting, and weight loss and are often hypotensive.

Diagnosis and Differential

Supportive laboratory tests include hypoglycemia, hyponatremia, and hyperkalemia. Septic, cardiogenic, and hypovolemic shock should be considered in the differential diagnosis.

Emergency Department Care and Disposition

Patients in shock should be given IV crystalloid boluses and **hydrocortisone** 100 to 300 mg IV every 6 to 8 hours while being worked up for other causes of shock. A serum cortisol level should be drawn before treatment, if time permits.

SYNDROME OF INAPPROPRIATE ANTI-DIURETIC HORMONE

The syndrome of inappropriate antidiuretic hormone (SIADH) is a clinical syndrome characterized by hyponatremia, inappropriately concentrated urine (>100 mOsm/L), and excessive urine sodium (>20 mEq/L) in the face of hypotonic plasma (<260 mOsm/L) and euvolemia. It can be caused by cancer (ectopic secretion of antidiuretic hormone) or its treatment (cytotoxicity of the paraventricular or supraoptic nucleus). Malignancies associated with SIADH include primary and metastatic brain cancer, small cell lung carcinoma, pancreatic adenocarcinoma, and prostate carcinoma.

Clinical Features

Symptoms are due mainly to hyponatremia, which includes anorexia, nausea, vomiting, headache, altered mentation, and seizure.

Diagnosis and Differential

Hypothyroidism, renal failure, cirrhosis, and adrenal crisis should be excluded. Hyponatremia in the proper context should raise the suspicion of SIADH. Serum osmolality, urine osmolality, and volume status should be determined before treatment.

Emergency Department Care and Disposition

Mild hyponatremia can be treated with water restriction (<500 mL/d). Sodium levels below 115 mEq/L associated with seizure activity should be treated with **3% normal saline** 1 mL/kg/h to raise the sodium concentration by not more than 2 mEq/L/h to avoid central pontine myelinolysis. Usually no more than 300 mL of hypertonic saline is required to improve the symptoms of hyponatremic encephalopathy. Patients should be monitored in an intensive care unit. Second-line drugs include **furosemide** 40 mg IV and **demeclocycline** 300 to 600 mg.

NEUTROPENIC FEVER

Fever, defined as recurrent temperatures above 38°C or a single temperature above 38.3°C in the presence of neutropenia, defined as an absolute neutrophil count (ANC) lower than 500 cells/mL, is a true medical emergency. Risks of death for patients increase as their ANC decreases, especially if the ANC is lower than 100 cells/mL.

Clinical Features

Febrile neutropenic patients initially may have minimal symptoms and findings but can succumb rapidly to sepsis and death. Infectious agents can be viral (cytomegalovirus, herpes simplex virus, or varicella zoster virus [VZV]), bacterial (*Staphylococcus, Streptococcus enterococci, Haemophilus influenzae, Escherichia coli, Klebsiella,* or *Pseudomonas aeruginosa*), or fungal (*Candida* or *Aspergillosis*).

Diagnosis and Differential

The sites of infection include central venous access catheter (exit site, tunnel, abscess, or line sepsis), skin, mouth, sinuses, chest or lung, abdomen (typhlitis or hepatosplenic candidiasis), perianal region (abscess), and central nervous system (meningitis, encephalitis, or brain abscess). Cultures should be taken from all lumens, skin and line sites, urine, sputum, and stool and sent for bacterial, fungal, and viral studies, as indicated. A chest radiograph may appear normal in neutropenic febrile patients with pneumonia because neutrophils are required for an infiltrate to appear. Others findings on the chest radiograph include radiation- or chemotherapy-induced changes and pulmonary hemorrhage or infarction. A complete blood count, chemistry, liver panel, coagulation panel, and urinalysis are also required in the workup.

Emergency Department Care and Disposition

Resuscitative measures should be initiated for hemodynamically unstable patients. Initial empiric antibiotic therapy should include an antipseudomonal agent such as **ceftazidime** (2 g IV), **cefepime** (2 g IV), or **imipenem** (500 mg IV), and an **aminoglycoside. Vancomycin** (1 g IV) is often added to cover methicillin-resistant *Staphylococcus aureus* and penicillin-resistant *Streptococcus pneumoniae.*

HYPERVISCOSITY SYNDROME

Clinical Features

Hyperviscosity syndrome refers to the condition of impaired blood rheology due to abnormal elevations of paraproteins (eg, Waldenström macroglobulinemia), pathologic erythrocytosis, or leukocytosis (eg, hematocrit >60%, white blood cell count >100 × 10^9/L). An elevated hematocrit (polycythemia) can be due to primary overproduction of red blood cells by the bone marrow (polycythemia vera) or as a paraneoplastic syndrome associated with renal cell carcinoma and hepatomas, among others. At levels above 60%, patients can develop symptoms such as headache, fatigue, and blurred vision and thrombotic complications such as stroke or mesenteric ischemia. Acute and chronic leukemias can produce white blood cell counts higher than 100,000/µL. Patients also may present with bleeding, abdominal pain, dyspnea, and altered mentation. Funduscopic examination may show the classic "sausage link effects."

Diagnosis and Differential

Hyperviscosity syndrome is usually suspected from history and physical examination, aided by findings of "rouleaux" formation (stacks of red blood cells) on routine smear. Serum viscosity may be 4 to 5 (normal, 1.4-1.8). Protein electrophoresis is diagnostic.

Emergency Department Care and Disposition

Patients who present with hyperviscosity syndrome should undergo a 2-unit **phlebotomy** and have 2 to 3 L crystalloid infused, followed by **plasmapheresis, leukapheresis,** or **chemotherapy,** as clinically indicated. Definitive care is individualized in consultation with the hematologist or oncologist.

NAUSEA AND VOMITING

Nausea and vomiting in cancer patients frequently result from cancer therapy (side effects of chemotherapy or radiation-induced enteritis), the cancer itself (infiltration of the gastrointestinal tract with neoplastic cells), or conditions causing nausea and vomiting as in the general population.

Clinical Features

Cancer patients present with a recent history of chemotherapy and may show signs of dehydration or infection.

Diagnosis and Differential

Increased intracranial pressure, bowel obstruction, infection, or cardiopulmonary disease should be excluded.

Emergency Department Care and Disposition

Nausea and vomiting in cancer patients receiving chemotherapy can be treated with dopamine receptor antagonists **(metoclopramide or promethazine), dexamethasone,** benzodiazepines **(lorazepam),** or a histamine antagonist **(diphenhydramine).** Serotonin antagonists **(ondansetron, dolasetron, or granisetron)** are the drugs of choice. In addition to antiemetics, dehydration and electrolyte abnormalities should be corrected with **IV crystalloid** and electrolyte replacement.

PAIN CONTROL

Pain in cancer patients can be broadly categorized into somatic pain (eg, bone pain from metastatic disease), visceral pain (eg, injury to the sympathetically innervated organs induced by cancer cells), and neuropathic pain (eg, infiltration or compression of central or peripheral nerves by cancer cells). The first 2 categories are also known as nociceptive and are usually responsive to narcotic analgesics. Treatment for neuropathic pain usually requires a multidisciplinary approach.

Clinical Features

Different cancer pain syndromes have been recognized. Radiation- and chemotherapy-induced mucositis causes pain due to injury of the mucosae in the upper (mouth) and lower (colorectal) portions of the gastrointestinal tract. A number of chemotherapeutic agents (eg, vinca alkaloids) can cause chemotherapy-induced polyneuropathy. Radiation also can cause radiation neuropathy, plexopathy, and myelopathy.

Diagnosis and Differential

Acute spinal cord compression, cauda equina syndrome, pathologic fractures, bowel obstruction, infection, and metastatic disease should be excluded in the evaluation.

Emergency Department Care and Disposition

Cancer patients with significant pain should be treated aggressively. Parenteral narcotic analgesics are preferred initially for all pain syndromes, with the recognition of its limited efficacy for neuropathic pain. The underlying cause of pain then should be identified and treated. Patients with intractable pain or inadequate social support should be admitted to the hospital for pain control.

For further reading in *Emergency Medicine: A Comprehensive Study Guide,* 6th ed., see Chap. 225, "Emergency Complications of Malignancy," by Paul Blackburn.

16 | NEUROLOGY

141 | Headache and Facial Pain

Jason Graham

HEADACHE

Clinical Features

Headaches represent up to 4% of all emergency department (ED) visits. The most important aspect in providing emergency care to a patient with a headache is to differentiate life-threatening from benign causes.

Patients with *subarachnoid hemorrhage* (SAH) (see Chaps. 142 and 161) most commonly complain of the sudden onset of a severe headache that is located in the occipital or neck region. The headache may be associated with nausea and vomiting. The history may define onset of headache with activities that elevate the blood pressure, such as exertion, defecation, intercourse, or coughing. Fifty percent of patients with SAH will have normal vital signs, normal level of consciousness, and no neck stiffness.

Subdural hematomas (see Chap. 161) should be suspected in any patient with a remote history of trauma and headache. Pain may be localized to the area of trauma or at another site as a result of a contrecoup injury. High-risk patients include alcoholics, those taking anticoagulants, and the elderly.

Meningitis (see Chap. 149) should be suspected in any patient presenting with headache, fever, and neck pain. The headache is usually diffuse in location and severity. Nuchal rigidity and photophobia may be present.

Migraine headaches are frequently the cause for patients to present to the ED. Aura-free migraine headaches account for approximately 80% of cases. Migraines are typically of gradual onset that become more severe. Pain is usually unilateral and exacerbated by physical activity, light, or loud noises. Nausea and vomiting are usually associated with the onset of the headache. Virtually any neurologic sign or symptom may occur with a migraine headache. Any change from the patient's typical migraine should raise the suspicion for other causes of headache.

Patients with *brain tumors* may describe the headache as bilateral, unilateral, constant, or intermittent. The headache may be worse in the morning, associated with nausea and vomiting, and positional.

Hypertensive headaches typically will become more severe as the diastolic pressure rises. Care must be taken to consider other causes of hypertension, such as pheochromocytoma, stroke, intracerebral process, preeclampsia, or any other cause of life-threatening headache. Distinction must be made from a hypertensive emergency, in which end-organ damage is present.

Tension headaches are usually bilateral, nonpulsatile, and not worsened by physical activity. Patients may complain of pain radiating from the neck up to the occiput.

Cluster headaches are rare and usually resolve without treatment. They can be of sudden onset, severe, and short acting. Headaches usually are unilaterally located in the temple, orbit, or supraorbital region. The pain is not exacerbated by movement, and patients typically will be pacing or unable to get into a position of comfort. Clinical findings associated with cluster headaches include conjunctival injection, lacrimation, nasal congestion, miosis, ptosis, and facial swelling.

Ophthalmic disorders, such as glaucoma, iritis, and optic neuritis, also may cause headache. Patients may complain of a headache that is localized to the globe, orbit, or retroorbital region.

Diagnosis and Differential

The most important tool in making the diagnosis in the patient with a headache is the history. Characteristics of headaches such as sudden onset, most severe, or associated with neurologic deficits, trauma, seizure, syncope, or fever should immediately direct the physician to evaluate for a potentially life-threatening cause of the headache. Prior history of a similar headache, family history, coexisting medical conditions, medications, immunosuppression, and location of pain are also important to assess.

A thorough physical examination, especially the neurologic examination, can complement the history in ruling out significant underlying pathology in most patients with headache. Areas to concentrate on include the funduscopic examination, palpation of the temporal region, sinuses, teeth, distribution of the fifth cranial nerve, meningeal signs, and unilateral "drift" in an outstretched, supinated arm. Tables 141-1 and 141-2 review the primary and secondary causes of headache syndromes and the differential diagnosis of headache, respectively.

Available modalities for further evaluation of the headache patient in the ED include computed tomography (CT), lumbar puncture, and magnetic resonance imaging. For a patient with a worrisome history or physical examination, CT scan of the head without contrast is usually the next step in the workup. The sensitivity of CT for detection of an SAH is approximately 93%. The sensitivity may be even higher if the scan is performed within the first 12 hours of hemorrhage; CT sensitivity falls to approximately 80% after 24 hours. If SAH is suspected and the head CT is negative, then the clinician must perform a lumbar puncture to screen for xanthochromia in the cerebrospinal fluid (CSF). A negative spectrophotometric test for CSF xanthochromia in a patient with longer than 12 hours of headache is nearly 100% sensitive. Xanthochromia may remain present for up to 2 weeks after a bleed. Persistently bloody CSF from tube 1 to tube 4 should raise the suspicion of SAH regardless of the presence of xanthochromia. In these cases, central nervous system vascular imaging or neurosurgical consultation should be obtained.

Emergency Department Care and Disposition

1. For patients with SAH, rebleeding and vasospasm are the major complications. Lowering the systolic blood pressure to 160 mm Hg or maintaining a mean arterial pressure of 110 mm Hg is associated with a decreased risk of rebleeding and mortality rate. **Nimodipine** (60 mg orally every 6 hours) reduces the incidence and severity of vasospasm and should be given to all patients with SAH. Nausea and vomiting should be treated promptly with antiemetics. Neurosurgical consultation is indicated.
2. Care of the patient with migraine headache consists of general comfort measures, abortive medications, and prophylactic therapy. General comfort measures include placing the patient in a darkened, quiet room and providing a cool, damp cloth for the forehead. Abortive medications used in the treatment of the patient with migraine headache include **dihydroergotamine mesylate, sumatriptan, and phenothiazine derivatives.**

TABLE 141-1 Primary and Secondary Causes of Headache

Primary headache syndromes
  Migraine
  Tension type
  Cluster
Secondary headache syndromes
  Vascular
    Subarachnoid hemorrhage
    Intraparenchymal hemorrhage
    Subdural or epidural hematoma
    Ischemic (stroke, transient ischemic attack)
    Cavernous sinus thrombosis
    Arteriovenous malformation
    Temporal arteritis
    Carotid or vertebral artery dissection
  CNS infection
    Meningitis (bacterial, viral, other)
    Encephalitis
    Cerebral abscess
  Non-CNS infection
    Focal or systemic
    Sinusitis
    Herpes zoster of face or scalp
  Other CNS
    Tumor (benign or malignant)
    Pseudotumor cerebri
  Ophthalmic
    Glaucoma
    Iritis
    Optic neuritis
  Drug-related and toxic or metabolic
    Nitrates and nitrites
    Chronic analgesic use and abuse
    Hypoxia or high altitude
  Hypercapnia
    Hypoglycemia
    Monosodium glutamate
    Carbon monoxide poisoning
    Alcohol withdrawal
  Miscellaneous
    Malignant hypertension
    Preeclampsia
    Fever
    Post-lumbar puncture
    Dental (referred)

Key: CNS = central nervous system.

Doses and considerations in the use of these agents are listed in Table 141-3.

3. Treatment of tension headaches consists of relaxation techniques, **nonsteroidal anti-inflammatory drugs (NSAIDs),** and other types of pain control. Severe tension headaches may be treated with the same medications as migraine headaches.

4. Cluster headaches will resolve with the administration of **high-flow oxygen** in 70% of patients. **Dihydroergotamine mesylate, NSAIDs, and**

TABLE 141-2 Differential Diagnosis of the Patient with Headache

Type of headache	History/physical findings
Migraine headache	Young at onset; lasts >60 min; unilateral, pulsating, throbbing; ± visual aura; nausea and vomiting; precipitated by foods, drugs, alcohol, exercise or orgasm; family history
Cluster headache	Onset in 20 s; predominantly male; brief episodes of pain (45–60 min); orbital/retroorbital pain; periodic and seasonal (spring/autumn); nasal congestion and conjunctival injection/tearing associated
Tension-type headache	Onset at any age; dull, nagging, persistent pain; progressively worse throughout day
Subarachnoid headache	Sudden onset, "worst headache ever"; loss of consciousness; meningismus; vomiting; occipital-nuchal location
Hypertensive headache	Throbbing, occipital
Meningitis	Entire head; fever; meningismus
Mass lesions	
Subdural hematoma	Depressed mental status; variable quality headache
Epidural hematoma	History of trauma, consciousness with headache followed by unconsciousness; fracture across groove of middle meningeal artery
Brain tumor	Pain on awakening or with Valsalva maneuver; new headache associated with nausea and vomiting
Brain abscess	Findings similar to those of mass lesions; fever
Sinusitis	Stabbing or aching pain, worse by bending or coughing, decreased in supine position
Toxic/metabolic headache	Bi-cranial; headache remits after removal from offending agent/environment
Postconcussion headache	History of trauma within hours to days; vertigo, nausea, vomiting, mood alterations, concentration difficulty associated
Pseudotumor cerebri	Obese, young female; irregular menstrual cycles/amenorrhea; papilledema
Acute glaucoma	Nausea, vomiting, orbital pain; edematous/cloudy cornea; midposition pupil; conjunctival injection; increased intraocular pressure

sumatriptan also may be effective; however, oral medications may be ineffective because of the length of time required for absorption and the short duration of the headache.

5. For patients with a hypertensive headache, reduction of blood pressure may be performed with a wide range of medications, including nitroglycerin, nitroprusside, or β-blockers (see Chap. 27). Care should be taken to decrease the mean arterial pressure by no more than 25% over the first hour. Patients who show no signs of end-organ damage and whose headache has resolved, blood pressure has normalized, and neurologic examination remains normal may be discharged with close follow-up in the next 24 hours.

6. Patients diagnosed with a subdural hematoma should receive an emergent neurosurgical consultation. See Chap. 161 for further discussion on therapy.

TABLE 141-3 Agents Used in the Emergency Department Treatment of Migraine Headache

Agent	Route	Considerations
Ergotamine	Inhalation, rectal	Contraindicated in coronary artery disease, hypertension, pregnancy
Chlorpromazine	0.1 mg/kg IV	May cause extrapyramidal effects, excellent antiemetic
Prochlorperazine	10 mg IV	May cause extrapyramidal effects, excellent antiemetic
Metoclopramide	10–20 mg IV	May cause extrapyramidal effects, excellent antiemetic
DHE	0.75–1.0 mg IV over 2 min	Contraindicated in coronary artery disease, hypertension, pregnancy
Sumatriptan	6 mg SC	Contraindicated in coronary artery disease, hypertension, pregnancy
Ketorolac	60 mg IM	Only moderately effective

Key: DHE = dihydroergotamine mesylate, IM = intramuscularly, IV = intravenously, SC = subcutaneously.

7. The emergency physician should administer empiric antibiotic therapy to any patient with suspected bacterial meningitis. Antibiotic therapy should not be delayed for the lumbar puncture. (See Chap. 149 for further discussion on therapy.)
8. Discharge instructions should include avoidance of the use of machinery or driving for patients who have received mentation-altering medications. Referral to a primary care physician is important because headache is often a chronic problem requiring ongoing care that is not best delivered in an ED. Discharge with combination analgesics that combine different mechanisms of action, thus leading to a lower dose of both analgesics, is recommended. These include acetaminophen or aspirin plus butalbital, with or without caffeine. Ergotamine is available sublingually, if not contraindicated.
9. Admission for management of pain associated with headache is rare. Reasonable indications for admission are: (*a*) migraine lasting for days associated with vomiting and dehydration, (*b*) chronic headache unresponsive to outpatient therapy, (*c*) headache secondary to suspected intracranial pathology (SAH, tumor, meningitis, etc), (*d*) underlying significant medical or surgical pathology, and (*e*) headache that significantly interferes with activities of daily living.

FACIAL PAIN

Temporal Arteritis

Temporal arteritis is a vasculitis affecting branches of the external carotid artery. Women are affected 4 times more frequently than men, and it occurs almost exclusively in patients older than 50 years. Headache is the most common complaint in patients with this disorder and is usually localized to the unilateral temple region. The pain usually is described as severe and throbbing. Systemic signs and symptoms may be present and include fever, malaise, weight loss, anorexia, diplopia, blurred vision, and polymyalgia. Physical examination may demonstrate tenderness to palpation of the temporal artery.

The diagnosis of temporal arteritis is established with at least 3 of 5 criteria: at least 50 years of age, new onset headache, temporal artery tenderness or diminished pulse of temporal artery, erythrocyte sedimentation rate greater than 50 mm/h, or abnormal temporal artery biopsy. The most serious complication of temporal arteritis is vision loss secondary to ischemic optic neuritis. Treatment with prednisone (40-60 mg/d) should be initiated immediately upon suspicion of temporal arteritis. Evaluation by an ophthalmologist should be made within 24 hours for definitive diagnosis.

Temporomandibular Disorder

Temporomandibular disorder (TMD) is a painful syndrome involving the temporomandibular joint, surrounding muscles, and ligaments. Patients often will complain of joint crepitance and pain with chewing, locking of the jaw with opening, and limited jaw movements. A small percentage of headaches may be traced to underlying TMD. Treatment of TMD consists of NSAIDs or narcotic analgesics. Follow-up should be made with a dentist.

Trigeminal neuralgia (Tic Douloureux)

Trigeminal neuralgia is often characterized as a sharp, electric-like pain that is brief and present in the unilateral trigeminal nerve distribution. Paroxysms of pain are integral in the diagnosis and the patient should be completely pain free in the interim. The pain typically lasts only a few seconds. The neurologic examination will be normal. Initial medical treatment may include carbamazepine, which has been shown to be very effective. Pain control is rarely an issue because the pain only lasts a few seconds. Referral to a neurologist should be made.

For further reading in *Emergency Medicine: A Comprehensive Study Guide,* 6th ed., see Chap. 227, "Headache and Facial Pain," by Christopher J. Denny and Michael J. Schull.

Stroke and Transient
Ischemic Attack

J. Stephen Huff

The term *stroke* refers to the clinical picture resulting from any disease process that disrupts blood flow to a region of the brain.

CLINICAL FEATURES

The clinical presentation of stroke is variable and depends on the area of brain injured and the degree of injury (Table 142-1). Transient ischemic attack (TIA) is a neurologic deficit that resolves within 24 hours, although most resolve within minutes. In the past, TIAs were not thought to result in permanent tissue injury; however, follow-up studies have indicated that more than 60% may be associated with radiologic changes of infarction, even in the absence of clinically detectable neurologic deficit.

Ischemic stroke involving the anterior cerebral artery typically causes leg weakness greater than arm weakness contralateral to the vascular occlusion. Patients may perseverate with speech or motor actions. A stroke involving the territory of the middle cerebral artery presents with contralateral weakness and numbness, typically with the arm affected more than the leg. The face is variably affected. A gaze preference toward the side of the infarct may be present. If the dominant hemisphere (left in most patients regardless of handedness) is involved, aphasia (receptive, expressive, or both) is often present. Inattention, neglect, or extinction on double-simultaneous stimulation (cortical sensory loss) may help to localize the lesion to the nondominant hemisphere.

The posterior circulation supplies blood to the brainstem, cerebellum, and visual cortex. Signs and symptoms attributable to a stroke in this distribution may be dramatic or subtle. They may include findings such as dizziness, vertigo, diplopia, dysphagia, ataxia, cranial nerve palsies, or bilateral limb weakness, singly or in combination. Occlusion of the basilar artery causes severe quadriplegia, coma, and the locked-in syndrome. The hallmark of a brainstem stroke is crossed neurologic deficits (ie, ipsilateral cranial nerve deficits with contralateral motor weakness). The lateral medullary syndrome (Wallenberg syndrome) is a specific posterior stroke syndrome resulting from occlusion of a vertebral artery and/or the posterior inferior cerebellar artery. Presenting signs include ipsilateral loss of facial pain and temperature sensation, with contralateral loss of these senses on the body, and gait or limb ataxia. Deficits of cranial nerves V, IX, X, or XI ipsilateral to the stroke may be present. Nausea and vomiting may be severe. An important subset of posterior circulation strokes are those involving the cerebellum. Early symptoms may include vertigo, headache, inability to walk, or nausea and vomiting. Cranial nerve abnormalities may be present.

Lacunar infarcts are fragments caused by large vessel syndromes and may be pure motor or sensory deficits; they are caused by infarction of small penetrating arteries and are commonly associated with chronic hypertension. Lesions are located primarily in the pons, deep white matter, internal capsule, and the basal ganglia.

TABLE 142-1 Stroke Syndromes

Ischemic stroke syndromes

Transient ischemic attack: resolves within 24 h (most within 30 min), 5–6% risk of stroke per year

Dominant hemispheric infarct: contralateral weakness or numbness, contralateral visual field cut, gaze preference, dysarthria, aphasia

Nondominant hemispheric infarct: contralateral weakness or numbness, visual field cut, constructional apraxia, dysarthria

Anterior cerebral artery infarct: contralateral weakness or numbness (leg more than arm), dyspraxia, speech perseveration, slow responses

Middle cerebral artery infarct: most common area involved, contralateral weakness or numbness (arm or face more than leg)

Posterior cerebral artery infarct: often go unrecognized by patient, minimal motor involvement, light-touch and pinprick sensation significantly affected

Vertebrobasilar syndrome: dizziness, vertigo, diplopia, dysphagia, ataxia, cranial nerve palsies, bilateral limb weakness, crossed neurologic deficits

Basilar artery occlusion: quadriplegia, coma, locked-in syndrome

Cerebellar infarct: "drop attack" associated with vertigo, headache, nausea, vomiting, and/or neck pain, cranial nerve abnormalities

Lacunar infarct: pure motor or sensory deficits

Arterial dissection: often associated with severe trauma, headache and neck pain hours to days prior to onset of neurologic symptoms

Hemorrhagic stroke syndromes

Intracerebral hemorrhage: similar to cerebral infarction with lethargy, headache, nausea, vomiting, significant hypertension

Cerebellar hemorrhage: dizziness, vomiting, truncal ataxia, inability to walk, rapidly progress to coma, herniation and death

Subarachnoid hemorrhage: severe headache, vomiting, decreased level of consciousness

Intracranial hemorrhages may be clinically indistinguishable from cerebral infarction and may present with any of the anatomic syndromes discussed previously. Headache, nausea, and vomiting may precede the neurologic deficit; the patient's condition may quickly deteriorate. Bleeding may occur in the putamen, thalamus, pons, or cerebellum (in order of decreasing frequency). Patients with subarachnoid hemorrhage (SAH) may develop focal findings related to location of an aneurysm. Patients typically present with a severe, constant headache, often occipital or nuchal in location. A recent history suggestive of a warning leak, or "sentinel hemorrhage," may be obtained in many patients. Vomiting often occurs with the onset of headache, and patients may have altered consciousness. Onset of headache is usually sudden, and a careful history may indicate onset with activity associated with elevated blood pressures such as exertion, defecation, intercourse, or coughing.

DIAGNOSIS AND DIFFERENTIAL

Although strokes are the most common cause of focal neurologic deficits, other causes must be considered (Table 142-2). All patients with neurologic deficits should be checked for hypoglycemia. Diagnostic tests that may indicate immediate emergency department interventions include an electrolyte panel, electrocardiogram, and computed tomography (CT).

TABLE 142-2 Differential Diagnosis of Acute Stroke

Hypoglycemia

Postictal paralysis (Todd paralysis)
Bell's palsy
Hypertensive encephalopathy
Epidural or subdural hematoma
Brain tumor or abscess
Complicated migraine
Encephalitis
Diabetic ketoacidosis
Hyperosmotic coma
Meningoencephalitis
Wernicke encephalopathy
Multiple sclerosis
Meniere disease
Drug toxicity (lithium, phenytoin, carbamazepine)

An emergent noncontrast CT scan is essential to quickly differentiate hemorrhage from ischemia. Most acute ischemic strokes will not be visualized by routine CT for at least 6 hours. Some hypodensity indicating infarction usually appears within 24 to 48 hours. CT identifies almost all parenchymal hemorrhages larger than 1 cm in diameter and up to 95% of subarachnoid hemorrhages (if obtained within 12 hours of symptom onset). If subarachnoid hemorrhage is still strongly suspected after a nondiagnostic CT scan, lumbar puncture is indicated.

Other diagnostic tests that may be of assistance in selected patients include a complete blood count, toxicologic tests, cardiac enzymes, echocardiogram, carotid duplex scanning, angiogram, and magnetic resonance imaging, or magnetic resonance imaging angiography.

EMERGENCY DEPARTMENT CARE AND DISPOSITION

1. Priority should be given to airway management and oxygenation. Patients should be placed on a cardiac monitor, and intravenous (IV) access should be established. Dextrose-containing solutions should be avoided except in patients with proven hypoglycemia.

2. A cautious approach to the management of elevated blood pressure is recommended in acute ischemic stroke. In general, only persistent, severe hypertension (systolic blood pressure >220 mm Hg systolic or mean arterial pressure >130 mm Hg) should be treated. Recommended agents include **labetalol** or **enalapril.**

3. In hypertensive patients being considered for thrombolytic therapy, the use of labetalol is recommended to reduce blood pressure to below 185/115 mm Hg; requirements for more aggressive treatment of hypertension exclude the use of recombinant tissue-type plasminogen activator (rt-PA) in stroke patients. However, after the use of rt-PA in acute stroke, aggressive treatment is warranted to maintain the blood pressure below 185/115 mm Hg.

4. The US Food and Drug Administration approved the use of IV **rt-PA (Activase/alteplase)** in acute ischemic stroke in 1996. The use of rt-PA for treatment of acute stroke requires medical staff and institutional commitments. Thrombolytic therapy in stroke is not recommended when the

time of onset cannot be ascertained reliably. Strokes recognized upon awakening should be timed from when the patient was last known to be without symptoms. The use of intraarterial delivery of thrombolytics remains investigational.

5. A review of rt-PA inclusion and exclusion criteria (Table 142-3) should be performed, and an emergent noncontrast head CT and neurologic consultation arranged. Any hemorrhage on CT scan excludes the use of rt-PA; detection of a large area of hypodensity may indicate an acute stroke and may suggest that onset was at least several hours previously. The total dose of rt-PA is 0.9 mg/kg IV, with a maximum dose of 90 mg;

TABLE 142-3 Criteria for Use of rt-PA in Acute Ischemic Stroke and Management of Patients After Use of rt-PA

Inclusion	Exclusion
Age 18 or older	Minor stroke syndromes
Clinical diagnosis of ischemic stroke	Rapidly improving neurologic signs
Well-established time of onset <3 h	Prior intracranial hemorrhage
	Blood glucose <50 or >400
	Seizure at onset of stroke
	Gastrointestinal or genitourinary bleeding within preceding 21 d
	Recent myocardial infarction
	Major surgery within 14 d
	Pretreatment SBP >185 mm Hg or DBP >110 mm Hg
	Previous stroke or head injury within 90 d
	Current use of oral anticoagulants
	Use of heparin within preceding 48 h
	Platelet count 100,000 mL
	Suspected aortic or vascular dissection or lumbar puncture (LP)

Management
Monitor arterial blood pressure during the first 24 h after starting treatment, every 15 min for 2 h after starting infusion, then every 30 min for 6 h, and then every 60 min for 24 h total.

If SBP is 180–230 mm Hg or DBP is 105–120 mm Hg for ≥2 readings 5–10 min apart:
  Give IV labetalol 10 mg over 1–2 min. The dose may be repeated or doubled every 10–20 min up to a total dose of 150 mm Hg.
  Monitor blood pressure every 15 min during labetalol treatment and observe for hypotension.

If SBP >230 mm Hg or if DBP is 121–140 mm Hg for ≥2 readings 5–10 min apart:
  Give IV labetalol 10 mg over 1–2 min. The dose may be repeated or doubled every 10–20 min up to a total dose of 150 mm Hg.
  Monitor blood pressure every 15 min during labetalol treatment and observe for hypotension.
  If no satisfactory response, infuse sodium nitroprusside 0.5–1.0 μg/kg/min; continuous arterial pressure monitor is advised.

If DBP >140 mm Hg for ≥2 readings 5–10 min apart:
  Infuse sodium nitroprusside 0.5–1.0 μg/(kg · min); continuous arterial pressure monitor is advised.

Key: DBP = diastolic blood pressure, IV = intravenously, LP = lumbar puncture, rt-PA = recombinant tissue type plasminogen activator, SBP = systolic blood pressure.

10% of the dose is administered as a bolus, with the remaining amount infused over 60 minutes. No aspirin or heparin should be administered in the initial 24 hours after treatment. Intracerebral bleeding should be suspected as the cause of any neurologic worsening until repeat CT imaging is obtained.

6. Antiplatelet strategies form the cornerstone for secondary stroke prevention in most stroke and TIA patients. **Aspirin** (50–300 mg orally) remains the initial choice in the patient with a first-ever stroke or TIA. Aspirin use, however, will interfere with any subsequent consideration for use of rt-PA. **Dipyridamole** and **clopidogrel** are other antiplatelet activity agents.

7. Although frequently used in the past for stroke treatment, the benefit of unfractionated heparin in any stroke syndrome remains unproven. However, its use may be considered in patients with recent TIAs who are at high risk for stroke, including patients with (*a*) known high-grade stenosis in the appropriate vascular distribution for the symptoms, (*b*) a cardioembolic source such as atrial fibrillation or valvular disease (except infective endocarditis), (*c*) TIAs of increasing frequency (crescendo TIAs), and (*d*) TIAs despite antiplatelet therapy.

8. Early **neurosurgical consultation** may be needed for patients with cerebellar infarction or hemorrhage. Cerebellar swelling with compressions of the brainstem may lead to rapid deterioration. Emergency posterior fossa decompression in selected patients may be lifesaving.

9. Management of blood pressure in intracranial hemorrhage remains controversial. Current recommendations are that only severe hypertension (ie, systolic blood pressure >220 mm Hg or diastolic blood pressure >120 mm Hg) be treated. When treated, blood pressure should be lowered gradually to pre-hemorrhage levels by using **labetalol** or **nitroprusside.** For patients with evidence of increased intracranial pressure (ICP), **head elevation** to 30° and **mannitol** (0.25–1.0 g/kg IV) are standard recommendations. Neurosurgical consultation for ICP monitoring should be considered in patients with a Glasgow Coma Scale score below 9 and in all patients whose condition is thought to be deteriorating because of elevated ICP.

10. In patients with SAH, risk of rebleeding is greatest in the first 24 hours. Rebleeding and vasospasm are the major complications. In patients with elevated blood pressures, lowering systolic blood pressure to 160 mm Hg or maintaining a mean arterial pressure of 110 mm Hg is associated with lower risk of rebleeding and a decreased mortality rate. **Nimodipine** 60 mg orally every 6 hours reduces the incidence and severity of vasospasm and should be given to all patients with SAH. **Phenytoin** loading to decrease possible seizures is often recommended. Nausea and vomiting should be treated promptly with antiemetics.

11. Patients with new onset ischemic strokes or hemorrhages should be admitted for monitoring and observation, even if they are not candidates for interventional therapy. Patients with new onset TIAs should be evaluated for possible cardiac sources of emboli or high-grade stenosis in the carotid arteries. Because of the proven efficacy of carotid endarterectomy, patients should be considered for admission unless high-grade stenosis of the carotid artery can be excluded promptly by imaging (ultrasound or magnetic resonance angiography). Current practice suggests that an alternative to admission may be prompt outpatient evaluation and

follow-up. Patients without high-grade stenosis may be discharged on antiplatelet therapy with close follow-up. The patient and family members should be given clear instructions to return for further treatment if the patient experiences worsening or new symptoms.

For further reading in *Emergency Medicine: A Comprehensive Study Guide,* 6th ed., see Chap. 228, "Stroke, Transient Ischemic Attack, and Other Central Focal Conditions," by Phillip A. Scott and Caroline A. Timmerman.

143 | Altered Mental Status and Coma

C. Crawford Mechem

Mental status is the clinical state of emotional and intellectual functioning of the individual. Presentations of altered mental status frequently encountered by emergency physicians include delirium, dementia, and coma.

DELIRIUM

Clinical Features

Delirium is a transient disorder characterized by impairment of attention and cognition. Wake and sleep cycles are disturbed, and the patient manifests a fluctuating course of confusion. Delirium is a constellation of signs and symptoms due to an underlying cause as opposed to being a distinct disease entity. Delirium may begin abruptly, but by definition lasts for less than 1 month. Attention, perception, thinking, and memory are distorted to different degrees. Alertness is reduced, as manifested by a difficulty in maintaining attention and concentration. Activity levels may be increased, decreased, or alternate between the 2 extremes of agitation and somnolence. Evidence of organic disease such as tachycardia, hypertension, tremor, asterixis, sweating, or emotional outbursts may be present. Hallucinations, more commonly visual, also may be noted.

Delirium, dementia, and psychiatric causes have features that might aid the clinician in distinguishing between them (Table 143-1). The distinction often can be made based on time course of onset and assessment of the patient's mental status.

Diagnosis and Differential

Historical and physical examination findings are needed to confirm the diagnosis. History is often obtained from family or caregivers who can confirm the time course of symptoms. The acute onset of attention deficits and cognitive abnormalities with fluctuating severity through the day and worsening at night is virtually diagnostic of delirium. The physical examination is directed at finding a precipitating process.

The ordering of ancillary tests should be guided by the specific case. Laboratory work such as fingerstick serum glucose level, basic chemistries, blood urea nitrogen (BUN), creatinine, urinalysis, complete blood count (CBC), blood cultures, liver function tests, thyroid function studies, arterial blood gas analysis, serum drug level of any daily medications, cerebrospinal fluid (CSF) analysis, ethanol level, and toxicologic screening are appropriate. A chest radiograph, echocardiogram, and computed tomography (CT) of the head also may be indicated.

The differential diagnosis of delirium in the elderly is listed in Table 143-2.

Emergency Department Care and Disposition

1. Treatment is directed at the underlying cause. The patient must be protected while diagnostic workup is in progress. Institutional confinement or

679

TABLE 143-1 Features of Delirium, Dementia, and Psychiatric Psychosis

Characteristic	Delirium	Dementia	Psychiatric
Onset	Sudden	Insidious	Sudden
Course over 24 h	Fluctuating	Stable	Stable
Consciousness	Reduced	Alert	Alert
Attention	Disordered	Normal	May be disordered
Cognition	Disordered	Impaired	May be impaired
Orientation	Impaired	Often impaired	May be impaired
Hallucinations	Visual and/or auditory	Often absent	Usually auditory
Delusions	Transient, poorly organized	Usually absent	Sustained
Movements	Asterixis, tremor may be present	Often absent	Absent

restraint policies should be adhered to, when indicated. Environmental manipulation such as adequate lighting and psychosocial support may put the patient at ease.

2. Sedation is often necessary to relieve severe agitation. **Haloperidol** 5 to 10 mg orally or parenterally is a frequent first choice. This may be repeated at 20- to 30-minute intervals as needed. The dose should be reduced in the elderly. **Lorazepam** 0.5 to 2 mg orally or parenterally may be used in conjunction with haloperidol, and the dose should be dictated by the patient's age and weight.

3. Unless a readily reversible cause for the acute mental status change is identified and corrected, and there is a return to baseline mental status, most patients should be admitted for further evaluation and treatment.

DEMENTIA

Clinical Features

Dementia is characterized by slowly progressing impairment of cognitive function while alertness remains intact. Most cases are idiopathic and are classified as Alzheimer disease. The other large category is vascular dementia. However, multiple other disease processes can progress to dementia. A rapid evolution of symptoms should prompt the emergency physician to search for another process simulating dementia or a comorbidity that may be hastening the progression of dementia.

Impairment of memory and orientation with preservation of motor function and speech is characteristic of the onset of Alzheimer disease. Short-term memory is more frequently affected, whereas long-term memory may be preserved. The progression of symptoms may include memory loss, difficulty naming objects, forgetting items, loss of reading ability, difficulty in social interactions, disorientation, speech difficulties, anxiety, depression, inability to care for oneself, and personality change. Patients with vascular dementia share many of the same symptoms of Alzheimer disease. However, on physical examination, they may have exaggerated or asymmetric reflexes, gait abnormalities, or focal extremity weakness.

TABLE 143-2 Important Medical Causes of Delirium in Elderly Patients

Infection	Pneumonia
	Urinary tract infection
	Meningitis or encephalitis
	Sepsis
Metabolic/toxic	Hypoglycemia
	Alcohol ingestion
	Electrolyte abnormalities
	Hepatic encephalopathy
	Thyroid disorders
	Alcohol or drug withdrawal
Neurologic	Stroke or transient ischemic attack
	Seizure or postictal state
	Subarachnoid hemorrhage
	Intracranial hemorrhage
	Mass CNS lesion
	Subdural hematoma
Cardiopulmonary	Congestive heart failure
	Myocardial infarction
	Pulmonary embolism
	Hypoxia or CO_2 narcosis from COPD
Drug related	Antiemetics
	Antihistamines
	Antiparkinsonian agents
	Antipsychotics
	Antispasmodics
	Muscle relaxants
	Tricyclic antidepressants
	Digoxin
	Sedative-hypnotics
	Narcotic analgesics

Key: CNS = central nervous system, COPD = chronic obstructive pulmonary disease.

Diagnosis and Differential

The history of memory problems is generally one of slow, steady progression. Abrupt changes increase the likelihood of a vascular etiology. Physical examination does not determine the diagnosis of dementia but may help to identify associated causes. Focal neurologic deficits may suggest vascular dementia or a mass lesion. Increased motor tone, muscle rigidity, or a movement disorder may suggest Parkinson disease.

Diagnostic testing should be directed at finding a potentially treatable etiology or a comorbidity that is exacerbating the patient's baseline condition. Laboratory work may include fingerstick serum glucose level, CBC, basic chemistries, BUN, creatinine, calcium, glucose, liver function tests, serum vitamin B_{12} level, thyroid function studies, urinalysis, and serology for syphilis. Additional studies that may be helpful in specific cases include erythrocyte sedimentation rate, serum folate, testing for the human immunodeficiency virus, and chest radiograph. CSF analysis is not required in all cases but should be considered if the diagnosis is in question. A head CT scan should be performed at some point during the patient's evaluation.

Diagnosis of probable vascular dementia requires signs of cerebrovascular disease. There must be a temporal relation between stroke and dementia, with dementia developing within 3 months of stroke.

The differential diagnosis of dementia includes delirium and a variety of other disease processes (Table 143-3).

Emergency Department Care and Disposition

1. Approximately 10% to 20% of patients have a treatable form of dementia, implying that the underlying process cannot be reversed in most cases. However, all types of dementia may benefit from environmental or psychosocial interventions. Treatment is best coordinated with caregivers who are in a position to monitor the patient's behavior pattern over time.

TABLE 143-3　Classification of Dementia by Cause

Degenerative
Alzheimer disease
Huntington disease
Parkinson disease, others
Vascular
Multiple infarcts
Hypoperfusion (cardiac arrest, profound hypotension, others)
Subdural hematoma
Subarachnoid hemorrhage
Infectious
Meningitis (sequelae of bacterial meningitis, fungal, TB)
Neurosyphilis
Viral encephalitis (herpes, HIV), Creutzfeldt-Jakob disease
Inflammatory
Lupus
Demyelinating disease, others
Neoplastic
Primary tumors, metastatic disease
Carcinomatous meningitis
Paraneoplastic syndromes
Traumatic
Traumatic brain injury
Subdural hematoma
Toxic
Alcohol
Medications (anticholinergics, polypharmacy)
Metabolic
B_{12} or folate deficiency
Thyroid disease
Uremia, others
Psychiatric
Depression
Hydrocephalus
Normal pressure hydrocephalus (communicating hydrocephalus)
Noncommunicating hydrocephalus

Key: HIV = human immunodeficiency virus, TB = tuberculosis.

2. Antipsychotic medications have been used to manage psychotic and nonpsychotic behavior among Alzheimer patients, but are associated with adverse effects. These medications therefore should be reserved for patients with persistent psychotic features or disruptive or violent behavior. Treatment of vascular dementia is limited to management of risk factors, including hypertension.

3. Most patients with a new diagnosis of dementia will require admission for further evaluation and management. However, patients with longstanding symptoms, consistent caregivers, and reliable follow-up may be discharged for outpatient evaluation after life-threatening conditions have been excluded. The existence of comorbidity, a rapidly progressive or atypical course, or an unsafe or uncertain home situation warrants admission.

COMA

Clinical Features

Coma may be defined as an eyes-closed state with inappropriate responses to environmental stimuli. Alertness, self-awareness, language, reasoning, spatial relationship integration, and emotions are impaired. The clinical features of coma vary with the depth of coma and the etiology. The causes of coma may be divided into 2 large categories: diffuse central nervous system (CNS) dysfunction (toxic-metabolic etiologies) and structural coma. Structural coma may be further divided into hemispheric (supratentorial) and posterior fossa comas. Toxic and metabolic causes of coma result from a wide range of clinical conditions. In most cases, physical examination findings will be symmetric without focal deficits, reflecting the diffuse insult to the brain. Pupils are, in general, small but reactive. Coma resulting from lesions of the hemispheres or supratentorial masses often presents with progressive hemiparesis and asymmetry of muscle tone and reflexes. Eyes may be conjugately deviated toward the side of the lesion. Posterior fossa (or infratentorial) lesions often cause abrupt coma, abnormal extensor posturing, loss of pupillary reflexes, and impaired extraocular movements.

Diagnosis and Differential

Diagnosis, stabilization, and treatment of the comatose patient often occur simultaneously. History is crucial in determining the etiology of coma. Valuable sources of information may include prehospital personnel, caregivers, family, bystanders, and old medical records. Establishing the time course over which the coma developed is important. An abrupt onset suggests a potentially catastrophic process such as an intracranial hemorrhage. A more gradual progression of symptoms may result from a metabolic process or tumor.

Physical examination of comatose patients can be challenging. Vital signs including temperature and oxygen saturation should be carefully assessed. A detailed physical examination may show signs of trauma or evidence of a toxidrome. A detailed neurologic examination may not be feasible. However, assessment of cranial nerves through pupillary examination and testing of corneal and oculovestibular reflexes may suggest a focal CNS lesion that is potentially treatable with surgery. Extensor or flexor posturing are nonspecific but suggest profound CNS dysfunction.

Diagnostic tests should be directed at identifying the underlying etiology. Laboratory work such as fingerstick serum glucose level, basic chemistries,

TABLE 143-4 Differential Diagnosis of Coma

Coma from causes affecting the brain diffusely
Encephalopathies
Hypoxic
Metabolic
Hypoglycemia
Hyperosmolar state (eg, hyperglycemia)
Electrolyte abnormalities (eg, hyper- or hyponatremial, hypercalcemia)
organ system failure
Hepatic encephalopathy
Uremia/renal failure
Endocrine (eg, Cushing, Addison, hypothyroid, etc)
Hypertensive encephalopathy
Toxins
Drug reactions (eg, neuroleptic malignant syndrome)
Environmental causes: hypothermia, hyperthermia
Deficiency state: Wernicke encephalopathy
Sepsis
Coma from primary CNS disease or trauma
Direct CNS trauma
Vascular disease
Intraparenchymal hemorrhage (hemispheric, basal ganglia, brainstem, cerebellar
Subarachnoid hemorrhage
Infarction
Hemispheric, brainstem
CNS infections
Neoplasms
Seizures
Nonconvulsive status epilepticus
Postictal state

Key: CNS = central nervous system.

urinalysis, BUN, creatinine, CBC, blood cultures, liver function tests, arterial blood gas analysis, serum drug level of any daily medications, CSF analysis, and toxicologic screening are appropriate. CT scanning of the head should be obtained even if the pretest probability is low because some intracranial processes may be corrected by emergency surgery.

The differential diagnosis of coma includes generalized disease processes that also affect the brain and primary CNS disorders (Table 143-4).

Emergency Department Care and Disposition

1. Treatment of coma involves identification of the etiology and initiation of specific therapy. Stabilization of airway, ventilation, and circulation is the top priority. **Endotracheal intubation** may be indicated to protect the airway. Readily reversible causes such as hypoglycemia, hypoxia, and opiate overdose should be sought.
2. If elevated intracranial pressure is suspected, urgent **neurosurgical consultation** should be requested. Standard methods should be used to decrease intracranial pressure (see Chap. 161).

3. Patients with readily reversible causes of coma, such as insulin-induced hypoglycemia, may be discharged if treatment is initiated, the patient returns to baseline mental status, the cause of the episode is clear, and the patient has reliable home care and follow-up. In all other cases, admission is warranted for further evaluation and treatment.

For further reading in *Emergency Medicine: A Comprehensive Study Guide,* 6th ed., see Chap. 229, "Altered Mental Status and Coma," by J. Stephen Huff.

144 | Ataxia and Gait Disturbances

C. Crawford Mechem

Ataxia is the failure to produce smooth, intentional movements. Gait disturbances include ataxia and other conditions. Ataxia and gait disturbances are symptoms of underlying illness as opposed to being disease entities in themselves.

CLINICAL FEATURES

Ataxia and gait disturbances result from systemic illnesses and conditions affecting the nervous system. Systemic illnesses include intoxication (ethanol, anticonvulsants, sedative-hypnotics, or heavy metals) or metabolic conditions (hyponatremia or inborn errors of metabolism). Neurologic causes include peripheral and central nervous system (CNS) pathology. Ataxia may be categorized into 2 types. *Motor ataxias* are usually due to cerebellar processes. *Sensory ataxia* results from failure of transmission of proprioceptive information to the CNS, usually from disorders of peripheral nerves, spinal cord, or cerebellar input tracts.

A thorough history and physical examination are needed to determine the underlying etiology. Onset of symptoms and their rate of progression determine acuity. For example, an abrupt onset of gait disturbance and a severe headache may reflect a catastrophic CNS event requiring immediate intervention. Thus, associated symptoms such as headache, nausea, fever, weakness, or paresthesias should be sought. The patient should be asked about current medications, ethanol use, and family history of similar conditions. In children, any history of musculoskeletal pathology, metabolic disorders, recent immunizations, or viral illnesses including varicella should be elicited.

A general physical examination should be performed to evaluate for systemic illness. This is followed by a detailed neurologic examination and gait testing. The patient should be observed while sitting upright, rising to a standing position, walking, and turning. Gait abnormalities may be manifested by asking the patient to walk at a normal speed, on the heels and on the toes, and tandem toe-to-toe walking. A *cerebellar* or *motor ataxic* gait is wide-based, with unsteady, irregular steps. The gait of sensory ataxia involves abrupt movement of the legs and slapping impact of the feet. An *apraxic* gait is one in which the patient has lost the ability to initiate the process of walking despite normal motor function. An *equine* gait is characterized by foot drop due to peroneal muscle weakness. A *festinating* gait is narrow-based, with small, shuffling steps that become more rapid, a gait common in Parkinson disease. A *senile* gait is slow with a short stride and wide base, commonly seen in the elderly and in those with neurodegenerative disorders. A *functional* gait is one in which the patient is seemingly unable to walk steadily, even though sensory and motor pathways and cerebellar function are intact, and is usually a manifestation of conversion disorder.

The cerebellum is tested by having the patient perform smooth, voluntary movements and rapidly alternating movements. Abnormalities include *dysmetria*, characterized by inaccurate fine movements. *Dyssynergia* is the breakdown of movements into parts as assessed by finger-to-nose testing. *Dysdiadochokinesia* is characterized by clumsy rapid movements, identified by having the patient pat the thigh with the palm and then the back of the hand in rapidly alternating movements. This should be performed on both sides. The heel-to-shin test also assesses cerebellar function. In cerebellar disease, there is an action tremor, and the knee is initially overshot. In posterior column disease, there is difficulty locating the knee, and the heel weaves from side to side or falls off the shin. The Romberg test assesses sensation and distinguishes sensory from motor ataxia. The patient stands upright with feet close together, arms outstretched, and eyes open. Inability to maintain a steady posture confirms the presence of ataxia. The patient then closes the eyes. If the ataxia worsens, the test is positive, suggesting a sensory ataxia. If there is no change with eyes closed (negative Romberg test), a motor ataxia is suggested, with possible localization to the cerebellum.

Sensory examination should include position or vibration testing and sensation to pinprick. Abnormal deep tendon reflexes, such as asymmetry or spasticity, may suggest an alternative diagnosis. Nystagmus suggests a cause in the CNS rather than in the spinal cord or peripheral nerves.

DIAGNOSIS AND DIFFERENTIAL

The extent of patient evaluation will be dictated by the acuity of symptom onset. Patients with an acute gait disturbance and children warrant an in-depth initial evaluation. Neuroimaging, such as computed tomography or magnetic resonance imaging, is appropriate in the proper clinical setting, as is neurology consultation. Ordering of laboratory studies such as electrolytes or a B_{12} level should be case specific. A lumbar puncture is warranted if an infectious etiology is suspected. For patients with ataxia, efforts should be directed at determining whether it is motor or sensory and whether the etiology is a systemic illness or nervous system pathology. In the latter case, distinguishing a central from a peripheral etiology is important.

EMERGENCY DEPARTMENT CARE AND DISPOSITION

Treatment is directed at the suspected etiology.

1. **Thiamine** 100 mg intravenously should be administered to patients, such as alcoholics, suspected of having Wernicke disease, which is suggested by findings of ataxia, altered mental status, and ophthalmoplegia.
2. **Vitamin B_{12}** replacement is appropriate for patients with suspected deficiency manifesting such as posterior column dysfunction.
3. Disposition depends on the presumptive diagnosis, likely progression, and consideration of patient safety. Patients unable to walk or care for themselves should be admitted. In the case of a slowly progressing process in which the patient can be safely cared for at home, referral for further outpatient evaluation may be appropriate once life-threatening processes have been excluded.

For further reading in *Emergency Medicine: A Comprehensive Study Guide*, 6th ed., see Chap. 230, "Ataxia and Gait Disturbances," by J. Stephen Huff.

145 | Vertigo and Dizziness

Andrew K. Chang

Dizziness is a common but nonspecific complaint encountered in the emergency department (ED). When interviewing patients who present with the chief complaint of dizziness, it is important not to suggest meanings to them. Instead, the emergency physician should ask patients to explain in their own words what they mean by the word *dizzy*. Patients generally provide an answer that falls into 1 or more of the following 4 categories of dizziness: vertigo, near syncope, disequilibrium, and psychogenic dizziness.

CLINICAL FEATURES

Vertigo

Vertigo is defined as an illusion of movement and is classically described as "the room is spinning." Other descriptions (such as rocking, tilting, somersaulting, and descending in an elevator) also qualify as vertigo.

Vertigo is classified as peripheral or central. *Peripheral vertigo* means peripheral to the brainstem (eg, the eighth cranial nerve and the vestibular apparatus). Although the onset is usually abrupt and intense, the causes of peripheral vertigo are not typically life threatening. Conversely, the causes of *central vertigo* (involving the brainstem and cerebellum) are usually more serious. The major concern in the management of patients with vertigo is to determine a peripheral or central cause. Table 145-1 reviews the differences between peripheral and central vertigo.

Benign paroxysmal positional vertigo (BPPV) is the most common cause of vertigo. It is associated with position change (with a latency of 1 to 5 seconds between movement and symptoms), subsides in less than 1 minute, and fatigues over the course of the day. The episodic vertigo in BPPV typically resolves spontaneously after days to weeks as the otoliths dissolve (but can be cured immediately at the bedside with the use of the Epley maneuver). Patients with BPPV sometimes state that their vertigo is continuous. These patients may be having such frequent attacks that they think their vertigo is continuous when in fact they are having many discrete episodes of BPPV, each typically lasting less than 1 minute. One helpful way to differentiate BPPV from vestibular neuritis and labyrinthitis is to ask whether the patient is experienc-

TABLE 145-1 Differentiating Factors between Peripheral and Central Causes of Vertigo

Factors	Peripheral	Central
Onset	Sudden	Gradual
Severity	Intense	Less intense
Pattern	Paroxysmal	Constant
Associated nausea/diaphoresis	Frequent	Infrequent
Fatigue of symptoms and signs	Yes	No
Hearing loss/tinnitus	May occur	Does not occur
Central nervous system symptoms/signs	Absent	Usually present

ing vertigo during the interview. A patient with BPPV should be asymptomatic while providing the history (assuming there is no head movement).

Near Syncope

Near syncope is the feeling that one is going to faint. This is due to global hypoperfusion of the brain. Patients often have associated autonomic warning signs, such as pallor, diaphoresis, and nausea. Observers may comment that the patient looks like he is about to faint. If the patient is unable to lie down (making it easier for the heart to perfuse the brain), then the patient will convert from near syncope to true syncope. If the patient is still unable to lie in a horizontal position, the body will start to make antigravity movements that a lay person may interpret as a seizure.

Disequilibrium

Disequilibrium is the sense of imbalance or unsteadiness while ambulating. Patients may state that they feel like they are going to fall. Patients with this type of dizziness are often asymptomatic while lying down or sitting but become symptomatic while standing or walking. The most common etiology is cervical spondylosis, which leads to a myelopathy and poor proprioception in the legs. Other causes include extrapyramidal and cerebellar diseases.

Psychogenic Dizziness

Psychogenic dizziness is generally attributed to anxiety states. These patients typically have great difficulty describing their dizziness in words other than the word *dizzy,* leading the emergency physician into the trap of suggesting meanings. As discussed previously, this is usually counterproductive.

The physical examination in the dizzy patient should include a complete assessment of the auditory, neurologic, and cardiac systems. For patients with vertigo, a Hallpike test and head-thrust test also should be performed.

DIAGNOSIS AND DIFFERENTIAL

BPPV may occur at any age but is most common in the elderly and those with a history of head trauma. Otoliths, which are normally attached to a membrane in the utricle, become dislodged and enter the posterior semicircular canal (the most dependent of the 3 semicircular canals). When the patient moves the head, these particles move and drag endolymph with them, causing the inappropriate stimulation of linear receptors in the canal. The Hallpike test is used to confirm the diagnosis of BPPV. In this test, the patient begins seated with the head turned 45° to one side. The patient is then assisted to a supine position with the head hanging over the edge of the bed an additional 30° to 45°. Patients with BPPV will exhibit a latent and short-lived nystagmus with the rapid component toward the affected ear. The patient is then returned to the sitting position (the nystagmus often reverses upon resuming the upright position). The other side is then tested. It is a common fallacy that this test needs to be done rapidly. The side that is symptomatic serves as the starting point for the curative Epley maneuver.

The head-thrust test is also used to evaluate patients with peripheral vertigo. This is a simple bedside test of the horizontal vestibuloocular reflex. It is performed by grasping the patient's head and applying a brief, small-amplitude, high-acceleration head turn, first to one side and then to the other.

The patient fixates on the examiner's nose, and the examiner watches for corrective rapid eye movements (saccades) that are a sign of decreased vestibular response. "Catch-up" saccades occurring in one direction but not the other indicates a peripheral vestibular lesion on that side.

Imaging studies usually are not necessary in peripheral vertigo as long as there is no suspicion of eighth nerve or cerebellopontine angle tumor.

Vestibular neuritis is characterized by the sudden onset of severe, often incapacitating vertigo. Episodes may last for days to weeks. Hearing is not affected. A viral etiology is suspected, and patients may have concurrent or recent symptoms of an upper respiratory infection. Labyrinthitis, although commonly viral, also can be due to bacterial infection from otitis media, meningitis, and mastoiditis. Hearing loss differentiates this entity from vestibular neuritis.

Ménière disease is thought to be caused by distention in the endolymphatic system with occasional ruptures and leakage of fluid from the endolymph into the perilymph. Symptoms typically last for hours instead of seconds. Roaring tinnitus and a sense of fullness and diminished hearing in the affected ear are typical. Because the diagnosis requires multiple episodes of attacks with progressive hearing loss, Ménière syndrome cannot be diagnosed on the first presentation of vertigo.

Perilymphatic fistula causes vertigo when an opening in the round or oval window allows pneumatic changes to be transmitted to the vestibule. Trauma, including barotrauma, and infection may cause a perilymph fistula, and symptoms are typically associated with situations resulting in pneumatic fluctuation such as flying, diving, or sneezing.

Tumors of the eighth cranial nerve and cerebellopontine angle such as meningioma, acoustic neuroma, and acoustic schwannoma also may present as vertigo with hearing loss. These tumors may be associated with ipsilateral facial weakness and impaired corneal reflexes and cerebellar signs.

Vertigo may occur after closed head injury due to direct labyrinthine trauma or dislodgement of otoliths leading to BPPV. In the former, the onset is typically immediate and may be constant with associated nausea and vomiting. The vertigo tends to resolve over weeks. Posttraumatic vertigo may be associated with basilar skull fracture.

Ototoxicity from a multitude of drugs and chemicals may induce vertigo and hearing loss. Common offenders causing peripheral toxicity include aminoglycosides, cytotoxic agents, quinidine, and quinine-related antimalarial agents. Anticonvulsants, antidepressants, neuroleptics, hydrocarbons, alcohol, and phencyclidine may cause centrally mediated vertigo.

Cerebellar hemorrhage or infarction is a central cause of vertigo. As is characteristic of central vertigo, the vertigo is of moderate intensity and may or may not be associated with nausea and vomiting. Truncal ataxia is typical, with abnormal Romberg and gait-testing apparent.

Lateral medullary infarction of the brainstem, or Wallenberg syndrome, causes vertigo and ipsilateral facial numbness, loss of the corneal reflex, Horner syndrome, and pharyngeal and laryngeal paralysis. Contralateral loss of pain and temperature sensation in the extremities also occurs.

Vertebrobasilar insufficiency (VBI) may result in vertigo due to brainstem transient ischemic attacks in patients with the typical risk factors for cerebrovascular disease. The vertigo may be sudden in onset and last minutes to hours but should not last longer than 24 hours. Associated focal brainstem signs are also likely to be present, as may syncope. Unlike other causes of central vertigo, VBI may be induced by movement of the head resulting in decreased vertebral artery blood flow.

Central vertigo also can be associated with migraine syndrome as a part of the aura or headache or as the migraine equivalent. Basilar migraine is defined as a migraine that has an aura with symptoms similar to VBI.

Other causes of central vertigo include multiple sclerosis with demyelination of isolated areas of the brainstem and fourth ventricular neoplasms.

EMERGENCY DEPARTMENT CARE AND DISPOSITION

1. With peripheral vertigo, patients typically present to the ED very symptomatic, often with vomiting and inability to ambulate. The most effective medications are usually the antihistaminic and anti-serotonergic medications. **Promethazine** 25 to 50 mg intravenously (IV), intramuscularly, or rectally, **meclizine** 25 mg orally, and **ondansetron** 4 mg IV are effective in providing symptomatic relief.

2. **Benzodiazepines** prevent the process of vestibular rehabilitation and should be used as second-line agents. **Scopolamine** is a pure anticholinergic medication that works by blocking the conflict signal size. However, because scopolamine takes about 4 to 8 hours to start working, it is not useful acutely in the ED setting.

3. Patients with BPPV should be treated with the **Epley maneuver** (canalith repositioning maneuver). This maneuver is easily performed at the patient's bedside and takes only a few minutes. By moving the otoliths out of the posterior semicircular canal and back into the utricle, where they belong, the patient potentially can be cured right at the bedside. The affected ear is determined by the side on which the Hallpike test is positive. The patient is seated and the head is turned 45° toward the affected ear. The patient is gently brought to the recumbent position with the head hanging 30° to 45° below the examining table. The head is gently rotated 45° to the midline. The head is then rotated another 45° to the unaffected side. The patient rolls onto the shoulder of the unaffected side while rotating the head another 45°. The patient is returned to the sitting position, and the head is retuned to the midline. Each portion of the maneuver should be performed slowly and evenly.

4. Because of their likely viral etiology, some experts recommend treating vestibular neuritis and labyrinthitis with oral **steroids** and **acyclovir.**

5. Most patients with peripheral vertigo may be discharged home with primary care or specialty follow-up. Patients with perilymph fistula, labyrinthitis of suspected bacterial etiology, and Ménière disease should be referred for follow-up with an emergent otolaryngologic specialist. Patients with intractable symptoms may require admission for IV antiemetics and hydration.

6. Patients with central vertigo require imaging studies and specialty referral. Posterior fossa hemorrhage is an emergency for which immediate **neurosurgical consultation** must be obtained. Similarly, suspected tumors should have urgent neurosurgical consultation and appropriate imaging studies. Other ischemic cerebrovascular incidents, suspected multiple sclerosis, and vertiginous migraine should have neurologic consultation for inpatient or outpatient workup.

7. In all cases, it must be remembered that antivertigo medications can have undesirable anticholinergic side effects such as drowsiness and urinary retention. The emergency physician should avoid the knee-jerk reflex of prescribing meclizine for all patients who present with dizziness. In patients without true vertigo, these medications may exacerbate the dizziness experienced by the patient.

For further reading in *Emergency Medicine: A Comprehensive Study Guide,* 6th ed., see Chap. 231, "Vertigo and Dizziness," by Brian Goldman.

146 | Seizures and Status Epilepticus in Adults

C. Crawford Mechem

A *seizure* is an episode of abnormal neurologic function caused by inappropriate electrical discharge of brain neurons. *Epilepsy* is a clinical condition in which an individual is subject to recurrent seizures. The term ordinarily is not applied to seizures caused by reversible conditions such as alcohol withdrawal, hypoglycemia, or other metabolic derangements. *Primary* or *idiopathic* seizures are those without a clear cause. *Secondary* or *symptomatic* seizures are the result of another identifiable neurologic condition, such as a mass lesion.

CLINICAL FEATURES

Seizures may be classified in 2 major groups: *generalized* and *partial* (focal) (Table 146-1). A subclass of generalized seizures are *absence* (petit mal) seizures. Classic absence seizures are seen in school-aged children. They usually resolve as the child matures. Generalized seizures are believed to be caused by a nearly simultaneous activation of the entire cerebral cortex. Partial seizures are due to electrical discharges in a localized, structural lesion of the brain. The discharges may remain local or spread to nearby regions or the entire cortex (generalized). Partial seizures may be *simple,* in which consciousness is not affected, or *complex,* in which consciousness is altered. Complex partial seizures are often due to focal discharges in the temporal lobe (also termed *temporal lobe seizures*).

Eclampsia refers to the combination of seizures, hypertension, edema, and proteinuria in pregnant women beyond 20 weeks' gestation or up to 8 weeks postpartum.

Status epilepticus has historically been defined as continuous seizure activity lasting for at least 30 minutes or 2 or more seizures without intervening return to baseline. It has been suggested that the defining duration of seizure activity be reduced to 5 minutes. *Nonconvulsive status epilepticus* is associated with minimal or imperceptible convulsive activity and is confirmed by electroencephalogram.

Generalized seizures begin with abrupt loss of consciousness and loss of postural tone. The patient may then become rigid, with extension of the trunk and extremities. Apnea, cyanosis, and urinary incontinence are common. As the rigid (tonic) phase subsides, symmetric rhythmic (clonic) jerking of the trunk and extremities develop. After the attack, the patient is flaccid and unconscious. A typical episode lasts from 60 to 90 seconds. Consciousness returns gradually, and postictal confusion may persist for several hours.

Absence seizures are very brief, usually lasting only a few seconds. Patients suddenly lose consciousness without losing postural tone. They appear confused or withdrawn, and current activity ceases. They may stare and have twitching of their eyelids. They do not respond to voice or other stimulation, do not exhibit voluntary movement, and are not incontinent. The attacks end abruptly, and there is no postictal period.

Simple partial seizures remain localized and consciousness is not affected. The likely location of the initial cortical discharge can be deduced from the

TABLE 146-1 Classification of Seizures

Generalized seizures (consciousness always lost)
Tonic-clonic seizures (grand mal)
Absence seizures (petit mal)
Myoclonic seizures
Tonic seizures
Clonic seizures
Atonic seizures
Partial (focal) seizures
Simple partial (no alteration of consciousness)
Complex partial (consiousness impaired)
Partial seizures (simple or complex) with secondary generalization
Unclassified (due to inadequate information)

clinical features at onset. Unilateral tonic or clonic movements limited to one extremity suggest a focus in the motor cortex, whereas tonic deviation of the head and eyes suggests a frontal lobe focus. Visual symptoms often result from an occipital focus, whereas olfactory or gustatory hallucinations may arise from the medial temporal lobe. Such sensory phenomena, or auras, are often the initial symptoms of attacks.

Complex partial seizures are focal seizures in which consciousness is affected. Because of their effect on thinking and behavior, they are occasionally called *psychomotor seizures.* They are commonly misdiagnosed as psychiatric problems. Symptoms may include automatisms, which are typically simple, repetitive, purposeless movements such as lip smacking or fiddling with clothing. Visceral symptoms, such as a sensation of "butterflies" rising up from the epigastrium, and olfactory, gustatory, visual, or auditory hallucinations may develop. Fear, paranoia, depression, or elation also may be noted.

DIAGNOSIS AND DIFFERENTIAL

The first step in diagnosis is determining whether the episode was indeed a true seizure. A careful history should be obtained from the patient and witnesses. Important historical information includes the rapidity of onset, presence of a preceding aura, progression of motor activity, whether the activity was local or generalized, and whether the patient became incontinent. The duration of the episode and whether there was postictal confusion also should be determined. If the patient has a known seizure disorder, the regular pattern of seizures, medications taken and any dosage changes, and the possibility of medication noncompliance should be sought. Contributing factors such as sleep deprivation, alcohol withdrawal, infection, and use or cessation of other drugs should be investigated. In patients with first-time seizures, a more detailed history should be obtained. This should include any recent or remote head trauma or headaches; current pregnancy or recent delivery; a history of metabolic derangements or hypoxia; systemic illness such as cancer, coagulopathy, or human immunodeficiency virus; drug ingestion or withdrawal; and alcohol use (Table 146-2).

The physical examination should include a search for any injuries resulting from the seizure, such as fractures, sprains, strains, posterior shoulder dislocation, tongue lacerations, and aspiration. In addition, clues to the cause of the seizure should be sought. A directed neurologic examination and frequent reassessments, with particular attention to level of consciousness, should be performed. Profound obtundation that improves with time is reassuring,

TABLE 146-2 Causes of Secondary Seizures

Trauma (recent or remote)*

Intracranial hemorrhage (subdural, epidural, subarachnoid, intraparenchymal)*

Structural abnormalities*
  Vascular lesion (aneurism, interiovenous malformation)
  Mass lesions (primary or metastatic neoplasms)
  Degenerative diseases
  Congenital abnormalities

Infection (meningitis, encephalitis, abscess)

Metabolic disturbances
  Hypo- or hyperglycemia*
  Hypo- or hypermatremia
  Hyperosmolar states
  Uremia
  Hepatic failure
  Hypocalcemia, hypomagnesemia (rare)

Toxins and drugs (many)
  Cocaine, lidocaine
  Antidepressants
  Theophylline
  Alcohol withdrawal*
  Drug withdrawal

Eclampsia of pregnancy (may occur up to 8 weeks postpartum)

Hypertensive encephalopathy

Anoxic-ischemic injury (cardiac arrest, severe hypoxemia)

*Most common etiologies.

whereas progressive deterioration warrants prompt intervention. Any localized neurologic deficits should be sought. A transient focal deficit after a focal seizure is referred to as *Todd's paralysis* and should resolve within 48 hours. However, a focal neurologic lesion as a precipitant of the seizure should be considered.

Ordering of laboratory studies should be guided by the particular case. In a patient with a known seizure disorder who has had a typical seizure, only a fingerstick serum glucose level and an anticonvulsant level may be needed. Interpretation of anticonvulsant levels is guided by the clinical context. The therapeutic level of a drug is that level that controls seizures without intolerable side effects, regardless of the normal range provided by the laboratory. In patients with a new onset seizure, more extensive testing is warranted and should include serum electrolytes, calcium, magnesium, blood urea nitrogen, creatinine, pregnancy test, and a toxicology screen. A total creatine kinase level should be ordered if rhabdomyolysis is suspected. An elevated anion-gap metabolic acidosis may be observed if blood is drawn shortly after the seizure. The acidosis generally will clear within 30 to 60 minutes.

There are specific indications for neuroimaging of seizure patients. In patients with a febrile seizure or seizure typical of their documented epilepsy, neuroimaging is rarely necessary. In patients with a first-time seizure or a change in their established seizure pattern, a noncontrast computed tomography of the head is warranted to investigate for hemorrhage or a structural lesion. Because many processes such as tumors or vascular anomalies are poorly visualized without contrast, a follow-up contrast computed tomography or magnetic resonance imaging may be arranged. Ordering of other radiographic studies will be guided by the specific case.

The differential diagnosis of seizures includes the various causes of syncope, hyperventilation syndrome, migraines, movement disorders, and narcolepsy. Also included are pseudoseizures or nonepileptic seizures, which are psychogenic and may be difficult to distinguish from true seizures.

EMERGENCY DEPARTMENT CARE AND DISPOSITION

1. Certain measures should be taken for all seizure patients. These include ensuring a patent airway and stabilizing vital signs. **Oxygen** should be administered and pulse oximetry initiated. Suction and airway adjuncts must be readily available. Intravenous (IV) access should be obtained.
2. **Endotracheal intubation** should be considered for prolonged seizures or if gastrointestinal decontamination is indicated. If rapid sequence intubation is performed, a short-acting paralytic agent should be used so that ongoing seizure activity can be observed. If longer-acting paralytics are required, electroencephalographic monitoring should be initiated.
3. Specific therapy is rarely necessary for active seizures because they are usually self-limited. The patient should be protected from harm until the seizure terminates. During the postictal period, the patient should be observed for improvement of mental status.

	Time Frame
Establish/maintain airway ↓	
IV, oxygen, monitor ↓	
Dextrose 25–50 g IV if indicated ↓	0–5 min
Consider thiamine 100 mg IV and magnesium 1–2 g IV for alcoholic or malnourished patients ↓	
Lorazepam 2 mg per min IV up to 0.1 mg per kg (*or* diazepam 5 mg IV q5 min up to 20 mg) ↓	
Phenytoin 20 mg/kg IV at 50 mg per min *or* fosphenytoin 20 mg/kg PE IV at 150 mg per min ↓	10–20 min
Additional phenytoin 5–10 mg/kg IV *or* additional fosphenytoin 5–10 mg/kg PE IV ↓	
Phenobarbital up to 20 mg/kg IV at 50–75 mg per min IV ↓	
and/or ↓	30 min
General anesthesia with Midazolam 0.2 mg/kg slow IVP then 0.75–10 μg/kg per min *or* propofol 1–2 mg/kg IV then 1–15 mg/kg per h *or* pentobarbital 10–15 mg/kg IV over 1 h then 0.5–1.0 mg/kg per h	

FIG. 146-1. Guidelines for management of status epilepticus. (Adapted from Lowenstein DH, Alldredge BK: Status epilepticus. *New Engl J Med.* 1998; 338:970.)

4. Patients in status epilepticus require prompt intervention. Morbidity is usually due to hypoxemia, hyperthermia, circulatory collapse, and neuronal injury. Treatment must be systematic, and the patient must be closely monitored for signs of respiratory or circulatory compromise. IV **thiamine** (100 mg) and **glucose** (25–50 g) should be given if hypoglycemia is confirmed. The anticonvulsants most frequently used are the **benzodiazepines (lorazepam, phenytoin, fosphenytoin,** and **phenobarbital** (Fig. 146-1). Phenytoin may be administered immediately after benzodiazepines or as a single agent in patients with less frequent seizures. Fosphenytoin is a pro-drug of phenytoin that has the advantages of fewer infusion site reactions, more rapid administration, and intramuscular injection. Phenobarbital is third-line agent in patients who cannot tolerate phenytoin or who do not respond to full doses of benzodiazepines and phenytoin. Respiratory and circulatory depression is common with its use.

5. Eclamptic patients should be administered **magnesium sulfate,** 4 to 6 g IV followed by an infusion of 1 to 2 g/h, in addition to the above regimen.

6. Status epilepticus refractory to the above measures is best controlled by induction of general anesthesia using agents such as **midazolam, propofol,** or **pentobarbital.**

7. Patients with a known seizure disorder who present after their typical seizure may be discharged once they return to baseline and serum anticonvulsant levels are addressed. When necessary, IV loading is preferable to the oral route because of the more rapid establishment of a therapeutic level (Table 146-3). The appropriate outpatient maintenance regimen should be resumed. Patients should be discharged with a reliable family member or friend and follow-up arranged. They should be advised to avoid activities in which seizure activity could threaten their safety or that of those around them.

TABLE 146-3 Properties of Commonly Used Anticonvulsant Drugs

Drug	Oral dose, mg/d*	Therapeutic level, μg/mL†	Days to reach steady state‡	Serum half-life, h
Phenytoin	300–600 divided TID	10–20	5–10	7–42
Carbamazepine	400–1200 divided TID or QID	6–12	2–4	12–17
Phenobarbital	60–200 QD	10–40	14–21	48–144
Primidone	750–2000 divided TID or QID	5–12	4–7	10–21
Valproic acid	15–60 mg/kg/d divided BID or TID	50–150	2–4	12–18

*Average therapeutic dose. Initiation dosing may be different. Daily dose is individualized. Drug–drug interactions may dramatically change daily doses in patients receiving multiple drugs.
†See text for definition of therapeutic and toxic levels.
‡Indicates time required to establish stable serum levels after any change in dose.
Key: BID = twice daily, qd = once daily, QID = 4 times a day, TID = 3 times a day.

8. Patients with a new onset seizure also may be discharged for further out-patient evaluation if they return to baseline and life-threatening conditions have been excluded. Disposition of such patients is ideally made in consultation with a neurologist or primary care physician. Indications for admission after a new onset seizure include persistent altered mental status, central nervous system infection or mass, eclampsia, underlying metabolic derangements not readily corrected in the emergency department, associated head trauma, absence of reliable caretakers at home, and inability to arrange a close follow-up appointment for further evaluation and therapy adjustment.

For further reading in *Emergency Medicine: A Comprehensive Study Guide,* 6th ed., see Chap. 232, "Seizures and Status Epilepticus in Adults," by Christina Lynne Catlett.

147 | Acute Peripheral Neurological Lesions

Howard E. Jarvis III

A systematic approach to evaluating neurologic symptoms includes localizing the problem anatomically and distinguishing peripheral from central etiology. The latter distinction is not always clear. Peripheral nerve disorders may affect sensory, motor, and autonomic functions. Diminished or absent reflexes are typically seen. Hyporeflexia occasionally occurs with acute central lesions, but hyperreflexia and spasticity ultimately develop.

MYOPATHIES

Polymyositis is an inflammatory myopathy characterized by chronic or subacute proximal, symmetric weakness. Patients may have dysphagia and muscular pain, and a few may progress to respiratory failure. Sensation is normal, as are reflexes, except with very severe weakness. Laboratory studies may show an elevated erythrocyte sedimentation rate, creatine kinase level, and leukocytosis. The differential diagnosis includes Lambert-Eaton syndrome, endocrinopathies, toxic myopathies, dermatomyositis, and others. Admission usually is warranted to monitor the airway and clinical progression and to complete the evaluation.

Dermatomyositis has similar laboratory findings and clinical manifestations, with the addition of a violaceous rash, often on the face and hands. Treatment is aimed at immunosuppression. Numerous other etiologies of myopathy include environmental (eg, alcohol), occupational, drugs (eg, steroids, zidovudine [AZT], or cholesterol-lowering agents), and infection (eg, trichinosis and viral agents).

DISORDERS OF THE NEUROMUSCULAR JUNCTION

Botulism is caused by *Clostridium botulinum* toxin and occurs in 3 forms: food borne, wound, and infantile. In the United States, the principal source is improperly prepared or stored food. In infantile botulism, organisms arise from ingested spores, often in honey, and produce a systemically absorbed toxin. Wound botulism should be considered in patients with a wound or a history of intravenous drug use and progressive, symmetric descending paralysis. Clinical features appear 1 to 2 days after ingestion and may be preceded by nausea, vomiting, and diarrhea. Early complaints commonly involve the eye or bulbar musculature and progress to descending weakness and respiratory insufficiency. Absent light reflex is a diagnostic clue, and mentation is normal. Infants may present with poor suck, listlessness, constipation, regurgitation, and weakness. Treatment includes respiratory support, gastrointestinal and wound decontamination, antibiotics (infants only), immune serum (adults and infants), and admission.

(*Myasthenia gravis* is discussed in Chap. 148.)

ACUTE PERIPHERAL NEUROPATHIES

Guillain-Barré syndrome (GBS) affects all ages and usually follows a viral illness, especially gastroenteritis. It may be rapidly progressive. Although numerous variants exist, extremity weakness, more pronounced initially in the legs, is typical. Bulbar musculature may be involved. Respiratory failure and lethal autonomic fluctuations may occur. Although subjective sensory complaints are common, objective sensory deficits are rare. The absence of deep tendon reflexes is classic. Cerebrospinal fluid (CSF) analysis typically shows a high protein level and a normal glucose level and cell count. The differential diagnosis includes diphtheria, botulism, lead poisoning, tick paralysis, Lyme disease, spinal cord compression, and porphyria. Emergency department (ED) treatment includes respiratory support, admission to a monitored setting, and neurologic consultation.

Acute intermittent porphyria is a rare autosomal dominant disorder involving the triad of weakness, psychosis, and abdominal pain. Occasionally they occur together, but each may occur independently. Seizures may be seen. Certain medications may trigger flares, such as phenytoin, barbiturates, sulfonamides, and estrogen. Neurologic findings include weakness and diminished reflexes, particularly in the lower extremities. Sensory abnormalities may occur. The differential diagnosis includes causes of pain and lower extremity weakness, such as spinal cord compression (brisk reflexes and up-going toes) and aortic aneurysm or dissection. ED treatment includes discontinuation of the offending drug, supportive care, glucose infusions, vitamin B_6, and hematin (4 mg/kg/d for 1-2 weeks).

ENTRAPMENT NEUROPATHIES

(*Carpal tunnel syndrome* is discussed in Chap. 183.) Other common nerve entrapments include ulnar (which can mimic C8 radiculopathy), deep peroneal (causing foot drop and numbness between the first and second toes), and meralgia paresthetica (entrapment of the lateral cutaneous nerve of the thigh). Meralgia paresthetica may follow weight loss and pelvic or gynecologic surgery and causes lateral thigh numbness. These and other entrapments often cause numbness or weakness and require referral to a specialist.

PLEXOPATHIES

Brachial neuritis causes severe shoulder, back, or arm pain, followed by weakness in the arm or shoulder girdle, and is bilateral in up to one third of cases. Patients have weakness in various distributions of the brachial plexus. Sensory deficits are less profound, and reflexes in the involved arm are diminished. The differential diagnosis includes multiple radiculopathies, Pancoast tumors, and neoplastic or inflammatory infiltration of the plexus, although a history of pain followed by weakness that plateaus in 1 to 2 weeks makes other diagnoses unlikely. A chest radiograph should be ordered to screen for mass lesions involving the plexus. The CSF should be analyzed to exclude other etiologies. ED treatment consists of conservative management, and close neurologic follow-up is indicated. If other etiologies are excluded, admission is elective.

Lumbar plexopathy, or diabetic amyotrophy, presents in diabetics with acute back pain followed within days by ipsilateral progressive leg weakness. Decreased strength (and possibly reflexes) in a variety of patterns, with relatively symmetric sensation, is found. Bowel and bladder functions are not affected. Plain radiographs and magnetic resonance imaging are ultimately needed. The differential diagnosis includes cauda equina and conus medullaris syndromes and arteriovenous malformation compression. Abdominal computed tomography aids in excluding aortic aneurysm and psoas muscle masses. Patients should be admitted for further evaluation of weakness.

HIV-ASSOCIATED PERIPHERAL NEUROLOGIC DISEASE

Infection with the human immunodeficiency virus (HIV) and its complications and treatments cause a variety of peripheral nerve disorders. The most common, drug-induced and HIV neuropathies, are chronic and do not cause acute symptoms. Patients with HIV have a higher rate of mononeuritis multiplex and a myopathy resembling polymyositis. In early infection, they are more prone to GBS. In the later stages of acquired immunodeficiency syndrome, they may develop cytomegalovirus radiculitis, with acute weakness, primarily lower extremity involvement, and variable bowel or bladder dysfunction. Primarily lower extremity weakness, hyporeflexia, and sensory deficits are seen. Rectal tone may be decreased. Magnetic resonance imaging (indicated to exclude mass lesion) shows swelling and clumping of the cauda equina. Admission is required; treatment, which should precede definitive diagnosis, consists of **ganciclovir** 5 mg/kg intravenously every 12 hours for 14 days.

OTHER CONDITIONS

Mononeuritis multiplex is caused by a vasculitis and involves multiple deficits in a stepwise fashion, usually involving both sides of the body. For example, a left foot drop may follow a right wrist drop. This must be differentiated from multiple compression neuropathies, and it requires urgent referral to a neurologist, with treatment usually in collaboration with a rheumatologist.

Bell's palsy causes seventh cranial nerve dysfunction, and patients may complain of facial weakness, articulation problems, difficulty keeping an eye closed, or inability to keep food in the mouth on one side. Physical examination findings demonstrate weakness on one side of the face, including the forehead, and no other focal neurologic findings. The differential diagnosis includes stroke, Lyme disease, GBS, parotid tumors, middle ear lesions, cerebellopontine angle tumors, eighth cranial nerve lesions, HIV, and vascular disease. The ear should be inspected for ulcerations caused by cranial herpes zoster activation (Ramsey-Hunt syndrome), which should be treated with oral **acyclovir.** If muscle strength is retained in the forehead, the lesion most likely is central (ie, in the brainstem or above); this would exclude Bell's palsy, and computed tomography of the head is indicated. Treatment is controversial, although most neurologists favor a short course of **prednisone** (50 mg/d for 7 days). Steroids are withheld if paresis has been present for longer than 1 week. **Acyclovir** (200 mg 5 times a day for 10 days) may be beneficial. Patients should apply **Lacrilube** to prevent corneal drying at night. Close follow-up with a neurologist or ENT specialist is indicated.

Lyme disease is caused by exposure to the tick-borne pathogen *Borrelia burgdorferi,* and prior tick exposure or exposure to areas endemic to deer ticks may be noted. In addition to initial arthralgias and fatigue, multiple neurologic manifestations may develop, including seventh cranial nerve palsy. Unless there is encephalitis, a rare complication, mental status is normal. Peripheral nerves and the nerve root are affected. Patients may describe acute or subacute progression of limb weakness and sensory loss, sometimes with radicular pain. Selected deep tendon reflexes may be diminished. Serum and CSF Lyme antibodies are suggestive of disease. CSF pleocytosis and increased protein with normal glucose are the most common laboratory abnormalities. Duration and route of antibiotic administration depend on the severity of clinical findings.

For further reading in *Emergency Medicine: A Comprehensive Study Guide,* 6th ed., see Chap. 233, "Acute Peripheral Neurological Lesions," by Michael M. Wang.

148 | Chronic Neurologic Disorders

Mark B. Rogers

An awareness of chronic neurologic disorders and their treatments are necessary to address certain complications, most notably respiratory failure.

AMYOTROPHIC LATERAL SCLEROSIS

Clinical Features

Amyotrophic lateral sclerosis (ALS) is caused by upper and lower motor neuron degeneration, leading to rapidly progressive muscle wasting and weakness. Upper motor neuron dysfunction causes limb spasticity, hyperreflexia, and emotional lability. Lower neuron dysfunction causes limb muscle weakness, atrophy, fasciculations, dysarthria, dysphagia, and difficulty in mastication. Symptoms are often *asymmetric* and more prominent in the upper extremities. Patients initially may have cervical or back pain consistent with an acute compressive radiculopathy. Respiratory muscle weakness progresses from dyspnea on exertion to dyspnea at rest, eventually leading to respiratory distress and failure.

Diagnosis and Differential

Most patients with ALS will go to the emergency department with the diagnosis established. The clinical diagnosis is suggested by symptoms of upper and lower motor neuron dysfunctions without other central nervous system (CNS) dysfunction. Electromyography is the most useful test. Other illnesses that should be considered include myasthenia gravis, diabetes, dysproteinemia, thyroid dysfunction, vitamin B_{12} deficiency, lead toxicity, vasculitis, and CNS and spinal cord tumors.

Emergency Department Care and Disposition

Emergency care is required for acute respiratory failure, aspiration pneumonia, choking episodes, or injuries related to falls. The treatment goal is to optimize pulmonary function, which may require nebulizer treatments, steroids, antibiotics, or endotracheal intubation. Admission is indicated for impending respiratory failure, pneumonia, inability to handle secretions, and worsening disease process that may require long-term placement.

MULTIPLE SCLEROSIS

Clinical Features

Multiple sclerosis (MS) is due to multifocal areas of CNS demyelination that cause motor, sensory, visual, and cerebellar dysfunctions. Three clinical courses are seen: relapsing and remitting (80% of cases), relapsing and progressive, and chronically progressive.

Deficits associated with MS are described as a heaviness, weakness, stiffness, or extremity numbness. Lower extremity symptoms are usually more severe. *Lhermitte's sign* is described as an electric shock sensation, a vibration,

703

or dysesthetic pain going down the back into the arms or legs from neck flexion. Physical examination may show decreased strength, increased tone, hyperreflexia, clonus, decrease in vibratory sense and joint proprioception, and reduced pain and temperature sense. Increases in body temperature, associated with exercise, hot baths, or fever, may worsen symptoms.

Rarely, acute transverse myelitis may occur. Cerebellar lesions may cause an intention tremor, saccadic dysmetria, and truncal ataxia. Brainstem lesions may cause vertigo. Cognitive and emotional problems are common, including dementia, poor motivation, and mood disorders.

Optic neuritis is the first presenting symptom in up to 30% of cases and may cause an afferent papillary defect (Marcus-Gunn pupil). Acute or subacute central vision loss occurs over several days and is usually unilateral. Retrobulbar or extraocular muscle pain usually precedes vision loss. The pain usually resolves in days; however, visual disturbances may last months. Funduscopy is usually normal, but the optic disc may appear pale. Visual acuity may worsen with increased body temperature. Other visual disturbances include nystagmus, diplopia, and internuclear ophthalmoplegia (INO). INO causes abnormal adduction and horizontal nystagmus, often bilaterally. Acute bilateral INO is strongly suggestive of MS.

Dysautonomia causes vesicourethral, gastrointestinal tract, and sexual dysfunctions. Urinary retention, urgency, frequency, detrusor-external sphincter dyssynergia, and stress or overflow incontinence can occur. Constipation or fecal incontinence may be seen.

Diagnosis and Differential

The diagnosis of MS is clinical and is suggested by 2 or more episodes, lasting days to weeks, causing neurologic dysfunction that implicates different sites in the white matter. Magnetic resonance imaging of the head may demonstrate various abnormalities, including discrete lesions in the supratentorial white matter or periventricular areas. Cerebrospinal fluid protein and γ-globulin levels are often elevated.

The differential diagnosis includes systemic lupus erythematosus, Lyme disease, neurosyphilis, and human immunodeficiency virus.

Emergency Department Care and Disposition

Treatment is directed at addressing the complications of acute MS exacerbation.

1. Those with severe motor or cerebellar dysfunction may be treated with steroids. A short-term (up to 5 days), high-dose course of pulsed intravenous (IV) **methylprednisolone** (250 mg every 6 hours), followed by oral prednisone tapered over 2 to 3 weeks, may be beneficial.

2. Fever must be reduced to minimize symptoms. A careful search for a source of infection should be initiated. Respiratory infections and distress must be managed aggressively. With any MS exacerbation, patients should be evaluated for acute cystitis and pyelonephritis, and any infection associated with postvoid residuals larger than 100 mL requires intermittent catheterization.

3. Admission is indicated for those at risk for further complications, respiratory compromise, depression with suicidal ideation, and those requiring IV antibiotics or steroid therapy. Referral to a neurologist is essential for subtle new onset symptoms.

MYASTHENIA GRAVIS

Clinical Features

Myasthenia gravis (MG) is an autoimmune disease caused by antibody destruction of the acetylcholine receptors at the neuromuscular junction, which results in variable muscle weakness. The thymus is abnormal in 75% of patients, and thymectomy resolves or improves symptoms in most patients. Most MG patients have generalized weakness, specifically of the proximal extremities, neck extensors, and facial or bulbar muscles. Ptosis and diplopia are the most common symptoms. Approximately 10% of patients will have ocular muscle weakness only, but most will develop dysarthria, dysphagia, and limb weakness. Symptoms usually worsen as the day progresses or with muscle use (eg, prolonged chewing or reading) and then improve with rest. There is usually no deficit in sensory, reflex, and cerebellar function. Elderly MG patients may be misdiagnosed with ischemic stroke with new onset of facial weakness.

Extreme weakness in the respiratory muscles may cause respiratory failure. This life-threatening condition, termed *myasthenic crisis,* may be seen before the diagnosis of MG.

Diagnosis and Differential

MG should be considered based on clinical findings, such as ocular, bulbar, and proximal limb muscle weaknesses, that worsen during the day and improve with rest. The diagnosis is confirmed through administration of edrophonium (an acetylcholinesterase inhibitor), electromyogram, and serum testing for acetylcholine receptor antibodies.

Performed at the bedside, the edrophonium (Tensilon) test confirms the diagnosis and can differentiate inadequate treatment from overmedication (cholinergic crisis). Edrophonium is preferred because of its rapid onset (30 seconds) and short duration (5-10 minutes). First, a test dose of 1 to 2 mg IV is given and, if symptoms such as muscle weakness or respiratory depression worsen (cholinergic crisis), then the test is stopped. Emergent intubation may be necessary. Otherwise, up to 10 mg IV of edrophonium is administered and, if symptoms improve transiently (10 min), then the test is considered positive, indicating myasthenic crisis. Edrophonium rarely causes heart block.

The differential diagnosis includes Lambert-Eaton syndrome, drug-induced disorders (eg, penicillamine, aminoglycosides, and procainamide), ALS, botulism, thyroid disorders, and other CNS disorders (intracranial mass lesions).

Emergency Department Care and Disposition

MG is treated with aggressive airway management, acetylcholinesterase inhibitors, and high-dose steroids with plasmapheresis or IV immunoglobulins.

1. With myasthenic crisis, supplemental **oxygen** should be administered. If the patient is unable to handle secretions or is in respiratory failure, the airway should be secured by endotracheal intubation. Depolarizing paralytic agents (eg, succinylcholine) and long-acting nondepolarizing agents should be avoided.

2. If the Tensilon test is positive (myasthenic crisis), then **neostigmine** can be given (0.5-2 mg IV or subcutaneously or 15 mg orally); it is effective

within 30 minutes and its effects last 4 hours. Any patient with severe MG should receive **high-dose steroid therapy,** which mandates admission to an intensive care unit due to possible increased weakness. MG patients treated for other conditions should receive their usual cholinergic inhibitors (usually pyridostigmine 60-90 mg orally every 4 hours). A neurologist should always be consulted for disposition, admission, and arrangement for plasmapheresis or IV immunoglobulin therapy.

LAMBERT-EATON MYASTHENIC SYNDROME

Lambert-Eaton myasthenic syndrome is an autoimmune disorder that causes fluctuating proximal limb muscle weakness and fatigue and is seen mainly in older men with lung cancer. Unlike MG, strength is improved with sustained activity. Patients complain of myalgias, stiffness, paresthesias, metallic tastes, and autonomic symptoms (eg, impotence and dry mouth). Eye movements are unaffected.

Treatment of the underlying neoplasm greatly improves symptoms. Electromyography is abnormal, and serum tests are specific for antibodies to voltage-gated calcium channels. Pyridostigmine and immunosuppressive drugs (eg, corticosteroids and azathioprine) may reduce symptom severity. Immunoglobulin therapy or plasmapheresis may be necessary.

PARKINSON DISEASE

Clinical Features

Parkinson disease (PD) presents with 4 classic signs: resting tremor, cogwheel rigidity, bradykinesia or akinesia, and impaired posture and equilibrium. Other signs include facial and postural changes, voice and speech abnormalities, depression, and fatigue. Initially, most complain of a unilateral resting arm tremor, described as "pill rolling," which improves with intentional movement.

Diagnosis and Differential

The diagnosis is clinical and based on the 4 classic clinical signs. Inquiries should be made concerning family history of neurologic disorders, medications, and exposure to toxins or street drugs. Parkinsonism can result from street drugs, toxins, neuroleptic drugs, hydrocephalus, head trauma, and other rare neurologic disorders. Drug-induced PD most commonly presents with akinesia. No laboratory test or neuroimaging study is pathognomonic.

Emergency Department Care and Disposition

Most patients with PD will go to the emergency department with the diagnosis established. They will be on medications that increase central dopamine (eg, levodopa, carbidopa, and amantadine), anticholinergics (eg, benztropine), and dopamine receptor agonists (eg, bromocriptine). Medication toxicity includes psychiatric or sleep disturbances, cardiac dysrhythmias, orthostatic hypotension, dyskinesias, and dystonia. With significant motor or psychiatric disturbances (eg, hallucinations or frank psychosis) or decreased drug efficacy, a "drug holiday" for 1 week should be initiated.

POLIOMYELITIS AND POSTPOLIO SYNDROME

Clinical Features

Poliomyelitis is caused by an enterovirus that causes paralysis via motor neuron destruction and muscle denervation and atrophy. Most symptomatic patients have only a mild viral syndrome and no paralysis. Symptoms include fever, malaise, headache, sore throat, and gastrointestinal symptoms. Spinal polio results in *asymmetric* proximal limb weakness and flaccidity, absent tendon reflexes, and fasciculations; sensory deficits are usually not seen. Maximal paralysis occurs within 5 days and is followed by muscle wasting. Autonomic dysfunction is common. Paralysis will resolve within the first year in nearly all patients. Other sequelae include bulbar polio (speech and swallowing dysfunction) and encephalitis.

Postpolio syndrome is the recurrence of motor symptoms after a latent period of several decades. Symptoms may include muscle fatigue, joint pain, or weakness of new and previously affected muscle groups. These patients may have new bulbar, respiratory, or sleep difficulties.

Diagnosis and Differential

Polio should be considered in a patient with an acute febrile illness, aseptic meningitis, and asymmetric flaccid paralysis with loss of deep tendon reflexes and normal sensation. Cerebrospinal fluid may show an elevated white blood cell count (mostly neutrophils) and positive cultures for poliovirus. Throat and rectal swabs are higher-yield tests. The diagnosis of postpolio syndrome is based on a prior history of paralytic polio with recovery and presentation with new symptoms not attributable to other causes.

The differential diagnosis includes Guillain-Barré syndrome, peripheral neuropathies (eg, mononucleosis, Lyme disease, or porphyria), abnormal electrolyte level, toxins, inflammatory myopathies, and other viruses (eg, Coxsackie, mumps, echo, and various enteroviruses).

Emergency Department Care and Disposition

Treatment is supportive. With severe cases of post–polio syndrome, problems such as dyspnea, respiratory dysfunction, sleep disorders, and psychiatric disorders need to be addressed. Disposition should be made in consultation with a neurologist.

For further reading in *Emergency Medicine: A Comprehensive Study Guide,* 6th ed., see Chap. 234, "Chronic Neurologic Disorders," by Edward P. Sloan.

149 | Meningitis, Encephalitis, and Brain Abscess

O. John Ma

MENINGITIS

Clinical Features

In classic and fulminant cases of bacterial meningitis, the patient presents with fever, headache, stiff neck, photophobia, and altered mental status. Seizures may occur in up to 25% of cases. The presenting picture, however, may be more nonspecific, particularly in the very young and the elderly. Confusion and fever may be symptoms of meningeal irritation in the elderly. It is important to inquire about recent antibiotic use, which may cloud the clinical picture in a less florid case. Other key historical data include living conditions (eg, army barracks or college dormitories), trauma, immunocompetence, immunization status, and recent neurosurgical procedures.

Physical examination must include assessment for meningeal irritation with resistance to passive neck flexion, Brudzinski sign (flexion of hips and knees in response to passive neck flexion), and Kernig sign (contraction of hamstrings in response to knee extension while hip is flexed). The skin should be examined for the purpuric rash characteristic of meningococcemia. Paranasal sinuses should be percussed and ears examined for evidence of primary infection in those sites. Focal neurologic deficits, which are present in 25% of cases, should be documented. Fundi should be assessed for papilledema, indicating increased intracranial pressure.

Diagnosis and Differential

When the diagnosis of bacterial meningitis is considered, performing a lumbar puncture (LP) is mandatory. At a minimum, cerebrospinal fluid (CSF) should be sent for Gram stain and culture, cell count, protein, and glucose. Typical CSF results for meningeal processes are listed in Table 149-1. Additional studies to be considered are latex agglutination or counter-immune electrophoresis for bacterial antigens in potentially partly-treated bacterial cases, India ink, or serum cryptococcal antigen in immunocompromised patients, acid-fast stain and culture for mycobacteria in tuberculous meningitis, *Borrelia* antibodies for possible Lyme disease, and viral cultures in suspected viral meningitis. Other laboratory tests should include a complete blood count, blood cultures, partial thromboplastin and prothrombin times, serum glucose, sodium, and creatinine levels.

LP can be performed safely if intracranial mass lesions and coagulopathy are unlikely based on clinical grounds. Patients who are immunocompetent, have no history of central nervous system disease, have had no recent seizure (<1 week), and have no papilledema or focal neurologic deficits are safe candidates for LP without prior neuroimaging.

The differential diagnosis includes subarachnoid hemorrhage, meningeal neoplasm, brain abscess, viral encephalitis, cerebral toxoplasmosis, and other infectious meningitides.

TABLE 149-1 Typical Spinal Fluid Results for Meningeal Processes

Parameter (normal)	Bacterial	Viral	Neoplastic	Fungal
OP (<170 mm CSF)	>300 min	200 mm	200 mm	300 mm
WBC (<5 mononuclear)	>1,000/μL	<1,000/μL	<500/μL	<500/μL
%PMNs (0)	>80%	1–50%	1–50%	1–50%
Glucose (>40 mg/dL)	<40 mg/dL	>40 mg/dL	<40 mg/dL	<40 mg/dL
Protein (<50 mg/dL)	>200 mg/dL	<200 mg/dL	>200 mg/dL	>200 mg/dL
Gram stain (−)	+	−	−	−
Cytology (−)	−	−	+	+

Key: OP = opening pressure, PMNs = polymorphonuclear cells, WBC = white blood cells.

Emergency Department Care and Disposition

1. Emergent respiratory and hemodynamic support are given top priority.
2. Upon presentation of the patient with suspected bacterial meningitis, the LP should be performed expeditiously. Empiric antibiotic therapy should be initiated as preparations for LP are made. Antibiotic therapy administered up to 2 hours before LP will not decrease the diagnostic sensitivity if CSF bacterial antigen assays are obtained with CSF cultures. However, if the patient has focal neurologic deficits or papilledema, computed tomography (CT) of the head should be performed before LP to determine the possible risks for transtentorial or tonsillar herniation associated with LP. In these cases, empiric antibiotic therapy must be initiated before patient transport to the radiology suite for CT scanning. Antibiotic therapy should *always* be initiated in the emergency department (ED) and never be delayed for neuroimaging or LP.
3. Empiric treatment for bacterial meningitis is based on the likelihood of certain pathogens and risk factors (Table 149-2). For the patient who is severely allergic to penicillin, the combination of **chloramphenicol** 1 g intravenously (IV), **vancomycin** 1 g IV, and **rifampin** 300 mg orally or IV is recommended.
4. Steroid therapy (**dexamethasone** 10 mg IV 15 minutes before antibiotic administration) has proven to be beneficial in adults. Its precise role in the ED, where emergency physicians rarely manage known cases of bacterial meningitis and appropriately administer antibiotics before confirmed diagnosis, remains unclear.
5. Other general management measures are important. Hypotonic fluids should be avoided. Serum sodium levels should be monitored to detect the syndrome of inappropriate antidiuretic hormone or cerebral salt wasting. Hyperpyrexia should be treated with **acetaminophen.** Coagulopathy needs to be corrected by using specific replacement therapies. Seizures should be treated with **benzodiazepines** and, if needed, **phenytoin** loading. Evidence of marked intracranial pressure should be treated with **head elevation** and **mannitol.**

TABLE 149-2 Guidelines for Empiric Treatment of Bacterial Meningitis* with No Organisms on Gram Stain

Patient category	Potential pathogens	Empiric therapy
Age		
18–50 y	*Streptococcus pneumoniae, Neisseria meningitidis*	Ceftriaxone 2 g IV q12h plus vancomycin or rifampin if *S pneumoniae* resistance possible
>50 y	*S pneumoniae, N meningitidis, Listeria monocytogenes,* aerobic gram-negative bacilli	Ceftriaxone 2 g IV q12h plus ampicillin 2 g IV q4h plus vancomycin or rifampin if *S pneumoniae* resistance possible
Special circumstances		
CSF leak with history of closed head trauma	*Staphylococcus pneumoniae, Haemophilus influenzae,* group B streptococcus	Ceftriaxone 2 g IV q12h
History of recent penetrating head injury, neurosurgery, CSF shunt	*Staphylococcus aureus, S epidermidis,* diphtheroids, aerobic gram-negative bacilli	Vancomycin 25 mg/kg IV load (not >500 mg/h infused) then 19 mg/kg at intervals dictated by Matzke nomogram plus ceftazidime 2 g IV q8h
Immunocompromised host	*S pneumoniae, N meningitidis, L monocytogenes,* aerobic gram-negative bacilli	Vancomycin 25 mg/kg IV load (not >500 mg/h infused) then 19 mg/kg at intervals dictated by Matzke nomogram plus ampicillin 2 g IV q4h plus ceftazidime 2 g IV q8h

*For pediatric meningitis treatment, see Chap. 118.

Key: CSF = cerebrospinal fluid, IV = intravenously, q = every.

6. Viral meningitis, without evidence of encephalitis, can be managed on an outpatient basis provided the patient is nontoxic in appearance, can tolerate oral fluids, and has reliable follow-up within 24 hours. However, it remains a diagnosis of exclusion; unless the diagnosis of viral meningitis is obvious, admission is warranted.

ENCEPHALITIS

Clinical Features

Viral encephalitis is a viral infection of brain parenchyma producing an inflammatory response. It is distinct from, although often coexists with, viral meningitis. In North America, viruses that cause encephalitis are the arboviruses (including the West Nile virus), herpes simplex virus (HSV), herpes zoster, Epstein-Barr virus, cytomegalovirus, and rabies.

Encephalitis should be considered in patients presenting with any or all of the following features: new psychiatric symptoms, cognitive deficits (aphasia, amnestic syndrome, or acute confusional state), seizures, and movement disorders. Signs and symptoms of headache, photophobia, fever, and meningeal irritation may be present. Assessment for neurologic findings and cognitive deficits is crucial. Motor and sensory deficits are not typical. Encephalitides may show special regional trophism. HSV involves limbic structures of the temporal and frontal lobes, with prominent psychiatric features, memory disturbance, and aphasia. Some arboviruses predominantly affect the basal ganglia, causing chorea-athetosis and parkinsonism. Involvement of the brainstem nuclei leads to hydrophobic choking characteristic of rabies encephalitis.

Symptoms of West Nile virus infection include fever, headache, muscle weakness, and lymphadenopathy. Most infections are mild and last only a few days. More severe symptoms and signs consist of high fever, neck stiffness, altered mental status, tremors, and seizures. In rare cases (mostly involving the elderly), the infection can lead to encephalitis and death.

Diagnosis and Differential

ED diagnosis can be suggested by findings on CT or magnetic resonance imaging and LP. Neuroimaging, in particular magnetic resonance imaging, not only excludes other potential lesions, such as brain abscess, but also may display findings highly suggestive of HSV encephalitis if the medial temporal and inferior frontal gray matter is involved. On LP, findings of aseptic meningitis are typical. For the West Nile virus, the most widely used screening test is the IgM ELISA assay for detecting acute antibody.

The differential diagnosis includes brain abscess; Lyme disease; subacute subarachnoid hemorrhage; bacterial, tuberculous, fungal, or neoplastic meningitis; bacterial endocarditis; postinfectious encephalomyelitis; toxic or metabolic encephalopathies; and primary psychiatric disorders.

Emergency Department Care and Disposition

1. The patient with suspected viral encephalitis should be admitted. Of the viruses causing encephalitis, only HSV has been shown by clinical trial to be responsive to antiviral therapy. The agent of choice is **acyclovir** 10 mg/kg IV every 8 hours for 14 days.
2. Potential complications of encephalitis, such as seizures, disorders of sodium metabolism, increased intracranial pressure, and systemic consequences of a comatose state, should be managed with standard methods.

3. There is no specific treatment for the West Nile virus infection. In more severe cases, intensive supportive therapy is indicated. The primary prevention step is advocating the use of insect repellant containing DEET when people go outdoors during dawn or dusk.

BRAIN ABSCESS

Clinical Features

A brain abscess is a focal pyogenic infection. It is composed of a central pus-filled cavity ringed by a layer of granulation tissue and an outer fibrous capsule. Because patients typically are not acutely toxic, the presenting features of brain abscess are nonspecific. For this reason, the initial diagnosis can be difficult in the ED. Presenting signs and symptoms include headache, neck stiffness, fever, vomiting, confusion, or obtundation. The presentation may be dominated by the origin of the infection (eg, ear or sinus pain). Meningeal signs and focal neurologic findings, such as hemiparesis, seizures, and papilledema, are present in less than half the cases.

Diagnosis and Differential

Classically, brain abscess can be diagnosed by CT of the head with contrast, which demonstrates one or several thin, smoothly contoured rings of enhancement surrounding a low-density center and in turn surrounded by white matter edema. LP is contraindicated when brain abscess is suspected and after the diagnosis has been established. Other routine laboratory studies are usually nonspecific. Blood cultures should be obtained.

The differential diagnosis includes cerebrovascular disease, meningitis, brain neoplasm, subacute cerebral hemorrhage, and other focal brain infections, such as toxoplasmosis.

Emergency Department Care and Disposition

1. Decisions on antibiotic therapy for brain abscess should depend on the likely source of the infection. In a suspected otogenic case, initial therapy should consist of a third-generation cephalosporin, such as **ceftriaxone** or **cefotaxime** 2 g IV, or **trimethoprim-sulfamethoxazole plus chloramphenicol or metronidazole.**
2. In a suspected sinogenic or odontogenic case, initial therapy should consist of **high-dose penicillin** 4 million U IV and **metronidazole** 1 g IV. This antibiotic regimen is also appropriate when a hematogenous source is suspected.
3. In a suspected cardiac case, initial therapy should consist of **vancomycin** 15 mg/kg IV with **metronidazole** 1 g IV or **chloramphenicol.** When communication with the exterior is suspected, as in penetrating trauma or postneurosurgical procedure, initial therapy should consist of **nafcillin** 2 g IV or **vancomycin. Ceftazidime** 2 g IV should be added if gram-negative aerobes are suspected. In cases in which no clear etiology exists, initial empiric therapy should consist of a **third-generation cephalosporin** and **metronidazole.**
4. Neurosurgical consultation and admission are warranted because many cases will require surgery for diagnosis, bacteriology and, often, definitive treatment.

For further reading in *Emergency Medicine: A Comprehensive Study Guide,* 6th ed., see Chap. 235, "Meningitis, Encephalitis, and Brain Abscess," by Keith E. Loring, David C. Anderson, and Alan J. Kozak.

17 | EYE, EAR, NOSE, THROAT, AND ORAL EMERGENCIES

150 | Ocular Emergencies

Steven Go

INFECTIONS

Stye (External Hordeolum)

A stye is an acute infection of an oil gland at the lash line that appears as a pustule. Warm, wet compresses 4 times daily and **erythromycin ointment** twice daily for 7 to 10 days generally will allow the lesion to express itself and resolve. If not, a referral to an ophthalmologist is appropriate.

Chalazion (Internal Hordeolum)

A chalazion is an acute or chronic noninfectious inflammation of the eyelid secondary to meibomian gland blockage in the tarsal plate. It appears as an erythematous, tender nodule at the lid margin or within the lid itself. A chalazion is prone to periods of quiescence with periodic flares. Treatment is approached in the same manner as a stye, although refractory lesions may improve with **doxycycline** orally (PO) for 14 to 21 days. A recurrent or persistent chalazion should be referred to an ophthalmologist for incision and curettage.

Bacterial Conjunctivitis

Bacterial conjunctivitis presents as monocular or binocular eyelash matting, mild to moderate mucopurulent discharge, and conjunctival inflammation. Fluorescein staining of the cornea should be performed in patients with suspected conjunctivitis to avoid missing abrasions, ulcers, and dendritic lesions. For patients older than 2 months, treatment consists of broad-spectrum antibiotic drops given 4 times daily for 5 to 7 days. Non-contact lens wearers should receive topical **trimethoprim-polymyxin B.** Contact lens wearers should receive topical antibiotic coverage for *Pseudomonas,* such as **ciprofloxacin, ofloxacin,** or **tobramycin.** The lens should be discarded and not replaced until the infection has completely resolved. In patients younger than 2 months, **sulfacetamide 10%** 1 drop 4 times daily for 5 to 7 days may be used. Gentamicin currently has fallen out of favor due to the high incidence of ocular irritation.

A severe purulent discharge with a hyperacute onset (within 12–24 hours) should prompt an emergent consult with an ophthalmologist for an aggressive workup for possible gonococcal conjunctivitis. *Neisseria gonorrhea* infections may be confirmed by Gram stain (gram-negative intracellular diplococci). Emergency department (ED) care for *N gonorrhea* infections include culture, antibiotics (**ceftriaxone** 1 g intramuscularly or **ciprofloxacin** 1 drop every 2 hours; for corneal involvement, use **ceftriaxone** 1 g intravenously [IV] every 12 hours, **tobramycin** 1 drop every 1 hour, or **doxycycline** 100 mg PO twice daily), frequent saline solution washes, and urgent ophthalmologic consultation.

Viral Conjunctivitis

Viral conjunctivitis presents as a monocular or binocular watery discharge, chemosis, and conjunctival inflammation. It is often associated with viral respiratory symptoms and a palpable preauricular node. Fluorescein staining may show occasional superficial punctate keratitis but otherwise should be clear. Treatment consists of cool compresses 4 times daily, **naphazoline/ pheniramine** 1 drop 3 to 4 times daily, as needed, for conjunctival congestion or itching, and ophthalmology follow-up in 7 to 14 days. If a clear distinction between viral and bacterial etiologies cannot be made, consideration should be made to add topical antibiotics until reexamination by an ophthalmologist; however, routine use of antibiotics is discouraged. All cases of viral conjunctivitis are extremely contagious, and appropriate precautions against transmission must be taken.

Allergic Conjunctivitis

Allergic conjunctivitis presents as a monocular or binocular pruritus, watery discharge, and chemosis with a history of allergies. There should be no lesions with fluorescein staining, and preauricular nodes should be absent. Conjunctival papillae are seen on slit lamp examination. Treatment consists of elimination of the inciting agent, cool compresses 4 times daily, **artificial tears** 4 to 8 times daily, and **naphazoline/pheniramine** 1 drop 4 times daily. **Diphenhydramine** 25 mg PO 3 to 4 times daily may be helpful in moderate to severe cases. Severe cases may require a mild topical steroid such as **fluorometholone 0.1%** 1 drop 4 times daily for 7 to 14 weeks.

Herpes Simplex Virus

Herpes simplex virus (HSV) infection may involve the eyelids, conjunctiva, or cornea. The hallmark dendrite of herpes keratitis appears as a linear branching, epithelial defect with terminal bulbs that stain brightly with fluorescein dye during slit lamp examination. It is essential that HSV infection not be confused with conjunctivitis; hence, the necessity of a slit lamp fluorescein examination in these patients. If the outbreak involves only the eyelids or conjunctiva, antiviral medications such as **trifluorothymidine 1%** drops or **vidarabine 3%** ointment 5 times daily should be prescribed. In addition, **topical erythromycin ointment** twice daily and warm soaks 3 times daily to skin lesions can help prevent secondary bacterial infections. If corneal involvement is present, then the **trifluorothymidine 1%** drops dosage must be increased to 9 times a day. If **vidarabine 3%** ointment is being used instead, the dosage remains 5 times daily. If an anterior-chamber reaction is present, a cycloplegic agent such as **scopolamine 0.25%** 1 drop 3 times daily can be used. **Acyclovir** 800 mg PO 5 times daily or **famciclovir** 500 mg 3 times daily for 7 to 10 days may be considered if the diagnosis is made within the first 3 days of the HSV outbreak. Topical steroids are to be strictly avoided. All treatment should be performed in consultation with an ophthalmologist, and follow-up within 1 to 2 days should be scheduled.

Herpes Zoster Ophthalmicus

Shingles in a trigeminal distribution with ocular involvement is termed *herpes zoster ophthalmicus* (HZO). The presence or eventual development of HZO should be suspected in any patient whose shingles involve the top of the nose (Hutchinson sign). Photophobia and pain secondary to iritis are often present. Slit lamp examination may show a "pseudo-dendrite," a poorly staining mucus plaque without epithelial erosion. **Acyclovir** 800 mg PO 5 times a day or **famciclovir** 500 mg 3 times daily for 7 to 10 days should be prescribed if the skin lesions are younger than 3 days. In addition, **erythromycin ointment** and warm compresses should be applied to skin lesions. Ocular involvement requires **erythromycin ointment** to the eye twice daily. For comfort, oral narcotic analgesia, cycloplegic agents (**scopolamine 0.25%** 1 drop 3 times daily or **cyclopentolate 1%** 1 drop 3 times daily), and cool compresses are helpful. If iritis is present, **prednisolone acetate 1%** 1 drop every 1 to 6 hours is effective. However, because topical steroid use in patients with herpes simplex keratoconjunctivitis may be catastrophic, it is imperative that there be no corneal lesions present on slit lamp examination before topical steroids are used. In severe cases, admission and **acyclovir IV** may be required. For this reason, all cases of suspected HZO require ophthalmologic consultation. All patients younger than 40 years with HZO should undergo a medical evaluation for a possible immunocompromised state.

Periorbital Cellulitis (Preseptal Cellulitis)

Periorbital cellulitis is a superficial infection of the eyelids that does not extend past the orbital septum. The eyelids become warm, indurated, and erythematous, but the eye itself is not involved. The most important step in managing periorbital cellulitis is to exclude *orbital cellulitis* (see below). This may be done clinically by documenting that there is no painful eye movement, no restriction of ocular motility, no acuity deficit, no impairment of pupillary function, and no proptosis. If orbital cellulitis cannot be excluded clinically, then computed tomography (CT) is required. Simple periorbital cellulitis in adults and in children older than 5 years is treated with **amoxicillin/clavulanate** (40 mg/kg PO divided in 3 doses in children or 500 mg PO 3 times daily in adults). For children younger than 5 years or in the presence of comorbidities or toxicity in adults, hospital admission for IV **ceftriaxone** and **vancomycin** may be required. Because of the risk of bacteremia and meningitis in children younger than 5 years with periorbital cellulitis, pediatric and ophthalmology consultations are strongly recommended in these patients.

Orbital Cellulitis (Postseptal Cellulitis)

Orbital cellulitis is a potentially sight- and life-threatening ocular infection deep to the orbital septum, typically as a result of spread from the ethmoid sinuses. Signs of orbital cellulitis include those of periorbital cellulitis plus any of the following: painful eye movement, restriction of ocular motility, fever, decreased vision, and proptosis. An emergent CT of the orbits and sinuses (axial and coronal views, with and without contrast) should be obtained. Ophthalmologic consultation and admission for **cefuroxime** IV (vancomycin IV or a cephalosporin IV in penicillin-allergic patients) is required.

Corneal Ulcer

A corneal ulcer is a serious infection of the corneal stroma. It is commonly associated with trauma, especially in patients who use extended-wear contact lenses and those who wear lenses while sleeping. Ulcers cause pain, redness, tearing, and photophobia. Slit lamp examination shows a staining corneal defect with a surrounding white hazy infiltrate. Occasionally, a hypopyon may be seen. Topical **ofloxacin** or **ciprofloxacin** should be instilled every 1 hour.

Topical cycloplegics, such as **cyclopentolate 1%** 1 drop 3 times daily, aid in pain relief. Eye patching is contraindicated because of the risk of *Pseudomonas* infection. An ophthalmologist should see the patient within 12 to 24 hours.

TRAUMA

Subconjunctival Hemorrhage

This injury represents a disruption of conjunctival blood vessels, typically secondary to trauma, sneezing, gagging, and the Valsalva maneuver. It requires no treatment and usually resolves within 2 weeks. Its primary clinical importance rests in the fact that it can be a sign of significant eye injury when accompanied by trauma. For example, a dense, circumferential subconjunctival hemorrhage ("bloody chemosis") mandates a workup to exclude an occult globe rupture.

Conjunctival Abrasions

Superficial conjunctival abrasions are treated with **erythromycin ointment** twice daily for 2 or 3 days. In the presence of abrasions, an ocular foreign body should be excluded.

Corneal Abrasion

Traumatic abrasions may cause superficial or deep epithelial defects resulting in tearing, photophobia, blepharospasm, and pain. Administration of a topical anesthetic often will facilitate the examination. **Proparacaine** is preferred over tetracaine because it causes less pain upon administration and provides comparable anesthesia. A corneal abrasion will fluoresce green during a fluorescein stain examination when using the cobalt blue light on the slit lamp. A careful search for an ocular foreign body (including lid eversion) must be done in the presence of an abrasion. Once the diagnosis of a simple abrasion is made, a cycloplegic (**cyclopentolate 1%** or **homatropine 5%** 1 drop 3 times daily) likely will provide pain relief. Simple abrasions are treated with topical antibiotics (eg, **tobramycin, erythromycin,** or **bacitracin/polymyxin ointment** 3 times daily). **Ciprofloxacin, ofloxacin,** or **tobramycin** 1 drop every 4 hours may be used instead. Contact lens abrasions are at risk for *Pseudomonas* infection and should be treated with **ofloxacin** or **ciprofloxacin** 1 drop 4 times daily. A cycloplegic also should be prescribed for comfort. Narcotic analgesia should be considered for severe pain. Tetanus status should be updated. Patching corneal abrasions traditionally has been recommended; however, excellent patient comfort can be achieved without it. More importantly, patching does not hasten the healing of abrasions and can greatly harm the patient if the lesions prone to infection (eg, contact lens abrasions or corneal ulcers) are patched. Prescribing topical anesthetics is absolutely contraindicated because repeated use may cause catastrophic corneal damage. All abrasions should be reexamined in 24 hours by an ophthalmologist.

Conjunctival Foreign Bodies

Foreign bodies of the conjunctiva are removed under topical anesthesia with a moistened sterile swab. Eversion of the upper lid is performed to rule out foreign matter in the superior conjunctival fornix.

Corneal Foreign Bodies

Superficial foreign bodies of the cornea are removed under slit lamp microscopy with a fine needle, an eye spud, or an ophthalmic burr. Topical anesthesia is used (also instilled in the unaffected eye to depress reflex blinking). For obvious reasons, this procedure should be attempted only in a sober, cooperative patient. Any corneal foreign body deep within the corneal stroma or in the central visual axis should be removed by an ophthalmologist. Metallic foreign bodies often leave an epithelial "rust ring" that may be removed immediately with an eye burr; however, it is often easier to remove in 24 to 48 hours. A corneal abrasion will result from foreign body removal and is treated in the standard manner. All patients should be referred to an ophthalmologist within 24 hours.

Lid Lacerations

All lid lacerations, except for the most superficial, generally should be evaluated and repaired by an ophthalmologist because of the high risk of associated ocular and nasolacrimal injuries and the possibility of a poor cosmetic and functional outcome from a suboptimal repair. Lid margin lacerations require closure under magnification by an ophthalmologist. For medial lid lacerations, injury to the lacrimal canaliculi and puncta must be excluded. Fluorescein instilled into the tear layer that appears in an adjacent laceration confirms the injury. Upper lid lacerations that involve the levator mechanism and all through-and-through lid lacerations must be repaired in the operating room. If an ophthalmologist is not immediately available to evaluate a high-risk lid laceration, it is not unreasonable to prescribe oral and topical antibiotics and gentle cold compresses with referral for ophthalmic evaluation within 24 hours, as long as any sight-threatening lesions have been excluded.

Blunt Ocular Trauma

An eye speculum is useful in visualization of the bluntly injured eye. Once the eye is visualized, the integrity of the globe and visual acuity must be assessed immediately. Signs such as an abnormal anterior chamber depth, an irregular pupil, or blindness indicate a ruptured globe until proven otherwise, and an emergent ophthalmology referral is indicated. If the globe and vision are preserved, signs of hyphema and blowout fracture should be sought. A complete slit lamp examination and a funduscopic examination (preferably dilated with **tropicamide 1%** 1 drop plus **phenylephrine 2.5%** 1 drop in non-whites) should be performed. A CT of the orbit and face is the test of choice to confirm the presence of an orbital fracture. Traumatic iritis in the absence of a corneal injury can be treated with **prednisolone acetate 1%** 1 drop every 6 hours and **cyclopentolate 1%** 1 drop every 8 hours. The care of the blunt trauma eye patient should be discussed with an ophthalmologist, and the patient should follow up with the ophthalmologist within 48 hours even if no significant injuries are initially found.

Hyphema

A hyphema is the presence of blood in the anterior chamber and often is a sign of significant trauma. It also can occur spontaneously in sickle cell patients and in patients with coagulopathies. The patient should be placed upright to allow the blood to settle inferiorly, with a protective eye shield in place, except during examination and medication administration. After ruptured globe is excluded, the patient should be evaluated for other eye injuries and treated appropriately. The pupil should be dilated with **atropine 1%** to prevent pupillary movement from tearing-damaged blood vessels. Increased intraocular pressure (IOP) is associated with hyphemas and can threaten sight. Therefore, after ruptured globe is excluded, IOP should be measured. If the IOP is greater than 30 mm Hg, **timolol 0.5%** 1 drop should be given. If increased IOP persists, **apraclonidine 0.5%** 1 drop should be added. **Acetazolamide** 500 mg PO is used in refractory cases. If the IOP is greater than 24 mm Hg in a sickle cell patient or in a patient with a spontaneous hyphema, **timolol 0.5%** 1 drop alone should be used because acetazolamide can cause red cells to sickle in the anterior chamber. **Mannitol** 1 to 2 g/kg IV may be used in either type of patient if initial measures are ineffective. In any case, emergent evaluation by an ophthalmologist is indicated. Because of the risk of rebleed in 3 to 5 days and the potential necessity of surgical intervention, any disposition decisions should be made by an ophthalmologist at the bedside, regardless of the size of the hyphema.

Blowout Fractures

Orbital blowout fractures commonly involve the inferior wall and medial wall. The resultant entrapment of the inferior rectus muscle may cause restriction of movement, with a resultant diplopia on upward gaze. Other signs include paresthesia in the distribution of the infraorbital nerve and subcutaneous emphysema, particularly when sneezing or blowing the nose. Recent data suggest that plain radiographs are of little utility in these patients; therefore, if a blowout fracture is suspected, CT of the orbit with 1.5-mm cuts should be performed, with additional studies as indicated. Because of the high incidence of associated ocular trauma (30%), an aggressive effort should be made to exclude associated injuries. Antibiotic prophylaxis (eg, **cephalexin** 250 mg PO 4 times daily for 10 days) is recommended due to sinus involvement. Isolated blowout fractures, with or without entrapment, require early referral to an ophthalmologist.

Penetrating Trauma or Ruptured Globe

Globe penetration or rupture is a catastrophic injury that must be identified immediately. Suggestive findings include a severe subconjunctival hemorrhage, shallow or deep anterior chamber as compared with the other eye, hyphema, teardrop-shaped pupil, limitation of extraocular motility, extrusion of globe contents, or a significant reduction in visual acuity. A penetrating injury should be suspected when the history of a high-speed foreign body (eg, the patient was hammering or grinding without eye protection) or a penetrating injury in proximity of the orbit is present. A bright-green streaming appearance to fluorescein instilled into the tear layer (Seidel test) is pathognomonic, although it may be absent if the wound has sealed. **Once a globe injury is suspected, any further manipulation or examination of the eye must be avoided.** In such cases, the patient should be placed upright and kept non-PO. A protective metallic eye shield should be put in place, and a first-generation cephalosporin should be administered (**cephazolin** 1 g IV) with an antiemetic (to prevent Valsalva). Tetanus status should be updated. A CT of the orbit is the test of choice to screen for an intraocular foreign body. An ophthalmologist should be called immediately if a globe rupture or a penetrating injury is strongly suspected.

Chemical Ocular Injury

Acid and alkali burns are managed in a similar manner. The eye should be **flushed immediately** at the scene and sterile **normal saline** or **Ringer lactate irrigation solution** should be continued in the ED immediately upon arrival (even before visual acuities or patient registration) until the pH is normal (7.0). A topical anesthetic and a Morgan lens are used in this procedure. After the first 2 L of irrigation, the pH may be checked in the lower cul-de-sac with litmus paper or the pH square on a urine dipstick 5 to 10 minutes after ceasing irrigation (to allow time for equilibration). Required irrigation volumes to reach normal pH may exceed 8 to 10 L, depending on the caustic substance. A persistently abnormal pH should prompt removal of any crystallized particles in the fornices with a moistened cotton-tipped applicator. Once the pH is normal, the fornices should be inspected thoroughly for any residual particles and re-swept with a moistened cotton-tipped applicator to remove them and any necrotic conjunctiva. The pH should be rechecked in 10 minutes to make sure that no additional corrosive is leaching out from the tissues. A thorough slit lamp examination, with lid eversion, should be done to assess the amount of damage and any associated injuries. IOP should be measured because it can become elevated with significant burns. A cycloplegic (**cyclopentolate 1%** or **homatropine 5%**) 1 drop 3 times daily will alleviate ciliary spasm, and **erythromycin ointment** applied every 1 to 2 hours while awake should be prescribed. Most patients will require narcotic pain medications. If there are signs of a severe injury, such as a pronounced chemosis, conjunctival blanching, corneal edema or opacification, or increased IOP, the patient should be seen in the ED by an ophthalmologist. Certain specialized burns, such as those due to hydrofluoric acid, also should be seen immediately. Otherwise, a telephone consult with the ophthalmologist to arrange close follow-up within 24 hours is acceptable.

Cyanoacrylate (Super Glue or Crazy Glue) Exposure

Cyanoacrylate glue easily adheres to the eyelids and corneal surface. Its primary morbidity stems from corneal injuries from the hard particles that form. Initial manual removal is facilitated by heavy application of **erythromycin ointment,** with special care to avoid damaging underlying structures. After the easily removable pieces are removed, the patient should be discharged with **erythromycin ointment** to be applied 5 times a day to soften the remaining glue. Complete removal of the residual glue can be accomplished by the ophthalmologist at a follow-up visit within 48 hours.

Ultraviolet Keratitis

Ultraviolet keratitis ("welder flash") results from excess ultraviolet exposure, typically from tanning booths, welding flashes, or prolonged sun exposure (especially during eclipses). Severe pain and photophobia develop 6 to 12 hours after exposure. Conjunctival hyperemia and superficial punctate keratitis are seen. Treatment is the same as for a corneal abrasion.

ACUTE VISUAL REDUCTION OR LOSS

Acute Angle Closure Glaucoma

Acute angle closure glaucoma classically presents with eye pain or headache, cloudy vision, colored halos around lights, conjunctival injection, a fixed mid-dilated pupil, and increased IOP of 40 to 70 mm Hg (normal range, 10-20 mm Hg). Nausea and vomiting are also common. Sudden attacks in patients with narrow anterior chamber angles can be precipitated in movie theaters, while reading, and after ill-advised use of dilatory agents or inhaled anticholinergics. Treatment to decrease the IOP must be started emergently. Immediate medications to administer include: **timolol 0.5%** 1 drop, **apraclonidine 0.5%** 1 drop, or **prednisolone acetate 1%** 1 drop every 15 minutes for 4 doses and then every 1 hour. If IOP is greater than 50 mm Hg or if vision loss is severe, then **acetazolamide** 500 mg IV should be considered. If IOP does not decrease and vision does not improve in 1 hour, **mannitol** 1 to 2 g/kg IV should be given. **Pilocarpine 1% to 2%** 1 drop every 15 minutes for 2 doses in the affected eye and **pilocarpine 0.5%** 1 drop in contralateral eye may be given once the IOP is below 40 mm Hg as long as the patient has a natural lens in place. Pilocarpine is contraindicated in aphakic and pseudophakic patients or when there is mechanical closure of the angle. Symptoms of pain and nausea should be treated, and the IOP should be monitored hourly. All cases require immediate ophthalmologic consultation.

Optic Neuritis

Optic neuritis refers to inflammation at any point along the optic nerve and presents with acute vision loss, with a particular reduction in color vision. It is often painful (>50%), especially with extraocular movements. A decrease in color vision can be diagnosed by the "red desaturation test." During this test, the patient looks at a dark red object with 1 eye, and then the color vision in the other eye is tested. The affected eye will see the object as pink or light red. An afferent pupillary defect (APD) often also can be detected. In anterior optic neuritis, the optic disc appears swollen (papillitis); there are no ophthalmoscopic findings in retrobulbar cases. An ophthalmologist should direct evaluation and treatment. Steroids have not been shown to improve visual outcome, but recent data have associated treatment with IV steroids with a slightly lower 2-year risk of development of multiple sclerosis.

Central Retinal Artery Occlusion

Central retinal artery occlusion presents as a sudden, painless, severe monocular loss of vision, often associated with a history of amaurosis fugax. Occlusion of the central retinal artery will cause complete visual loss, whereas arterial branch obstruction will cause abrupt loss of a partial visual field. Classic signs include nearly complete or complete vision loss (94% with counting fingers to light perception only), a marked APD, superficial opacification or whitening of the retina in the posterior pole, and a bright red macula "cherry red spot." Segmentation of the blood column in the arterioles ("boxcarring") sometimes can be seen. A thorough evaluation to uncover the embolic source (commonly carotid or cardiac) is required, and giant cell arteritis must be excluded. An ophthalmologist should be contacted immediately once the diagnosis is made. In an attempt to dislodge the embolus, firm pressure should be applied to the globe through closed eyelids for 15 seconds, followed by a sudden release. This may be repeated several times. **Acetazolamide** 500 mg IV or **timolol 0.5%** 1 drop is used to reduce IOP. Inhalation of carbogen has not been demonstrated to improve outcomes. Further management should be directed by an ophthalmologist who may perform anterior-chamber paracentesis to lower IOP.

Central Retinal Vein Occlusion

Central retinal vein occlusion causes acute, painless monocular vision loss. Examination shows optic disc edema, cotton wool spots, and retinal hemorrhages in all 4 quadrants. This pattern is described as "blood-and-thunder fundus." IOP should be measured. There is no immediate treatment for central retinal vein occlusion, but predisposing drugs (eg, oral contraceptives or diuretics) should be discontinued. Ophthalmologic follow-up is required. Aspirin therapy is often recommended, but it has not been demonstrated to be efficacious.

Giant Cell Arteritis (Temporal Arteritis)

Giant cell arteritis (GCA) is a systemic vasculitis that can cause a painless ischemic optic neuropathy. Patients are typically women older than 50 years, often with a history of polymyalgia rheumatica. Associated symptoms include headache, jaw claudication, scalp or temporal artery tenderness, fatigue, fever, and anorexia. One third of cases have associated neurologic events such as transient ischemic attacks or stroke. An APD is frequently present, and funduscopic examination may show flame hemorrhages. A sixth cranial nerve palsy may occur. When GCA is suspected, a sedimentation rate and C-reactive protein should be ordered; both are elevated in CGA. Most biopsy-proven cases have a sedimentation rate in the range of 70 to 110 seconds. If CGA is not treated, bilateral vision loss can develop. Therefore, if there is strong suspicion of GCA or vision loss is present, the patient should be admitted for **methylprednisolone** 250 mg IV every 6 hours. For less suspicious patients with no vision loss, they may be discharged with **prednisone** 80 to 100 mg/d PO with close follow-up. Steroids should not be delayed pending results of a biopsy. Antiulcer medications should be prescribed to be given with systemic steroids.

For further reading in *Emergency Medicine: A Comprehensive Study Guide,* 6th ed., see Chap. 238, "Ocular Emergencies," by John D. Mitchell.

151 | Face and Jaw Emergencies

Robert J. French

FACIAL INFECTIONS

Impetigo

Impetigo is a superficial epidermal infection. There are 2 different presentations of impetigo: bullous and nonbullous. Bullous impetigo is caused by *Staphylococcus aureus*. It presents as a vesicle that rapidly enlarges to form a bulla (2 to 5 cm) that collapses, leaving a honey-colored central crust. Nonbullous impetigo is caused by *Streptococcus pyogenes* and *S aureus*. This form presents as a vesicle, develops into a pustule, and eventually forms the characteristic honey-colored crust. Symptoms of mild itching are present, but systemic symptoms are infrequent.

Antibiotic treatment should cover both pathogens. **Mupirocin ointment 2%** applied topically 3 times daily is the treatment of choice for localized infections. A 7- to 10-day course of oral antibiotics is indicated for more diffuse infections. Oral antibiotic regimens include **dicloxacillin** 12 to 25 mg/kg/d divided 4 times daily, **cephalexin** 25 to 50 mg/kg/d divided 4 times daily, or **amoxicillin/clavulanate** 45 mg/kg/d divided twice daily. Clindamycin or azithromycin are appropriate alternatives for individuals with a penicillin allergy.

Erysipelas

Erysipelas is a superficial cellulitis, usually limited to the epidermis and dermis, with prominent lymphatic involvement. It is almost always due to *S pyogenes* and rarely *S aureus*. The face, ears, and lower legs are common sites of infection. Erysipelas is painful and presents as a fiery red, edematous, indurated lesion with a sharply demarcated palpable border. Streptococcal bacteremia occurs in 5% of patients.

Mild early cases of erysipelas secondary to *S pyogenes* can be treated orally with **penicillin V** 250 to 500 mg 4 times daily. When *S aureus* cannot be excluded, **dicloxacillin** 250 to 500 mg 4 times daily or **cephalexin** 250 to 500 mg 4 times daily is indicated. For severe cases of facial erysipelas, nafcillin or oxacillin 2 g intravenously every 4 hours is appropriate. Diabetic patients may require broader coverage with ampicillin-sulbactam, amoxicillin-clavulanate, or a second- or third-generation cephalosporin. In penicillin-allergic patients, clindamycin, erythromycin, azithromycin, clarithromycin, gatifloxacin, or moxifloxacin can be prescribed.

Facial Cellulitis

Cellulitis is a painful, acute, spreading infection of the skin that extends deeper than erysipelas and involves the subcutaneous tissue. In contrast to erysipelas, the borders are not elevated and are less clearly defined. It commonly occurs secondary to violation of the skin barrier. If there is no obvious portal of entry, then contiguous spread from deep space infection or lymphatic or hematogenous seeding should be considered. The pathogen usually is *S pyogenes* or *S aureus*. In children (and rarely in adults), *Haemophilus influenza*, *Streptococcal pneumoniae*, and anaerobic and oral commensals may play a role in facial cellulitis. In streptococcal cellulitis, the skin is red, progression is rapid, and toxicity is more common. Staphylococcal skin infections are red, may blister, progress more indolently, and form an abscess more commonly. In children with *H influenza* cellulitis, the skin often has a violaceous tinge, and there is an absence of integument violation. These patients appear acutely ill and have a high fever, white blood cell count greater than 15,000/μL, and up to 90% positive blood cultures. In adults, *H influenza* facial cellulitis is often preceded by pharyngitis and fever.

Empiric antibiotic treatment should begin early and provide coverage for both *S pyogenes* and *S aureus*. Treatments include **cefazolin, cephalexin,** and **dicloxacillin.** If *H influenza* is clinically suspected, appropriate agents are **ampicillin/sulbactam, amoxicillin/clavulanate,** or a **second- or third-generation cephalosporin.** Patients with a penicillin allergy can be treated with clindamycin, erythromycin, azithromycin, clarithromycin, gatifloxacin, or moxifloxacin. Patients with severe infections or signs of toxicity should be admitted. Immunocompromised patients should be treated aggressively and have a lower threshold for admission. Patients who are treated as outpatients need to be followed up in 24 to 48 hours.

SALIVARY GLAND DISORDERS

Viral Parotitis

Mumps, a paramyxovirus, is the most common cause of viral parotitis in children younger than 15 years. The virus is spread by airborne droplets. Symptoms begin after an incubation period of 2 to 3 weeks and consist of fever, malaise, headache, myalgias, arthralgias, and anorexia. These prodromal symptoms continue for 3 to 5 days and are followed by parotid gland enlargement. Bilateral parotid enlargement occurs in 75% of cases and lasts up to 5 days. The gland is tense and painful, but erythema and warmth are absent. There is no discharge from the parotid (Stensen) duct. Diagnosis is clinical.

Treatment is supportive and consists of analgesics and antipyretics. The patient is contagious for 9 days after the onset of parotid gland swelling. Epididymoorchitis is the most common extrasalivary gland involvement in postpubertal males, affecting 20% to 30% of patients. It can precede or follow parotitis. Epididymoorchitis may present as the sole manifestation of mumps. Oophoritis occurs in only 5% of females.

Suppurative Parotitis

Suppurative parotitis is a potentially fatal bacterial infection that occurs in patients with diminished salivary flow. Retrograde transmission of bacteria leads to infection. Factors and conditions that lead to decreased salivary flow include recent anesthesia, dehydration, prematurity, advanced age, sialolithiasis, medications (eg, diuretics, β-blockers, antihistamines, phenothiazines, and tricyclic antidepressants), and certain disorders (eg, diabetes, human immunodeficiency virus, hypothyroidism, and Sjögren syndrome). Symptoms progress rapidly and consist of fever, trismus, and severe pain over the parotid gland. Physical examination shows induration, erythema, and tenderness to palpation over the cheek and angle of the mandible. In contrast to mumps, pus may be expressed from the parotid (Stensen) duct. Bilateral parotid gland involvement is found in 25% of cases.

Treatment consists of hydration, local massage, heat, sialogogs (eg, lemon drops or orange juice), and β-lactamase- or penicillinase-resistant antibiotics.

Amoxicillin/clavulanate or **ampicillin/sulbactam** contains β-lactamase inhibitors. **Dicloxacillin, oxacillin,** and **second-generation cephalosporins** are penicillinase resistant. Some investigators recommend adding **metronidazole** to enhance anaerobic coverage. In penicillin-allergic patients, clindamycin or a combination of cephalexin and metronidazole should be used. ENT consultation is required in severe cases or treatment failures.

Sialolithiasis

Eighty percent of salivary calculi (sialoliths) occur in the submandibular (Wharton) duct, and most of the remainder occur in the parotid duct. Patients present with unilateral pain, swelling, and tenderness of the involved gland. The stone may be palpable and the gland will be firm. Submandibular calculi are usually radiopaque and can be visualized on intraoral radiographs. Sialolithiasis is often difficult to distinguish from suppurative sialoadenitis, and at times the 2 may coexist.

Treatment initially consists of analgesic, massage, and sialogogs. If concurrent infection is suspected, treatment with antibiotics is indicated. Palpable stones can be milked form the duct. Persistently retained calculi can be removed electively by an otolaryngologist via dilatation or incision of the ductal orifice.

Masticator Space Abscess

The masticator space consists of 4 contiguous potential spaces bounded by the muscles of mastication. These spaces include the masseteric, pterygomandibular, superficial temporal, and deep temporal spaces. Infection in these spaces is polymicrobial and commonly associated with an odontogenic source. Abscesses in these spaces result in swelling over the buccal, submandibular, or sublingual areas. Signs and symptoms depend in part on the abscess location and include fever, facial swelling, pain, erythema, fever, and trismus. Contrast-enhanced computed tomography can help differentiate cellulitis from abscess and, if an abscess is present, its extent can be detailed. Because these spaces ultimately communicate with the tissue planes that extend into the mediastinum, early treatment is imperative.

Well-appearing patients with minimal symptoms and no palpable abscess are candidates for outpatient treatment. Therapy includes analgesics and oral antibiotics (**clindamycin** or **amoxicillin/clavulanate**) for 10 to 14 days. Follow-up is required in 24 hours. Patients with significant trismus, potential airway compromise, palpable abscess, diffuse cellulitis, or sepsis should be admitted. Clindamycin 600 mg intravenously every 6 to 8 hours is recommended. Alternative agents include ampicillin-sulbactam, cefoxitin, or combination therapy with penicillin and metronidazole. In severe cases, emergent ENT consultation is needed for operative drainage.

MANDIBLE DISORDERS

Temporomandibular Joint Dysfunction

The temporomandibular joint combines a hinge and gliding movement. Anatomic internal derangement or systemic disease can cause dysfunction of this joint. Patients present with unilateral dull pain in the region of the temporomandibular joint or localized over 1 of the muscles of mastication. The pain worsens over the course of the day and in severe cases can cause trismus.

Physical examination findings include reduced mandible range, with a maximum interincisor distance narrower than 35 mm. Tenderness to palpation over the condylar head may be present when opening and closing the mouth.

Treatment consists of warm compresses, soft diet, analgesics, and muscle relaxants. Patients should be referred to a dental specialist for evaluation and consideration for occlusal splint therapy.

Mandible Dislocation

The mandible can be dislocated in an anterior, posterior, lateral, or superior direction. Anterior dislocation is most common. Patients with acute mandible dislocations present with severe pain, difficulty swallowing, and malocclusion. In anterior dislocations, pain is localized anterior to the tragus, and a history of extreme mouth opening is typical. All other mandibular dislocations require significant trauma. The diagnosis of a nontraumatic anterior dislocation is made clinically. In other dislocations, or if there is a history of trauma, radiographs are needed.

Reduction may be attempted in closed anterior dislocations without fracture. Patients with open or nonreducible dislocations, associated fractures, or nerve injury should be emergently referred to an oral maxillofacial surgeon. After successful reduction, patients are placed on a soft diet and instructed not to open their mouths wider than 2 cm for 2 weeks.

For further reading in *Emergency Medicine: A Comprehensive Study Guide,* 6th ed., see Chap. 240, "Face and Jaw Emergencies," by Robert Haddon and W. Franklin Peacock IV.

OTOLOGIC EMERGENCIES

Otitis Externa

Otitis externa (OE), or "swimmer's ear," is characterized by pruritus, pain, and tenderness of the external ear. Erythema and edema of the external auditory canal (EAC) also may be present and may cause hearing loss of the involved ear. Clear or purulent otorrhea may be present. Pain is elicited with movement of the pinna or tragus. Risk factors for development of OE include swimming, trauma of the EAC, and any process that elevates the pH of the EAC.

The most common organisms implicated in OE are *Pseudomonas aeruginosa* and *Staphylococcus aureus. Bacteroides* species and polymicrobial infection may account for a significant number of cases. Otomycosis, or fungal OE, accounts for approximately 10% of cases, especially in tropical climates. *Aspergillus* and *Candida* are the most common fungal pathogens.

The treatment of OE includes analgesics, cleaning the EAC, acidifying agents, topical antimicrobials, and occasionally topical **steroid preparations. Floxin otic, Cortisporin otic suspension,** and **Cipro HC otic** are commonly used to treat OE. If significant swelling of the EAC is present, a wick or piece of gauze may be inserted into the EAC to allow passage of topical medications.

Malignant OE is a potentially life-threatening infection of the EAC with variable extension to the skull base. *Pseudomonas aeruginosa* is the most common causative organism. Elderly patients, diabetics, and patients with the human immunodeficiency virus are most commonly affected. Diagnosis of malignant OE requires a high index of suspicion. Computed tomography (CT) is necessary to determine the extent and stage of the disease. Emergent otolaryngologic (ENT) consultation, intravenous (IV) **aminoglycoside** and **anti-pseudomonal penicillin, cephalosporin,** or **fluoroquinolone** therapy, and admission to the hospital are mandatory.

Otitis Media

The incidence and prevalence of otitis media (OM) peak in the preschool years and decline with advancing age. The most common bacterial pathogens in acute OM are *Streptococcus pneumoniae, Haemophilus influenzae,* and *Moraxella catarrhalis.* The predominant organisms involved in chronic OM are *S aureus, P aeruginosa,* and anaerobic bacteria.

Patients with OM present with otalgia, with or without fever; occasionally, hearing loss and otorrhea are present. The tympanic membrane (TM) may be retracted or bulging and will have impaired mobility on pneumatic otoscopy. The TM may appear red as a result of inflammation or may be yellow or white due to middle ear secretions.

A 10-day course of **amoxicillin** is the preferred initial treatment for OM. Alternative agents include trimethoprim/sulfamethoxazole, azithromycin, or cefuroxime. Cefuroxime or amoxicillin/clavulanate may be given for OM unresponsive to first-line therapy after 72 hours. Antibiotic coverage should be extended to 3 weeks for patients with OM with effusion. Analgesics should be prescribed for patients with any degree of pain. Patients should follow up with a primary care physician for reexamination and to assess the effectiveness of therapy.

Complications of OM include TM perforation, conductive hearing loss, acute serous labyrinthitis, facial nerve paralysis, acute mastoiditis, lateral sinus thrombosis, cholesteatoma, and intracranial complications. TM perforation and conductive hearing loss are most often self-limiting and often require no specific intervention. Facial nerve paralysis is uncommon but requires emergent ENT consultation.

Acute Mastoiditis

Acute mastoiditis occurs as infection spreads from the middle ear to the mastoid air cells. Patients present with otalgia, fever, and postauricular erythema, swelling, and tenderness. Protrusion of the auricle with obliteration of the postauricular crease may be present. CT will delineate the extent of bony involvement. Emergent **ENT consultation, cefotaxime** 1.0 g IV every 4 hours, and admission to the hospital are necessary. Surgical drainage ultimately may be required.

Lateral Sinus Thrombosis

This condition arises from extension of infection and inflammation into the lateral and sigmoid sinuses. Headache is common and papilledema, sixth nerve palsy, and vertigo may be present. Diagnosis may be made with CT, although magnetic resonance imaging or angiography may be necessary. Therapy consists of emergent ENT consultation, combination of IV **nafcillin, ceftriaxone,** and **metronidazole** therapy, and hospital admission.

Bullous Myringitis

Bullous myringitis is a painful condition of the ear characterized by bulla on the TM and deep EAC. Numerous pathogens have been reported in the etiology, including viruses, *Mycoplasma pneumoniae,* and *Chlamydia psittaci.* The diagnosis is made by clinical examination. The treatment consists of pain control, warm compresses, and oral antibiotics if an associated middle ear effusion is present.

Trauma to the Ear

Lacerations to the ear should be copiously irrigated, and any injury to the perichondrium should be closed with 5-0 or 6-0 absorbable suture. ENT or plastic surgery should be consulted for significant injuries, especially in avulsion injuries with tissue loss.

A hematoma can develop from any type of trauma to the ear. Improper treatment of ear hematomas can result in stimulation of the perichondrium and development of asymmetric cartilage formation. The resultant deformed auricle has been termed *cauliflower ear.* Immediate incision and drainage of the hematoma with a compressive dressing is necessary to prevent reaccumulation of the hematoma.

Thermal injury to the auricle may be caused by excessive heat or cold. Superficial injury of either type is treated with cleaning, topical non–sulfa-containing antibiotic ointment, and a light dressing. Frostbite is treated with rapid rewarming by using saline soaked gauze at 38°C to 40°C. The rewarming process will be quite painful and may necessitate analgesics or conscious sedation. Any second- or third-degree burn requires immediate ENT or burn center consultation.

Foreign Bodies in the Ear

On examination, the foreign body is usually visualized, and signs of infection or TM perforation should be sought. Live insects should be immobilized with **2% lidocaine** distilled into the ear canal before removal. Foreign bodies may be removed with forceps and direct visualization or with the aid of a hooked probe or suction catheter. Irrigation is often useful for small objects; however, organic material may absorb water and swell. ENT consultation is required for cases of foreign body with TM perforation or if the object cannot be safely removed.

Tinnitus

Tinnitus is the perception of sound without external stimuli. It may be constant, pulsatile, high or low pitched, hissing, clicking, or ringing in nature. Objective tinnitus can be heard by the examiner, whereas the more common subjective tinnitus cannot. Causes of tinnitus include sensorineural hearing loss, hypertension, conductive hearing loss, head trauma, medications (aspirin, nonsteroidal antiinflammatory drugs, aminoglycoside, loop diruetics, and chemotherapeutics), temporomandibular joint disorders, depression, acoustic neuromas, multiple sclerosis, benign intracranial hypertension, Ménière disease, Cogan syndrome, arteriovenous malformations, arterial bruits, enlarged eustachian tube, palatum clonus, and stapedial muscle spasm. Accurate diagnosis usually requires referral to an otolaryngologist. Pharmacologic treatment with antidepressant medications may alleviate tinnitus in which no correctable cause can be found.

Hearing Loss

Causes of sudden hearing loss include idiopathic (most common), infectious (mumps, Epstein-Barr virus, herpes, cytomegalovirus, syphilis, and labyrinthitis), vascular or hematologic (leukemia, sickle cell disease, polycythemia, Berger disease, and cerebral aneurysm), metabolic (diabetes and hyperlipidemia), rheumatologic (temporal arteritis and Wegener granulomatosis), conductive (OE, OM, ruptured tympanic membrane, neoplasm, and osteonecrosis), Ménière disease, Cogan syndrome, acoustic neuroma, cochlear rupture, and ototoxic medications. Indictors of poor prognosis include severe hearing loss on presentation and the presence of vertigo. If the cause is not readily determined by history and physical examination, otolaryngologic consultation is necessary.

NASAL EMERGENCIES AND SINUSITIS

Epistaxis

Epistaxis is classified as anterior or posterior. Posterior epistaxis is suggested if an anterior source is not visualized, if bleeding occurs from both nares, or if blood is seen draining into the posterior pharynx after anterior sources have been controlled.

Anterior and posterior epistaxes requires an initial evaluation to identify and control the source.

1. A quick history should determine the duration and severity of the hemorrhage and the contributing factors (trauma, anticoagulant use, infection, bleeding diathesis, etc).
2. The patient should blow the nose to dislodge any clots.
3. A quick inspection is made to identify obvious anterior sources. A Frazier suction catheter will help keep the passage clear.
4. Cotton swabs or pledgets moistened with a topical anesthetic or vasoconstrictor are inserted into the nasal cavity with bayonet forceps. **Four percent lidocaine** provides excellent results when mixed with **1:1000 epinephrine, 1% phenylephrine,** or **0.05% oxymetazoline.**
5. Direct external pressure is then applied for 15 minutes. Active bleeding into the pharynx despite direct pressure suggests inadequate pressure, drainage from a clot in the posterior nasal cavity, or true posterior epistaxis.
6. If this approach fails, it should be repeated 1 or 2 more times. If still unsuccessful and the source of bleeding is anterior, an anterior pack may be inserted or local cautery may be attempted if the source of bleeding is easily identified and is a discrete area of bleeding.
7. **Chemical cautery with silver nitrate** is the standard of care for emergency department (ED) cautery of anterior epistaxis. After hemostasis is achieved, the mucosa is cauterized by firmly rolling the tip of a silver nitrate applicator over the area until it turns silvery-black. A small surrounding area also should be cauterized to control local arterioles. Overzealous use of cautery is discouraged because it may cause septal perforation and unintended local tissue necrosis.
8. **Anterior nasal packing** may be performed with gauze or commercial devices. One popular device is the Merocel nasal sponge (Merocel Corp, Mystic, CT), a compact, dehydrated sponge available in several lengths to control anterior and posterior epistaxes. The sponge is rapidly inserted along the floor of the nasal cavity and then expands upon contact with blood or secretions. A film of antibiotic ointment applied to the sponge will ease insertion and reduce chances of infection. After insertion, expansion is hastened by rehydrating the sponge with sterile water from a catheter-tipped syringe after the sponge has been inserted. A mixture of lidocaine and a topical vasoconstrictor also may be used to hydrate the sponge and provide topical anesthesia and vasoconstriction. The longer sponges used to control posterior hemorrhages have been associated with some morbidity and should be used only when indicated; they are not indicated for the control of isolated anterior epistaxis. All nasal packs are removed in 2 to 3 days by an ENT physician.
9. If packing or local cautery fails to control anterior bleeding, ENT consultation is necessary.
10. **Posterior epistaxis** may be treated with a dehydrated posterior sponge pack, as outlined above, or a commercial balloon tamponade device. The balloon devices use independently inflatable anterior and posterior balloons to quickly control refractory epistaxis at these sites; the instructions for insertion are included in the balloon kit. To protect against potentially serious complications, all patients with posterior packs require ENT consultation for possible hospital admission. Posterior packs are removed in 2 to 3 days after placement.

11. Complications of nasal packing include dislodgment of the pack, recurrent bleeding, sinusitis, and toxic shock syndrome. All patients with nasal packs should be started on antibiotic prophylaxis with **cephalexin** or **amoxicillin/clavulanate.** Penicillin-allergic patients may be given clindamycin or trimethoprim/sulfamethoxazole.

Nasal Fractures

Nasal fracture is a clinical diagnosis suggested by the injury mechanism, swelling, tenderness, crepitance, gross deformity, and periorbital ecchymosis. Radiographic diagnosis usually is not necessary in the ED. Intermittent ice application, analgesics, and over-the-counter decongestants are the normal treatment. Follow-up in 2 to 5 days for reexamination and possible fracture reduction is prudent.

The nose should be examined for a septal hematoma, which is a collection of blood beneath the perichondrium of the nasal septum. Septal hematomas appear as bluish, fluid-filled sacs (or grapelike clusters) on the nasal septum. If left untreated, a septal hematoma may result in abscess formation or necrosis of the nasal septum. The treatment is local **incision and drainage** with subsequent placement of an anterior nasal pack.

A fracture of the cribriform plate may violate the subarachnoid space and cause cerebrospinal fluid rhinorrhea. Symptoms may be delayed for several weeks. If a cribriform plate injury is suspected, CT and immediate neurosurgical consultation should be obtained.

Nasal Foreign Bodies

Nasal foreign bodies should be suspected in patients with unilateral nasal obstruction, foul rhinorrhea, or persistent unilateral epistaxis. After topical vasoconstrictors and anesthetic agents have been used, the foreign body should be removed under direct visualization. Tools for removal include forceps, suction catheters, hooked probes, and balloon-tipped catheters. For pediatric patients, one technique is to apply positive pressure via a puff of air to the patient's mouth, with a finger occluding the unobstructed nostril. ENT consultation is required for any unsuccessful removal.

Sinusitis

Maxillary sinusitis presents with pain in the infraorbital area, whereas frontal sinusitis causes pain in the supraorbital and lower forehead region. Ethmoid sinusitis, which is especially serious in children because of its tendency to spread to the central nervous system, often produces a dull, aching sensation in the retroorbital area. Sphenoid sinusitis is uncommon and has vague signs and symptoms. Chronic sinusitis often produces local discomfort and a chronic, purulent exudate.

Unfortunately, the physical findings of sinusitis are neither sensitive nor specific. The diagnosis of sinusitis is often clinical. Radiographs may show sinus opacification, air/fluid levels, or mucosal thickening of at least 6 mm, but they generally are not required in the ED. Treatment includes nasal decongestant sprays, such as oxymetazoline or phenylephrine, for no longer than 3 days. Antibiotic choices for 14- to 21-day regimens include **ampicillin, trimethoprim/sulfamethoxazole, clarithromycin, second-generation cephalosporins,** and **amoxicillin/clavulanate.** Complications of sinusitis include osteomyelitis, meningitis, intracranial abscess, Pott's puffy tumor, periorbital cellulitis, orbital cellulitis, and cavernous sinus thrombosis.

For further reading in *Emergency Medicine: A Comprehensive Study Guide,* 6th ed., see Chap. 239, "Common Disorders of the External, Middle, and Inner Ear," by Anne Tintinalli and Michael Lucchesi; and Chap. 241, "Nasal Emergencies and Sinusitis," by Thomas A. Waters and W. Frank Peacock.

153 | Oral and Dental Emergencies
Steven Go

OROFACIAL PAIN

Tooth Eruption

Eruption of the primary teeth ("teething") in children may be associated with pain, irritability, and drooling. Although fever and diarrhea also have been traditionally associated with teething, it is important that more ominous causes of these symptoms be excluded first. Adequate hydration, by giving the child a frozen, damp towel to suck on, and **acetaminophen** 15 mg/kg orally (PO) every 6 hours usually will control symptoms. Topical benzocaine has the potential to depress the gag reflex of infants who unfortunately also possess a strong predilection for putting foreign objects into their mouths. Therefore, the routine use of benzocaine is to be discouraged unless careful parental supervision is constantly available. Adults may experience pain and local inflammation with the eruption of the third molars ("wisdom teeth"). **Penicillin VK** 500 mg PO 4 times daily or **clindamycin** 300 mg PO 4 times daily, **ibuprofen** 800 mg PO 3 times daily, and warm saline mouth rinses will help temporize symptoms until an oral surgeon can remove the teeth.

Dental Caries and Periradicular Pathology

The most common cause of toothache is periapical pathology. Pain can be localized to a single tooth or be diffuse, with pain radiating to various aspects of the head and neck. Examination sometimes finds a grossly decayed tooth, although frequently there is no visible pathology. Localization may be accomplished by percussing individual teeth with a metallic object. Treatment includes **penicillin VK** 500 mg PO 4 times daily or **clindamycin** 300 mg PO 4 times daily, **ibuprofen** 800 mg PO 3 times daily, **oxycodone** 5 mg/**acetaminophen** 325 mg 1 to 2 tablets PO 4 times daily for 48 hours, warm saline mouth rinses, and referral to a dentist. If a fluctuant oral abscess is present, then an incision and drainage should be performed in addition to the above treatments.

Facial Cellulitis

Odontogenic infections can spread readily to the facial spaces. Therefore, it is imperative to exclude deep-space involvement whenever a dental infection is encountered.

Ludwig's angina is a cellulitis involving the submandibular spaces and the sublingual space that can spread to the neck and mediastinum, causing airway compromise, overwhelming infection, and even death. Early diagnosis is imperative, with special focus on preserving the patient's airway. When the diagnosis is suspected, **ampicillin/sulbactam** 3 g intravenously (IV) or **ticarcillin/clavulanate** 3.1 g IV, or **clindamycin** 900 mg IV with **metronidazole** 15 mg/kg IV should be administered, and an emergent oral and maxillofacial surgical consultation should be obtained.

If dental infections spread to the infraorbital space, a *cavernous sinus thrombosis* may result. This condition may present with limitation of lateral gaze, meningeal signs, sepsis, and coma. The antibiotic treatment for cavernous sinus thrombosis is similar to that of Ludwig angina. Anticoagulation with heparin also has been shown to be efficacious to prevent further thrombosis. Surgical intervention, if any, should be directed toward draining the site of the infection as opposed to the cavernous sinus thrombosis itself.

Postextraction Alveolar Osteitis

Periosteitis is pain experienced within 24 to 48 hours after a tooth extraction and responds well to analgesics alone. Postextraction alveolar osteitis ("dry socket") occurs when the clot from the socket is displaced, typically on the second or third postoperative day. It presents with severe pain and foul odor and taste. Dental radiographs should be taken to exclude a retained foreign body or root. Treatment consists of **saline irrigation** of the socket, followed by packing the socket with **eugenol-impregnated gauze. Penicillin VK** 500 mg PO 4 times daily or **clindamycin** 300 mg PO 4 times daily should be prescribed in severe cases, with daily packing changes and dental follow-up in 24 hours.

Periodontal Abscess

A periodontal abscess results from plaque and debris entrapped between the tooth and gingiva. Small abscesses resolve with **oral antibiotics, analgesics,** and **chlorhexidine mouth rinses** twice daily. Appropriate antibiotic choices include **penicillin VK** 500 mg PO 4 times daily or **clindamycin** 300 mg PO 4 times daily. Larger abscesses require incision and drainage. All patients need prompt dental referral.

Acute Necrotizing Ulcerative Gingivitis

Acute necrotizing ulcerative gingivitis presents with pain, ulcerated or "punched out" interdental papillae, gingival bleeding, fever, and malaise. The associated fetid breath gives acute necrotizing ulcerative gingivitis its nickname of "trench mouth." It occurs mainly in patients with lowered resistance due to the human immunodeficiency virus, malnourishment, and perhaps stress. Treatment consists of **metronidazole** 250 mg PO 3 times daily and **chlorhexidine mouth rinses** twice daily. Symptomatic improvement is dramatic within 24 hours, and the patient should be referred for workup of predisposing factors.

SOFT TISSUE LESIONS OF THE ORAL CAVITY

Oral Candidiasis

Sixty percent of adults harbor candidal organisms. Risk factors include extremes of age, immunocompromised states, use of intraoral prosthetic devices, concurrent antibiotic use, and malnutrition. Typical lesions consist of removable white, curd-like plaques on an erythematous mucosal base. Treatment consists of oral antifungal agents such as **clotrimazole troches** 10 mg 5 times daily, **nystatin oral suspension** 500 000 U PO 4 times daily, or **fluconazole** 200 mg PO twice daily.

Aphthous Stomatitis

Aphthous stomatitis is a common pattern of intraoral ulceration triggered by cell-mediated immunity. These painful lesions, which are frequently multiple, involve the labial and buccal mucosa and measure from 2 mm to several centimeters in diameter. Treatment consists of **betamethasone syrup** or **dexamethasone 0.01% elixir** used as a mouth rinse. Resolution is often complete within 2 days.

Herpes Gingivostomatitis

Herpes gingivostomatitis causes painful ulcerations of the gingiva and mucosal surfaces. Fever, lymphadenopathy, and tingling often precede the eruption of numerous vesicles, which then rupture and form ulcerative lesions. If **acyclovir** 400 mg PO 3 times daily or **valacyclovir** 500 mg PO twice daily for 5 days is initiated during the prodromal phrase, the clinical duration and severity may be attenuated.

Herpangina and Hand, Foot, and Mouth Disease

Herpangina and hand, foot, and mouth disease are caused by infection with coxsackievirus A species. Herpangina presents with high fever, sore throat, headache, and malaise, followed by eruption of oral vesicles, which rupture to form painful, shallow ulcers. The soft palate, uvula, and tonsillar pillars are typically affected, whereas the buccal mucosa, tongue, and gingiva are spared (which helps distinguish it from herpes infection). Hand, foot, and mouth disease causes vesicles initially to form on the soft palate, gingiva, tongue, and buccal mucosa. The vesicles then rupture, leaving painful ulcers surrounded by red halos. Lesions also may appear on the buttocks, palms, and soles. Both infections last approximately 5 to 10 days. Treatment is supportive and consists of hydration and acetaminophen or ibuprofen. Topical anesthetics should be used with great caution in young infants due to its potential to depress the gag reflex. Infected children should be kept home from school until the lesions resolve.

OROFACIAL TRAUMA

Dentoalveolar Trauma

In all dentoalveolar trauma, a search for associated injuries should be undertaken (including retained fragments in surrounding tissue), and the patient should be warned of the possibility of occult damage to the neurovascular bundle, with subsequent pulp necrosis or root resorption.

Dental Fractures

The Ellis system is used to classify the anatomy of fractured teeth. *Ellis class 1* fractures involve only the enamel of the tooth. These injuries may be smoothed with an emery board or referred to a dentist for cosmetic repair. *Ellis class 2* fractures involve the creamy yellow dentin underneath the white enamel. The patient complains of air and temperature sensitivities. To decrease the chances of contamination, the exposed dentin must be thoroughly dried and promptly covered with **zinc oxide/eugenol paste, calcium hydroxide paste,** or **glass ionomer cement.** All patients should see a dentist within 24 hours. In patients younger than 12 years, the protective dentinal layer is thin. A visible blush of pulp under this thin dentinal layer thus indicates that the pulp is at risk and should be treated like an Ellis class 3 fracture. *Ellis class 3* fractures are tooth-threatening fractures that involve the pulp and can be identified by a red blush of the dentin or a visible drop of blood after wiping the tooth. Ideally, a dentist should evaluate the patient immediately. If a dentist is not immediately available, the tooth may be covered temporarily with **zinc oxide/eugenol paste, calcium hydroxide paste,** or **glass ionomer cement** until the dentist is seen within 24 hours. Oral analgesics may be needed, but topical anesthetics are contraindicated. The use of prophylactic antibiotics is controversial.

Concussions, Luxations, and Avulsions

Concussion injuries involve tenderness to percussion with no mobility. Dental trauma with tenderness to percussion and mobility without evidence of dislodgment is called *subluxation,* which has a higher incidence of future pulp necrosis. Management for these 2 entities includes **nonsteroidal antiinflammatory drugs,** soft diet, and referral to a dentist.

Extrusive luxation occurs when a tooth is partly avulsed from the alveolar bone. Treatment involves gentle repositioning of the tooth to its original location and **splinting with zinc oxide** (Coe-Pak) periodontal dressing. A dentist should evaluate these patients within 24 hours. When the tooth is laterally displaced with a fracture of the alveolar bone, the condition is called *lateral luxation.* Although manual relocation is possible, the treatment of such injuries is best done in consultation with a dentist. If the alveolar bone fracture is significant, splinting by a dentist in the emergency department (ED) is required. An *intrusive luxation* occurs when the tooth is forced below the gingival and often has a poor outcome. Treatment is similar to that of subluxations.

Dental *avulsion* is an emergency in which a tooth has been completely removed from the socket. *Primary teeth* in children are not replaced because of potential damage to the permanent teeth. *Permanent teeth* that have been avulsed for less than 3 hours must be **reimplanted immediately** to attempt to save the periodontal ligament fibers. At the scene, an avulsed tooth should be handled by the crown only, rinsed with water, and reimplanted immediately. If reimplantation at the scene is not possible due to risk of aspiration, the tooth should be rinsed and placed in a nutrient solution, such as **Hank's solution, sterile saline,** or **milk,** and the tooth should be transported immediately with the patient to the ED. An effective, but somewhat unsettling, way to safely transport the avulsed tooth of the child is underneath the parent's tongue. Upon arrival in the ED, the socket can be gently irrigated with sterile normal saline before reimplantation. If the root of the avulsed tooth is moist upon arrival to the ED, the tooth should be reimplanted immediately. If the root has been dry between 20 and 60 minutes, it should be rinsed and soaked in Hank solution for 30 minutes before reimplantation. If the root has been dry longer than 60 minutes, the tooth should be soaked in **citric acid** (for 5 minutes), then 2% **stannous fluoride,** and then **doxycycline** (for 5 minutes) before reimplantation. Once replaced, the patient may gently bite on gauze while waiting to be seen by a dentist in the ED. Early consultant with a dentist is imperative, but reimplantation should not be delayed while awaiting the arrival of the specialist. If a patient arrives with an empty socket and the tooth cannot be located, adjacent tissue should be searched. Radiographs may be necessary to exclude displaced or aspirated teeth.

Soft Tissue Trauma

Dental trauma should be stabilized before repairing soft tissue trauma. In addition, a thorough search for retained foreign bodies should take place before repair, and tetanus status should be updated.

Most *intraoral mucosal lacerations* will heal by themselves; however, they should be repaired if they are gaping (typically wider than 2 cm) or if flaps are present. Good anesthesia is essential. The wound should be inspected for foreign bodies, especially tooth fragments, and devitalized tissue débrided as necessary. The wound is copiously irrigated and closed with a few 5-0 absorbable sutures, taking care to bury the knots. The repair of through-and-through lacerations is controversial. Some advocate first repairing the intraoral laceration and then irrigating the wound before closing the external laceration, using superficial and deep sutures, if necessary. Others close the external laceration only. The patient should be instructed to eat a soft diet with gentle rinses after each meal. Adequate analgesic medication should be prescribed. Antibiotics generally are not indicated, and 48-hour dental follow-up is appropriate.

Tongue lacerations that gape widely, actively bleed, are flap shaped, or involve muscle should be closed. Smaller lacerations heal by themselves. An assistant will be required to hold the tongue with gauze to allow repair. Lacerations may be repaired with 4-0 absorbable sutures, taking care to carefully approximate wound edges as precisely as possible to avoid subsequent formation of clefts, which can have cosmetic and functional consequences. A bite block may be useful to prevent bites to health care providers during repair. It may not be possible to safely repair a frightened child or uncooperative patient without conscious sedation. Such cases may best be left to a specialist. Aftercare is similar to that of other intraoral lacerations.

Lip lacerations are potentially complex because of the possible involvement of the vermillion border (the transition between lip tissue and the skin of the face), which must be aligned precisely to avoid a noticeable cosmetic defect. Before repair, adequate anesthesia must be achieved, preferably by an infraorbital nerve block (upper lip) or mental nerve block (lower lip) to avoid distortion of tissue. Gross debris and devitalized tissue should be removed. If the deep muscular layers of the lip are involved, they should be closed first by deep 5-0 absorbable sutures. If the vermillion border is involved, it should be approximated with a 6-0 nonabsorbable monofilament suture. The use of surgical loupes may be useful in ensuring meticulous alignment of this critical landmark. Once alignment has been achieved, the rest of the wound may be closed. If the laceration extends into the oral cavity, the intraoral portion of the wound is repaired in the same way as other intraoral mucosal lesions. Aftercare is similar to that of other oral lacerations, with the addition of **penicillin VK** 500 mg PO 4 times daily or **clindamycin** 300 mg PO 4 times daily for 5 days. A cosmetic surgeon should repair extensive lip lacerations or those that involve the philtrum or the oral commissures. Specialized consultation also should be sought for pediatric lip lacerations.

Laceration of the *maxillary labial frenulum* usually does not require repair. The *lingual frenulum* is very vascular and usually should be repaired with 4-0 absorbable sutures.

HEMORRHAGE

Postoperative Bleeding

Bleeding after dental extraction usually is controlled by direct pressure for 20 minutes applied by biting on gauze. If bleeding persists, packing with Gelfoam, Avitene, or Surgicel into the socket may be effective. Sutures should be used to hold these packing agents in place, but the gingiva should not be closed under tension due to the risk of gingival flap necrosis. Failure of these measures warrants a screening coagulation profile and consultation with an oral surgeon.

For further reading in *Emergency Medicine: A Comprehensive Study Guide,* 6th ed., see Chap. 242, "Oral and Dental Emergencies," by Ronald W. Beaudreau.

154 | Neck and Upper Airway Disorders

Robert J. French

PHARYNGITIS AND TONSILLITIS

Clinical Features

Pharyngotonsillitis in adults is often due to an infectious etiology, most commonly viral. Other infectious causes include bacteria, fungi, and parasites. Group A β-hemolytic streptococcus (GABHS) causes up to 15% of acute pharyngitis cases, typically with sudden onset of sore throat, painful swallowing, chills, and fever. Headache, vomiting, and abdominal pain are commonly associated symptoms. It is often difficult to differentiate pharyngitis caused by GABHS from other etiologies on clinical grounds alone. Clinical criteria for GABHS pharyngitis include (*a*) tonsillar exudate, (*b*) tender anterior cervical adenopathy, (*c*) history of fever, and (*d*) absence of cough.

Emergency Department Care and Disposition

1. Empiric antibiotic therapy may be started when clinical likelihood of GABHS is high. Alternatively, a rapid streptococcal antigen test can guide treatment decisions.
2. **Penicillin** remains the antibiotic of choice for treatment of GABHS pharyngotonsillitis. A single dose of benzathine penicillin 1.2 million U intramuscularly or penicillin V 500 mg orally (PO) 2 or 3 times daily for 10 days is first-line treatment for GABHS.
3. In penicillin-allergic patients, a 10-day course of erythromycin is the recommended alternative. Oral cephalosporins and clindamycin are additional alternative agents for GABHS pharyngitis.
4. Treatment with antibiotics is recommended in patients with GABHS to help prevent suppurative and nonsuppurative poststreptococcal sequelae. Suppurative complications include cervical lymphadenitis, peritonsillar abscess, retropharyngeal abscess, sinusitis, and otitis media. Virulent strains of GABHS are associated with the nonsuppurative complications of acute rheumatic fever and poststreptococcal glomerulonephritis. Treatment with appropriate antibiotics, resulting in eradication of GABHS infection, can help prevent acute rheumatic fever.
5. **Dexamethasone** 10 mg PO or intramuscularly may be used in patients with severe symptoms.

PERITONSILLAR ABSCESS

Clinical Features

Peritonsillar abscess (PTA) is the most frequent deep-space infection of the head and neck. It is caused by a collection of purulent material between the palatine tonsil capsule and the superior constrictor and palatopharyngeus muscle. Although GABHS is the most common cause of PTA, mixed aerobic and anaerobic bacteria are often present. Symptoms of PTA include fever, malaise, sore throat, odynophagia, dysphagia, "hot potato voice," sore throat, otalgia, and different degrees of trismus. Signs include unilateral tonsillar enlargement with inferomedial displacement, palatal and uvula edema, contralateral deflection of the uvula, tender ipsilateral anterior lymphadenopathy, drooling, and dehydration.

Diagnosis and Differential

The differential diagnosis includes tonsillitis, peritonsillar cellulitis, infectious mononucleosis, retropharyngeal abscess, tumor, and internal carotid artery aneurysm. Differentiating peritonsillar cellulitis from abscess may be challenging. Trismus is uncommon in peritonsillar cellulitis. Digital or cotton-tip applicator palpation for fluctuance may help differentiate PTA from cellulitis. Complications of PTA include airway obstruction, aspiration of ruptured abscess contents, septicemia, retropharyngeal abscess, and mediastinitis.

Emergency Department Care and Disposition

1. **Aspiration of purulent material** with an 18- or 20-gauge needle is diagnostic and therapeutic for PTA and will effectively treat 85% of these patients. This procedure should be performed by individuals skilled in the technique.
2. After needle aspiration, antibiotic therapy is recommended to eradicate offending organisms. **Penicillin V** 500 mg PO 4 times daily for 10 days is the treatment of choice. In penicillin-allergic patients, clindamycin 300 to 450 mg PO 4 times daily is recommended.
3. Broader-spectrum agents, such as **amoxicillin/clavulanate** or **cefuroxime plus metronidazole,** can be used if there is inadequate clinical improvement.

RETROPHARYNGEAL ABSCESS

Clinical Features

Retropharyngeal abscess is most common in children younger than 5 years but also can occur in adults. Due to anatomic and pathophysiologic differences, retropharyngeal abscess in children is typically more localized than that in adults. Patients present with fever, sore throat, odynophagia, dysphagia, neck stiffness, neck pain, muffled voice, stridor, and respiratory distress. These patients gravitate toward a supine position, with the neck in slight extension to minimize compression of the upper airway. Sitting them up can increase their dyspnea. Physical examination may show tender cervical lymphadenopathy, neck swelling, torticollis, pharyngeal erythema, and edema. Movement of the trachea or larynx side to side ("tracheal rock") commonly causes pain.

Diagnosis and Differential

The lateral soft tissue neck radiograph may demonstrate thickening in the prevertebral space. A contrast-enhanced computed tomography (CT) of the neck can help differentiate cellulitis from abscess and help define the extent of the infection. Cultures from retropharyngeal abscesses are usually polymicrobial, with aerobic and anaerobic organisms.

Emergency Department Care and Disposition

1. Emergency department treatment consists of airway management, emergent otolaryngologic consultation, and antibiotics.

2. In adults, **clindamycin** 600 to 900 mg intravenously (IV) every 8 hours or **ampicillin/sulbactam** 3 g IV every 6 hours is used.

PARAPHARYNGEAL ABSCESS

Parapharyngeal abscess (PPA) occurs secondary to odontogenic and pharyngeal tonsillar infections or as a result of direct extension from an adjacent deep neck abscess. This space is shaped like an inverted pyramid and extends from the base of the skull to the hyoid. The styloid process arbitrarily divides this space into anterior and posterior compartments. Patients with anterior space infection will present with trismus and bulging of the lateral pharyngeal wall. Posterior space infections are more ominous and can result in palsies of cranial nerves IX to XII, Horner's syndrome, internal jugular vein thrombosis, and carotid artery rupture, or pseudoaneurysm formation. The lateral soft tissue neck radiograph is less sensitive in detection of PPA than in detection of retropharyngeal space infections. Contrast-enhanced neck CT accurately diagnose and delineate the extent of the PPA. Doppler ultrasound or angiography may be required if vascular encroachment is a concern. The management and treatment are similar to those followed for retropharyngeal space infections.

EPIGLOTTITIS

Clinical Features

Epiglottitis can lead to rapid, unpredictable airway obstruction. Once a disease primarily of childhood, it is now most often seen in adults, with a mean age of 46 years. Supraglottic inflammatory changes are most commonly secondary to *Haemophilus influenza* type b infection. Adults present with a 1- to 2-day history of worsening dysphagia, odynophagia, and dysphonia. The throat pain is disproportionate to clinical examination findings. Other signs include anxiety, fever, tachycardia, cervical adenopathy, and pain with gentle palpation of the trachea or larynx. Clinical indicators of imminent airway obstruction include dyspnea, drooling, aphonia, and stridor.

Diagnosis and Differential

All diagnostic procedures should be deferred in the unstable patient, and attention should focus on airway patency. Lateral soft tissue neck radiographs may show an edematous epiglottis ("thumbprint sign") with loss of the vallecula and ballooning of the hypopharynx. Direct fiberoptic laryngoscopy classically shows a "cherry red" epiglottis. Differential diagnosis includes pharyngitis, infectious mononucleosis, croup, deep-space neck abscess, diphtheria, pertussis, laryngeal trauma, foreign body aspiration, and laryngospasm.

Emergency Department Care and Disposition

1. Patients with suspected epiglottitis require immediate otolaryngology consultation, and the emergency physician must be prepared to establish a definitive airway.
2. Initial airway management consists of supplemental **humidified oxygen** and comfortable patient positioning. **Helium and oxygen** can be given as a temporizing measure.

3. The stable pediatric patient is treated with **endotracheal intubation,** preferably in the operating room. Stable adults are often managed without intubation. If airway intervention is needed and the clinical situation permits, awake nasotracheal fiberoptic intubation is the preferred method.
4. Patients with signs of impending airway obstruction can be treated with a bag-valve mask while preparing for a definitive airway.
5. Orotracheal intubation can be attempted but will be difficult secondary to anatomic distortion. If intubation is unsuccessful, patients younger than 8 years may require needle cricothyroidotomy and those older than 8 years may require surgical cricothyroidotomy.
6. **Cefuroxime** 0.75 to 1.5 g IV every 8 hours is the recommended first-line treatment and should be initiated in the emergency department. Cefotaxime, ceftriaxone, or ampicillin/sulbactam is an acceptable alternative.

ODONTOGENIC ABSCESS

Suppurative odontogenic infections are polymicrobial, consisting of *Streptococcus* sp and oral anaerobes. Untreated, they can erode cortical bone and spread into soft tissue. Ludwig's angina is an odontogenic infection of the submandibular, sublingual, and submandibular spaces. Patients present with edema of the upper midline neck, dysphagia, trismus, and marked edema of the floor of the mouth. The tongue can rapidly become elevated and displaced posteriorly, leading to airway compromise. Early signs and symptoms of airway compromise may be subtle. Anxiety, drooling, and stridor suggest impending airway collapse. Sublingual and submandibular abscesses may extend into deep-neck spaces, including the prevertebral, parapharyngeal, and retropharyngeal spaces. Contrast-enhanced CT is used to diagnose the location of the deep-neck space abscess.

Emergency Department Care and Disposition

1. Awake nasotracheal fiberoptic intubation or tracheotomy should be performed if there is concern for airway compromise.
2. Treatment of odontogenic abscesses includes operative drainage and IV antibiotics. Emergent otolaryngologic consultation is warranted.
3. First-line antibiotic treatment in adults is (*a*) **clindamycin** 600 to 900 mg IV every 8 hours or (*b*) **penicillin G** 24 million U/d IV divided every 4 to 6 hours plus **metronidazole** 1.0 g IV, followed by 500 mg every 6 hours. Alternative agents include (*a*) cefoxitin 2.0 g IV every 8 hours or (*b*) ampicillin-sulbactam 3.0 g IV every 6 hours.

ACUTE UPPER AIRWAY OBSTRUCTION

Foreign bodies can cause partial or complete airway obstruction. Size, shape, and location of the foreign body dictate symptoms. Lodging at the laryngeal inlet or subglottic region (upper airway) can cause acute airway obstruction, with choking crisis, stridor, and subsequent respiratory arrest. Foreign bodies that are distal to the trachea (lower airway) are less likely to cause acute obstructive symptoms but may present instead with cough, wheezing, dyspnea, or pneumonia.

In the stable patient, foreign body detection can be aided by direct inspection of the oropharynx with indirect or direct laryngoscopy or fiberoptic nasopharyngoscopy. In the patient with critical upper airway obstruction, a quick attempt at removal with Magill forceps under direct laryngoscopy is indicated. If the foreign body is visualized but cannot be removed, a surgical airway may be required. If the foreign body is not visualized and the patient is unstable, endotracheal intubation should be performed. The endotracheal tube is passed distal to the carina, thereby forcing the foreign body into the right (usually) or left mainstem bronchus. The endotracheal tube is then pulled back and secured at its normal position. Ventilation of the unobstructed lung is achieved while preparation is made for emergent bronchoscopy.

ANGIOEDEMA OF THE UPPER AIRWAY

Clinical Features

Angioedema of the upper airway can progress rapidly and lead to airway obstruction. Patients with airway involvement can present with "throat tightness," dyspnea, cough, hoarseness, and stridor. Causes include (*a*) C1-esterase inhibitor deficiency, (*b*) immunoglobulin E–mediated type 1 allergic reaction, (*c*) adverse reaction to angiotensin-converting enzyme (ACE) inhibitor therapy, and (*d*) idiopathic reaction. The incidence of ACE inhibitor-related angioedema is 0.1% to 0.2%. Sixty percent of these cases occur within 1 week of starting the drug, but ACE inhibitor-related angioedema can occur months to years after initiation of treatment.

Emergency Department Care and Disposition

1. In adults, 0.3 mL (0.3 mg) of **epinephrine** 1:1000 is administered subcutaneously. This can be repeated every 15 to 20 minutes, as needed.
2. Additional medications that should be administered include **diphenhydramine** 50 mg IV, **methylprednisolone** 125 mg IV, and an **H$_2$-histamine antagonist**.
3. Fiberoptic nasopharyngoscopy is used to assess possible laryngeal edema. Patients with laryngeal edema, potential for airway compromise, or worsening symptoms despite maximal therapy require admission.
4. Patients taking an ACE inhibitor should permanently discontinue its use.

LARYNGEAL TRAUMA

Laryngeal injuries may result from blunt or penetrating trauma. Patients may present with hoarseness, dyspnea, dysphagia, stridor, hemoptysis, and aphonia. Physical examination may show anterior neck tenderness, laryngeal swelling, tracheal displacement, or subcutaneous emphysema. Asphyxia, secondary to laryngotracheal separation, can occur at the scene in patients with high-impact mechanisms. Minor laryngeal injuries may progress due to edema and expanding hematomas, and close observation is needed. A strong suspicion for cervical spine injury is appropriate. Emergent otolaryngologic consultation is warranted. In stable patients, bedside nasopharyngoscopy can evaluate airway integrity. This can be followed by spiral neck CT to delineate the extent of the injury. In unstable patients with massive laryngeal trauma, immediate tracheostomy should be performed. If this cannot be done, endotracheal intubation or fiberoptic intubation should be attempted.

For further reading in *Emergency Medicine: A Comprehensive Study Guide,* 6th ed., see Chap. 243, "Neck and Upper Airway Disorders," by Carol G. Shores.

18 | DISORDERS OF THE SKIN

| # Dermatologic Emergencies

Michael Blaivas

EXFOLIATIVE DERMATITIS

Clinical Features

Exfoliative dermatitis, a cutaneous reaction to a drug, chemical, or underlying systemic disease state, occurs when most or all of the skin is involved with a scaling erythema leading subsequently to exfoliation. The underlying mechanism is largely unknown. Etiologies responsible for exfoliative dermatitis include (in decreasing order of incidence): generalized flares of pre-existing skin disease (psoriasis, atopic and seborrheic dermatitides, lichen planus, pemphigus foliaceus, etc), contact dermatitis, malignancy, and medications or chemicals.

Patients may present with acute, acute on chronic, or chronic disease. The acute onset form is encountered most often in cases involving medications, contact allergens, or malignancy, whereas the chronic variety usually is related to an underlying cutaneous disease. Patients may complain of pain, pruritus, tightening of the skin, a chilling sensation of the skin, fever, nausea, vomiting, weight loss, and fatigue. The physical examination may show generalized warmth and erythroderma, scaling with desiccation, exfoliation of the skin, fever, and other signs of systemic toxicity. Chronic findings include dystrophic nails, thinning of body hair, alopecia, and hypo- or hyperpigmentation. Acute complicating factors include fluid and electrolyte losses, secondary infection, and excessive heat loss with hypothermia. High-output congestive heart failure (CHF) may be noted due to extensive cutaneous vasodilation in poorly compensated individuals.

Diagnosis and Differential

Diffuse erythema with desiccation or exfoliation must be considered exfoliative dermatitis until proven otherwise. The diagnosis is made with careful clinical evaluation and skin biopsy. A careful search for etiologic factors is mandatory. Dermatologic consultation is typically necessary if disease is suspected. Dermatologic syndromes to consider in the differential diagnosis include acute generalized exanthematous pustulosis, toxic epidermal necrolysis, primary blistering disorders, Kawasaki disease, the toxic infectious erythemas, and the general ichthyoses (dry skin conditions).

Emergency Department Care and Disposition

1. Management should focus on airway, breathing, and circulation support with appropriate correction of any life-threatening abnormality. After resuscitation has been completed, treatment of secondary infection, correction of electrolyte disorders, control of body temperature, and management of CHF are clinical issues to address.
2. Dermatologic treatment includes oral **antihistamines,** systemic **corticosteroids,** oatmeal baths, and bland lotions. For patients with a new presentation or a significant recurrence of exfoliative dermatitis, admission with dermatologic consultation is advised. For patients with chronic disease

747

with mild recurrence who are not systemically ill, outpatient treatment with prompt dermatologic follow-up is reasonable.

ERYTHEMA MULTIFORME

Clinical Features

Erythema multiforme (EM) is an acute inflammatory skin disease with significant associated morbidity and mortality. EM presents across a spectrum of disease, ranging from a mild papular eruption (EM minor) to the severe vesiculobullous form with mucous membrane involvement and systemic toxicity (EM major or the Stevens-Johnson syndrome) (See Color Plate in this section). EM strikes all ages, with the highest incidence in young adults (20 to 40 years), affects males twice as often as females, and occurs commonly in the spring and fall. Etiologies include infection (most commonly mycoplasma and herpes simplex), drugs (most commonly antibiotics and anticonvulsants), malignancy, rheumatologic disorders, physical agents, and pregnancy. No causal agent is identified in 50% of cases. Medications (adults) and infections (children) are the major etiologic factors.

Symptoms include malaise, arthralgias, myalgias, fever, diffuse pruritus, and a generalized burning sensation that may be noted days before skin abnormalities. Signs noted on examination primarily involve the skin and mucosal surfaces, including erythematous papules (which appear first) and maculopapules, target lesion (evolve in 24 to 48 hours), urticarial plaques, vesicles, bullae, vesiculobullous lesions, and mucosal (oral, conjunctival, respiratory, and genitourinary) erosions. Significant systemic toxicity also may be noted on initial presentation. Patients are at risk for significant fluid and electrolyte deficiencies and for secondary infection. Recurrence is noted, especially involving cases in which infection or medication is involved.

Diagnosis and Differential

The diagnosis of EM is based on the simultaneous presence of lesions with multiple morphologies at times with mucous membrane involvement. The target lesion is highly suggestive of EM. Urticarial plaques are frequently misdiagnosed as allergic reaction. The differential diagnosis includes herpetic infections, vasculitis, toxic epidermal necrolysis, primary blistering disorders, Kawasaki's disease, and toxic infectious erythemas.

Emergency Department Care and Disposition

1. Patients may present in extremis; as such, attention to the standard resuscitative therapies is required.
2. Patients with localized papular disease without systemic manifestation and mucous membrane involvement may be managed on an outpatient basis with dermatologic consultation. **Topical steroids** to noneroded skin and oral **analgesics** and **antihistamines** are recommended.
3. For patients with extensive disease or systemic toxicity, inpatient therapy in a critical care setting with immediate dermatologic consultation is advised. In addition to intensive management of potential fluid, electrolyte, infectious, nutritional, and thermoregulatory issues, parenteral analgesics and antihistamines are required. **Systemic steroids** are recommended by some authorities. **Diphenhydramine** and **lidocaine rinses** are useful

for painful oral lesions; cool **Burrow's solution** (aqueous aluminum sulfate/calcium acetate) compresses are applied to blistered regions. Ophthalmologic care is advised if any eye complaints or findings are noted.

TOXIC EPIDERMAL NECROLYSIS

Clinical Features

Toxic epidermal necrolysis (TEN) is an explosive, potentially fatal, inflammatory skin disease, striking all ages and both sexes equally. Potential etiologies include medications, chemicals, infections, and immunologic factors (See Color Plate in this section). Medications by far constitute the major etiologic group; infectious triggers are much less commonly involved as compared with EM. TEN is felt to be part of a spectrum of disease including Stevens-Johnson syndrome and EM.

Patients may complain of malaise, anorexia, myalgias, arthralgias, fever, painful skin, and upper respiratory infection symptoms; these symptoms may be present for 1 to 2 weeks before the development of skin abnormality. Physical examination findings include a warm and tender erythema, flaccid bullae, positive Nikolsky sign, erosions with exfoliation, mucous membrane (oral, conjunctival, respiratory, and genitourinary) lesions, and systemic toxicity. Nikolsky sign is positive when the superficial layers of skin slip free from the lower layers with a slight rubbing pressure; large areas of the skin will blister and peel away leaving wet, red, and painful areas. Acute and chronic complications are similar to those encountered in EM major patients. Infection, hypovolemia, and electrolyte disorders are typical causes of death, an end result in as many as 30% of cases. Predictors of poor prognosis include advanced age, extensive disease, leucopenia, azotemia, and thrombocytopenia.

Diagnosis and Differential

The diagnosis is often possible at presentation based on the clinical features. Definitive diagnosis is made via skin biopsy. The differential diagnosis includes toxic infectious erythemas, exfoliative drug eruptions, primary blistering disorders, Kawasaki disease, and EM major (Stevens-Johnson syndrome).

Emergency Department Care and Disposition

1. TEN is best cared for in a critical care setting such as a burn unit.
2. Attention to adequate cardiorespiratory function is essential; correction of fluid, electrolyte, and infectious complications are early treatment considerations. Any airway compromise should be monitored and addressed.
3. Immediate **dermatologic consultation** is required.

TOXIC INFECTIOUS ERYTHEMAS

Clinical Features

A number of infectious syndromes caused by toxigenic bacteria with toxin-mediated dermatologic manifestations have been described, including toxic shock syndrome (TSS), streptococcal toxic shock syndrome (STSS), and staphylococcal scaled skin syndrome (SSSS). TSS is a multisystem illness presenting with fever, shock, and erythroderma followed by desquamation associated with toxigenic *Staphylococcus aureus*. STSS, a syndrome caused by

Streptococcus organisms, is characterized by multiple organ system involvement, with fever, hypotension, and skin findings. Most cases of STSS are associated with soft tissue infections; cellulitis, myositis, and fascitis are the most common presenting diagnoses. SSSS develops in previously healthy children usually younger than 2 years in outbreaks and sporadic cases. The toxin exfoliatin is responsible for the erythroderma and desquamation, and the patient's immune response to the antigenic toxin results in fever and irritability.

The manifestations of TSS range from a mild, trivial disease, often misdiagnosed as a viral syndrome, to a rapidly progressive, potentially fatal, multisystem illness. Criteria for the diagnosis of TSS are defined in the case definition.

Major Criteria

1. Fever: temperature higher than 102°F
2. Rash: erythroderma (localized or diffuse) followed by peripheral desquamation
3. Mucous membrane: hyperemia of oral and vaginal mucosa and of conjunctiva
4. Hypotension: history of dizziness, orthostatic changes, or hypotension

Multisystem Manifestations

1. Central nervous system: altered mentation without focal neurologic signs
2. Cardiovascular: distributive shock, CHF, and dysrhythmias
3. Pulmonary: adult respiratory distress syndrome
4. Gastrointestinal: vomiting and diarrhea
5. Hepatic: elevations in bilirubin, alkaline phosphatase, and the transaminases
6. Renal: Serum urea nitrogen and/or creatinine elevations; abnormal urinary sediment; and oliguria
7. Hematologic: thrombocytopenia or thrombocytosis, anemia, leukopenia, or leukocytosis
8. Musculoskeletal: myalgias, arthralgias, or rhabdomyolysis
9. Metabolic: hypocalcemia and hypophosphatemia
10. Absence of other etiologic agents

The diagnosis of TSS requires the presence of all 4 major criteria and 3 or more indications of multisystem involvement. TSS is also identified by its sudden, violent onset and rapid progression to multisystem dysfunction.

The clinical presentation of STSS is similar to that of TSS; in fact, similar criteria may be used for the diagnosis. Most STSS cases have associated soft tissue infection (in contrast to TSS); an exhaustive search for the site of infection is warranted.

The presentation of SSSS can be divided into 3 phases: (*a*) erythroderma (initial), (*b*) exfoliative, and (*c*) desquamation and recovery. Initially, the sudden appearance of a tender erythroderma usually is diffuse, although localized disease is noted. The involved skin may have a sandpaper texture similar to the rash of scarlet fever. The exfoliative stage begins on the second day of the illness with a wrinkling and peeling of the previously erythematous skin; Nikolsky sign is found. Large, flaccid, fluid-filled bullae and vesicles then appear. These lesions easily rupture and are shed in large sheets; the underlying tissue resembles scalded skin and rapidly desiccates. During the exfoliative phase, the patient is often febrile and irritable. After 3 to 5 days of illness, the involved skin desquamates, leaving normal skin in 7 to 10 days.

Diagnosis and Differential

For TSS and STSS, fever and hypotension with associated erythroderma should suggest the diagnosis. The differential diagnosis is broad and includes scarlet fever, Rocky Mountain spotted fever, leptospirosis, rubeola, meningococcemia, SSSS, Kawasaki disease, TEN, Stevens-Johnson syndrome, gramnegative sepsis, and exfoliative drug eruptions. Infants and toddlers with fever and diffuse erythroderma suggest SSSS. The differential diagnosis for SSSS includes TEN, TSS, exfoliative drug eruptions, staphylococcal scarlet fever, and localized bullous impetigo.

Emergency Department Care and Disposition

1. Management of patients with TSS and STSS is dictated by the severity of the illness. If the patient presents in extremis, airway control, ventilatory status, and hemodynamic status should be addressed emergently.
2. Any potential source of infection and associated toxin should be identified and removed; **broad-spectrum antibiotic therapy** is indicated.
3. Patients must be checked for evidence of organ system dysfunction. The vast majority of patients with TSS require hospital admission; the patient who is critically ill is best managed in the intensive care setting.
4. Management of the patient with SSSS includes **fluid resuscitation,** correction of electrolyte abnormalities, and identification and treatment of the source of the toxigenic *Staphylococcus* with the appropriate anti-staphylococcal antibiotic, preferably a **penicillinase-resistant penicillin.** The newborn may be treated with topical sulfadiazine or its equivalent.

BULLOUS DISEASES

Clinical Features

Pemphigus vulgaris (PV) is a generalized, mucocutaneous, autoimmune, blistering eruption with a grave prognosis characterized by intraepidermal acantholytic blistering. Bullous pemphigoid (BP) is a generalized mucocutaneous blistering disease of the elderly, with an average age of 70 years at the time of initial diagnosis. PV and BP are characterized by the presence of unique antigen and autoantibody systems.

The primary lesions of PV are vesicles or bullae that vary in diameter from smaller than 1 cm to several centimeters, commonly first affecting the head, trunk, and mucous membranes. The blisters are usually clear and tense, originating from normal skin or atop an erythematous or urticarial plaque. Within 2 to 3 days, the bullae become turbid and flaccid, with rupture soon following, producing painful, denuded areas. These erosions are slow to heal and prone to secondary infection. Nikolsky sign is positive in PV and absent in other autoimmune blistering diseases. Mucous membranes are affected in 95% of PV patients (See Color Plate in this section).

BP is characterized by tense blisters (up to 10 cm in diameter) arising from normal skin or from erythematous or urticarial plaques; frequent sites of involvement include intertriginous and flexural areas. Ulceration with tissue loss follows blister formation. Lesions of the oral cavity occur in BP in 40% of cases, but with less consistency and severity than in PV. Involvement in the mouth is often overlooked.

Diagnosis and Differential

Diagnosis is suspected with the appearance of the blistering lesions and confirmed by skin biopsy and immunofluorescence testing. The differential diagnosis of PV and BP includes all of those diseases that can present with primary skin blistering, including TEN, EM, other autoimmune blistering diseases, burns, severe contact dermatitis, bullous diabeticorum, and friction blisters.

Emergency Department Care and Disposition

1. Patients with PV should be hospitalized with early dermatologic consultation; **high-dose parenteral** steroids and other therapies are best administered to the elderly in the hospital.
2. Blisters or eroded skin should be treated as burns with **silver sulfadiazine cream** or antibiotic ointments with clean dressings; pain originating from oral lesions may be partly relieved with soothing mouth washes (1:1 mixture of diphenhydramine elixir with Mylanta) or with viscous Lidocaine. Close observation and rapid treatment with appropriate antibiotics for superficial infection are imperative.
3. Treatment with **corticosteroids** results in the complete recovery of some PV patients and control of the disease in others if the therapy is continued. BP is also managed by systemic steroids.

MENINGOCOCCEMIA

Clinical Features

Meningococcemia is a potentially fatal infectious illness caused by *Neisseria meningitides.* It has a wide clinical spectrum, including pharyngitis, meningitis, and bacteremia. Illness typically affects patients younger than 20 years. Epidemics are seen with very virulent strains.

Infection develops 2 to 10 days after exposure and presents with severe headache, fever, altered mental status, nausea, vomiting, myalgias, arthralgia, and neck stiffness. Dermatologic manifestations include petechia, urticaria, hemorrhagic vesicles, and macules (See Color Plate in this section). Fulminant disease is seen in fewer than 5% of patients.

Diagnosis and Differential

Diagnosis relies on clinical suspicion based on presentation of an ill-appearing patient with petechial rash and associated symptoms. Cerebrospinal fluid cultures may be positive. The differential diagnosis includes Rocky Mountain spotted fever, TSS, gonococcemia, bacterial endocarditis, vasculitis, viral and bacterial infections, and disseminated intravascular coagulation.

Emergency Department Care and Disposition

1. **Ceftriaxone** 2 g intravenously and **vancomycin** 1 g intravenously should be administered empirically as soon as the disease is suspected.
2. Hospital admission is necessary.

For further reading in *Emergency Medicine: A Comprehensive Study Guide,* 6th ed., see Chap. 246, "Serious Generalized Skin Disorders," by William J. Brady, Andrew D. Perron, and Daniel J. DeBehnke.

156 | Other Dermatologic Disorders

Michael Blaivas

PHOTOSENSITIVITY

Clinical Features

Patients with *sunburn* have an inflammatory response to ultraviolet (UV) radiation and may present with minimal discomfort or extreme pain with extensive blistering. A tender, warm erythema is seen in sun-exposed areas; vesiculation may occur, representing a second-degree burn injury. *Exogenous photosensitivity* results from the topical application or the ingestion of an agent that increases the skin's sensitivity to UV light. The topical photosensitizers usually result in a cutaneous eruption at the site of application once UV light is applied. Furocoumarins such as lime juice, various fragrances, figs, celery, and parsnips when topically applied are the most common group of agents causing photo-eruptions; other topical photosensitizers include PABA esters and topical psoralens. Numerous medications also can result in eruption, which frequently involves all sun-exposed areas. The exogenous photo-eruption is similar to a severe sunburn reaction, often with blistering.

Diagnosis and Differential

Sunburn should be suspected in a patient who has frequented the outdoors with significant UV light exposure. The diagnosis of exogenous photosensitivity is based on identifying the offending agent. A linear appearance to the rash suggests an externally applied substance.

Emergency Department Care and Disposition

1. Sunburns are treated symptomatically with tepid baths, oral analgesics, and burn wound care including topical antibiotics to blistered areas.
2. Prevention is of great importance, and appropriate-strength sunscreen should be used.
3. Initial management of exogenous photosensitivity is similar to the sunburn reaction, including the avoidance of the sun until the eruption has cleared. Any causative agent should be discontinued, if possible.

CONTACT DERMATITIS

Clinical Features

Contact dermatitis may be a primary irritant reaction or an allergic-mediated event. Certain allergens may be applied to facial skin via an aerosolization or direct physical contact. Agents capable of causing an aerosolized reaction include rhus (poison ivy and oak) when the plant has been burned. Allergic contact dermatitis resulting from an aerosolized allergen presents with erythema or scaling, at times accompanied by blistering. The involvement is diffuse, with upper and lower eyelids affected. Examples of directly applied agents include nickel, nail polishes, toothpaste, preservatives in cosmetics, contact lens solutions, eyeglasses, and hair care products, among others.

Diagnosis and Differential

Direct application of the allergen produces similar findings on the most sensitive skin areas, such as the eyelids. This is in contrast to the sun-exposed areas of photosensitivity.

Emergency Department Care and Disposition

1. **Corticosteroids** (topical or oral depending on the severity) are often required. Only low-potency topical corticosteroids (hydrocortisone 2.5%) should be used on the face; cream or ointment should be used initially.
2. Extensive and severe periocular involvement requires oral **prednisone.**
3. Oral **antihistamines** are also useful in reducing pruritus.

ALOPECIA

Clinical Features

The causes of hair loss are numerous and typically are divided into scarring and nonscarring alopecia. The causative syndromes include the nonscarring (secondary syphilis, alopecia areata, contact dermatitis, thyroid disorders, or related to medication) and scarring (tinea capitis, zoster infection, discoid lupus, sarcoidosis, scleroderma, or malignancy) syndromes. *Tinea capitis* is a dermatophyte infection of the scalp and is most commonly seen in children. Areas of alopecia with broken hair shafts and peripheral scaling are noted; the alopecia is patchy and usually nonscarring. Areas of boggy, tender, indurated plaques with superficial pustules and overlying alopecia may be noted. *Alopecia areata* presents with a patchy alopecia; loose, round patches of hair are lost, leaving behind normal scalp that lacks scaling or scarring. Any hair-bearing area may be affected, but the scalp is the most common site of involvement. Alopecia areata usually resolves spontaneously within 2 to 6 months, particularly if the initial involvement is mild; extensive disease is less likely to resolve. *Telogen effluvium* is hair loss resulting from major stressors such as pregnancy, major surgery, or illness. Occurrence is delayed by 2 to 3 months after the stressor, and recovery is spontaneous.

Diagnosis and Differential

Diagnosis of tinea capitis is based on a potassium hydroxide preparation or positive fungal culture. Diagnosis of alopecia areata is based on clinical examination.

Emergency Department Care and Disposition

1. **Griseofulvin** (15 mg/kg/d divided twice daily for 6 weeks) is the first-line agent; topical treatment alone is not effective. The patient should be reevaluated after 6 weeks of treatment. **Nizoral shampoo** at least 3 times per week is recommended in addition to griseofulvin.
2. Other family members, especially children, also should be evaluated.
3. No specific therapy based in the emergency department is available for *Alopecia areata.* If the disease is extensive or rapidly progressive, dermatology referral is recommended.

Color Plates

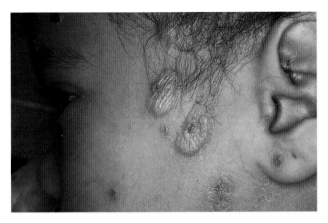

Bullous Impetigo A child with impetiginous lesions on the face. Note the formation of bullae. *(Courtesy of Anne W. Lucky, MD.)*

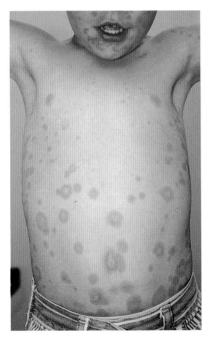

Erythema Multiforme Note the symmetric distribution of the target macules. *(Courtesy of Michael Redman, PA-C.)*

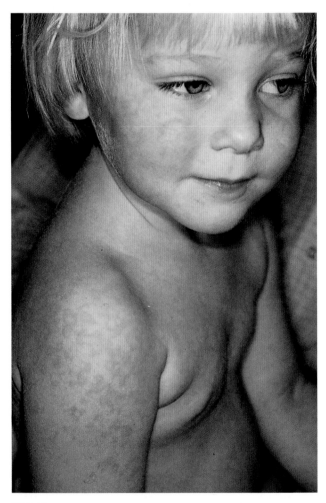

Fifth Disease Toddler with the classic slapped-cheek appearance of fifth disease caused by parvovirus B19. Also note the lacy reticular macular rash on the shoulder and upper extremity. *(Courtesy of Anne W. Lucky, MD.)*

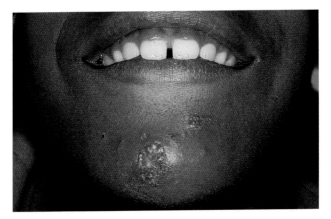

Impetigo Young girl with crusting impetiginous lesions on her chin. *(Courtesy of Michael J. Nowicki, MD.)*

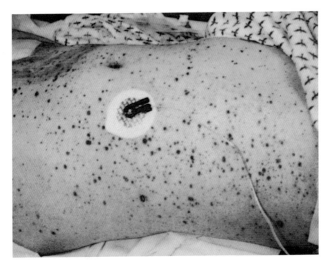

Meningococcemia Diffuse petechiae in a patient with meningococcemia. *(Courtesy of Richard Straight, MD.)*

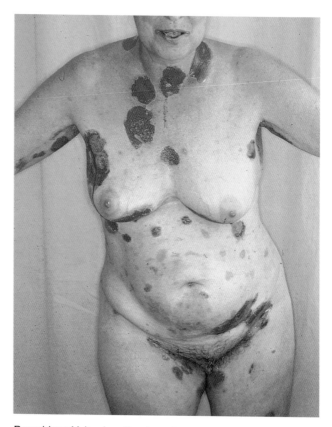

Pemphigus Vulgaris Classic vesiculobullous lesions of pemphigus vulgaris throughout the chest and abdomen. *(Courtesy of James J. Nordlund, MD.)*

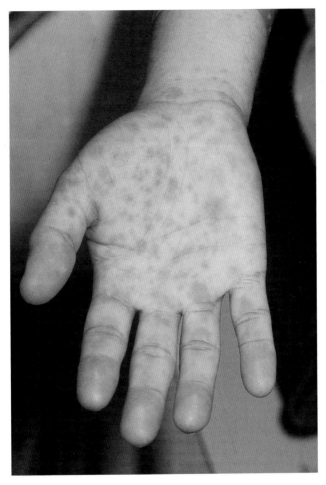

Rocky Mountain Spotted Fever   These erythematous macular lesions will evolve into a petechial rash that will spread centrally. *(Courtesy of Daniel Noltkamper, MD.)*

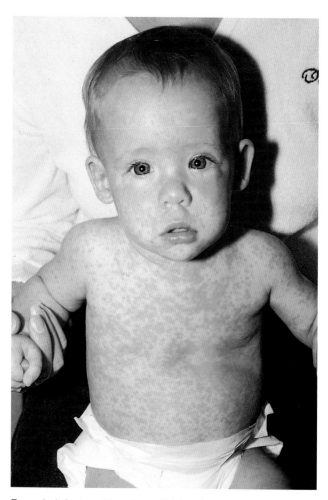

Roseola Infantum (Exanthem Subitum) Toddler with maculopapular eruption of roseola. *(Courtesy of Raymond C. Baker, MD.)*

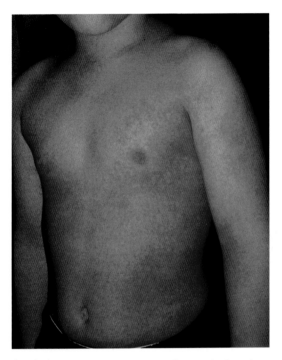

Scarlatina Erythematous scarlatiniform rash of scarlet fever. *(Courtesy of Lawrence B. Stack, MD.)*

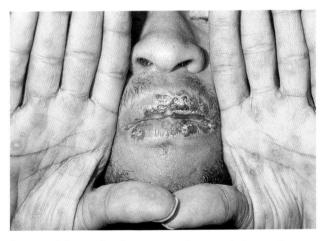

Stevens-Johnson Syndrome Note the target lesions on the hands of this patient, as well as the mucosal involvement on the lips. *(Courtesy of Alan B. Storrow, MD.)*

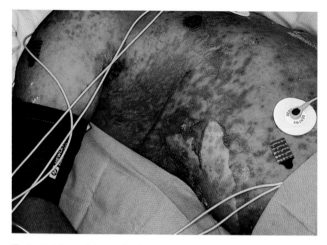

Toxic Epidermal Necrolysis The initial bullae have coalesced, leading to extensive exfoliation of the epidermis. *(Courtesy of Keith Batts, MD.)*

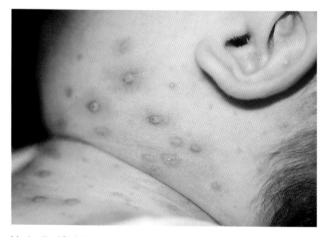

Varicella (Chickenpox) Multiple umbilicated cloudy vesicles of varicella. *(Courtesy of Lawrence B. Stack, MD.)*

TINEA INFECTIONS

Clinical Features

Tinea pedis is a fungal infection of the feet, also known as *athlete's foot.* *Tinea manuum,* a dermatophyte infection of the hand, is often unilateral and frequently associated with tinea pedis. Tinea pedis may present in several distinct forms. The most common form is the interdigital presentation manifested by maceration and scaling in the web spaces between the toes; ulcerations may be present in severe cases with secondary infection. The second type, which is the form seen in tinea manuum, is characterized by chronic, dry scaling with minimal inflammation on the palmar or plantar surfaces; it often extends to the medial and lateral aspects of the feet but not to the dorsal surface. Maceration between the toes is common. Onychomycosis may be present. The third type of fungal infection presents as an acute, painful, pruritic vesicular eruption on the palms or soles; erythema is a prominent feature, whereas the nails and web spaces are usually spared. *Tinea cruris,* a fungal infection of the groin, commonly called *jock itch,* is very common in males. Erythema with a peripheral annular, scaly edge is seen; the rash extends onto the inner thighs and the buttocks and spares the penis and scrotum, a feature that is important in distinguishing tinea cruris from other eruptions in the groin, as most other eruptions will affect the scrotum.

Diagnosis and Differential

Identification of fungal elements on a potassium hydroxide preparation or with fungal culture may be required if the diagnosis is uncertain. Typically, the diagnosis is made clinically. The differential diagnosis can include psoriasis and chronic dermatitis.

Emergency Department Care and Disposition

1. Nonbullous tinea pedis and manuum can be treated with topical antifungal agents such as **clotrimazole, miconazole, ketoconazole,** or **econazole.** Treatment should be continued for 1 week after clearing has occurred.
2. Nail infections also should be treated with oral antifungal agents (**itraconazole, fluconazole,** or **terbinafine**).
3. Bullous tinea pedis often does not respond to topical treatment; oral antifungal treatment is necessary.
4. Treatment of tinea cruris is with antifungal creams such as **clotrimazole, ketoconazole,** or **econazole** twice daily. Antifungal powders should be used on a daily basis to prevent recurrences.
5. Follow-up with a primary care physician or dermatologist is recommended.

PSORIASIS

Clinical Features

Psoriasis vulgaris presents with erythema, scales, and fissures as discrete plaques on the palms and soles. More extensive disease also can be seen. In pustular psoriasis erythema, some scaling and numerous pustules are seen on the palms and soles.

Diagnosis and Differential

The diagnosis is usually made clinically. Biopsy may be helpful. Hand and foot dermatitis, lichen simplex chronicus, and Reiter syndrome are in the differential diagnosis for vulgaris. Pustular psoriasis includes tinea pedis or manuum, dyshidrosis, *Staphylococcus aureus,* or herpes infections.

Emergency Department Care and Disposition

Topical corticosteroids, tar preparations, and lubrication are beneficial. Symptoms may be slow to respond, and referral to dermatology is recommended.

ACNEIFORM ERUPTIONS

Clinical Features

Although typical acne vulgaris is unlikely to be a presenting complaint, other similar eruptions may be seen. *Acne fulminans* is a severe form of cystic acne with ulcerating cysts and may include systemic symptoms such as fever, myalgias, arthralgia, malaise, and anorexia. *Pyoderma faciale* is an inflammatory cystic acneiform eruption on the central face. It is found mostly in women and frequently results in scarring. Dissecting cellulitis of the scalp and neck is an inflammatory scarring process seen mostly in young black males. Sinus tracts extend from suppurative nodules. *Acne keloidalis* is a perifollicular inflammatory process of the scalp. It is more common in blacks than in whites, and males predominate.

Diagnosis and Differential

The diagnosis is made clinically. Cellulitis should be considered.

Emergency Department Care and Disposition

1. Treatment of acne fulminans and pyoderma faciale includes systemic **corticosteroids** and **isotretinoin** (teratogenic).
2. Treatment for dissecting cellulitis of the scalp and acne keloidalis includes topical and systemic antibiotics, topical or oral corticosteroids, isotretinoin, and excision of the lesions.

HERPES ZOSTER INFECTION

Clinical Features

Herpes zoster results from activation of latent varicella zoster virus causing chickenpox. Pain or dysesthesia precedes the eruption by 3 to 5 days. Eruptions can occur anywhere on the body and commonly involve thoracic dermatomes. Erythematous papules progress to clusters of vesicles with an erythematous base. In 10% of cases, branches of the trigeminal nerve are involved. Lesions involving the nose should lead to significant concern for ophthalmic involvement and development of keratitis, which can lead to blindness.

Diagnosis and Differential

The differential diagnosis includes herpes simplex, impetigo, and contact dermatitis. A Tzanck prep and viral culture can confirm a diagnosis typically made on history and physical examination.

Emergency Department Care and Disposition

1. Antivirals such as **acyclovir** or **valacyclovir** are beneficial if administered within 72 hours after the eruption of the lesions.
2. Domeboro solution compresses provide symptomatic treatment.

HUMAN SCABIES

Clinical Features

Human scabies is an infestation of the skin by *Sarcoptes scabiei.* Scabies can affect anyone and is transmitted by close physical contact or linens and clothing. Scabetic mites burrow into the stratum corneum, with the time from infestation to clinical symptoms taking 3 to 4 weeks. The eruptions are very pruritic. Hands, feet, elbows, knees, umbilicus, groin, and genitals may be involved. Excoriations and pruritic papules may be the only visible clues. In crusted scabies, hyperkeratosis develops on the hands and feet, with nails frequently affected.

Diagnosis and Differential

Diagnosis is based on high clinical suspicion and positive scabies preparation. The differential diagnosis includes other bites, body lice, atopic dermatitis, neurotic excoriations, and delusions of parasitosis.

Emergency Department Care and Disposition

1. Topical scabicides are applied from the neck down to the feet. **Permethrin 5% cream** and **lindane 1% lotion** are equally effective. Lindane is neurotoxic in infants, children, and pregnant women. All household and sexual contacts should be treated.
2. Oral antihistamines and topical corticosteroids help relieve symptoms.

PEDICULOSIS

Clinical Features

Pediculosis capitis is an infestation of the hair and scalp with the mite pediculus capitis and occurs most commonly in school-age children and those attending day care. The infestation is much more common in whites than in blacks. The louse is spread via close personal contact, clothing, and bed linens. Itching can be mild or intense. Excoriation may be seen in the posterior neck and occiput. *Pediculus corporis,* body lice, is less commonly seen. It typically occurs in overcrowded conditions with poor hygiene. Bites are typically not felt by individuals, but red urticarial papules are left. Areas not covered by clothing are typically spared. *Phthirus pubis* is pubic lice and is sexually transmitted.

Diagnosis and Differential

Diagnosis of pediculosis capitis is made by visualization of lice and nits (firmly attached to hair shafts) on physical examination. Diagnosis of body and pubic lice is made on examination.

Emergency Department Care and Disposition

Permethrin 1% rinse is first-line therapy for head, body, and pubic lice. It should be applied to the scalp for 10 minutes. Fifty percent vinegar solution rinse followed by combing can remove nits. All contacts should be examined and treated as necessary.

For further reading in *Emergency Medicine: A Comprehensive Study Guide,* 6th ed., see Chap. 247, "Disorders of the Face and Scalp"; Chap. 248, "Disorders of the Hands, Feet, and Extremities"; and Chap. 250, "Infestations," by Dean Morrell and Lisa May.

19 | TRAUMA

157 | Initial Approach to the Trauma Patient

J. Christian Fox

Trauma is the leading cause of death up to the age of 44 years. All emergency physicians must be skilled in trauma resuscitation and initiating a team approach to patient management in concert with the emergency department staff and the surgeon on call.

CLINICAL FEATURES

Trauma patients sustain infinite types and combinations of injuries. Many will present with obviously abnormal vital signs, neurologic deficits, or other gross evidence of injury. These signs must prompt a thorough search for the specific underlying injuries and rapid interventions to correct the abnormalities. Nonspecific signs such as tachycardia, tachypnea, or mild alterations in consciousness must similarly be presumed to signify serious injury until proven otherwise, and these must be evaluated and treated aggressively. Further, without signs of significant trauma, the mechanism of injury may suggest potential problems, and these also should be pursued diligently.

DIAGNOSIS AND DIFFERENTIAL

The diagnosis in trauma begins with a brief history from the patient or the paramedics. Information that should be gathered includes the mechanism and sites of apparent injury, blood loss at the scene, damage to any vehicles, or descriptions of weapons involved. The primary survey (A-B-C-D-E: airway, breathing, circulation, disability, exposure), including the assessment of a complete set of vital signs, is characterized by the orderly identification and concomitant treatment of the most life-threatening injuries. First, airway patency and breathing are assessed by means of examination of the head and neck for gag reflex, pooling of secretions, airway obstruction, tracheal deviation, quality of breath sounds, flail chest, crepitation, sucking chest wounds, and fractures of the sternum. Problems such as tension pneumothorax, pneumothorax, hemothorax, and malpositioned endotracheal tube should be remedied before proceeding any further. Ensuring cervical spine immobilization in the appropriate clinical setting is a key component during the airway assessment. Circulatory status is evaluated via vital signs and cardiac monitoring. Sites of obvious bleeding, indications of shock, and signs of cardiac tamponade (Beck's triad of hypotension, jugular venous distention, and muffled heart sounds) are all identified. Intravenous (IV) access sites should be secured. The primary survey concludes with a brief neurologic examination for disability by using the Glasgow Coma Scale, pupil size and reactivity, and motor function assessment. The patient is then completely exposed to identify other injuries.

The secondary survey is a rapid but thorough head-to-toe examination to identify all injuries and to set priorities for care. Resuscitation and frequent monitoring of vital signs continue throughout this process. Evidence of significant head injury (eg, skull and facial fractures) is sought and the pupils are rechecked. The neck, chest, and abdominal examinations are completed, and

761

the stability of the pelvis is assessed. Thereafter, radiographs of the cervical spine, chest, and pelvis are obtained, as appropriate for the scenario. A gastric tube should be inserted (orally in the setting of facial fractures) to decompress the stomach and assess for hemorrhage. The genitourinary system is evaluated by external inspection and rectal examination; a urethrogram should be ordered if urethral injury (blood at the meatus or the finding of a displaced prostate) is suspected. Otherwise, a Foley catheter is placed, and the urine should be checked for blood; a pregnancy test should be ordered for female patients of childbearing age. Vaginal blood on a bimanual examination is an indication for a speculum examination. To maintain cervical spine immobilization, patients are log-rolled for a close examination of the back. Extremities are checked for soft tissue injury, fractures, and pulses. A more thorough neurologic examination is completed, with careful checking of motor and sensory function.

After the secondary survey, laboratory studies are ordered as needed. Additional radiologic studies may be ordered (eg, cystogram, IV pyelogram, aortogram) as indicated. Computed tomography (CT) of the head, chest, or abdomen should be considered. For blunt trauma patients, the focussed assessment with sonography for trauma (FAST) examination is preferred to CT to evaluate the hemodynamically unstable patient for hemoperitoneum, hemopericardium, or hemothorax. In some centers where the FAST examination is not available, a diagnostic peritoneal lavage can be performed in the unstable patient to evaluate for hemoperitoneum.

EMERGENCY DEPARTMENT CARE AND DISPOSITION

1. The emergency department management of trauma patients begins before patient arrival. A team captain and assistants with defined roles are assigned, a prehospital history is acquired, and at least 2 U of O-negative blood is obtained. Equipment for cardiac monitoring, airway management, IV fluid administration, and laboratory evaluation should be ready.

2. Airway patency is confirmed at the outset of the primary survey. A chin lift initially may help in opening the airway; suctioning may remove foreign material, blood, loose tissue, or avulsed teeth. Nasopharyngeal or oropharyngeal airways can be useful adjuncts. **Endotracheal intubation** via a rapid sequence technique is indicated for patients with altered mental status, including severe agitation, or those who for any reason are unable to maintain a patent airway on their own. Patients with evidence of intracranial injury on examination may benefit from endotracheal intubation for airway protection. In cases of extensive facial trauma or when endotracheal intubation is not possible, **cricothyrotomy** or another advanced airway technique may be used to secure the airway.

3. Patients should be administered **100% oxygen** via mask or endotracheal tube. Suspected tension pneumothorax is treated immediately with **needle decompression** followed by **tube thoracostomy.** For large hemothoraces, consideration may be given to **autotransfusion** and immediate operative exploration for initial chest tube output larger than 1,500 mL of blood. For intubated patients who are noted to have unilateral decreased or absent breath sounds, proper tube placement must be confirmed or reestablished. The presence of a flail chest may mandate endotracheal intubation to ventilate patients adequately. Sucking chest wounds require placement of an **occlusive dressing** followed by **chest tube placement.**

4. Circulation requires placement of at least 2 large-bore peripheral IV lines, with central lines initially used only if adequate peripheral access cannot be accomplished. If the patient is hypotensive, then 2 L warm crystalloid should be administered to treat shock; this may be followed by administering **O-negative** or **type-specific blood** as required. Severe external hemorrhage should be managed with **compression** at the bleeding site.

5. Bleeding from scalp lacerations should be controlled with Raney clips. Tamponade of severe epistaxis may be achieved with balloon compression devices.

6. Reduction of fractures may prevent distal neurovascular compromise; all fractures should be splinted. Open fractures should be treated with **cephalexin** 2 g IV, with consideration given to additional antibiotic coverage for particularly contaminated injuries. Patients with pelvic fractures and signs of persistent hemorrhage may benefit from **pelvic arteriography and embolization.**

7. **Tetanus prophylaxis** must be assured; an antibiotic such as **cefotetan** 2 g IV is indicated for possible ruptured abdominal viscus and vaginal or rectal lacerations.

8. Intravenous **mannitol** 0.25 to 1.0 g/kg should be considered for acute neurologic deterioration.

9. Upon completion of the secondary survey, typical options for disposition of patients are to move to the operating room, admit to the hospital, or transfer to another facility. Ideally, the trauma surgeon or surgeon on call is present for the secondary survey and can assume primary responsibility at that point. If transfer is to be made, the resuscitating physician must relay all pertinent information to the accepting physician. Advanced life-support personnel must accompany patients during transport.

For further reading in *Emergency Medicine: A Comprehensive Study Guide*, 6th ed., see Chap. 251, "Initial Approach to Trauma," by Edward E. Cornwell III.

158 | Pediatric Trauma

Charles J. Havel Jr.

Trauma is the most common cause of death in children older than 1 year. Although the priorities for the management of adult and pediatric trauma patients are similar, differences in anatomy, physiology, and psychology mandate modifications to trauma evaluation and management specific to children.

CLINICAL FEATURES

Head trauma is the most frequent injury resulting in pediatric trauma death. Overall, motor vehicle crash is the most common mechanism of injury, and it is the leading mechanism of traumatic death in children older than 1 year. Homicide accounts for up to 25% of pediatric trauma deaths, with infants 10 times more likely to die in this manner than children 5 to 9 years of age.

Emergency physicians must be aware of the manifestations and consequences of trauma unique to pediatric patients, particularly as they present during the primary survey.

Airway Airway management in children can be particularly challenging. Anatomic differences responsible for this challenge include a relatively larger tongue and more cephalad location of the larynx.

Breathing As obligate nose breathers, infants younger than 6 months with facial trauma or bleeding into the nasopharynx will demonstrate significant respiratory distress. A difference in the mechanics of breathing in children results in the early appearance of tachypnea and accessory muscle use in dyspneic patients. Nasal flaring, grunting, and retractions are other signs that should be noted in the evaluation of respiratory status.

Circulation The physiology of shock in children causes tachycardia to be the most sensitive and earliest sign of volume loss; conversely, hypotension is a late and ominous finding. Other important signs of significant blood loss are increased capillary refill time, decreased degree of responsiveness, decreased urine output, narrowed pulse pressure, and decreased skin temperature.

Disability Evaluation of infants must include assessment of the anterior fontanelle. Determination of coma scoring in younger children is performed by using formal age-specific adaptations of the classic Glasgow Coma Scale.

Exposure The ratio of surface area to mass is greater in children than in adults, thus putting them at greater risk for hypothermia after injury. It is advisable to have external warming devices such as warming lights easily available. Also, administration of warmed intravenous (IV) fluids is indicated.

DIAGNOSIS AND DIFFERENTIAL

Head Injury

"Simple" scalp injuries, particularly in younger children, may result in significant blood loss due to the high degree of vascularity of the scalp. The circulatory status of children with these injuries should be assessed carefully. In

764

the setting of head trauma, evaluating changes in mental status can be challenging due to variations in developmental age and a heightened level of anxiety commonly observed in pediatric patients. Early signs of intracranial injury also may be subtle or nonspecific in children. Up to 50% of children with parietal skull fractures and 75% with occipital fractures will have associated intracranial bleeding. Consequently, liberal use of noncontrast computed tomography (CT) is warranted.

Spine Injuries

The increased flexibility of the spine in children is responsible for the relatively lower incidence of spinal fracture in these patients. It is also responsible for the phenomenon of spinal cord injury without radiographic abnormality (SCIWORA). This entity initially may present with minimal symptoms followed by delayed progression of disability.

"Clearing the spine," especially the cervical spine, in pediatric patients by physical examination alone and without radiographs is somewhat controversial. Applying the same criteria as for adult patients can be difficult, particularly in the very young.

Chest Trauma

The relatively compliant chest wall of the child means that considerable force may be transmitted to intrathoracic structures, resulting in serious injury with a paucity of external signs. As a corollary, radiographic identification of any rib fracture carries great significance as a sensitive indicator of underlying lung injury, even if early imaging is otherwise unremarkable. Chest radiographs are therefore an essential tool in the evaluation of any child with trauma to the torso.

Abdominal and Genitourinary Trauma

The physical examination in children has been shown to be unreliable in determining the severity of injury in up to 45% of pediatric trauma patients. Advanced imaging, usually CT, is indicated in patients with a suspicious mechanism of injury, those who are symptomatic, or those with more than 20 red blood cells per high-power field on urinalysis. Identification of a pelvic fracture, particularly an anterior ring fracture, should prompt investigation for associated urethral or bladder injury.

Burns

Careful documentation of the depth and extent of injury must be performed with the recognition that the Rule of Nines may be inaccurate in estimating burn surface area in children. Carbon monoxide levels should be obtained in patients with thermal injuries sustained in closed spaces.

Nonaccidental Trauma (Child Abuse)

The possibility of abuse should be kept in mind when evaluating pediatric trauma patients, especially when the described mechanism of injury is inconsistent with the injuries sustained. Other markers for abuse include the presence of retinal hemorrhages, specific pattern injuries, and unexplained bruising or skeletal fractures in various stages of resolution or healing.

EMERGENCY DEPARTMENT CARE AND DISPOSITION

It is essential that complete, organized, and rigorous primary and secondary surveys be completed for all pediatric patients with significant mechanism of injury. Many problems identified are managed in similar fashion to those in adult patients. Several issues deserve special discussion.

1. All patients initially should be administered **100% oxygen.** Suctioning, jaw thrust or chin lift maneuvers, and placement of a nasal or an oral airway are measures to be considered.
2. In patients requiring definitive airway management, **orotracheal intubation** is the route of choice; nasotracheal intubation should be avoided due to potential swelling and injury to the nasopharynx. Choosing an appropriate endotracheal tube size is conveniently done by using the following formula:

$$\text{internal diameter (mm)} = (16 + \text{age of patient in years})/4$$

3. In children younger than 8 years, the narrowest portion of the airway is subglottic and a tube that fits through the vocal cords may not pass through this region. Patients in this age range should have an **uncuffed endotracheal tube** placed. **Rapid sequence intubation** using pretreatment with 100% oxygen, lidocaine 1.0 mg/kg IV, atropine 0.02 mg/kg IV (minimum dose, 0.1 mg; maximum dose, 1.0 mg), and appropriate sedation and pharmacologic paralysis is indicated for patients with head injuries or those who are uncontrollably combative.
4. Securing an airway in the setting of severe facial trauma is best achieved by **transtracheal catheter ventilation.** Identification of the cricothyroid membrane can be difficult, and the cricoid cartilage is easily damaged, so cricothyrotomy is not recommended in small children. If prolonged ventilation is required before surgical creation of a tracheostomy, a tracheostomy tube or shortened endotracheal tube can be placed over a guidewire by using the catheter in a Seldinger-type procedure.
5. Vascular access can be difficult in children, especially with accompanying hypotension. Early employment of **intraosseous cannulation,** particularly in young children and infants, is warranted. Resuscitative fluids should be administered in 20-mL/kg boluses of crystalloid; if there is no improvement or deterioration occurs after an initial response, 10-mL/kg boluses of packed red blood cells should be administered. Burn patients should be resuscitated according to a standard burn formula, such as the Parkland formula.
6. Neurologic injuries present special challenges given the high anxiety levels in pediatric patients. Sedation or analgesia with **morphine sulfate** and **midazolam,** each at 0.05 to 0.1 mg/kg IV (or similar agents), is appropriate after completion of the neurologic examination and may be required to facilitate imaging.
7. Aggressive treatment of hypoxia and hypotension accompanying severe head injury is integral to achieving a good outcome. Patients should be tracheally intubated, the P_{CO_2} maintained at 30 to 35 mm Hg, the head of the bed elevated to 30°, and the head and neck positioned at neutral. **Mannitol** at 0.25 to 1.0 g/kg and **furosemide** at 1.0 mg/kg IV can be used to treat cerebral edema. Posttraumatic seizures are more common in children than in adults; prophylaxis with **fosphenytoin** 18 mg/kg phenytoin equivalents (PE) may be considered.

TABLE 158-1 Indications for Transfer to a Pediatric Trauma Center

Mechanism of injury	Ejected from a motor vehicle
	Prolonged extrication
	Death of other occupant in motor vehicle
	Fall from greater distance than three times the child's height
Anatomic injury	Multiple severe trauma
	More than three long-bone fractures
	Spinal fractures or spinal cord injury
	Amputations
	Severe head or facial trauma
	Penetrating head, chest, or abdominal trauma

8. **Spinal immobilization** must be achieved in infants and younger children, with allowance for their relatively larger heads, by placement of padding behind the shoulders. For neurologic deficit attributable to blunt closed spinal cord injury, steroids should be administered within 8 hours. Dosing consists of a bolus of **methylprednisolone** 30 mg/kg IV over 15 minutes followed 45 minutes later by an IV infusion at 5.4 mg/kg/h for 48 hours.

9. Children should be hospitalized with any of the following injuries: skull fractures or evidence of intracranial injury on CT, spinal trauma, significant chest trauma, abdominal trauma with internal organ injury, or significant burns. Guidelines for referral to a pediatric trauma center are listed in Table 158-1. Social service consultation and reporting to child protective services are indicated if there is any suspicion of nonaccidental trauma (see Chap. 188).

For further reading in *Emergency Medicine: A Comprehensive Study Guide,* 6th ed., see Chap. 252, "Pediatric Trauma," by William E. Hauda II.

159 | Geriatric Trauma

O. John Ma

With the rapid growth in the size of the elderly population, the incidence of geriatric trauma is expected to increase. Emergency physicians need to stay abreast with many of the unique injury mechanisms and clinical features associated with geriatric trauma patients and apply special management principles when caring for them.

CLINICAL FEATURES

Falls are the most common cause of injury in patients older than 65 years. Syncope, which has been implicated in many cases, may be secondary to dysrhythmias, venous pooling, autonomic derangement, hypoxia, anemia, or hypoglycemia. Motor vehicle crashes rank as the most common mechanism for fatal incidents in elderly persons through age 80 years. Also, elderly pedestrians struck by a motor vehicle are much more likely to die than are younger pedestrians. Violent assaults account for 4% to 14% of trauma admissions in this age group. Just as in pediatric trauma cases, emergency physicians should have a heightened suspicion for elder or parental abuse.

Because elderly patients may have a significant medical history that affects their trauma care, obtaining a precise history is vital. Often, the time frame for obtaining information about the traumatic event, past medical history, medications, and allergies is quite short. Family members, medical records, and the patient's primary physician may be helpful in gathering information regarding the traumatic event and the patient's previous level of function. Medications, such as cardiac agents, diuretics, psychotropic agents, and anticoagulants, must be carefully listed.

On physical examination, frequent monitoring of vital signs is essential. Emergency physicians should be wary of a "normal" heart rate in the geriatric trauma victim. A normal tachycardic response to pain, hypovolemia, or anxiety may be absent or blunted in the elderly trauma patient. Medications such as β-blockers may mask tachycardia and delay appropriate resuscitation.

Special attention should be paid to anatomical variation that may make airway management more difficult. These variations include the presence of dentures, cervical arthritis, or temporomandibular joint arthritis. A thorough secondary survey is essential to uncover less serious injuries. These "minor" injuries may not be severe enough to cause problems during the initial resuscitation but cumulatively may cause significant morbidity and mortality. Seemingly stable geriatric trauma patients can deteriorate rapidly and without warning.

DIAGNOSIS AND DIFFERENTIAL

Head Injury

When evaluating the elderly patient's mental status during the neurologic examination, it would be a grave error to assume that alterations in mental status are due solely to any underlying dementia or senility. Elderly persons have a much lower incidence of epidural hematomas than do the general population; however, there is a higher incidence of subdural hematomas. More liberal indications for computed tomography (CT) are justified.

Cervical Spine Injuries

The pattern of cervical spinal injuries in the elderly is different from that in younger patients because there is an increased incidence of C1 and C2 fractures with the elderly. When the elderly trauma patient presents with neck pain, emergency physicians need to place special emphasis on maintaining cervical immobilization until the cervical spine is properly assessed. Because underlying cervical arthritis may obscure fracture lines, the elderly patient with persistent neck pain and negative plain radiographs should undergo CT of the neck.

Chest Trauma

In blunt trauma, there is an increased incidence of rib fractures due to osteoporotic changes. The pain associated with rib fractures and any decreased physiologic reserve may predispose patients to respiratory complications. More severe thoracic injuries, such as hemopneumothorax, pulmonary contusion, flail chest, and cardiac contusion, can quickly lead to decompensation in elderly individuals whose baseline oxygenation status may already be diminished. Arterial blood gas analysis may provide early insight into elderly patients' respiratory function and reserve.

Abdominal Trauma

The abdominal examination in elderly patients is notoriously unreliable as compared with that in younger patients. Even with an initially benign physical examination, emergency physicians must have a high index of suspicion for intraabdominal injuries in patients who have associated pelvic and lower rib cage fractures. For older patients, the adhesions associated with previous abdominal surgical procedures may increase the risk of performing diagnostic peritoneal lavage. Therefore, the focused assessment with sonography for trauma examination may assist in evaluating for hemoperitoneum and the need for exploratory laparotomy in hemodynamically unstable patients. For patients who are stable, CT with contrast is a valuable diagnostic test. It is important to ensure adequate hydration and baseline assessment of renal function before the contrast load for CT. Some patients such as diuretics may be volume depleted due to medications. This hypovolemia coupled with contrast administration may exacerbate any underlying renal pathology.

Orthopedic Injuries

Hip fractures occur primarily in 4 areas: intertrochanteric, transcervical, subcapital, and subtrochanteric. Intertrochanteric fractures are the most common, followed by transcervical fractures. Emergency physicians must be aware that pelvic and long bone fractures are often the sole etiology for hypovolemia in elderly patients. Timely orthopedic consultation, evaluation, and treatment with open reduction and internal fixation should be coordinated with the diagnosis and management of other injuries.

Long bone fractures of the femur, tibia, and humerus may produce a loss of mobility, with a resulting decrease in the independent lifestyle of elderly patients. Early orthopedic consultation for intramedullary rodding of these fractures may result in increased early mobilization.

The incidence of Colles fractures and humeral head and surgical neck fractures in elderly patients are increased by falls on the outstretched hand or elbow. Localized tenderness, swelling, and ecchymosis to the proximal humerus are characteristic of these injuries. Early orthopedic consultation and treatment with a shoulder immobilizer or surgical fixation should be arranged.

EMERGENCY DEPARTMENT CARE AND DISPOSITION

As in all trauma patients, the primary survey should be assessed expeditiously.

1. The main therapeutic goal is maintaining adequate oxygen delivery. **Prompt tracheal intubation** and use of mechanical ventilation should be considered in patients with more severe injuries, respiratory rates faster than 40 breaths/min, or when the Pao_2 is lower than 60 mm Hg or the $Paco_2$ is higher than 50 mm Hg. Although nonventilatory therapy helps to prevent respiratory infections and is always desirable, early mechanical ventilation may avert the disastrous results associated with hypoxia.

2. Geriatric trauma patients can decompensate with over-resuscitation just as quickly as they can with inadequate resuscitation. Elderly patients with underlying coronary artery disease and cerebrovascular disease are at a much greater risk of suffering the consequences of ischemia to vital organs when they become hypotensive after sustaining trauma. During the initial resuscitative phase, crystalloid, although the primary option, should be administered judiciously because elderly patients with diminished cardiac compliance are more susceptible to volume overload. Strong consideration should be made for early and more liberal use of **packed red blood cell transfusion.** This practice early in the resuscitation would enhance oxygen delivery and help minimize tissue ischemia.

3. **Early invasive monitoring** has been advocated to help physicians assess the elderly patient's hemodynamic status. One study found that urgent invasive monitoring provides important hemodynamic information early, aids in identifying occult shock, limits hypoperfusion, helps prevent multiple organ failure, and improves survival. Survival was improved because of enhanced oxygen delivery through the use of adequate volume loading and inotropic support.

4. If the insertion of invasive monitoring lines is impractical in the emergency department, every effort should be made by emergency physicians to expedite care of elderly trauma patients and prevent unnecessary delays. In the evaluation of blunt trauma patients, the chest radiograph, cervical spine series, and pelvic radiographs are necessary diagnostic tests during the secondary survey. Although it is vital to be thorough in the diagnosis of occult orthopedic injuries, expending a great deal of time in the radiology suite may compromise patient care. Only a few radiologic studies, such as emergent head and abdominal CT scans, should take precedence over obtaining vital information from invasive monitoring. Elderly trauma patients will benefit most from an expeditious transfer to the intensive care unit for invasive monitoring; in that setting, patients can be assessed for subtle hemodynamic changes that may compromise those with limited physiologic reserve.

5. Emergency physicians, in consultation with the trauma surgeon, should have a low threshold for having the geriatric trauma patient admitted for further evaluation and observation.

For further reading in *Emergency Medicine: A Comprehensive Study Guide,* 6th ed., see Chap. 253, "Geriatric Trauma," by O. John Ma and Stephen W. Meldon.

160 | Trauma in Pregnancy
C. Crawford Mechem

Trauma is the leading cause of nonobstetric morbidity and mortality in pregnant women. Fetal survival is highly dependent on stabilization of the mother. Successful outcomes for mother and fetus require a collaborative effort among prehospital providers, emergency physician, trauma surgeon, obstetrician, and neonatologist.

CLINICAL FEATURES

Physiologic changes of pregnancy make determination of severity of injury problematic. Heart rate increases 10 to 20 beats/min in the second trimester while systolic and diastolic blood pressures drop 10 to 15 mm Hg. Blood volume can increase 45%, but red cell mass increases to a lesser extent, leading to a physiologic anemia of pregnancy. It may be difficult to determine whether tachycardia, hypotension, or anemia is due to blood loss or normal physiologic changes. Due to the hypervolemic state, the patient may lose 30% to 35% of her blood volume before manifesting signs of shock. Pulmonary changes in pregnancy include elevation of the diaphragm and decreases in residual volume and function residual capacity. Tidal volume increases, resulting in hyperventilation with associated respiratory alkalosis. Renal compensation causes the serum pH to remain unchanged.

Anatomic changes with pregnancy affect the types of injuries seen in the mother. After 12 weeks' gestation, the enlarging uterus emerges from the pelvis and by 20 weeks reaches the level of the umbilicus. Its blood flow increases, making severe maternal hemorrhage from uterine trauma more likely. The uterus also can compress the inferior vena cava when the patient is supine, leading to the "supine hypotension syndrome." As pregnancy progresses, the small intestines are pushed cephalad, increasing their likelihood of injury in penetrating trauma to the upper abdomen. Decreased intestinal motility is associated with gastroesophageal reflux, thus predisposing the patient to vomiting and aspiration. The bladder moves into the abdomen in the third trimester, thereby increasing its susceptibility to injury. Splenic injury remains the most common cause of abdominal hemorrhage in the pregnant trauma patient.

Abdominal trauma affects the fetus and the mother. Fetal injuries are more likely to be seen in the third trimester, often associated with pelvic fractures or penetrating trauma. Uterine rupture is rare but is associated with a fetal mortality rate of close to 100%. More common complications of trauma include preterm labor and abruptio placentae. Second only to maternal death, abruptio placentae is the most common cause of fetal death. It presents with abdominal pain, vaginal bleeding, uterine contractions, and signs of disseminated intravascular coagulation. Fetal–maternal hemorrhage occurs in more than 30% of cases of significant trauma and may result in rhesus (Rh) isoimmunization of Rh-negative women.

DIAGNOSIS AND DIFFERENTIAL

Because maternal stability and survival offer the best chance for fetal well-being, no critical interventions or diagnostic procedures should be withheld

771

out of concern for potential adverse effects on the fetus. In addition to the standard trauma evaluation, special attention should be directed to the gravid abdomen, looking for evidence of injury, tenderness, or uterine contractions. If abdominal or pelvic trauma is suspected, a sterile pelvic examination is indicated, looking for genital trauma, vaginal bleeding, or ruptured amniotic membranes. Fluid with a pH of 7 in the vaginal canal suggests amniotic rupture, as does a branch-like pattern, or "ferning," on drying of vaginal fluid on a microscope slide.

Initial laboratory studies include a complete blood count, blood type, Rh status, and coagulation studies including fibrin split products and fibrinogen to determine the presence of disseminated intravascular coagulation. The ordering of radiographs adheres to the fundamental principles of trauma management. However, shielding the uterus when possible and limiting radiographs to those that will significantly affect the patient's care are prudent measures. Adverse fetal effects from radiation are negligible from doses lower than 0.1 Gy, which is an exposure far greater than that received from most trauma radiographs. Abdominal and pelvic computed tomography, pelvic angiography, and pelvic fluoroscopy result in the highest doses of radiation. In the case of computed tomography, exposure may be decreased by reducing the number of cuts obtained. Bedside ultrasonography is a highly sensitive and specific, radiation-free alternative for imaging the abdomen. In addition to evaluating fetal heart rate, ultrasonography can assess gestational age, fetal activity or demise, placental location, and amniotic fluid volume. Magnetic resonance imaging and ventilation-perfusion scanning have not been associated with adverse fetal outcome. Diagnostic peritoneal lavage remains a valid modality for evaluating the pregnant abdominal trauma patient. However, an open supraumbilical technique should be used.

Auscultation of fetal heart tones for determining fetal viability and identifying fetal distress should be performed early in the evaluation. A Doppler stethoscope or ultrasound facilitates this assessment. A normal fetal heart rate is in the range of 120 to 160 beats/min. Fetal bradycardia is most likely from hypoxia due to maternal hypotension, respiratory compromise, or placental abruption. Fetal tachycardia is most likely due to hypoxia or hypovolemia. Absence of fetal heart tones in the setting of trauma precludes fetal viability. In the setting of blunt abdominal trauma, external fetal monitoring is indicated for all patients beyond 20 weeks' gestation and is more predictive than ultrasound for abruptio placentae. Four hours is the recommended initial period of monitoring and is extended to 24 hours in case of documented uterine irritability. Beyond the viable gestational age of 23 weeks, fetal tachycardia, lack of beat-to-beat or long-term variability, or late decelerations on tocodynamometry are diagnostic of fetal distress and may be indications for emergent cesarean section.

EMERGENCY DEPARTMENT CARE AND DISPOSITION

As is the case of all trauma patients, initial priorities remain the ABCs of resuscitation directed at the mother. Care should be coordinated with surgical and obstetric consultants.

1. All pregnant trauma patients should receive supplemental **oxygen.**
2. Large-bore, peripheral intravenous lines with **crystalloid** infusions should be initiated. For patients beyond 20 weeks' gestation who must remain supine, a wedge may be placed under the right hip, tilting the patient 30°

to the left, thus reducing the likelihood of supine hypotension syndrome. Otherwise, the patient should be kept in a left lateral decubitus position whenever possible.

3. Early gastric intubation should be performed to reduce the risk of aspiration.

4. **Vasopressors** can have deleterious effects on uterine perfusion and should be avoided.

5. **Tetanus prophylaxis** is not contraindicated in pregnancy and should be administered when indicated.

6. **D immune globulin** 300 μg intramuscularly should be administered to all non-sensitized D-negative pregnant patients after abdominal trauma.

7. **Tocolytics** have a variety of side effects, including fetal and maternal tachycardia. They should be administered only in consultation with an obstetrician.

8. Indications for emergent laparotomy in the pregnant patient remain the same as those in the nonpregnant patient. In addition, emergent cesarean section has been associated with a 75% fetal survival rate when the gestational age is at or older than 26 weeks, fetal heart tones are present on admission, and the procedure is performed at the earliest sign of fetal distress. Perimortem cesarean section also has been associated with favorable fetal outcomes. It should be considered only after optimal resuscitation efforts have been initiated in patients beyond 23 weeks of pregnancy. Improved outcomes are associated with delivery within 5 minutes of maternal death.

The decision to admit or discharge a pregnant trauma patient is based on the nature and severity of the presenting injuries and is often made after consultation with surgical and obstetric consultants. Patients who display evidence of fetal distress or increased uterine irritability during initial observation should be admitted. Patients who are discharged should be instructed to seek medical attention immediately if they develop abdominal pain or cramps, vaginal bleeding, leakage of fluid, or perception of decreased fetal activity.

For further reading in *Emergency Medicine: A Comprehensive Study Guide,* 6th ed., see Chap. 254, "Trauma in Pregnancy," by Nelson Tang and Drew White.

161 | Head Injury

O. John Ma

Head injuries account for approximately one third of all trauma-related deaths in persons younger than 45 years. An initial impact injury to the brain produces different degrees of mechanical neuronal and axonal injury. Secondary brain injury occurs from potentially treatable factors such as intracranial hemorrhage and masses, cerebral edema, ischemia, hypoxia (P_{O_2} <60 mm Hg), hypotension (systolic blood pressure <90 mm Hg), anemia (hematocrit <30%), and increased intracranial pressure (ICP). Optimal emergency department (ED) management is paramount in helping to minimize secondary brain injury, thus decreasing the overall mortality and morbidity.

CLINICAL FEATURES

Traumatic brain injury (TBI) results from direct or indirect forces to the brain. Direct injury is caused by the force of an object striking the head or a penetrating injury. Indirect injuries result from acceleration and deceleration forces that result in the movement of the brain within the skull.

TBI can be classified as mild, moderate, and severe. Mild TBI includes patients with a Glasgow Coma Scale (GCS; Table 161-1) score of at least 14. Patients may be asymptomatic with only a history of head trauma or may be confused and amnestic of the event. They may have experienced brief loss of consciousness and complain of a diffuse headache, nausea, and vomiting. Patients at high risk in this subgroup include those with a skull fracture, large subgaleal swelling, focal neurologic findings, coagulopathy, age older than 60 years, or drug or alcohol intoxication.

Moderate TBI (GCS 9–13) accounts for approximately 10% of all patients with head injuries. Overall, 40% of moderate TBI patients have a positive computed tomographic (CT) scan and 8% require neurosurgical intervention. Roughly 10% of these patients will deteriorate and progress to severe TBI.

Severe TBI (GCS <9) accounts for approximately 10% of head injury patients. The mortality of severe TBI approaches 40%. The immediate clinical priority in these patients is to prevent secondary brain injury, identify other life-threatening injuries, and identify treatable neurosurgical conditions.

Out-of-hospital medical personnel often may provide critical parts of the history, including mechanism and time of injury, presence and length of unconsciousness, initial mental status, seizure activity, vomiting, verbalization, and movement of extremities. For an unresponsive patient, family and friends should be contacted to gather key information, including past medical history, medications (especially anticoagulants), and recent use of alcohol or drugs.

Clinically important features of the neurologic examination that should be addressed include assessing the mental status and GCS; pupils for size, reactivity, and anisocoria; cranial nerve function; motor, sensory, and brainstem functions; deep tendon reflexes; and noting any development of decorticate or decerebrate posturing.

Skull Fractures

Isolated, linear, nondepressed fractures with an intact scalp are common and do not require treatment. However, life-threatening intracranial hemorrhage

TABLE 161-1 The Glasgow Coma Scale for All Age Groups*

	4 y to Adult	Child <4 y	Infant
Eye opening			
4	Spontaneous	Spontaneous	Spontaneous
3	To speech	To speech	To speech
2	To pain	To pain	To pain
1	No response	No response	No response
Verbal response			
5	Alert and oriented	Oriented, social, speaks, interacts	Coos, babbles
4	Disoriented conversation	Confused speech, disoriented, consolable, aware	Irritable cry
3	Speaking but nonsensical	Inappropriate words, inconsolable, unaware	Cries to pain
2	Moans or unintelligible sounds	Incomprehensible, agitated, restless, unaware	Moans to pain
1	No response	No response	No response
Motor response			
6	Follows commands	Normal, spontaneous movements	Normal, spontaneous moves
5	Localizes pain	Localizes pain	Withdraws to touch
4	Movement or withdrawal to pain	Withdraws to pain	Withdraws to pain
3	Decorticate flexion	Decorticate flexion	Decorticate flexion
2	Decerebrate extension	Decerebrate extension	Decerebrate extension
1	No response	No response	No response
3–15			

*Glasgow Coma Scale reporting should be modified for intubated and paralyzed patients.

may result if the fracture causes disruption of the middle meningeal artery or a major dural sinus. Depressed skull fractures are classified as open or closed depending on the integrity of the overlying scalp. Although basilar skull fractures can occur at any point in the base of the skull, the typical location is in the petrous portion of the temporal bone. Findings associated with a basilar skull fracture include hemotympanum, cerebrospinal fluid otorrhea or rhinorrhea, periorbital ecchymosis ("raccoon eyes"), and retroauricular ecchymosis (Battle sign).

Brain Concussion

Concussion is a diffuse head injury usually associated with transient loss of consciousness that occurs immediately after a nonpenetrating blunt impact to the head. It generally occurs when the head, while moving, strikes or is struck by an object. The duration of unconsciousness is typically brief (seconds to minutes). Symptoms of amnesia and confusion are clinical hallmarks. Complete recovery is typical, although persistent headache and problems with memory, anxiety, insomnia, and dizziness can continue in some patients for weeks after the injury.

Brain Contusion and Intracerebral Hemorrhage

Common locations for contusions are the frontal poles, the subfrontal cortex, and the anterior temporal lobes. Contusions may occur directly under the site of impact or on the contralateral side (contrecoup lesion). The contused area is usually hemorrhagic, with surrounding edema, and occasionally associated with subarachnoid hemorrhage. Neurologic dysfunction may be profound and prolonged, with patients demonstrating mental confusion, obtundation, or coma. Focal neurologic deficits are usually present. Combination of parenchymal hemorrhage and contusion can produce an expanding mass lesion; when present in the anterior temporal lobe, uncal herniation can occur without a diffuse increase in ICP.

Traumatic Subarachnoid Hemorrhage

This condition results from the disruption of subarachnoid vessels and presents with blood in the cerebrospinal fluid. Patients may complain of diffuse headache, nausea, or photophobia. Traumatic subarachnoid hemorrhage may be the most common CT abnormality in patients with moderate or severe TBI. Some cases may be missed if the CT scan is obtained less than 6 hours after injury.

Epidural Hematoma

An epidural hematoma results from an acute collection of blood between the inner table of the skull and the dura. Approximately 80% of the time, it is associated with a skull fracture that lacerates a meningeal artery, most commonly the middle meningeal artery. Underlying injury to the brain may not necessarily be severe. In the classic scenario (20% of cases), the patient experiences loss of consciousness after a head injury. The patient may present to the ED with clear mentation, signifying the "lucid interval," and then begin to develop mental status deterioration in the ED. A fixed and dilated pupil on the side of the lesion with contralateral hemiparesis are classic late findings. The high pressure arterial bleeding of an epidural hematoma can lead to herniation within hours of injury.

Subdural Hematoma

A subdural hematoma (SDH), which is a collection of venous blood between the dura matter and the arachnoid, results from tears of the bridging veins that extend from the subarachnoid space to the dural venous sinuses. A common mechanism is sudden acceleration and deceleration. Patients with brain atrophy, such as in alcoholics or the elderly, are more susceptible to an SDH. In acute SDH, patients present within 14 days of the injury and most become symptomatic within 24 hours of injury. After 2 weeks, patients are defined as having a chronic SDH. Symptoms may range from a headache to lethargy or coma. It is important to distinguish between acute and chronic SDHs by history, physical examination, and CT scan.

Herniation

Diffusely or focally increased ICP can result in herniation of the brain at several locations. *Transtentorial (uncal) herniation* occurs when an SDH or temporal lobe mass forces the ipsilateral uncus of the temporal lobe through the tentorial hiatus into the space between the cerebral peduncle and the tentorium. This results in compression of the oculomotor nerve and parasympathetic paralysis of the ipsilateral pupil, causing it to become fixed and dilated. The cerebral peduncle is simultaneously compressed, resulting in contralateral hemiparesis. The increased ICP and brainstem compression result in progressive deterioration in the level of consciousness. Occasionally, the contralateral cerebral peduncle is forced against the free edge of the tentorium on the opposite side, resulting in paralysis ipsilateral to the lesion—a false localizing sign. The posterior cerebral artery can be compressed against the free edge of the tentorium, resulting in infarction of the occipital lobe. If the herniation continues untreated, there is progressive brainstem deterioration leading to hyperventilation, decerebration, and then to apnea and death. *Cerebellotonsillar herniation* through the foramen magnum occurs much less frequently. Resultant medullary compression causes bradycardia, respiratory arrest, and death. *Cingulate* or *subfalcial herniation* occurs when one cerebral hemisphere is displaced underneath the falx cerebri into the opposite supratentorial space. This is rarely clinically diagnosed.

Penetrating Injuries

Gunshot wounds and penetrating sharp objects can result in penetrating injury to the brain. The degree of neurologic injury will depend on the energy of the missile, whether the trajectory involves a single or multiple lobes or hemispheres of the brain, the amount of scatter of bone and metallic fragments, and whether a mass lesion is present.

DIAGNOSIS AND DIFFERENTIAL

Approximately 4% of patients with a severe TBI will have an associated cervical spine fracture. Cervical spine radiographs should be obtained on all trauma patients who present with altered mental status, midline cervical tenderness, intoxication, neurologic deficit, or severe distracting injury.

All patients with a GCS of 14 or less should undergo an emergent head CT scan without contrast after stabilization. Patients with a GCS of 15 should undergo a CT scan if they experienced loss of consciousness, nausea or vomiting, posttraumatic seizure, amnesia, continued diffuse headache, a history of coagulopathy, or intoxication without significant improvement after a period of observation. Other indications for CT include clinical neurologic deterioration during observation, presence of distracting injuries, persistent focal neurologic or mental status deficit, and skull fractures in the vicinity of the middle meningeal artery or major venous sinuses.

Routine skull radiographs are not indicated. Anteroposterior and lateral skull radiographs may be obtained for penetrating wounds of the skull or for suspected depressed skull fracture. Skull radiographs may help localize the position of a foreign body within the cranium and may determine the amount of bony depression. If CT of the head are to be obtained, bone windows can be obtained, thus eliminating the need for skull films.

Laboratory work for significant head injury patients should include type and crossmatching, complete blood count, electrolytes, glucose, arterial blood gas analysis, directed toxicologic studies, prothrombin time, partial thromboplastin time, platelets, and dissemination intravascular coagulation panel.

EMERGENCY DEPARTMENT CARE AND DISPOSITION

1. Standard protocols for evaluation and stabilization of trauma patients should be initiated (see Chap. 157). A careful search for other significant injuries should be made because up to 60% of patients with severe TBI have associated major injuries.
2. The patient should be administered **100% oxygen,** and cardiac monitoring and 2 intravenous (IV) lines should be secured. For patients with severe TBI, **endotracheal intubation** (via rapid sequence intubation) to protect the airway and prevent hypoxemia is the top priority. When properly performed, rapid sequence intubation assists in preventing increased ICP and has a low complication rate. When performing rapid sequence intubation, it is imperative to provide adequate cervical spine immobilization and use an adequate sedation or induction agent.
3. Because hypotension can lead to depressed cerebral perfusion pressure, restoration of an adequate blood pressure is vital. Resuscitation with **IV crystalloid fluid** to a mean arterial pressure (MAP) of 90 mm Hg is indicated; if hypertensive, a 25% to 30% reduction in MAP should be achieved. Once an adequate blood pressure is maintained, IV fluids should be administered cautiously to prevent cerebral edema. Hypotonic and glucose-containing solutions should be avoided.
4. Once a head CT scan demonstrating intracranial injury has been identified, immediate **neurosurgical consultation** is indicated. Patients with new neurologic deficits from an acute epidural or SDH require emergent neurosurgical consultation for definitive operative care.
5. All patients who demonstrate signs of increased ICP should have the head of the **bed elevated 30°** (provided that the patient is not hypotensive), adequate volume resuscitation to a MAP of 90 mm Hg, and maintenance of adequate arterial oxygenation. After these steps, **mannitol,** 0.25 to 1.0 g/kg IV bolus, should be administered.
6. Hyperventilation is no longer recommended as a prophylactic intervention to lower ICP because of its potential to cause cerebral ischemia. Hyperventilation should be reserved as a last resort for decreasing ICP; if used, it should be implemented as a temporary measure, and the P_{CO_2} monitored closely to maintain the range of 30 to 35 mm Hg.
7. When all other methods to control the ICP have failed, patients with signs

of impending brain herniation may need emergency decompression by trephination ("burr holes"). CT scanning before attempting trephination is recommended to localize the lesion and direct the decompression site.

8. For posttraumatic seizures, prophylactic anticonvulsants should be administered in consultation with the neurosurgeon. Seizures should be treated with **benzodiazepines,** such as lorazepam, and **fosphenytoin** at a loading dose of 18 to 20 mg/kg (phenytoin equivalents) IV.

9. Patients with a basilar skull fracture or penetrating injuries (gunshot wound or stab wound) should be admitted to the neurosurgical service and started on prophylactic (eg, ceftriaxone 1 g every 12 hours) antibiotic therapy.

10. The use of **nimodipine** (2 mg/h) in patients with traumatic subarachnoid hemorrhage reduces the likelihood of death or severe disability by 55%.

11. Patients with an initial GCS of 15 that is maintained during the observation period, normal serial neurologic examinations, and a normal CT scan may be discharged home. Those with a positive CT scan require neurosurgical consultation and admission. Patients with an initial GCS of 14 and a normal CT scan should be observed in the ED for at least 6 hours. If their GCS improves to 15 and they remain completely neurologically intact, they can be discharged home. All patients who experience a head injury should be discharged home with a reliable companion who can observe the patient for at least 24 hours, carry out appropriate discharge instructions, and follow the Head Injury sheet instructions.

For further reading in *Emergency Medicine: A Comprehensive Study Guide,* 6th ed., see Chap. 255, "Head Injury," by Thomas D. Kirsch and Christopher A. Lipinski.

Spine and Spinal Cord Injuries

Jeffrey N. Glaspy

Spinal cord injuries (SCIs) are devastating, life-changing events. They occur 4 times more frequently in men than in women. Motor vehicle crashes account for about 90% of these injuries. The most commonly injured segment of the spine is the cervical region.

CLINICAL FEATURES

Damage to the spinal cord results in 2 types of injury. The first is direct mechanical injury with resultant hemorrhage, edema, and ischemia. Within hours a secondary tissue degeneration phase begins with release of membrane destabilizing enzymes and inflammatory mediators, which induces lipid peroxidation and hydrolysis. SCIs are complete or incomplete lesions. The severity of injury determines the prognosis for recovery of function. Lesions cannot be deemed complete until spinal shock has resolved, which usually occurs over a 24- to 48-hour period.

Not all patients with SCI have neurologic deficits on initial presentation. Many unstable spinal fractures may present without spinal cord or nerve root trauma. Symptomatic patients may complain of paresthesias, dysesthesias, weakness, or other sensory disturbances with or without specific physical examination findings. More severely injured patients may have an obvious neurologic deficit on physical examination.

Patients may present with spinal shock, in which hypotension and bradycardia are the most common findings. Although hypotension in spinal shock is due to a transection of sympathetic tone, hypovolemic shock must be considered the cause of the hypotension until proven otherwise. Patients with spinal shock generally have pink, warm extremities and adequate urine output. Other signs of autonomic dysfunction may accompany spinal shock, such as gastrointestinal ileus, urinary retention, fecal incontinence, priapism, and loss of the normal ability to regulate body temperature.

DIAGNOSIS AND DIFFERENTIAL

An injury to the spine or spinal cord should be considered in any patient with a traumatic mechanism that may result in damage to these structures. The mechanism of injury is useful in determining the most likely spinal injury or SCI (Table 162-1). Any neurologic complaints, even if transitory, must raise suspicion for an SCI. Palpation of the entire spine will identify any potential areas for spinal injury. A complete neurologic examination should include motor strength and tone (corticospinal tract), pain and temperature sensations (spinothalamic tract), proprioception and vibration sensations (dorsal columns), reflexes, perianal sensation and wink, and bulbocavernosus reflex.

Patients with any 1 of the following characteristics must have radiographs taken of the traumatized portion of the spine: (*a*) midline bony spinal tenderness, crepitus, or stepoff; (*b*) physical examination findings of a neurologic deficit; (*c*) altered mental status; (*d*) presence of additional painful or distracting injuries; and (*e*) complaint of paresthesias or numbness (Table 162-2).

TABLE 162-1 Cervical Spine Injuries: Mechanism of Injury

Flexion
  Anterior subluxation (hyperflexion sprain)
  Bilateral interfacetal dislocation
  Simple wedge (compression) fracture
  Clay-shoveler's (coal-shoveler's) fracture
  Flexion teardrop fracture

Flexion–rotation
  Unilateral interfacetal dislocation

Pillar fracture
  Fracture/separation (pedicolaminar fracture)

Vertical compression
  Jefferson burst fracture of atlas
  Burst (bursting, dispersion, axial-loading) fracture

Hyperextension
  Hyperextension dislocation
  Avulsion fracture of anterior arch of atlas
  Extension teardrop fracture
  Fracture of posterior arch of atlas
  Laminar fracture
  Traumatic spondylolisthesis ("hangman's" fracture)

Lateral flexion
  Uncinate process fracture

Injuries caused by diverse or poorly understood mechanisms
  Occipitoatlantal dissociation
  Occipital condylar fractures
  Dens fractures

For the cervical spine, at least 3 radiographic views (lateral, odontoid, and anteroposterior) are necessary. These views will identify most bony injuries but cannot exclude ligamentous or occult bony injuries. A complete and systematic survey of the cervical spine radiographic series includes: (*a*) determining that all 7 cervical vertebral bodies and the superior margin of T1 are adequately visualized; (*b*) inspecting the alignment of the 4 lordotic curves: the anterior longitudinal line, the posterior longitudinal line, the spinolaminar line, and the tips of the spinous processes; (*c*) checking for any abrupt angulation greater than 11° at a single interspace; (*d*) examining for fanning of the spinous processes; (*e*) inspecting each vertebral body for fracture; (*f*) checking the atlantooccipital relation for signs of dislocation; (*g*) determining the width of the predental space: wider than 3 mm in adults or 4 mm in children

TABLE 162-2 NEXUS Criteria for Cervical Spine Radiography

According to NEXUS low-risk criteria, cervical spine radiography is indicated for trauma patients unless they exhibit *all* of the following criteria:

1. No posterior midline cervical spine tenderness
2. No evidence of intoxication
3. Normal level of alertness
4. No focal neurologic deficit
5. No painful distracting injuries

may suggest transverse ligament injury; (*h*) examining the anteroposterior diameter of the spinal canal; (*i*) inspecting the width of the prevertebral soft tissues; (*j*) checking the odontoid view for a fracture of the odontoid and inspecting the relation of the lateral masses; and (*k*) examining the antero-posterior view for alignment of the spinous processes and checking for any other sign of rotation.

Because occult fractures and ligamentous injuries may be missed on plain radiographs, clinical clearance of the cervical spine must be performed after a negative cervical spine series. To clinically clear the cervical spine, patients must have no midline tenderness in the cervical region. After painless palpation, the patient is asked to turn the head 45° to both sides and to flex the neck. If the patient experiences any pain or paresthesias during this procedure, the process should be stopped immediately and the patient should be placed back in cervical spinal immobilization. Patients with painful distracting injuries, altered mental status, or intoxication should not undergo clinical clearance of the cervical spine.

The characteristics and stability of common cervical spine fractures are summarized in Table 162-3. A Jefferson fracture is a burst fracture of C1 and usually occurs with an axial load injury. On the odontoid view, the lateral masses of C1 will be displaced. If the displacement of the lateral masses on each side added together is greater than 7 mm, rupture of the transverse ligament is likely.

Type I fractures of the odontoid include avulsions of the tip of the odontoid and is considered a stable fracture. Type II fractures occur at the junction of the odontoid and the body of C2 and are the most common odontoid fracture. Type III fractures occur through the superior portion of C2 at the base of the dens.

A hangman's fracture is located in the pedicles of C2, with anterior displacement of C2 on C3. These are caused by hyperextension injuries and are unstable fractures.

Hyperflexion injuries include anterior subluxation, clay-shoveler's fracture, simple wedge fractures, flexion teardrop fracture, and bilateral interfacetal dislocation. Unilateral facet dislocations result from flexion and rotation injuries. Extension and rotation injuries include pillar fractures and pedico-laminar fractures. Burst fractures result from vertical compression injuries and are unstable fractures. Hyperextension injuries include hyperextension dislocations, extension teardrop fractures, and laminar fractures. Uncinate process fractures result from lateral flexion injuries.

Radiographs of the thoracic and lumbar spine is the initial technique used for imaging. Discovery of a spinal injury at any level must prompt imaging of the remainder of the spine. Additional imaging modalities may be indicated for patients with positive findings on initial plain films at any level or in those in whom spinal injury is still suspected despite a negative initial radiographic evaluation. These additional modalities are flexion and extension views (of the cervical spine) for evaluation of ligamentous injury, computed tomography with or without contrast myelography, or magnetic resonance imaging.

For patients with obvious SCI, the differential diagnosis includes complete lesions and a number of incomplete lesions or syndromes. The difference between complete and incomplete lesions is crucial; prognosis for complete lesions is poor, whereas patients with incomplete lesions can be expected to have at least some degree of improvement. The characteristics of some of the more common incomplete syndromes are listed in Table 162-4. SCI without radiographic abnormality is an entity that is seen most commonly in the pediatric population. Spine injury or SCI in children should raise a suspicion for child abuse.

TABLE 162-3 Characteristics of Common Cervical Spine Fractures and Injuries Arranged in Descending Order from the Most Unstable Fractures to the Least Unstable

Type of fracture	Mechanism	Other facts	Stability
Occipitoatlantal dislocation	Skull is displaced from the cervical spine	Frequently results in death	Most unstable
Transverse ligament disruption	Diverse mechanism, possibly a blow to the occiput	Identified by examination of predental space (>3 mm)	Highly unstable
Odontoid fracture	Diverse mechanism	Classified as type I, II, or III	Depends on type of fracture
Flexion teardrop	Extreme flexion	Complete disruption of all ligamentous structures at the level of injury	Unstable
Bilateral facet dislocation	Hyperflexion	Disruption of all ligamentous structures occurs	Unstable
Burst fracture	Direct axial load	Fracture fragments may displace into spinal cord	Unstable
Hyperextension dislocation	Hyperextension	Complete tear of anterior longitudinal ligament and intervertebral disk, with disruption of posterior ligamentous complex	Unstable

(continued)

TABLE 162-3 Characteristics of Common Cervical Spine Fractures and Injuries Arranged in Descending Order from the Most Unstable Fractures to the Least Unstable (continued)

Type of fracture	Mechanism	Other facts	Stability
Hangman's fracture (traumatic spondylolisthesis of the axis)	Hyperextension	Located in pedicles of C2, with C2 displacing anteriorly on C3	Unstable
Extension teardrop	Hyperextension	Anterior longitudinal ligament avulses inferior portion of anterior vertebral body	Unstable in extension
Jefferson fracture (burst fracture of C1)	Axial load	Lateral masses of C1 are displaced on odontoid view	Likely unstable
Unilateral facet dislocation	Flexion and rotation	Anteroposterior view shows the rotation	Mechanically stable unless associated with fracture
Anterior subluxation (aka hyperflexion sprain)	Hyperflexion	Failure of posterior ligamentous structures	Potentially unstable
Simple wedge fracture	Hyperflexion	Posterior ligaments may be disrupted	Unstable if posterior element disruption occurs
Pillar fracture	Extension and rotation	Impaction of a superior vertebrae on the inferior articular mass occurs	Stable
Spinous process fracture	Hyperflexion	Intense flexion against contracted posterior erector spinal muscles	Isolated fractures are stable

TABLE 162-4 Spinal Cord Syndromes

Syndrome	Etiology	Symptoms	Prognosis
Anterior cord	Direct anterior cord compression Flexion of cervical spine Thrombosis of anterior spinal artery	Complete paralysis below the lesion with loss of pain and temperature sensation Preservation of proprioception and vibratory function	Poor
Central cord	Hyperextension injuries Disruption of blood flow to the spinal cord Cervical spinal stenosis	Quadriparesis—greater in the upper extremities than the lower extremities. Some loss of pain and temperature sensation, also greater in the upper extremities	Good
Brown-Séquard	Transverse hemisection of the spinal cord Unilateral cord compression	Ipsilateral spastic paresis, loss of proprioception and vibratory sensation and contralateral loss of pain and temperature sensation	Good
Cauda equina	Peripheral nerve injury	Variable motor and sensory loss in the lower extremities, sciatica, bowel/bladder dysfunction and "saddle anesthesia"	Good
Spinal shock	Partial or complete injury usually at the T6 level and above	Areflexia, loss of sensation, and flaccid paralysis below the level of the lesion; a flaccid bladder and loss of rectal tone; bradycardia and hypotension	Complete lesions have a poor prognosis Incomplete lesions have some degree of recovery

EMERGENCY DEPARTMENT CARE AND DISPOSITION

Blunt and penetrating injuries to the spine are treated with similar goals in mind. These goals include identification and stabilization of identified injuries and prevention of secondary injuries.

1. Airway assessment and management with **inline cervical immobilization** is the first and most pressing treatment in the emergency department. For patients with cervical spine injury (especially for injuries of C5 and above), a low threshold for endotracheal intubation should be maintained. Diaphragmatic weakness or paralysis can lead to hypoventilation or hypoxemia. The patient should be placed on **high-flow oxygen** and have 2 large-bore intravenous (IV) lines established. Fluid resuscitation facilitates spinal cord resuscitation; obvious bleeding must be controlled, and a rapid assessment of other life-threatening injuries must ensue.

2. Patients should be log-rolled (while maintaining inline spinal immobilization that prevents secondary injury to the spine and preserves residual spinal cord function) to identify any obvious fractures or associated injuries. Patients should be removed from hard backboards to prevent skin breakdown and pressure sores. A thorough neurologic examination must be performed and any abnormalities noted. Strong consideration should be given to computed tomography or ultrasonography to exclude associated abdominal injuries, especially in hypotensive patients.

3. Neurosurgical or orthopedic consultation should be obtained as soon as an injury is identified. Treatments should be initiated to promote the best possible chance for spinal cord recovery. Spinal shock should be treated with oxygen, IV fluids, and, if necessary, vasopressors, such as **norepinephrine** or **dopamine.** For blunt mechanism of SCI, **methylprednisolone** should be given. The dose is 30 mg/kg IV over 15 minutes, followed by 45 minutes with no medication, and then 5.4 mg/kg/h for 23 hours.

4. Any patient with a significant injury to the spine or spinal cord or any patient with significant associated injury should be admitted to the hospital. Further, any patient with intractable pain, nerve root injury, or intestinal ileus should be admitted. For patients who are adequately evaluated and found to have no indications for admission, discharge home with appropriate follow-up in 3 to 5 days is reasonable. These patients should be given analgesics (nonsteroidal anti-inflammatory drugs or narcotics) and given specific return precautions.

For further reading in *Emergency Medicine: A Comprehensive Study Guide,* 6th ed., see Chap. 256, "Spinal cord Injuries," by Bonny J. Baron and Thomas M. Scalea; and Chap. 272, "Injuries to the Spine," by James L. Larson Jr.

163 | Maxillofacial Trauma

C. Crawford Mechem

Despite the concern for cosmetic sequelae, the greatest complication in patients with maxillofacial trauma is airway compromise. Management requires a coordinated approach by emergency physicians and surgical specialists to ensure a favorable outcome.

CLINICAL FEATURES AND DIAGNOSIS

In patients who have sustained maxillofacial trauma, important points that should be obtained in the history include mechanism of injury, loss of consciousness, facial paresthesias, malocclusion, and visual changes, such as diplopia. Monocular diplopia suggests lens dislocation or corneal or retinal injury, whereas binocular diplopia implies dysfunction of the extraocular muscles or nerves.

The physical examination should begin with a close inspection of the face to evaluate for elongation or asymmetry. The muscles of facial expression should be assessed. Ecchymoses around the eyes (raccoon eyes) or over the mastoids (Battle sign) suggest basilar skull fracture. A posttraumatic Bell's palsy may be the result of a temporal bone fracture.

Next, the entire face should be palpated, with special attention given to bony suture lines. Subcutaneous air is pathognomonic for a sinus or nasal fracture. Simultaneous palpation of the zygomatic arches will demonstrate any asymmetry. Soft tissue tenderness may be distinguished from bony tenderness by intraoral palpation with a gloved hand.

Facial stability is assessed by grasping the maxillary arch with the mouth open. LeFort fractures are diagnosed by rocking the maxillary arch while feeling the central face for movement with the opposite hand (Fig. 163-1). In *LeFort I*, a transverse fracture separates the body of the maxilla from the lower portion of the pterygoid plate and nasal septum. With stress of the maxilla, only the hard palate and upper teeth move. A pyramidal fracture of the central maxilla and the palate defines a *LeFort II*. Facial tugging moves the nose but not the eyes. *LeFort III*, or cranial-facial disjunction, occurs when the facial skeleton separates from the skull. The entire face shifts with tugging. A *LeFort IV* fracture includes the frontal bone and the midface.

A sensory examination of the face should be performed. Anesthesia may be due to nerve contusion or bony fracture. Damage to the infraorbital nerve, often from a blowout or orbital rim fracture, may result in anesthesia of the ipsilateral upper lip, nasal mucosa at the vestibule, lower eyelid, and maxillary teeth. Lower lip and lower teeth anesthesia may occur with mandible fractures.

An eye examination should be performed, including visual acuity. If the patient is unable to see the Snellen eye chart, the ability to count fingers or perceive light should be documented. The pupils are examined for reactivity, alignment, and shape. A tear-drop shape may suggest globe rupture or penetration. A swinging-light test is performed to check for a Marcus-Gunn pupil, which initially dilates (rather than constricts) when first illuminated, indicating damage to the retina or optic nerve. The eyes are checked for hyphema, preferably with the patient in a seated position. The presence of subconjunctival hemorrhage or eyelid trauma should be noted. Penetrating trauma to the

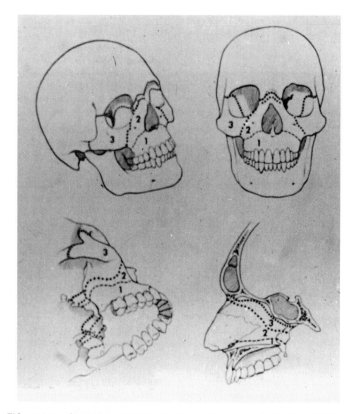

FIG. 163-1.   Schematic of midfacial fracture lines: Le Fort I, II, and III are represented by Figures 257-1, 2, and 3 respectively. [Reprinted with permission from Dingman RO, Natvig P: Surgery of Facial Fractures. Philadelphia: Saunders, 1964, p 248.]

medial third of the lids may cause damage to the lacrimal apparatus. Extraocular muscles are tested. Diplopia, especially on upward gaze, may be due to fractures of the zygomatic arch or orbital floor. Pain with extraocular motions may suggest an occult orbital fracture. The distance between the medial canthi, normally 35 to 40 mm, should be measured. Widening, or *telecanthus,* suggests serious nasoethmoidal–orbital complex trauma, as does medial canthus tenderness. Widening of the distance between the pupils, or hypertelorism, results from orbital dislocation and often is associated with blindness.

The nose should be examined for deformity, crepitus, or subcutaneous air. Septal hematoma may be observed, appearing as a bluish, bulging mass on a widened septum. Cerebrospinal fluid (CSF) rhinorrhea is suggested by clear nasal drainage mixed with blood that forms a double ring, or halo sign, when dropped on a paper towel or bed sheet. However, this finding is not specific for CSF. The ears should be examined for subperichondrial hematoma, and the canals should be inspected for lacerations, CSF leak, hemotympanum, or tympanic membrane rupture. The mouth should be inspected for lacerations, malocclusion, tooth trauma, or lip or gingival anesthesia, often due to fracture-induced nerve injury. To assess for mandibular fracture, the physician may have the patient bite down on a tongue blade and then twist the blade in an attempt to break it. A patient with a mandible fracture will open the mouth, whereas a patient with an intact mandible will break the tongue blade.

DIAGNOSIS AND DIFFERENTIAL

Diagnosis of many maxillofacial injuries is made clinically, as described in the previous section. The choice and timing of radiographs depend on the stability of the patient. Associated head, chest, and abdominal injuries take precedence. Patients who are stable, reliable, and have access to follow-up may have facial radiographs done as an outpatient. However, if compliance is in question, emergency department studies may be appropriate. Plain films are excellent as screening studies. However, facial computed tomography (CT) is frequently required to make the definitive diagnosis and guide surgical management.

EMERGENCY DEPARTMENT CARE AND DISPOSITION

1. Initial management should focus on **airway control.** A chin lift or jaw thrust without neck extension often restores airway patency. In severe mandible fractures, loss of bony support may result in posterior displacement of the tongue. To prevent airway obstruction, the tongue should be pulled forward with a gauze pad, towel clips, or a suture passed through the tip. Once the cervical spine has been cleared, the patient should be allowed to sit up and use a tonsil-tip suction catheter.

2. When **endotracheal intubation** is required, the oral route is preferred because of concern for naso-cranial intubation or severe epistaxis with the nasal route. Rapid sequence intubation carries the risk of inability to ventilate the patient if intubation is unsuccessful. Alternative strategies include awake intubation or use of sedatives, such as benzodiazepines or ketamine, at doses that minimize respiratory depression. If patients are given paralytics, equipment for emergent cricothyroidotomy should be at the bedside, and the neck should be prepped. The laryngeal mask airway may be used as a bridge to intubation or surgical airway, provided the hypopharynx remains intact.

3. Hemorrhage may be controlled with **direct pressure.** Blind clamping should be avoided because of the risk of damaging the facial nerve or parotid duct. Pharyngeal bleeding may require packing around a cuffed endotracheal tube. In LeFort fractures, bleeding may be controlled by manually realigning the fragments. Severe epistaxis requires direct pressure or nasal packing. In massive nasopharyngeal bleeding, passing a Foley catheter along the floor of the nose and inflating the balloon may be lifesaving.

CARE OF SPECIFIC FACIAL FRACTURES

Frontal Sinus and Frontal Bone Fractures

These injuries usually result from blunt trauma to the frontal bone and frequently are associated with intracranial injury. Young children have a high incidence of frontal bone injuries due to the prominence of the bone. Late complications include cranial empyema and mucopyocele. Consultation with an ear, nose, and throat specialist or neurosurgeon may be warranted. Antibiotics covering sinus pathogens should be administered; these include **first-generation cephalosporins, amoxicillin/clavulanate,** or **trimethoprim/sulfamethoxazole.** Depressed fractures or posterior wall involvement warrant admission for intravenous antibiotics. Those with isolated fractures of the anterior wall may be treated on an outpatient basis.

Nasoethmoidal-Orbital Injuries

These fractures usually result from trauma to the bridge of the nose or medial orbital wall. If the medial canthus is tender, evidence of CSF rhinorrhea should be sought. If present, a CT of the facial bones should be ordered. If a nasoethmoidal-orbital fracture is noted, a maxillofacial surgeon should be consulted.

Blowout fractures are the most common orbital fracture and occur when a blunt object strikes the globe, causing rupture of the orbital floor. Suggestive physical examination findings include enophthalmos, infraorbital anesthesia, diplopia on upward gaze, and a stepoff deformity on palpation of the infraorbital rim. If a blowout fracture is diagnosed clinically or with plain films, a CT scan should be obtained to determine the surface area of the broken floor. Indications for surgery include enophthalmos or persistent diplopia. However, this may be delayed for 1 to 2 weeks. Antibiotics covering sinus pathogens are often recommended for patients with subcutaneous emphysema. The patient is also advised to minimize nose blowing to prevent accumulation of subcutaneous air.

The oculomotor and ophthalmic divisions of the trigeminal nerve course through the superior orbital fissure. An orbital fracture involving this canal leads to the *superior orbital fissure syndrome,* which is characterized by paralysis of extraocular motions, ptosis, and periorbital anesthesia. When the orbital apex is involved, the patient may develop these symptoms and blindness. The swinging-light test and visual acuity determination are crucial in making this diagnosis. Patients with this syndrome require emergent ophthalmologic consultation.

Nasal Fractures

Cosmesis and the ability to breathe are usually the main concerns in patients with nasal fractures. Nasal films are rarely ordered because they do not change emergency department management. A septal hematoma is treated by local anesthesia with benzocaine or cocaine, followed by incision of the inferior border with a no. 11 blade, which allow it to drain. Packing the nose will prevent reaccumulation. The patient should seek follow-up in 2 to 3 days. All other patients with suspected nasal fracture should be referred for reevaluation by an ear, nose, and throat specialist in 5 to 7 days.

Zygomatic Fractures

Zygoma fractures occur in 2 major patterns, *tripod fractures* and *isolated zygomatic arch fractures.* Tripod fractures involve the infraorbital rim, diastasis of the zygomaticofrontal suture, and disruption of the zygomaticotemporal junction at the arch. Plain films are usually adequate to diagnose isolated zygomatic arch fractures, whereas a facial CT is warranted if a tripod fracture is suspected. Tripod fractures require admission for open reduction and internal fixation. Patients with isolated fractures of the zygomatic arch can have elective outpatient repair.

Maxillary Fractures

These are high-energy fractures and are often seen in victims of multisystem trauma. Patients frequently require endotracheal intubation for airway control. Visual acuity should be tested, especially with LeFort III fractures, in which the incidence of blindness is high. A CT scan of the face can be obtained in conjunction with neuroimaging. Patients with complex fractures require admission for open reduction and internal fixation.

Mandibular Fractures and Temporomandibular Dislocation

Patients with open fractures require admission and intravenous antibiotics. **Penicillin, clindamycin,** or a **first-generation cephalosporin** is recommended. Many patients with closed fractures may be managed as outpatients. A Barton bandage, an Ace bandage wrapped around the jaw and head, may be worn for comfort.

To reduce a temporomandibular dislocation, the physician stands behind the seated patient and presses downward and backward on the posterior molars or the mandibular ridge by using the thumbs wrapped in gauze. Intravenous benzodiazepines may be helpful in relieving muscle spasm. A Barton bandage is applied, and the patient is discharged on a liquid diet with close follow-up.

For further reading in Emergency Medicine: A Comprehensive Study Guide, 6th edition, see chapter 257, "Maxillofacial Trauma," by Nael Hasan and Stephen Colucciello.

164 | Neck Trauma

Walter N. Simmons

Due to the high concentration of vascular, aerodigestive, and spinal structures in the neck, any trauma to this region has the potential for significant morbidity and mortality. Patients with apparently minor neck injuries under initial inspection may experience serious complications. Vital structures at risk include the trachea, major blood vessels, a variety of neural elements including the cervical spinal cord, and the upper portion of the gastrointestinal tract.

CLINICAL FEATURES

Patients with neck trauma may demonstrate a variety of clinical presentations, ranging from asymptomatic to cardiopulmonary arrest. Blunt and penetrating laryngeal or pharyngeal trauma can cause dysphonia, stridor, hemoptysis, hematemesis, dysphagia, neck emphysema, and dyspnea progressing to respiratory arrest. It is not uncommon for an expanding hematoma in the neck to cause significant mass effect that leads to airway compromise. Patients may present with signs of shock (diaphoresis, tachycardia, and hypotension) after experiencing significant blood loss. Neurologic injury demonstrated by subjective complaints of pain and paresthesias or more objective findings of hemiplegia, quadriplegia, and coma may be observed. Significant esophageal injury initially may be associated with complaints of dysphagia and hematemesis. Strangulation may cause the presence of petechiae of the skin above the site of injury or in the subconjunctivae.

DIAGNOSIS AND DIFFERENTIAL

All patients with neck trauma should be evaluated quickly for hemodynamic stability, obvious aerodigestive injury, and violation of the platysma muscle. Probing of neck wounds in the emergency department is not indicated; full exploration should occur in the operating room, where the capacity for proximal and distal vascular control is optimal. Laboratory testing for blood type and crossmatching, complete blood cell count, and coagulation studies are indicated for all patients in whom there is even a weak suspicion for serious injury. Plain radiographs can identify cervical spine injury, the presence of any penetrating foreign body, air in the soft tissues, and soft tissue swelling. A chest radiograph is warranted for any suspected thoracic cavity penetration. Additional diagnostic procedures to be considered, in conjunction with surgical consultation, include arteriography or duplex sonography for suspected arterial injury, computed tomography (CT) of the larynx or cervical spine, endoscopy of the airway and esophagus, or contrast studies of the esophagus.

Penetrating wounds are classified by the zone of injury (Table 164-1). Stable patients with zone I injuries should undergo angiography, esophagram, and/or esophagoscopy. Those with zone III injuries should undergo angiography. Controversy surrounds the management of stable patients with zone II injuries. They may undergo immediate surgical exploration or be evaluated with angiography, esophagram, or esophagoscopy. Patients with any symptoms suggestive of laryngotracheal injury require laryngoscopy and bronchoscopy. Helical CT may be useful in stable patients to visualize the trajectory of penetrating injuries and its proximity to vital structures.

TABLE 164-1 Zones of the Neck

Zone I	Base of the neck to the cricoid cartilage
Zone II	Cricoid cartilage to the angle of the mandible
Zone III	Angle of the mandible to the base of the skull

The differential diagnosis relates to the various structures at risk for injury. Airway injury may be encountered in cases involving blunt trauma and penetrating mechanisms of injury. Vascular injury is most common with penetrating trauma, although major vessel injury can occur due to blunt trauma and may simulate an acute stroke. Neurologic injuries include generalized brain ischemia (seen primarily with strangulation), spinal cord trauma, nerve root damage, and peripheral nerve damage. Cervical spine injury initially may present without neurologic deficit, but the spine can be cleared clinically in selected blunt trauma and gunshot wound victims. The remainder of patients must have their cervical spine cleared by plain films or CT. Gastrointestinal injuries are often occult and generally require evaluation by endoscopy or contrast radiography.

EMERGENCY DEPARTMENT CARE AND DISPOSITION

1. Standard trauma protocols for evaluation and stabilization of trauma patients should be initiated (see Chap. 157). High-flow oxygen, cardiac and respiratory monitoring, and intravenous access should be quickly established.
2. Management of the airway is of the utmost concern. Any patient with acute respiratory distress, airway compromise from blood secretions, evidence of expanding hematoma on the neck, massive subcutaneous emphysema, tracheal shift, impending respiratory arrest, or severe alteration in mental status necessitates the establishment of a definitive airway. **Endotracheal intubation** is indicated for these patients. In cases in which oral or nasal intubation is not possible or is contraindicated, **cricothyrotomy or transtracheal jet insufflation** should be performed.
3. The cervical spine should be immobilized and assessed, as clinically appropriate.
4. Injuries in proximity to the base of the neck predispose patients to simultaneous injury to the chest. The chest also must be assessed for injuries such as pneumothorax and hemothorax, which are seen primarily in penetrating trauma. **Needle decompression** is performed to relieve tension pneumothorax, and **tube thoracostomy** is indicated for pneumothorax and hemothorax.
5. **Direct pressure** often can control active hemorrhage. Blind clamping of blood vessels is contraindicated due to the complex vital anatomy compressed into a relatively small space and the danger of causing further injury with a misguided surgical instrument. Fluid resuscitation should begin with crystalloid followed by blood products, if needed.
6. Minor penetrating wounds that do not violate the platysma muscle require standard, meticulous wound care and closure. These patients should be observed for several hours in the emergency department. If asymptomatic and hemodynamically stable after 4 to 6 hours, these patients may be discharged home with close follow-up.

7. Wounds that violate the platysma muscle mandate surgical consultation. These patients are admitted for surgical exploration or for further diagnostic evaluation of any significant deep structure injury.

8. Patients with blunt neck trauma initially may present with subtle signs of injury and may develop significant symptoms on a delayed basis, particularly those with a strangulation mechanism. After a period of observation, asymptomatic patients may be discharged with close follow-up, although a low threshold for admission should be maintained. Hoarseness, dysphagia, and dyspnea are indications for more extensive evaluation. Any initial symptoms of airway, vascular, or neurologic injury demand evaluation and stabilization in addition to urgent surgical consultation and admission.

For further reading in *Emergency Medicine: A Comprehensive Study Guide,* 6th ed., see Chap. 258, "Penetrating and Blunt Neck Trauma," by Bonny J. Baron.

165 | Cardiothoracic Trauma

Jeffrey N. Glaspy

Thoracic trauma accounts for 25% of civilian trauma deaths. Penetrating injuries frequently result in pneumothorax or hemothorax. Hemothorax accompanies pneumothorax in 75% of cases. Blunt trauma causes injury by several mechanisms: compression (organ rupture), direct trauma (fractures and soft tissue injuries), and acceleration and deceleration forces (vessel shear and tear).

GENERAL PRINCIPLES AND CONDITIONS

All patients should be assessed with initial consideration for airway, breathing, and circulation. Cervical spine immobilization should be maintained via inline stabilization until a spinal injury can be safely and completely excluded. In all cases of significant respiratory distress, the airway should be secured, and adequate oxygenation and ventilation should be provided. Indications for endotracheal intubation include the need to protect airway patency, failure of oxygenation or ventilation, and planned procedures necessitating intubation (general anesthesia or bronchoscopy).

The patient's breathing and oxygenation should be rapidly assessed. High-flow oxygen may help prevent secondary injury from hypoxia. Tracheal position and breath sounds should be examined. The presence of bowel sounds in the chest should suggest the possibility of a diaphragmatic injury. Inequality of breath sounds may suggest a pneumothorax, hemothorax, or an improperly placed endotracheal tube. It is essential to recognize tension pneumothorax, cardiac tamponade, flail chest, open pneumothorax, and massive hemothorax. The patient should be completely exposed. Any associated hemorrhage must be controlled and any associated injuries must be stabilized. Strong consideration must be given to associated abdominal and pelvic injuries. Life-threatening injuries must be rapidly recognized and stabilized.

If subclavian venous cannulation is required, it should be placed on the side of the injury. In patients with cardiac arrest due to chest trauma, external cardiac compression is of no value and may be harmful secondary to additional trauma to thoracic and abdominal organs or vessels. If cardiac compression is deemed potentially beneficial, emergency department (ED) thoracotomy and internal cardiac compression are warranted.

CHEST WALL INJURIES

Clinical Features and Diagnosis and Differential

Small open chest wounds (sucking chest wounds) can act as one-way valves by allowing air to enter during inspiration but none to exit during expiration. This will result in an expanding pneumothorax. These injuries should be covered immediately by a sterile petroleum gauze dressing, and a chest tube should be placed at a separate site to relieve the pneumothorax. Injuries with large amounts of chest wall tissue loss will require mechanical ventilation and surgical repair.

Patients with subcutaneous emphysema should be presumed to have a pneumothorax, even if the initial chest radiograph does not show a pneumothorax. If severe subcutaneous emphysema is palpated, then a major bronchial injury should be suspected. Clavicular fractures occasionally may injure the subclavian vein, producing a large hematoma or venous thrombosis.

Rib fractures should be assumed to be present in any patient with localized tenderness over 1 or more ribs after chest trauma. Up to 50% of rib fractures may not be apparent on initial radiographs. Fractures of the first or second ribs suggest high-force injuries and frequently are associated with other significant injuries.

Flail chest refers to segmental fractures (ie, fractures in 2 or more locations on the same rib) in 3 or more adjacent ribs. This injury is characterized by paradoxical inward movement of the involved portion of the chest wall during spontaneous inspiration and outward movement during expiration. Sternal fractures should alert the physician of possible underlying soft tissue injuries, especially to the heart or great vessels.

Emergency Department Care and Disposition

1. Bleeding from chest wall injuries is best controlled by **direct pressure.** Probing of these wounds is not recommended in the ED. If significant subcutaneous emphysema is present, a pneumothorax should be presumed to be present, and a chest tube should be inserted, especially if endotracheal intubation is imminent.
2. For rib fractures, adequate **analgesia** (with nonsteroidal anti-inflammatory drugs and narcotic analgesics) and pulmonary toilet are the mainstays of treatment. Patients with multiple rib fractures should be admitted for 24 to 48 hours if they cannot cough and clear secretions, are elderly, or have preexisting pulmonary disease. Intercostal nerve blocks, intrapleural administration of anesthetics, and epidural analgesia should be considered in patients with intractable pain.
3. The preferred treatment of flail chest injuries is analgesia to allow the patient to fully expand the underlying lung, with a goal of improving ventilation and pulmonary toilet. Indications for **ventilatory support** include 3 or more associated injuries, severe head trauma, comorbid pulmonary disease, fracture of 8 or more ribs, or age older than 65 years. Surgical repair of flail chest is controversial.
4. Patients with sternal fractures should have a screening electrocardiogram (ECG) for blunt myocardial injury.

LUNG INJURIES

Clinical Features and Diagnosis and Differential

The diagnosis of a tension pneumothorax should be made on physical examination and not by radiograph. Signs and symptoms include dyspnea, hypoperfusion, distended neck veins, decreased or absent breath sounds on the affected side, hyperresonant percussion on the affected side, and deviation of the trachea away from the affected side. Tension pneumothorax needs to be recognized and treated immediately.

Pulmonary contusions are defined as direct damage to the lung resulting in hemorrhage and edema in the absence of a pulmonary laceration. These injuries are a significant source of morbidity and mortality. Two sources of injury occur in pulmonary contusion. The first is the direct tissue injury, and the second results from fluid administration during resuscitation. The radiographic diagnosis of pulmonary contusion may be delayed for up to 6 hours.

Hemothorax should be considered in the severely traumatized patient with unilateral decreased breath sounds. Volumes of blood as low as 200 to 300 mL are usually visualized on an upright chest radiograph. However, volumes in excess of 1 L may be missed on a supine chest radiograph. If a pneumothorax is suspected but not seen on the initial chest radiograph, an expiratory chest film may facilitate diagnosis. Subcutaneous emphysema in the neck or the presence of a crunching sound (Hamman sign) over the heart during systole suggests the presence of pneumomediastinum. Although readily seen on computed tomography (CT), this diagnosis may be missed on chest radiograph. It is essential to look for injury to the larynx, trachea, major bronchi, pharynx, or esophagus.

Emergency Department Care and Disposition

1. When a tension pneumothorax is suspected, **immediate needle thoracostomy** with a 14-gauge intravenous (IV) catheter in the second intercostal space, midclavicular line is mandatory. This procedure converts a tension pneumothorax into an open pneumothorax and often significantly improves that patient's clinical condition. Lack of improvement should signal another cause of hypoperfusion. Subsequent placement of a chest tube is required.

2. The treatment of pulmonary contusions includes maintenance of adequate ventilation, pain control, and adequate pulmonary toilet. Patients with more than 25% of total lung involvement frequently require mechanical ventilation. However, **mechanical ventilation,** with the use of **positive end-expiratory pressure** may be required, even if less than 25% of the lung volume is involved.

3. If a hemothorax or nontension pneumothorax is suspected in a patient with severe respiratory distress, a **chest tube** should be inserted before obtaining a chest radiograph. **Tube thoracostomy,** with a 36- or 40-French chest tube, is the mainstay of treatment of a hemothorax. Ongoing assessment of blood loss from chest tubes is essential. Indications for **thoracotomy** include initial drainage of 1,500 mL of blood, drainage of 100 mL of blood per hour for 6 or more hours, persistent air leakage or failure of the lung to completely reexpand after tube thoracostomy, and clinical judgment of the thoracic surgeon in the face of a hemodynamically unstable patient. Chest tube drainage of occult pneumothorax (one seen on CT scan but not on plain film) is not required, unless the patient requires mechanical ventilation. A chest radiograph should be obtained in all patients after insertion of a chest tube. Persistent air leakage and failure of the lung to completely expand may indicate the need for thoracotomy. Small pneumothoraces that have not expanded on serial chest radiographs taken 6 to 12 hours apart usually do not require chest tube insertion; however, admission for serial examination is recommended.

TRACHEOBRONCHIAL INJURIES

Most injuries to major bronchi are due to deceleration shearing forces on mobile bronchi from the more fixed proximal structures, although compression against vertebral bodies or forced expiration against a closed glottis also may damage bronchi. Dyspnea, hemoptysis, subcutaneous emphysema, Hamman sign, and sternal tenderness are the most common presenting signs and symptoms, although approximately 10% are asymptomatic. On chest radiograph, a large pneumothorax, pneumomediastinum, deep cervical emphysema, or endotracheal tube balloon that appears round suggest tracheobronchial injury. Most tracheobronchial injuries occur within 2 cm of the carina or at the origin of lobar bronchi.

Management includes assuring **adequate ventilation** and referral for **immediate bronchoscopy** to evaluate and treat the injury. Injuries of the cervical trachea usually occur at the junction of the trachea and cricoid cartilage and are caused by direct trauma. Inspiratory stridor is common and indicates 70% to 80% obstruction. Orotracheal intubation, preferably over a bronchoscope, should be attempted. If gentle intubation is not possible, a formal tracheostomy should be performed.

DIAPHRAGMATIC INJURIES

Most diaphragmatic injuries are caused by penetrating trauma. The incidence of left- versus right-side diaphragmatic injuries may be equal, although left-side injuries are more commonly diagnosed, because right-side lesions may be masked due to the liver blocking herniation of abdominal contents. Evidence of intrathoracic injury from a penetrating abdominal wound should alert the physician to the likely possibility of diaphragmatic disruption. With blunt trauma, any abnormality of the diaphragm or lower lung fields on chest radiograph should arouse suspicion for diaphragmatic tear. CT and upper gastrointestinal series may diagnose less obvious diaphragmatic injuries. However, many of these injuries are diagnosed only on laparotomy or thoracotomy. The treatment of these injuries is surgical repair of the diaphragm.

PENETRATING INJURIES TO THE HEART

Clinical Features and Diagnosis and Differential

Blunt and penetrating cardiac injuries have the potential to cause cardiac tamponade. The presentation is similar to tension pneumothorax and includes the Beck triad of hypotension, distended neck veins, and muffled heart tones. Bedside ultrasonography can quickly and accurately facilitate the diagnosis of cardiac tamponade. Other causes of Beck's triad include tension pneumothorax, myocardial dysfunction, and systemic air embolism.

A hypotensive patient with penetrating chest injury anywhere near the heart should be considered to have sustained a cardiac injury until proven otherwise. Penetrating wounds to the heart are usually rapidly fatal, with fewer than 25% of patients reaching the hospital alive. Factors affecting survival include the weapon used, the size of myocardial injury, the chamber injured, coronary artery damage, the presence of tamponade, associated injuries, and the time taken to reach the hospital.

Chest radiographs are rarely helpful in diagnosing acute cardiac injury, and changes in ECG are usually nonspecific. Bedside ultrasonography and transesophageal echocardiography are rapid and sensitive modalities for diagnosing pericardial effusion. Pericardiocentesis has limited value in the evaluation of patients with possible cardiac injury due to a high incidence of false positive and false negative aspirates. Pericardiocentesis should be reserved for patients in extremis, when the possibility of tamponade must be excluded in a matter of seconds. In the hemodynamically stable patient, when echocardiography is not available, a subxiphoid pericardial window can be performed in the operating room under general anesthesia.

Emergency Department Care and Disposition

1. The initial management of patients with penetrating cardiac injury includes airway, breathing. and circulation. Two large-bore IV catheters should be placed, with one catheter in a leg vein in the event that the superior vena cava or one of its major branches is injured. Patients in shock who do not respond to adequate fluid resuscitation and who are suspected of having a cardiac injury should undergo **emergent thoracotomy.**
2. The immediate treatment of cardiac tamponade is **pericardiocentesis,** with subsequent surgical repair. An initial fluid bolus should be given to increase filling pressure in the right atrium; however, this effect is transitory, and decompression of the tamponade by pericardiocentesis or surgery will be needed.
3. A patient with penetrating thoracic trauma who loses vital signs just before arriving at the ED may require **emergent thoracotomy** to assess for and treat pericardial or cardiac wall injury.

BLUNT INJURIES TO THE HEART

Clinical Features and Diagnosis and Differential

The most common mechanism of injury causing blunt cardiac trauma is a deceleration injury, such as motor vehicle crashes (even at speeds slower than 20 mph), falls, direct blows to the chest, crush injuries, blast injuries, and athletic trauma. Blunt cardiac trauma may result in rupture of an outer chamber wall, septal rupture, valvular injuries (with the aortic valve being the most common), direct myocardial injury (contusion), laceration or thrombosis of coronary arteries, and pericardial injury. Blunt cardiac injury can be difficult to detect. A history of moderate to severe chest or upper abdominal injury, even without abnormalities on physical examination, should raise the suspicion of cardiac injury.

Blunt myocardial injury (BMI) is a term used to include myocardial contusion and myocardial concussion. The areas most commonly affected include the anterior right ventricular wall, the anterior interventricular septum, and the anterior-apical left ventricle. The most common clinical features of BMI include tachycardia out of proportion to blood loss, arrhythmias (especially premature ventricular contractions and atrial fibrillation), and conduction defects. Screening tests, such as ECG and cardiac isoenzymes, usually do not accurately indicate the severity of injury, nor are they predictive of major morbidity or mortality. Chest radiography has its greatest value in the recognition of associated injuries. A normal cardiac troponin I in a patient without other clinical findings is reasonably predictive of absence of serious BMI. Echocardiography is best reserved for patients who demonstrate cardiac dysrhythmias or dysfunction.

Emergency Department Care and Disposition

1. Although occasional patients with BMI will require treatment for heart failure or rhythm and conduction disturbances, specific treatment or intervention is rarely required. Patients should be treated with supplemental **oxygen** and given **analgesics** as needed. Nitrates should be avoided unless the patient has preexisting coronary artery disease. IV fluids and inotropic agents (dopamine or dobutamine) may be used for hypotension once cardiac tamponade has been excluded.

2. For patients with BMI, an initial ECG may identify dysrhythmias or injury patterns. If the initial ECG is normal, continuous cardiac monitoring should be performed for 4 to 6 hours. If there are no identified dysrhythmias and the patient is otherwise uninjured, then the patient may be discharged home. If the ECG is abnormal, but there is no hemodynamic instability, the patient should be admitted to a monitored setting, with repeat ECG in 12 to 24 hours.

3. Upon discharge from the hospital, patients with cardiac injury should have close follow-up to evaluate for posttraumatic pericarditis, ventricular septal defect, valvular defects, and ventricular aneurysms.

PERICARDIAL INFLAMMATION SYNDROME

Although the cause of this syndrome is unclear, pericardial inflammation syndrome should be suspected in patients who develop chest pain, fever, and pleural or pericardial effusions 2 to 4 weeks after cardiac trauma or surgery. A friction rub may be present, and ECG may show ST-segment changes consistent with pericarditis. Treatment is primarily symptomatic. with nonsteroidal anti-inflammatory agents as a first line therapy. Occasionally, glucocorticoids may be required.

PENETRATING TRAUMA TO THE GREAT VESSELS

Clinical Features and Diagnosis and Differential

Simple lacerations of the great vessels may cause exsanguination, tamponade, hemothorax, air embolism, and development of an arteriovenous fistula or false aneurysm. The size of the knife, its length, and the angle of penetration may suggest the vessels or organs most likely to be injured. Projectile missile wounds may enter a major vessel and embolize to distant locations. Assessment of bilateral upper extremity pulses should be noted, and the entire chest should be auscultated for bruits, which may represent a false aneurysm or arteriovenous fistula.

On chest radiograph, widening of the upper mediastinum may indicate injury to the brachiocephalic vessels. A "fuzzy" foreign body may indicate motion artifact caused by a foreign body within or adjacent to pulsatile vascular structures. In stable patients, CT can localize hematomas adjacent to major vascular structures. The use of contrast helps further evaluate these structures and may demonstrate a vascular defect or false aneurysm. A preoperative arteriogram will help visualize the arch of the aorta and its major branches. Water-soluble contrast swallows or endoscopy may help diagnose esophageal injuries, but these studies require a hemodynamically stable patient.

Emergency Department Care and Disposition

1. If the patient did not have "signs of life" in the field, then no resuscitative efforts are warranted; however, if the patient "lost vital signs" immediately before arriving in the ED, then **ED thoracotomy** is indicated.

2. Early **endotracheal intubation** should be performed in patients with penetrating injuries to the thoracic inlet. This approach avoids problems with expanding hematomas that may occlude the airway.

3. In patients with severe shock (systolic blood pressure <60 mm Hg), **immediate surgery** is indicated. With mild to moderate shock (systolic blood pressure 60 to 90 mm Hg), infusion of 2 to 3 L crystalloid should be rapidly administered while the need for emergent surgery is evaluated.

BLUNT TRAUMA TO THE GREAT VESSELS

Clinical Features and Diagnosis and Differential

About 80% to 90% of patients with blunt trauma to the thoracic great vessels (especially the aorta) die at the scene; 50% of the remaining patients die within 24 hours if not treated promptly.

Preexisting vascular disease (atherosclerosis or medial necrosis) does not appear to predispose patients to traumatic aortic rupture. Approximately 90% of patients with blunt aortic injuries who reach the hospital alive have their aortic injury in the isthmus, between the left subclavian artery and the ligamentum arteriosum. Other common sites of injury are the innominate or left subclavian artery at their origins or a subclavian artery over the first rib.

Most patients initially will be asymptomatic after an aortic injury. Therefore, this injury should be suspected in anyone with a sudden, severe deceleration or a high-speed impact from the side. About 33% of patients with blunt trauma to the aorta have no external evidence of thoracic injury. Physical examination findings that suggest aortic injury include an acute onset of upper extremity hypertension, difference in pulse amplitude in the upper and lower extremities, and the presence of a harsh systolic murmur over the precordium or interscapular area.

Up to 33% of patients with traumatic rupture of the aorta initially will present with a normal chest radiograph. Radiographic abnormalities associated with traumatic aortic rupture include superior mediastinal widening, deviation of the esophagus and/or trachea at T-4, obscuration of the aortic knob and/or descending aorta, displacement of the left mainstem bronchus more than 40° below horizontal, widening of the paratracheal stripe, displacement of the paraspinal lines, obscuration of the medial aspects of the left upper lobe, apical cap, and fracture of the first or second rib.

Transesophageal echocardiography is a highly sensitive diagnostic modality for evaluating traumatic aortic rupture. It also can be performed on hemodynamically unstable patients in the ED. However, due to variability of findings and operator availability, its role in the acute evaluation of aortic injury has not been defined. Newer-generation helical CT scans may offer a rapid and available diagnostic modality for traumatic aortic injury; however, angiography remains the gold standard.

Very few patients with injury to the ascending aorta survive long enough for the diagnosis to be established and the repair to be completed. If there is an associated valvular injury, a murmur of aortic insufficiency may be heard. Injuries to the descending aorta are uncommon. Descending aortic injuries present with paraplegia, mesenteric ischemia, anuria, or lower extremity ischemia.

Blunt injuries to the innominate artery are second in frequency only to rupture of the aorta at the isthmus in patients reaching the hospital alive. These injuries are associated with rib fractures, flail chest, hemopneumothorax, fractured extremities, head injuries, facial fractures, and abdominal injuries. Diminished right radial or brachial pulse is found in 50% of patients. Chest radiographic findings are similar to those for traumatic aortic disruption. CT angiography is widely used as an initial screening tool, but aortography is generally required to make the diagnosis.

Subclavian artery injuries are caused most often by fractures to the first rib or clavicle. Absence of a radial pulse on the affected side is the most important sign. A pulsatile mass or bruit at the base of the neck is suggestive of injury to the subclavian artery. Associated injury to the brachial plexus occurs in 60% of patients. Horner syndrome often indicates avulsion of nerve roots from the spinal cord. Chest radiograph may show a widened superior mediastinum without obscuration of the aortic knob.

Emergency Department Care and Disposition

1. Patients with traumatic aortic injury should not be allowed to develop a systolic blood pressure over 120 mm Hg or to perform a Valsalva maneuver. Fluid administration should be monitored carefully, and administration of sedatives, vasodilators, analgesics, and β-blockers may be required to reduce the systolic blood pressure. A nasogastric tube should be inserted cautiously to avoid gagging or coughing in the patient.
2. Although surgical repair is the accepted standard of care, aggressive medical control of blood pressure with delayed repair and prolonged observation may be alternatives to patients at high risk for surgery. Endovascular stenting may provide a less invasive approach to surgical repair.

ESOPHAGEAL AND THORACIC DUCT INJURIES

Injury to the thoracic esophagus is rare. If suspected, a swallow study with water-soluble contrast should be obtained. If this study is negative, then a follow-up barium swallow is recommended. Flexible esophagoscopy is another diagnostic study that may be considered. Immediate esophageal repair is the treatment of choice. If repair is delayed beyond 24 hours, local edema and tissue necrosis make repair unlikely. Mortalities for esophageal injury are 5% to 25% if repaired within 12 hours and 25% to 66% if treated after 24 hours. Most injuries to the thoracic duct result in chylothorax on the right side. Drainage, usually with a chest tube, is the treatment of choice. Patients also should be kept NPO (nothing by mouth).

For further reading in *Emergency Medicine: A Comprehensive Study Guide,* 6th ed., see Chap. 259, "Thoracic Trauma," by Timothy G. Buchman, Bruce L. Hall, William M. Bowling, and Gabor D. Kelen.

166 | Abdominal Trauma

O. John Ma

The primary goal in the evaluation of abdominal trauma is to promptly recognize conditions that require immediate surgical exploration. A prolonged examination to pinpoint specific injuries is potentially detrimental to the patient. The most critical mistake is to delay surgical intervention when it is needed.

CLINICAL FEATURES

Solid Visceral Injuries

Injury to the solid organs causes morbidity and mortality, primarily as a result of acute blood loss. The spleen is the most frequently injured organ in blunt abdominal trauma and is commonly associated with other intraabdominal injuries. The liver also is commonly injured in blunt and penetrating injuries. Tachycardia, hypotension, and acute abdominal tenderness are the primary physical examination findings. Kehr's sign, representing referred left shoulder pain, is a classic finding in splenic rupture. Lower left rib fractures should heighten clinical suspicion for splenic injury. Some patients with solid organ injury occasionally may present with minimal symptoms and nonspecific findings on physical examination. This is commonly associated with younger patients and those with distracting injuries, head injury, or intoxication. A single physical examination is insensitive for diagnosing abdominal injuries. Serial physical examinations on an awake, alert, and reliable patient are important for identifying intraabdominal injuries.

Hollow Visceral Injuries

These injuries produce symptoms by the combination of blood loss and peritoneal contamination. Perforation of the stomach, small bowel, or colon is accompanied by blood loss from a concomitant mesenteric injury. Gastrointestinal contamination will produce peritoneal signs over time. Patients with head injury, distracting injuries, or intoxication may not exhibit peritoneal signs initially.

Small bowel and colon injuries are most frequently the result of penetrating trauma. However, a deceleration injury can cause a bucket-handle tear of the mesentery or a blow-out injury of the antimesenteric border. Suppurative peritonitis may develop from small bowel and colonic injuries. Inflammation may take 6 to 8 hours to develop.

Retroperitoneal Injuries

The diagnosis of retroperitoneal injuries can be difficult. Signs and symptoms may be subtle or absent at initial presentation. Duodenal injuries most often are associated with high-speed vertical or horizontal decelerating trauma. These injuries may range in severity from an intramural hematoma to an extensive crush or laceration. Duodenal ruptures are usually contained within the retroperitoneum. Clinical signs of duodenal injury are often slow to develop. Patients may present with abdominal pain, fever, nausea, and vomiting, although these symptoms may take hours to become clinically obvious.

Pancreatic injury often accompanies rapid deceleration injury or a severe crush injury. The classic case is a blow to the midepigastrium from a steering wheel or the handlebar of a bicycle. Pancreatic injuries can present with subtle signs and symptoms, making the diagnosis elusive. Leakage of activated enzymes from the pancreas can produce retroperitoneal autodigestion, which may become superinfected with bacteria and produce a retroperitoneal abscess.

Diaphragmatic Injuries

Presentation of diaphragm injuries is often insidious. Only occasionally is the diagnosis obvious when bowel sounds can be auscultated in the thoracic cavity. On chest radiograph, herniation of abdominal contents into the thoracic cavity or a nasogastric tube coiled in the thorax confirms the diagnosis. In most cases, however, the only finding on chest radiograph is blurring of the diaphragm or an effusion. This injury is diagnosed most often on the left.

(Urologic injuries may occur from abdominal trauma and are discussed in Chap. 168.)

DIAGNOSIS AND DIFFERENTIAL

Plain Radiographs

For blunt abdominal trauma, routine use of plain abdominal radiographs is not a cost-effective and prudent method for evaluating the trauma patient. A chest radiograph is helpful in evaluating for herniated abdominal contents in the thoracic cavity and for evidence of free air under the diaphragm. An anteroposterior pelvis radiograph is important for identifying pelvic fractures, which can produce significant blood loss and be associated with intraabdominal visceral injury.

Diagnostic Peritoneal Lavage

Diagnostic peritoneal lavage (DPL) remains an excellent screening test for evaluating abdominal trauma. Its advantages include its sensitivity, availability, relative speed with which it can be performed, and low complication rate. Disadvantages include the potential for iatrogenic injury, its misapplication for evaluation of retroperitoneal injuries, and its lack of specificity. Laparotomy based solely on a positive DPL results in a nontherapeutic laparotomy approximately 30% of the time.

For blunt trauma, indications for DPL include (*a*) patients who are too hemodynamically unstable to leave the emergency department for computed tomography (CT) and (*b*) unexplained hypotension in patients with an equivocal physical examination.

In penetrating trauma, DPL should be performed when it is not clear that exploratory laparotomy should be performed. DPL is useful in evaluating patients sustaining stab wounds in whom local wound exploration indicates that the superficial muscle fascia has been violated. Also, it may be useful in confirming a negative physical examination when tangential or lower chest wounds are involved.

In blunt abdominal trauma, the DPL is considered positive if more than 10 mL of gross blood is aspirated immediately, the red blood cell count is higher than 100,000 cells/μL, the white blood cell count is higher than 500 cells/μL, bile is present, or if vegetable matter is present.

The only absolute contraindication to DPL is when surgical management is clearly indicated, in which case the DPL would delay patient transport to the operating room. Relative contraindications include patients with advanced hepatic dysfunction, severe coagulopathies, previous abdominal surgeries, or a gravid uterus.

Ultrasonography

The focused assessment with sonography for trauma (FAST) examination, like DPL, is an accurate screening tool for abdominal trauma. The underlying premise behind the use of the FAST examination is that clinically significant injuries will be associated with the presence of free fluid accumulating in dependent areas. Advantages of the FAST examination are that it is accurate, rapid, noninvasive, repeatable, portable, and involves no contrast material or radiation exposure to the patient. There is limited risk for patients who are pregnant, coagulopathic, or have had previous abdominal surgery. The FAST examination can be performed in less than 4.0 minutes. One major advantage of the FAST examination is the ability to evaluate for free pericardial and pleural fluid.

Disadvantages include the inability to determine the exact etiology of the free intraperitoneal fluid and the operator-dependent nature of the examination. Other disadvantages of the FAST examination are the difficulty in interpreting the views in patients who are obese or have subcutaneous air or excessive bowel gas and the inability to distinguish intraperitoneal hemorrhage from ascites. The FAST examination also cannot evaluate the retroperitoneum as well as CT scanning.

Computed Tomography

Abdominal CT has a greater specificity than do DPL and ultrasonography, thus making it the initial diagnostic test of choice at most trauma centers. Oral and intravenous (IV) contrast material should be given to provide optimal resolution.

Advantages of CT include its ability to precisely locate intraabdominal lesions preoperatively, to evaluate the retroperitoneum, and to identify injuries that may be managed nonoperatively and its noninvasiveness. The disadvantages of CT are its expense, time required to perform the study, need to transport the trauma patient to the radiology suite, and the need for contrast materials.

EMERGENCY DEPARTMENT CARE AND DISPOSITION

1. Standard protocols for evaluation and stabilization of trauma patients should be initiated (see Chap. 157).
2. Patients should be administered **100% oxygen** and have cardiac monitoring and 2 large-bore IV lines secured.
3. For hypotensive abdominal trauma patients, resuscitation with **IV crystalloid fluid** is indicated. **Transfusion with O-negative or type-specific packed red blood cells** should be considered in addition to crystalloid resuscitation.
4. Laboratory work for patients with abdominal trauma should be based on the mechanism of injury (blunt vs penetrating); it may include type and crossmatching, complete blood count, electrolytes, arterial blood gas,

TABLE 166-1 Indications for Laparotomy

	Blunt		Penetrating
Absolute	Anterior abdominal injury and hypotension Abdominal wall disruption Peritonitis Free air on chest x-ray CT-diagnosed injury requiring surgery (eg, pancreatic transection, duodenal rupture	Absolute	Injury to abdomen, back, and flank with hypotension Abdominal tenderness Gastrointestinal evisceration Positive DPL High suspicion for transabdominal trajectory (GSW) CT-diagnosed injury requiring surgery (eg, ureter or pancreas)
Relative	Positive DPL or FAST in stable patient Solid visceral injury in stable patient Hemoperitoneum on CT without clear source	Relative	Positive local wound exploration (SW)

Key: CT = computed tomography, DPL = diagnostic peritoneal lavage, FAST = focused assessment with sonography for trauma, GSW = gunshot wound, SW = stab wound.

directed toxicologic studies, prothrombin time, partial thromboplastin time, platelets, hepatic enzymes, and lipase.

5. Table 166-1 lists the indications for exploratory laparotomy. When a patient presents to the emergency department with an obvious high-velocity gunshot wound to the abdomen, DPL or the FAST examination should not be performed because it will only delay transport of the patient to the operating room. If organ evisceration is present, it should be covered with a moist, sterile dressing before surgery.

6. For an equivocal stab wound to the abdomen, surgical consultation for local wound exploration is indicated. If the wound exploration demonstrates no violation of the anterior fascia, the patient can be discharged home safely.

7. For the hemodynamically stable, blunt trauma patient with a positive FAST examination, further evaluation with CT may be warranted before admission to the surgical service.

For further reading in *Emergency Medicine: A Comprehensive Study Guide,* 6th ed., see Chap. 260, "Abdominal Injuries," by Thomas M. Scalea and Sharon Boswell.

167 | Penetrating Trauma to the Flank and Buttock

Robert A. Schwab

Penetrating trauma to the flank and buttock present a diagnostic challenge to the emergency physician due to the potential for retroperitoneal injuries and injuries to intraperitoneal organs, vessels, and nerves. Management priorities include resuscitation, identification of the need for immediate laparotomy, and use of diagnostic modalities to identify occult injuries.

PENETRATING TRAUMA TO THE FLANK

Clinical Features

The organs most commonly injured by penetrating trauma to the flank include the liver, kidney, colon, duodenum, and pancreas. Presentations may be dramatic, with hemodynamic instability and frank shock, but more commonly the patient will present with stable vital signs and a relatively innocuous-appearing injury. Key historical features include the mechanism of injury and type of weapon, time since injury, postinjury symptoms, in particular hematemesis, and general medical history. Physical examination should begin with inspection for evidence of exsanguinating hemorrhage, evisceration, or frank peritoneal signs. Perfusion of the lower extremities should be assessed. Digital rectal examination can identify occult bowel injuries if intraluminal bleeding is significant. Auscultation of the lung fields may help identify thoracic or diaphragmatic injuries.

Diagnosis and Differential

Wound exploration should be reserved for apparently superficial stab wounds in a hemodynamically stable patient. Exploration of injuries extending through fascia or muscle is not recommended. Useful diagnostic adjuncts include chest radiography, which can demonstrate free intraperitoneal air or pneumothorax, and plain abdominal or pelvic films, which can assist in determining the missile pathway and can detect fractures. Diagnostic peritoneal lavage and bedside ultrasonography can detect intraperitoneal bleeding with a high degree of accuracy. None of these diagnostic modalities can detect retroperitoneal injuries; therefore, the most useful diagnostic modality in penetrating injuries to the flank is computed tomography (CT). Performed with oral, intravenous, and rectal contrast media, CT is highly sensitive and specific for the detection of intraperitoneal and retroperitoneal injuries.

Useful laboratory assessments include a complete blood count, coagulation studies, type and crossmatch, liver function studies, amylase and lipase, and urinalysis.

Emergency Department Care and Disposition

1. Standard resuscitation principles apply; patients should receive 2 large-bore intravenous (IV) lines, supplemental oxygen, cardiac monitoring, and nasogastric tube insertion. A urinary catheter should be placed unless there

807

is high suspicion of urethral injury. Surgical consultation should be obtained immediately.

2. After resuscitation, the emergency physician's next priority is to identify indications for immediate operative intervention. These indications include hemodynamic instability, signs of peritonitis, evisceration, gross blood on rectal examination, and gunshot wound with a transpelvic or transperitoneal pathway.

3. If no immediate indication for laparotomy is found, CT should be used to determine the need for operation and to detect occult injuries. Free intraperitoneal air or major organ, vessel, or nerve injury identified by imaging may require operation, but good outcomes with decreased morbidity are achieved through the use of selective management with early CT scanning.

4. Broad-spectrum antibiotics (eg, Zosyn 3.375 g IV) should be administered for suspected gastrointestinal (GI) tract injuries. Tetanus immunization should be given according to guidelines.

5. All patients should be admitted for observation with the exception of those sustaining very superficial stab wounds whose diagnostic evaluation shows no significant injury. Safe discharge requires a reliable patient and family without transportation or language barriers to impede follow-up care. Reevaluation within 48 hours is mandatory.

PENETRATING TRAUMA TO THE BUTTOCK

Clinical Features

Injuries to the GI and genitourinary tracts are of greatest concern for this mechanism of trauma, but injuries to pelvic bony and vascular structures can lead to significant morbidity, as can injuries to major nerves (sciatic and femoral). Key historical features include the mechanism of injury and type of weapon, time since injury, postinjury symptoms, in particular hematuria or hematochezia, and general medical history. Physical examination should be directed toward detection of evisceration, exsanguinating hemorrhage, or peritonitis followed by careful assessment for genitourinary or rectal injuries. Inspection of the urethral meatus and genitalia followed by digital rectal examination is mandatory. Genitourinary trauma can present with hematuria and scrotal or penile hematomas. Pelvic stability should be assessed by palpation, and distal extremity perfusion should be ensured.

Diagnosis and Differential

Wound exploration of injuries extending through fascia or muscle is not recommended. Useful diagnostic adjuncts include plain abdominal or pelvic films, which can assist in determining missile pathway and can detect fractures. Proctosigmoidoscopy should be performed for penetrating buttock injuries; bleeding or other evidence of injury is an indication for operative management. The most useful imaging modality in penetrating injuries to the buttock is CT, which is highly sensitive and specific for the detection of intraperitoneal and retroperitoneal injuries.

Useful laboratory assessments include a complete blood count, coagulation studies, type and crossmatch, liver function studies, amylase and lipase, and urinalysis.

Emergency Department Care and Disposition

1. Standard resuscitation principles apply; patients should receive 2 large-bore IV lines, supplemental oxygen, cardiac monitoring, and nasogastric tube insertion. A urinary catheter should be inserted after careful evaluation for urethral injury. Surgical consultation should be obtained immediately.

2. After resuscitation, the emergency physician's next priority is to identify indications for immediate operative intervention. These indications include hemodynamic instability, signs of peritonitis, evisceration, gross blood on rectal examination, gunshot wound with a transpelvic or transperitoneal pathway, or a gunshot wound with an entrance wound above the level of the greater trochanters.

3. If no immediate indication for laparotomy is found, CT should be used to determine the need for operation and to detect occult injuries. Broad-spectrum antibiotics (eg, Zosyn 3.375 g IV) should be administered for suspected GI tract injuries. Tetanus immunization should be given according to guidelines.

4. All patients should be admitted for observation with the exception of those sustaining very superficial stab wounds whose diagnostic evaluation shows no significant injury. Safe discharge requires a reliable patient and family without transportation or language barriers to impede follow-up care. Reevaluation within 48 hours is mandatory.

For further reading in *Emergency Medicine: A Comprehensive Study Guide,* 6th ed., see Chap. 261, "Penetrating Trauma to the Flank and Buttock," by Alasdair K. T. Conn.

168 | Genitourinary Trauma

C. Crawford Mechem

Injuries to the genitourinary system occur in 2% to 5% of adult trauma patients, usually in the setting of blunt trauma. Although rarely life threatening, they often are associated with more serious injuries and require prompt and thorough management.

CLINICAL FEATURES

The history and physical examination should raise suspicion for genitourinary injuries. Patients with any abdominal trauma, including penetrating trauma in the vicinity of genitourinary structures, are at risk. High-velocity deceleration predisposes to renal pedicle injuries, including lacerations and thromboses of the renal artery and vein. Fractures of the lower ribs or lower thoracic or lumbar vertebrae often are associated with renal or ureteral injuries, and pelvic fractures and straddle injuries are associated with urethral or bladder trauma.

Because genitourinary trauma is rarely life threatening, the initial evaluation should focus on more emergent injuries. However, during the secondary survey, a careful abdominal and genitourinary examination should be performed. Flank ecchymoses, tenderness, or masses suggest renal injuries. The perineum should be inspected for blood or lacerations, which may denote an open pelvic fracture. The presence of a penile, scrotal, or perineal hematoma or blood at the penile meatus suggests urethral injury. If blood at the meatus is present, then no attempt at inserting a urethral catheter should be made due to the concern for converting a partial urethral laceration into a complete transection. A rectal examination should be performed, assessing sphincter tone, checking for blood, and determining the position of the prostate. A high-riding prostate or one that feels boggy suggests injury to the membranous urethra. In men, the scrotum should be examined for ecchymoses, lacerations, or testicular disruption. In women, the vaginal introitus should be inspected for lacerations and hematomas, which often are associated with pelvic fractures. If there is evidence of injury in this area, or if injury is suspected, a bimanual examination should be performed. If blood is present, a speculum examination is warranted to check for vaginal lacerations.

DIAGNOSIS AND DIFFERENTIAL

The approach to evaluation depends on whether the mechanism of injury is blunt or penetrating, the patient's age and hemodynamic stability, whether there is hematuria, and if so, whether it is gross or microscopic. Microscopic hematuria is defined as more than 5 red blood cells per high-power field. This is based on a 10-mL urine specimen centrifuged for 5 minutes at 2000 rpm. In general, blood at the urethral meatus should be excluded, and the urine should be evaluated for hematuria before passage of a urinary catheter is considered. If placement of a catheter is urgent and injury to the urethra has not been excluded, then the suprapubic approach may be used.

Analysis of the first-voided urine may help localize the injury. Initial hematuria suggests injury to the urethra or prostate, whereas terminal hematuria is associated with bladder neck trauma. Continuous hematuria is often due to injury to the bladder, ureter, or kidney. In blunt trauma, the degree of hematuria does not correlate with severity of injury. However, in hemodynamically stable patients, isolated microscopic hematuria rarely represents significant injury. Exceptions to this include associated transient hypotension, a rapid deceleration mechanism that may cause renal pedicle or vascular injury, or pediatric cases. In stable children, injury is unlikely if the urine contains fewer than 50 red blood cells per high-power field.

The choice of imaging study will be dictated by the hemodynamic status of the patient and suspicion for associated injuries (Table 168-1). Blunt trauma patients who have sustained a rapid deceleration mechanism, demonstrated hemodynamic instability, have gross hematuria, or demonstrated microscopic hematuria with associated injuries should undergo abdominal computed tomography (CT). This modality has the advantage of simultaneously imaging other organs. CT, however, should be performed only on hemodynamically stable patients. Patients who are unstable should undergo a one-shot intravenous pyelogram (IVP) in the emergency department or operating room. If the patient's systolic blood pressure is 70 mm Hg or lower, dye-induced nephrotoxicity may result. An IVP also can be used in stable patients if CT is unavailable, but the resolution may be poor. IVP remains the mainstay of diagnosing ureteral injuries, which is identified by extravasation of contrast dye. In many centers, spiral CT scanners are also being used for this purpose and have the advantage of visualizing the entire retroperitoneal space.

In penetrating trauma, there is no correlation between degree of hematuria and severity of injury. Therefore, penetrating trauma patients with the potential for genitourinary injury should be imaged by CT or IVP, depending on their stability, before exploratory laparotomy.

Cystography is commonly used to diagnose suspected bladder injuries. It is performed by instilling contrast medium retrogradely into the bladder and looking for extravasation, preferably under fluoroscopy. Urethral injuries also are investigated by retrograde cystography. A non-lubricated urinary catheter is passed 2 to 3 cm into the distal urethra, the balloon is inflated with 1 to 3 mL water, and 20 to 30 mL contrast material is injected. An oblique film is obtained, looking for extravasation. Urethral injuries should

TABLE 168-1 Selection of Diagnostic Imaging for Suspected Renal System Injury

Imaging study	Suspected injury
Retrograde urethrogram or cystogram	Urethral injury
CT (with IV contrast)	Renal injury (staging) Ureteral injury
Cystogram, plain film (retrograde)	Bladder injury
CT cystogram (retrograde)	Bladder injury
"One-shot" IVP	Unstable patients taken to operating room
IVP	Alternative to CT in unstable patients Ureteral injury
Angiogram or venogram	Pedicle injuries, venous disruption
Retrograde pyelogram	Renal pelvis disruption

Key: IVP = intravenous pyelogram.

not be investigated in the case of pelvic trauma until it is certain that pelvic angiography or embolization is not required.

EMERGENCY DEPARTMENT CARE AND DISPOSITION

Standard protocols for evaluation and stabilization of trauma patients should be initiated (see Chap. 157). Emphasis should be placed on identifying life-threatening injuries. Patients with isolated microscopic hematuria and no other injuries may be discharged with repeat urinalysis in 1 to 2 weeks.

MANAGEMENT OF SPECIFIC INJURIES

Kidney

Contusions account for more than 90% of renal injuries, with renal lacerations, pedicle injuries, and shattered kidneys making up the rest. Renal contusions and lacerations not involving the collecting system are usually managed nonoperatively. In the absence of other injuries, these patients may be discharged with repeat urinalysis in 1 to 2 weeks. Patients with pedicle injuries or lacerations involving the collecting system should be admitted. Many of these patients have associated injuries requiring surgical repair. In the case of isolated injury, however, patients may be managed nonoperatively with frequent reassessment. They should be put at bedrest, kept well hydrated, and have frequent hematocrit determinations and frequent urinalyses to assess degree of hematuria. Patients with shattered kidneys require operative repair, as do any patients with uncontrolled renal hemorrhage, multiple kidney lacerations, renal vascular injuries, a pulsatile or expanding hematoma on abdominal exploration, or penetrating injuries.

Ureter

Ureteral injuries are the rarest of the genitourinary injuries and usually result from penetrating trauma. If the ureter is completely transected, hematuria may be absent. Ureter injuries should be managed operatively.

Bladder

Bladder contusions are treated expectantly. Incomplete bladder lacerations may be managed by catheter placement and observation. Bladder rupture is intra- or extraperitoneal. Intraperitoneal rupture usually results from a burst injury of a full bladder and is managed operatively. Extraperitoneal rupture often is associated with a pelvic ring fracture. Symptoms include abdominal pain and tenderness, hematuria, and inability to void. Management involves urethral catheter drainage alone. Penetrating bladder injuries are managed operatively.

Urethra

Urethral injuries in males involve the posterior (prostatomembranous) urethra and the anterior (bulbous and penile) urethra. Posterior injuries are associated with pelvic fractures. Anterior injuries result from direct trauma or instrumentation. In females, urethral injuries are often associated with pelvic fractures and commonly present with vaginal bleeding. Anterior contusions are managed conservatively, with or without a urethral catheter. Partial anterior urethral lacerations are managed with an indwelling catheter or with suprapubic cystotomy. Complete lacerations are repaired with end-to-end anastomosis. Partial lacerations of the posterior urethra are managed with urethral or suprapubic drainage. Complete lacerations are managed surgically or with suprapubic drainage alone.

Testicles and Scrotum

Blunt testicular injuries consist of contusions or rupture. Testicular ultrasound can help to determine the type and extent of injury. Contusions may be managed conservatively with nonsteroidal anti-inflammatory drugs, ice, elevation, scrotal support, and urologic follow-up. Testicular rupture or penetrating trauma requires operative repair to improve outcome. Scrotal skin avulsion is managed by housing the testicle in the remaining scrotal skin, which usually will return to normal size in several months.

Penis

Injuries range from small contusions to degloving injuries or amputations. Lacerations and amputations require operative debridement and reconstruction or reimplantation. A fractured penis, due to traumatic rupture of the corpus cavernosum, is managed by immediate surgical drainage of blood clot and repair of the torn tunica albuginea and any associated urethral injuries. Penile skin avulsion is managed with split-thickness skin grafting after debridement. Zipper injury to the penis results when the penile skin is trapped in the trouser zipper. Mineral oil and lidocaine infiltration are useful in freeing the penile skin from the zipper. Otherwise, wire-cutting or bone-cutting pliers are used to cut the median bar (diamond) of the zipper, thus causing the zipper to fall apart. Contusions to the perineum or penis are treated conservatively with cold packs, rest, and elevation. If the patient is unable to void, catheter drainage may be required.

For further reading in *Emergency Medicine: A Comprehensive Study Guide,* 6th ed., see Chap. 262, "Genitourinary Trauma," by Frederick Levy and Gabor D. Kelen.

Emergency physicians play a crucial role in caring for patients who have sustained penetrating extremity injuries through prompt recognition of arterial, nerve, soft tissue, and bony injuries; initiation of treatment crucial to limb rescue; and early consultation with appropriate surgical specialists.

CLINICAL FEATURES

After the initial trauma evaluation and resuscitation are complete, a careful history should be obtained, including the type of weapon used. The patient should be asked about past medical history and any history of vascular disease or neuromuscular deficits. A thorough physical examination should be performed to determine the presence of injuries warranting immediate operative repair and which diagnostic studies may be needed.

The size and shape of wounds or soft tissue injuries should be noted, and any obvious bony deformity should be examined carefully. The extremity should be checked for evidence of compartment syndrome. Wounds near or overlying joints should be assessed for penetration of the joint capsule. Vascular integrity of the affected extremity should be evaluated by assessing distal pulses, which can be compared with those on the unaffected side. The color, temperature, and capillary refill of the involved extremity may be indicators of subtle vascular injury.

The presence of "hard signs" of arterial injury should be determined; these include absent or diminished distal pulses, obvious arterial bleeding, large expanding or pulsatile hematoma, audible bruit, palpable thrill, or distal ischemia. Distal ischemia is suggested by pain, pallor, paralysis, paresthesias, and coolness. "Soft signs" of arterial injury also should be sought. These are the presence of a small and stable hematoma, injury to an anatomically related nerve, unexplained hypotension, history of hemorrhage no longer present, proximity of injury to major vessels, or a complex fracture. A final component of the clinical assessment of the injured extremity is a careful neuromuscular examination investigating for evidence of motor or sensory deficits.

DIAGNOSIS AND DIFFERENTIAL

Diagnostic tests that can assist the emergency physician in evaluating penetrating extremity wounds include ankle brachial indices (ABIs) and radiologic studies. Measurement of ABIs objectively verifies diminished extremity pulses noted on physical examination. Doppler devices are used to measure ABI to a diagnostic accuracy of up to 95%. However, the sensitivity and specificity vary depending on whether an abnormal ratio is set at 0.9 or at 1.0. In addition, ABIs do not reliably detect nonocclusive arterial injuries such as intimal flaps and pseudoaneurysms.

ABIs are performed by placing the patient in a supine position and measuring the systolic blood pressure in all 4 extremities. To measure an ankle systolic pressure, a standard adult blood pressure cuff is wrapped around the ankle just above the malleoli. The cuff is inflated to approximately 30 mm Hg above the systolic pressure, and the Doppler flowmeter is used to detect the systolic pressure over the anterior tibial artery just distal to the blood pressure cuff as it is slowly deflated. The systolic blood pressure is also measured in both upper extremities using the Doppler device. The ABI measurement is then calculated by dividing the ankle systolic pressure by the greater of the 2 upper extremity pressures. An ABI measurement greater than 1.0 is normal. An ABI measurement between 0.5 and 0.9 is indicative of injury to a single artery segment, whereas an ABI measurement less than 0.5 indicates severe arterial injury or injury to multiple arterial segments. A difference of greater than 20 mm Hg between upper extremity systolic pressures indicates upper extremity arterial injury. Underlying medical conditions, such as preexisting peripheral vascular disease or severe hypothermia, can affect the accuracy of ABI measurement.

Plain radiographs, including anteroposterior and lateral views, of the involved extremity should be obtained when fractures or retained foreign bodies are a possibility. The joints above and below the injury should be included. In the cases of shotgun wounds, the extremity distal to the wound should be imaged because of the risk of embolized shot pellets. Computed tomography may be required to detect fractures and to determine whether intraarticular fractures, fragments, or foreign bodies are present.

Arteriography can be used to delineate the extent, nature, and location of vascular injuries in special situations such as shotgun wounds, multiple or severe fractures, chronic vascular disease, thoracic outlet wounds, or extensive soft tissue injury. It has become the gold standard in the evaluation of patients with wounds in proximity to major neurovascular bundles.

EMERGENCY DEPARTMENT CARE AND DISPOSITION

1. Once the patient's airway, breathing, and circulatory status are assessed and stabilized, attention can be directed to the extremity injury. The general principles of wound management, including tetanus prophylaxis, apply. There is no proven role for prophylactic antibiotics unless the wound is contaminated or the patient has an underlying immunocompromising condition.
2. Although present in fewer than 6% of cases, hard signs of arterial injury require surgical evaluation and arteriography or immediate exploration in the operating room. Soft signs of vascular injury require inpatient observation.
3. Wound exploration in the emergency department is reserved for those patients with suspected foreign bodies in the wound, for ligamentous involvement, or for control of minor venous bleeding.
4. Patients with evidence of compartment syndrome, nerve injuries, or orthopedic injuries should be evaluated by the appropriate surgical subspecialist.
5. Patients with no signs of vascular, bony, or nerve injury; minimal soft tissue defect; and no signs of developing compartment syndrome over a 3- to 12-hour period of observation can be discharged home.

For further reading in *Emergency Medicine: A Comprehensive Study Guide,* 6th ed., see Chap. 263, "Penetrating Trauma to the Extremities," by Alan M. Kumar and Richard D. Zane.

20 | INJURIES TO THE BONES, JOINTS, AND SOFT TISSUE

Initial Evaluation and Management of Orthopedic Injuries

Michael P. Kefer

A delay in diagnosis of many orthopedic injuries can potentially increase the chance of significant complications and poor functional outcome.

CLINICAL FEATURES

Knowing the precise mechanism of injury or listening carefully to the patient's symptoms is important in diagnosing fracture or dislocation. Pain may be referred to an area distant from the injury (eg, hip injury presenting as knee pain). If key aspects of the history and physical examination are not appreciated, then all necessary radiographs may not be obtained and the diagnosis may be missed.

The physical examination includes (*a*) inspection for deformity, edema, or discoloration; (*b*) assessment of active and passive ranges of motion of joints proximal and distal to the injury; (*c*) palpation for tenderness or deformity; and (*d*) assessment of neurovascular status distal to the injury. Careful palpation can prevent missing a crucial diagnosis due to referred pain. The neurovascular status should be documented early, before performing reduction maneuvers.

Radiologic evaluation is based on the history and physical examination, not simply on where the patient reports pain. Radiographs of all long bone fractures should include the joint proximal and distal to the fracture to evaluate for coexistent injury. A negative radiograph does not exclude a fracture. This commonly occurs with scaphoid, radial head, or metatarsal shaft fractures. The emergency department diagnosis is often clinical and is not confirmed until 7 to 10 days after the injury, when enough bone resorption has occurred at the fracture site to detect a lucency on the radiograph.

An accurate description of the fracture to the orthopedic consultant is crucial and should include the following details:

- Closed versus open: whether the skin overlying the fracture is intact (closed) or not (open).
- Location: midshaft, junction of proximal and middle or middle and distal thirds, or distance from the bone end. Intraarticular involvement with disruption of the joint surface may require surgery. Anatomic bony reference points should be used when applicable (eg, humerus fracture just above the condyles is described as the supracondylar, as opposed to the distal, humerus).
- Orientation of fracture line: transverse, spiral, oblique, comminuted (shattered), and segmental (single large segment of free floating bone).
- Displacement: amount and direction the distal fragment is offset in relation to the proximal fragment.
- Separation: the degree 2 fragments have been pulled apart. Unlike displacement, alignment is maintained.
- Shortening: reduction in bone length due to impaction or overriding fragments.

- Angulation: angle formed by the fracture segments. This term describes the degree and direction of deviation of the distal fragment.
- Rotational deformity: degree the distal fragment is twisted on the axis of the normal bone. It is usually detected by physical examination and not seen on the radiograph.
- Fractures combined with dislocation or subluxation: associated disruption of proper joint alignment should be described as *fracture-dislocation* or *fracture-subluxation* to clearly communicate the more serious nature of the injury.

Complications resulting from neurovascular deficit may be immediate or delayed. Compartment syndrome that presents with the 5 classic signs of pain, pallor, paresthesias, pulselessness, and paralysis is well advanced. Long term complications of fracture include malunion, nonunion, avascular necrosis, arthritis, and osteomyelitis.

EMERGENCY DEPARTMENT CARE AND DISPOSITION

1. Swelling should be controlled with application of cold packs and elevation. Analgesics should be administered as necessary. Objects, such as rings or watches, that may constrict the injury should be removed as swelling progresses. The patient should be kept NPO (nothing by mouth) if anesthesia will be required.
2. Prompt reduction of fracture deformity with steady, longitudinal traction is indicated to (*a*) alleviate pain; (*b*) relieve tension on associated neurovascular structures; (*c*) minimize the risk of converting a closed fracture to an open fracture when a sharp, bony fragment tents overlying skin; and (*d*) restore circulation to a pulseless distal extremity. Whether the procedure is performed by the emergency physician or the orthopedist depends on the practice environment. Of the above indications, however, distal vascular compromise is the most critical with respect to time. Postreduction radiographs should be obtained to confirm proper anatomic repositioning.
3. Open fractures are treated immediately with prophylactic antibiotics to prevent osteomyelitis. A common regimen is a first-generation cephalosporin and an aminoglycoside. Irrigation and debridement in the operating room are indicated.
4. The fracture or relocated joint should be immobilized. Fiberglass or plaster splinting material is commonly used. The chemical reaction that causes the material to set is an exothermic reaction that begins upon contact with water. The amount of heat liberated is directly proportional to the setting process, which in turn is directly proportional to the temperature of the water. Severe burns, therefore, can result from the splinting material because the peak temperature to the skin is the sum of the water temperature plus the heat released by the exothermic reaction. The use of water slightly warmer than room temperature is a safe practice. Padding is necessary under the splint to prevent pressure sores and irritation. An adequate length to immobilize the injury should be used. Splints for midshaft fractures should be long enough to immobilize the joint above and below the fracture.
5. Crutches should be prescribed for the patient who has a lower extremity injury that requires non–weight bearing. Ideal crutch height is one hand width below the axilla. The pressure of the crutch pads is borne by the sides of the thorax, not the axilla, to avoid injury to the brachial plexus.

Walkers and canes are appropriate for partial weight-bearing conditions, and they may be alternatives for patients too weak to use crutches.
6. The patient who is discharged home is instructed to keep the injured extremity elevated above heart level and to seek immediate reevaluation if increased swelling, cyanosis, pain, or decreased sensation develops.

For further reading in *Emergency Medicine: A Comprehensive Study Guide,* 6th ed., see Chap. 267, "Initial Evaluation and Management of Orthopedic Injuries," by Jeffrey S. Menkes.

171 | Hand and Wrist Injuries
Michael P. Kefer

For hand and wrist injuries, the key therapeutic concepts are preservation of function by proper splinting and appropriate referral. Padded aluminum splinting adequately immobilizes flexion and extension movements as occur at the distal interphalangeal (DIP) and proximal interphalangeal (PIP) joints. Plaster or fiberglass splinting is required to control rotary motion, as occurs at the metacarpal phalangeal (MCP) joint and wrist. Open fracture or open joint injury usually is treated in the operating room, and immediate intravenous antibiotics are indicated. Fracture or dislocation that compromises neurovascular function requires immediate reduction.

HAND INJURIES

Tendon Injuries

Knowing the position of the hand at the time of injury predicts where, along its course, a tendon is injured. Extensor tendon repair often can be performed by the emergency physician. Flexor tendon repair should be performed by the hand surgeon. It is common for the emergency care of tendon lacerations to consist of closing the skin and splinting until definitive repair by the hand surgeon, which can occur up to 4 weeks later. Follow-up and rehabilitation of all tendon injuries are necessary.

Boutonniere Deformity

Boutonniere deformity results from an injury at the dorsal surface of the PIP joint that disrupts the extensor hood apparatus. Lateral bands of the extensor mechanism become flexors of the PIP joint and hyperextensors of the DIP joint. An extensor hood injury is easily missed on emergency department presentation. Reexamination after 7 days is indicated. Treatment consists of splinting the PIP joint in extension and referral to an orthopedist.

Gamekeeper Thumb

This injury results from forced radial abduction at the MCP joint, with injury to the ulnar collateral ligament of the thumb. This is the most critical of the collateral ligament injuries because it affects pincer function. A complete tear is diagnosed when abduction stress causes greater than 40° of radial angulation. Treatment consists of a thumb spica splint and referral for surgical repair.

DIP Joint Dislocations

These injuries are uncommon because of the firm attachment of skin and fibrous tissue to underlying bone. A radiograph is indicated to distinguish dislocation from fracture and dislocation. Dislocations are usually dorsal. Reduction is performed under digital block anesthesia. The dislocated phalanx is distracted, slightly hyperextended, and then repositioned. Inability to reduce the joint may be from an entrapped volar plate, profundus tendon, or avulsion fracture.

PIP Joint Dislocations

Dorsal dislocation results from rupture of the volar plate. The method of reduction is the same as that described for DIP joint dislocations. An irreducible joint from an entrapped volar plate may require surgical reduction. Lateral dislocation results from rupture of the collateral ligaments. Dorsal and lateral reduced injuries should be splinted at 30° flexion and referred. Volar dislocation is rare.

MCP Joint Dislocations

These are usually dorsal dislocations that require surgical reduction due to volar plate entrapment. Closed reduction is attempted with the wrist flexed and pressure applied to the proximal phalanx in a distal and volar direction. The joint should be splinted in flexion.

Distal Phalanx Fractures

A tuft fracture is the most common injury. If associated with subungual hematoma, drainage is recommended. Transverse fractures with displacement are always associated with nail bed laceration, which may require repair. Avulsion fracture of the base results in a mallet finger. If less than one third of the articular surface is involved, a dorsal extension splint should be applied. If greater than one third of the articular surface is involved, then internal fixation is recommended.

Middle and Proximal Phalanx Fractures

This diagnosis is often suspected if the fingertips of the closed hand do not point to the same spot on the wrist and the plane of the nail bed of the involved digit is not aligned with those of the other digits. Treatment of nondisplaced fractures is a gutter splint in the position of function and referral. Treatment of displaced fractures usually requires surgical intervention. Rotational malalignment is a common problem and requires correction.

Metacarpal Fractures

A fourth or fifth metacarpal neck fracture, the boxer fracture, is the most common metacarpal fracture. Angulations of 20° in the ring finger and 40° in the fifth finger can be tolerated, but ideally, angulation greater than 20° should be reduced. Second and third metacarpal fractures causing angulation greater than 15° should be reduced. Treatment consists of a gutter splint with the wrist extended 20° and the MCP joint flexed 90° and referral.

First metacarpal base fractures with intraarticular involvement (Bennett and Rolando fractures) should be immobilized in a thumb spica splint and referred for surgical repair.

Compartment Syndrome

Crush injuries to the hand are especially at risk for compartment syndrome. Patients will complain of pain that is out of proportion to the physical examination findings. Examination shows that the hand at a resting position is extended at the MCP joint and slightly flexed at the PIP joint. This is associated with pain with passive stretch of the involved compartment and tense edema. This condition is a surgical emergency.

High Pressure Injection Injury

This injury occurs when substances under high pressure, such as grease, paint, or hydraulic fluid, are injected into the hand. Oil-based paint causes the most severe tissue reaction and can result in ischemia, leading to amputation. Radiographs of the hand and forearm are indicated to evaluate for radiopaque substances and subcutaneous air. This is a surgical emergency.

WRIST INJURIES

Scapholunate Dissociation

This injury is a commonly missed diagnosis in the emergency department. The patient presents with wrist tenderness that may be localized to the scapholunate joint. The radiograph demonstrates a space between the scaphoid and lunate that is wider 3 mm. Early referral for ligamentous repair is indicated.

Lunate and Perilunate Dislocations

The most common carpal bone dislocations are lunate and perilunate. In both injuries, lateral wrist radiograph visualizes the dislocation as loss of the normal alignment of the radius, lunate, and capitate (the "3 Cs" sign). With a lunate dislocation, the lunate dislocates anterior to the radius, but the remainder of the carpus aligns with the radius. On posteroanterior radiograph, the lunate has a triangular shape, which is the pathognomonic "piece of pie" sign. With a perilunate dislocation, the lunate remains aligned with the radius, but the remainder of the carpus is dislocated, usually dorsal to the lunate. There is usually concomitant fracture of the scaphoid and the proximal portion of the scaphoid remains with the lunate, whereas the distal portion dislocates with the carpus. Prompt referral for closed reduction or surgical repair is indicated.

Scaphoid Fracture

This is the most common carpal fracture. The patient is tender in the anatomic snuff box. The wrist radiograph is commonly negative, so the diagnosis is based on physical examination findings. Treatment of the patient with snuff box tenderness is thumb spica splint and referral. Without proper treatment, there is risk of avascular necrosis of the scaphoid bone.

Triquetrum Fracture

Triquetrum fracture is a dorsal avulsion or body fracture. There is tenderness dorsally, just distal to the ulnar styloid. The wrist radiograph is often negative, so diagnosis is based on physical examination findings. Treatment consists of a volar splint and referral.

Lunate Fracture

This is the most important of the carpal fractures because it occupies two thirds of the articular surface of the radius. There is risk of avascular necrosis. Tenderness is present over the lunate fossa (distal to the rim of the radius at the base of the third metacarpal). Wrist radiograph is commonly negative, so diagnosis is based on physical examination findings. Treatment consists of a thumb spica splint and referral.

Trapezium Fracture

Trapezium fracture results in painful thumb movement. Tenderness is present at the apex of the anatomic snuff box and the base of the thenar eminence. Treatment consists of a thumb spica splint and referral.

Pisiform Fracture

The pisiform is a sesamoid bone within the flexor carpi ulnaris tendon. There is tenderness at its bony prominence at the base of the hypothenar eminence. Treatment consists of a volar splint at 30° flexion with ulnar deviation to relieve tension on the tendon and referral.

Hamate Fracture

Hamate fracture most commonly involves the hook, which is palpable in the soft tissue of the radial aspect of the hypothenar eminence. Treatment consists of a volar splint and referral.

Capitate Fracture

Isolated capitate fracture is rare. It usually is associated with scaphoid fracture. The capitate is also at risk of avascular necrosis. Treatment consists of a thumb spica splint and referral.

Trapezoid Fracture

Trapezoid fracture is extremely rare and difficult to see on radiographs. Treatment consists of a thumb spica splint and referral.

Radial Styloid Fracture

The major carpal ligaments on the radial side of the wrist insert on the radial styloid. Therefore, fracture can produce carpal instability and is associated with scapholunate dissociation. Early orthopedic referral is indicated.

Ulnar Styloid Fracture

Ulnar styloid fracture may result in radial ulnar joint instability. Treatment consists of an ulnar gutter splint with the wrist in the neutral position and ulnar deviation.

Colles and Smith Fractures

These fractures involve the distal radius at the metaphysis. With a Colles fracture, the distal radius is displaced dorsally, causing a dinner-fork deformity. With a Smith fracture, the distal radius is displaced volarly, causing a garden-spade deformity. Treatment is hematoma block, placement of the hand in a finger trap, and closed reduction.

For further reading in *Emergency Medicine: A Comprehensive Study Guide*, 6th ed., see Chap. 268, "Injuries to the Hand and Digits," by Robert L. Muelleman and Michael C. Wadman; and Chap. 269, "Wrist Injuries," by Dennis T. Uehara, Dean Wolanyk, and Robert Escarza.

172 | Forearm and Elbow Injuries
Sandra L. Najarian

ELBOW DISLOCATIONS

Clinical Features

Most dislocations are posterior and result from a fall on an outstretched hand. On examination, the patient holds the elbow in 45° of flexion. The olecranon is directed posteriorly and often is obscured by significant swelling. It is essential to assess neurovascular status because the brachial artery and ulnar nerve are most prone to injury. The brachial and radial pulses and the ulnar, median, and radial nerves must be evaluated thoroughly.

Diagnosis and Differential

Radiographs of the elbow confirm the diagnosis. On the lateral view, the ulna and radius are displaced posteriorly. On the anteroposterior (AP) view, the ulna and radius may be displaced medially or laterally, but these bones maintain their normal relation to each other. Associated fractures should be noted.

Emergency Department Care and Disposition

Appropriate treatment of elbow dislocations requires adequate reduction and recognition of neurovascular complications, associated fractures, and postreduction instability.

1. After adequate sedation, **reduction of the elbow dislocation** is accomplished by gentle traction on the wrist and forearm. An assistant applies countertraction on the arm. Any medial or lateral displacement is corrected with the other hand. Distal traction is applied to wrist while downward pressure is applied to the proximal forearm to help disengage the coronoid process from the olecranon fossa. Successful reduction is noted by a palpable "clunk."
2. Neurovascular status must be reassessed after reduction and a period of observation. Postreduction films should be obtained.
3. A **long-arm posterior splint** is used to immobilize the elbow in 90° of flexion. The risk of subsequent edema is significant, and cylindrical casts should not be placed.
4. Close orthopedic follow-up must be arranged. Patients with instability in extension, neurovascular compromise, or open dislocations require immediate orthopedic consultation.

ELBOW FRACTURES

The most common fracture of the elbow is the radial head fracture, usually resulting from a fall on an outstretched hand. Intercondylar fractures result from a force directed against the elbow and occur most commonly in adults. Supracondylar fractures are extraarticular fractures that occur most commonly in children. In 95% of these fractures, an extension force causes posterior displacement. Olecranon fractures are also common and often result from direct trauma.

Clinical Features

Radial head fractures result in lateral elbow pain and tenderness and inability to fully extend the elbow. Patients with intercondylar and supracondylar fractures will have significant swelling and tenderness and limited range of motion. Supracondylar fractures may resemble a posterior elbow dislocation because the olecranon is prominent posteriorly. Evaluation of neurovascular compromise is essential because neurovascular injuries are common with supracondylar fractures. The anterior interosseus nerve, a motor branch of the median nerve, is most prone to injury. Asking the patient to make a circle or an "OK" sign with the thumb and index finger tests this nerve. Acute vascular injuries are usually secondary to transient vasospasm, which results in a decreased or absent radial pulse. Olecranon fractures result in localized swelling and tenderness and limited mobility.

Diagnosis and Differential

AP and lateral radiographs of the elbow should be obtained. Radial head fractures may not present with a visible fracture line; a posterior fat pad sign may be the only evidence of injury. Careful inspection for a fracture line separating the condyles and the humerus signifies an intercondylar fracture. In supracondylar fractures, the AP radiograph shows a transverse fracture line, and the lateral view shows an oblique fracture line and displacement of the distal fragment proximally and posteriorly. A posterior and anterior fat pad sign also may be seen on the lateral view. In olecranon fractures, it is important to note any displacement (>2 mm).

Emergency Department Care and Disposition

1. Immobilization in a splint and orthopedic referral are appropriate for nondisplaced fractures. Minimally displaced radial head fractures may be treated with a sling and early range of motion.
2. Immediate **orthopedic consultation** is warranted for all displaced fractures, open fractures, and evidence of neurovascular compromise. Supracondylar fractures are often treated with closed reduction and percutaneous pinning. Displaced intercondylar fractures and olecranon fractures often require open reduction and internal fixation. Patients with significant swelling and displaced fractures should be admitted for observation of neurovascular status.

FOREARM FRACTURES

Fractures of the ulna and radius usually occur from significant trauma, such as a motor vehicle crash or a fall from height. Isolated fractures of the ulna usually occur from a direct blow to the forearm. Radius fractures usually result from direct trauma or from a fall on an outstretched hand.

Clinical Features

Examination of both bone fractures shows swelling, tenderness, and deformity of the forearm. Open fractures of the forearm are common. Isolated ulna or radius fractures present with localized swelling and tenderness over the fracture site. Monteggia fracture-dislocation, a fracture of the proximal ulna shaft with a radial head dislocation, presents with significant pain and swelling over the elbow. In contrast, Galeazzi fracture-dislocation, a fracture of the distal radius with an associated distal radioulnar joint dislocation, causes localized swelling and tenderness over the distal radius and wrist.

Diagnosis and Differential

AP and lateral radiographs of the forearm easily confirm the diagnosis. The amount of displacement, angulation, and shortening needs to be evaluated. Any rotational angulation should be noted. A sudden change in the width of a bone or a change in the normal orientation of various bony prominences suggests rotational deformity. Isolated ulna fractures are considered displaced if there is greater than $10°$ of angulation or greater than 50% displacement. The radial head dislocation in a Monteggia fracture can be subtle. Normally, the radial head aligns with the capitellum in all radiographic views of the elbow. The radial head dislocation is in the same direction as the apex of the ulnar fracture. In a Galeazzi fracture, the distal radioulnar joint dislocation may be difficult to identify. An increase in the distal radioulnar joint space may be seen on the AP view; on the lateral view, the ulnar is displaced dorsally.

Emergency Department Care and Disposition

1. Nondisplaced isolated fractures may be immobilized in a long-arm cast and given close orthopedic referral.
2. Most of these injuries will have significant displacement and require **orthopedic consultation** and management. Closed reduction is often adequate for both bone fractures in children. Open reduction and internal fixation is usually required for displaced fractures in adults and for Monteggia and Galeazzi fracture-dislocations.

BICEPS AND TRICEPS RUPTURES

Clinical Features

Proximal long-head biceps ruptures are most common and usually occur from a sudden or prolonged contraction against resistance. Patients often describe a snap or pop and complain of pain in the anterior shoulder. Swelling, tenderness, and crepitus over the bicipital groove can be seen on examination. The distally retracted biceps will appear as a "ball" in the mid-arm when the elbow is flexed. There is minimal loss of strength in elbow flexion because of the function of the brachialis and supinators. In contrast, strength in supination and elbow flexion is notably weaker in distal biceps ruptures. Examination also shows swelling, ecchymosis, and tenderness in the antecubital fossa. The distal biceps tendon is no longer palpable in the antecubital fossa.

Triceps ruptures almost always occur distally as a result of a direct blow to the olecranon or a fall on an outstretched hand causing a forceful flexion of the extended forearm. On examination, swelling and tenderness are noted proximal to the olecranon. Extension of the forearm is weak. Triceps function can be assessed with a modified Thompson test. With the arm supported, the elbow flexed at $90°$, and the forearm hanging in a relaxed position, squeezing the triceps should produce extension of the forearm. This is absent in a complete triceps rupture.

Diagnosis and Differential

Diagnosis is mainly clinical. Radiographs should be obtained to exclude an associated avulsion fracture.

Emergency Department Care and Disposition

Treatment includes a sling, ice, analgesia, and orthopedic referral for definitive management. Surgical repair is indicated for young, active individuals with complete ruptures.

For further reading in *Emergency Medicine: A Comprehensive Study Guide,* 6th ed., see Chap. 270, "Injuries to the Elbow and Forearm," by Arthur F. Proust, Jason H. Bredenkamp, and Dennis T. Uehara.

173 | Shoulder and Humerus Injuries

Robert J. French

The shoulder consists of 4 joints: sternoclavicular, acromioclavicular, glenohumeral, and scapulothoracic. Injury to muscular, ligamentous, or osseous components causes loss of motion, instability, and pain.

STERNOCLAVICULAR JOINT INJURIES

Clinical Features

The sternoclavicular joint is the most frequently moved, nonaxial joint of the body as virtually all movements of the upper extremity are transferred proximally to this joint. Sternoclavicular injury results from direct trauma to the joint or forceful rolling of the shoulder forward or backward. Injuries include sternoclavicular sprains or dislocations. The sternoclavicular joint is the least commonly dislocated major joint in the body. Anterior dislocations are more common than posterior dislocations. Posterior dislocations are more ominous due to potential injury of the mediastinal contents. Sternoclavicular sprains cause localized pain and swelling. Patients with sternoclavicular dislocations have severe pain that is exacerbated by movement or supine position. Anterior dislocations can be diagnosed clinically by visual and palpable prominence of the medial clavicle head. In posterior dislocations, the medial clavicle head is less visible and nonpalpable. The expected medial clavicle depression may be obscured by local edema, resulting in a missed or delayed diagnosis. Patients with posterior dislocations may present with hoarseness, dysphagia, dyspnea, upper extremity paresthesias, and weakness. Plain radiographs cannot reliably differentiate sprains from dislocations. Computerized tomography can accurately diagnose sternoclavicular joint dislocations.

Emergency Department Care and Disposition

1. Treatment of sternoclavicular sprains is symptomatic with ice, analgesics, and sling.
2. Closed reduction of anterior sternoclavicular dislocations can be attempted, and, if successful, the patient is placed in a figure-of-eight clavicle splint. These reductions often prove to be unstable.
3. For nonreducible anterior dislocations and all posterior dislocations, urgent orthopedic consultation is required.

CLAVICLE FRACTURES

Clavicle fractures account for almost 50% of significant shoulder girdle injuries and are the most common fracture in children. Patients typically present with pain, swelling, deformity, and localized tenderness. Although rare, injuries to the lung and neurovascular bundle can occur. Routine clavicle views visualize 80% of fractures in the middle third of the clavicle, 15% in the distal third, and 5% in the medial third.

Treatment consists of analgesics and immobilization, preferably by sling, for 4 to 8 weeks. Orthopedic consultation is needed for open fractures, neurovascular compromise, skin tenting, or interposition of soft tissue. Fractures with marked displacement or shortening are at greater risk of nonunion; therefore, early orthopedic follow-up is required.

ACROMIOCLAVICULAR JOINT INJURIES

Clinical Features

Injury to the acromioclavicular joint occurs most commonly in young males secondary to sport-related activities. The mechanism of injury is usually direct trauma to the point of the shoulder with the arm adducted. This mechanism, in conjunction with pain, tenderness, and deformity at the acromioclavicular joint, help establish this clinical diagnosis. These injuries are classified as types I through VI based on severity of injury to the acromioclavicular and coracoclavicular ligaments. Types III through VI represent complete acromioclavicular and coracoclavicular ligament disruption with different orientations of the displaced clavicle.

Diagnosis and Differential

Acromioclavicular radiographs help determine the severity of injury and associated fractures. An acromioclavicular ligament sprain or partial tear is a type I injury, and radiographs will be normal. Type II injuries, associated with disruption of the acromioclavicular ligament, result in 25% to 50% elevation of the clavicle above the acromial process. Type III injuries, characterized by complete disruption of the acromioclavicular and coracoclavicular ligaments, show 100% superior displacement of the clavicle and coracoclavicular space widening. In type I and type II injuries, the coracoclavicular distance is 1.1 to 1.3 cm. A coracoclavicular gap differential wider than 5 mm between the injured and uninjured shoulders is diagnostic of a type III injury.

Emergency Department Care and Disposition

1. Treatment of type I and II injuries consists of rest, ice, analgesics, and immobilization for 1 to 3 weeks. Once pain free, the patient can begin range-of-motion and strengthening exercises.
2. Treatment of type III injuries is controversial, with proponents for conservative or operative management. The recent trend favors conservative management, as in type I and II injuries.
3. More severe injuries, types IV through VI, generally are managed operatively.

GLENOHUMERAL JOINT DISLOCATION

Clinical Features

Dislocation of the glenohumeral joint is the most common major joint dislocation. The glenohumeral joint can dislocate anteriorly, posteriorly, inferiorly, and superiorly. Anterior dislocations account for 95% to 97% of all dislocations. The most common mechanism for anterior dislocation is an indirect force levered on the joint capsule from a combination of abduction, extension, and external rotation. The patient typically is in severe pain and holds the arm in slight abduction and external rotation. The shoulder has a "squared-off" and shortened appearance. The axillary nerve is the most common neurovascular structure injured in anterior dislocations and can be assessed by pinprick sensation over the skin of the lateral shoulder.

Anteroposterior and lateral scapular "Y" or axillary views are often obtained. Although associated fractures can be identified radiographically in up to 50% of patients with glenohumeral dislocation, most of these fractures are compression fractures of the humeral head (Hill-Sachs lesion), which require no additional treatment. Other associated injuries include anterior glenoid rim fractures (Bankard lesion), greater tuberosity avulsion fractures, and rotator cuff tears.

Emergency Department Care and Disposition

1. **Modified hippocratic technique.** This method uses traction and counter-traction. The patient is supine with the arm abducted and the elbow flexed 90°. A sheet is placed across the thorax of the patient and tied around the waist of the assistant. Another sheet is placed around the patient's flexed elbow and the physician's waist. The physician gradually applies traction while the assistant provides countertraction. Gentle internal and external rotation may aid reduction.

2. **Stimson technique.** The patient is placed prone on a gurney with the dislocated extremity hanging over the side and a 10-lb weight attached at the wrist. Reduction occurs in 20 to 30 minutes if complete muscle relaxation is achieved.

3. **Milch technique.** With the patient supine, the physician slowly abducts and externally rotates the arm to the overhead position. With the elbow fully extended, gentle traction is applied. If reduction is not achieved, the humeral head can be manipulated into the glenoid fossa with the physician's free hand.

4. **Scapular manipulation technique.** The first step is to apply traction to the arm held in 90° of forward flexion. This can be accomplished in the prone position by using the Stimson technique or in a seated position with an assistant applying traction. The arm should be positioned in slight external rotation. The scapular tip is then pushed as far medially as possible while stabilizing the superior aspect of the scapula with the other hand. A small amount of dorsal displacement of the scapula tip is recommended. Scapular manipulation accomplishes reduction by repositioning the glenoid fossa rather than the humeral head.

5. **External rotation technique.** The patient is supine with the arm adducted to the side. The elbow is flexed to 90°, and the arm is slowly and gently externally rotated. No traction is applied. Reduction is subtle and usually occurs before reaching the coronal plane.

6. **Aronen technique.** This technique is most useful when reduction is easy to achieve, as in recurrent dislocations or immediately after injury before muscle spasm and swelling have occurred. This technique can be taught to patients with recurrent dislocations, as self-reduction may be the only method available to them in certain situations (solo sailing, cross-country skiing, etc). In this technique, the patient is seated on a gurney with the ipsilateral leg and knee in flexion. Patients are instructed to clasp their hands around the ipsilateral knee and then relax the shoulder muscles, thereby allowing the weight of the lower limb to provide gentle inline traction. Countertraction is applied by the patients' upper body weight and their own paraspinous muscles. Taping the clasped hands together can aid reduction.

7. After reduction, the neurovascular status should be reassessed, and postreduction radiographs should be obtained. A shoulder immobilizer or a sling

and swath should be applied, and orthopedic follow-up should be arranged. The shoulder should be immobilized for 3 to 6 weeks in younger patients and 1 or 2 weeks in older patients (>40 years). Early range-of-motion exercises reduce the risk of adhesive capsulitis.

Posterior dislocations account for 1% to 2% of glenohumeral dislocation. They occur with convulsive seizures, direct trauma to the anterior shoulder, or falls on an outstretched arm. They are less clinically apparent than anterior dislocations. In posterior dislocations, the arm is held across the chest in adduction and internal rotation. Abduction is severely compromised, and external rotation is completely blocked. The anterior shoulder appears flat with a prominent coracoid process, and the posterior aspect appears full. Anteroposterior radiographs in posterior glenohumeral dislocations show a loss of the elliptical half-moon shape overlap seen on normal films. The humeral head takes on a "light bulb" or "drum stick" appearance due to its internally rotated configuration. In these injuries, the scapular "Y" view or other lateral projection will confirm this diagnosis. Reduction is performed in the supine patient by applying axial traction along the long axis of the humerus, anteriorly directed pressure on the posterior humeral head, and a small amount of external rotation.

Inferior dislocations (luxatio erecta) are extremely rare, accounting for 0.5% of glenohumeral dislocations. The mechanism of injury is a forceful hyperabduction or an inferior directed axial load on the abducted shoulder. The patient presents with the arm locked overhead. Reduction consists of traction in an upward and outward direction in line with the humerus.

SCAPULA INJURIES

Clinical Features

Fractures of the scapula are a rare occurrence, accounting for fewer than 1% of all fractures. Due to the excessive forces needed to fracture this protected bone, associated injuries of the ipsilateral lung, thoracic cage, and shoulder girdle are a major concern. Because these fractures are associated with more significant injuries, the diagnosis often is delayed or missed. Patients will present with localized tenderness over the scapula and the arm held in adduction. They should be evaluated for other injuries during the primary and secondary surveys. Plain radiographs confirm the diagnosis.

Emergency Department Care and Disposition

1. A thorough investigation for associated intrathoracic injuries is mandated. Careful consideration should be made for admission of patients with scapula fracture for observation.
2. The fracture is managed nonoperatively with a sling for immobilization, ice, analgesics, and early range-of-motion exercises.
3. Surgical intervention may be warranted for displaced glenoid articular fractures, angulated glenoid neck fractures, and certain acromion or coracoid fractures.

HUMERUS FRACTURES

Clinical Features

Fractures of the proximal humerus are a relatively common injury and are seen typically in elderly patients with osteoporosis after a fall on an outstretched hand. Humeral shaft fractures occur most commonly in young men and osteoporotic women after direct or indirect trauma to the humeral shaft. Patients with proximal humerus and humeral shaft fractures present with localized pain, swelling, tenderness, ecchymosis, and crepitus. The arm is held closely against the chest wall. In proximal humerus fractures, a thorough neurovascular examination can identify injuries of the axillary nerve, axillary artery, or brachial plexus. Shortening of the upper extremity may be noted in displaced humeral shaft fractures. In shaft fractures, a careful neurovascular examination may show injuries to the brachial artery or vein or to the radial, ulna, or median nerves. The most commonly injured nerves in proximal humerus fractures and humeral shaft fractures are the axillary nerve and the radial nerve, respectively. The diagnosis of proximal humerus and humeral shaft fractures is made radiographically.

Emergency Department Care and Disposition

1. Treatment consists of analgesics, immobilization, and orthopedic referral for simple fractures. Immobilization can be achieved with a sling and swath or a shoulder immobilizer.
2. Urgent orthopedic consultation is indicated for multipart proximal humerus fractures, significantly displaced or angulated shaft fractures, open fractures, or any fracture with neurovascular compromise.

For further reading in *Emergency Medicine: A Comprehensive Study Guide,* 6th ed., see Chap. 271, "Injuries to the Shoulder Complex and Humerus," by Dennis T. Uehara and John P. Rudzinski.

174 | Pelvis, Hip, and Femur Injuries

E. Parker Hays Jr

Pelvic fractures are associated with a high morbidity and mortality because of (*a*) the large forces required to fracture the bony pelvis; (*b*) concomitant abdominal, thoracic, and head injuries; and (*c*) the possibility of major hemorrhagic loss from highly vascular pelvic bones and proximate major blood vessels. Hip fractures are common in elderly osteoporotic patients after falls. In younger patients, hip and femur fractures are usually due to violent mechanisms.

PELVIC FRACTURES

Clinical Features

Pelvic fractures should be suspected whenever there is trauma to the torso or a fall from a height. Pain, crepitus, or instability on palpation of the pelvis suggests a fracture. Hematoma over the inguinal ligament or perineum, gross hematuria, or vaginal or rectal bleeding should increase suspicion. Hypotension may be secondary to abdominal or thoracic injuries or blood loss from disrupted pelvic bones or vessels.

Diagnosis and Differential

Radiographs confirm suspected pelvis fractures. The anteroposterior (AP) pelvic view is the most useful; additional views include oblique hemi-pelvis, inlet (to evaluate AP displacement), and outlet (to evaluate superior–inferior displacement) views. Computed tomography provides more detailed information. Many classifications for pelvic fractures exist; the Young system is helpful because classifications are based on mechanism and directional forces and can predict the likelihood of severe hemorrhage (Table 174-1). Four main patterns (suggested by the alignment of pubic rami fractures, pubic symphysis diastasis, and sacroiliac joint displacement) have been identified: lateral compression, AP compression, vertical shear, and combination mechanisms. The alignment of pubic rami fractures suggests the direction of injurious force. Horizontal fracture lines suggest lateral compression injury, whereas vertical fractures point to an AP compression mechanism. Complications often correlate with, and can be anticipated by, the fracture pattern.

Emergency Department Care and Disposition

1. Standard protocols for evaluation and stabilization of trauma patients should be initiated (see Chap. 157). A careful search for other significant injuries should be made because there is a strong association with other major injuries.
2. Patients should receive **100% oxygen** and have cardiac monitoring and 2 large-bore intravenous (IV) lines established. Blood should be sent for type and crossmatching. Hypotension should be treated aggressively with the infusion of **packed red blood cells.**
3. If the pelvis is unstable, it should be wrapped circumferentially with a bed sheet that is pulled to provide enough tension to reduce pelvic volume and

TABLE 174-1 Injury Classification Keys According to the Young System

Category	Distinguishing characteristics; severe hemorrhage incidence (%)
LC	Transverse fracture of pubic rami, ipsilateral, or contralateral to posterior injury I: Sacral compression on side of impact II: Crescent (iliac wing) fracture on side of impact (36) III: LC-1 or LC-2 injury on side of impact; contralateral open-book (APC) injury (60)
APC	Symphyseal diastasis and/or longitudinal rami fractures: I: Slight widening of pubic symphysis and/or anterior SI joint; stretched but intact anterior SI, sacrotuberous, and sacrospinous ligaments; intact posterior SI ligaments II: Widened anterior SI joint; disrupted anterior SI, sacrotuberous, and sacrospinous ligaments; intact posterior SI ligaments (28) III: Complete SI joint disruption with lateral displacement; disrupted anterior SI, sacrotuberous, and sacrospinous ligaments; disrupted posterior SI ligaments (53)
VS	Symphyseal diastasis or vertical displacement anteriorly and posteriorly, usually through the SI joint, occasionally through the iliac wing and/or sacrum (75)
CM	Combination of other injury patterns, LC/VS being the most common (58)

Key: APC = anterior-posterior compression, CM = combination mechanisms, LC = lateral compression, SI = sacroiliac, VS = vertical shear.

stem hemorrhage. An orthopedic surgeon should be consulted early to provide **external fixation** for persistent hemodynamic instability. **Angiography** for embolization of pelvis vessels is another option with continued major blood loss.

4. Intraabdominal solid organ injuries and other sources of blood loss should be considered. If diagnostic peritoneal lavage is performed, a supraumbilical approach should be taken to avoid disruption of pelvic hematoma.

5. A Foley catheter should not be placed if urethral injury is suspected until a retrograde urethrogram is performed. Rectal examination (and bimanual pelvic examination for women) should be performed to assess for rectal and gynecologic injuries. If blood is found on pelvic examination, a speculum examination should be performed to evaluate for vaginal lacerations (which may occur with anterior pelvic fractures). Vaginal lacerations mandate operative debridement and irrigation; patients should receive **cefotetan** 1 g IV in the emergency department. Rectal injuries are treated with irrigation and diverting colostomy; patients should receive **cefotetan** 2 g IV in the emergency department.

Stable Pelvic Avulsion and Single Bone Fractures

The mechanism and clinical findings of avulsion and single bone fractures are summarized in Table 174-2. Avulsion fractures involve a single bone that is avulsed during forceful muscular contraction. Fracture of a single ischial bone or pubic ramus can occur in the elderly with direct trauma from a fall. In general, if other injuries are not present, these injuries are stable (no com-

TABLE 174-2 Pelvic Avulsion and Single Bone Fractures

Fracture	Mechanism of injury	Clinical findings/ associated injuries
Iliac wing (Duverney) fracture	Direct trauma, usually lateral to medial	Swelling, tenderness over iliac wing; abdominal pain; ileus; acetabular fractures; serious injury infrequent
Single ramus of pubis or ischium	Fall or direct trauma in the elderly; exercise-induced stress fracture in the young or in pregnant women	Local pain and tenderness; inability to ambulate; rectal injury
Ischium body	Violent, external trauma or from fall in sitting position; least common fracture	Local pain and tenderness; pain with hamstring movement; rectal injury
Sacral fracture	Transverse fractures from direct AP trauma; upper transverse fractures from fall in flexed position	Pain on rectal examination; sacral root injury with upper transverse fractures
Coccyx fracture	Fall in sitting position; more common in women	Pain, tenderness over sacral region; pain on compression during rectal exam
Anterior superior iliac spine	Forceful sartorius muscle contraction (eg, adolescent sprinters)	Pain with hip flexion and abduction
Anterior inferior iliac spine	Forceful rectus femoris muscle contraction (eg, adolescent soccer players)	Pain in groin; pain with hip flexion
Ischial tuberosity	Forceful contraction of hamstrings	Pain with sitting or flexing the thigh

Key: AP = anteroposterior.

promise to pelvic ring integrity) and treated with analgesia, rest, crutches, and primary physician or orthopedic follow-up in 1 to 2 weeks.

Acetabular Fractures

Acetabular fractures account for 20% of pelvic fractures and result from lateral force across the hip or force through the femur (eg, knee versus dashboard). They are commonly associated with femur and hip fractures, knee injuries, and especially hip dislocations. If acetabular fracture is seen on AP pelvis radiograph or suspected clinically, oblique views (Judet views) of the hip should be obtained. Significant hip pain with weight bearing after trauma and normal radiograph suggests the possibility of occult fracture, especially of the femoral neck or acetabulum, and may warrant computed tomography or magnetic resonance imaging. Orthopedic consultation and admission should be obtained for acetabular fractures. Nondisplaced fractures are treated with bedrest, whereas displaced fractures may require open reduction and repair.

HIP FRACTURES

Hip fractures are common in elderly patients who present after a fall. The affected leg is classically shortened and externally rotated. Morbidity is high and often related to underlying medical conditions. Complications include infection, venous thromboembolism, avascular necrosis, and nonunion.

The position of the extremity, ecchymoses, deformity, and range of motion should be evaluated. Heel percussion may elicit pain. Posteroanterior, lateral, and frog-leg views should be obtained.

Hip fractures are classified as intracapsular (femoral head and neck) or extracapsular (intertrochanteric and subtrochanteric). Intracapsular fractures may compromise blood supply to the femoral head, with resultant avascular necrosis.

Femoral head fractures are most commonly associated with hip dislocations. Femoral neck fractures are common in elderly patients with osteoporosis. Patients complain of pain in the groin and inner thigh. The leg is shortened and held in external rotation. Skeletal traction is contraindicated in femoral neck fractures because it may further compromise femoral head blood flow. Nondisplaced neck fractures are treated with pin fixation; displaced fractures are treated with open reduction or prosthesis placement.

Stress fracture of the femur should be suspected if there is significant pain without radiographic abnormality. Radiographs may show a fracture, but a bone scan is more sensitive for subtle fractures. Stress fractures are treated conservatively with protected weight bearing (eg, crutches) while awaiting a bone scan in 1 to 2 days or follow-up radiograph in 10 to 14 days.

Intertrochanteric fractures occur in the elderly after a fall with rotational forces. The leg is shortened and externally rotated. Treatment includes nonemergent operative fixation.

Subtrochanteric fractures may be seen in elderly osteoporotic patients and young patients after major trauma. Symptoms include pain, deformity, and swelling. Immobilization with a traction apparatus is recommended, with eventual operative fixation.

Greater trochanter fractures may occur in adults (true fracture) or children (avulsion of the apophysis). Pain is present on abduction and extension. Treatment is controversial and may include conservative treatment or operative fixation based on the patient's age and displacement of fragment.

Lesser trochanter avulsions are most common in young athletes, after avulsion of the iliopsoas muscle. There is pain during flexion and internal rotation. If there is more than 2 cm of displacement, operative fixation with screws is recommended.

HIP DISLOCATIONS

Hip dislocations are most often the result of massive forces during trauma. Most (90%) are posterior and 10% are anterior. Both types are treated with early closed reduction (<6 hours) to decrease the incidence of avascular necrosis.

Posterior dislocations, which occur when a posterior force is applied to the flexed knee, may coexist with acetabular fractures. The leg is shortened, internally rotated, and adducted. AP, lateral, and oblique views will evaluate the status of the acetabulum and the femoral head. Treatment includes early closed reduction using the **Allis maneuver** (hip flexion to 90° and then internal and external rotation with traction) or the **Stimson maneuver** (patient prone, with the leg hanging over the edge of stretcher, and application of gentle traction).

Anterior dislocations occur during forced abduction. The leg is held in abduction and external rotation. Treatment includes early closed reduction with strong, inline traction and flexing and externally rotating the leg with abduction once the femoral head clears the acetabulum.

FEMORAL SHAFT FRACTURES

Femoral shaft fractures most often occur in men after falls, industrial accidents, motor vehicle crashes, and gunshot wounds. Because the femur has a rich vascular supply and is surrounded by soft tissue, it can accommodate 1 L or more of blood, which can contribute to hypotension and shock after a fracture. Distal neurovascular function should be thoroughly evaluated because sciatic nerve injury can occur. Diagnosis is confirmed radiographically. Treatment involves immediate immobilization with **Hare or Sager traction** (relatively contraindicated in open fractures and sciatic nerve injury) or a Thomas splint. Open fractures should be grossly decontaminated, and **cefazolin** 1 g IV and tetanus toxoid should be administered. Definitive repair is by operative fixation or traction (in children).

For further reading in *Emergency Medicine: A Comprehensive Study Guide,* 6th ed., see Chap. 273, "Trauma to the Pelvis, Hip, and Femur," by Mark T. Steele and Stefanie R. Ellison.

175 | Knee and Leg Injuries

Jeffrey N. Glaspy

Knee injuries are most often the result of ligamentous and cartilaginous injuries but may include bony fractures and dislocations. The Pittsburgh Knee Rules provide a guideline for obtaining radiographs of the knee. Radiographic evaluation is recommended if the patient has sustained a blunt trauma mechanism and is (*a*) younger than 12 years or older than 50 years or (*b*) unable to walk 4 weight-bearing steps in the emergency department.

FRACTURES

Patella Fractures

Patella fractures occur from direct trauma or from forceful contraction of the quadriceps tendon. Physical examination shows tenderness, swelling, effusion, and often a palpable defect of the patella. The extensor mechanism of the knee should be evaluated. Nondisplaced patellar fractures with intact extensor mechanisms are treated with knee immobilization, ice, analgesics, elevation, and referral for casting. Fractures that are displaced more than 3 mm or are associated with disruption of the extensor mechanism require early orthopedic referral for operative repair.

Femoral Condyle Fractures

Femoral condyle fractures usually result from direct trauma with an axial load or from a blow to the distal femur. Signs and symptoms include pain, swelling, deformity, rotation, shortening, and inability to ambulate. Associated injuries should be identified and include popliteal artery injury, ipsilateral hip dislocation or fracture, quadriceps mechanism injury, and neurologic injury, especially the deep perineal nerve. Orthopedic consultation is required as most fractures will require operative repair.

Tibial Spine Fractures

Tibial spine fractures are caused by direct anterior or posterior force against the flexed proximal tibia. Anterior spine fracture is about 10-fold more common than is posterior spine fracture. Physical examination shows tenderness, swelling, inability to extend the knee, and a positive Lachman sign. Nondisplaced fractures are treated with knee immobilization in full extension. Displaced fractures require operative repair.

Tibial Plateau Fractures

Tibial plateau fractures result from varus or valgus forces combined with axial loading. The lateral plateau is more commonly fractured. Symptoms include pain, swelling of the knee, and decreased range of motion. Radiographic evaluation may show a fracture or only a lipohemarthrosis. Computed tomography may be helpful in evaluating the fracture. Ligamentous instability is common and occurs in about one third of cases. Early orthopedic consultation is necessary due to the need for precise reconstruction of the articular surface.

Tibial Fractures

Fractures to the tibia may result from direct trauma or from rotational or torsional stress. Patients present with pain, swelling, and crepitance. A complete neurovascular evaluation is essential as is a search for possible compartment syndrome. Radiographs of the tibia and of the ankle and knee are required to exclude associated fractures. Treatment depends on the location and extent of injury. Most tibial fractures require emergent orthopedic consultation. Indications for emergent operative repair include open fractures, vascular compromise, or compartment syndrome.

Fibular Fractures

Fibular fractures most commonly involve the distal fibula at the ankle. Isolated shaft fractures usually occur from direct trauma. Proximal fibular fractures may result from external rotation injuries, whereas distal fibular fractures may result from internal rotation injuries. Patients with isolated fibular fracture may be able to bear weight. Treatment includes splinting, ice, elevation, and non–weight bearing pending follow-up with an orthopedic specialist or primary care physician.

DISLOCATIONS

Patella Dislocation

Patella dislocation usually results from a twisting injury on an extended knee. Associated tearing of the medial joint capsule may occur. Radiographs should be obtained to exclude associated fracture. Reduction is accomplished after conscious sedation by flexing the hip, hyperextending the knee, and sliding the patella back into place. Knee immobilization and orthopedic or primary care follow-up are necessary.

Knee Dislocation

Knee dislocations result from various large force mechanisms and are associated with tremendous ligamentous and capsular injuries. Posterior knee dislocations are most common, although anterior, medial, lateral, rotational, or combined injuries may occur. Because of instability, reduction often occurs spontaneously. A severely unstable knee in multiple directions is suspicious for a spontaneously reduced knee dislocation. There is a high incidence of associated popliteal artery and peroneal nerve injuries. Therefore, determining pre- and postreduction neurovascular status is essential. Radiographs should be obtained to exclude associated fractures. Early reduction of the dislocation is essential. Any patient with absent or diminished pulse, foot ischemia, or bruit requires emergent arteriography or vascular surgery consultation for surgical exploration. All patients should be admitted for serial vascular examinations.

TENDON, LIGAMENTOUS, AND MENISCAL INJURIES

Patellar Tendon Rupture

Patellar tendon rupture is more common in patients younger than 40 years with a history of patellar tendonitis or steroid injections. This injury often occurs after forceful contraction of the quadriceps muscle. On physical examination, patients will have a defect inferior to the patella and an inability to extend the knee. On lateral radiograph, a high or low riding patella may be seen. Treatment consists of knee immobilization and orthopedic consultation for operative repair.

Quadriceps Tendon Rupture

Quadriceps tendon rupture is more common in individuals older than 40 years after sudden contraction of the quadriceps muscle (landing after a jump). Symptoms include sharp pain at the proximal knee with ambulation. If the tear is complete, the patient may be unable to extend the flexed knee. There may be a palpable defect, with tenderness and swelling at the suprapatellar region with distal migration of the patella. Radiographs are useful in excluding a patellar or femoral avulsion fracture. Treatment consists of knee immobilization and orthopedic consultation for possible operative repair.

Achilles Tendon Rupture

Rupture of the Achilles tendon occurs with forceful plantar flexion of the foot. Risk factors include rheumatoid arthritis, lupus, quinolone antibiotics, previous steroid injections of the Achilles, and poor athletic conditioning. The diagnosis is made clinically with a positive Thompson test (no plantar flexion of the foot with squeezing of the calf) and inability to toe walk. Treatment includes splinting in plantar flexion, non-weight bearing, analgesics, elevation, and referral to an orthopedist for possible surgical repair.

Ligamentous Injuries

Anterior cruciate ligament injuries often result from a deceleration, hyperextension, or internal rotation of the tibia on the femur. Patients often will report hearing a "pop," and marked swelling may occur minutes to hours after the injury. The Lachman test is the most sensitive test for anterior cruciate ligament injuries. Other tests include the anterior drawer test and the lateral pivot shift test.

Isolated posterior cruciate ligament injuries are rare. The mechanism of injury is usually an anterior-to-posterior force applied to the tibia or lower leg. Injuries to this ligament are examined with the posterior drawer test.

Injuries to the medial collateral ligament and medial capsular structures are investigated by abduction (or valgus) stress testing with the knee in 30° of flexion. If instability exists in flexion, the test should be repeated in full extension (if possible). Medial instability in full extension indicates a severe lesion involving the cruciate ligaments and posterior capsule.

Injuries to the lateral collateral ligament and the lateral capsule are investigated by adduction (or varus) stress testing with the knee in 30° of flexion. If instability exists in flexion, then the test should be repeated in full extension (if possible). Lateral instability in full extension indicates a severe lesion involving the cruciate ligaments and the posterolateral corner of the capsule. Perineal nerve injuries may be associated with lateral injuries.

Although most ligamentous injuries present with hemarthrosis, serious ligamentous injuries may present with minimal pain and no hemarthrosis due to disruption of the capsule. Treatment of most ligamentous injuries consists of knee immobilization, ice, elevation, analgesics, and referral to an orthopedist. For severe ligamentous injuries with an unstable knee, immediate orthopedic consultation may be prudent to plan for operative intervention.

Meniscal Injuries

Cutting, squatting, or twisting maneuvers may cause injury to a meniscus. The medial meniscus is injured more often than the lateral meniscus. Symptoms of meniscal injuries include painful locking of the knee, a popping or clicking sensation, or a sensation of the knee giving out. The McMurray test and other tests for meniscal injuries are not sensitive. Definitive diagnosis can be made by outpatient magnetic resonance imaging or arthroscopy. Treatment of meniscal injuries includes knee immobilization, analgesics, ice, elevation, and orthopedic referral.

OVERUSE INJURIES

Patellar Tendonitis

This condition, known as "jumper's knee," presents with pain over the patellar tendon that is exacerbated when running up hills or standing from a sitting position. Treatment consists of ice, nonsteroidal anti-inflammatory drugs, and quadriceps-strengthening exercises.

Chondromalacia Patellae

This condition is caused by patellofemoral malalignment, which places lateral stress on the articular cartilage. It is most common in young, active women and presents with anterior knee pain that worsens with stair climbing or rising from a sitting position. Diagnosis is assisted with the patellar compression test and the apprehension test. Treatment includes rest, nonsteroidal anti-inflammatory drugs, and quadriceps-strengthening exercises.

Shin Splints

Shin splints present with pain over the anterior or lateral tibia on exertion. Radiographs are helpful in excluding a stress fracture. Treatment includes cessation of the activity for 2 to 3 weeks.

For further reading in *Emergency Medicine: A Comprehensive Study Guide,* 6th ed., see
Chap. 274, "Knee Injuries," by Mark T. Steele and Jeffrey N. Glaspy; and Chap. 275, "Leg Injuries," by Paul R. Heller.

176 | Ankle and Foot Injuries

Michael C. Wadman

Ankle and foot injuries usually require conservative management to ensure a good outcome. Certain injuries, however, may result in long-term pain and disability if not evaluated and managed appropriately.

ANKLE INJURIES

LIGAMENTOUS SPRAINS

Clinical Features

Sprains result from abnormal motion of the talus within the mortise, leading to stretching or disruption of the ligaments. Typically, the patient is able to bear weight immediately after the injury, with subsequent increase in pain and swelling as the patient continues to ambulate. Physical examination shows tenderness and swelling over the involved ligament, with a corresponding lack of tenderness over the bony prominences of the ankle. The lateral ankle is injured more frequently, with the anterior talofibular ligament the most commonly injured ligament. Isolated sprain of the medial deltoid ligament is rare, and an associated fibular fracture or syndesmotic ligament injury may be present.

Diagnosis and Differential

To exclude other injuries, evaluation of the injured ankle begins with examination of the joints above and below the injury. The Achilles tendon should be palpated for tenderness or a defect and the Thompson test (squeeze the calf while observing for resultant plantar flexion) should be performed. The proximal fibula should be palpated for tenderness resulting from a Maisonneuve fracture or fibulotibialis ligament tear. The fibula should be squeezed toward the tibia to evaluate for syndesmotic ligament injury. Also, the calcaneus, tarsals, and the base of the fifth metatarsal should be palpated to evaluate for foot fractures causing ankle pain that may not be readily apparent on standard ankle radiography. For the ankle, the active and passive ranges of motion should be assessed, with any discrepancy suggesting a soft tissue injury. The posterior aspects of the medial and lateral malleoli should be palpated from 6 cm proximally to the distal tips. If tenderness is isolated to the posterior aspect of the lateral malleolus, then a peroneal tendon subluxation may be present. If the examination is normal and the patient is able to ambulate with normal weight transfer, then a clinically significant fracture is unlikely.

The Ottawa Ankle Rules (Fig. 176-1) are simple guidelines that have been validated extensively in numerous clinical trials. When applied properly, they can help the emergency physician identify a subset of patients who can be safely treated without undergoing radiographic studies.

The classification of ankle sprains most clinically useful in emergency practice describes injuries as stable and potentially unstable or unstable. Instability is suspected based on physical examination and radiography. The examiner may perform the anterior drawer and talar tilt tests to assess stability. While holding the distal tibia, the examiner grasps the posterior heel and attempts to move it anteriorly. Any movement greater than 5 mm in relation to

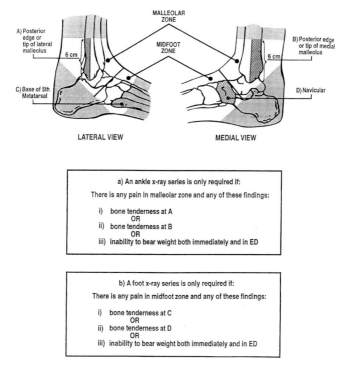

FIG. 176-1.   Ottawa Ankle Rules for ankle and midfoot injuries.
Key: ED = emergency department.

the uninjured side is a positive test for instability. Likewise, relative movement greater than 10° is considered a positive talar tilt test. If the examiner is unable to perform reliable stress testing due to excessive swelling or pain, then the injury is considered potentially unstable. Radiographically, any asymmetry in the gap between the talar dome and the malleoli on the talus view suggests joint instability.

Emergency Department Care and Disposition

1. Initial treatment consists of **rest, ice, compression, and elevation (RICE)** for 24 to 72 hours and analgesics. The patient with a stable joint and the ability to easily bear weight needs only analgesics, an elastic compression bandage, and a 1-week follow-up if the pain persists.
2. If unable to bear weight, the patient with a stable joint may benefit from an **ankle brace** (allowing dorsoplantar flexion while preventing eversion or inversion) and a 1-week follow-up for repeat examination.
3. Patients with unstable joints should be immobilized in a **posterior splint** and referred to an orthopedist.

FRACTURES

Emergency department decision making is facilitated by the Henderson scheme, which groups ankle fractures into 3 classifications based on radiologic appearance: unimalleolar, bimalleolar, and trimalleolar. Bimalleolar and trimalleolar fractures usually require open reduction and internal fixation. Emergency department care includes posterior splinting, elevation, and ice application while initiating appropriate consultation for definitive treatment. Unimalleolar fractures are usually treated with posterior splinting, non–weight bearing, and orthopedic follow-up. Minimally displaced, small (<3 mm) avulsion factures of the fibula are treated like ankle sprains.

Open fractures require wet sterile dressing coverage, splinting, administration of tetanus toxoid, as necessary, and a first-generation cephalosporin (eg, cefazolin 1 g intravenously). If gross contamination is noted, tetanus immunoglobulin and an aminoglycoside (eg, gentamicin) should be added to the treatment regimen.

DISLOCATIONS

Ankle dislocations most commonly occur in the posterior plane and frequently involve associated fractures. Most dislocations are treated urgently by an orthopedist, but the absence of dorsalis pedis or posterior tibial pulses and a cool, dusky foot require immediate reduction by the examining physician. Reduction is performed by applying longitudinal traction on the heel and foot and rotation opposite that of the mechanism of injury while an assistant stabilizes the proximal leg. Longitudinal traction is then applied with rotation in the direction opposite of the mechanism of injury followed by postreduction neurovascular examination, radiographic evaluation, and orthopedic consultation.

FOOT INJURIES

Clinical Features

Foot injuries most commonly result from direct or twisting forces, with twisting-type mechanisms resulting in more minor avulsion-type injuries. Physical examination begins with an assessment of the ankle as outlined previously, followed by inspection and palpation of the Achilles tendon, calcaneus, dorsum of the midfoot, metatarsals, and phalanges, with special attention to the base of the fifth metatarsal and the area over the base of the second metatarsal.

Diagnosis and Differential

A normal physical examination combined with the ability to easily transfer weight while ambulating essentially excludes fracture. Abnormal findings mandate a standard 3-view foot radiographic series and an additional axial calcaneal view for tenderness about the heel. Computed tomography may best define a subtle diastasis at the Lisfranc joint.

Acute Soft Tissue Injuries

Open soft tissue injuries to the foot, such as gunshot wounds to the foot and lawnmower injuries, commonly involve extensive soft tissue damage that requires consultation and operative debridement.

Crush Injuries and Compartment Syndrome

A crushed foot that becomes tensely swollen and is associated with complaints of pain out of proportion to physical examination findings suggests the possibility of compartment syndrome. Typically, pain is not relieved by elevation of the foot and is increased with passive dorsiflexion of the great toe. Distal neurovascular examination may yield normal results. Diagnosis is made by measurement of intracompartmental pressure.

Hindfoot Injuries

Small avulsion fractures of the talus usually are treated with posterior splinting and orthopedic follow-up. Major fractures of the talar neck and body and subtalar dislocations require immediate orthopedic consultation. Calcaneus fractures frequently result when a patient falls from a height and may accompany other fractures of the lower extremities and vertebral column. Compression fractures of the calcaneus may result in subtle radiographic findings that require the measurement of the Böhler angle (formed at the intersection of a line along the superior cortex of the body of the calcaneus with a line from the dome to the anterior tubercle on the lateral view) to improve diagnostic accuracy. An angle smaller than 20° increases the likelihood of fracture. Treatment consists of posterior splinting, elevation, analgesics, and orthopedic consultation.

Midfoot Injuries

Tarsal bones fractures are uncommon and treated conservatively. Isolated fractures of the cuboid and cuneiforms suggest injury to the Lisfranc joint (the ligamentous tarsometatarsal complex). Most Lisfranc joint injuries are associated with a fracture, especially the base of the second metatarsal. Point tenderness over the midfoot and laxity between the first and second metatarsals in a dorsal-to-plantar direction suggest the diagnosis. On the plain anteroposterior radiograph of the foot, a gap wider than 1 mm between the bases of the first and second metatarsals is diagnostic, but computed tomography is the imaging modality of choice. All Lisfranc joint injuries require orthopedic consultation for possible open reduction and internal fixation.

Forefoot

Most nondisplaced metatarsal shaft fractures need only conservative management, with the exception of keeping fractures of the first metatarsal non–weight bearing. Displaced shaft fractures of the middle metatarsals are treated with closed reduction and cast immobilization, whereas displaced fracture of the first metatarsal usually requires open reduction and internal fixation. Fifth metatarsal fractures, including the pseudo-Jones avulsion fractures at the tuberosity of the metatarsal base, are likewise treated conservatively. The true Jones fracture (transverse fracture at the fifth metatarsal base) is frequently complicated by non-union and is treated in a non–weight-bearing cast and orthopedic follow-up.

Phalangeal fractures, if nondisplaced, are easily treated with buddy taping and a stiff-sole cast shoe. Displaced fractures and dislocations are treated with digital block, reduction by manual traction, and buddy taping.

For further reading in *Emergency Medicine: A Comprehensive Study Guide,* 6th ed., see Chap. 276, "Ankle Injuries," and Chap. 277, "Foot Injuries," by John A. Michael and Ian G. Stiell.

177 | Compartment Syndromes

Gary M. Gaddis

Compartment syndromes may lead to muscle necrosis and are caused by continued elevated pressures within the closed tissue space of one or more anatomic muscle compartments.

CLINICAL FEATURES

Elevated pressure in a muscle compartment compromises blood flow to that compartment's muscle(s). This may cause muscle and nerve necrosis if pressures are sufficiently great for a long enough time. Elevated compartment pressure can be caused by decreased compartment size or distensibility, increased compartment volume, or both. Constrictive dressings, casts, and decreased tissue compliance due to thermal injury or frostbite can decrease available compartment size. Increased compartment volume may be due to edema or hemorrhage within the compartment after blunt or penetrating injuries. Virtually any muscle mass enclosed by fascia may be at risk for the development of a compartment syndrome. Compartment syndromes are more common in anatomic regions where there is relatively less ability to expand due to bony or dense connective tissue boundaries, such as the anterior and lateral compartments of the leg.

Conscious patients who develop compartment syndromes usually experience deep, severe, constant, poorly localized pain over the involved muscle compartment. Palpation of the affected compartment, active contraction, or passive stretching of muscles in the affected compartments will exacerbate the pain. Hypoesthesia can appear shortly after the onset of pain when elevated compartment pressures compromise neurologic function. Sensory changes precede motor weakness or paralysis. Absent pulses, pallor, and excessive coolness are unlikely to appear until well after occurrence of pain and neurologic compromise. Muscle necrosis and permanent posttraumatic muscle contracture (Volkmann's ischemia) are the end result of an untreated compartment syndrome.

DIAGNOSIS AND DIFFERENTIAL

A high index of suspicion for compartment syndrome should exist in any patient with injury to or compression of extremity. Missing the diagnosis of compartment syndrome by attributing pain solely to the other injuries can lead to morbidity. Suspicion of the diagnosis is even more important in unconscious patients because they cannot express that they are in pain.

The mainstay of diagnosis is measurement of compartment pressure. Most muscle compartments normally have pressures lower than 10 mm Hg, and such pressures are often near 0 mm Hg. The presence of an abnormally elevated pressure confirms the diagnosis.

The differential diagnosis for a compartment syndrome would include other causes of pain, such as fracture or hematoma. Other possible neurologic or vascular compromises must be considered when symptoms advance beyond pain only.

848

EMERGENCY DEPARTMENT CARE AND DISPOSITION

Initial stabilization of injuries and measurement of compartment pressures dictate subsequent treatment and disposition. Compartment pressures should be measured by an emergency physician or surgical consultant experienced in the technique.

1. Patients with compartment pressures lower than 10 mm Hg do not require further therapy.
2. Compartment pressures of 15 to 20 mm Hg require reevaluation in 12 to 24 hours, with serial compartment pressure measurements in persistently symptomatic patients. Clinical judgment must be exercised with regard to whether to discharge patients based on their likelihood to follow discharge instruction and return for close follow-up.
3. Compartment pressures higher than 20 mm Hg can compromise capillary blood flow; these patients require **hospital admission or surgical consultation** because persistent pressures in this range can damage nerve and muscle.
4. Compartment pressures higher than 30 to 40 mm Hg place nerve and muscle at risk for necrosis and are grounds for **immediate fasciotomy.** Ice cooling and limb elevation should be avoided because both techniques can decrease perfusion to muscle. Bedrest and serial neurovascular checks are the conservative treatments when immediate fasciotomy is not indicated. The goal of treatment is the avoidance of muscle necrosis, rhabdomyolysis, and nerve damage in the affective areas.

For further reading in *Emergency Medicine: A Comprehensive Study Guide,* 6th ed., see Chap. 278, "Compartment syndromes," by Paul Haller.

178 | Rhabdomyolysis

Gary M. Gaddis

Rhabdomyolysis syndromes involve skeletal muscle injury and necrosis, followed by release of intracellular contents, most notably myoglobin (which leads to nephrotoxicity) and skeletal muscle biomarker enzymes, such as creatine phosphokinase (CPK). Rhabdomyolysis is most strongly associated with alcohol and drug abuse, trauma, strenuous physical activity, heat-related illness, toxin ingestion, and certain infections.

CLINICAL FEATURES

A patient's history compatible with risk factors for this illness should increase suspicion for rhabdomyolysis syndromes because classic signs of rhabdomyolysis may be absent in up to 50% of cases.

Historical clues that strongly suggest the patient may be at risk for rhabdomyolysis include:

1. Recent immobility with probable prolonged muscle compression or abnormally increased muscular activity due to drug intoxication (such as after alcohol, cocaine, amphetamine, or phencyclidine [PCP] use).
2. Unaccustomed muscular activity such as strenuous exercise by those with poor fitness (especially when done in the heat), seizures, dystonia, or delirium tremens.
3. Electrical or lightning injury.
4. Injuries that might cause compartment syndromes and/or prolonged muscular compression, such as traumatic crush injuries, heat stroke, and acutely casted long bone fractures.
5. Diseases such as sickle cell disease, dermatomyositis, and polymyositis.

Classically, rhabdomyolysis syndromes are of acute onset, and patients present with myalgias, muscle stiffness, weakness, malaise, and low-grade fever. Dark urine is expected when significant myoglobinuria occurs. These classic findings may be absent in up to 50% of patients with rhabdomyolysis syndromes. Nonspecific symptoms such as nausea, vomiting, abdominal pain, palpitations, and mental status changes due to acute uremia may be present.

Most commonly, muscles involved are the postural muscles of the calves, thighs, and lower back. Involved muscles are often tender to palpation, but observable swelling of these muscles may be subtle or absent until the patient is rehydrated. Muscle involvement may be localized or diffuse.

Complications of rhabdomyolysis are numerous. Acute renal failure (ARF), which may be oliguric (most commonly) or nonoliguric, is the most serious complication. Up to 10% of ARFs may be due to rhabdomyolysis. Ferrihemate, a breakdown product of myoglobin, is nephrotoxic. The probability of ARF with rhabdomyolysis is not directly related to the degree of elevation of CPK or with the degree of myoglobinuria. However, the degree of elevation of CPK correlates with the extent of muscular injury. Hypovolemia and aciduria (pH <5.6) potentiate ARF. Hyperkalemia may be present due to myonecrosis or ARF. Hyperuricemia is common with crush injuries. Phosphate levels initially rise with myo-cellular injury and then fall. Hypocalcemia is common early in rhabdomyolysis due to precipitation with anions such as phosphate; subsequently, hypercalcemia is common. Peripheral neuropathy may accompany compartment syndromes consequent to muscle swelling, and disseminated intravascular coagulation may occur in severe rhabdomyolysis syndromes.

DIAGNOSIS AND DIFFERENTIAL

A 5-fold or greater increase of serum CPK above the upper limit of normal level is the hallmark for the diagnosis of rhabdomyolysis. The CPK-MB fraction, originating primarily in cardiac muscle, should not exceed 5% of the total CPK value. In general, serum CPK levels rise 2 to 12 hours after muscle injury. Peak levels occur in 24 to 72 hours and then decline about 39% per day thereafter. If CPK levels fail to fall in this manner, ongoing muscular necrosis should be suspected.

Myoglobin released after muscle necrosis will be present in the urine if plasma concentrations exceed 1.5 mg/dL. Reddish-brown urine is observed at or above about 100 mg/dL of myoglobinuria. Myoglobin contains the heme ring, so it causes positive urine dipstick tests in the absence of microhematuria. Whenever the urine dipstick test is positive and very few or no blood cells are present on microscopic examination, rhabdomyolysis should be suspected. Radioimmunoassays are sensitive for the presence of myoglobinuria but are not required for the diagnosis. Serum myoglobin levels may return to normal within 1 to 6 hours of injury, so the absence of myoglobinuria or myoglobinemia does not rule out the diagnosis of rhabdomyolysis.

Patients with suspected rhabdomyolysis should have serum electrolytes (especially potassium), blood urea nitrogen, creatinine, calcium, phosphorus, and uric acid levels checked. Urinalysis and a complete blood count should be obtained. A disseminated intravascular coagulation profile should be obtained when rhabdomyolysis is confirmed or strongly suspected. Magnetic resonance imaging with gadolinium enhancement occasionally may be useful to localize the site of rhabdomyolysis and to direct treatment of underlying causes when the site of myonecrosis may be unclear.

The differential diagnosis includes other causes of muscle ischemia or pain, such as sickle cell disease, toxin exposures, inflammatory myopathies, and infectious myalgias.

EMERGENCY DEPARTMENT CARE AND DISPOSITION

1. Rehydration is the mainstay of therapy. Volume deficits should be corrected with intravenous **(IV) normal saline (NS) or 5% dextrose (D_5) in NS** to maintain a urine output of at least 2 mL/kg/h. This generally initially requires approximately 2.5 mL/kg/h of crystalloid infusion after an initial 1- to 2-L bolus of NS; this bolus should be initiated by paramedics before arrival to the hospital. Solutions containing potassium or lactate should be avoided.
2. Cardiac monitoring is required. Electrolyte derangements are common, especially hyperkalemia and hypocalcemia. Invasive hemodynamic monitoring to prevent fluid overload may be prudent for patients with significant cardiac or renal disease. A Foley catheter is required to monitor urine output.
3. Serial measurements of urinary pH, venous pH, electrolytes, CPK, calcium, phosphorus, serum urea nitrogen, and creatinine must be performed.

4. The use of **sodium bicarbonate** (1 mEq/kg IV bolus) should be considered. A bicarbonate infusion can be prepared by adding 2 or 3 ampules of sodium bicarbonate to 1 L of D_5W solution and then initiating an infusion rate of 100 mL/h. The target, a urine pH above 6.5, may be associated with decreased renal injury via decreased ferriheme production, but hypocalcemia can be exacerbated by bicarbonate administration.

5. **Diuresis** can be enhanced by **20% mannitol** after fluid replacement, although no controlled studies exist to support its theoretical benefit. If used, the initial dose is 25 g followed by 5 g/h; an alternate regimen is to administer an initial dose of 1 g/kg over 30 minutes. Mannitol should be administered only after sufficient volume replacement has occurred and oliguria is absent. Use of loop diuretics such as furosemide has become controversial because loop diuretics acidify the urine, whereas mannitol does not.

6. Hyperkalemia should be treated to prevent cardiac complications. **Sodium polystyrene sulfate** (15-25 g orally with 50 mL sorbitol or 20 g rectally in 200 mL 20% sorbitol) is often effective. **Sodium bicarbonate** and **calcium chloride** (10 mL over 10-20 minutes) should be used to treat or prevent cardiac toxicity. **Glucose** (D_{50}, 1 ampule IV) and **insulin** (5–10 U regular insulin IV) may be less effective with rhabdomyolysis than with other causes of hyperkalemia. **Dialysis** is a viable treatment option when hyperkalemia is accompanied by renal insufficiency or failure.

7. For hypocalcemia, calcium chloride (10 mL) is seldom required unless profound signs and symptoms of this disorder occur.

8. Hypercalcemia can be treated by furosemide (20-40 mg IV) and saline infusion.

9. Hyperphosphatemia merits oral phosphate binders such as **sodium polystyrene sulfonate** (dosed as above) when serum levels exceed 7 mg/dL.

10. Hypophosphatemia should be treated if serum levels fall below 1 mg/dL. Phosphate salts can be infused with the crystalloid solution.

11. All patients with rhabdomyolysis require hospital admission to a monitored bed. In addition to treatment of the underlying etiology of the disease, a nephrology consultation should be obtained for all cases of renal insufficiency or failure.

For further reading in *Emergency Medicine: A Comprehensive Study Guide,* 6th ed., see Chap. 279, "Rhabdomyolysis," by Francis L. Counselman.

21 | NONTRAUMATIC MUSCULOSKELETAL DISORDERS

179 | Neck and Thoracolumbar Pain

Thomas K. Swoboda

Neck and back pain are common complaints for patients presenting to the emergency department. Causes of these symptoms are numerous, including trauma, degenerative disease, infection, neoplasms, inflammatory processes, congenital malformations, and psychiatric conditions.

CLINICAL FEATURES

A thorough history that includes symptom duration and location, neurologic complaints, systemic complaints, history of trauma, and family history will help determine the severity of the condition causing the pain. In all patients with neck and back pain, it is important to discern patients with localized pain arising from muscles, joints, and ligaments from those patients with neurologic symptoms consistent with a neuropathy, radiculopathy (symptoms associated with a single nerve root), or a myelopathy (symptoms associated with a cord lesion, stenosis, or compression). Most patients with neck and back pain often complain of localized stiffness and limited range of motion. Commonly they have one position that will exacerbate symptoms and another position that relieves symptoms.

A physical examination must include a thorough musculoskeletal examination and focused neurologic examination to identify causes that are life threatening or associated with permanent disability. Patients with neck pain may not have localized tenderness. When the pain radiates in a dermatomal pattern down the shoulder and arm, the patient has a cervical radiculopathy. Local neurogenic symptoms and signs such as sensory changes, motor weakness, reflex changes, or loss of coordination also may be noted. Systemic neurologic findings (such as hyperreflexia or Babinski sign) with sexual or sphincter dysfunction may be noted in cervical myelopathy.

Pain originating from the thoracic spine is less common than pain from cervical or lumbar regions. Localized pain and tenderness may not be present during examination. Resulting radicular pain in the chest or abdomen is more common. Neurologic findings consistent with spinal cord pathology are rare but require further workup, particularly for metastatic disease.

Pain from the lumbosacral area can result from musculoskeletal, neurogenic, and more remote causes. Localized bony and muscle pain or local percussion tenderness suggests a musculoskeletal etiology. Radicular pain can be seen with musculoskeletal and neurologic causes. Neurologic deficits are the result of spinal or extraspinal causes. Systemic complaints such as fever, chills, night sweats, and malaise in association with abnormal abdominal, neurologic, or rectal examinations are highly indicative of a life-threatening or permanently disabling extraspinal cause.

DIAGNOSIS AND DIFFERENTIAL

A thorough history and review of symptoms are essential when developing a differential diagnosis. Patients younger than 18 years and older than 50 years have a greater likelihood for a serious cause of neck or back pain. Duration of symptoms, pain location, trauma history, neurologic symptoms, systemic symptoms, and specific pain features, such as factors that alleviate or worsen the pain, are important features to ascertain.

In patients presenting with acute trauma, understanding the mechanism of injury is essential in determining severity of the injury. While resuscitating the trauma patient, a focused examination identifying any neurologic deficit after the ABCs is required. Particular attention must be paid to areas where there is bony tenderness, crepitus, stepoff, or complaints of pain from the patient. Radiographic imaging of the spine should be obtained, as warranted. In stable patients with a history consistent with a nontraumatic cause, a complete examination can be performed before any imaging is considered.

In patients with cervical pain, active and passive movements of the neck should be assessed, with any limited or painful movements noted. Techniques to test for radicular symptoms such as the *Spurling sign* (gentle pressure applied to the patient's head during extension with lateral rotation) and the *abduction relief sign* (relief of symptoms by having the patient place the hand of the affected extremity on top of the head) also should be done. An examination of distal upper extremity pulses and a thorough neurologic examination of both upper extremities are essential. For patients with previously undiagnosed findings, a 3-view cervical spine radiograph should be performed. Patients with suspected new onset radiculopathy or myelopathy require magnetic resonance imaging (MRI).

In patients with recent trauma, it is important to exclude vertebral fracture. Patients without localized bony spinal tenderness and with normal radiographs or computed tomography (CT) images should be treated for cervical soft tissue injury. These patients may have accompanying nonspecific symptoms such as dizziness, tinnitus, dysphagia, and dysesthesia, but they do not require further studies provided that they have no focal neurologic deficits.

Patients with symptoms of radiculopathy will have neck pain with radiation in a dermatomal pattern. Sensory and motor changes in a dermatomal distribution also may be seen (Table 179-1). It is important to distinguish these symptoms from findings of myelopathy, which are upper extremity hyperreflexia, lower extremity hyperreflexia, positive Babinski sign, or sphincter changes. Patients who have acute cervical disk herniation may have a radiculopathy or myelopathy. Extension and lateral flexion of the neck will worsen radicular symptoms, whereas symptoms of myelopathy will not be affected. MRI or CT myelogram will be required to confirm the diagnosis because cervical radiographs are often negative, even with large disk herniations. Patients with chronic degenerative disk disease may develop cervical spondylosis and progress to spinal stenosis. They can present with a continuum of symptoms ranging from simple pain and stiffness to myelopathy. Metastatic cancer should be considered in patients with chronic neck pain even without a past history of cancer. Unremitting pain at night is highly suggestive of a malignancy. Lung, breast, and prostate cancers and lymphoma and multiple myeloma can involve the cervical spine. Myofascial pain syndrome (MPS) can be confused with radiculopathy. MPS patients have pain in the neck, scapula, and shoulder in a nondermatomal distribution ("trigger point"). MPS patients frequently have psychological distress and personality characteristics causing conversion of emotional distress into complaints of pain.

Direct trauma and hyperflexion injuries frequently cause painful thoracic fractures. Pathologic vertebral body fractures, commonly seen in elderly

TABLE 179-1 Symptoms and Signs of Cervical Radiculopathies

Disk space	Nerve root	Pain complaint	Sensory change	Motor weakness	Altered reflex
C1–2	C1–2	Neck, scalp	Scalp	None	None
C4–5	C5	Neck, shoulder, upper arm	Shoulder, thumb	Spinati, deltoid, biceps	Biceps
C5–6	C6	Neck, shoulder, upper scapula, proximal forearm, thumb	Thumb, index finger, lateral forearm	Deltoid, biceps, pronator teres, wrist extensors	Biceps, brachioradialis
C6–7	C7	Neck, posterior arm, dorsal and proximal forearm, chest, medial scapula, middle finger	Middle finger, forearm	Triceps, pronator teres	Triceps
C7–T1	C8	Neck, posterior arm, proximal forearm, medial scapula, medial hand, ring and little fingers	Ring, little fingers	Triceps, flexor carpi ulnaris, hand intrinsic muscles	Triceps

females with osteoporosis, are generally stable. Metastatic lesions to the thoracic spine may present with myelopathy and sphincter changes. CT or MRI can distinguish between disk herniation, vertebral fracture, and metastasis. Osteoarthritis in the thoracic spine can cause radicular pain with localized stiffness. It also can progress to thoracic spinal stenosis. Before the appearance of its characteristics rash, herpes zoster can present with an acute thoracic radiculopathy similar to that seen in osteoarthritis. Diabetic neuropathies can have a similar presentation.

In patients with low back pain, examination of the back, abdomen, rectum, and lower extremities, with a focus on neurologic and vascular components, should be performed. Any signs of lumbar radiculopathies or sciatica (Table 179-2) should be identified. Patients with radicular symptoms that are not severe or progressing rapidly should be scheduled for a nonurgent MRI. Any additional imaging, such as ultrasound or CT of the abdomen or additional laboratory studies, are indicated in patients who have low back pain and other clinical findings. Abdominal aortic aneurysm should always be considered in select patients who present with nonspecific low back pain and an unremarkable musculoskeletal examination.

The vast majority of patients with lumbar back pain do not have symptoms of radiculopathy or myelopathy. Only 1% of all patients with back pain have sciatica, most commonly caused by disk herniation, although it can be caused by intraspinal tumor, infection, foraminal stenosis, or epidural compression. Patients with sciatica generally complain more about the symptoms associated with the radiculopathy than about any pain in the back. Those patients with sciatica without further risk factors for serious disease do not need further diagnostic workup in the emergency department. Low back and lower extremity pain that occurs when walking and is relieved with rest can be caused by spinal stenosis or peripheral vascular disease. An MRI of the lumbar spine and possibly arteriography may be needed to determine the diagnosis. Patients with low back pain, which is associated neurologic deficits, urinary retention with overflow incontinence, and sciatica in one or both legs have an epidural compression of the spinal cord until proven otherwise. These patients require aggressive evaluation and treatment. Low back pain may be the presenting symptom of several serious intraabdominal conditions including pyelonephritis, peptic ulcer disease, pancreatic disease, diverticulitis, abdominal aortic aneurysm, and pelvic inflammatory disease.

TABLE 179-2 Symptoms and Signs of Lumbar Radiculopathies

Disk space	Nerve root	Pain complaint	Sensory change	Motor weakness	Altered reflex
L2–3	L3	Medial thigh, knee	Medial thigh, knee	Hip flexors	None
L3–4	L4	Medial lower leg	Medial lower leg	Quadriceps	Knee jerk
L4–5	L5	Anterior tibia, great toe	Medial foot	Extensor hallicus longus	Biceps femoris
L5–S1	S1	Calf, little toe	Lateral foot	Foot plantar flexors	Achilles

EMERGENCY DEPARTMENT CARE AND DISPOSITION

1. Any patient with significant trauma or a life- and limb-threatening condition requires aggressive and urgent evaluation, resuscitation, and treatment as appropriate. Patients with suspected epidural compression should be treated with **dexamethasone** (10-100 mg intravenously) before any imaging tests are done. Prompt consultation with appropriate specialists should be obtained. Any patient with intractable pain, signs of progression of neurologic deficits, or myelopathy should be admitted to the hospital.

2. The vast majority of patients can be sent home with medications for symptomatic relief. Treatment with nonsteroidal anti-inflammatory drugs (**ibuprofen** 600 mg 4 times daily or **naproxen** 250-500 mg twice daily) for 5 to 7 days can be started. Patients with renal disease or peptic ulcer disease and the elderly instead should be treated with acetaminophen. A muscle relaxant such as **diazepam** 5 mg 3 times daily also may be helpful. A limited amount of opioid analgesic can be provided for patients with moderate to severe pain. Applications of cold or heat to sore areas also may provide relief.

3. Patients should be encouraged to resume normal activities as quickly as possible. Close follow-up with a primary physician is suggested to monitor for any new neurologic findings.

For further reading in *Emergency Medicine: A Comprehensive Study Guide,* 6th ed., see Chap. 281, "Neck Pain," by William J. Frohna; and Chap. 282, "Thoracic and Lumbar Pain Syndromes," by David Della-Giustina and Marco Coppola.

Andrew D. Perron

Shoulder pain is a common musculoskeletal complaint, especially in patients older than 40 years. Occupational, recreational, and normal daily activities stress the shoulder joint and may result in pain from acute injury or, more commonly, chronic overuse conditions. Complicating the evaluation of shoulder pain is that the origin of pain may be from pathology intrinsic to the shoulder joint or from extrinsic disorders causing referred pain.

CLINICAL FEATURES

The pain of musculoskeletal shoulder pathology often is described by patients as an aching sensation, particularly in the setting of a more chronic process. Nighttime pain is a common feature of intrinsic shoulder pathology. Specific motions may exacerbate it, and this history is helpful in making a specific diagnosis. Decreased range of motion, crepitus, weakness, or muscular atrophy may be associated with certain conditions. Any systemic symptoms (eg, shortness of breath, fever, or radiation of pain from the chest or abdomen) should raise suspicion for extrinsic and potentially life-threatening problems.

DIAGNOSIS AND DIFFERENTIAL

The primary diagnostic maneuver is a thorough history and physical examination. Examination of the shoulder joint should include range of motion and muscle strength testing, palpation for local tenderness or other abnormality, and identification of any neurovascular deficit. Specific tests for impingement and individual tests of rotator cuff muscle function are often helpful in intrinsic disease. Plain radiographic studies of the shoulder joint are rarely diagnostic but may be helpful to exclude bony abnormalities in selected patients or to evaluate for abnormal calcifications. In patients in whom extrinsic causes of shoulder pain are suspected, further diagnostic testing may be indicated, such as laboratory studies, additional radiographs, and an electrocardiogram.

The differential diagnosis includes a variety of intrinsic musculoskeletal disorders, and individual patients may exhibit considerable overlap in their symptoms manifesting a combination of specific conditions. *Impingement syndrome* is a term that has been adopted to encompass many painful shoulder syndromes that result most frequently from repetitive overhead use of the arm. The pathologic entities included in this syndrome are subacromial tendonitis and bursitis, supraspinatus tendonitis, rotator cuff tendonitis, and the painful arc syndrome. Impingement syndrome is a painful overuse condition characterized by positive findings with impingement testing and relief of pain with anesthetic injection of the subacromial space. *Subacromial bursitis* is generally seen in patients younger than 25 years and will present with positive impingement tests with different degrees of tenderness at the lateral proximal humerus or in the subacromial space. *Rotator cuff tendonitis* is distinguished by an incidence primarily in individuals 25 to 40 years of age and findings of tenderness of the rotator cuff with mild to moderate muscular weakness. In more chronic disease, crepitus, decreased range of motion, and osteophyte formation visible on plain radiograph also may be apparent. *Ro-*

tator cuff tears occur primarily in patients older than 40 years and are associated with muscular weakness (especially with abduction and external rotation) and cuff tenderness. Ninety percent will be chronic tears with a history of minimal or no trauma; in severe disease, muscular atrophy may be present. Acute tears may occur in patients of any age and result from significant force producing a tearing sensation with immediate pain and disability. In patients between the ages of 30 and 50 years, abnormal calcifications on x-ray in the clinical setting of a painful shoulder with rotator cuff tenderness and often crepitus suggest the diagnosis of calcific tendonitis. *Osteoarthritis* is characteristically associated with degenerative disease in other joints (primary) or previous fracture or other underlying disorder (secondary). The hallmark of *adhesive capsulitis* is significantly painful and limited range of motion often, but not always, associated with a period of immobilization. Radiographs should be obtained to exclude posterior glenohumeral dislocation.

Other causes of shoulder pain that should be considered are a number of extrinsic conditions. *Pancoast tumor* may compress the brachial plexus and thus manifest itself as shoulder pain. *Degenerative disease of the cervical spine, brachial plexus disorders, and suprascapular nerve compression* are neurologic processes that should be sought in patient evaluation. Vascular pathology, notably *axillary artery thrombosis,* also may cause shoulder pain. Acute cardiac, aortic, pulmonary, and abdominal pathology may cause pain referred to the shoulder, and the clinician must remain alert to this possibility.

EMERGENCY DEPARTMENT CARE AND DISPOSITION

1. For intrinsic disease, the primary goals of emergency department care are to reduce pain and inflammation and prevent progression of disease. For most conditions, this translates to relative rest of the joint assisted by use of a sling (full immobilization is not suggested), **nonsteroidal anti-inflammatory drugs,** opioid analgesics as needed, and the application of cold packs. Range-of-motion exercises should be encouraged as soon as pain allows to prevent loss of flexibility and maintain strength.

2. **Joint space injection** with glucocorticoids (eg, triamcinolone 20-40 mg) with or without a local anesthetic such as lidocaine should be used judiciously in view of the potential deleterious effects on soft tissues, tendon rupture with direct injection, and a recommended limitation of 3 injections into a single area. For all intrinsic disorders, follow-up with a primary care physician with expertise in joint disease or orthopedic referral is suggested within 7 to 14 days. Physical therapy referral for stretching and strengthening also may be valuable.

3. In extrinsic disease, the treatment and referral pattern will depend on the diagnosis. Neurologic problems will require analgesia and anti-inflammatory medications and may require neurology or neurosurgical follow up. Vascular causes of shoulder pain must be evaluated carefully and, with axillary artery thrombosis, immediate consultation made to initiate thrombolysis. Treatment of other extrinsic conditions depends on the specific diagnosis.

For further reading in *Emergency Medicine: A Comprehensive Study Guide,* 6th ed., see Chap. 283, "Shoulder Pain," by David Della-Giustina, Benjamin Harrison, and D. Monte Hunter.

181 | Acute Disorders of the Joints and Bursae

Andrew D. Perron

Acute disorders of the joints and bursae are common emergency conditions that involve a wide spectrum of ages, acuities, and etiologies. Mismanagement of certain pathologic entities can lead to significant morbidity for the patient.

CLINICAL FEATURES

Multiple pathways can cause disruption of the normal joint milieu leading to acute joint complaints. These pathways include degeneration of articular cartilage (osteoarthritis), deposition of immune complexes (rheumatoid arthritis), crystal-induced inflammation (gout and pseudogout), seronegative spondyloarthropathies (ankylosing spondylitis and Reiter's syndrome), and bacterial and viral invasion (septic arthritis). These pathologic events invariably lead to pain, the most common complaint of patients with a joint problem. Important historical factors to elicit include a determination of previous joint or bursal disease; presence of constitutional symptoms; and whether the pain is acute, chronic, or acute on chronic. Determining the number and distribution of joints affected can help narrow the differential diagnosis (Table 181-1).

On physical examination, arthritis should be distinguished from more focal periarticular inflammatory processes such as cellulitis, bursitis, and tendonitis. True arthritis produces joint pain exacerbated by active and passive motions.

DIAGNOSIS AND DIFFERENTIAL

The most useful tool for evaluation of joint disorders in the emergency department is evaluation of synovial fluid, which routinely should be sent for culture, Gram stain, cell count, and crystal evaluation (Table 181-2). Except in pediatric septic arthritis, where the erythrocyte sedimentation rate has been shown to have a 90% sensitivity, the serum white blood cell count and erythrocyte sedimentation rate lack the sensitivity and specificity to be reliable discriminators in disorders of the joints and bursae.

Radiographs should be obtained when the differential diagnosis includes trauma, tumor, osteomyelitis, ankylosing spondylitis, or avascular necrosis. More sophisticated modalities such as computed tomography, magnetic resonance imaging, and radioisotope scanning are used in isolated cases.

EMERGENCY DEPARTMENT CARE AND DISPOSITION OF SPECIFIC CONDITIONS

Septic arthritis is a condition that can rapidly lead to irreversible joint destruction if inadequately treated. It typically presents as a monoarticular arthritis and may be associated with fever, chills, or malaise, although absence of these symptoms does not exclude the diagnosis. The synovial fluid confirms the diagnosis. Therapy requires admission for parenteral antibiotics

TABLE 181-1 Classification of Arthritis by Number of Affected Joints

Number of joints	Differential considerations
1 = Monoarthritis	Trauma-induced arthritis
	Infection/septic arthritis
	Crystal-induced (gout, pseudogout)
	Osteoarthritis (acute)
	Lyme disease
	Avascular necrosis
	Tumor
2–3 = Oligoarthritis	Lyme disease
	Reiter syndrome
	Ankylosing spondylitis
	Gonococcal arthritis
	Rheumatic fever
>3 = Polyarthritis	Rheumatoid arthritis
	Systemic lupus erythematosus
	Viral arthritis
	Osteoarthritis (chronic)

and repeated needle aspiration, arthroscopy, or open surgical drainage. Specific patient demographics can help guide empiric antibiotic therapy in septic arthritis (Table 181-3).

Traumatic hemarthrosis is associated with intraarticular fracture or ligamentous injury. Aspiration of large effusions may decrease pain and increase range of motion. Treatment is supportive. Spontaneous hemarthrosis may be associated with coagulopathies requiring specific clotting factor replacement. It is usually not recommended to aspirate spontaneous hemarthroses.

Crystal-induced synovitis generally affects middle-age to elderly patients. Gout (uric acid crystals) typically affects the great toe, tarsal joints, and knee, whereas pseudogout (calcium pyrophosphate crystals) typically affects the knee, wrist, ankle, and elbow. Pain with gout usually evolves over hours, whereas the pain associated with pseudogout occurs over a day or more. Either condition may be precipitated by trauma, surgery, significant illness, dietary or alcohol indiscretions, or certain medications. The synovial fluid is inflammatory with negative birefringent needle-shaped (gout) or weakly positive birefringent rhomboid (pseudogout) crystals. Treatment is with nonsteroidal anti-inflammatory drugs (eg, oral indomethacin 50 mg 3 times daily for 3 to 5 days) and opioid analgesics. Although not routinely necessary, colchicine (0.6 mg/h orally until resolution of symptoms or intolerable gastrointestinal side effects) may be used as a complementary therapy.

Osteoarthritis is a chronic, symmetric, polyarticular destruction of joints (including the distal interphalangeal) distinguished by a lack of constitutional symptoms. Patients may present with acute monoarticular exacerbations with small, noninflammatory synovial fluid collections and characteristic joint space narrowing on radiographs. Treatment involves rest and analgesics.

Lyme arthritis is a monoarticular or symmetric oligoarticular arthritis (especially of the large joints) with brief exacerbations followed by complete remission occurring weeks to years after the primary infection. Synovial fluid is inflammatory with usually negative cultures. Treatment with appropriate antibiotics (doxycycline, erythromycin, or amoxicillin) for 3 to 4 weeks is effective.

TABLE 181-2 Examination of Synovial Fluid

	Normal	Noninflammatory	Inflammatory	Septic
Clarity	Transparent	Transparent	Cloudy	Cloudy
Color	Clear	Yellow	Yellow	Yellow
WBC/μL	<200	<200–2,000	200–50,000	>50,000
PMNs (%)*	<25	<25	>50%	>50%
Culture	Negative	Negative	Negative	>50% positive
Crystals	None	None	Multiple or none	None
Associated conditions		Osteoarthritis, trauma, rehumatic fever	Gout, pseudogout, spondyloarthropathies, RA, Lyme disease, SLE	Nongonococcal or gonococcal septic arthritis

*The WBC and PMNs are affected by a number of factors, including disease progression, affecting organism, and host immune status. The joint aspirate WBC and %PMNs should be considered part of a continuum for each disease, particularly septic arthritis, and should be correlated with other clinical information.

Key: PMN = polymorphonuclear leucocytes, RA = rheumatoid arthritis, SLE = systemic lupus erythematosus, WBC = white blood cell count.

TABLE 181-3 Commonly Encountered Organisms in the Septic Arthritis Patient

Patient/ condition	Expected organisms	Antibiotic considerations
Neonates and infants	*Staphylococcus,* gram-negative bacteria, group B *Streptococcus, Candida*	Nafcillin* plus aminoglycoside or third-generation cephalosporin, ampicillin-sulbactam
Children <5 y	*Staphylococcus, Haemophilus influenzae*	Nafcillin* plus cefuroxime, ampicillin-sulbactam
Older children and healthy adults	*Staphylococcus, Gonococcus, Streptococcus*	Nafcillin* plus third-generation cephalosporin, ampicillin-sulbactam
Involvement of the foot	*Staphylococcus, Pseudomonas*	Nafcillin* plus ceftazidime or aminoglycoside
Intravenous drug users	*Staphylococcus,* gram-negative bacilli	Nafcillin* plus aminoglycoside, ampicillin-sulbactam
Sickle cell patients	*Salmonella*	Ciprofloxacin, ofloxacin, or ceftriaxone

*First-generation cephalosporin may be substituted for penicillinase-resistant penicillin. Vancomycin should be employed for treatment of suspected methicillin-resistant staphylococci.

Gonococcal arthritis is an immune-mediated infectious arthritis that typically affects adolescents and young adults. Fever, chills, and a migratory tenosynovitis or arthralgias typically precede mono- or oligoarthritis. Vesiculopustular lesions on the distal extremities are characteristic. Synovial fluid is usually inflammatory and often culture negative; cultures of the pharynx, urethra, cervix, and rectum increase the culture yield. The patient should be admitted for pain control and parenteral antibiotic therapy. Orthopedic consultation is advised.

Reiter's syndrome is a seronegative reactive spondyloarthropathy characterized by acute asymmetric oligoarthritis (especially of the lower extremities) preceded 2 to 6 weeks by an infectious illness such as urethritis (*Ureaplasma* or *Chlamydia*) or enteric infection (*Salmonella* or *Shigella*). The classic triad of arthritis, conjunctivitis, and urethritis is not required for diagnosis. Synovial fluid is inflammatory. Treatment is symptomatic, and antibiotics have not been found to be useful.

Ankylosing spondylitis is a seronegative spondyloarthropathy that primarily affects the spine and pelvis and may be associated with morning stiffness and constitutional symptoms such as fatigue and weakness. Hereditary predilection (HLA-B27 antigen or absence of rheumatoid factor) is significant. Radiographic findings include sacroiliitis and squaring of the vertebral bodies (bamboo spine). Treatment is symptomatic.

Rheumatoid arthritis is a chronic, symmetric, polyarticular joint disease (with sparing of the distal interphalangeal) associated with morning stiffness, depression, fatigue, and generalized myalgias. Pericarditis, myocarditis, pleural effusion, pneumonitis, and mononeuritis multiplex may occur. Synovial fluid is inflammatory. Treatment of an acute exacerbation involves immobilization, nonsteroidal anti-inflammatory drugs, and, occasionally, corticosteroids. Antimalarials, gold, and methotrexate are used for long-term therapy.

Bursitis refers to an inflammatory process involving any of the more than 150 bursae throughout the human body and may be caused by infection, trauma, rheumatologic diseases, or crystal deposition. Certain repetitive activities also may precipitate bursitis: "carpet layer's knee" (prepatellar bursitis) or "student's elbow" (olecranon bursitis). A suspicion for septic bursitis, especially in olecranon bursitis, necessitates aspiration of bursal fluid. Septic bursal fluid characteristically is purulent in appearance, with more than 15,000 leukocytes/mm3 and positive culture. Treatment principles include drainage, rest, compressive dressing, analgesics, and antibiotics for septic bursitis.

For further reading in *Emergency Medicine: A Comprehensive Study Guide,* 6th ed., see Chap. 286, "Acute Disorders of the Joint and Bursae," by John H. Burton.

182 | Emergencies in Systemic Rheumatic Diseases

Michael P. Kefer

RHEUMATIC EMERGENCIES ASSOCIATED WITH RISK OF MORTALITY

Respiratory System

Death may result from airway obstruction, respiratory muscle failure, or pulmonary tissue involvement.

Airway Obstruction

Relapsing polychondritis presents with the abrupt onset of pain, redness, and swelling of the ears or nose. The tracheobronchial cartilage is involved in approximately 50% of cases. Hoarseness and throat tenderness over the cartilage are noted. Repeated attacks can lead to airway collapse. Treatment of an exacerbation involves administering high-dose steroids and hospital admission for observation.

Rheumatoid arthritis (RA) may involve the cricoarytenoid joints, causing pain with speaking, hoarseness, or stridor. The cricoarytenoid joints may fix in a closed position, which may mandate emergency tracheostomy.

Respiratory Muscle Failure

Dermatomyositis and polymyositis may lead to respiratory failure from respiratory muscle involvement in poorly controlled disease.

Pulmonary Tissue Involvement

Pulmonary hemorrhage complicates Goodpasture disease, systemic lupus erythematosus (SLE), Wegener granulomatosis, and other vasculitic conditions. Pulmonary fibrosis complicates ankylosing spondylitis, scleroderma, and other conditions. Pleural effusion complicates RA and SLE.

Heart

Pericarditis occurs in RA and SLE. Myocardial infarction may occur from coronary artery involvement in Kawasaki disease or polyarteritis nodosa. Pancarditis occurs in acute rheumatic fever. Valvular heart disease occurs in ankylosing spondylitis, relapsing polychondritis, and rheumatic fever. Involvement may extend into the conduction system.

Adrenal Glands

Glucocorticoids are often used in the treatment of rheumatic conditions. Doses required may result in adrenal suppression. As a result, these patients may be unable to respond to the physiologic stress of an acute illness or injury and proceed to develop adrenal insufficiency. In this situation, treatment with stress-dose steroids is indicated.

RHEUMATIC PRESENTATIONS ASSOCIATED WITH RISK OF MORBIDITY

Cervical Spine and Spinal Cord

Patients with rheumatologic involvement of the cervical spine may be at high risk for serious cervical spine or spinal cord injury from otherwise trivial trauma, such as manipulation during endotracheal intubation if extreme caution is not exercised. Ligamentous destruction of the transverse ligament of C2, with resultant symptoms of cord compression, may complicate RA. Cervical spine inflexibility from ankylosing spondylitis predisposes to injury out of proportion to the mechanism. Anterior spinal artery syndrome may result from rheumatologic conditions causing vasculitis, aortic dissection, or embolism.

Eye

Rheumatologic involvement ranges from mild irritation to complete blindness. Temporal arteritis is a cause of sudden blindness and should be considered in any patient older than 50 years who presents with new onset headache, visual change, or jaw or tongue claudication. Laboratory investigation shows an elevated erythrocyte sedimentation rate (>50 mm/h) and C-reactive protein (>2.45 mg/dL). Treatment with prednisone 60 mg/d should be initiated immediately based on clinical and laboratory findings. Temporal artery biopsy for definitive diagnosis must be obtained within the first week of treatment to be accurate.

Dry eyes (and dry mouth) from Sjögren syndrome may occur alone or in combination with many rheumatologic conditions. Episcleritis is a self-limited, painless infection of the episcleral vessels. It is included the differential diagnosis of the red eye in patients with RA. Scleritis is also seen in patients with RA and presents with marked ocular tenderness. The eye has a purple discoloration. The potential for visual impairment and scleral rupture mandate emergent ophthalmologic consult and high-dose steroids.

Hypertension

Hypertension can complicate any rheumatologic condition that affects the kidneys directly, as in polyarteritis nodosa, scleroderma, or SLE, or indirectly from nephrotoxic drugs used to treat the underlying disorder.

Kidney

Renal insult is due to the primary disease process, the drugs used to treat the disease, or both. Nephritis is a common complication of SLE, Wegener granulomatosis, and systemic vasculitis. Renal dysfunction from malignant hypertension occurs with scleroderma. Nephrotic syndrome in patients with SLE predisposes to renal vein thrombosis. Renal insufficiency from prostaglandin inhibition by nonsteroidal anti-inflammatory drugs is more frequent in the elderly. It also may result from rhabdomyolysis in the patient with florid myositis or from sclerosis in the patient with scleroderma.

For further reading in *Emergency Medicine: A Comprehensive Study Guide,* 6th ed., see Chap. 284, "Emergencies in Systemic Rheumatic Diseases," by Richard C. Chandler and Mary Chester Morgan-Wasko.

183 | Infectious and Noninfectious Disorders of the Hand

Michael P. Kefer

Rest and elevation are the mainstays of treatment for many inflammatory conditions of the hand. This method helps to decrease inflammation, avoid secondary injury, and prevent spread of any existing infection. The optimal position for splinting of the hand is the position of function: wrist in 15° extension, metacarpal phalangeal joint in 50° to 90° flexion, proximal interphalangeal joint in 10° to 15° flexion, and distal interphalangeal joint in 10° to 15° flexion.

HAND INFECTIONS

Infections of the hand are often polymicrobial. Skin organisms are frequently involved. Infections from animal bite wounds may be infected with *Pasteurella multocida* and human bite wounds with *Eikenella corrodens*. Abscesses always require surgical drainage. Table 183-1 summarizes the common infections of the hand, the likely organisms involved, and recommended antibiotic therapy.

Cellulitis is a superficial infection presenting with localized warmth, erythema, and edema. The examiner must exclude the involvement of deeper structures by demonstrating absence of tenderness on deep palpation and range of motion of the hand. Emergency department (ED) care consists of antibiotics, splinting in the position of function, elevation, and close follow-up.

Flexor tenosynovitis is diagnosed on examination by the presence of the 4 cardinal signs: (*a*) tenderness over the flexor tendon sheath, (*b*) symmetric swelling of the finger, (*c*) pain with passive extension, and (*d*) flexed position of the involved digit. ED care consists of splinting, elevation, intravenous (IV) antibiotics, and orthopedic consultation for drainage.

Deep space infections involve the web or midpalmar space. Web space infection occurs after penetrating injury to the web space. Clinically, dorsal and volar swelling of the web space with separation of the affected digits is noted. Midpalmar space infection occurs from spread of a flexor tenosynovitis or penetrating wound to the palm causing infection of the radial or ulnar bursa of the hand. ED care of deep space infections consists of splinting, elevation, IV antibiotics, and orthopedic consultation for drainage.

Closed fist injury is essentially a human bite wound to the metacarpal phalangeal joint that results from punching an individual in the teeth. Risk of infection spreading along the extensor tendons is high. Wounds penetrating the skin should be explored, irrigated, and allowed to heal by secondary intention. When inspecting for extensor tendon injury, it is essential to consider the position of the hand at the time of injury. ED care consists of IV antibiotics, splinting, and hand surgery consultation for disposition. Extensor tendon repair is delayed until the risk of infection has passed.

Paronychia is an infection of the lateral nail fold. ED care of a small paronychia consists of inserting a number 11 blade into the nail fold, parallel to the nail, to drain the abscess. In an advanced infection or one where pus is seen beneath the nail, the corner of the paronychia should be incised and the

TABLE 183-1 Initial Antibiotic Coverage for Common Hand Infections

Infection	Initial antibiotic	Likely organisms	Comments
Cellulitis	First-generation cephalosporin (cephalexin) or antistaphylococcal penicillin (amoxicillin/clavulanate, dicloxacillin)	S pyogenes, S aureus	Consider vancomycin for intravenous drug abusers
Felon/paronychia	First-generation cephalosporin (cephalexin) or antistaphylococcal penicillin (amoxicillin/clavulanate, dicloxacillin)	Polymicrobial, S aureus anaerobes	Antibiotics indicated for infections with associated localized cellulitis
Flexor tenosynovitis	β-Lactamase inhibitor (ampicillin/sulbactam) or first-generation cephalosporin (cefazolin) and penicillin	S aureus, streptococci, anaerobes, gram-negatives	Parenteral antibiotics are indicated; consider ceftriaxone for N gonorrhoeae
Deep space infection	β-Lactamase inhibitor (ampicillin/sulbactam) or first-generation cephalosporin (cefazolin) and penicillin	S aureus, streptococci, anaerobes, gram-negatives	Inpatient management
Animal bites (including human)	β-Lactamase inhibitor or first-generation cephalosporin and penicillin	S aureus, streptococci, Eikenella corrodens (human), Pasteurella multocida (cat), anaerobes and gram negatives	All animal bite wounds should receive prophylactic oral antibiotics
Herpetic whitlow	None, unless secondary bacterial contamination is present	Herpes simplex	Consider acyclovir; no surgical drainage is indicated

nail fold lifted. A portion of the nail may have to be removed and packing placed for adequate drainage. Injury to the nail bed should be avoided. The wound should be rechecked in 24 to 48 hours; the packing should be pulled off and warm soaks initiated.

Felon is an infection of the pulp space of the fingertip. Pain results from the accumulation of pus in the fibrous septae of the finger pad. ED care consists of drainage by the lateral approach to protect the neurovascular bundle. An incision should begin 5 mm distal to the distal interphalangeal joint crease and continue just palmar to and parallel with the paronychia, stopping distally at the phalangeal tuft. The incision should be deep enough to extend across the entire finger pad to divide the septae at the bony insertions. Unless there is a pointing abscess, the radial aspect of the index and middle fingers and the ulnar aspect of the thumb and small finger should be avoided. The wound should be packed loosely. The hand should be splinted in the position of function. The wound should be rechecked in 24 to 48 hours; the packing should be pulled off and warm soaks initiated.

Herpetic whitlow is a viral infection of the fingertip involving intracutaneous vesicles. Clinically, it may present similar to a felon. ED care consists of immobilization, elevation, and protection with a dry dressing to prevent autoinoculation and transmission. Antiviral agents may shorten the duration.

NONINFECTIOUS CONDITIONS

Tendonitis and tenosynovitis are usually due to overuse. Examination demonstrates tenderness over the involved tendon. ED care consists of immobilization and nonsteroidal anti-inflammatory drugs (NSAIDs).

Trigger finger is a tenosynovitis of the flexor sheath of the digit and may result in stenosis of the sheath. Impingement and snap release of the tendon occurs as the finger is extended from a flexed position. Steroid injection may be effective in early stages. Definitive treatment is surgery.

De Quervain tenosynovitis involves the extensor pollicis brevis and abductor pollicis tendons. Pain occurs at the radial aspect of the wrist and radiates into the forearm. The Finkelstein test is diagnostic: the patient grasps the thumb in the fist and deviates the hand ulnarly, thereby reproducing the pain. ED care consists of a thumb spica splint, NSAIDs, and referral.

Carpal tunnel syndrome results from compression of the median nerve by the transverse carpal ligament. The cause is usually edema secondary to overuse, pregnancy, or congestive heart failure. Pain in the median nerve distribution of the hand tends to be worse at night. On examination, pain may be reproduced by tapping over the nerve at the wrist (Tinel sign) or by holding the wrist flexed maximally for longer than 1 minute (Phalen sign). Treatments consists of a wrist splint and NSAIDs. Advanced cases require surgical decompression.

Dupuytren contracture results from fibrous changes in the subcutaneous tissues of the palm, which may lead to tethering and joint contractures. Referral to a hand surgeon is indicated.

Ganglion cyst is a cystic collection of synovial fluid within a joint or tendon sheath. Treatment consists of NSAIDs and referral.

For further reading in *Emergency Medicine: A Comprehensive Study Guide,* 6th ed., see Chap. 285, "Nontraumatic Disorders of the Hand," by Mark W. Foure.

184 | Soft Tissue Problems of the Foot

Mark B. Rogers

PLANTAR WARTS

Plantar warts are contagious and caused by the human papillomavirus. The diagnosis is clinical and treatment options exist; however, many lesions spontaneously resorb within 2 years. Referral to a dermatologist or podiatrist is suggested.

ONYCHOCRYPTOSIS (INGROWN TOENAIL)

Clinical Features

Ingrown toenails occur when part of the nail plate penetrates the nail sulcus and subcutaneous tissue. This is most commonly due to the curvature of the nail and often is associated with external trauma or self-treatment. Inflammation, swelling, and infection of the medial or lateral toenail are present, usually involving the great toe. Patients with underlying diabetes, arterial insufficiency, cellulites, ulceration, or necrosis are at risk for amputation if treatment is delayed.

Emergency Department Care and Disposition

1. If infection is not present, elevation of the nail with a wisp of cotton between the nail plate and the skin, daily foot soaks, and avoiding pressure on the area are often sufficient.
2. After a digital block, a spicule of the offending nail also can be removed and the nail groove débrided. If granulation tissue or infection is present, **partial removal of the nail** is indicated.
3. After a digital block, one fourth or less of the nail should be cut longitudinally, including the nail beneath the cuticle, with a nail splitter or scissors. The cut portion then should be grasped by hemostats and removed by using a rocking motion. The nail groove should be débrided and nonadherent gauze with antibiotic ointment should be applied. A bulky dressing should be placed and the wound checked in 24 to 48 hours.

BURSITIS

There are many bursae in the foot, any of which may become painful due to various causes. Noninflammatory bursae are induced by pressure over the bony prominences. Inflammatory bursae are due to gout, syphilis, or rheumatoid arthritis. Suppurative bursae are due to pyogenic organisms, usually from adjacent wounds. Complications include a hygroma, calcified bursae, fistula, and ulcer formation. Diagnosis is dependent on aspirated bursa fluid. Fluid should be sent for cell count, crystal analysis, Gram stain, culture, protein, glucose, and lactate levels. Treatment depends on the cause. Patients should avoid pressure to the area and be non–weight bearing. Septic bursitis should be treated with **nafcillin** or **oxacillin.** Repeated aspiration or incision and drainage may become necessary.

PLANTAR FASCIITIS

The plantar fascia is connective tissue that anchors the plantar skin to the bone and protects the arch of the foot. Inflammation of the plantar aponeurosis usually is caused by overuse or in those unaccustomed to activity. The patient has point tenderness over the anterior-medial calcaneus that is worse on arising and after activity. Plantar fasciitis is usually self-limited. Treatment includes rest, ice, and **nonsteroidal anti-inflammatory drugs** (NSAIDs). Glucocorticoid injections are not recommended in the emergency department. Severe cases may need a short-leg walking cast and should be referred to a podiatrist.

TARSAL TUNNEL SYNDROME

Tarsal tunnel syndrome involves compression of the posterior tibial nerve as it courses inferior to the medial malleolus and causes foot and heel pain. The causes include running, restrictive footwear (eg, ski boots or skates), edema of pregnancy, posttraumatic fibrosis, ganglion cysts, osteophytes, and tumors. Pain is worse at night and located at the medial malleolus, the heel, sole, and distal calf. Tinel sign is positive, and eversion and dorsiflexion worsen symptoms. Ultrasound, computed tomography, and magnetic resonance imaging (MRI) may aid in diagnosis. Differential diagnosis includes plantar fasciitis and Achilles tendonitis; however, the pain of tarsal tunnel syndrome involves the more medial heel and arch and worsens with activity. Treatment includes **NSAIDs,** rest, and possible orthopedic referral.

GANGLIONS

A ganglion is a benign synovial cyst attached to a joint capsule or tendon sheath. The anterolateral ankle is a typical site. Ganglions may appear suddenly or gradually enlarge or diminish in size and may be painful or asymptomatic. A firm, usually nontender, cystic lesion is seen on examination. The diagnosis is clinical, but MRI or ultrasound can be used if in doubt. Treatment includes **aspiration and injection of glucocorticoids,** but most require surgical excision.

TENDON LESIONS

Tendon lesions usually require orthopedic consultation. Tenosynovitis or tendonitis usually occurs due to overuse and present with pain over the involved tendon. Treatment includes ice, rest, and NSAIDs.

Tendon laceration should be explored and repaired if the ends are visible in the wound; however, due to the high complication rate, specialty consultation is recommended. After repair, extensor tendons are immobilized in dorsiflexion and flexor tendons in equinus.

Achilles tendon rupture presents with pain, a palpable defect in the area of tendon, inability to stand on tiptoes, and absence of plantar flexion with squeezing of the calf (Thompson sign). Treatment is generally surgical in younger patients and conservative (casting in equines) in the elderly. Anterior tibialis tendon rupture results in a palpable defect and mild foot drop. Surgery usually is not necessary. Posterior tibialis tendon rupture is usually chronic and insidious and presents with a flattened arch and swelling over the medial ankle. Examination may show weakness on inversion, a palpable defect, and inability to stand on tiptoes. Treatment may be conservative or surgical.

Flexor hallices longus rupture presents with loss of plantar flexion of the great toe and must be surgically repaired in athletes. Disruption of the peroneal retinaculum occurs with a direct blow during dorsiflexion, causing localized pain behind the lateral malleolus and clicking while walking as the tendon is subluxed. The treatment is surgery.

PLANTAR INTERDIGITAL NEUROMA (MORTON'S NEUROMA)

Neuromas are thought to occur from entrapment of the plantar digital nerve due to tight-fitting shoes, typically those worn by women. Patients present with burning, cramping, or aching over the area of the metatarsal head and improve after shoe removal. Diagnosis is clinical, but ultrasound or MRI may help. Conservative treatment includes wide shoes with inserts and glucocorticoid injections. Surgery may be needed.

IMMERSION FOOT (TRENCH FOOT)

Immersion foot results from prolonged exposure to moist, nonfreezing ($<60°F$ or $<15°C$), and occlusive environment. It is classically seen in military recruits and the homeless. At first, the involved area is pale, anesthetic, pulseless, and immobile but not frozen. With rewarming, one sees hyperemia (lasting up to weeks) with severe burning pain and return of sensation. Edema, bullae, and hyperhidrosis may develop. The differential includes cellulites and fungal infections. Treatment includes **admission for bedrest, leg elevation, and air drying at room temperature.**

PLANTAR FIBROMATOSIS

Plantar fibromatosis (Dupuytren contracture of the plantar fascia) involves small, asymptomatic, palpable, slowly growing, firm masses on the non–weight-bearing plantar surface of the foot. Toe contractures do not occur, lesions tend to reabsorb spontaneously, and treatment is conservative.

FOOT ULCERS

Clinical Features

Foot ulcers are classified as ischemic or neuropathic. Diabetics are most prone to both types and are more apt to develop infections. Ischemic ulcers are due to vascular compromise of the larger vessels. The examination shows a cool foot, dependent rubor, pallor on elevation, atrophic shiny skin, and diminished pulses. Neuropathic ulcers are pressure ulcers due to poor sensation. The ulcers appear well demarcated, with surrounding white callus-like material. The foot (in the absence of severe vascular disease) has normal temperature, color, and pulses. Decreased touch, pressure, and proprioception are common.

Emergency Department Care and Disposition

1. Treatment of an ischemic ulcer requires vascular surgery. Noninfected neuropathic ulcers require relief of pressure and referral to an appropriate foot care specialist.
2. Treatment of an infected ulcer initially consists of debridement, pressure relief via bedrest or total contact casting, and **broad-spectrum antibiotics**

(eg, ampicillin or sulbactam 3 g intravenously every 6 hours). Cultures of purulent drainage should be obtained.
3. Radiographs should be obtained to exclude gas in the soft tissue, foreign body, osteomyelitis, or Charcot foot. Palpation of bone in an infected ulcer correlates strongly with osteomyelitis. Serum glucose levels should be checked. Consultation with a vascular surgeon and admission are often warranted.

For further reading in *Emergency Medicine: A Comprehensive Study Guide,* 6th ed., see Chap. 287, "Soft Tissue Problems of the Foot," by Franz R. Melio.

22 | PSYCHOSOCIAL DISORDERS

185 | Clinical Features of Behavioral Disorders

Lance H. Hoffman

Patients commonly present to the emergency department with psychiatric complaints. These presentations may be related primarily to the psychiatric disorder itself or as a consequence of the psychiatric disorder in the form of an injury or illness. Psychiatrists use a diagnostic system composed of 5 axes to describe various domains of patient information. Axes I to V correspond to clinical syndromes of mental disorders, personality and developmental disorders, general medical conditions, psychosocial and environmental stressors, and a measure of overall functioning, respectively.

CLINICAL PSYCHIATRIC SYNDROMES

Cognitive Disorders

Dementia

Dementia is a disorder consisting of a pervasive disturbance in cognition-impairing memory, abstraction, judgment, personality, and higher critical functions such as language. Its onset is typically gradual, and the patient's normal level of consciousness is maintained. Individuals familiar with the affected person usually notice memory disturbances before impairment in other cognitive areas. Medical illnesses, adverse drug effects, or a change in the patient's environment may contribute to acutely diminished functioning in a patient with dementia. Further, the patient's impaired ability to communicate makes the identification of medical illness by the clinician more challenging. Metabolic and endocrine disorders, adverse drug effects and interactions, and depression are potentially reversible causes of dementia.

Delirium

Delirium is characterized by a global impairment in cognitive functioning that is usually acute in onset with a fluctuating severity of symptoms. The patient experiences a diminished level of consciousness, inattention, and sensory misperceptions. Visual hallucinations are common and typically result in a strong emotional response. Most causes of delirium are reversible and include infection, electrolyte abnormalities, toxic ingestions, and head injury. Treatment should be directed toward correcting the underlying cause.

Substance-Induced Disorders

Intoxication is an exogenous substance-induced syndrome that results in maladaptive behavior and impaired cognitive functioning and psychomotor activity. The individual's judgment, perception, attention, and emotional control may be affected. Repeated use of such a substance is defined as substance abuse and may lead to physical or psychological dependence on the substance. *Substance withdrawal* entails a collection of symptoms specific to substance of abuse that result from the reduction or cessation of use of that substance. These symptoms promptly subside with further use of the exogenous substance.

Psychotic Disorders

Psychotic disorders are characterized by the presence of hallucinations or delusions. Hallucinations are false perceptions experienced in a sensory modality in an alert individual. Auditory hallucinations are most commonly associated with psychiatric causes of psychosis, whereas hallucinations involving other sensory modalities are more commonly associated with medical causes of psychosis. Delusions are fixed false beliefs that are not changed by presenting facts to the contrary and are not shared by others of similar cultural background. Common delusions include persecution or grandiosity.

Schizophrenia

Schizophrenia is a chronic disease characterized by functional deterioration; the presence of hallucinations, delusions, disorganized speech or behavior, or catatonic behavior ("positive symptoms"); the presence of blunted affect, emotional withdrawal, lack of spontaneity, anhedonia, or impaired attention ("negative symptoms"); cognitive impairment expressed as loose associations or incoherence; and the relative absence of a mood disorder. Patients may present to the emergency department for worsening psychosis, suicidal ideations, bizarre or violent behavior, or adverse effects of medications. Older antipsychotic medications, such as haloperidol, effectively treat the "positive symptoms," and newer antipsychotic medications, such as olanzapine and clozapine, effectively treat "positive" and "negative" symptoms.

Schizophreniform Disorder

The diagnosis of schizophreniform disorder is made when an individual experiences symptoms and demonstrates signs consistent with schizophrenia for a period shorter than 6 months.

Brief Psychotic Disorder

A brief psychotic disorder is a psychosis that lasts shorter than 4 weeks and is a response to a traumatic life experience, such as sexual assault or death of a loved one.

Mood Disorders

Major Depression

Major depression consists of a persistent dysphoric mood or a pervasive loss of interest and pleasure in usual activities (anhedonia) lasting longer than 2 weeks. Associated psychologic symptoms include feelings of guilt over past events, self-reproach, worthlessness, hopelessness, and recurrent thoughts of death or suicide. Vegetative symptoms affecting physiologic functioning include a loss of appetite and weight, sleep disturbances, fatigue, inability to concentrate, and psychomotor agitation or retardation. The diagnosis should be entertained in any patient presenting with multiple vague complaints. The lifetime risk of suicide in patients with this disorder is 15%. Consequently, all patients suspected of having major depression should be questioned about suicidal thoughts, and an appropriate psychiatric consultation and referral are mandatory for those with suicidal thoughts.

Bipolar Disorder

Bipolar disorder is characterized by recurrent, cyclic episodes of manic and depressive symptoms, with depressive episodes being more common than manic episodes. Manic individuals experience an elated mood that can quickly deteriorate to irritability and hostility should their expectations not be met. They tend to act energetically and expansively, while demonstrating a decreased need for sleep, poor impulse control, racing thoughts, and pressured speech. They have grandiose ideas about how they will attain positions of power. Complications of this disorder include suicide, substance abuse, and marital and occupational disruptions. Valproic acid and lithium salts are commonly prescribed as chronic mood stabilizers.

Anxiety Disorders

Panic Disorder

Panic disorder consists of recurrent episodes of severe anxiety and sudden, extreme autonomic symptoms that peak within 10 minutes and last for up to 1 hour. It is a diagnosis of exclusion because these symptoms can mimic those of life-threatening cardiovascular and pulmonary disorders. Benzodiazepines, such as alprazolam and lorazepam, are effective in treating acute episodes of anxiety.

Generalized Anxiety Disorder

The diagnosis of generalized anxiety disorder can be made when a patient experiences persistent worry or tension without discrete panic attacks for at least 6 months.

Specific Phobia

A specific phobia consists of symptoms of anxiety, recognized as excessive by the person, prompted by the exposure to, or the anticipated exposure to, a specific stimulus.

Posttraumatic Stress Disorder

Posttraumatic stress disorder is an anxiety reaction to a severe, psychosocial stressor, typically perceived as life threatening. The individual experiences repetitive, intrusive memories of the event. In addition, nightmares, feelings of guilt and depression, and substance abuse are common.

Obsessive-Compulsive Disorder

Individuals with obsessive-compulsive disorder experience intrusive thoughts or images that create anxiety (obsessions). To control these thoughts and anxiety, the individual engages in repetitive behaviors or rituals (compulsions).

For further reading in *Emergency Medicine: A Comprehensive Study Guide,* 6th ed., see Chap. 288, "Behavioral Disorders: Clinical Features," by Douglas A. Rund.

Emergency Assessment and Stabilization of Behavioral Disorders

Lance H. Hoffman

In individuals with behavioral disorders who present to the emergency department, differentiating between medical and psychiatric illness as the cause for the abnormal behavior is important in determining the appropriate treatment and disposition for the patient. Patients requiring emergency stabilization are those who are suicidal, homicidal, or violent or have a rapidly progressive medical condition resulting in the abnormal behavior.

CLINICAL FEATURES

Suicidal patients may be referred for emergency care by the police, family members, friends, crisis intervention groups, or the individuals themselves. Patients presenting in this manner are often forthcoming about their intentions for self-harm. In addition, emergency medical personnel may transport a suicidal patient to the emergency department after a suicide attempt has been made. In this situation, the intentions of the patient may be more difficult to infer, especially if a nontraumatic suicide attempt has been made and the patient has an altered level of consciousness. In contrast, self-inflicted traumatic injuries, including shootings, stabbings, or hangings, are more easily identified as a suicide attempt.

Patients with schizophrenia, substance abuse, and depression are at higher risk of being suicidal. A high index of suspicion for depression should be maintained in patients presenting to the emergency department with vague, seemingly unrelated, somatic complaints, and this should prompt an inquiry into the patient's mood and thoughts for self-harm. Additional suicidal risk factors include advanced age, male sex, divorce or death of a spouse, unemployment, chronic medical illness, prior suicide attempt (especially if the attempt was violent or highly lethal), and poor social support with social isolation. Medication overdose is the most common type of suicide attempt.

Homicidal or violent patients tend to pose little diagnostic dilemma to the clinician. These patients may openly assert their harmful intentions. Their language may contain profanity, escalate in volume, and be rapid or pressured. Mannerisms suggestive of a potentially violent patient include restlessness, pacing in the examination room, clenched fists, acts of violence directed toward inanimate objects in the room, and hypervigilance.

Patients possessing a rapidly progressive medical condition as the etiology of their abnormal behavior may present to the emergency department in a variety of ways. These individuals may be suicidal or homicidal and potentially violent. They also may present with an acute psychosis or altered level of consciousness. Individuals older than 40 years presenting with an acute alteration of behavior without a prior psychiatric diagnosis have a higher likelihood of possessing a medically reversible etiology for their altered behavior.

DIAGNOSIS AND DIFFERENTIAL

A variety of reversible medical conditions might result in the acute onset of a behavioral abnormality. These can include hypoglycemia, hypoxemia, hypertensive encephalopathy, meningitis or encephalitis, head trauma (including intracranial hemorrhage), seizure, intracranial neoplasm, stroke, acute organ system failure, delirium secondary to infection, endocrinopathy (thyroid, parathyroid, or adrenal), and substance intoxication, poisoning, or withdrawal. It is important to obtain a third-party account of the patient's behavior as it compares with the patient's normal behavior and level of functioning. This also will give the clinician a better understanding of the acuity of onset. Important historical information includes the presence of previous psychiatric illness, fever, head trauma, infections, ingestion of medications or legal and illegal substances, disorientation or confusion, impaired speech, syncope or loss of consciousness, headaches, and difficulty performing routine tasks.

A mental status examination should always be included as part of the evaluation of a patient experiencing a behavioral abnormality. Important components of the mental status examination are documentation of the patient's physical appearance, affect, orientation, speech pattern, behavior, level of consciousness, attention, language, memory, judgment, thought content, and perceptual abnormalities. Impaired language performance can indicate the presence of a central nervous system abnormality. Visual hallucinations tend to be more suggestive of a medical etiology, whereas auditory hallucinations tend to support a psychiatric etiology. If the patient is unable to draw a clock face correctly with the hands reading a specific time designated by the examiner, then a medical etiology of the behavioral abnormality is likely.

Patients with behavioral disorders should receive a complete physical examination beginning with a set of vital signs. This is especially important because the differential diagnosis of behavioral abnormalities is so varied. All abnormal vital signs should be investigated and corrected before attributing the patient's abnormal behavior to a psychiatric etiology. Special attention should be devoted to discovering signs of trauma, infection, substance abuse, endocrine disorders, and disorders of the central nervous system.

The patient's laboratory evaluation should be directed toward discovering or confirming suspected abnormalities based on the patient's history, mental status examination, and physical examination. Determining the patient's capillary glucose concentration and oxygen saturation on room air is critical in rapidly excluding hypo- or hyperglycemia and hypoxemia, respectively, as potential causes of the patient's altered behavior. Obtaining a urinalysis is important in the elderly individual because urinary tract infections may result in delirium in this population. Additional tests that can be useful include a complete blood count, serum electrolytes, creatinine, ammonia level, hepatic enzymes, free thyroxine level, thyroid-stimulating hormone, ethanol, urine drug screen and pregnancy test, arterial blood gas analysis, cerebrospinal fluid analysis, electrocardiogram, and computed tomography or magnetic resonance imaging of the brain. Salicylate and acetaminophen levels also are useful in the suicidal patient.

EMERGENCY DEPARTMENT CARE AND DISPOSITION

1. Patients demonstrating violent behavior toward themselves or others in the emergency department should be immediately restrained by physical and chemical means. Physical restraint should be accomplished by security

personnel who have training in subduing individuals. Five people are typically employed, with 1 person assigned to each of the patient's extremities and the leader controlling the head.

2. The violent patient should be chemically sedated to avoid self-injury by struggling against restraints. **Lorazepam** 1 to 2 mg intramuscularly, as a starting dose, is a safe and effective benzodiazepine sedative that can be titrated to the desired effect. **Haloperidol** 2.5 to 5 mg intramuscularly is a neuroleptic sedating agent that can be used alone or with benzodiazepines. Cardiac dysrhythmias resulting in cardiac arrest have rarely been described with this class of medication when used in patients with a prolonged QT interval by electrocardiogram or sympathomimetic intoxication.

3. Suicidal and homicidal or violent patients should be disrobed, gowned, and searched for potentially dangerous items.

4. The clinician should approach the violent patient with a nonthreatening voice and posture while avoiding excessive eye contact. The room's exit should be easily accessible to the patient and the clinician. Enforceable limits as to what constitutes acceptable behavior by the patient must be set by the clinician.

5. Suicidal patients should be approached in an empathetic and nonthreatening manner, with the physician clarifying that the goal is to help the individual.

6. After an appropriate history, mental status examination, physical examination, and laboratory evaluation have excluded a medical cause for an individual's altered behavior, a psychiatric consultation should be obtained. Patients judged to be at high risk to themselves or others or who are unable to effectively care for themselves while alone should be admitted to a psychiatric facility for definitive care.

7. Patients whose evaluation demonstrates a medical etiology for their behavioral change should receive appropriate medical therapy specific to the disorder, whether it mandates hospital admission or outpatient treatment. Hospital admission is necessary if the disorder is not readily reversible, is likely to recur or progress, or if the patient's behavior remains such that independent living would be dangerous.

For further reading in *Emergency Medicine: A Comprehensive Study Guide,* 6th ed., see Chap. 289, "Behavioral Disorders: Emergency Assessment and Stabilization," by Douglas A. Rund.

187 | Panic and Conversion Disorders

Lance H. Hoffman

Patients commonly present to the emergency department for somatic symptoms related to a psychiatric etiology. Panic disorder, one of the anxiety disorders, and conversion disorder, one of the somatoform disorders, are two such diagnoses that should be considered when an organic etiology for the patient's symptoms is not found.

PANIC DISORDER

Clinical Features

Panic disorder is one of the anxiety disorders in which the patient experiences acute, recurrent episodes of intense anxiety and fear, resulting in a persistent fear regarding the implications of having another such episode. Women are 2 to 3 times more likely than men to suffer from this disorder. A typical panic attack begins unexpectedly with symptom severity peaking within 10 minutes of symptom onset and lasting for approximately 1 hour. Different somatic and cognitive symptoms dominate these panic attacks. Somatic symptoms that are commonly described include palpitations, chest tightness or pain, dyspnea, generalized weakness or dizziness, nausea, and paresthesias. Cognitive symptoms include feelings of anxiety, derealization, and depersonalization and a fear of losing control or dying. The frequency and severity of these episodes differ across individuals. Findings of autonomic hyperactivity are commonly found on physical examination.

Diagnosis and Differential

Panic disorder is a diagnosis of exclusion because its symptoms and signs mimic those of several potentially life-threatening disorders. Performing a thorough history and physical examination is crucial to excluding life-threatening disorders as the etiology of the patient's symptoms. Medical diagnoses that should be considered include substance intoxication or withdrawal, anaphylaxis, acute exacerbation of asthma or chronic obstructive pulmonary disease, pulmonary embolism, unstable angina, acute myocardial infarction, cardiomyopathy, heart failure, and adverse medication reactions. Psychiatric diagnoses that should be considered include social or specific phobia, posttraumatic stress disorder, obsessive-compulsive disorder, and depression. Victims of intimate partner violence or sexual abuse or assault may present similarly to the emergency department.

Emergency Department Care and Disposition

1. Treatment of this disorder may begin after first excluding life-threatening causes of the patient's symptoms.
2. Benzodiazepines are the mainstay of therapy for controlling symptoms acutely. **Alprazolam** 0.25 to 0.5 mg orally or **lorazepam** 1 to 2 mg orally or intravenously is effective.

3. The patient should be questioned specifically about suicidal thoughts and criteria for major depression because patients with panic disorder and co-morbid depression have a lifetime suicide risk of 19.5%.
4. Referral to a psychiatrist as an outpatient is warranted if symptoms are controlled in the emergency department and the patient has no suicidal thoughts. Otherwise, psychiatric consultation and admission are necessary.

CONVERSION DISORDER

Clinical Features

Conversion disorder is a somatoform disorder in which a person unconsciously and acutely produces a symptom suggestive of a physical disorder that results in a change or loss of physical functioning as a response to a stressor or conflict. By definition, the symptom cannot be explained by a known organic etiology or culturally sanctioned response pattern, and it cannot be limited to pain or sexual dysfunction. The symptom typically involves a loss of neurologic functioning. A loss of motor function, such as paralysis or pseudoseizure, is described more commonly than a loss of sensory function, such as blindness or numbness. Women are affected much more commonly than men.

Diagnosis and Differential

An organic explanation for the patient's symptom must be excluded before the diagnosis of conversion disorder can be made. Different physical examination maneuvers have been described to assist the clinician in differentiating neurologic symptoms caused by a psychological etiology from an organic etiology. For instance, in a patient with conversion disorder experiencing arm paralysis or coma, if the affected arm is dropped by the examiner from a position directly over the patient's face, then the patient's arm will not strike the patient's face. Further, an opticokinetic drum will produce nystagmus in a patient with conversion disorder experiencing blindness.

A high index of suspicion must be maintained for organic etiologies that might explain the symptom. Between 25% and 50% of patients previously diagnosed with conversion disorder go on to develop an organic condition that might have explained the symptom. Such diseases include systemic lupus erythematosus, polymyositis, multiple sclerosis, Lyme disease, and drug toxicity. In addition, conversion disorder differs from other somatoform disorders such as somatization disorder, in which multiple organ systems are affected, and hypochondriasis, in which the patient continues to worry about an undiscovered medical illness despite evidence to the contrary.

Emergency Department Care and Disposition

1. An organic etiology to the symptom should be excluded through the appropriate use of laboratory and imaging modalities.
2. After presenting the normal test results, the patient should be reassured that a serious medical illness is not present. The patient should not be directly confronted that the symptom has no organic etiology because this may worsen the symptom.
3. The physician should suggest to the patient that the symptom often spontaneously resolves in cases in which the test results are normal.
4. Psychiatric or neurologic consultation in the emergency department is

warranted if the symptom does not resolve and precludes discharging the patient home. Otherwise, an outpatient psychiatric referral is acceptable because approximately 25% of patients will experience a second episode in the next 1 to 6 years.

For further reading in *Emergency Medicine: A Comprehensive Study Guide,* 6th ed., see Chap. 292, "Panic Disorder," by Linda M. Nicholas, Ann E. Maloney, and Susan L. Siegfreid; and Chap. 293, "Conversion Disorder," by Gregory P. Moore and Kenneth C. Jackimeczyk.

23 | ABUSE AND ASSAULT

188 | Child and Elderly Abuse

Kristine L. Bott

CHILD ABUSE

The spectrum of child abuse includes physical abuse, sexual abuse, emotional abuse, parental substance abuse, neglect, and Munchausen syndrome by proxy (MSBP). The physical stigmata of abuse may be characteristic or subtle. Recognition of abuse is aided by knowledge of normal child development.

Clinical Features

Child neglect in early infancy results in the syndrome of failure to thrive (FTT). Overall physical care and hygiene are frequently poor. These infants have little subcutaneous tissue, the ribs protrude prominently through the skin, and the skin over the buttocks hangs in loose folds. Muscle tone is usually increased but may be decreased. Behavioral characteristics include wariness, irritability, and avoidance of eye contact. Children older than 2 to 3 years with environmental neglect are termed *psychosocial dwarfs*. They manifest the classic triad of short stature, bizarre voracious appetite, and a disturbed home situation. They are frequently hyperactive with delayed speech.

Several injury patterns should be recognized as suggestive of physical abuse. Bruises over multiple areas, especially the lower back, buttocks, thighs, cheeks, ears, neck, ankles, wrists, and mouth, should cause suspicion. Belt buckles, cords, or other blunt instruments produce well-demarcated bruises. Bites produce a characteristic oval pattern. Scald burns do not follow a typical splash configuration, but rather a "stocking and glove" distribution caused by immersion in hot water. Skeletal injuries may present with unexplained swelling of an extremity. Abused children with head injuries may appear well or may exhibit vomiting, irritability, apnea, or seizures. Injuries to the abdomen may present with vomiting, abdominal pain and distension, and diminished bowel sounds. Abused children may be overly affectionate with medical staff, may be submissive and compliant, and often do not resist painful medical procedures, such as blood draws.

MSBP is an uncommon form of child abuse in which a caretaker fabricates illness in a child to secure prolonged contact with health care providers. These patients may present with bleeding, vomiting, seizures, altered mental status, apnea, or other symptoms as a result of the intentional administration of ipecac, warfarin, or other substances. Sexually abused children may have vaginal or urethral discharge, vaginal bleeding, or dysuria or may exhibit excessive masturbation, genital fondling, encopresis, nightmares, or sexually oriented or provocative behavior.

Diagnosis and Differential

A history that is inconsistent with the nature or extent of the injury, keeps changing as to the circumstances surrounding the injury, or develops a discrepancy between the story the child gives and the story the caretaker gives should raise the index of suspicion for abuse. Any serious injury or anogenital complaint should be examined carefully. All FTT infants should have weight, height, and head circumference measured and plotted on the appropriate growth chart. These infants typically will gain weight normally once admitted to the hospital, thus confirming the diagnosis. Children with suspected sexual abuse should have genital and rectal examinations performed. Careful examination of the perineum and hymen for tears and concavities can confirm the diagnosis. Swabs of the vagina, rectum, and oral cavity should be performed, with cultures for gonorrhea and chlamydia included. Erythema of the hymen and perineum suggests irritation and is not specific for abuse. It is important to note that a normal examination does not exclude the diagnosis of sexual abuse.

Children with suspected physical abuse should have a complete blood cell count, coagulation studies, platelets, and a skeletal survey. Inflicted injuries are suggested by spiral fractures of a long bone, metaphyseal chip fractures, multiple fractures at different stages of healing, and unusual fracture sites. Infants and children with suspected head or abdominal trauma should be evaluated with computed tomography. Rarely, conditions such as leukemia, aplastic anemia, and osteogenesis imperfecta can mimic physical abuse.

Emergency Department Care and Disposition

Abused infants and children should be treated medically according to their injuries. Infants with FTT and MSBP should be admitted. A full social services assessment should be obtained in all cases of suspected neglect and physical and sexual abuse. All 50 states have mandatory reporting laws that require a verbal report be filed with law enforcement or a child protection agency. Failure to report may result in misdemeanor charges and lead to a fine or imprisonment. The child may be placed in temporary custody, with the final disposition dependent on a court hearing.

ELDERLY ABUSE

Elder abuse affects 3% of the US elderly population. It continues to be underrecognized and underreported.

Clinical Features

Elderly victims frequently live with their abuser who may be dependent on them financially, socially, or emotionally. They are often isolated from other family and friends. Abuse is strongly associated with personality problems of the caregiver who may have a history of mental illness, substance abuse, or personality disorder. Abused patients often have poor personal hygiene, inappropriate or soiled clothing, malnutrition, and worsening decubiti. They may abuse alcohol or drugs. Specific injuries suggestive of abuse include unexplained fractures or dislocations; unexplained lacerations, abrasions, and bruises; burns in unusual locations; and unexplained injuries to the head or face. Abused patients have been found to have significantly greater cognitive impairment than nonabused elderly patients. They often have a history of problematic behavior such as nocturnal shouting, incontinence, wandering, or paranoia.

Diagnosis and Differential

Most mistreatment of elderly patients occurs in residential settings and can be difficult to recognize. This difficulty is confounded by the fact that patients are often reluctant to disclose their abuse due to embarrassment or fear of abandonment, retaliation, or nursing home placement. The diagnosis should be considered in elderly patients with dementia, frequent falls, and dehydration or malnutrition. The following findings are suggestive of an abusive relationship between the patient and the caretaker: (*a*) the patient appears fearful of his or her companion, (*b*) there are conflicting accounts of the injury of illness between the patient and the caretaker, (*c*) there is an absence of assistance toward the patient from the caretaker, (*d*) the caretaker displays an attitude of anger or indifference toward the patient, (*e*) the caretaker is overly concerned with the cost of treatment, and (*f*) the caretaker denies the physician private interaction with the patient. Whenever suspected, the patient should be questioned directly about abuse.

Emergency Department Care and Disposition

Management of elder abuse involves treatment of medical conditions and immediate intervention. Admission is indicated when medically necessary or when the patient cannot be safely discharged back to the current living situation. A social services consultation should be obtained, and adult protective services should be notified. Forty-two states have mandatory reporting laws directed toward health care and social service workers, which require reporting of abuse despite the victim's wishes. When appropriate, caretakers should be provided with supportive services such as home health services, Meals on Wheels, transportation, and mental health services.

For further reading in *Emergency Medicine: A Comprehensive Study Guide,* 6th ed., see Chap. 297, "Child Abuse and Neglect," by Carol D. Berkowitz; and Chap. 300, "Abuse in the Elderly and Impaired," by Ellen H. Taliaferro.

189 | Sexual Assault and Intimate Partner Violence and Abuse

Stefanie R. Ellison

Sexual assault accounts for 1% of all violent crimes reported in the *2001 United States Uniform Crimes Report*. Most episodes of sexual assault are committed by a person known to the victim. Until recently, male sexual assault was underrecognized and underreported. The incidence in men is estimated to be 10% of all sexual assaults.

Intimate partner violence and abuse (IPVA) is defined as a pattern of assaultive behavior that may include physical injury, sexual assault, psychological abuse, stalking, deprivation, intimidation, and threats. IPVA occurs in every race, ethnicity, culture, geographic region, and religious affiliation and occurs in gay, lesbian, and heterosexual relationships.

CLINICAL FEATURES

A brief, tactfully obtained history should include the following elements: (*a*) who (whether the assailant was known and the number of attackers), (*b*) what happened (including physical assault and injuries), (*c*) when (time since assault), (*d*) where (actual or attempted vaginal, oral, or anal penetration and whether ejaculation occurred; use of condoms or foreign bodies), (*e*) whether the patient has showered, douched, or changed clothes since the attack, and (*f*) suspicion of drug-facilitated sexual assault (whether there is a period of amnesia, intoxication greater than expected for the amount of alcohol consumed, or history of waking in a different location with genital pain).

Past medical history pertinent to the sexual assault victim should include last menstrual period, birth control method, and last consensual intercourse (this may affect laboratory analysis of evidence). Allergies and prior medical history should be obtained for sexually transmitted disease (STD) and pregnancy prophylaxes and prior sexual assault.

The history for the IPVA victim can be more difficult to obtain. Between 4% and 15% of women are seen in emergency departments (EDs) because of symptoms related to IPVA. Risk factors for IPVA include female sex, age between 16 and 24 years, low socioeconomic status, separated relationship status, and children younger than 3 years in the home. When a victim reveals a history of IPVA, it should be documented in the patient's own words. Recent and remote abuse, including dates, locations, details of abuse, and witnesses, should be documented. Injuries inconsistent with the patient's history, multiple injuries in various stages of healing, delay in the time of injury occurrence and presentation, a visit for vague complaints without evidence of injury, or suicide attempts should trigger suspicions of IPVA. Patients also may complain initially of chronic pain syndromes, gynecologic or psychiatric difficulties, and alcohol and substance abuse. The victim of IPVA also may appear frightened when the partner is present.

Physical Examination

The examinations for sexual assault and IPVA should include a general medical examination, including general appearance and demeanor. Patients who

894

present to the ED may request only a forensic examination for sexual assault; however, trauma is present in 45% to 67% of cases, with genital injury in 9% to 45%. Injuries should be described and documented, including photographs of injuries, if available. In the sexual assault victim, a pelvic examination should include documentation of vaginal discharge, abrasions, cervical abrasions, and lacerations. The rectum also should be examined for lacerations and abrasions. Anoscopy has proven to be a better tool for detection of trauma. Toluidine blue can detect small lacerations by staining the deeper dermis; it can be applied with gauze and removed with lubrication before the speculum examination. A colposcope also increases documentation of genital injuries, especially to the posterior fourchette.

In the IPVA victim, characteristic injuries include fingernail scratches, bite marks, cigarette burns, rope burns, and forearm bruising or nightstick fractures, suggesting a defensive posture. Central injuries to the head, neck, face, and thorax should be identified and documented. Abdominal injuries are common in the pregnant IPVA patient.

Evidence Examination

Evidence collection in sexual assault is credible only within the first 72 hours after the assault. After 72 hours, a history, physical examination, and documentation of injuries should be provided with STD prophylaxis. The evidence should be labeled clearly with the victim's name, type and source of evidence, date and time, and name of the examiner collecting the evidence.

DIAGNOSIS AND DIFFERENTIAL

Sexual assault is a legal determination, not a medical diagnosis. The legal definition contains 3 elements: carnal knowledge, nonconsent, and compulsion or fear of harm. Because of the legal considerations, careful documentation and evidence collection are important. Informed consent should be obtained, and a system to preserve the "chain of evidence" should be maintained. A prepackaged sexual assault, or "rape," kit with directions for sample collection should be used. Diagrams for documentation of genital and physical injuries can be useful. If a sexual assault kit is not available, smears from the vagina and cervix are made, labeled, and air dried. A wet mount from the same areas should be microscopically examined for sperm. A vaginal aspirate using 5 to 10 mL normal saline should be obtained and tested for acid phosphatase. Premoistened rectal and buccal swabs should be obtained to check for the presence of sperm. A Wood lamp should be used to examine for areas where semen may be collected on the body. If anal penetration occurred, a rectal aspirate and rectal swab should be taken and slides made, labeled, and air dried in the same manner as for the vaginal swabs. Additional forensic laboratory evaluation may include glycoprotein p30 testing and genetic typing.

EMERGENCY DEPARTMENT CARE AND DISPOSITION FOR SEXUAL ASSAULT

The health care provider initially should address life-threatening injuries and the psychological needs of the sexual assault patient.

Pregnancy Prophylaxis

1. A pregnancy test should be obtained. Approximately 5% of all sexual assault victims will become pregnant as a result of the assault.

2. Oral pregnancy prophylaxis options include **levonorgestrel** (Plan B) 1 tablet initially followed by 1 tablet in 12 hours, **ethinyl estradiol and levonorgestrel** (Preven) 2 tablets initially followed by 2 tablets in 12 hours, or **ethinyl estradiol and norgestrel** (Ovral) 2 tablets initially followed by 2 tablets in 12 hours.

STD Prophylaxis

1. The 2002 guidelines of the Center for Disease Control (CDC) for gonorrhea are a single dose of **ceftriaxone** 125 mg intramuscularly, **cefixime** 400 mg orally, **ciprofloxacin** 500 mg orally, or **ofloxacin** 400 mg orally. Ceftriaxone 125 mg intramuscularly is recommended in pregnancy.
2. Recommended regimens for chlamydia prophylaxis are a single dose of **azithromycin** 1 g orally, **doxycycline** 100 mg orally twice daily for 7 days, **erythromycin** base 500 mg orally 4 times daily for 7 days, or **amoxicillin** 500 mg orally 3 times for 7 days.
3. Recommended regimens for trichomoniasis and bacterial vaginosis prophylaxis are a single dose of **metronidazole** 2 g orally, **metronidazole** 250 mg 3 times daily for 7 days, or **clindamycin** 300 mg orally twice daily for 7 days. If pregnant and symptomatic, metronidazole 2 g orally may be used with close follow-up.
4. Recommended treatment regimens for hepatitis B prophylaxis is vaccination at the time of initial evaluation and follow-up doses at 1 to 2 months and at 4 to 6 months.

Prophylaxis or Counseling for the Human Immunodeficiency Virus

1. Rates of human immunodeficiency virus (HIV) are 0.008% to 0.032% from receptive, unprotected anal intercourse and 0.005% to 0.0015% from vaginal intercourse with HIV-positive assailants. Circumstances should guide treatment with known assailant positivity, high viral load exposures, vaginal trauma, and ejaculate on membranes, which represent a moderate to high risk for HIV seroconversion.
2. Postexposure prophylaxis also should consider expense and side effects of the medications and the need to arrange follow-up with a primary physician with experience in HIV treatment. Per CDC guidelines, treatment is currently "recommended" for victims with "moderate" risk exposures. Routine prophylaxis is not recommended, and counseling and follow-up should be provided.

Follow-up Care

The patient should be counseled by a social worker or sexual assault counselor at the time of the assault. Follow-up medical care is needed to reexamine physical injuries and to examine the effectiveness of pregnancy and STD prophylaxes.

EMERGENCY DEPARTMENT CARE AND DISPOSITION FOR THE IPVA VICTIM

1. The first goal of treatment should be to address any life-threatening injuries to the patient while simultaneously ensuring the safety of the victim and any children involved while they are in the ED. IPVA experts (trained social workers or IPVA advocates) can assist with providing information about IPVA and assisting the victims with available options for their families.

2. Safety assessment should identify indicators of a potentially lethal situation. Risk indicators include increasing frequency or severity of violence, the threat or use of weapons, obsession with the victim, taking hostages, stalking, homicidal or suicidal threats, and substance abuse by the assailant, especially with crack cocaine or amphetamines.
3. The most dangerous period for victims is during the time of abuse disclosure and during an attempt to leave the relationship. Hospital admission is an option in high-risk situations if a safe location cannot be established before discharge.

For further reading in *Emergency Medicine: A Comprehensive Study Guide,* 6th ed., see Chap. 298, "Female and Male Sexual Assault," by Patricia R. Salber; and Chap. 299, "Intimate Partner Violence and Abuse," by Kim M. Feldhaus.

Index

Note: Page numbers in *italics* denote figures; those followed by "t" denote tables.

A

AAA. *See* Abdominal aortic aneurysm
Aapraxic gait, 687
Abciximab, 654
  for acute coronary syndromes, 132t,
    136
ABCs of resuscitation, 3
Abdominal aortic aneurysm (AAA),
    162–163
  acute rupture of, 162
  aortoenteric fistula, 162
  chronic contained rupture of, 162
  diagnosis and differential of,
    162–163
  as incidental finding, 162
  management of, 163
  pain of, 212
Abdominal distention, neonatal, 322
Abdominal emergencies in children,
    351–354
  clinical features of, 351
  diagnosis and differential of,
    351–354, 352t
  management of, 354
  traumatic injuries, 765
Abdominal pain, 199–203. *See also*
  Pelvic pain
  of acute pancreatitis, 212, 250
  of appendicitis, 214
  biliary colic, 247–249
  in children, 351–354
  classification of, 199, 215–216
  clinical features of, 199–202
  of Crohn disease, 221
  diagnosis and differential of, 202
  of diverticulitis, 225
  of ectopic pregnancy, 286
  in elderly patients, 201–202
  in helminthic infections, 432t
  of intestinal obstruction, 217
  intraabdominal vs. extraabdominal
    sources of, 199
  management of, 202–203
  nonspecific, 216
  of peptic ulcer disease, 212
  of pseudomembranous colitis, 224
  of ruptured aortic aneurysm, 162
Abdominal palpation, 200
  rebound tenderness on, 200
Abdominal radiography, 202

Abdominal trauma, 803–806
  clinical features of, 803–804
  diagnosis and differential of,
    804–805
  diaphragmatic, 804
  duodenum, 803
  geriatric, 769
  liver, 803
  management of, 805–806
  pancreas, 804
  pediatric, 765
  retroperitoneal, 803–804
  small bowel and colon, 803
  spleen, 803
  stomach, 803
Abduction relief sign, 856
ABG. *See* Arterial blood gas analysis
ABI (ankle brachial index), 814–815
Abortion
  induced, complications of, 309
  spontaneous, 294–295
    diagnosis and differential of, 294
    incomplete vs. complete, 294
    inevitable, 294
    management of, 294–295
    missed, 294
    septic, 294
    threatened, 294
Abruptio placentae, 295, 771
Abscess
  anorectal, 230–231
  Bartholin gland, 450
  cutaneous, 450–451
  masticator space, 726
  odontogenic, 743
  parapharyngeal, 742
  periodontal, 735
  peritonsillar, 372–373, 740–741
  pilonidal, 450
  postoperative intraabdominal, 255
  from puncture wound, 113
  retroperitoneal, 804
  retropharyngeal, 373, 741–742
  scrotal, 272
  staphylococcal soft tissue, 451
  tubo-ovarian, 305–306
Abuse
  of children, 765, 891–892
  of elderly persons, 892–893
  by intimate partner, 894–897

Acalculous cholecystitis, 247–248
Acarbose, 555, 607
Accelerated idioventricular rhythm (AIVR), 18, *19*
ACE inhibitors. *See* Angiotensin-converting enzyme inhibitors
Acetabular fractures, 837
Acetaminophen
  for acute mountain sickness, 580
  for acute pain, 68
  for enteroviral infection, 378
  for febrile child, 314
  for fever in meningitis, 709
  for neck and back pain, 859
  overdose of, 467, 507–509
    clinical features of, 507
    diagnosis and differential of, 507–509
    management of, 472t, 509
    Rumack-Matthew nomogram for, *508,* 508–509
  for pain crisis in sickle cell disease, 392
  for teething pain, 734
  for thyroid storm, 615t
  for toothache, 734
  use in pregnancy, 292t
  for varicella, 380
Acetaminophen with codeine, for headache in children, 362
Acetazolamide
  for acute mountain sickness, 579
  for intraocular pressure elevation, 720, 722
  toxicity of, 518
N-Acetylcysteine (NAC)
  for acetaminophen overdose, 472t, 509
  for herbal toxicity, 548
Achilles tendon injury, 107, 842, 844, 873
Acid burns, 590–591
Acid–base disorders, 40–45
  assessment of, 40
  clinical problem solving in, 41
  metabolic acidosis, 41–43, 42t, 43t
  metabolic alkalosis, 43–44
  respiratory acidosis, 44
  respiratory alkalosis, 44–45
Acne fulminans, 756
Acne keloidalis, 756
Acquired immunodeficiency syndrome (AIDS). *See* Human immunodeficiency virus infection
Acrodynia, 540
Acromioclavicular joint injuries, 831

Actifoam, 84
Activated charcoal, 472t, 474
  for acetaminophen overdose, 509
  for anticholinergic toxicity, 476
  for antidepressant overdose
    bupropion, 482
    mirtazapine, 482
    monoamine oxidase inhibitors, 485
    selective serotonin reuptake inhibitors, 483
    trazodone or nefazodone, 481
    tricyclics, 480
    venlafaxine, 483
  for antipsychotic overdose, 487
  for β-blocker toxicity, 515
  for calcium channel blocker toxicity, 517
  for cocaine "body packers," 502
  for cyanide poisoning, 551
  for digitalis glycoside toxicity, 514
  for hallucinogen intoxication, 504
  for hypoglycemic agent overdose, 556
  for lithium overdose, 488
  for mercury poisoning, 541
  for methemoglobinemia, 554
  for opioid overdose, 500
  for phenytoin toxicity, 522
  for plant or mushroom poisoning, 603
  for salicylate overdose, 506
  for sedative-hypnotic overdose
    barbiturates, 490
    benzodiazepines, 491
    nonbenzodiazepines, 493
  for theophylline toxicity, 513
  for vitamin A overdose, 547
Activated partial thromboplastin time (aPTT), 625t
Acute chest syndrome, in sickle cell disease, 392–393
Acute coronary syndromes, 129–136. *See also* Angina pectoris, unstable; Myocardial infarction, acute
  clinical features of, 129–130
  diagnosis and differential of, 130–131, 131t
  management of, 131–136
Acute intermittent porphyria, 700
Acute mountain sickness (AMS), 578–580
  clinical features of, 578–579
  diagnosis and differential of, 579
  management of, 579–580

Acute necrotizing ulcerative gingivitis, 735
Acute renal failure (ARF), 259–263
    clinical features of, 259
    diagnosis and differential of, 259–261, 261t
    etiologies of, 260t
    management of, 261–263
    oliguric vs. nonoliguric, 259
    rhabdomyolysis and, 850
    risk factors for, 259
Acute rheumatic fever, 389–390
Acute transverse myelitis, 704
Acyclovir
    for febrile infant, 316t
    for herpes simplex virus infection, 411, 417
        conjunctivitis, 335, 716
        encephalitis, 711
        genital, 405
        gingivostomatitis, 736
        in transplant recipients, 458
    for herpes zoster, 412, 418, 701, 757
    for herpes zoster ophthalmicus, 716
    use in pregnancy, 291t
    for varicella, 380
Adenosine
    for supraventricular tachycardia, 15, 17
        in children, 29–30
    for Wolff-Parkinson-White syndrome, 25
Adenovirus enteric infection, 349t
Adhesive capsulitis of shoulder, 861
Adhesive tapes for wound closure, 92
Adolescents. *See* Pediatric patients
Adrenal crisis, 617–618
    in cancer patients, 661
Adrenal insufficiency, 617–618
    clinical features of, 617
    corticosteroid-induced, 867
    diagnosis and differential of, 617–618
    management of, 618
Adrenocorticotropic hormone (ACTH), 617
    inadequate secretion of, 617
    for infantile spasms, 347
Adynamic ileus, 217
    postoperative, 255
Aeromonas infection, 108
β-Agonists
    for asthma and chronic obstructive pulmonary disease, 193
        in children, 341

    in pregnancy, 289
    for bronchiolitis, 342
AIDS dementia complex, 415
AIDS indicator conditions, 413, 414t. *See also* Human immunodeficiency virus infection
Air embolism, 582, 583
Airflow obstruction
    in asthma and chronic obstructive pulmonary disease, 192
    in bronchitis, 179
    in croup, 369
    in epiglottitis, 370
    wheezing due to, 176–177
Airway angioedema, 744
Airway injuries, 792–794
Airway obstruction
    in cancer, 657
    in rheumatic diseases, 867
Airway support, advanced, 3–8. *See also* Intubation
    alternative techniques for, 8
    for children, 26–28, 764, 766
    cricothyrotomy, 7, 7–8
    for geriatric patients, 768, 770
    initial approach, 3
    nasotracheal intubation, 6
    orotracheal intubation, 3–4
        rapid sequence induction for, 5
    techniques to open airway, 3
    for trauma patients, 762
        with maxillofacial injuries, 789
AIVR (accelerated idioventricular rhythm), 18, *19*
Albendazole
    for ascariasis, 433
    for cysticercosis, 436
    for pinworm, 433
Albumin, 648
Albuterol
    for asthma and chronic obstructive pulmonary disease, 193
        in children, 341
        in pregnancy, 289
    for bronchiolitis, 342
    for bronchitis, 179
    for bronchospasm, 61
    for hyperkalemia, 38
    for pediatric pneumonia, 338
Alcohol
    intoxication with, 494
    use in pregnancy, 290
    withdrawal from
        chlordiazepoxide for, 252
        in pregnancy, 290

Alcoholic ketoacidosis, 612–613
  clinical features of, 612
  diagnosis and differential of, 612
  management of, 612–613
Alcoholic liver disease, 239, 243–246
  clinical features of, 243
  diagnosis and differential of, 244
  management of, 245–246
Alkali injuries, 530–532, 590–591
Alkaline reflux gastritis, postoperative,
  256
Allergic conjunctivitis, 716
Allergic reactions, 60–61
  to blood products, 651t
  contact dermatitis, 753–754
  to foods, 60–61
  to local anesthetics, 71
Alloimmune hemolytic anemia, 643
Alopecia, 754
Alprazolam, for panic disorder, 881,
  885
ALS (amyotrophic lateral sclerosis),
  703
ALTE (apparent life-threatening event)
  in neonate, 323–324
Alteplase. *See* Tissue plasminogen
  activator
Altered mental status, 679–685, 680t
  in children, 359–361
    clinical features of, 359
    diagnosis and differential of, 359,
      360t
    management of, 359–361
  coma, 683–685
  delirium, 679–680, 681t
  dementia, 680–683, 682t
  in meningitis, 708
Altitude-related syndromes, 578–580
  clinical features of, 578–579
  diagnosis and differential of, 579
  management of, 579–580
Alveolar osteitis, postextraction, 735
Alzheimer disease, 680, 683
Amantadine, for influenza, 410–411
Amebiasis, 349t
AMI. *See* Myocardial infarction, acute
Amiloride toxicity, 518
ε-Aminocaproic acid (EACA), for
  bleeding, 639
Aminoglycoside overdose, 550
Amiodarone
  for atrial flutter, 13
  for dilated cardiomyopathy, 150
  for supraventricular tachycardia, 15
  for ventricular fibrillation, 21
  for ventricular tachycardia, 19

  for wide-complex tachycardia, 17
Amitriptyline, for chronic pain, 78
Amniotic fluid embolism, 298
Amoxicillin
  for chlamydial infection, 896
  for endocarditis prophylaxis, 147t,
    420, 421t
  for febrile children, 313–314, 316
  for Lyme disease, 438
  for otitis media, 330, 728
  for pneumonia in children, 339t
  for sinusitis, 336
  for streptococcal pharyngitis, 333
  for urinary tract infection, 269
    in children, 398
    in pregnancy, 289
Amoxicillin-clavulanate
  for bite wound prophylaxis, 85, 114,
    115, 117, 118
  for cellulitis, 449, 725, 870t
  for cutaneous abscesses, 451
  for felon, 870t
  for frontal sinus and frontal bone
    fractures, 790
  for impetigo, 375, 724
  for masticator space abscess, 726
  for otitis media, 330
  for paronychia, 870t
  for periorbital cellulitis, 717
  for peritonsillar abscess, 741
  for pneumonia, 181
  for sinusitis, 336, 732
  for suppurative parotitis, 726
  for urinary tract infection, 269
    in children, 398
Amphetamine toxicity, 468t, 500–502
Amphotericin B
  for cryptococcosis, 417
  for sporotrichosis, 451
  for transplant recipients, 458
Ampicillin
  for caustic ingestion, 531
  for cholecystitis, 249
  for diarrhea, 349t, 350
  for diverticulitis, 226
  for endocarditis prophylaxis, 147t,
    420, 421t
  for febrile infant, 316t, 320
  for intraabdominal infection in
    transplant recipients, 458
  for meningitis, 710t
  for pneumonia in children, 339t
  for postpartum endometritis, 298
  for posttransplant meningitis, 458
  for sinusitis, 732
  for ulcerative colitis, 223

Ampicillin (*Cont.*):
  for urinary tract infection
    in children, 398
    in pregnancy, 289
Ampicillin/sulbactam
  for appendectomy, 215
  for cellulitis, 336, 725
    periorbital and orbital, 337
  for cirrhosis and liver failure, 245
  for deep space infections of hand,
    870t
  for dog bites, 116
  for flexor tenosynovitis, 870t
  for foot ulcers, 875
  for human bites, 115
  for intestinal obstruction, 218
  for intraabdominal infection in
    transplant recipients, 458
  for Ludwig angina, 734
  for pelvic inflammatory disease,
    306t
  for peritonsillar abscess, 373
  for pneumonia, 182
  for retropharyngeal abscess, 373,
    742
  for septic abortion, 294
  for sinusitis, 336
  for suppurative parotitis, 726
Amputation of finger tip, 103
Amrinone, for β-blocker toxicity,
  516
AMS. *See* Acute mountain sickness
Amyl nitrate, 472t
Amyotrophic lateral sclerosis (ALS),
  703
Analgesics
  for abdominal pain, 203
  for acute pain, 67–69
    acetaminophen, 68
    dosing for, 69t
    nonsteroidal anti-inflammatory
      drugs, 68
    opiates, 68–69
  for acute pancreatitis, 251
  for appendicitis pain, 215
  for biliary colic, 249
  for bone metastases, 656
  for burns, 589
  for cancer pain, 77t, 664
  for chronic pain, 75–78, 77t
  for corneal abrasion, 718
  for headache, in children, 362
  for headaches, 668–671, 671t
  for neck and back pain, 859
  oral rinses, 378
  overdose of, 505–511

  for pain crisis in sickle cell disease,
    392, 642
  for postherpetic neuralgia, 412
  in pregnancy, 292t
  procedural, 67–71 (*See also*
    Procedural sedation and
    analgesia)
  for renal colic, 277
  for rib fractures, 796
  for shoulder pain, 861
  for temporomandibular disorder,
    672
  for toothache, 734
  for wounds, 119
Anaphylaxis, 60–61
Anastomotic leaks after
  gastrointestinal surgery, 255
Ancylostoma duodenale infection,
  433–434
Anemia, 621–627
  acquired hemolytic, 643–645
  clinical features of, 621
  diagnosis and differential of,
    621–627, 622t, *623,* 624t–626t
  in helminthic infections, 432t
  hereditary hemolytic, 641–643
    glucose-6-phosphate
      dehydrogenase deficiency,
      642–643
    hereditary spherocytosis, 643
    sickle cell disease, 391–396,
      641–642
    variants of sickle cell disease,
      396, 642
  management of, 627
Anesthesia
  local and regional, 71–73
  for nasotracheal intubation, 6
  for rapid sequence induction, 5
    in children, 26–28
  topical, 73
  for wound care, 84
Aneurysm, abdominal aortic (AAA),
  162–163
  acute rupture of, 162
  aortoenteric fistula, 162
  chronic contained rupture of, 162
  diagnosis and differential of,
    162–163
  as incidental finding, 162
  management of, 163
  pain of, 212
Angina pectoris. *See also* Chest pain
  diagnosis of, 123–125, 130
    echocardiography, 124–125
    electrocardiography, 123–124

Angina pectoris (*Cont.*)
    provocative tests, 125, 131
    serum markers, 124, *124*
  pain of, 125–126, 129
  stable, 125, 129
  unstable, 125, 129
  variant (Prinzmetal), 125, 129
Angioedema, 60
  of upper airway, 744
Angioplasty, for acute coronary
    syndromes, 131
  primary, 135
  rescue, 136
Angiotensin-converting enzyme (ACE)
    inhibitors
  for acute coronary syndromes, 136
  angioedema of upper airway
    induced by, 744
  for aortic regurgitation, 146
  for dilated cardiomyopathy, 150
  for restrictive cardiomyopathy, 151
  toxicity of, 520
  use in pregnancy, 291t
Angiotensin II receptor antagonist
    toxicity, 520
Angle closure glaucoma, acute,
    721–722
Animals
  bites from, 115–117
    antibiotics for, 870t
    cat, 116–117
    dog, 115–116
    rabies from, 423–425
    rodents, livestock, exotic and
      wild animals, 117
  diseases transmitted by, 437–446
    (*See also* Zoonoses)
Anion gap, 41–43, 42t
Anistreplase (APSAC), 654
Ankle brachial index (ABI), 814–815
Ankle injuries, 844–846
  dislocations, 846
  fractures, 845–846
  lacerations, 107
  ligamentous sprains, 844–845
  Ottawa Ankle Rules for, 844, *845*
Ankylosing spondylitis, 865
Annelida, 576–577
Anorectal anatomy, 227, *228*
Anorectal disorders, 227–233
  abscesses, 230–231
  cryptitis, 230
  fissure in ano, 230
  fistula in ano, 231
  hemorrhoids, 227–229
  in HIV infection, 416

  pilonidal sinus, 232
  pruritus ani, 233
  rectal foreign bodies, 231–232
  rectal prolapse, 231
  tumors, 232
Anoscopy, 227
Anovulatory dysfunctional uterine
    bleeding, 283–284
Ant stings, 567–568
Antacids, for peptic ulcer disease, 213
Anterior cerebral artery occlusion, 673
Anterior cord syndrome, 785t
Anterior cruciate ligament injury, 842
Anthraquinone, for constipation, 238
Anthrax, 444–445
  as biological weapon, 454t
  clinical features of, 444
  diagnosis and differential of, 444
  management of, 445
Antibiotic prophylaxis
  for appendectomy, 215
  for infective endocarditis, 147t,
    420–421, 421t
  for marine animal injuries, 576–577
  for meningitis, 671
  for open fractures, 763, 820, 839,
    846
  for trauma patients, 763
  for urinary catheterization, 275
  for wounds, 85–86, 118
    cat bites, 116–117
    dog bites, 115
    human bites, 114
    puncture wounds, 112–113
    topical, 118
Antibiotic therapy. *See also* specific
    drugs
  for acute chest syndrome in sickle
    cell disease, 393
  for acute necrotizing ulcerative
    gingivitis, 735
  for acute rheumatic fever, 390
  for anthrax, 445
  for asthma and chronic obstructive
    pulmonary disease, 194
  for bacterial tracheitis, 371
  for bacterial vaginosis, 302
  for bite injuries, 870t
    cats, 117
    dogs, 115–116
    human, 115
    other animals, 117
  for brain abscess, 712
  for bullous impetigo, 374
  for burns, 589
  for caustic ingestion, 531

Antibiotic therapy (*Cont.*)
  for cellulitis, 336–337, 449, 725,
    870t
  for chancroid, 405
  for chlamydial infection, 402, 896
  for cholecystitis, 249
  for cirrhosis and liver failure, 245
  for conjunctivitis, 334–335
  for corneal abrasion, 718
  for corneal ulcer, 717
  for Crohn disease, 222
  for cutaneous abscesses, 451
  diarrhea associated with, 224–225,
    254, 349t
  for diverticulitis, 226
  for epiglottitis, 370, 742
  for erysipelas, 375, 450
  for esophageal perforation, 208
  for febrile children, 313–316, 316t,
    320
  for febrile neutropenia, 662
  for foot ulcers, 874–875
  for frontal sinus and frontal bone
    fractures, 790
  for gas gangrene, 447, 448
  for gonococcal infection, 402–403
  for hand infections, 870t
  for *Helicobacter pylori* infection,
    213
  for impetigo, 375, 724
  for infectious diarrhea, 236
    in children, 349t, 350
  for inflammation from wisdom
    teeth, 734
  for intestinal obstruction, 218
  for lateral sinus thrombosis, 729
  for Ludwig angina, 734
  for Lyme disease, 438, 863
  for lymphogranuloma venereum,
    406
  for mandibular fractures, 791
  for masticator space abscess, 726
  for mastitis, 298
  for mastoiditis, 729
  for meningitis, 316t, 318, 709, 710t
  for meningococcemia, 752
  for necrotizing fasciitis, 448
  for odontogenic abscess, 743
  for orbital cellulitis, 717
  for otitis externa, 332, 728
  for otitis media, 330, 728–729
  overdose of, 550
  for pelvic inflammatory disease,
    306, 306t
  for penetrating injuries of flank,
    808

  for perforated or strangulated
    hernia, 220
  for periodontal abscess, 735
  for periorbital cellulitis, 717
  for peritonitis, 266
  for peritonsillar abscess, 373, 741
  for pharyngitis, 333, 740
  for plague, 446
  for *Pneumocystis carinii*
    pneumonia, 417
  for pneumonia, 181–182
    in children, 339, 339t
  for postextraction alveolar osteitis,
    735
  for postpartum endometritis, 298
  for pseudomembranous colitis,
    224–225
  for retropharyngeal abscess, 373,
    742
  for Rocky Mountain spotted fever,
    377, 440
  for scarlet fever, 377
  for sepsis in children, 316t, 318,
    320
  for septic abortion, 294
  for septic arthritis, 387
  for septic shock, 55
  for sinusitis, 336, 732
  for staphylococcal scalded skin
    syndrome, 751
  for streptococcal toxic shock
    syndrome, 409
  for suppurative parotitis, 725–726
  for syphilis, 404
  for tetanus, 423
  for tooth decay, 734
  for toxic shock syndrome, 408
  for transplant recipients, 458
  for trichomoniasis, 302
  for tularemia, 442–443
  for ulcerative colitis, 223
  for urinary tract infection, 269
    in pregnancy, 289
  use in pregnancy, 289, 291t
Anticardiolipin antibody, 633
Anticholinergic toxicity, 476–478
  clinical features of, 468t, 476
  diagnosis and differential of, 476
  management of, 476–478
  substances associated with, 477t
Anticoagulation. *See also*
    Antithrombotic therapy
  for acute coronary syndromes, 132t,
    133–134
  for atrial fibrillation, 13, 14
  for atrial flutter, 12

Anticoagulation (*Cont.*)
bleeding induced by
heparin, 630
warfarin, 628, 629t
for deep venous thrombosis, 168
for dilated cardiomyopathy, 150
oral drugs for, 653
parenteral drugs for, 653
in pregnancy, 292t
for pulmonary embolism, 157
Anticonvulsants
for seizures, 697, 697t
in children, 345–347
use in pregnancy, 290, 291t
Antidepressants
for chronic pain, 77t, 78
toxicity of, 479–486
bupropion, 482
mirtazapine, 482
monoamine oxidase inhibitors, 484–486, 485t, 486t
selective serotonin reuptake inhibitors, 482–483
serotonin syndrome, 469t, 479
trazodone and nefazodone, 481
tricyclics, 479–481
venlafaxine, 483
Antidiarrheal agents, 222, 236
Antidotes for poisons, 467, 472t–473t, 536t
Antiemetics, 236–237, 249, 252
for chemotherapy-induced nausea/vomiting, 663
for children, 350
for patients with abdominal pain, 203
use in pregnancy, 292t, 295
for vertigo, 691
Antifungal therapy. *See also* specific drugs
for candidal infections, 303, 417
for cryptococcosis, 417
for onychomycosis, 755
for posttransplant infections, 458
for sporotrichosis, 451
for tinea infections, 754, 755
Antihistamines. *See also* specific drugs
for contact dermatitis, 754
for erythema multiforme, 748
for exfoliative dermatitis, 747
Antihypertensive agents, 160–161
toxicity of, 518–520
use in pregnancy, 291t
Antimalarial drugs, 427–430, 428t–429t

toxicity of, 549–550
Antimycobacterial drugs
for children, 186t
for *Mycobacterium avium* complex, 417
for tuberculosis, 185, 186t, 417
Antiparkinsonian agents, 706
Antiphospholipid antibodies, 633
Antiplatelet agents
for acute coronary syndromes, 132t, 133, 136
for stroke, 677
Antipsychotics
for dementia, 683
toxicity of, 486–487
Antiretroviral therapy, 418
after sexual assault, 896
Antithrombin III, 648
Antithrombotic therapy, 59, 653–655
for acute myocardial infarction, 131, 132, 132t, 134–135, 654–655
bleeding due to, 628, 630
contraindications to, 134t, 655t
for deep venous thrombosis or pulmonary embolism, 157–158, 655
direct thrombin inhibitors for, 654
fibrinolytic agents for, 654
inhibitors of platelet activation for, 654
inhibitors of platelet aggregation for, 654
for ischemic stroke, 655, 675–677, 676t
oral anticoagulants for, 653
parenteral anticoagulants for, 653
for pulmonary embolism, 157–158
Antivenom Fab, 472t
Antiviral therapy
for cytomegalovirus infection, 417
for febrile infant, 316t
for herpes simplex virus infection, 411, 417
conjunctivitis, 335, 716
encephalitis, 711
genital, 405
gingivostomatitis, 736
in transplant recipients, 458
for herpes zoster, 412, 418, 701, 757
for herpes zoster ophthalmicus, 716
for HIV infection, 418
for influenza, 410–411
for posttransplant infections, 458
use in pregnancy, 291t
for varicella, 380
AOM. *See* Otitis media, acute

Aortic aneurysm, abdominal (AAA),
162–163
acute rupture of, 162
aortoenteric fistula, 162
chronic contained rupture of, 162
diagnosis and differential of,
162–163
as incidental finding, 162
management of, 163
Aortic dissection, 163–165
classification of, 164
clinical features of, 163–164
diagnosis and differential of, 164
with hypertension, 160
management of, 165
pain of, 126, 145, 163
risk factors for, 163–164
Aortic incompetence, 143t, 145–146
Aortic stenosis, 143t, 144–145
Aortic trauma, 800–802
blunt, 801–802
penetrating, 800
Aortoenteric fistula, 162
Apathetic thyrotoxicosis, 614
Aphthous stomatitis, 735–736
Aplastic anemia, in sickle cell disease,
394
Apnea, neonatal, 322
Apparent life-threatening event
(ALTE) in neonate, 323–324
Appendicitis, 214–216
in children, 215, 353
clinical features of, 214
complications of, 214
diagnosis and differential of,
214–215
in elderly persons, 215
management of, 215–216
aPPT (activated partial thromboplastin
time), 625t
Apraclonidine, for intraocular pressure
elevation, 720, 722
APSAC (anistreplase), 654
ARF. *See* Acute renal failure
Aronen technique, for glenohumeral
joint dislocation, 832
Arrhythmias. *See* Dysrhythmias
Arsenic poisoning, 539–540
clinical features of, 539
diagnosis and differential of,
539–540
management of, 536t, 540
Arterial blood gas (ABG) analysis
airway management and, 3
in chronic obstructive pulmonary
disease, 193

in cyanosis, 177
for dyspnea, 173
in hypercapnia, 175
in pneumonia, 181
for wheezing, 177
Arterial occlusion, 168–169
anterior cerebral artery, 673
basilar artery, 673
central retinal artery, 673
clinical features of, 168
diagnosis and differential of,
168–169
management of, 169
middle cerebral artery, 673
posterior cerebral artery, 673
posterior inferior cerebellar artery,
673
stroke due to, 673–678
vertebral artery, 673
Arterial–alveolar oxygen gradient,
175
Arthritis
classification of, 863t
gonococcal, 865
Lyme, 863
osteoarthritis, 863
poststreptococcal reactive, in
children, 390
in Reiter syndrome, 865
rheumatoid, 865
juvenile, 390
septic, 113, 862–863, 865t
in children, 387
ASA. *See* Aspirin
Ascaris lumbricoides infection, 433
Ascites, cirrhotic, 246
Aspergillus infection, otitis externa,
728
Aspiration of foreign bodies, 371–372,
743–744
clinical features of, 371–372
diagnosis and differential of, 372
management of, 372
Aspiration pneumonia, 180
Aspirin (ASA)
for acute coronary syndromes, 132t,
133
for acute mountain sickness, 580
for acute pain, 68
antiplatelet activity of, 654
for cardiogenic shock, 58
for juvenile rheumatoid arthritis,
390
for Kawasaki disease, 382
overdose of, 467, 469t, 505–507
for stroke, 677

Assisted reproductive technology, complications of, 285, 309
Asthma, 192–195
  bronchitis and, 179
  "cardiac," 193
  in children, 340–342
  clinical features of, 192, 340
  diagnosis and differential of, 192–193, 340–341
  drugs to avoid in, 195
  management of, 193–195, 341–342
  in pregnancy, 289
Asystole, 24
Ataxia, 686–687, *687*
  clinical features of, 686–687
  diagnosis and differential of, 687
  management of, 687
  motor, 687
  sensory, 687
Atelectasis, postoperative, 253
Atenolol
  for acute coronary syndromes, 132t
  for hypertrophic cardiomyopathy, 151
  for mitral valve prolapse, 144
Athlete's foot, 755
Atovaquone-proguanil, for malaria, 427, 429t
Atrial fibrillation, *13*, 13–14
  aortic stenosis and, 145
  mitral incompetence and, 143
  mitral stenosis and, 142
Atrial flutter, *12*, 12–13
  in Wolff-Parkinson-White syndrome, 25
Atrioventricular (AV) block, 21–24
  in acute myocardial infarction, 130
  first-degree, 21
  second-degree Mobitz I (Wenckebach), 21–22, *22*
  second-degree Mobitz II, *22*, 22–23
  third-degree (complete), 21, *23*, 23–24
Atrophic vaginitis, 304
Atropine
  for asystole, 24
  for bradycardia, 9, 62
  for clonidine toxicity, 519
  for digitalis glycoside toxicity, 514
  for junctional rhythms, 16
  for ketamine-induced hypersalivation, 70
  for monoamine oxidase inhibitor overdose, 485
  overdose of, 468t
  for pesticide poisoning, 536t
  for pulseless electrical activity, 24
  for pupillary dilation, 720
  during rapid sequence induction, 5
    in children, 26
  for second-degree Mobitz I AV block, 22
  for second-degree Mobitz II AV block, 23
  for third-degree AV block, 24
Autoimmune hemolytic anemia, 643
AV block. *See* Atrioventricular block
Axillary nerve testing, 831–832
Azathioprine
  adverse effects of, 459t
  for Crohn disease, 222
  for hemolytic anemia, 644
  for ulcerative colitis, 224
Azithromycin
  for cellulitis, 336, 725
  for chancroid, 405
  for chlamydial infection, 402, 896
  for endocarditis prophylaxis, 147t, 421t
  for erysipelas, 450
  for Lyme disease, 438
  for otitis media, 330
  for pharyngitis, 333
  for pneumonia, 181
  for tularemia, 443
  use in pregnancy, 291t

B

B-type natriuretic peptide, 58
Babinski sign, 856
Bacillus anthracis infection, 444–445, 454t
Bacitracin/polymyxin, for corneal abrasion, 718
Back pain, 855–859
  articular, 76t, 77t
  clinical features of, 855
  diagnosis and differential of, 855–858, 858t
  management of, 859
  myofascial, 76t, 77t
  neurogenic, 76t, 77t
Bacteremia in children
  fever and, 313–314, 315
  occult, 315–316
Bacterial tracheitis, 371
Bacterial vaginosis (BV), 302
  prophylaxis after sexual assault, 896
Bacteriuria
  asymptomatic, 269
  urinary tract infection, 267–269

Bacteroides infection, otitis externa, 728

Bag-valve-mask ventilation, 3–5
  for children, 26

BAL. *See* British Anti-Lewisite

Balanoposthitis, 273

Bankard lesion, 832

Barbiturates
  abstinence syndrome, 490
  overdose of, 489–490
    clinical features of, 489
    diagnosis and differential of, 489
    management of, 489–490
  for procedural sedation, 70
  side effects of, 70

Barotrauma, 581–583

Bartholin gland abscess, 450

Barton bandage, 791

Basilar artery occlusion, 673

Battle sign, 787

Beck triad, 798

Bed bug bites, 571

Beef tapeworm, 435

Beestings, 567

Behavioral disorders. *See* Psychosocial disorders

Bell palsy, 701

Belladonna suppositories, for male urinary retention, 275

Benign paroxysmal positional vertigo (BPPV), 688–691
  clinical features of, 688–689
  diagnosis and differential of, 689
  Epley maneuver for, 691

Benzocaine, for teething pain, 734

Benzodiazepines. *See also* specific drugs
  for drug- or toxin-induced seizures, 474, 476, 480, 482, 483, 485, 487, 488
  for hallucinogen intoxication, 502, 504
  overdose of, 490–491
    clinical features of, 490–491
    diagnosis and differential of, 491
    flumazenil for, 68, 491
    management of, 491
  for panic disorder, 881, 885
  for procedural sedation, 69–70
  for serotonin syndrome, 479
  side effects of, 69
  for stimulant overdose, 501
  use in pregnancy, 290
  use with opiates, 69
  for vertigo, 691
  withdrawal from, 491

Betamethasone, for aphthous stomatitis, 736

Bethesda inhibitor assay (BIA), 634

Biceps rupture, 828–829

Bigeminy, 16

Biliary colic, 213, 247
  clinical features of, 247
  diagnosis and differential of, 248
  management of, 248–249
  postoperative, 255

Bilirubin level, 239–241

Bioterrorism attack, 452–455
  agents in, 453–455, 454t
    anthrax, 444–445
    botulism, 453
    Ebola and Marburg, 455
    plague, 445–446
    ricin, 455
    smallpox, 453
    tularemia, 442–443
  detection of, 452
  management issues for, 455
  response actions for, 452–453
  response planning for, 452

Biotin, for biotinidase deficiency, 347

Bipolar disorder, 880–881

Bisacodyl, for constipation, 238

Bismuth subsalicylate, for *Helicobacter pylori* infection, 213

Bite wounds, 114–117
  antibiotic prophylaxis for, 85
  cats, 116–117
  dogs, 115–116
  human, 114–115
  infection risk from, 83
  rodents, livestock, exotic and wild animals, 117

Bites and stings, 567–574
  ants, 568
  bed bugs, 571
  blister beetle, 571
  chiggers, 570
  coral snake, 574
  fleas, 570–571
  gila monster, 574
  Hymenoptera, 567
  kissing bugs, 571
  lice, 571
  pit vipers, 571–573
  puss caterpillar, 571
  scabies, 570
  scorpions, 569–570
  spiders, 568–569
  tarantula, 569

Black widow spider bite, 569

Blackwater fever, 427

Bladder injuries, 812
Bleeding
    after dental extraction, 738–739
    in disseminated intravascular
        coagulation, 630–632, 631t, 632t
    due to circulating anticoagulants,
        633
    due to heparin use or fibrinolytic
        therapy, 630
    due to platelet abnormalities, 628
    due to warfarin use or vitamin K
        deficiency, 628, 629t
    dysfunctional uterine, 283
    epidural hematoma, 776
    evaluation of patient with, 621–627
    gastrointestinal, 53, 54, 204–205
    in hemophilias, 634–639
    hemoptysis, 190–191
    hemothorax, 797
    in HIV infection, 633
    intracerebral, 776
    within joints, 863
    in liver disease, 628–629
    in mitral stenosis, 142
    nasal, 730–732
    post-conization, 309
    postpartum, 298
    in renal disease, 629
    shock due to, 51
    subconjunctival, 718
    subdural hematoma, 777
    thrombolytic-induced, 135
    in trauma patients, 762–763
        with maxillofacial injuries, 789
    vaginal, in non-pregnant patient,
        283–284
    variceal, 204–205, 208, 246
    from vascular access site for
        hemodialysis, 265–266
    in von Willebrand disease, 639–640
    from wounds, 84
Bleeding time (BT), 624t
Blindness, 721–723
Blister beetles, 571
β-Blockers
    for acute coronary syndromes, 132t,
        133
    for aortic incompetence, 146
    for chloral hydrate–induced
        dysrhythmias, 493
    for dilated cardiomyopathy, 150
    for hypertension, 160, 161
    for hypertrophic cardiomyopathy,
        151
    for mitral valve prolapse, 144
    for thyroid storm, 615t

    toxicity of, 515–516
    use in pregnancy, 291t
"Blood-and-thunder fundus," 723
Blood pressure. *See also*
        Hypertension; Hypotension
    drug-induced changes in, 470t–471t
    hypertensive emergencies, 159–161
    in pregnancy, 771
    in shock, 49–50
Blood transfusion. *See* Transfusion
        therapy
Blood type and crossmatch, 646
Blood volume, 646
    in pregnancy, 771
Blowout fracture, 720
Body lice, 571, 757–758
Body surface area (BSA) of burns,
        586, 586–587, *587,* 587t
Body temperature
    drug-induced changes in, 470t–471t
    heat-related illness, 564–566
    hypothermia and frostbite, 561–563,
        562t
Böhler angle, 847
Boils, 451
Bone metastases, 656
Borrelia burgdorferi infection, 437–438
Botulism, 699
    as biological weapon, 453, 454t
Boutonniere deformity, 822
Boyle law, 581
BP. *See* Bullous pemphigoid
BPD (bronchopulmonary dysplasia),
        323, 340
BPPV. *See* Benign paroxysmal
        positional vertigo
Brachial neuritis, 700
Brachioradial delay, in aortic stenosis,
        145
Bradycardia
    in children, 29
    in neurogenic shock, 62
    sinus, 9–10
    in spinal shock, 780
Brain abscess, 711–712
Brain concussion, 776
Brain contusion, 776
Brain herniation, 777
Brain injury, traumatic, 774–779, 776.
        See also Head trauma
Brain tumors, headache and, 667
Braxton-Hicks contractions, 299
Breast surgery complications, 255
Breathing
    in children, 764
    neonatal, 322

Brief psychotic disorder, 880
British Anti-Lewisite (BAL)
    for arsenic poisoning, 536t, 540
    for lead poisoning, 538t
    for mercury poisoning, 541
Bronchial injuries, 797–798
Bronchiolitis, 340, 342–343
    clinical features of, 342
    diagnosis and differential of, 342
    management of, 342–343
    obliterative, in lung transplant
        recipient, 461, 462
Bronchitis
    chronic, 192–195
    uncomplicated acute, 179
Bronchodilators
    for asthma, 193–195, 341–342
    for bronchiolitis, 342–343
    for bronchitis, 179
Bronchopneumonias, 180
Bronchopulmonary dysplasia (BPD),
    323, 340
Brown recluse spider bite, 568
Brown-Séquard syndrome, 785t
Brudzinski sign, 314, 708
BSA (body surface area) of burns,
    586, 586–587, *587,* 587t
BT (bleeding time), 624t
Bubonic plague, 445–446, 454t
Bullous impetigo, 374, *374,* 724
Bullous myringitis, 180, 729
Bullous pemphigoid (BP), 751–752
    clinical features of, 751
    diagnosis and differential of, 752
    management of, 752
Bumetanide
    for pulmonary edema, 140
    toxicity of, 518
Bupivacaine, 71
Bupropion toxicity, 482
Burn injuries, 586–592
    burn unit referral criteria for, 589,
        590t
    chemical, 590–592
    pediatric, 765
    thermal, 586–590
"Burp" maneuver, 4
"Burr holes," for increased intracranial
    pressure, 779
Burrow solution, for erythema
    multiforme, 748
Bursitis, 860, 865
    of foot, 872
Burst fracture of cervical spine,
    783t
Buspirone overdose, 492

Butoconazole, for *Candida* vaginitis,
    303
Buttock trauma, penetrating, 808–809
Button battery ingestion, 210, 532
BV (bacterial vaginosis), 302
    prophylaxis after sexual assault, 896

C

CABG (coronary artery bypass graft)
    surgery, 59, 131, 136
Calcaneus fractures, 847
Calcitonin
    for hypercalcemia, 39
        of malignancy, 660
    for reflex sympathetic dystrophy,
        77t, 78
Calcitriol, for hypocalcemia, 38
Calcium balance
    hypercalcemia, 38–39
    hypocalcemia, 38
Calcium channel blockers
    toxicity of, 516–517
        clinical features of, 516
        diagnosis and differential of,
            516–517
        management of, 517
    use in pregnancy, 291t
Calcium chloride
    for calcium channel blocker
        toxicity, 517
    for caustic exposures, 531
    for hyperkalemia, 36, 852
    for hypermagnesemia, 40
    for hypocalcemia, 38, 852
    for poisoning, 472t
Calcium gluconate
    for calcium channel blocker
        toxicity, 517
    for caustic exposures, 531
    for hydrofluoric acid burns, 591
    for hyperkalemia, 36
    for hypocalcemia, 38
        in neonates, 347
    for poisoning, 472t
Calcium sign, 164
Campylobacter jejuni infection, 349t
Cancer complications, 656–664
    acute spinal cord compression,
        656–657
    adrenal crisis, 661
    bone metastases, 656
    hypercalcemia of malignancy,
        659–660
    hyperviscosity syndrome, 662–663
    malignant pericardial effusion with
        tamponade, 658

Cancer complications (*Cont.*)
nausea and vomiting, 663
pain, 77t, 663–664
superior vena cava syndrome, 658–659
syndrome of inappropriate antidiuretic hormone, 661
thromboembolism, 659
tumor lysis syndrome, 660–661
upper airway obstruction, 657
Candesartan toxicity, 520
Candida infection
in HIV disease, 416
management of, 417
oral, 323, 416, 417, 735
otitis externa, 728
vaginal, 302–303
Capitate fracture, 825
Capnography, 3, 4
Captopril
for hypertension, 161
toxicity of, 520
Carbamate insecticide poisoning, 468t, 536t
Carbamazepine
for seizures, 697t
in children, 346
use in pregnancy, 291t
Carbon monoxide poisoning, 588, 598–600
clinical features of, 598
diagnosis and differential of, 598–599
management of, 590, 599–600, 599t
Carboxyhemoglobinemia, 553–554, 598–599
cyanosis and, 177–178, 178t
Carbuncle, 451
Cardiac enzymes
in acute myocardial infarction, 58, 124, *124*, 131
in blunt cardiac trauma, 799
in myocarditis, 152
Cardiac injuries, 798–800
blunt, 799–800
penetrating, 798–799
Cardiac monitoring, 3, 132
Cardiac pacing
for asystole, 24
for β-blocker toxicity, 516
for junctional rhythms, 16
for second-degree Mobitz I AV block, 22
for second-degree Mobitz II AV block, 23

for sinus bradycardia, 9–10
for third-degree AV block, 24
Cardiac standstill, 24
Cardiac syncope, 137, 138
Cardiac tamponade, 153–154
cardiac trauma with, 798
clinical features of, 153–154
diagnosis and differential of, 154
etiologies of, 153
malignant pericardial effusion with, 658
management of, 154, 799
nontraumatic, 153–154
pain of, 126
uremic pericarditis and, 264
Cardiac transplant patients, 460–461
Cardiogenic shock, 57–59
in acute myocardial infarction, 57, 130, 136
in children, 329
Cardiomyopathy, 149–152
dilated, 149–150
hypertrophic, 150–151
restrictive, 151
right ventricular, 152
uremic, 264
Cardiopulmonary resuscitation (CPR)
advanced airway support, 3–8
management of dysrhythmias, 9–25
in pediatric patients, 26–31
defibrillation and cardioversion, 30
drugs, 29
dysrhythmia management, 29–30
fluids, 29, 32
length-based equipment chart for, 27t
neonates, 30–31
rapid sequence induction, 26–28
securing airway, 26
vascular access, 28–29
Cardiothoracic trauma, 795–802
cardiac injuries, 798–800
blunt, 799–800
penetrating, 798–799
chest wall injuries, 795–796
in children, 765
diaphragmatic injuries, 798, 804
esophageal injuries, 802
evaluation of, 795
in geriatric patients, 769
injuries of great vessels, 800–802
blunt, 801–802
penetrating, 800
lung injuries, 796–797
neck injuries and, 793

Cardiothoracic trauma (*Cont.*)
  pericardial inflammation syndrome,
    800
  thoracic duct injuries, 802
  tracheobronchial injuries, 797–798
Cardiovascular disease, 121–169
  cardiomyopathy, 149–152
  chest pain, 123–128
  congestive heart failure and
    pulmonary edema, 140–141
  end-stage renal disease and, 264
  hypertensive emergencies, 159–161
  myocardial infarction and unstable
    angina, 129–136
  myocarditis, 152
  nontraumatic cardiac tamponade,
    153–154
  pediatric, 325–329
    clinical presentations of, 325,
      325t
    congestive heart failure, 327–329,
      328t
    with cyanosis and shock,
      325–327
  pericarditis, 152–155
  peripheral vascular disorders,
    166–169
  pulmonary embolism, 156–158
  syncope, 137–139
  valvular heart disease, 142–148
Cardioversion
  for atrial fibrillation, 13, 14
  for atrial flutter, 13, 25
  in children, 30
  in pregnancy, 288
  for supraventricular tachycardia, 15
  for ventricular tachycardia, 17, 19
  for Wolff-Parkinson-White
    syndrome, 25
Carnett sign, 200
Carotid sinus massage, 15
Carpal tunnel syndrome, 700, 871
Carvedilol, for dilated
  cardiomyopathy, 150
Cat bites, 116–117
  rabies from, 423–425
Cauda equina syndrome, 785t
Causalgia, 75, 76t, 77t
Caustic agent exposure, 530–532
  clinical features of, 530
  diagnosis and differential of,
    530–531
  management of, 531–532
Cavernous sinus thrombosis, 734–735
Cefadroxil, for endocarditis
  prophylaxis, 147t

Cefazolin
  for cellulitis, 336, 449, 725
    periorbital and orbital, 337
  for deep space infections of hand,
    870t
  for endocarditis prophylaxis, 147t,
    421
  for flexor tenosynovitis, 870t
  for open fractures, 839, 846
  for toxic shock syndrome, 408
  for urinary tract infection in
    pregnancy, 289
  for wound infections in transplant
    recipients, 458
Cefdinir
  for otitis media, 330
  for sinusitis, 336
Cefepime
  for febrile neutropenia, 662
  for pneumonia, 182
  for urinary tract infection in
    children, 398
Cefixime
  for gonococcal infection, 402, 896
  for urinary tract infection in
    children, 398
Cefotaxime
  for acute chest syndrome in sickle
    cell disease, 393
  for brain abscess, 712
  for cholecystitis, 249
  for cirrhosis and liver failure,
    245
  for epiglottitis, 370
  for esophageal perforation, 208
  for febrile infant, 313, 316t, 320
  for mastoiditis, 729
  for perforated or strangulated
    hernia, 220
  for pneumonia, 182
    in children, 339t
    nosocomial, 458
  for posttransplant meningitis, 458
  for septic arthritis, 387
  for septic shock, 55
  for urinary tract infection in
    children, 398
Cefotetan
  for pelvic inflammatory disease,
    306t
  for trauma patients, 763
Cefoxitin
  for human bites, 115
  for pelvic inflammatory disease,
    306t
  for postpartum endometritis, 298

Cefpodoxime
  for otitis media, 330
  for pneumonia, 181
  for sinusitis, 336
Cefprozil
  for sinusitis, 336
  for streptococcal pharyngitis, 333
Ceftazidime
  for brain abscess, 712
  for cholecystitis, 249
  for febrile neutropenia, 662
  for infected puncture wound, 113
  for pneumonia in children, 339t
  for septic shock, 55
Ceftizoxime, for cholecystitis, 249
Ceftriaxone
  for acute chest syndrome in sickle
    cell disease, 393
  for bacterial tracheitis, 371
  for brain abscess, 712
  for cellulitis, 449
  for chancroid, 405
  for cholecystitis, 249
  for cirrhosis and liver failure, 245
  for epiglottitis, 370
  for erysipelas, 450
  for esophageal perforation, 208
  for febrile infant, 313–316, 316t
  for gonococcal infection, 402, 403,
    896
    conjunctivitis, 334, 715
    pharyngitis, 333
  for lateral sinus thrombosis, 729
  for Lyme disease, 438
  for meningitis, 710t
  for meningococcemia, 752
  for otitis media, 330
  for pelvic inflammatory disease,
    306t
  for perforated or strangulated
    hernia, 220
  for periorbital cellulitis, 717
  for pneumonia, 181, 182
  for septic shock, 55
  for sinusitis, 336
  for streptococcal toxic shock
    syndrome, 409
  for urinary tract infection, 269
    in children, 398
Cefuroxime
  for cat bite prophylaxis, 117
  for epiglottitis, 370, 742
  for Lyme disease, 438
  for orbital cellulitis, 717
  for peritonsillar abscess, 741
  for pneumonia, 181

  in children, 339t
  for streptococcal pharyngitis, 333
Cefuroxime axetil, for otitis media,
  330
Cellulitis, 448–449
  in children, 336–337
  clinical features of, 336, 449
  diagnosis and differential of, 336,
    449
  facial, 724–725, 734–735
  of hand, 869, 870t
  from human bite injury, 114, 115
  management of, 336–337, 449
  orbital, 337, 717
  periorbital, 337, 717
  from puncture wound, 113
Central cord syndrome, 785t
Central retinal artery occlusion, 722
Central retinal vein occlusion, 723
Cephalexin
  for balanoposthitis, 273
  for cellulitis, 336, 725, 870t
  for cutaneous abscesses, 451
  for diverticulitis, 226
  for dog bites, 116
  for endocarditis prophylaxis, 147t,
    421
  for erysipelas, 375, 724
  for felon, 870t
  for impetigo, 374, 375, 724
  for mastitis, 298
  for open fractures, 763
  for paronychia, 870t
  for suppurative parotitis, 726
  for urinary tract infection, 269
    in children, 398
    in pregnancy, 289
  for wound prophylaxis, 85, 113, 118
Cephalic tetanus, 422
Cephalosporin use in pregnancy, 291t
Cerebellar gait, 687
Cerebellopontine angle tumors, 690
Cerebellotonsillar herniation, 777
Cerebral edema
  high-altitude, 578–580
  pediatric diabetic ketoacidosis and,
    355, 356, 610
Cerebrospinal fluid rhinorrhea, 788
Cervical conization, bleeding after,
  309
Cervical radiculopathy, 856, 857t
Cervical spine immobilization, 795,
  796
Cervical spine injury, 792–794
  airway management in patients
    with, 3, 4, 793

Cervical spine injury (*Cont.*)
clinical clearance of, 782
diagnosis and differential of,
780–782
fractures, 782, 783t–784t
in geriatric patients, 769
head trauma and, 777
mechanisms of, 781t
radiographic evaluation of,
780–782, 781t
rheumatic diseases and, 868
Cestodes, 435–436
dwarf tapeworm, 435
pork tapeworm, 435–436
CFI (clenched fist injury), 114–115,
869
Chalazion, 715
Chancre, in syphilis, 403
Chancroid, 405
Charcot triad, 248
Cheek lacerations, 98, *98*
Chelation therapy
for arsenic poisoning, 536t, 540
for iron poisoning, 472t, 525–526
for lead poisoning, 538–539
for mercury poisoning, 541
Chemical burns, 590–592
clinical features of, 590–591
diagnosis and differential of, 591
management of, 591–592
ocular, 544, 591, 721
Chemical pneumonitis, 527–528
Chest pain, 123–128
of acute chest syndrome in sickle
cell disease, 392
of acute myocardial infarction, 123,
126, 129–130
of acute pericardial tamponade, 126
of angina, 125, 129
unstable, 125
variant, 126
of aortic dissection, 126, 145, 163
of aortic stenosis, 144
clinical features of, 123
diagnosis of, 123–125, 130–131
echocardiography, 124–125, 131
electrocardiography, 123–124,
130, 131t
provocative tests, 125, 131
serum markers, 124, *124*, 131
differential diagnosis of, 125, 125t,
131
of dilated cardiomyopathy, 149
of esophageal perforation, 207
evaluation and management of,
127–128
gastrointestinal causes of, 127
of hypertrophic cardiomyopathy,
150
of mitral valve prolapse, 144
musculoskeletal causes of, 127
myofascial, 76t, 77t
of pericarditis, 126, 152–153
physical examination of, 123
of pulmonary embolism, 126, 156
Chest radiography (CXR)
in acute chest syndrome of sickle
cell disease, 392
in aortic dissection, 164
in aortic incompetence, 145–146
in asthma, 340
in bronchiolitis, 342
in cardiac tamponade, 154
of diaphragmatic injuries, 798, 804
in dilated cardiomyopathy, 149
in esophageal perforation, 207
of hemothorax, 797
in hypertensive emergencies,
159–160
in Loeffler syndrome, 433
in mitral incompetence, 143
in mitral stenosis, 142
in penetrating injuries of great
vessels, 800
in pericarditis, 153
in plague, 445
in pneumonia, 181, 338
of pulmonary contusions, 796
in restrictive cardiomyopathy, 151
in Rocky Mountain spotted fever,
439
of tracheobronchial injuries,
797–798
in tuberculosis, 185
Chest trauma. *See* Cardiothoracic
trauma
Chest tube placement
for hemothorax, 797
for pneumothorax, 188–189, 762,
793, 797
Chest wall injuries, 795–796
CHF. *See* Congestive heart failure
Chickenpox, 380, *380*
Chigger bites, 570
Chilblains, 561–562
Child abuse, 765, 891–892
burns due to, 586
clinical features of, 891
diagnosis and differential of,
891–892
fractures due to, 384–385
management of, 892

Child abuse (*Cont.*)
  of neonate, 320
  sexual, 892
Chin lift maneuver, 3, 762
  in children, 26
Chlamydia infection
  C. pneumoniae, 180
  C. trachomatis, 397, 401–402
    clinical features of, 401
    conjunctivitis, 334
    diagnosis and differential of,
      401–402
    lymphogranuloma venereum,
      405–406
    management of, 402
    pelvic inflammatory disease, 305
    prophylaxis after sexual assault,
      896
    urinary tract infection, 269
Chloral hydrate
  overdose of, 492–493
  for procedural sedation, 70
  side effects of, 70
Chloramphenicol
  for brain abscess, 712
  for gas gangrene, 447
  for meningitis, 709
  for plague, 446
  for Rocky Mountain spotted fever,
    377, 440
  for tularemia, 442
Chlordiazepoxide, for alcohol
  withdrawal, 252
Chlorhexidine mouth rinse
  for acute necrotizing ulcerative
    gingivitis, 735
  for periodontal abscess, 735
Chloroquine
  for malaria, 427, 428t
  toxicity of, 549–550
Chlorpromazine, for migraine, 671t
Cholecystitis, 247–249
  acalculous, 247–248
  clinical features of, 247
  diagnosis and differential of, 248
  management of, 248–249
  postoperative, 255
  risk factors for, 247
Cholestyramine, for diarrhea, 222
Cholinergic overdose, 468t
Chondromalacia patellae, 843
Chronic obstructive pulmonary disease
  (COPD), 192–195
  clinical features of, 192
  diagnosis and differential of,
    192–193

drugs to avoid in, 195
  management of, 193–195
Chvostek sign, 38
Cimetidine, for peptic ulcer disease,
  213
Cingulate herniation, 777
Ciprofloxacin
  for anthrax, 445
  for chancroid, 405
  for conjunctivitis, 715
  for corneal abrasion, 718
  for corneal ulcer, 717
  for Crohn disease, 222
  for diarrhea, 236
  for diverticulitis, 226
  for dog bites, 115, 116
  for gonococcal infection, 402, 715,
    896
  for human bites, 115
  for kidney stones, 277
  for otitis externa, 332
  for salmonellosis, 417
  for tuberculosis, 186t
  for tularemia, 443
  for urinary tract infection, 269
  for wound prophylaxis, 86, 108,
    112–113
Circulating anticoagulants, 633
Cirrhosis, 243–246
  clinical features of, 243
  diagnosis and differential of, 244
  jaundice and, 239
  management of, 245–246
CK-MB. *See* Creatine kinase-MB
Clarithromycin
  for cellulitis, 449, 725
  for endocarditis prophylaxis, 147t
  for Lyme disease, 438
  for *Mycobacterium avium* complex,
    417
  for pneumonia, 181
  for sinusitis, 732
  use in pregnancy, 291t
Clavicular fracture, 796, 830–831
  in children, 385
Clenched fist injury (CFI), 114–115,
  869
Clindamycin
  for bacterial vaginosis, 302, 896
  for cellulitis, 725
  for cholecystitis, 249
  for cutaneous abscesses, 451
  for diverticulitis, 226
  for dog bites, 115
  for endocarditis prophylaxis, 147t,
    420, 421t

Clindamycin (*Cont.*)
 for erysipelas, 375
 for esophageal perforation, 208
 for gas gangrene, 447, 448
 for human bites, 115
 for impetigo contagiosum, 375
 for inflammation from wisdom
  teeth, 734
 for intraabdominal infection in
  transplant recipients, 458
 for Ludwig angina, 734
 for mandibular fractures, 791
 for masticator space abscess, 726
 for necrotizing fasciitis, 448
 for odontogenic abscess, 743
 for pelvic inflammatory disease,
  306t
 for perforated or strangulated
  hernia, 220
 for periodontal abscess, 735
 for peritonsillar abscess, 373, 741
 for pneumonia, 182
 for postextraction alveolar osteitis,
  735
 for retropharyngeal abscess, 373,
  742
 for septic abortion, 294
 for septic shock, 55
 for streptococcal toxic shock
  syndrome, 409
 for suppurative parotitis, 726
 for tooth decay, 734
 for trichomoniasis, 896
 for ulcerative colitis, 223
 use in pregnancy, 291t
 for wound prophylaxis, 85
Clonazepam, for status epilepticus,
 346
Clonidine
 for hypertensive urgency, 161
 for opioid withdrawal, 500
  in pregnancy, 290
 for tetanus, 423
 toxicity of, 518–519
Clopidogrel
 for acute coronary syndromes, 132t,
  136
 for stroke, 677
Closed fist injury, 114–115, 869
Clostridial myonecrosis, 447–448
Clostridium botulinum infection, 699
 as biological weapon, 453, 454t
Clostridium difficile infection, 349t
Clotrimazole
 for balanoposthitis, 273
 for candidal infection

  oral, 417, 735
  vaginal, 303
 for tinea infections, 755
Cluster headaches, 667
 management of, 669–670
CMV. *See* Cytomegalovirus infection
Co-trimoxazole, for urinary tract
 infection, 269
Coagulation factors, 621
 assays of, 626t
 deficiencies of
  bleeding due to, 621
  in hemophilias, 634–639
  replacement therapy for, 649t
Cocaine
 cardiac effects of, 129, 500–501
 ingestion of bags of, 211, 501, 502
 intoxication with, 468t, 500–502
 use in pregnancy, 290, 500–501
Coccyx fracture, 837t
Codeine
 for cough, 191
 dosage of, 69t
Cognitive disorders, 679–683, 879
Coins
 aspiration of, 372
 ingestion of, 210
Cold agglutinin syndrome, 643
Cold-related injuries, 561–563, 562t
Colitis
 pseudomembranous, 224–225
 ulcerative, 222–224
Colles fracture, 769, 825
Colon injuries, 803
Colonic polyps, 354
Colonoscopy complications, 256
Colorado tick fever, 443–444
Coma, 683–685
 clinical features of, 683
 diagnosis and differential of,
  683–684, 684t
 management of, 684–685
 myxedema, 615–616
Compartment syndromes, 848–849
 clinical features of, 820, 848
 diagnosis and differential of, 848
 foot injuries with, 846–847
 hand injuries with, 823
 management of, 9848
 penetrating trauma to extremities
  and, 814
 pit viper bite and, 573
Complex regional pain syndromes,
 75–78, 76t, 77t
Computed tomography (CT)
 abdominal, 202

Computed tomography (CT) (*Cont.*)
  abdominal aortic aneurysm on, 163
  abdominal injuries on, 805
  aortic dissection on, 164
  appendicitis on, 215
  cholecystitis on, 248
  diverticulitis on, 226
  in genitourinary trauma, 811, 811t
  for head injury, 777–778
    pediatric, 765, 767t
  kidney stones on, 276
  for pediatric seizures, 344
  pulmonary embolism on, 157
  for stroke, 674–675
  subarachnoid hemorrhage on, 668
  in trauma patients, 762
Concussion
  brain, 776
  myocardial, 799
Conduction disturbances, 21–24
Congenital heart disease, 325, 326
Congestive heart failure (CHF)
  in children, 327–329
    clinical features of, 327
    diagnosis and differential of,
      327–328, 328t
    management of, 328–329
  dilated cardiomyopathy and, 149
  end-stage renal disease and, 264
  infective endocarditis and, 419
  long-term treatment of, 141
  myocarditis and, 152
  prerenal failure due to, 261
  pulmonary edema and, 140–141
Conjunctival abrasions, 718
Conjunctival foreign bodies, 718
Conjunctivitis, 334–335, 714–715
  allergic, 716
  bacterial, 715
  in children, 334–335
  clinical features of, 334
  diagnosis and differential of, 334
  management of, 334–335
  viral, 715–716
Constipation, 237–238
  clinical features of, 237
  diagnosis and differential of, 237
  management of, 237–238
  neonatal, 322
Constrictive pericarditis, 154–155
  clinical features of, 154
  diagnosis and differential of, 154
  etiologies of, 154
  management of, 155
  vs. restrictive cardiomyopathy, 151
Contact dermatitis, 753–754

Continuous "running" percutaneous
  sutures, 89, *89*
Contusions
  bladder, 812
  brain, 776
  myocardial, 799
  penile, 813
  pulmonary, 796–797
  renal, 812
  testicular, 813
Conversion disorder, 886–887
  clinical features of, 886
  diagnosis and differential of, 886
  management of, 886–887
Cooling procedures
  for burns, 589
  for heat stroke, 565
Coombs test, 622t
COPD. *See* Chronic obstructive
  pulmonary disease
Copperhead bite, 572–573
Coral snake bite, 574
Corneal abrasion, 718
Corneal foreign bodies, 719
Corneal ulcer, 717–718
Coronary artery bypass graft (CABG)
  surgery, 59, 131, 136
Corticosteroids. *See also* specific
  drugs
  for acneiform eruptions, 756
  adrenal suppression by, 618, 867
  for aphthous stomatitis, 736
  for asthma and chronic obstructive
    pulmonary disease, 193–194, 341
  for bronchiolitis, 343
  for bullous pemphigoid, 752
  for caustic ingestion, 531
  for cold injuries, 562
  for contact dermatitis, 754
  for Crohn disease, 222
  for croup, 369
  for erythema multiforme, 748
  for exfoliative dermatitis, 747
  for Hymenoptera sting, 567
  for meningitis, 709
  for multiple sclerosis, 704
  for myasthenia gravis, 706
  for pemphigus vulgaris, 752
  for pharyngitis with airway
    obstruction, 333
  for *Pneumocystis carinii*
    pneumonia, 417
  for temporal arteritis, 672
  for thyroid storm, 615t
  for ulcerative colitis, 223–224
  use in pregnancy, 291t

Cosyntropin stimulation test, 617
Coughing
in acute bronchitis, 179
of blood, 190–191
in chronic bronchitis, 192
codeine for, 191
in croup, 369
in influenza, 410
in tuberculosis, 184
COX-2 (cyclooxygenase-2) inhibitor toxicity, 510–511
Coxsackievirus infection, 377, 736
CPK (creatine phosphokinase), in rhabdomyolysis, 850, 851
Crack cocaine, 501
Creatine kinase-MB (CK-MB)
in acute myocardial infarction, 58, 124, *124*, 131
in electrical injuries, 593
in end-stage renal disease, 264
Creatine phosphokinase (CPK), in rhabdomyolysis, 850, 851
Cricoarytenoid joints, in rheumatoid arthritis, 867
Cricoid pressure for orotracheal intubation, 4, 5
in children, 28
Cricothyrotomy, *7,* 7–8, 762, 793
Crohn disease, 221–222
clinical features of, 221
diagnosis and differential of, 221–222
management of, 222
Crotaline envenomation, 572–573
Crotamiton, for chigger bites, 570
Croup, 369–370
clinical features of, 369
diagnosis and differential of, 369
management of, 369–370
Crutches, 820–821
Crying in infants, excessive, 319–320, 320t
Cryoprecipitate, 647
for disseminated intravascular coagulation, 630
for fibrinolytic-induced bleeding, 630
for hemophilia, 635
in liver disease, 629
in renal disease, 629
for thrombolytic-induced hemorrhage, 135
for von Willebrand disease, 640
Cryptitis, 230
Cryptococcosis
in HIV infection, 415

management of, 417
Crystal-induced synovitis, 863
CT. *See* Computed tomography
Cuff cellulitis after hysterectomy, 308–309
Cullen sign, 255
CXR. *See* Chest radiography
Cyanide poisoning, 551–552
antidote for, 472t
clinical features of, 551
diagnosis and differential of, 551
management of, 551–552, 552t
Cyanoacrylate tissue adhesives, 92–93, 106
eye exposure to, 721
Cyanosis, 177–178
in children, 325–327
clinical features of, 326
diagnosis and differential of, 326–327
management of, 327
neonates, 322–323
clinical features of, 177
diagnosis and differential of, 177–178, 178t
management of, 178
Cyclooxygenase-2 (COX-2) inhibitor toxicity, 510–511
Cyclopentolate
for chemical ocular injury, 721
for corneal abrasion, 718
for corneal ulcer, 718
for herpes zoster ophthalmicus, 717
Cyclophosphamide, for hemolytic anemia, 644
Cyclosporine
adverse effects of, 459t, 460
for ulcerative colitis, 223
Cyproheptadine, for serotonin syndrome, 479
Cyst
ganglion
of foot, 873
of hand, 871
infected sebaceous, 450
ovarian, 284
Cysticercosis, 435–436
Cystitis, 267–269. *See also* Urinary tract infection
Cystography, 811, 811t
Cytomegalovirus (CMV) infection
in HIV disease, 413, 414
radiculitis, 701
retinitis, 416
management of, 417
in transplant recipients, 456, 458

D

D-dimer assay, 626t
  for deep venous thrombosis, 167
  for pulmonary embolism, 157, 659
Dalteparin, for deep venous
    thrombosis, 168
Dantrolene, for monoamine oxidase
    inhibitor overdose, 486
DCM. *See* Dilated cardiomyopathy
DCS (decompression sickness),
    582–583
DDAVP. *See* Desmopressin
De Quervain tenosynovitis, 871
Deafness, 730
Debridement of wounds, 85
Decompression sickness (DCS),
    582–583
Decontamination of poisoned patient,
    474. *See also* Activated charcoal;
    Chelation therapy
  after caustic ingestion, 531
  after cyanide exposure, 551
  after hazardous materials exposure,
    542–543
  after hydrocarbon and volatile
    substance exposure, 529
Deep dermal sutures, 89–90, *90*
Deep venous thrombosis (DVT),
    166–168, 167t
  clinical features of, 166
  diagnosis and differential of,
    166–167
  management of, 167–168, 655
  predictors of, 166, 167t
  in pregnancy, 288–289
  risk factors for, 166
Deferoxamine, for iron poisoning,
    472t, 525–526
Defibrillation, 21
  in children, 30
Dehydration, 32
  in children, 348, 366–368
    clinical features of, 366–367,
      366t
    diagnosis and differential of, 367
    fluid and electrolyte therapy for,
      367–368
Delayed wound closure, 91
Delirium, 679–680, 879
  clinical features of, 679
  diagnosis and differential of, 679,
    680t, 681t
  management of, 679–680
Delivery of infant, emergency,
    299–301
  with breech presentation, 301

  with cord prolapse, 300
  diagnosis and differential for, 299
  episiotomy for, 299
  after maternal trauma, 773
  postpartum care after, 301
  with shoulder dystocia, 301
  technique for, 299–300
Demeclocycline, for syndrome of
    inappropriate antidiuretic hormone,
    662
Dementia, 680–683, 879
  clinical features of, 680
  diagnosis and differential of, 680t,
    681–682, 682t
  management of, 682–683
Dental avulsion, 737
Dental caries, 734
Dental concussion, 737
Dental fractures, 736–737
Dental luxations, 737
Dental procedures
  endocarditis prophylaxis for, 147t,
    421t
  postextraction alveolar osteitis, 735
  postextraction hemorrhage, 738–739
Dental soft tissue trauma, 737
Dentoalveolar trauma, 736
Depacon. *See* Valproate
Depression, 879
Dermal toxin exposure, 544
Dermatitis
  contact, 753–754
  exfoliative, 747–748
Dermatomyositis, 699, 867
Desmopressin (DDAVP)
  for bleeding, 629
    in hemophilia A, 639
    in von Willebrand disease, 639
  for central diabetes insipidus, 35
Dexamethasone
  for aphthous stomatitis, 736
  for caustic ingestion, 531
  for chemotherapy-induced
    nausea/vomiting, 663
  for croup, 369
  for high-altitude syndromes, 579,
    580
  for meningitis, 709
  for pharyngitis, 740
  for pharyngitis with airway
    obstruction, 333
  for spinal cord compression, 657,
    859
  for superior vena cava syndrome,
    658
  for thyroid storm, 615t

Dextrose solutions, 32
  for calcium channel blocker
    toxicity, 517
  for hypoglycemia, 358, 472t, 556,
    607
DHE (dihydroergotamine)
  for cluster headaches, 669
  for migraine, 668, 671t
Diabetes insipidus, 34–35
Diabetes mellitus, 607–611
  hyperosmolar hyperglycemic state
    in, 610–611
  hypoglycemia in, 607–608
  ketoacidosis in, 608–610
  in pregnancy, 288
Diabetic ketoacidosis (DKA), 42t,
  608–610
  in children, 355–356
  clinical features of, 355, 608
  diagnosis and differential of, 355,
    608
  vs. hyperosmolar hyperketotic state,
    610
  management of, 355–356, 609–610
  in pregnancy, 288
Dialysis
  for acute renal failure, 262
  for barbiturate overdose, 490
  complications of, 264–266
  for hemolytic-uremic syndrome,
    645
  for hypercalcemia of malignancy,
    660
  for hyperkalemia, 36, 38, 852
  for lithium overdose, 488
  for metformin-induced lactic
    acidosis, 556
  for methanol or ethylene glycol
    toxicity, 497
  for pediatric hypernatremia, 35
  for poisoned patient, 475
  for salicylate overdose, 507
  for theophylline toxicity, 513, 513t
  for tumor lysis syndrome, 660
Diaphragmatic injuries, 798, 804
Diarrhea, 234–237
  in children, 348–350, 351
    neonates, 321–322
  clinical features of, 234–235
  in Crohn disease, 221
  diagnosis and differential of,
    235–236
  drug-induced, 224–225, 254
  in helminthic infections, 432t
  in HIV infection, 416
  infectious, 235, 236

  management of, 222, 236–237
  in pseudomembranous colitis, 224
  in ulcerative colitis, 222–223
Diazepam
  for febrile seizures, 347
  for neck and back pain, 859
  for procedural sedation, 70
  for status epilepticus, 345, *696*
  for stimulant overdose, 501
  for toxin-induced seizures, 480
Diazoxide, for sulfonylurea overdose,
  556
DIC. *See* Disseminated intravascular
  coagulation
Dicloxacillin
  for cellulitis, 336, 449, 725, 870t
  for dog bites, 116
  for erysipelas, 724
  for felon, 870t
  for impetigo, 374, 375, 724
  for mastitis, 298
  for paronychia, 870t
  for suppurative parotitis, 726
  for wound prophylaxis, 85, 118
Digital blocks, *72*, 72–73
Digital intubation, 8
Digital nerve injuries, 103
Digitalis glycoside toxicity, 514–515
  clinical features of, 514
  diagnosis and differential of, 514
  with hyperkalemia, 37, 514
  management of, 16, 514–515
Digoxin
  for atrial fibrillation, 14
  for atrial flutter, 13
  for dilated cardiomyopathy, 150
  for pediatric heart failure, 329
  for supraventricular tachycardia, 15
Digoxin-specific Fab, 16, 37, 472t,
  515
Dihydroergotamine (DHE)
  for cluster headaches, 669
  for migraine, 668, 671t
Dilated cardiomyopathy (DCM),
  149–150
  clinical features of, 149
  diagnosis and differential of, 149
  management of, 150
Diltiazem
  for atrial fibrillation, 14
  for atrial flutter, 12
  for multifocal atrial tachycardia, 12
  for supraventricular tachycardia, 15
Dimercaprol
  for arsenic poisoning, 536t, 540
  for lead poisoning, 538t

Dimercaprol (*Cont.*)
  for mercury poisoning, 541
Dimercaptosuccinic acid (DMSA)
  for arsenic poisoning, 536t, 540
  for lead poisoning, 538
  for mercury poisoning, 541
DIP (distal interphalangeal) joint
    dislocations, 822
Diphenhydramine
  for allergic conjunctivitis, 335, 716
  for allergic reactions, 61
  for angioedema of upper airway,
      744
  for chemotherapy-induced
      nausea/vomiting, 663
  for erythema multiforme, 748
  for Hymenoptera sting, 567
  for "niacin flush," 548
  for pityriasis rosea, 382
  use in pregnancy, 292t
  for varicella, 380
Diphenoxylate and atropine, for
    diarrhea, 222, 236
Diphyllobothrium latum infection, 436
Diplopia, 788
Dipyridamole, for stroke, 677
Direct thrombin inhibitors, 654
Disc battery ingestion, 210, 532
Disequilibrium, 689
Dislocations
  ankle, 846
  distal interphalangeal joint, 822
  elbow, 826
  facet dislocation of cervical spine
    bilateral, 783t
    unilateral, 784t
  fracture–dislocation, 820
  glenohumeral joint, 831–833
  hip, 838–839
  knee, 841
  lunate, 824
  mandibular, 727
  metacarpophalangeal joint, 823
  occipitoatlantal, 783t
  patella, 841
  perilunate, 824
  proximal interphalangeal joint, 823
  sternoclavicular joint, 830
  temporomandibular, 791
Disseminated intravascular
    coagulation (DIC), 54, 56, 630–632
  clinical features of, 630
  conditions associated with, 631t
  diagnosis and differential of, 630,
      632t
  management of, 630–632

Distal interphalangeal (DIP) joint
    dislocations, 822
Diuretics
  for dilated cardiomyopathy, 150
  for mitral stenosis, 142
  for pulmonary edema, 140, 144, 145
  for restrictive cardiomyopathy, 151
  for rhabdomyolysis, 852
  toxicity of, 518
Diverticulitis, 225–226
  clinical features of, 225
  diagnosis and differential of,
      225–226
  management of, 226
Diving complications, 581–583
Diving reflex, in supraventricular
    tachycardia, 15
Dizziness, 688–692. *See also* Vertigo
  psychogenic, 689
DKA. *See* Diabetic ketoacidosis
DMSA. *See* Dimercaptosuccinic acid
Dobutamine
  for aortic incompetence, 146
  for mitral incompetence, 144
  for monoamine oxidase inhibitor
      overdose, 485
  for pulmonary edema, 140
  for right ventricular infarction, 136
  for shock, 52
    cardiogenic shock, 58, 329
    neurogenic shock, 62
Dog bites, 115–116
  rabies from, 423–425
Dolasetron, for chemotherapy-induced
    nausea/vomiting, 663
Domestic violence. *See* Intimate
    partner violence and abuse
Dopamine
  for acute renal failure, 262
  for aortic incompetence, 146
  for barbiturate overdose, 490
  for pediatric sepsis, 317
  for pulmonary edema, 140
  for shock, 52
    cardiogenic shock, 58, 329
    neurogenic shock, 62
    septic shock, 55
  for sinus bradycardia, 10
  for spinal shock, 786
  for toxic shock syndrome, 407
Dopamine agonist toxicity, 520
Doxazosin toxicity, 519
Doxycycline
  for anthrax, 445
  for cat bite prophylaxis, 117
  for chalazion, 715

Doxycycline (*Cont.*)
  for chlamydial infection, 402, 896
  for ehrlichiosis, 443
  for gonococcal conjunctivitis, 715
  for Lyme disease, 438
  for lymphogranuloma venereum,
    406
  for malaria, 427, 428t–429t
  for pelvic inflammatory disease,
    306t
  for plague, 446
  for pneumonia, 181
  for Rocky Mountain spotted fever,
    440
  for tularemia, 443
DPL (diagnostic peritoneal lavage),
  804–805
Dressings for wounds, 118
Dressler syndrome, 130, 152
"Drop attack," 137
Drowning, 584–585
Drug abuse, 499–504, 879
  cocaine, amphetamines, and other
    stimulants, 500–502
  hallucinogens, 502–504, 503t
  opioids, 499–500
  in pregnancy, 290
Drug allergy, 60–61
Drug-seeking behavior, 78–79, 78t
Dry drowning, 584
Dry eyes, 868
Dumping syndrome, postoperative,
  256
Duodenal injuries, 803
Dupuytren contracture, 871
Duroziez sign, 145
Duverney fracture, 837t
DVT. *See* Deep venous thrombosis
Dwarf tapeworm, 435
Dysbarism, 581–583
  clinical features of, 581–582
  diagnosis and differential of,
    582–583
  gas laws and, 581
  management of, 583
Dysdiadochokinesia, 686–687
Dysentery, 348
Dysfunctional uterine bleeding,
  283–284
Dyshemoglobinemias, 553–554
  clinical features of, 553
  diagnosis and differential of,
    553–554
  management of, 554
Dysmenorrhea, 285
Dysphagia, 206

Dyspnea, 173–174
  clinical features of, 173
  diagnosis and differential of, 173,
    174t
  disorders associated with
    aortic incompetence, 145
    aortic stenosis, 144
    dilated cardiomyopathy, 149
    hypertrophic cardiomyopathy,
      150
    mitral incompetence, 143
    mitral stenosis, 142
    mitral valve prolapse, 144
    pneumonia, 180
    pulmonary embolism, 156
    restrictive cardiomyopathy, 151
  management of, 174
Dysrhythmias, 9–25
  acute myocardial infarction and,
    130
  in cardiac transplant recipient, 461
  in children, 29–30
  cocaine-induced, 500, 502
  conduction disturbances, 21–24
    first-degree AV block, 21
    second-degree Mobitz I
      (Wenckebach) AV block,
      21–22, 22
    second-degree Mobitz II AV
      block, 22, 22–23
    third-degree (complete) AV
      block, 23, 23–24
  digitalis glycoside–induced, 514
  due to anticholinergic toxicity, 476
  due to antipsychotic overdose, 487
  due to electrical injuries, 594, 594t
  due to lightning injuries, 596t
  due to tricyclic antidepressant
    toxicity, 480
  preexcitation syndromes, 24–25, 25
  in pregnancy, 288
  preterminal rhythms, 24
    asystole, 24
    idioventricular rhythm, 24
    pulseless electrical activity, 24
  pulmonary edema and, 141
  supraventricular, 9–16
    atrial fibrillation, 13, 13–14
    atrial flutter, 12, 12–13
    junctional rhythms, 16, 16
    multifocal atrial tachycardia, 11,
      11–12
    premature atrial contractions,
      10–11, 11
    sinus bradycardia, 9–10
    sinus dysrhythmia, 9, 9

Dysrhythmias (*Cont.*)
  sinus tachycardia, 10
  supraventricular tachycardia, *14,* 14–16, *15*
  syncope due to, 137, 138
  theophylline-induced, 512, 513
  ventricular, 16–21
    aberrant vs. ventricular tachyarrhythmias, 16–17
    accelerated idioventricular rhythm, 18, *19*
    premature ventricular contractions, 17–18, *18*
    torsades de pointes, 20, *20*
    ventricular fibrillation, *20,* 20–21
    ventricular tachycardia, 19, *19*
Dysrhythmogenicity of right ventricular cardiomyopathy, 152
Dyssynergia, 686

E
EACA (ε-aminocaproic acid), for bleeding, 639
Ear trauma
  evaluation of, 788–789
  foreign bodies, 730
  lacerations, *97,* 97–98, 729
  pressure dressings for, 118
Eastern coral snake bite, 574
Ebola virus, 455
EBV (Epstein-Barr virus) infection
  infectious mononucleosis, 378–379
  pharyngitis, 332–333
ECG. *See* Electrocardiogram
Echinodermata, 576–577
Echocardiography
  in aortic dissection, 164
  in aortic incompetence, 146
  in aortic stenosis, 145
  cardiac injuries on, 798
  in cardiac tamponade, 154
  in cardiogenic shock, 58
  for chest pain, 124–125
  in children, 326
  in dilated cardiomyopathy, 149
  in hypertrophic cardiomyopathy, 151
  in mitral incompetence, 143–144
  in mitral stenosis, 142
  in mitral valve prolapse, 144
  in pericarditis, 153
  in restrictive cardiomyopathy, 151
  in traumatic aortic rupture, 801
Echovirus infection, 377
Eclampsia, 161, 296–298, 297t, 693, 697

Econazole, for tinea infections, 755
Ecstasy (3,4-methylenedioxymethamphetamine; MDMA), 503t
Ectopic pregnancy (EP), 286–287
  clinical features of, 286
  diagnosis and differential of, 286–287
  management of, 287
  risk factors for, 286
Edema
  cerebral
    high-altitude, 578–580
    pediatric diabetic ketoacidosis and, 355, 356, 610
  heat, 566
  pulmonary, 140–141
Edrophonium test, 705
EDTA (ethylene diamine tetraacetic acid), for lead poisoning, 538
Ehrlichiosis, 443
Eikenella infection
  antibiotic prophylaxis for, 85
  from human bites, 114
Elbow injuries, 826–827
  dislocations, 826
  fractures, 826–827
    in children, 385–386
  "nursemaid's" elbow, 386
Elder abuse, 892–893
  clinical features of, 892
  diagnosis and differential of, 892–893
  management of, 893
Electrical injuries, 593–595
  clinical features of, 593
  complications of, 594t
  diagnosis and differential of, 593
  indications for admission for, 595t
  management of, 593–595
Electrocardiogram (ECG). *See also* Dysrhythmias
  in antidepressant overdose
    selective serotonin reuptake inhibitors, 483
    trazodone, 481
    tricyclics, 480
    venlafaxine, 483
  in aortic incompetence, 145
  in aortic stenosis, 145
  in blunt myocardial injury, 799, 800
  in cardiac tamponade, 154
  in cardiac transplant recipient, 460
  in cardiogenic shock, 57
  cocaine effects on, 500
  in dilated cardiomyopathy, 149

Electrocardiogram (ECG) (*Cont.*)
  in hypercalcemia, 39, 660
  in hyperkalemia, 36
  in hypertensive emergencies, 159
  in hypertrophic cardiomyopathy,
    150–151
  in hypocalcemia, 38
  in hypokalemia, 35
  in hypomagnesemia, 39
  in hypothermia, 561
  in lithium toxicity, 488
  in mitral incompetence, 143
  in mitral stenosis, 142
  in myocarditis, 152
  in patient with chest pain, 123–124,
    127, 130, 131t
  in pericarditis, 126, 153
    constrictive, 154
  in phenytoin toxicity, 521
  in Prinzmetal angina, 126
  in pulmonary edema, 140, 141
  in restrictive cardiomyopathy, 151
  in syncope, 138
    pediatric, 365
Electrolyte disorders, 33–40
  from blood transfusion, 648
  hypercalcemia, 38–39
  hyperkalemia, 36–38, 37t
  hypermagnesemia, 40
  hypernatremia, 34–35, 35t
  hypocalcemia, 38
  hypokalemia, 35–36, 36t
  hypomagnesemia, 39–40
  hyponatremia, 33, 34t
  rhabdomyolysis and, 850–851
EM (erythema multiforme), 376,
  748–749
EMLA (lidocaine prilocaine), 73
Emphysema, 192
  subcutaneous, 795–796
Empyema, 180
Enalapril
  for dilated cardiomyopathy, 150
  for hypertension in ischemic stroke,
    675
  toxicity of, 520
Enalaprilat
  for hypertensive emergency, 160
  toxicity of, 520
Encephalitis, 711
  herpes simplex virus, 711
  West Nile virus, 440–441
End-stage renal disease (ESRD). *See*
  Renal failure
Endocarditis. *See* Infective
  endocarditis

Endocrine disorders, 605–618
  adrenal insufficiency and adrenal
    crisis, 617–618
  alcoholic ketoacidosis, 612–613
  diabetic emergencies, 607–611
  thyroid emergencies, 614–616
Endometriosis, 285
Endometritis, postpartum, 298
Endoscopy
  for caustic ingestions, 530
  for esophageal bleeding, 208
  for esophageal perforation, 207
  for gastrointestinal bleeding, 205
  for removal of ingested foreign
    bodies, 210, 211
Enemas, for constipation, 238
Enoxaparin, 653
  for acute coronary syndromes, 132t,
    134
  for deep venous thrombosis, 168
  for pulmonary embolism, 157, 659
  use in pregnancy, 292t
Entamoeba histolytica infection, 349t
Enterobacter urinary tract infection,
  268
Enterobius vermicularis infection,
  433
Enterovirus infection with rash,
  377–378
Entrapment neuropathies, 700
Environmental injuries, 559–603
  bites and stings, 567–574
  carbon monoxide poisoning,
    598–600
  chemical burns, 590–592
  dysbarism and diving
    complications, 581–583
  electrical injuries, 593–595
  frostbite and hypothermia, 561–563
  heat-related illness, 564–567
  high-altitude syndromes, 578–580
  lightning injuries, 595–597
  marine fauna envenomation,
    575–577
  near drowning, 584–585
  plant and mushroom poisonings,
    601–603
  thermal burns, 586–590
Eosinophilia, in helminthic infections,
  432t
EP. *See* Ectopic pregnancy
Epididymitis, 272
Epidural hematoma, 776
Epiglottitis, 742–743
  in children, 370
  clinical features of, 370, 742

Epiglottitis (*Cont.*)
  diagnosis and differential of, 370, 742
  management of, 370, 742–743
Epilepsy, 693. *See also* Seizures
Epinephrine
  adding to local anesthetics, 71, 84
  for allergic reactions, 61
  for angioedema of upper airway, 744
  for asthma, 193, 341
  for asystole, 24
  for β-blocker toxicity, 516
  for bronchiolitis, 342–343
  for cardiac arrest, 29
  for children, 29
  for croup, 369
  for epistaxis, 731
  for foreign body aspiration, 372
  for Hymenoptera sting, 567
  for idioventricular rhythm, 24
  for neonatal resuscitation, 30
  for pediatric sepsis, 317
  for priapism, 394
  for pulseless electrical activity, 24
  for sinus bradycardia, 10
  for ventricular fibrillation, 21
  for ventricular tachycardia, 17
Episcleritis, 868
Episiotomy, 299
Epistaxis, 730–732
Epley maneuver, 691
Epstein-Barr virus (EBV) infection
  infectious mononucleosis, 378–379
  pharyngitis, 332–333
Eptifibatide, 654
  for acute coronary syndromes, 132t, 136
Equine gait, 687
Equipment chart for children, length-based, 27t
Erethism, 540
Ergot alkaloids
  for cluster headaches, 669
  for migraine, 668, 671t
  use in pregnancy, 292t
Erysipelas, 375, 449–450, 724
Erythema infectiosum, 378, *379*
Erythema multiforme (EM), 376, 748–749
Erythema nodosum, 382
Erythromycin
  for acute rheumatic fever, 390
  for anthrax, 445
  for cellulitis, 725
  for chancroid, 405
  for chemical ocular injury, 721
  for chlamydial infection, 402, 896
  for conjunctival abrasions, 718
  for conjunctivitis, 334
  for corneal abrasion, 718
  for dog bite prophylaxis, 115
  for erysipelas, 375
  for eye exposure to cyanoacrylate glue, 721
  for herpes simplex conjunctivitis, 716
  for herpes zoster ophthalmicus, 717
  for impetigo contagiosum, 375
  for lymphogranuloma venereum, 406
  for pharyngitis, 740
  for pneumonia, 182
  for pneumonia in children, 339t
  for scarlet fever, 377
  for septic shock, 55
  for streptococcal toxic shock syndrome, 409
  for stye, 715
  use in pregnancy, 291t
Erythromycin ethylsuccinate
  for cellulitis, 337
  for streptococcal pharyngitis, 333
Escherichia coli infection
  in children, 349t
  hemolytic-uremic syndrome, 236
  pneumonia, 179
  urinary tract infection, 268
Esmolol
  for acute coronary syndromes, 133
  for hypertensive emergency, 160
  for supraventricular tachycardia, 15
  for thyroid storm, 615t
Esophageal disorders, 206–208
  bleeding, 204–205, 208
  due to button battery ingestion, 210, 532
  due to caustic ingestions, 530–532
  dysphagia, 206
  esophageal perforation, 207–208
  gastroesophageal reflux disease, 206–207
  in HIV infection, 416
  traumatic injuries, 802
Esophageal procedures, endocarditis prophylaxis for, 421t
ESRD (end-stage renal disease). *See* Renal failure
Estrogen
  for bleeding in renal disease, 629
  for dysfunctional uterine bleeding, 283–284
Ethacrynic acid toxicity, 518

Ethambutol
  for *Mycobacterium avium* complex, 417
  for tuberculosis, 185, 186t
  use in pregnancy, 291t
Ethanol. *See also* Alcohol
  for ethylene glycol or methanol poisoning, 472t, 497
Ethchlorvynol overdose, 492
Ethmoid sinusitis, 732
Ethosuximide, for seizures in children, 346
Ethylene diamine tetraacetic acid (EDTA), for lead poisoning, 538
Ethylene glycol intoxication, 495–498
  clinical features of, 496
  diagnosis and differential of, 496, 496t
  management of, 497–498
Etomidate
  dosage of, 69t
  for procedural sedation, 70
  for rapid sequence induction, 5
    in children, 28
  side effects of, 70
Evidence collection for sexual assault, 895
Exanthem subitum, 381, *381*
Exchange transfusion
  for hemolytic anemia, 644
  for sickle cell disease, 642
Exfoliative dermatitis, 747–748
  clinical features of, 747
  diagnosis and differential of, 747
  management of, 747–748
Exotic animal bites, 117
Exploratory laparotomy for abdominal trauma, 805, 806t
Extension teardrop fracture, 784t
Extensor tendon injuries
  forearm, 100, 100t
  hand, 102, *102*
External rotation technique, for glenohumeral joint dislocation, 832
Extremity injuries, penetrating, 814–815
  clinical features of, 814
  diagnosis and differential of, 814–815
  management of, 815
Eye examination, 787
Eye infections, 334–335, 715–718
Eyelid lacerations, 95, *95,* 719

F

Facet dislocation of cervical spine
  bilateral, 783t
  unilateral, 784t
Facial and scalp lacerations, 94–98
  cheeks and face, 98, *98*
  ear, *97,* 97–98, 729
  eyelids, 95, *95,* 719
  lips, *96,* 96–97, 738
  nose, 95–96
  scalp and forehead, *94,* 94–95
Facial cellulitis, 724–725, 734–735
Facial fractures, 787, *788*
Facial infections, 724–725
Facial pain, 671–672
Factor I deficiency, 649t
Factor II deficiency, 649t
Factor V deficiency, 649t
Factor VII deficiency, 649t
Factor VIII deficiency, 634–639, 649t
Factor VIII inhibitor, 633
Factor VIII products, 637t, 638t
Factor IX complex products, 637t, 638t
Factor IX deficiency, 634–639, 649t
Factor X deficiency, 649t
Factor XI deficiency, 649t
Factor XII deficiency, 649t
Factor XIII deficiency, 649t
Failure to thrive (FTT), 891–892
Falls, 768–770
Famciclovir
  for herpes simplex virus infection
    conjunctivitis, 716
    cutaneous, 417
    genital, 405
  for herpes zoster, 412, 418
  for herpes zoster ophthalmicus, 717
Famotidine, for peptic ulcer disease, 213
Fasciitis
  necrotizing, 253–255, 408–409, 448
  plantar, 873
Fasciotomy, 849
Febrile seizure, 347
Fecal blood, 237
Fecal impaction, 238
Feeding difficulties in neonates, 321
Feeding tube complications, 256
Felbamate, for seizures in children, 346
Felon, 870t, 871
Femoral fractures
  condylar, 840
  head and neck, 837
  shaft, 839
Fenoldopam
  for dopamine agonist toxicity, 520
  for hypertensive emergency, 160

Fenoldopam (*Cont.*)
  for monoamine oxidase inhibitor
    overdose, 485
Fentanyl
  for appendicitis pain, 215
  dosage of, 69t
  for rapid sequence induction, 5
Festinating gait, 687
Fetal distress, 299
Fetal monitoring, 299
Fetal–maternal hemorrhage, 771
Fetus
  emergency delivery of, 299–301
  injuries of, 771–773
Fever
  in helminthic infections, 432t
  in HIV infection, 413
  in malaria, 426
  in meningitis, 708, 709
  neutropenic, 662
  in pediatric patients, 313–314
    clinical features of, 313
    diagnosis and differential of,
      313–314
    management of, 314
    neonates, 313–314, 320
    occult bacteremia and, 313–314,
      315
    seizures and, 347
  postoperative, 253
FFP. *See* Fresh-frozen plasma
Fibrin degradation products, 626t
Fibrinolytic therapy, 59, 654. *See also*
  Antithrombotic therapy
  for acute coronary syndromes, 131,
    132, 132t, 134–135
    contraindications to, 134t
  bleeding induced by, 630
  for pulmonary embolism, 157–158
Fibroids, uterine, 285
Fibromyalgia, 76t, 77t
Fibular fractures, 841
Fifth disease, 289, 378
Finger and finger tip injuries, *103,*
  103–105, *104*
  digital blocks for, *72,* 72–73
  ring removal for, 105, *105*
Finkelstein test, 871
Fire ant stings, 568
Fish tapeworm, 436
Fishhook removal, *110,* 110–111, *111*
Fissure in ano, 230
Fistula(s)
  aortoenteric, 162
  after gastrointestinal surgery, 255
  in ano, 231

  perilymphatic, 690
Fitz-Hugh-Curtis syndrome, 305
Flail chest, 796
Flank trauma, penetrating, 807–808
Flatworms, 435–436
Flea bites, 570–571
Flexion teardrop fracture, 783t
Flexor hallucis longus rupture, 874
Flexor tendon injuries
  forearm, 100, 100t
  hand, 103
Flexor tenosynovitis, 869
Fluconazole
  for balanoposthitis, 273
  for candidal infection
    oral, 735
    vaginal, 303
  for cryptococcosis, 417
  for fungal esophagitis, 417
  for onychomycosis, 755
  for posttransplant fungal infections,
    458
Fluid and electrolyte therapy, 32
  for abdominal trauma, 805
  for acute pancreatitis, 251
  for acute renal failure, 261, 262
  for adrenal insufficiency, 618
  for alcoholic ketoacidosis, 612
  for antipsychotic overdose, 487
  for barbiturate overdose, 490
  for biliary colic, 249
  for burns, 589
  for calcium channel blocker
    toxicity, 517
  for cardiac tamponade, 154
  for children, 29, 32, 361, 366–368
  for diabetic ketoacidosis, 355–356,
    609
  for diverticulitis, 226
  for electrical injuries, 594
  for esophageal bleeding, 208
  for gastrointestinal bleeding, 205
  for head trauma patients, 778
  for hepatitis, 243, 245
  for hypercalcemia, 39
  for hyperemesis gravidarum, 295
  for hyperkalemia, 38
  for hypermagnesemia, 40
  for hypernatremia, 34–35
  for hyperosmolar hyperketotic state,
    610
  for hypoglycemia, 358
  for hypokalemia, 36
  for hyponatremia, 33
  for hypotension, 61
  for intestinal obstruction, 218

Fluid and electrolyte therapy (*Cont.*)
  for lithium overdose, 488
  for monoamine oxidase inhibitor
    overdose, 485
  for neurogenic shock, 62
  for pediatric sepsis, 317
  for poisoned patient, 474
  for pulmonary embolism, 157
  for rhabdomyolysis, 851
  for salicylate overdose, 506
  for septic shock, 55
  for shock, 51–52
  for toxic shock syndrome, 407
  for trazodone or nefazodone
    overdose, 481
  for tricyclic antidepressant toxicity,
    480–481
  for ulcerative colitis, 223
  for vomiting and diarrhea, 236
Flukes, 435
Flumazenil, for benzodiazepine
  reversal, 68, 491
Fluorometholone, for allergic
  conjunctivitis, 716
Folate, for methanol toxicity, 472t,
  497
Folliculitis, 451
Fomepizole, for methanol or ethylene
  glycol toxicity, 472t, 497
Food allergy, 60–61
Food bolus impaction, 209–210
Foot conditions, 872–875
  bursitis, 872
  ganglion cyst, 873
  immersion foot, 561–562, 874
  injuries, 846–847
    high pressure injection injuries,
      113
    lacerations, 107–108
  onychocryptosis, 872
  plantar fasciitis, 873
  plantar fibromatosis, 874
  plantar interdigital neuroma, 874
  plantar warts, 872
  tarsal tunnel syndrome, 873
  tendon lesions, 873–874
  ulcers, 874–875
Foot drop, 700, 701
Forearm
  extensor compartments in, 100, 100t
  flexor tendons in, 100, 101t
  fractures of, 827–828
  lacerations of, 100, *101*
Forehead lacerations, *94,* 94–95
Foreign bodies
  aspiration of, 371–372, 743–744

conjunctival, 718
corneal, 719
ear, 730
ingestion of, 209–211
nasal, 732
from puncture wounds, 112
rectal, 231–232
removal from soft tissue wounds,
  83–84, 109–111
upper airway obstruction from,
  743–744
urethral, 274
vaginal, 283, 304
Forensic examination for sexual
  assault, 895
Foscarnet, for cytomegalovirus
  infection, 417
Fosphenytoin
  for seizures, 697
    in children, 346, 766
    in neonates, 347
    posttraumatic, 766, 779
    status epilepticus, 345, *696*
  toxicity of, 521–523
    clinical features of, 521–522
    diagnosis and differential of, 522
    management of, 522–523
Fournier gangrene, 273
Fracture–dislocation, 820
Fractures, 769–770
  acetabulum, 837
  ankle, 845–846
  buckle, 384
  clavicle, 385, 796, 830–831
  clinical features of, 819–820
  Colles, 769, 825
  cortical, 384
  dental, 736–737
  description of, 819–820
  due to child abuse, 384–385
  Duverney, 837t
  elbow, 385–386, 826–827
  femoral condyle, 840
  fibular, 841
  foot, 847
  frontal sinus and frontal bone
    fractures, 789–790
  greenstick, 384
  hip, 769, 837
  humerus, 769, 833–834
  immobilization of, 820
  Jones, 847
  LeFort, 787, *788*
  management of, 763, 820–821
  mandible, 787, 791
  maxilla, 791

Fractures (*Cont.*)
  metacarpal, 823
  metatarsal, 847
  midfacial, 787, *788*
  nasal, 732, 787, 790
  open, 763, 820
  orbital blowout, 720, 787, 790
  patella, 840
  pediatric, 383–386
  pelvis, 763, 810, 835–837, 836t, 837t
  penile, 273, 813
  phalangeal
    of foot, 847
    of hand, 103, 104, 823
  plastic deformities, 384
  radius, 827–828
  reduction of, 820
  rib, 796
  Salter-Harris classification of, *383,* 383–384
  scapula, 833
  skull, 765, 774–776, 787
  Smith, 825
  spinal, 780–786, 783t–784t
  sternum, 796
  tibial, 841
  tibial plateau, 840
  tibial spine, 840
  toddler's, 385
  torus, 384
  tripod, 790–791
  ulnar, 827–828
  wrist, 824–825
  zygomatic, 790–791
Fracture–subluxation, 820
Francisella tularensis infection, 442–443, 454t
Fresh-frozen plasma (FFP), 647
  for bleeding in liver disease, 629
  for disseminated intravascular coagulation, 630
  for hemolytic anemia, 644
  for hemophilias, 635
  for thrombolytic-induced hemorrhage, 135, 630
Frontal sinus and frontal bone fractures, 789–790
Frostbite, 561–563
  classification of severity of, 561, 562t
  clinical features of, 561
  diagnosis and differential of, 562
  of ear, 729–730
  management of, 562–563, 563t
Frostnip, 561

FTT (failure to thrive), 891–892
Fulminant hepatic failure, 241, 243
Functional gait, 687
Furosemide
  for dilated cardiomyopathy, 150
  for hypercalcemia, 39, 660, 852
  for hyperkalemia, 38
  for hypermagnesemia, 40
  for hypernatremia, 35
  for hyponatremia, 33
  for increased intracranial pressure, in children, 766
  for mitral stenosis, 142
  for pediatric heart failure, 329
  for pulmonary edema, 140, 144, 145
  for syndrome of inappropriate antidiuretic hormone, 662
  toxicity of, 518
Furuncle, 451

G
G-6-PD (glucose-6-phosphate dehydrogenase) deficiency, 642–643
Gabapentin
  for chronic pain, 77t, 78
  for postherpetic neuralgia, 412
  for seizures in children, 346
Gait disturbances, 686–687
  clinical features of, 686–687
  diagnosis and differential of, 687
  management of, 687
Gallstones, 247–249
  clinical features of, 247–248
  diagnosis and differential of, 248
  risk factors for, 247
Gamekeeper thumb, 822
Ganciclovir, for cytomegalovirus infection, 417, 458, 701
Ganglion cyst
  of foot, 873
  of hand, 871
Gas gangrene, 447–448
  clostridial, 447–448
    clinical features of, 447
    diagnosis and differential of, 447
    management of, 447–448
  nonclostridial, 448
Gastric decontamination, 474. *See also* Activated charcoal
  for caustic ingestion, 531
  for hydrocarbon and volatile substance toxicity, 529
Gastric lavage, 474
  for calcium channel blocker toxicity, 517
  for iron poisoning, 525

Gastric lavage (*Cont.*)
  for mercury poisoning, 541
  for theophylline toxicity, 512
Gastric outlet obstruction, 212–213
Gastritis, 212–213
Gastroenteritis in children, 348–350
  clinical features of, 348, 349t
  diagnosis and differential of, 348
  fluid and electrolyte therapy for,
      366–368
  management of, 349–350
  microbiology of, 348, 349t
Gastroesophageal reflux disease
    (GERD), 206–207
Gastrointestinal bleeding, 204–205
  from aortoenteric fistula, 162
  in children, 351–354
  clinical features of, 204
  in Crohn disease, 221
  diagnosis and differential of, 204
  esophageal, 204–205, 208
  from hemorrhoids, 204, 227
  management of, 204–205
  in patients with liver disease, 246
  in peptic ulcer disease, 204, 212,
      213
  septic shock with, 53, 54
  in ulcerative colitis, 223
  upper vs. lower, 204
Gastrointestinal disorders, 197–256
  acute abdominal pain, 199–203
  acute pancreatitis, 250–252
  anorectal disorders, 227–233
  in anthrax, 444
  appendicitis, 214–216
  chest pain due to, 127
  cholecystitis and biliary colic,
      247–249
  complications of general surgical
      procedures, 253–256
  constipation, 237–238
  Crohn disease, 221–222
  diverticulitis, 225–226
  esophageal disorders, 206–208
  gastrointestinal bleeding, 204–205
  hernia, 219–220
  in HIV infection, 415–416
  intestinal obstruction, 217–218
  jaundice and hepatic disorders,
      239–246
  in neonates, 321–322
  peptic ulcer disease and gastritis,
      212–213
  pseudomembranous colitis, 224–225
  swallowed foreign bodies, 209–211
  traumatic injuries, 803

  ulcerative colitis, 222–224
  vomiting and diarrhea, 234–237
    in children, 348–350
Gastrointestinal procedures,
    endocarditis prophylaxis for, 421t
Gastrostomy tube complications,
    256
Gatifloxacin
  for cellulitis, 725
  for gonococcal infection, 402
  for pneumonia, 181
GBS (Guillain-Barré syndrome),
    699–700
GCA (giant cell arteritis), 671–672,
    723, 868
GCS (Glasgow Coma Scale), 584,
    761, 774, 775t, 777, 779
Gelfoam, 84
Generalized anxiety disorder, 881
Genital herpes, 404–405
Genital problems in male, 271–275
  epididymitis, 272
  Fournier gangrene, 273
  orchitis, 272
  penile, 273–274
  scrotal abscess, 272
  testicular torsion, 271
  urethral, 274
  urinary retention, 274–275
Genitourinary complications of
    surgery, 253
Genitourinary injuries, 810–814
  bladder, 812
  in children, 765
  clinical features of, 810
  diagnosis and differential of,
      810–812, 811t
  due to sexual assault, 895
  kidney, 812
  management of, 812–813
  penis, 813
  testicles and scrotum, 813
  ureter, 812
  urethra, 812–813
Genitourinary procedures, endocarditis
    prophylaxis for, 421t
Gentamicin
  for cellulitis, 336
    periorbital and orbital, 337
  for cholecystitis, 249
  for conjunctivitis, 335
  for diverticulitis, 226
  for endocarditis prophylaxis, 147t,
      421, 421t
  for febrile infant, 320
  for gas gangrene, 447, 448

Gentamicin (*Cont.*)
  for intraabdominal infection in
    transplant recipients, 458
  for pelvic inflammatory disease,
    306t
  for plague, 446
  for pneumonia
    in children, 339t
    nosocomial, 458
  for postpartum endometritis, 298
  for septic abortion, 294
  for septic shock, 55
  for tularemia, 442
  for ulcerative colitis, 223
  for urinary tract infection, 269
    in neonates, 398
    in pregnancy, 289
GERD (gastroesophageal reflux
  disease), 206–207
Geriatric patients
  abdominal pain in, 201–202
  abuse of, 892–893
  appendicitis in, 215
  traumatic injuries in, 768–770
    clinical features of, 768
    diagnosis and differential of,
      768–770
    management of, 770
    mechanisms of, 768
German measles, 380
Gestational trophoblastic disease
  (GTD), 294
GHB (γ-hydroxybutyrate), 491–492
Giant cell arteritis (GCA), 671–672,
  723, 868
Giardia lamblia infection, 349t
Gila monster bite, 574
Gilbert syndrome, 239
Gingivitis, acute necrotizing
  ulcerative, 735
Gingivostomatitis, herpes, 736
Glasgow Coma Scale (GCS), 584,
  761, 774, 775t, 777, 779
Glaucoma, acute angle closure,
  721–722
Glenohumeral joint dislocation,
  831–833
  clinical features of, 831–832
  management of, 832–833
Globe penetration or rupture, 720
Glucagon
  for β-blocker toxicity, 515
  for calcium channel blocker
    toxicity, 517
  for hypoglycemia, 358, 556, 697
  for hypotension, 61

  for poisoned patient, 473t, 474
  to relax lower esophageal sphincter,
    210
Glucocorticoids. *See* Corticosteroids
Glucose-6-phosphate dehydrogenase
  (G-6-PD) deficiency, 642–643
α-Glucosidase inhibitors, 555, 607
Glucosuria, 355
Glutethimide overdose, 492
Glycerin rectal suppositories, for
  constipation, 238
Glycoprotein IIb/IIIa antagonists, 654
  for acute coronary syndromes, 132t,
    136
Glycopyrrolate, for vomiting, 249
Gonococcal infection. *See Neisseria
  gonorrhoeae* infection
Goodpasture syndrome, 867
Gout, 863
Graft-versus-host disease, from blood
  transfusion, 649
Granisetron, for chemotherapy-
  induced nausea/vomiting, 663
Great vessels
  blunt injuries of, 801–802
  penetrating injuries of, 800
  transposition of, 326
Greater trochanteric fractures, 837
Griseofulvin, for tinea capitis, 754
Groin masses, 220
GTD (gestational trophoblastic
  disease), 294
Guanabenz toxicity, 518–519
Guanethidine, for thyroid storm, 615t
Guanfacine toxicity, 518–519
Guillain-Barré syndrome (GBS),
  699–700

H
H$_2$-receptor antagonists
  for angioedema of upper airway,
    744
  for peptic ulcer disease, 213
HACE (high-altitude cerebral edema),
  578–580
Haemophilus ducreyi infection, 405
Haemophilus influenzae infection
  cellulitis, 336, 337, 724–725
  epiglottitis, 370, 742
  otitis media, 330, 728
  pneumonia, 179, 180
  sinusitis, 335
Hair
  loss of, 754
  removal from wounds, 84–85
Hair tourniquet syndrome, 108

Hallucinations, from plant ingestion, 601
Hallucinogen intoxication, 502–504
  clinical features of, 502, 503t
  diagnosis and differential of, 502
  management of, 502–504
Haloperidol
  for agitated patient, 474
  for delirium, 680
  for hallucinogen intoxication, 502
  for violent patient, 884
Hamate fracture, 825
Hamman sign, 797
Hand conditions, 869–871
  infectious, 869–871, 870t
  noninfectious, 871
Hand-foot-and-mouth disease, 377–378, 736
Hand injuries, 822–824
  boutonniere deformity, 822
  compartment syndrome from, 823
  distal interphalangeal joint dislocations, 822
  dog bites, 115–116
  dorsal lacerations, 102
  finger and finger tip injuries, *103,* 103–105, *104*
    ring removal, 105, *105*
  gamekeeper thumb, 822
  high pressure injection injuries, 113–114, 824
  human bites, 114–115
  metacarpal fractures, 823
  metacarpophalangeal joint dislocations, 823
  palm lacerations, 100–101
  phalangeal fractures, 103, 104, 823
  proximal interphalangeal joint dislocations, 823
  specialist consultation for, 99
  tendons, 822
    extensor tendon lacerations, 102, *102*
    flexor tendon lacerations, 103
Hangman's fracture, 782, 784t
HAPE (high-altitude pulmonary edema), 578–580
Hare traction, 839
Hazardous materials exposure, 542–545
  bioterrorism agents, 452–455
  chemical burns from, 590–592
  decontamination for, 542–543
  dermal toxins, 544
  inhaled toxins, 543
  metabolic toxins, 544–545

myocardial toxins, 545
  neurotoxins, 544
  ocular, 544, 591
  post-incident response, 545
  sources of data about, 542
β-hCG (β-human chorionic gonadotropin) test for pregnancy, 286–287, 294
HCM. *See* Hypertrophic cardiomyopathy
HDCV (human diploid cell vaccine), 425
Head lice, 571, 757–758
Head-thrust test of vestibuloocular reflex, 689–690
Head trauma, 774–779
  benign paroxysmal positional vertigo and, 689
  brain concussion, 776
  brain contusion and intracerebral hemorrhage, 776
  brain herniation, 777
  clinical features of, 774–777
  diagnosis and differential of, 777–778
  epidural hematoma, 776
  geriatric, 768
  Glasgow Coma Scale in, 774, 775t
  pediatric, 764–767
    computed tomography for, 765, 767t
    diagnosis and differential of, 764–765
    management of, 766–767
    mechanisms of, 764
  penetrating, 777
  seizures and, 347
  severity of brain injury from, 774
  skull fractures, 774–776, 787
  subarachnoid hemorrhage, 776
  subdural hematoma, 776
Headache, 667–671
  brain tumor and, 667
  in children, 361–362
  clinical features of, 667–668
  cluster, 667, 669–670
  diagnosis and differential of, 668, 669t, 670t
  hypertensive, 667, 670
  management of, 668–671, 671t
  in meningitis, 667
  migraine, 667–669, 671t
  myofascial, 76t, 77t
  primary and secondary causes of, 361, 668, 669t

Headache (*Cont.*)
from subarachnoid hemorrhage,
667, 668, 674
from subdural hematoma, 667
from temporal arteritis, 671
tension, 667, 669
"thunderclap," 137
Hearing loss, sudden, 730
Heart disease. *See* Cardiovascular
disease
Heart failure. *See* Congestive heart
failure
Heart rate, drug-induced changes in,
470t–471t
Heart sounds and murmurs
in children, 325, 325t
in dilated cardiomyopathy, 149
in hypertrophic cardiomyopathy,
150
in infective endocarditis, 419
in restrictive cardiomyopathy, 151
in valvular heart disease, 143t
prosthetic valve disease, 146
Heart transplant patients, 460–461
Heart trauma, 798–800
blunt, 799–800
penetrating, 798–799
Heartburn, 206–207
Heat cramps, 566
Heat edema, 566
Heat exhaustion, 565
Heat rash, 566
Heat stroke, 564–565
Heat syncope, 565
Heat tetany, 566
Heel-to-shin test, 687
Helicobacter pylori infection, 212,
213
Helium-oxygen (Heliox)
for asthma, 194
for bronchiolitis, 343
for croup, 369
for epiglottitis, 370, 742
for foreign body aspiration, 372
HELLP syndrome, 296, 297, 644
Helminths, 431–436
blood and tissue nematodes, 434
cestodes (flatworms), 435–436
beef tapeworm, 435
dwarf tapeworm, 435
fish tapeworm, 436
pork tapeworm, 435–436
clinical features of, 431, 432t
diagnosis and differential of, 431
management of, 431
nematodes (roundworms), 432–434

ascariasis, 433
hookworm, 433–434
pinworm, 433
threadworm, 433
trichinosis, 434
whipworm, 434
trematodes (flukes), 435
schistosomiasis, 435
Hemarthrosis, traumatic, 863
Hematemesis, 204, 212
Hematochezia, 204, 208
Hematology
acquired bleeding disorders,
628–633
evaluation of anemia and bleeding
patient, 621–627
exogenous anticoagulants and
antiplatelet agents, 653–655
hemolytic anemias, 641–645
hemophilias, 634–639
hyperviscosity syndrome in cancer
patients, 662–663
transfusion therapy for, 646–652
von Willebrand disease, 639–640
Hematoma
epidural, 776
septal, 788
subdural, 667, 670, 777
subperichondrial, 788
subungual, 104
Hematuria, 267–270
diagnosis and differential of, 268
etiologies of, 269–270
management of, 270
traumatic injuries with, 810–811
Hemodialysis
for acute renal failure, 262
for barbiturate overdose, 490
for bleeding in renal disease, 629
complications of, 265
related to vascular access, 265–266
for hypercalcemia of malignancy,
660
for lithium overdose, 488
for metformin-induced lactic
acidosis, 556
for poisoning, 475
for salicylate overdose, 507
for theophylline toxicity, 513, 513t
for tumor lysis syndrome, 660
Hemoglobin, 621, 622t
defects of, 553–554
Hemolytic anemias, 641–645
acquired, 643–645
clinical features of, 643–644
diagnosis and differential of, 644

Hemolytic anemias (*Cont.*)
  management of, 644–645
  hereditary, 641–643
    glucose-6-phosphate
      dehydrogenase deficiency,
      642–643
    hereditary spherocytosis, 643
    sickle cell disease, 394–395,
      641–642
    variants of sickle cell disease,
      396, 642
Hemolytic disease of newborn, 643
Hemolytic transfusion reactions, 648,
  650t
Hemolytic-uremic syndrome (HUS),
  236, 354, 643, 645
Hemoperfusion
  for poisoning, 475
    barbiturates, 490
    nonbenzodiazepine sedative-
      hypnotics, 493
  for theophylline toxicity, 513, 513t
Hemophilias, 634–639
  classification of, 634
  clinical features of, 634
  diagnosis and differential of, 634
  management of, 634–639
    choice of products for, 635, 637t
    initial factor replacement
      guidelines, 635, 636t
    in patients with inhibitors, 635,
      638t
Hemoptysis, 190–191
  clinical features of, 190
  diagnosis and differential of, 190
  management of, 191
Hemorrhage. *See* Bleeding
Hemorrhagic stroke, 674, 674t
Hemorrhoids, 227–229
  bleeding from, 204, 227
  clinical features of, 227–229
  management of, 229, *229*
Hemostasis
  in end-stage renal disease, 265
  for maxillofacial injuries, 789
  tests of, 624t–626t
  for wound management, 84
Hemothorax, 761–762, 797
Henoch-Schönlein purpura (HSP),
  354, 388
Henry law, 581
Heparin, 653
  for acute coronary syndromes, 132t,
    133–134
  for arterial occlusion, 169
  for atrial fibrillation, 13, 14

for atrial flutter, 12
  bleeding induced by, 630
  for cavernous sinus thrombosis, 735
  for deep venous thrombosis, 168
  for disseminated intravascular
    coagulation, 630
  low-molecular-weight, 653
  protamine reversal of, 133, 266,
    473t, 630
  for pulmonary embolism, 157, 659
  for stroke, 677
  thrombocytopenia induced by, 168,
    630
  unfractionated, 653
  use in pregnancy, 292t
Hepatic encephalopathy, 245–246
Hepatic sequestration crisis, in sickle
  cell disease, 394
Hepatitis, 241–243
  alcoholic, 243–245
  clinical features of, 241–242
  diagnosis and differential of, 242
  etiologies of, 241
  hepatitis B prophylaxis after sexual
    assault, 896
  HIV infection and, 416
  jaundice and, 239
  management of, 242–243
  from needle-stick injury, 113
  pain of, 213
  viral, 241–243
Hepatorenal syndrome, 244
Herbal preparations, toxicity of,
  546–548
Herbicide poisoning, 533–537
Hereditary spherocytosis, 643
Hernia, 219–220, 220
  in children, 353
    neonates, 321
  clinical features of, 219, *219*
  diagnosis and differential of, 220
  inguinal, 220
  intestinal obstruction due to, 217,
    219
  management of, 220
  reducible vs. incarcerated, 220
  risk factors for, 219
  strangulation of, 220
  umbilical, 220
Heroin, 468t
Herpangina, 736
Herpes simplex virus (HSV) infection,
  411
  clinical features of, 411
  conjunctivitis, 334–335, 716
  encephalitis, 711

Herpes simplex virus (HSV) infection (*Cont.*)
  genital, 404–405
  gingivostomatitis, 736
  in HIV disease, 416, 417
  management of, 411, 417
  in transplant recipients, 458
Herpes zoster, 411–412, 756–757
  clinical features of, 412, 756
  diagnosis and differential of, 756
  in HIV disease, 416
  management of, 412, 418, 757
Herpes zoster ophthalmicus (HZO), 412, 418, 716–717
Herpesvirus 6 infection, 381
Herpetic whitlow, 870t, 871
HHS. *See* Hyperosmolar hyperglycemic state
High-altitude cerebral edema (HACE), 578–580
High-altitude pulmonary edema (HAPE), 578–580
High pressure injection injuries, 113–114, 824
Hip
  dislocation of, 838–839
  fractures of, 769, 837
  transient synovitis of, 388
Hiradenitis suppurativa, 450
Hirudin, 654
Histoplasmosis, in HIV infection, 415
HIV. *See* Human immunodeficiency virus infection
Hobo spider bite, 568
Homan sign, 166
Homatropine
  for chemical ocular injury, 721
  for corneal abrasion, 718
Homicidal patients, 882–884
Hookworm, 433–434
Hordeolum, 715
Horizontal mattress sutures, 91, *91*
Horner syndrome, 802
HSP (Henoch-Schönlein purpura), 354, 388
Human bites, 114–115, 870t
β-Human chorionic gonadotropin (β-hCG) test for pregnancy, 286–287, 294
Human diploid cell vaccine (HDCV), 425
Human immunodeficiency virus (HIV) infection, 413–418
  AIDS indicator conditions, 413, 414t
  appendicitis in, 215

  bleeding in, 633
  CD4 cell count and complications of, 413–414
  clinical features of, 413–416
  diagnosis and differential of, 416–417
  Kaposi sarcoma in, 416
  management of, 417–418
    antiretroviral therapy, 418
    for infectious complications, 417–418
    universal precautions, 417
  from needle-stick injury, 113
  peripheral neurologic disease in, 701
  Pneumocystis carinii pneumonia in, 180, 415
  in pregnancy, 290
  prophylaxis and counseling after sexual assault, 896
  risk factors for, 413
  tuberculosis in, 184–185, 415
Human rabies immune globulin, 424–425
Humerus fractures, 769, 833–834
HUS (hemolytic-uremic syndrome), 236, 354, 643, 645
Hydralazine
  for hypertension in pregnancy, 161, 297
  for priapism, 394
  toxicity of, 519–520
Hydration status of children, 348
Hydrocarbon toxicity, 527–529, 544
  clinical features of, 527–528, 527t
  diagnosis and differential of, 528
  management of, 528–529
Hydrochlorothiazide toxicity, 518
Hydrocodone, 69t
Hydrocortisone
  for adrenal insufficiency, 607, 618, 661
  for contact dermatitis, 754
  for hypercalcemia, 39
  for hypoglycemia, 358
  for myxedema coma, 616
  for otitis externa, 332
  for phimosis, 273
  for thyroid storm, 615t
  for ulcerative colitis, 223
Hydrofluoric acid burns, 590–591
Hydrogen sulfide exposure, 544–545
Hydromorphone
  dosage of, 69t
  for pain crisis in sickle cell disease, 392

Hydromorphone (*Cont.*)
  for renal colic, 277
Hydroxocobalamin, for cyanide
    poisoning, 552
γ-Hydroxybutyrate (GHB), 491–492
Hydroxyzine
  for allergic conjunctivitis, 335
  use with opiates, 69
Hymenolepis nana infection, 435
Hymenoptera stings, 567
Hyperamylasemia, 250
Hyperbaric oxygen therapy
  for carbon monoxide poisoning,
    590, 599–600, 599t
  for hydrocarbon and volatile
    substance poisoning, 529
Hyperbilirubinemia, 239–241
  neonatal, 323
Hypercalcemia, 38–39
  of malignancy, 659–660
  rhabdomyolysis and, 851, 852
  vitamin A–induced, 546, 548
  vitamin D–induced, 546, 548
Hypercapnia, 175–176
  in childhood asthma, 340
  in chronic obstructive pulmonary
    disease, 192, 193
  clinical features of, 175
  diagnosis and differential of, 175,
    176t
  management of, 176
  mechanisms of, 175
Hyperemesis gravidarum, 234, 295
Hyperextension dislocation of cervical
    spine, 783t
Hyperglycemia
  in diabetic ketoacidosis, 355, 608
  hyperosmolar hyperglycemic state,
    610–611
  septic shock with, 54
Hyperkalemia, 36–38, 37t
  from blood transfusion, 648
  due to digitalis toxicity, 37, 514
  management of, 37, 38, 852
  rhabdomyolysis and, 850, 852
  in tumor lysis syndrome, 660
Hypermagnesemia, 40
Hypernatremia, 34–35, 35t
Hyperosmolar hyperglycemic state
    (HHS), 610–611
  clinical features of, 610
  diagnosis and differential of, 610
  management of, 610–611
Hyperphosphatemia, rhabdomyolysis
    and, 850, 852
Hypersensitivity reactions, 60–61

Hypertelorism, 788
Hypertension
  classification of, 159
  drug-induced, 470t–471t
  headache and, 667
    management of, 670
  ischemic stroke with, 675
  in pregnancy, 159, 161, 296–298,
    297t
  in rheumatic diseases, 868
Hypertensive emergencies, 159–161
  in children, 161
  clinical features of, 159
  definition of, 159
  diagnosis and differential of,
    159–160
  management of, 160–161
  monoamine oxidase inhibitor-
    related, 484
Hypertensive urgency, 159
Hyperthyroidism
  apathetic thyrotoxicosis, 614
  in pregnancy, 288
  thyroid storm, 614–615, 615t
Hypertrophic cardiomyopathy (HCM),
    150–151
  clinical features of, 150
  diagnosis and differential of,
    150–151
  management of, 152
  syncope and, 137, 151
Hyperuricemia, rhabdomyolysis and,
    850
Hyperventilation syndrome, 44–45
Hyperviscosity syndrome in cancer
    patients, 662–663
Hypervitaminosis A, 546
Hypervitaminosis D, 546
Hyphema, 719–720
Hypocalcemia, 38
  from blood transfusion, 648
  rhabdomyolysis and, 850–852
Hypoglycemia
  autonomic response to, 555
  causes of, 556
  in children, 317, 357–358
    neonates, 347
  clinical features of, 357, 607
  in diabetic patients, 607–608
  diagnosis and differential of, 357t,
    358, 607
  drug-induced, 357, 556, 607
  idiopathic ketotic, 358
  management of, 358, 556,
    607–608
  in pregnancy, 288

Hypoglycemic agent toxicity, 555–557, 607–608
  clinical features of, 469t, 555–556
  diagnosis and differential of, 556
  management of, 556–557
Hypokalemia, 35–36, 36t
  from blood transfusion, 648
  in diabetic ketoacidosis, 356
Hypomagnesemia, 39–40
Hyponatremia, 33, 34t
  in diabetic ketoacidosis, 356
  in syndrome of inappropriate antidiuretic hormone, 661
Hypotension, 49–52
  in allergic reactions, 60–61
  in cardiac transplant recipient, 461
  in cardiogenic shock, 57
  drug-induced, 470t–471t
  hemodialysis-induced, 265
  in neurogenic shock, 62
  in septic shock, 54
  in spinal shock, 780
  supine, in pregnancy, 771
Hypothermia, 561–563
  clinical features of, 561, 562t
  diagnosis and differential of, 561
  due to icy-water submersion, 585
  management of, 562–563, 563t
  in septic shock, 53
Hypothyroidism, 615–616
Hypoxemia, 174–175
  in children, 329
  clinical features of, 174–175
  cyanosis and, 178t
  diagnosis and differential of, 175
  management of, 175
  mechanisms of, 174
Hypoxia, in chronic obstructive pulmonary disease, 192, 193
Hysterectomy, cuff cellulitis after, 308–309
Hysteroscopy complications, 308
HZO (herpes zoster ophthalmicus), 412, 418, 716–717

I

Ibuprofen
  for acute pain, 68
  for febrile child, 314
  for headache, in children, 362
  for inflammation from wisdom teeth, 734
  for neck and back pain, 859
  for pericarditis, 153
  for toothache, 734
  for transient synovitis of hip, 388

  use in pregnancy, 292t
Ibutilide, for atrial flutter, 13
ICP. *See* Intracranial pressure elevation
Idiopathic thrombocytopenic purpura, 628
Idioventricular rhythm, 24
IE. *See* Infective endocarditis
Iliac spine fracture, 837t
Iliac wing fracture, 837t
Imaging. *See* specific imaging modalities
Imipenem
  for cellulitis, 449
  for erysipelas, 450
  for febrile neutropenia, 662
  overdose of, 550
  for pneumonia, 182
    nosocomial, 458
  for septic shock, 55
Immersion foot, 561–562, 874
Immunizations in pregnancy, 292t
Immunosuppressive agents
  for Crohn disease, 222
  posttransplant complications related to, 459–460, 459t
  for ulcerative colitis, 223, 224
Impedance plethysmography, 167
Impetigo
  bullous, 374, *374,* 724
  contagiosum, 374–375, *375*
  facial, 724
Impingement syndrome, 860
In vitro fertilization, complications of, 285, 309
Indomethacin, for pain, 68
Infantile spasms, 347
Infants. *See* Neonates; Pediatric patients
Infections, 399–463. *See also* Abscess; Sepsis; specific infections
  from biological weapons, 452–455
  from blood transfusion, 648
  brain abscess, 711–712
  bronchitis, 179
  cellulitis, 336–337, 724–725
  dental, 734
  diarrhea and, 235, 236
    in children, 348–350, 349t
  encephalitis, 711
  endocarditis, 419–421
  eye, 334–335, 715–718
  facial, 724–725
  in febrile children, 313–314
    occult bacteremia, 315–316
  hand, 869–871, 870t
  helminthic, 431–436

Infections (*Cont.*)
  herpes simplex virus, 411
  herpes zoster, 411–412
  HIV and AIDS, 413–418
  influenza, 410–411
  malaria, 426–430
  from marine animal injuries, 575
  meningitis, 708–711
  myocarditis, 152
  pericarditis, 152
  from peritoneal dialysis, 266
  pneumonia, 179–182
    in children, 314, 338–339
  rabies, 423–425
  with rash, 374–382, 724
  severe acute respiratory syndrome,
    182–183
  sexually transmitted diseases,
    401–406
  in sickle cell disease, 395
  sinusitis, 335–336
  soft tissue, 447–451
  spontaneous bacterial peritonitis,
    244
  tetanus, 422–423
  tinea, 755
  toxic shock syndrome, 407–409
  in transplant recipients, 456–463,
    457t
  urinary tract, 267–269
    in children, 397–398
  vaginal, 302–303
  of vascular access device for
    hemodialysis, 265
  of wounds, 83
    dog bites, 115
    human bites, 114–115
    postoperative, 253–254
    puncture wounds, 112–113
  zoonotic, 437–446
Infectious mononucleosis, 378–379
Infective endocarditis (IE), 419–421
  clinical features of, 419
  diagnosis and differential of,
    419–420
  management of, 420–421
  microbiology of, 419
  native valve, 419
  prophylaxis for, 147t, 420–421, 421t
  prosthetic valve, 147, 419
  skin findings in, 419, 420t
Inferior vena cava filter, 168
Inflammatory bowel disease, 221–224
  Crohn disease, 221–222
  in pregnancy, 289
  ulcerative colitis, 222–224

Infliximab, for Crohn disease, 222
Influenza, 410–411
  clinical features of, 410
  diagnosis and differential of, 410
  management of, 410–411
Informed consent
  for evidence collection in sexual
    assault cases, 895
  for fibrinolytic therapy, 134
  for procedural sedation and
    analgesia, 68
Ingested foreign bodies, 209–211
  button batteries, 210, 532
  clinical features of, 209
  cocaine packets, 211
  coins, 210
  diagnosis and differential of, 209
  food bolus impaction, 209–210
  management of, 209–211
  retrieval of, 211
  sharp objects, 210
Ingrown toenail, 872
INH. *See* Isoniazid
Inhalation injuries, 543
  carbon monoxide, 588, 590,
    598–600
  smoke, 588
Innominate artery injuries, 801
Insect bites and stings, 567–571
Insecticide poisoning, 468t, 533–537
Insulin
  for calcium channel blocker
    toxicity, 517
  for diabetic ketoacidosis, 356, 609
  for hyperosmolar hyperketotic state,
    611
  hypoglycemia induced by, 555,
    607–608
  in multiorgan failure, 56
  overdose of, 469t
  in pregnancy, 288
Intercondylar fractures, 826–827
Interferon, for hepatitis, 243
Interphalangeal joint dislocations
  distal, 822
  proximal, 822
Interrupted percutaneous sutures,
  87–89, *88*
Intertrochanteric fractures, 837
Intestinal colic in infants, 320
Intestinal injuries, 803
Intestinal obstruction, 217–218
  in children, 353
  clinical features of, 217
  diagnosis and differential of,
    217–218

Intestinal obstruction (*Cont.*)
in helminthic infections, 432t
hernia and, 217, 219
management of, 218
postoperative, 255
vs. pseudoobstruction, 218
Intimate partner violence and abuse
(IPVA), 894–897
clinical features of, 894
diagnosis and differential of, 895
management of, 896–897
physical examination for, 894–895
in pregnancy, 290
risk factors for, 894
Intoxicated patients, 499–504, 879
Intraaortic balloon pump
counterpulsation
for cardiogenic shock, 58
for mitral incompetence, 144
for right ventricular infarction, 136
Intracerebral hemorrhage, 776
Intracranial pressure (ICP) elevation
brain herniation due to, 777
management of, 356, 610, 677, 709,
778–779
trephination for, 779
Intraocular pressure (IOP) elevation
in acute angle closure glaucoma,
722
due to central retinal artery
occlusion, 722
hyphema with, 720
Intraosseous line placement in
children, 28–29, 766
Intravenous immunoglobulins,
647–648
for Kawasaki disease, 382
Intravenous pyelography (IVP), 276,
811, 811t
Intubation, 3–6
alternative techniques for, 8
of children, 26, 766
of comatose patient, 684
of geriatric patients, 770
for hemoptysis, 191
nasotracheal, 6
orotracheal, 3–4
of poisoned patient, 473
preoxygenation for, 3, 4, 5, 26
for pulmonary edema, 140
rapid sequence induction for, 5
in children, 26–28
for transient analgesic-induced
respiratory depression, 68
of trauma patients, 762
with head injury, 778

with maxillofacial injuries, 789
with neck injuries, 4, 793
Intussusception, 217, 353
Iodine, for thyroid storm, 615t
IOP. *See* Intraocular pressure elevation
Ipratropium, for asthma, 194, 341
IPVA. *See* Intimate partner violence
and abuse
Iron poisoning, 524–526
clinical features of, 524
diagnosis and differential of,
524–525
management of, 525–526
Irrigation of wounds, 85
Ischemic heart disease. *See also*
Angina pectoris; Myocardial
infarction, acute
acute coronary syndromes,
129–136
in cardiac transplant recipient, 460
chest pain from, 123–128
clinical features of, 123
complications of, 130
diagnostic evaluation of, 123–125,
130–131
with hypertension, 160
mortality from, 129
physical examination for, 123
silent, 129
Ischemic stroke, 673, 674t
Ischium fracture, 837t
Isoniazid (INH)
overdose of, 549
for tuberculosis, 185, 186t, 417
use in pregnancy, 291t
Isopropanol intoxication, 494–495
Isoproterenol
for β-blocker toxicity, 516
for monoamine oxidase inhibitor
overdose, 485
Isotretinoin, for acneiform eruptions,
756
Itraconazole
for onychomycosis, 755
for sporotrichosis, 451
Ivermectin, for *Strongyloides
stercoralis* infection, 433
IVP (intravenous pyelography), 276,
811, 811t

J
Jaundice, 239–241
bilirubin level and, 239
in children, 351
neonates, 323
clinical features of, 239

Jaundice (*Cont.*)
diagnosis and differential of, 239–241
etiologies of, 240t
in helminthic infections, 432t
management of, 241
Jaw thrust maneuver, 3
in children, 26
Jefferson fracture, 782, 784t
Jellyfish stings, 575, 577
Jock itch, 755
Joint disorders, 862–865
ankylosing spondylitis, 865
clinical features of, 862, 863t
crystal-induced synovitis, 863
diagnosis and differential of, 862, 864t
gonococcal arthritis, 865
Lyme arthritis, 863
osteoarthritis, 863
Reiter syndrome, 865
rheumatoid arthritis, 865
juvenile, 390
septic arthritis, 113, 862–863, 865t
in children, 387, 862
traumatic hemarthrosis, 863
Jones fracture, 847
JRA (juvenile rheumatoid arthritis), 390
Junctional escape rhythms, 16, *16*
Juvenile rheumatoid arthritis (JRA), 390

K

Kaposi sarcoma, 416
Kawasaki disease, 382, 867
Kayexalate. *See* Sodium polystyrene sulfonate
Kehr sign, 803
Kerley B lines, 142
Kernig sign, 314, 708
Ketamine
for asthma, 194, 342
contraindications to, 70
dosage of, 69t
for procedural sedation, 70
for rapid sequence induction, 5
in children, 28
side effects of, 70
Ketoacidosis, 42t
alcoholic, 612–613
diabetic, 608–610
in children, 355–356
Ketoconazole, for tinea infections, 755
Ketonuria, 355
Ketorolac

for acute pain, 68
for biliary colic, 249
for migraine, 671t
Kidney stones, 276–277
clinical features of, 276
in Crohn disease, 221
diagnosis and differential of, 276–277
management of, 277
Kidney transplant patients, 462
Kidney trauma, 812
Kissing bug bites, 571
Klebsiella infection
pneumonia, 179, 180
urinary tract infection, 268
Knee injuries, 840–843
dislocations, 841
fractures, 840
ligamentous, 842
meniscal, 843
overuse syndromes, 843
tendon rupture, 841–842
wounds over, 107
Koplik spots, 378
Kussmaul respiration, 355, 608
Kussmaul sign, 151, 154

L

Labetalol
for aortic incompetence, 146
for hypertension, 160, 161
in children, 161
in hemorrhagic stroke, 677
in ischemic stroke, 675
in pregnancy, 297
for tetanus, 423
Labor
emergency delivery, 299–301
false, 299
monitoring of patients in, 299
preterm, 296
Labyrinthitis, 690, 691
Lacerations
ankle, 107
cheek, 98, *98*
dorsal hand, 102
ear, *97*, 97–98
extensor tendon, 102, *102*
eyelids, 95, *95*, 719
finger and finger tip, 103–104, *104*
flexor tendon, 103
foot, 107–108
forearm and wrist, 100, 100t, *101*, 101t
of great vessels, 800–801
intraoral, 738

Lacerations (*Cont.*)
  knee, 107
  lingual frenulum, 738
  lip, *96,* 96–97, 738
  maxillary labial frenulum, 738
  nose, 95–96
  palm, 100–101
  penile, 813
  renal, 812
  scalp and forehead, *94,* 94–95, 763
  scarring from, 119
  tongue, 738
  urethral, 813
  vaginal, 810
Lactated Ringer's solution, 32
Lactic acidosis, 42t, 49, 50
  metformin-induced, 556
Lactulose, for constipation, 238, 245
Lacunar infarcts, 673
Lambert-Eaton myasthenic syndrome, 706
Lamivudine, for hepatitis B, 243
Lamotrigine, for seizures in children, 346
Lansoprazole, for peptic ulcer disease, 213
Laparoscopy complications, 308
Laparotomy, for abdominal trauma, 805, 806t
Laryngeal trauma, 744, 792
Laryngoscopy, 4
Laryngotracheobronchitis
  membranous, 371
  viral, 369–370
Lateral collateral ligament injury, 842
Lateral medullary syndrome, 673, 690
Lateral sinus thrombosis, 729
Laxatives
  for constipation, 238
  for patients with hemorrhoids, 229
Lead poisoning, 538–539
  clinical features of, 538, 539t
  diagnosis and differential of, 538
  management of, 538–539
LeFort fractures, 787, *788*
Left ventricular outflow obstruction syndromes, 327
Legg-Calvé-Perthes disease, 388–389
Legionella pneumonia, 179–181
Leiomyomas, uterine, 285
Lesser trochanteric fractures, 837
LET (lidocaine epinephrine tetracaine), 73
Leucovorin, for methotrexate toxicity, 472t
Levofloxacin

  for chlamydial infection, 402
  for pelvic inflammatory disease, 306t
  for pneumonia, 181–182
    nosocomial, 458
  for urinary tract infection, 269
Levothyroxine, for myxedema coma, 616
LGV (lymphogranuloma venereum), 405–406
Lhermitte sign, 703–704
Lice, 571, 757–758
Lid lacerations, 95, *95,* 719
Lidocaine
  for antipsychotic overdose, 487
  for β-blocker toxicity, 516
  for digitalis glycoside toxicity, 514
  for digoxin toxicity, 16
  for episiotomy, 299
  for epistaxis, 731
  for erythema multiforme, 748
  for head-injured patients, 26
  for local anesthesia, 71
  for monoamine oxidase inhibitor overdose, 485
  for premature ventricular contractions, 18
  for status epilepticus, 345
  topical, 73
  for tricyclic antidepressant toxicity, 480
  for ventricular fibrillation, 21
  for ventricular tachycardia, 19
  for wide-complex tachycardia, 17
Lidocaine epinephrine tetracaine (LET), 73
Lidocaine prilocaine (EMLA), 73
Ligament injuries
  ankle, 844–845, *845*
  knee, 842
Lightning injuries, 595–597
  clinical features of, 595–596
  complications of, 596t
  diagnosis and differential of, 596
  management of, 596–597
Lima PROST, for cold injuries, 562
Lindane
  for chigger bites, 570
  for scabies, 757
Lingual frenulum laceration, 738
Lip lacerations, *96,* 96–97, 738
Lisfranc joint injuries, 847
Listeria monocytogenes meningitis, 458
Lithium toxicity, 487–488

Liver disease
  bleeding in, 628–629
  hepatitis, 241–243
  septic shock and, 53
Liver enzymes
  in alcoholic liver disease, 244
  in HIV infection, 416
  in viral hepatitis, 242
Liver failure, 241, 243, 245–246
Liver injuries, 803
Liver metastases, 239
Liver transplant patients, 462–463
Livestock bites, 117
Local anesthetics, 71–73
  for digital blocks, 72–73
  infiltration of, 73
Locked-in syndrome, 673
Loeffler syndrome, 433
Loperamide, for diarrhea, 222, 236
Lorazepam
  for chemotherapy-induced
    nausea/vomiting, 663
  for delirium, 680
  for panic disorder, 881, 885
  for seizures, 697
    drug- or toxin-induced, 474, 476,
      480
    in neonates, 347
    posttraumatic, 779
    status epilepticus, 345, *696*
  for stimulant overdose, 501
  for tetanus, 423
  for violent patient, 884
Losartan toxicity, 520
Low back pain, 855–859
Lower extremity lacerations, 106–108
  ankle, 107
  clinical features of, 106
  diagnosis and differential of, 106
  foot, 107–108
  hair tourniquet syndrome, 108
  knee, 107
  peripheral nerve testing for, 106,
    107t
  tendon function testing for, 107t
  wound care for, 106
    patient instructions, 108
LSD (lysergic acid diethylamide), 503t
Ludwig angina, 734, 743
Lumbar pain, 855–859
Lumbar plexopathy, 700–701
Lumbar puncture
  for meningitis, 318, 708–709
  for seizures, 345
Lumbar radiculopathy, 858, 858t
Lunate dislocation, 824

Lunate fracture, 824
Lung injuries, 796–797
Lung transplant patients, 461–462
Lupus anticoagulant, 633
Lyme disease, 437–438
  arthritis in, 863
  clinical features of, 437–438
  diagnosis and differential of, 438
  management of, 438
  neurologic symptoms of, 701–702
  vaccination against, 438
Lymphogranuloma venereum (LGV),
  405–406
Lysergic acid diethylamide (LSD),
  503t

M
MAC (Mycobacterium avium
  complex), in HIV infection, 413,
  414, 417
Magnesium balance
  hypermagnesemia, 40
  hypomagnesemia, 39–40
Magnesium citrate
  for caustic ingestion, 531
  for constipation, 238
Magnesium sulfate
  for asthma, 194, 341
  for β-blocker toxicity, 516
  for digitalis glycoside toxicity, 514
  for hypomagnesemia, 39–40, 609
  for multifocal atrial tachycardia, 11
  for neonatal seizures, 347
  for preeclampsia or eclampsia, 297,
    697
  for tetanus, 423
  for torsades de pointes, 20, 480, 487
  for ventricular fibrillation, 21
Magnetic resonance imaging
  for deep venous thrombosis, 167
  for pediatric seizures, 344
MAHA (microangiopathic hemolytic
  anemia), 643, 644
Major depression, 880
Malaria, 426–430
  cerebral, 427
  clinical features of, 426–427
  complications of, 426–427
  diagnosis and differential of, 427
  epidemiology of, 426
  etiology of, 426
  management of, 427–430,
    428t–429t
Mallory-Weiss tear, 204, 208, 234,
  351
Malrotation of gut, 321, 353

Mandible
  dislocation of, 727
  fractures of, 787, 791
Mannitol
  for acute neurologic deterioration,
    763
  for increased intracranial pressure,
    356, 610, 677, 709, 778
    in children, 766
  for increased intraocular pressure,
    720, 722
  for rhabdomyolysis, 262, 852
  toxicity of, 518
Mantoux test, 185
Marburg virus, 455
Marcus-Gunn pupil, 704, 787
Marijuana, 503t
Marine animal injuries, 575–577
  clinical features of, 575–576
  management of, 576–577
Massasauga bite, 572–573
Masticator space abscess, 726
Mastitis, 298
Mastoiditis, acute, 729
Mattress sutures
  horizontal, 91, *91*
  vertical, 90, *91*
Maxillary fractures, 791
Maxillary labial frenulum laceration,
  738
Maxillary sinusitis, 732
Maxillofacial trauma, 787–791
  clinical features and evaluation of,
    787–789
  diagnosis and differential of, 789
  frontal sinus and frontal bone
    fractures, 789–790
  LeFort fractures, 787, *788*
  management of, 789–791
  mandibular fractures, 791
  maxillary fractures, 791
  nasal fractures, 732, 787, 790
  nasoethmoidal-orbital injuries, 788,
    790
  temporomandibular dislocation,
    791
  zygomatic fractures, 790–791
McBurney point, 214
MCP (metacarpophalangeal) joint
  dislocations, 823
MCV (mean corpuscular volume),
  622t, *623*
MDMA (3,4-methylenedioxymeth-
  amphetamine; Ecstasy), 503t
Mean corpuscular volume (MCV),
  622t, *623*

Measles, 378
Mebendazole
  for ascariasis, 433
  for pinworm, 433
  for trichinosis, 434
Meckel diverticulum, 354
Meclizine
  use in pregnancy, 292t
  for vertigo, 691
Meconium aspiration, 31
Medial collateral ligament injury,
  842
Median nerve testing, 99, 99t, 100t
Medroxyprogesterone, for
  dysfunctional uterine bleeding,
  284
Mees lines, 539
Mefloquine
  for malaria, 427, 428t
  toxicity of, 549–550
Melena, 204, 208, 212
Memory impairment, 680–681
Ménière disease, 690, 691
Meningitis, 708–711
  antibiotic prophylaxis for, 671
  in children, 314, 318
  clinical features of, 708
  diagnosis and differential of, 708,
    709t
  headache from, 667
  management of, 709–711, 710t
  in transplant recipients, 458
  tuberculous, 708
Meningococcemia, 752
Meniscal injuries, 843
Menorrhagia, 283
Mental illness. *See* Psychosocial
  disorders
Mental status change, 679–685, 680t
  in children, 359–361
    clinical features of, 359
    diagnosis and differential of, 359,
      360t
    management of, 359–361
  coma, 683–685
  delirium, 679–680, 681t, 879
  dementia, 680–683, 682t, 879
Mental status examination, 883
Meperidine, 68–69
  for biliary colic, 249
Mepivacaine, 71
Meprobamate overdose, 492
Meralgia paresthetica, 700
6-Mercaptopurine
  for Crohn disease, 222
  for ulcerative colitis, 224

Mercury poisoning, 540–541
  clinical features of, 540
  diagnosis and differential of, 540
  management of, 541
Meropenem
  for nosocomial pneumonia, 458
  for septic shock, 55
Mesalamine
  for Crohn disease, 222
  for ulcerative colitis, 224
Mescaline, 503t
Metabolic acidosis, 41–43, 42t, 43t
  in alcoholic ketoacidosis, 612
  in diabetic ketoacidosis, 355, 608
  high anion-gap, differential
    diagnosis of, 496t, 608
  in septic shock, 54
  in shock, 49, 50
Metabolic alkalosis, 43–44
Metabolic toxin exposure, 544–545
Metacarpal fractures, 823
Metacarpophalangeal (MCP) joint
  dislocations, 823
Metallic needles, removal from soft
  tissue, 110
Metaproterenol, for asthma and
  chronic obstructive pulmonary
  disease, 193
Metatarsal fractures, 847
Metformin, hypoglycemia induced by,
  555–557, 607
Methadone, use in pregnancy, 290
Methamphetamine toxicity, 501
Methanol intoxication, 495–498
  clinical features of, 495–496
  diagnosis and differential of, 496,
    496t
  management of, 497–498
Methaqualone overdose, 492
Methemoglobinemia, 553–554
  cyanosis and, 177–178, 178t
Methimazole, for thyroid storm, 615t
Methohexital
  dosage of, 69t
  for procedural sedation, 70
Methyldopa
  toxicity of, 518–519
  use in pregnancy, 291t
Methylene blue, for
  methemoglobinemia, 473t, 554
3,4-Methylenedioxymethamphetamine
  (MDMA; Ecstasy), 503t
Methylprednisolone
  for allergic reactions, 61
  for angioedema of upper airway,
    744

for asthma and chronic obstructive
  pulmonary disease, 194
  in pregnancy, 289
  for caustic ingestion, 531
  for giant cell arteritis, 723
  for Hymenoptera sting, 567
  for multiple sclerosis, 704
  for neurogenic shock, 62–63
  for organ rejection, 461, 462, 463
  for spinal cord injury, 786
  in children, 767
  for superior vena cava syndrome,
    658
  for toxic shock syndrome, 408
  for ulcerative colitis, 223
Metoclopramide
  for migraine, 671t
  for patients with abdominal pain,
    203
  use in pregnancy, 292t, 295
  for vomiting, 237, 663
Metoprolol
  for acute coronary syndromes, 132t,
    133
  for atrial fibrillation, 14
  for atrial flutter, 13
  for hypertension, 161
  for premature ventricular
    contractions, 18
  for supraventricular tachycardia, 15
Metronidazole
  for acute necrotizing ulcerative
    gingivitis, 735
  for bacterial vaginosis, 302, 896
  for brain abscess, 712
  for Crohn disease, 222
  for diarrhea, 236, 349
  for diverticulitis, 226
  for esophageal perforation, 208
  for gas gangrene, 447, 448
  for *Helicobacter pylori* infection,
    213
  for intraabdominal infection in
    transplant recipients, 458
  for lateral sinus thrombosis, 729
  for Ludwig angina, 734
  for odontogenic abscess, 743
  for pelvic inflammatory disease,
    306t
  for peritonsillar abscess, 741
  for pseudomembranous colitis, 224
  for septic shock, 55
  for suppurative parotitis, 726
  for tetanus, 423
  for trichomoniasis, 302, 403, 896
  for ulcerative colitis, 223

Metronidazole (*Cont.*)
  use in pregnancy, 291t, 303, 403
MG. *See* Myasthenia gravis
Miconazole
  for *Candida* vaginitis, 303
  for tinea infections, 755
Microangiopathic hemolytic anemia
    (MAHA), 643, 644
Midazolam
  for children, 28, 766
    neonatal seizures, 347
  dosage of, 69t
  for procedural sedation, 69–70
  for rapid sequence induction, 5
    in children, 28
  for status epilepticus, 345, 346, *696,*
    697
  for tetanus, 423
Middle cerebral artery occlusion, 673
Miglitol, 555, 607
Migraine headache, 667
  management of, 668–669, 671t
  in pregnancy, 290
  transformed, 76t, 77t
  vertigo and, 691
Milch technique, for glenohumeral
    joint dislocation, 832
Miliary tuberculosis, 184
Milk of magnesia, for constipation,
    238
Milrinone, for cardiogenic shock, 58
Mineral oil, for constipation, 238
Minoxidil toxicity, 519–520
Mirtazapine toxicity, 482
Mitral incompetence, 143–144, 143t
Mitral stenosis, 142, 143t
Mitral valve prolapse, 143t, 144
Modified hippocratic technique, for
    glenohumeral joint dislocation,
    832
Monoamine oxidase inhibitors
    (MAOIs), 484–486
  drug interactions with, 484, 485t
  toxicity of, 484–486
    clinical features of, 484
    diagnosis and differential of, 484,
      486t
    management of, 484–486
Monocryl sutures, 87
Mononeuritis multiplex, 701
Monospot test, 379
Moraxella catarrhalis infection
  otitis media, 330, 728
  sinusitis, 335
Morphine, 68–69
  for abdominal pain, 203

for acute coronary syndromes, 132t,
    133
  for acute pancreatitis, 251
  for chest pain, 58
  for children, 766
    dosage of, 69t
  for headache in children, 362
  for hypercyanotic spells in children,
    327
  overdose of, 468t
  for pain crisis in sickle cell disease,
    392
  for pulmonary edema, 141
  for renal colic, 277
  for tetanus, 423
Morton's neuroma, 874
Motor ataxia, 687
Moxifloxacin
  for cellulitis, 725
  for pneumonia, 181
MPS (myofascial pain syndrome), 76t,
    77t, 856
MS. *See* Multiple sclerosis
MSBP (Munchausen syndrome by
    proxy), 891–892
Mucocutaneous lymph node
    syndrome, 382, 867
MUDPILES acronym, 496t, 608, 612
Multifocal atrial tachycardia, *11,*
    11–12
Multiple sclerosis (MS), 703–704
  clinical features of, 703–704
  diagnosis and differential of, 704
  management of, 704
Mumps, 725
Munchausen syndrome by proxy
    (MSBP), 891–892
Mupirocin, for impetigo, 374, 375,
    724
Musculoskeletal disorders, 817–875
  acute disorders of joints and bursae,
    862–866
  bone metastases, 656
  in children, 383–390
    acute rheumatic fever, 389–390
    acute suppurative arthritis, 387
    clavicle fracture, 385
    fractures associated with child
      abuse, 384–385
    Henoch-Schönlein purpura, 388
    juvenile rheumatoid arthritis,
      390
    Legg-Calvé-Perthes disease,
      388–389
    Osgood-Schlatter disease, 389
    patterns of injury, *383,* 383–384

Musculoskeletal disorders (*Cont.*)
    poststreptococcal reactive
      arthritis, 390
    radial head subluxation, 386
    slipped capital femoral epiphysis,
      386–387
    supracondylar and condylar
      fractures, 385–386
    transient synovitis of hip, 388
  emergencies in rheumatic diseases,
    867–868
  hand conditions, 869–871
  neck and thoracolumbar pain,
    855–859
  shoulder pain, 860–861
  soft tissue problems of foot,
    872–875
  traumatic, 817–852
    ankle and foot injuries, 844–847
    compartment syndromes,
      848–849
    evaluation and management of,
      819–821
    femoral shaft fractures, 839
    forearm and elbow injuries,
      826–829
    hand and wrist injuries, 822–825
    hip injuries, 838–839
    knee and leg injuries, 840–843
    pelvic fractures, 835–837
    rhabdomyolysis, 850–852
    shoulder and humerus injuries,
      830–834
Mushroom poisoning, 601–603, 602t
  clinical features of, 601
  diagnosis and differential of,
    601–603
  management of, 603
Myasthenia gravis (MG), 705–706
  clinical features of, 705
  diagnosis and differential of, 705
  management of, 705–706
Myasthenic crisis, 705
Mycobacterium avium complex
  (MAC), in HIV infection, 413, 414,
  417
Mycophenolate mofetil, 459t
Mycoplasma infection
  pneumonia, 180, 181
  with rash, 375–376
Myocardial infarction, acute (AMI),
  129–136
  cardiogenic shock and, 57, 130
  cocaine-precipitated, 129
  complications of, 130
  diagnosis of, 57–58, 123–125

    echocardiography, 124–125, 131
    electrocardiography, 123–124,
      130, 131t
    serum markers, 58, 124, *124,* 131
  dysrhythmias in, 130
  localization of, 130, 131t
  management of, 131–136, 132t
    angioplasty, 135, 136
    angiotensin-converting enzyme
      inhibitors, 136
    aspirin, 133
    β-blockers, 133
    cardiac intensive care, 136
    clopidogrel, 136
    coronary artery bypass graft, 59,
      131, 136
    fibrinolytic therapy, 134–135,
      134t, 654–655
    glycoprotein IIb/IIIa antagonists,
      136
    low-molecular-weight heparins,
      133–134
    morphine, 133
    nitroglycerin, 133
    oxygen therapy, 132
    right ventricular infarct, 136
    unfractionated heparin, 133
  pain of, 123, 126, 129–130
    vs. peptic ulcer disease, 213
  prognosis for, 130
  pulmonary edema and, 141
  right ventricular, 130, 136
  risk factors for, 129
Myocardial injuries, 798–800
  blunt, 799–800
  penetrating, 798–799
Myocardial ischemia. *See* Ischemic
  heart disease
Myocardial oxygen consumption, 129,
  131
Myocardial toxin exposure, 545
Myocarditis, 152
  in children, 328
Myofascial pain syndrome (MPS), 76t,
  77t, 856
Myoglobin
  in acute myocardial infarction, 124,
    124, 131
  in rhabdomyolysis, 850, 851
Myonecrosis, 447–448
  clostridial, 447–448
  nonclostridial, 448
Myopathies, 699
Myxedema coma, 615–616
  clinical features of, 615–616
  diagnosis and differential of, 616

Myxedema coma (*Cont.*)
  management of, 616

N

NAC (*N*-acetylcysteine)
  for acetaminophen overdose, 472t,
    509
  for herbal toxicity, 548
Nafcillin
  for brain abscess, 712
  for cellulitis, 336, 449
    periorbital and orbital, 337
  for epiglottitis, 370
  for erysipelas, 450
  for gas gangrene, 447
  for infected puncture wound, 113
  for lateral sinus thrombosis, 729
  for septic arthritis, 387
  for toxic shock syndrome, 408
  for wound infections in transplant
    recipients, 458
Nail bed injuries, 103–104, *104*
Naloxone, 68
  for clonidine toxicity, 519
  for neonatal narcotic respiratory
    depression, 30
  for opioid intoxication, 473t, 474,
    499–500
  for tricyclic antidepressant toxicity,
    480
Naphazoline/pheniramine, for
  conjunctivitis, 716
Naproxen
  for acute pain, 68
  for neck and back pain, 859
  use in pregnancy, 292t
Nasal bleeding, 730–732
Nasal foreign bodies, 732
Nasal fractures, 732, 787, 790
Nasal lacerations, 95–96
Nasal packing
  complications of, 732
  for epistaxis, 731
  for septal hematoma, 790
Nasal trauma, 787, 788
Nasoethmoidal-orbital injuries, 788,
  790
Nasogastric tube placement
  for acute pancreatitis, 251
  for caustic ingestion, 531
  for gastrointestinal bleeding, 204,
    205
  for incarcerated hernia, 220
  for intestinal obstruction, 218
Nasotracheal intubation, 6
Nateglinide, 607

Near drowning, 584–585
  clinical features of, 584
  diagnosis and differential of, 584
  management of, 584–585
Near syncope, 689
Necator americanus infection,
  433–434
Neck. *See also* Airway; Cervical spine
  anatomy of, *7*
  epiglottitis, 370, 742–743
  immobilization of, 795, 796
  parapharyngeal abscess, 742
  peritonsillar abscess, 372–373,
    740–741
  pharyngitis, 332–333, 740
  retropharyngeal abscess, 373,
    741–742
  traumatic injuries of, 744, 792–794
    clinical features of, 792
    diagnosis and differential of,
      792–793
    management of, 793–794
    zones of injury, 792, 793t
Neck pain, 855–859
  clinical features of, 855
  diagnosis and differential of,
    855–858, 857t
  management of, 859
Necrotizing fasciitis, 253–255,
  408–409, 448
Needle-stick injuries, 113
Needles, removal from soft tissue, 110
Nefazodone toxicity, 481
Neisseria gonorrhoeae infection,
  402–403
  arthritis, 865
  clinical features of, 402
  conjunctivitis, 334, 715
  diagnosis and differential of, 402
  management of, 402–403
  pelvic inflammatory disease, 305
  pharyngitis, 332–333
  prophylaxis after sexual assault, 896
Neisseria meningitidis infection, 752
Nematodes, 432–434
Neonates, 319–324. *See also* Pediatric
  patients
  abuse of, 320
  apparent life-threatening events in,
    323–324
  cardiorespiratory symptoms in,
    322–323
    apnea and periodic breathing, 322
    bronchopulmonary dysplasia, 323
    cyanosis and blue spells, 322–323
    noisy breathing and stridor, 322

Neonates (*Cont.*)
excessive crying of, 319–320, 320t
fever and sepsis in, 313–318, 320
gastrointestinal symptoms of,
321–322
abdominal distention, 322
constipation, 322
diarrhea, 321–322
feeding difficulties, 321
regurgitation, 321
surgical lesions, 321
vomiting, 321
hemolytic disease of newborn, 643
intestinal colic in, 320
jaundice in, 323
nonspecific signs of illness in, 319t
normal vegetative functions of, 319
oral thrush in, 323
premature, 319
preventing meconium aspiration in,
31
resuscitation of, 30–31
seizures in, 347
tetanus in, 422
urinary tract infection in, 397–398
Neostigmine, for myasthenia gravis,
705–706
Nephrostomy tube complications, 278
Nerve gas poisoning, 533
Nesiritide, for pulmonary edema, 140
Neuralgia
postherpetic, 76t, 77t
trigeminal, 672
Neuraminidase inhibitors, for
influenza, 410
Neurogenic shock, 62–63
Neurologic disorders, 665–712
acute peripheral nerve disorders,
699–702
altered mental status and coma,
679–685
amyotrophic lateral sclerosis, 703
ataxia and gait disturbances,
686–687
brain abscess, 711–712
central nervous system
vasoocclusive events in sickle cell
disease, 393
encephalitis, 711
end-stage renal disease and,
264–265
headache and facial pain, 667–672
in HIV infection, 415
Lambert-Eaton myasthenic
syndrome, 706
meningitis, 708–711

multiple sclerosis, 703–704
myasthenia gravis, 705–706
Parkinson disease, 706
poliomyelitis and postpolio
syndrome, 707
seizures and status epilepticus
in adults, 693–698
in children, 344–347
spinal trauma, 780–786
stroke and transient ischemic attack,
673–678
vertigo and dizziness, 688–692
Neuromuscular blockade
for monoamine oxidase inhibitor
overdose, 485
for rapid sequence induction, 5
in children, 28
for tetanus, 423
Neuromuscular junction disorders, 699
Neurotoxin exposure, 544
Neutropenic fever, 662
"Niacin flush," 546, 548
Nicardipine, for hypertensive
emergency, 160
Nifedipine
for aortic regurgitation, 146
for cold injuries, 562
for high-altitude pulmonary edema,
580
to relax lower esophageal sphincter,
210
Nikolsky sign, 749, 750
Nimodipine
for hypertensive emergency, 160
for subarachnoid hemorrhage, 668,
779
Nitrofurantoin
for urinary tract infection, 269
use in pregnancy, 289, 291t
Nitroglycerin (NTG)
for acute coronary syndromes, 129,
132t, 133
in cardiogenic shock, 58
for hypertensive emergency or
urgency, 160, 161
for pulmonary edema, 140
to relax lower esophageal sphincter,
210
Nitroprusside. *See* Sodium
nitroprusside
Nitrous oxide
contraindications to, 70–71
for procedural sedation, 70–71
Nizatidine, for peptic ulcer disease,
213
Nizoral shampoo, for tinea capitis, 754

Nonsteroidal anti-inflammatory drugs (NSAIDs)
  for acute pain, 68
  adverse effects of, 68
  antiplatelet activity of, 654
  for chronic pain, 75, 77t
  for crystal-induced synovitis, 863
  drug interactions with, 510
  for dysfunctional uterine bleeding, 284
  for headache, 669
  for juvenile rheumatoid arthritis, 390
  for musculoskeletal chest pain, 127
  for neck and back pain, 859
  for pain crisis in sickle cell disease, 392
  peptic ulcer disease and, 212, 213
  for pericardial inflammation syndrome, 800
  for pericarditis, 153
  for plantar fasciitis, 873
  for poststreptococcal reactive arthritis, 390
  for renal colic, 203, 277
  for shoulder pain, 861
  for tarsal tunnel syndrome, 873
  for temporomandibular disorder, 672
  toxicity of, 510–511
    clinical features of, 510
    diagnosis and differential of, 510
    management of, 510–511
  use in pregnancy, 292t
Norepinephrine
  for antipsychotic overdose, 487
  for barbiturate overdose, 490
  for chloral hydrate–induced dysrhythmias, 493
  for monoamine oxidase inhibitor overdose, 485
  for shock, 52
    cardiogenic shock, 58
    septic shock, 55
  for spinal shock, 786
  for trazodone or nefazodone overdose, 481
  for tricyclic antidepressant toxicity, 481
Norfloxacin, for gonococcal infection, 402
Normal saline (NS), 32
Northwestern brown spider bite, 568
Norwalk virus infection, 349t
Nose
  bleeding from, 730–732
  foreign bodies in, 732
  fractures of, 732, 787, 790
  lacerations of, 95–96
  packing of
    complications of, 732
    for epistaxis, 731
    for septal hematoma, 790
  traumatic injuries of, 787, 788
NS (normal saline), 32
NSAIDs. *See* Nonsteroidal anti-inflammatory drugs
NTG. *See* Nitroglycerin
"Nursemaid's" elbow, 386
Nystatin
  for balanoposthitis, 273
  for candidiasis, 417, 735

O

Obliterative bronchiolitis, in lung transplant recipient, 461, 462
Obsessive-compulsive disorder, 881
Obstetrics and gynecology, 281–309. *See also* Pregnancy
  comorbid diseases in pregnancy, 288–293
  complications of gynecologic procedures, 308–309
  ectopic pregnancy, 286–287
  emergencies during pregnancy and postpartum period, 294–298
  emergency delivery, 299–301
  pelvic inflammatory disease and tubo-ovarian abscess, 305–307
  vaginal bleeding and pelvic pain in non-pregnant patient, 283–285
  vulvovaginitis, 302–304
Occipitoatlantal dislocation, 783t
Octreotide
  for esophageal variceal bleeding, 205, 208
  for hypoglycemia, 473t, 607
  for sulfonylurea overdose, 556
Ocular trauma, 719–721
  blunt, 719
  chemical injury, 544, 591, 721
  evaluation of, 787–788
  globe penetration or rupture, 720
  with hyphema, 719–720
  orbital blowout fracture, 720, 787, 790
Odontogenic abscess, 743
Odontoid fracture, 782, 783t
OE. *See* Otitis externa
Ofloxacin
  for chlamydial infection, 402
  for conjunctivitis, 715

Ofloxacin (*Cont.*)
  for corneal abrasion, 718
  for corneal ulcer, 717
  for gonococcal infection, 402, 896
  for otitis externa, 332
  for pelvic inflammatory disease,
    306t
  for urinary tract infection, 269
Olecranon bursitis, 866
Olecranon fractures, 826–827
OME (otitis media with effusion), 331
Omeprazole, for peptic ulcer disease,
  213
Ondansetron
  for chemotherapy-induced
    nausea/vomiting, 663
  for iron poisoning, 525
  use in pregnancy, 292t, 295
  for vertigo, 691
  for vomiting, 237
Onychocryptosis, 872
Onychomycosis, 755
Ophthalmologic disorders, 715–723
  acute visual reduction or loss,
    721–723
  angle closure glaucoma, 721–722
  blunt ocular trauma, 719
  central retinal artery occlusion,
    722
  central retinal vein occlusion, 723
  chalazion, 715
  chemical ocular injury, 544, 591,
    721
  conjunctival abrasions, 718
  conjunctival foreign bodies, 718
  conjunctivitis, 334–335, 715–716
  corneal abrasion, 718
  corneal foreign bodies, 719
  corneal ulcer, 337, 717–718
  cyanoacrylate exposure, 721
  disorders associated with headache,
    668
  eyelid lacerations, 95, *95*, 719
  herpes zoster ophthalmicus, 412,
    418, 716–717
  hyphema, 719–720
  nasoethmoidal-orbital injuries, 788,
    790
  ocular complications of HIV
    infection, 416
  ocular disease in helminthic
    infections, 432t
  ocular exposure to caustic agent,
    531
  ocular herpes simplex virus
    infection, 716

Ophthalmologic disorders (*Cont.*)
  ocular symptoms of multiple
    sclerosis, 704
  optic neuritis, 722
  orbital blowout fracture, 720, 787,
    790
  orbital cellulitis, 337, 717
  penetrating trauma or ruptured
    globe, 720
  periorbital cellulitis, 337, 717
  in rheumatic diseases, 868
  stye, 715
  subconjunctival hemorrhage, 718
  temporal arteritis, 671–672, 723
  ultraviolet keratitis, 721
Opioids
  for acute pain, 68–69
  for cancer pain, 77t
  for chronic pain, 75
  for headache in children, 362
  neonatal respiratory depression
    induced by, 30
  overdose of, 468t, 499–500
    clinical features of, 499
    diagnosis and differential of, 499
    management of, 499–500
  for pain crisis in sickle cell disease,
    392
  side effects of, 68
  withdrawal from, 499–500
    in pregnancy, 290
Opium suppositories, for male urinary
  retention, 275
OpSite dressing, 118
Optic neuritis, 722
  multiple sclerosis and, 704
  temporal arteritis and, 672
Oral contraceptives
  for dysfunctional uterine bleeding,
    284
  for pregnancy prophylaxis after
    sexual assault, 896
Oral lacerations, 738
Oral procedures, endocarditis
  prophylaxis for, 421t
Oral rehydration therapy, for children,
  349–350, 349t, 368
Oral thrush
  in HIV infection, 416
  management of, 417
  neonatal, 323
Orbital blowout fracture, 720, 787,
  790
Orbital cellulitis, 717
  in children, 337
Orchitis, 272

Organic spines, removal from soft tissue, 110
Organophosphate poisoning, 468t, 533–537, 536t, 542–543
Orofacial pain, 734–735
  acute necrotizing ulcerative gingivitis, 735
  dental caries, 734
  facial cellulitis, 724–725, 734–735
  periodontal abscess, 735
  postextraction alveolar osteitis, 735
  tooth eruption, 734
Orofacial trauma, 736–738
  antibiotic prophylaxis for, 86
  dental avulsion, 737
  dental concussion, 737
  dental fractures, 736–737
  dental luxations, 737
  dentoalveolar injuries, 736
  infection risk from, 83
  intraoral mucosal lacerations, 738
  lip lacerations, 96, 96–97, 738
  tongue lacerations, 738
Oropharyngeal dysphagia, 206
Orotracheal intubation, 3–4
  rapid sequence induction for, 5
Orthostatic hypotension, 137, 138
Oseltamivir, for influenza, 410–411
Osgood-Schlatter disease, 389
Osmolarity, 32
Osteoarthritis, 863
  of shoulder, 861
Osteomyelitis, from puncture wound, 112, 113
Otitis externa (OE), 728
  in children, 331–332
  clinical features of, 331, 728
  diagnosis and differential of, 331
  management of, 332, 728
  microbiology of, 728
Otitis media, acute (AOM), 728–729
  in children, 330–331, 728
  clinical features of, 330, 728
  complications of, 729
  diagnosis and differential of, 330
  in infants, 314
  management of, 330–331, 728–729
Otitis media with effusion (OME), 331
Otologic disorders, 728–730
  acute mastoiditis, 729
  bullous myringitis, 180, 729
  ear trauma, 729–730
  foreign bodies in ear, 730
  lateral sinus thrombosis, 729
  otitis externa, 331–332, 728
  otitis media, 330–331, 728–729

  sudden hearing loss, 730
  tinnitus, 730
Ototoxic drugs, 690
Ottawa Ankle Rules, 844, 845
Ovarian cyst, 284
Ovarian hyperstimulation syndrome, 285, 309
Ovarian torsion, 284–285
Overdose of drug. See Toxicology and pharmacology
Oxacillin
  for cellulitis, 336
    periorbital and orbital, 337
  for septic arthritis, 387
  for septic shock, 55
  for suppurative parotitis, 726
  for toxic shock syndrome, 408
  for wound infections in transplant recipients, 458
Oxycel, 84
Oxycodone
  dosage of, 69t
  for toothache, 734
Oxygen saturation, 3
Oxygen therapy
  for acute coronary syndromes, 132
  for acute pancreatitis, 251
  for allergic reactions, 61
  for asthma and chronic obstructive pulmonary disease, 193, 289, 341
  for carbon monoxide poisoning, 599
  for caustic ingestion, 531
  for children with altered mental status, 361
  for cluster headaches, 669
  for croup, 369
  for cyanide poisoning, 551
  for cyanosis, 178
  for dysbarism, 583
  for epiglottitis, 370
  for high-altitude syndromes, 579, 580
  for hypoxemia, 175
  before intubation, 3, 4, 5, 26
  for near drowning, 584–585
  for pneumonia, 181
  for poisoned patient, 467
  for pulmonary edema, 140
  for pulmonary embolism, 157
  for septic shock, 55
  for shock, 51
  for trauma patients, 762, 766
Oxygenation
  cyanosis and, 177–178
  hypoxemia and, 174–175
Oxymetazoline, for epistaxis, 731

Oxytocin, for uterine atony, 298, 301

P

Packed red blood cells (PRBCs), 646
PACs (premature atrial contractions),
   10–11, *11*
Pain
   acute, 67–73
      frequency of, 67
      local and regional anesthesia for,
         71–73
      management in children, 67
      nonpharmacologic management
         of, 67
      systemic analgesia and sedation
         for, 67–71, 69t
      undertreatment of, 67
   acute abdominal, 199–203
      in children, 351–354, 352t
   of acute myocardial infarction, 123,
      126, 129–130
   of acute pancreatitis, 212, 250
   anginal, 125–126, 129
   of aortic dissection, 126, 145, 163
   of aortic stenosis, 144
   of appendicitis, 214
   assessment of, 67
   biliary colic, 247–249
   in cancer, 77t, 663–664
   chest, 123–128
   chronic, 75–79
      clinical features of, 75, 76t
      diagnosis and differential of, 75
      management of, 75–78, 77t
      in patients with drug-seeking
         behavior, 78–79, 78t
   of compartment syndrome, 848
   of Crohn disease, 221
   of dilated cardiomyopathy, 149
   of diverticulitis, 225
   of ectopic pregnancy, 286
   of endometriosis, 285
   of esophageal perforation, 207
   facial, 671–672
   headache, 667–671
   of herpes zoster, 412
   of hypertrophic cardiomyopathy,
      150
   of intestinal obstruction, 217
   of labor, 299
   of mitral valve prolapse, 144
   neck and thoracolumbar, 855–859
   orofacial, 734–735
   of ovarian cyst, 284
   of ovarian torsion, 284–285
   pelvic, 284–285

of pelvic inflammatory disease, 305
of peptic ulcer disease, 212
of pericardial tamponade, 126
of pericarditis, 126, 152–153
physiologic responses to, 67
postherpetic neuralgia, 412
of pulmonary embolism, 126, 156
renal colic, 276–277
shoulder, 860–861
in sickle cell disease, 391–392
of temporal arteritis, 671
of temporomandibular joint
   dysfunction, 672, 726
of tooth decay, 734
of tooth eruption, 734
toothache, 734
of trigeminal neuralgia, 672
Painful arc syndrome, 860
Palm lacerations, 100–101
Pamidronate, for hypercalcemia of
   malignancy, 660
Pancoast tumor, 861
Pancreatic injuries, 804
Pancreatitis, acute, 250–252
   in children, 354
   clinical features of, 250
   diagnosis and differential of, 250
   etiologies of, 251t
   gallstone, 248
   management of, 251–252
   pain of, 212, 250
   postoperative, 255
Panic disorder, 881, 885–886
   clinical features of, 885
   diagnosis and differential of, 885
   management of, 885–886
Paralytic ileus, 217
   postoperative, 255
Parapharyngeal abscess (PPA), 742
Paraphimosis, 273
Parasitic infections, 431
Parkinson disease, 681, 686, 706
Paronychia, 869–871, 870t
Parotitis, 725–726
   suppurative, 725–726
   viral, 725
Paroxysmal cold hemoglobinemia,
   643
Pasteurella multocida infection
   from animal bites, 116, 869
   antibiotics for, 85, 116
Patella
   dislocation of, 841
   fractures of, 840
Patellar tendon rupture, 841–842
Patellar tendonitis, 843

PCP (phencyclidine) intoxication, 502–504, 503t
PE. *See* Pulmonary embolism
Pediatric patients, 311–398
  abdominal emergencies in, 351–354
  abuse of, 765, 891–892
  airway management in, 26–28, 764
  altered mental status in, 359–361, 360t
  antimycobacterial drugs for, 186t
  appendicitis in, 215
  asthma in, 340–342
  bacterial tracheitis in, 371
  bronchiolitis in, 342–343
  cardiopulmonary resuscitation in, 26–31
  cellulitis in, 336–337
  conjunctivitis in, 334–335
  croup in, 369–370
  determining hydration status of, 348
  epiglottitis in, 370
  exanthems in, 374–382
  failure to thrive, 891–892
  fever in, 313–314
  foreign body aspiration by, 371–372
  Glasgow Coma Scale in, 775t
  headache in, 361–362
  heart disease in, 325–329
  hypertensive emergencies in, 161
  hypoglycemia in, 357–358
  ingestion of foreign bodies by, 209–211
  meningitis in, 314, 318
  musculoskeletal disorders in, 383–390
  neonatal problems, 319–324 (*See also* Neonates)
  occult bacteremia in, 315–316
  otitis externa in, 331–332
  otitis media in, 330–331
  pain management in, 67–69, 69t
  pelvic pain and vaginal bleeding in, 283–284
  peritonsillar abscess in, 372–373
  pharyngitis in, 332–333
  pneumonia in, 338–339
  restraint of, 67
  retropharyngeal abscess in, 373
  seizures in, 344–347
  sepsis in, 316–318, 317t
  shock in, 317, 764
  sickle cell disease in, 391–396
  sinusitis in, 335–336
  syncope and sudden death in, 363–365, 364t
  tooth eruption in, 734
  traumatic injuries in, 764–767
  vascular access in, 28–29, 766
  vomiting and diarrhea in, 348–350
Pediculosis, 571, 757–758
Pelvic arteriography and embolization, 763
Pelvic fractures, 763, 810, 835–837
  acetabular, 837
  clinical features of, 835
  diagnosis and differential of, 835
  management of, 835–837
  stable pelvic avulsion and single bone fractures, 836–837, 837t
  Young classification system for, 835, 836t
Pelvic inflammatory disease (PID), 305–307
  clinical features of, 305
  diagnosis and differential of, 305–306
  management of, 305t, 306–307, 306t
  risk factors for, 305
Pelvic pain, 284–285
  from endometriosis, 285
  from leiomyomas, 285
  from ovarian cyst, 284
  from ovarian hyperstimulation syndrome, 285
  from ovarian torsion, 284–285
  of pelvic inflammatory disease, 305
Pemphigus vulgaris (PV), 751–752
  clinical features of, 751–752
  diagnosis and differential of, 752
  management of, 752
Penciclovir, for herpes simplex virus infection, 411
Penetrating injuries
  of buttock, 808–809
  of extremities, 814–815
  of flank, 807–808
  genitourinary, 810–811
  of globe, 720
  of great vessels, 800
  of head, 777
  of heart, 798–799
Penicillin(s)
  for acute rheumatic fever, 390
  for anthrax, 445
  for brain abscess, 712
  for cat bites, 117
  for deep space infections of hand, 870t
  for dog bites, 115
  for erysipelas, 375, 450, 724
  for flexor tenosynovitis, 870t

Penicillin(s) (*Cont.*)
  for frostbite, 562
  for gas gangrene, 447, 448
  for inflammation from wisdom
    teeth, 734
  for mandibular fractures, 791
  for necrotizing fasciitis, 448
  for odontogenic abscess, 743
  overdose of, 550
  for periodontal abscess, 735
  for peritonsillar abscess, 741
  for pharyngitis, 740
  for postextraction alveolar osteitis,
    735
  for poststreptococcal reactive
    arthritis, 390
  for scarlet fever, 377
  for staphylococcal scalded skin
    syndrome, 751
  for streptococcal pharyngitis, 333
  for streptococcal toxic shock
    syndrome, 409
  for syphilis, 404
  for tooth decay, 734
  use in pregnancy, 291t
  for wound prophylaxis, 85–86, 118
Penile disorders, 273–274
  balanoposthitis, 273
  paraphimosis, 273
  penile entrapment, 273
  penile fracture, 273, 813
  Peyronie disease, 273
  phimosis, 273
  priapism, 273–274
  traumatic injuries, 813
Pentamidine, for *Pneumocystis carinii*
  pneumonia, 417, 458
Pentobarbital
  for neonatal seizures, 347
  for procedural sedation, 70
  for status epilepticus, *696*, 697
Peptic ulcer disease (PUD), 212–213
  bleeding due to, 204, 212, 213
  clinical features of, 212
  diagnosis and differential of,
    212–213
  management of, 213
  risk factors for, 212
Percutaneous sutures
  continuous "running," 89, *89*
  simple interrupted, 87–89, *88*
Percutaneous transluminal angioplasty,
  59
Pericardial effusion with tamponade,
  malignant, 658
Pericardial friction rub, 152, 264, 800

Pericardial inflammation syndrome,
  800
Pericardial "knock," 154
Pericardial tamponade. *See* Cardiac
  tamponade
Pericardial window, 798
Pericardiocentesis, 154, 658, 798, 799
Pericarditis, 152–155
  in children, 328
  clinical features of, 152–153
  constrictive, 154–155
    vs. restrictive cardiomyopathy,
      151
  diagnosis and differential of,
    152–153
  etiologies of, 152
  management of, 153
  after myocardial infarction, 130
  pain of, 126, 152–153
  in rheumatic diseases, 867
  uremic, 264
Perilunate dislocation, 824
Perilymphatic fistula, 690
Periodic breathing, neonatal, 322
Periodontal abscess, 735
Periorbital cellulitis, 717
  in children, 337
Periosteitis after tooth extraction, 735
Peripheral blood smear, 622t
Peripheral nerve testing
  in lower extremity, 106, 107t
  in upper extremity, 99, 99t, 100t
Peripheral neuropathy, 699–700
  end-stage renal disease and,
    264–265
  rhabdomyolysis and, 851
Peripheral vascular disorders, 166–169
  acute arterial occlusion, 168–169
  deep venous thrombosis and
    thrombophlebitis, 166–168, 167t
Peritoneal dialysis
  for acute renal failure, 262
  complications of, 266
Peritoneal lavage, diagnostic (DPL),
  804–805
Peritonitis
  due to peritoneal dialysis, 266
  spontaneous bacterial, 244
Peritonsillar abscess (PTA), 740–741
  in children, 372–373
  clinical features of, 372, 740–741
  diagnosis and differential of, 372,
    741
  management of, 372–373, 741
Permethrin
  for chigger bites, 570

Permethrin (*Cont.*)
  for lice, 571, 758
  for scabies, 570, 757
Peroneal retinaculum disruption, 874
Pesticide poisoning, 533–537
  clinical features of, 533–535
  diagnosis and differential of, 535
  management of, 535–537, 536t
Peyronie disease, 273
pH, 41. *See also* Acid–base disorders
Phalangeal fractures
  of foot, 847
  of hand, 103, 104, 823
Phalen sign, 871
Phantom limb pain, 76t, 77t
Pharyngeal trauma, 792
Pharyngitis, 740
  in children, 332–333
  clinical features of, 332, 740
  diagnosis and differential of,
    332–333
  management of, 333, 740
Phencyclidine (PCP) intoxication,
  502–504, 503t
Phenobarbital, for seizures, 697, 697t
  in children, 346
  drug- or toxin-induced, 480, 482,
    487, 488
  febrile, 347
  in neonates, 347
  status epilepticus, 345, *696*
Phenothiazine, use in pregnancy, 292t
Phenoxybenzamine toxicity, 519
Phentolamine
  for hallucinogen intoxication, 504
  for monoamine oxidase inhibitor
    overdose, 485
  for stimulant toxicity, 502
Phenylephrine, for epistaxis, 731
Phenytoin
  for digitalis glycoside toxicity, 16,
    514
  hypersensitivity to, 522
  for monoamine oxidase inhibitor
    overdose, 485
  for seizures, 697, 697t
    in children, 346
    drug-induced, 487
    in meningitis, 709
    status epilepticus, *696*
  toxicity of, 521–523
    clinical features of, 521–522
    diagnosis and differential of, 522
    management of, 522–523
    plasma level and, 522, 522t
  use in pregnancy, 291t, 522

Pheochromocytoma, 161
Phimosis, 273
Phlegmasia alba dolens, 166
Phlegmasia cerulea dolens, 166
Phobias, 881
Phosphorus, for diabetic ketoacidosis,
  609
Photosensitivity, 753
Physostigmine, for anticholinergic
  toxicity, 473t, 476–478
PID. *See* Pelvic inflammatory disease
Pillar fracture of cervical spine, 784t
Pilocarpine, for acute angle closure
  glaucoma, 722
Pilonidal abscess, 450
Pilonidal sinus, 232
Pinworm, 433
Pioglitazone, 607
PIP (proximal interphalangeal) joint
  dislocations, 822
Piperacillin/tazobactam
  for appendectomy, 215
  for cirrhosis and liver failure, 245
  for esophageal perforation, 208
  for intestinal obstruction, 218
  for perforated or strangulated
    hernia, 220
  for pneumonia, 182
    nosocomial, 458
Pisiform fracture, 825
Pit viper bite, 572–573
Pityriasis rosea, 382
Placenta previa, 295
Plague, 445–446
  as biological weapon, 454t
  clinical features of, 445
  diagnosis and differential of, 445
  management of, 446
Plant poisoning, 601–603
  clinical features of, 601
  diagnosis and differential of,
    601–603
  management of, 603
Plantar fasciitis, 873
Plantar fibromatosis, 874
Plantar interdigital neuroma, 874
Plantar warts, 872
Plasmodium infection. *See* Malaria
Platelet abnormalities, bleeding due to,
  628
Platelet count, 624t
Platelet inhibitors, 654
Platelet transfusion, 628, 647
  for disseminated intravascular
    coagulation, 630
  in liver disease, 629

Platelet transfusion (*Cont.*)
in renal disease, 629
for von Willebrand disease, 640
Pleural effusion
esophageal perforation and, 207
pneumonia and, 180
rheumatic diseases with, 867
Plexopathies, 700–701
Pneumocystis carinii pneumonia
in HIV infection, 180, 415
management of, 417, 458
prophylaxis for, in pregnancy, 290
in transplant recipients, 456, 458
Pneumonia, 179–182
aspiration, 180
in children, 314, 338–339
clinical features of, 338
diagnosis and differential of, 338
management of, 338–339, 339t
clinical features of, 180
diagnosis and differential of,
180–181
etiologies of, 179–180
in HIV infection, 180, 415
management of, 181–182
nosocomial, in transplant recipients,
458
postoperative, 253, 254
Pneumonic plague, 445–446, 454t
Pneumothorax, 188–189, 761–762
clinical features of, 188
diagnosis and differential of, 188
iatrogenic, 188
management of, 188–189, 762, 797
primary vs. secondary, 188
subcutaneous emphysema and,
795–796
tension, 188, 762, 793, 796–797
Poisoning, 467–475. *See also*
Toxicology and pharmacology
clinical features of, 467
agents that may alter presenting
signs or symptoms, 470t–471t
toxidromes, 467, 468t–469t
diagnosis and differential of, 467
management of, 467, 473–475
antidotes, 467, 472t–473t
decontamination, 474
Poliovirus infection, 377, 707
Polyarteritis nodosa, 867
Polycythemia vera, 178
Polyethylene glycol
for arsenic poisoning, 540
for iron poisoning, 525
for whole bowel irrigation, 474
Polymyositis, 699, 867

Polyps, colonic, 354
Polyvalent Crotalidae Immune Fab,
573
POPS (pulmonary over-pressurization
syndrome), 581–583
Pork tapeworm, 435–436
Portal hypertension, 354
Posterior cerebral artery occlusion,
673
Posterior cruciate ligament injury, 842
Posterior inferior cerebellar artery
occlusion, 673
Posterior tibialis tendon rupture, 873
Postherpetic neuralgia, 76t, 77t, 412
Postmenopausal women
atrophic vaginitis in, 304
vaginal bleeding in, 283
Postoperative complications, 253–256
after breast surgery, 255
clinical features of, 253–254
diagnosis and differential of, 254
after gastrointestinal surgery,
255–256
management of, 254–255
Postpartum care after emergency
delivery, 301
Postpartum disorders, 298
amniotic fluid embolism, 298
endometritis, 298
hemorrhage, 298
mastitis, 298
Postperfusion syndrome, 644
Postpolio syndrome, 707
Postrenal failure, 260t, 261–262
Postseptal (orbital) cellulitis, 717
in children, 337
Poststreptococcal reactive arthritis
(PSRA), 390
Posttransplant lymphoproliferative
disease (PTLD), 461, 462
Posttraumatic stress disorder, 881
Potassium balance
hyperkalemia, 36–38, 37t
hypokalemia, 35–36, 35t
Potassium iodide, for thyroid storm,
615t
Potassium therapy
for diabetic ketoacidosis, 609
for hypokalemia, 36, 356
PPA (parapharyngeal abscess), 742
PPD (purified protein derivative) test,
185
Pralidoxime, for cholinergic toxicity,
473t
Praziquantel
for cestode infections, 435–436

Praziquantel (*Cont.*)
  for schistosomiasis, 435
Prazosin toxicity, 519
PRBCs (packed red blood cells), 646
Prednisolone
  for asthma, 341
  for croup, 369
Prednisolone acetate
  for herpes zoster ophthalmicus, 717
  for intraocular pressure elevation,
    722
Prednisone
  for acute rheumatic fever, 389
  adverse effects of, 459t
  for allergic reactions, 61
  for asthma and chronic obstructive
    pulmonary disease, 193–194
    in children, 341
    in pregnancy, 289
  for Bell palsy, 701
  for cold injuries, 562
  for contact dermatitis, 754
  for Crohn disease, 222
  for croup, 369
  for hemolytic anemia, 644
  for idiopathic thrombocytopenic
    purpura, 628
  for multiple sclerosis, 704
  for pharyngitis with airway
    obstruction, 333
  for *Pneumocystis carinii*
    pneumonia, 417
  for temporal arteritis, 672, 723
  for ulcerative colitis, 223–224
Preeclampsia, 159, 296–298, 297t
Preexcitation syndromes, 24–25, *25*
Pregnancy. *See also* Postpartum
  disorders
  asthma in, 289
  diabetes in, 288
  diagnostic imaging in, 292–293
  domestic violence in, 290
  dysrhythmias in, 288
  ectopic, 286–287
  emergency delivery, 299–301
  HIV infection in, 290
  hypertension, preeclampsia, and
    eclampsia in, 159, 161, 296–298,
    297t
  hyperthyroidism in, 288
  inflammatory bowel disease in, 289
  medication use in, 290, 291t–292t
  migraine in, 290
  nausea and vomiting in, 234, 235,
    295
  pelvic inflammatory disease in, 305

  phlegmasia alba dolens in, 166
  physiologic changes of, 771
  preterm labor, 296
  prophylaxis after sexual assault,
    895–896
  seizures in, 290
  sickle cell disease in, 289
  substance abuse in, 290
  testing for, 286–287, 294
  threatened abortion and abortion,
    294–295
  thromboembolism in, 288–289
  trauma in, 771–773
    clinical features of, 771
    diagnosis and differential of,
      771–772
    fetal injuries and, 771
    management of, 772–773
  urinary tract infection in, 289
  vaginal bleeding in second half of,
    295–296
    abruptio placentae, 295, 771
    placenta previa, 295
    premature rupture of membranes,
      296
Premature atrial contractions (PACs),
  10–11, *11*
Premature rupture of membranes
  (PROM), 296
Premature ventricular contractions
  (PVCs), 17–18, *18*
  in acute myocardial infarction, 130
Prepatellar bursitis, 866
Prerenal failure, 259–261, 260t
Preseptal (periorbital) cellulitis, 717
  in children, 337
Preterm labor, 296
Preterminal rhythms, 24
  asystole, 24
  idioventricular rhythm, 24
  pulseless electrical activity, 24
Priapism, 273–274
  in sickle cell disease, 393–394
Prickly heat, 566
Primaquine
  for malaria, 427, 428t
  toxicity of, 549–550
Primidone, for seizures, 697t
  in children, 346
Prinzmetal angina, 125, 129
Procainamide
  for monoamine oxidase inhibitor
    overdose, 485
  for ventricular fibrillation, 21
  for ventricular tachycardia, 19
  for wide-complex tachycardia, 17

Procainamide (*Cont.*)
  for Wolff-Parkinson-White
    syndrome, 25
Procaine, 71
Procedural sedation and analgesia
  (PSA), 67–73
  discharge after, 71
  informed consent for, 68
  local and regional anesthesia, 71–73
  systemic, 67–71, 69t
Prochlorperazine
  for migraine, 671t
  for vomiting, 237
PROM (premature rupture of
  membranes), 296
Promethazine
  for iron poisoning, 525
  use in pregnancy, 295
  for vertigo, 691
  for vomiting, 236, 249, 252, 663
Proparacaine, for corneal abrasion,
  718
Propofol
  dosage of, 69t
  for procedural sedation, 70
  for rapid sequence induction in
    children, 28
  side effects of, 70
  for status epilepticus, 345, *696,
    697*
Propoxyphene, use in pregnancy, 292t
Propranolol
  for supraventricular tachycardia, 15
  for thyroid storm, 615t
Propylthiouracil
  for hyperthyroidism, 288
  for thyroid storm, 615t
Prostaglandin E₁
  for closure of ductus arteriosus, 327
  for cold injuries, 562
Prosthetic valve disease, 146–148
  clinical features of, 146
  diagnosis and differential of,
    146–147
  hemolysis, 645
  infective endocarditis, 147, 419
  management of, 147–148
Protamine, for heparin reversal, 133,
  266, 473t, 630
Proteus urinary tract infection, 268
Prothrombin time (PT), 625t
Proximal interphalangeal (PIP) joint
  dislocations, 822
Pruritus, 60
  ani, 233
  in helminthic infections, 432t

PSA. *See* Procedural sedation and
  analgesia
Pseudoephedrine, for priapism, 273,
  393
Pseudogout, 863
Pseudomembranous colitis, 224–225
Pseudomonas aeruginosa infection
  antibiotic prophylaxis for, 86, 113
  otitis externa, 728
  otitis media, 728
  pneumonia, 179, 182
  from puncture wounds, 112, 113
  urinary tract infection, 268
Psilocybin, 503t
Psoas sign, 214
Psoriasis, 755–756
PSRA (poststreptococcal reactive
  arthritis), 390
Psychiatric consultation, 884
Psychopharmacologic agent toxicity,
  479–488
  antipsychotics, 486–487
  lithium, 487–488
  monoamine oxidase inhibitors,
    484–486, 485t, 486t
  newer antidepressants, 481–483
  serotonin syndrome, 479
  tricyclic antidepressants,
    479–481
Psychosis, 680t, 880
Psychosocial disorders, 877–887
  bipolar disorder, 880–881
  clinical presentation of, 882
  conversion disorder, 886–887
  delirium, 679–680, 680t, 879
  dementia, 680–683, 680t, 879
  depression, 880
  diagnosis and differential of, 883
  generalized anxiety disorder, 881
  homicidal or violent patients,
    882–884
  management of, 883–884
  obsessive-compulsive disorder,
    881
  panic disorder, 881, 885–886
  posttraumatic stress disorder, 881
  psychotic disorders, 680t, 880
  schizophrenia, 879
  specific phobia, 881
  substance-induced disorders,
    499–504, 879
  suicidal patients, 882–884
Psychosocial dwarfs, 891
Psyllium, for constipation, 238
PT (prothrombin time), 625t
PTA. *See* Peritonsillar abscess

PTLD (posttransplant lymphoproliferative disease), 461, 462
Pubic lice, 571, 757–758
Pubis fracture, 837t
PUD. *See* Peptic ulcer disease
Pulmonary angiography, 156
Pulmonary disorders, 171–195. *See also* Respiratory disorders in children
in anthrax, 444
asthma and chronic obstructive pulmonary disease, 192–195
in children, 340–342
bronchitis, 179
contusions, 796–797
in helminthic infections, 432t
hemoptysis, 190–191
in HIV infection, 414–415
neonatal, 322–323
pneumonia, 179–182
in children, 338–339
pneumothorax, 188–189
respiratory distress, 173–178
in rheumatic diseases, 867
severe respiratory distress syndrome, 182–183
tuberculosis, 184–187
Pulmonary edema, 140–141
aortic incompetence and, 145, 146
aortic stenosis and, 145
from blood transfusion, 648
clinical features of, 140
diagnosis and differential of, 140
heart failure and, 140–141
high-altitude, 578–580
with hypertension, 160
management of, 140–141
mitral incompetence and, 143, 144
noncardiogenic, 140
Pulmonary embolism (PE), 156–158
clinical features of, 156
diagnosis and differential of, 156–157
inferior vena cava filter for prevention of, 168
management of, 157–158, 655
pain of, 126, 156
in pregnancy, 288–289
risk factors for, 156
syncope and, 137
Pulmonary over-pressurization syndrome (POPS), 581–583
Pulse oximetry, 3, 173, 179, 193, 339, 340, 342
Pulseless electrical activity, 24

Pulsus paradoxus, 154, 192
Puncture wounds, 112–113
animal bites, 115–117
antibiotic prophylaxis for, 112–113
clinical features of, 112
diagnosis and differential of, 112
high pressure injection injuries, 113–114, 824
human bites, 114–115
indications for hospital admission for, 113
with infection at presentation, 113
infection risk from, 112
management of, 112–113
needle-stick injuries, 113
Purified protein derivative (PPD) test, 185
Puss caterpillar stings, 571
PV. *See* Pemphigus vulgaris
PVCs (premature ventricular contractions), 17–18, *18*
in acute myocardial infarction, 130
Pyelonephritis, 267–269. *See also* Urinary tract infection
Pyloric stenosis, 353
Pyoderma faciale, 756
Pyrantel pamoate
for ascariasis, 433
for pinworm, 433
Pyrazinamide, for tuberculosis, 185, 186t, 417
Pyridostigmine, for myasthenia gravis, 706
Pyridoxine
for ethylene glycol poisoning, 473t, 497
for isoniazid toxicity, 549
for mushroom poisoning, 603
for neonatal seizures, 347
overdose of, 546
Pyrimethamine, for toxoplasmosis, 417, 458
Pyrimethamine-sulfadoxine, for malaria, 428t

Q
Quadriceps tendon rupture, 842
Quincke pulse, 145
Quinidine, for malaria, 429t, 430
Quinine
for malaria, 428t
toxicity of, 549–550

R
Rabies, 423–425
clinical features of, 424

Rabies (*Cont.*)
  diagnosis and differential of, 424
  management of, 424–425
Raccoon eyes, 776, 787
Radial fractures, 827–828
Radial head fractures, 826–827
Radial head subluxation, 386
Radial nerve testing, 99, 99t, 100t
Radial styloid fracture, 825
Radiculopathy, 855–859
  cervical, 856, 857t
  lumbar, 858, 858t
Ramsay-Hunt syndrome, 412, 701
Ranitidine
  for allergic reactions, 61
  for Hymenoptera sting, 567
  for peptic ulcer disease, 213
  for theophylline toxicity, 513
Rape. *See* Sexual assault
Rapid sequence induction (RSI), 5
  in children, 26–28
Rash. *See also* Skin disorders
  in bullous impetigo, 374, *374,* 724
  in chickenpox, 380, *380*
  in children, 374–382
  in contact dermatitis, 753–754
  in enteroviral infection, 377–378
  in erysipelas, 375, 449, 724
  in erythema infectiousum, 378, *379*
  in erythema multiforme, 748
  in erythema nodosum, 382
  heat-related, 566
  in herpes zoster, 412, 756
  in HIV infection, 413, 416
  in impetigo contagiosum, 374–375,
    375
  in infectious mononucleosis,
    378–379
  in Kawasaki disease, 382
  in Lyme disease, 437
  in measles, 378
  in mycoplasmal infection, 375–376
  in pityriasis rosea, 382
  in Rocky Mountain spotted fever,
    377, 439
  in roseola infantum, 381, *381*
  in rubella, 380
  in scarlet fever, *376,* 376–377
  of tinea infections, 755
  in toxic shock syndrome, 407
Rattlesnake bite, 572–573
Rectal anatomy, 227, *228*
Rectal examination, 227
  of children, 352
Rectal foreign bodies, 231–232
Rectal prolapse, 231

Rectal surgery complications, 256
Reflex sympathetic dystrophy (RSD),
  75–78, 76t, 77t
Regional anesthesia, 71–73
Regional enteritis, 221–222
Regurgitation, neonatal, 321
Rehydration therapy. *See also* Fluid
  and electrolyte therapy
  for children, 349–350, 349t, 368
  for rhabdomyolysis, 851
Reiter syndrome, 865
Relapsing polychondritis, 867
Renal colic, 276–277
  vs. abdominal aortic aneurysm, 163
  clinical features of, 276
  diagnosis and differential of,
    276–277
  management of, 203, 277
Renal disease
  bleeding in, 629
  kidney stones, 276–277
  rheumatic diseases and, 868
Renal failure
  acute, 259–263
    clinical features of, 259
    diagnosis and differential of,
      259–261, 261t
    etiologies of, 260t
    management of, 261–263
    oliguric vs. nonoliguric, 259
    rhabdomyolysis and, 850
    risk factors for, 259
  complications of, 264–266
    cardiovascular, 264
    dialysis-related, 265–266
    gastrointestinal, 265
    hematologic, 265
    neurologic, 264–265
  hypertension and, 160
  septic shock and, 52
Renal injuries, 812
Renal transplant patients, 462
Repaglinide, 555, 607
Reserpine, for thyroid storm, 615t
Respiratory acidosis, 44
Respiratory alkalosis, 44–45
  in shock, 50, 54
Respiratory complications of surgery,
  253
Respiratory depression
  induced by procedural sedation and
    analgesia, 68
  opioid-induced, 499
    in neonates, 30
Respiratory disorders in children
  asthma, 340–342

Respiratory disorders in children
(*Cont.*)
  bacterial tracheitis, 371
  bronchiolitis, 340, 342–343
  epiglottitis, 370
  foreign body aspiration, 371–372
  neonatal cardiorespiratory
    symptoms, 322–323
  peritonsillar abscess, 372–373
  pneumonia, 338–339
  retropharyngeal abscess, 373
  viral croup, 369–370
Respiratory distress, 173–178
  cyanosis, 177–178, 178t
  dyspnea, 173–174, 174t
  hypercapnia, 175–176, 176t
  hypoxemia, 174–175
  wheezing, 176–177, 177t
Respiratory procedures, endocarditis
  prophylaxis for, 421t
Respiratory syncytial virus infection,
  340, 342
Respiratory viral infections
  bronchitis, 179
  croup, 369–370
  pneumonia, 180, 338
  severe acute respiratory syndrome,
    182–183
Restraint of patient
  for pediatric procedures, 67
  for violent behavior, 883–884
Restrictive cardiomyopathy, 151
  clinical features of, 151
  diagnosis and differential of, 151
  management of, 151
Resuscitation
  advanced airway support, 3–8
  of geriatric patients, 768, 770
  management of dysrhythmias, 9–25
  of pediatric patients, 26–31
  of trauma patients, 761
Reteplase (rPA), 654
  for acute coronary syndromes, 132t,
    135
Reticulocyte count, 622t
Retinitis, cytomegalovirus, 416
Retrograde pyelography, 811t
Retrograde tracheal intubation, 8
Retrograde urethrography, 811t
Retroperitoneal abscess, 804
Retroperitoneal injuries, 803
Retropharyngeal abscess, 741–742
  in children, 373
  clinical features of, 373, 741
  diagnosis and differential of, 373,
    741

  management of, 373, 741–742
Rewarming procedures for
  hypothermia, 562–563, 563t
Rh (D) immune globulin, 294, 296,
  773
Rh isoimmunization, 771
Rhabdomyolysis, 850–852
  clinical features of, 850–851
  complications of, 850–851
  diagnosis and differential of, 851
  management of, 851–852
  risk factors for, 850
Rheumatic fever, acute, 389–390
Rheumatoid arthritis, 865
  emergencies in, 867–868
  juvenile, 390
Rib fractures, 796
Ricin, 455
Rickettsia rickettsii infection, 377,
  438–440
Rifabutin
  for *Mycobacterium avium* complex,
    417
  for tuberculosis, 417
Rifampin
  for meningitis, 709, 710t
  for tuberculosis, 185, 186t
Right bundle branch block, 17
Right ventricular cardiomyopathy,
  dysrhythmogenicity of, 152
Rimantadine, for influenza, 410–411
Ring removal technique, 105, *105*
Rocky Mountain spotted fever
  (RMSF), 377, 438–440
  clinical features of, 439
  complications of, 439
  diagnosis and differential of,
    439–440
  management of, 377, 440
  rash of, 377, 439
Rocuronium, for rapid sequence
  induction, 5
  in children, 28
Rodent bites, 117
Rodenticide poisoning, 533–537
Romberg test, 687, 690
Roseola infantum, 381, *381*
Rosiglitazone, 607
Rotator cuff tears, 860–861
Rotator cuff tendonitis, 860
Rotavirus infection, 349t
Roundworms, 432–434
Rovsing sign, 214
rPA (reteplase), 654
  for acute coronary syndromes, 132t,
    135

RSD (reflex sympathetic dystrophy), 75–78, 76t, 77t
RSI (rapid sequence induction), 5
in children, 26–28
Rubella, 380
Rule of 6s, for pediatric drug calculation, 29
"Rule of Nines" for burns, 586, *586*
Rumack-Matthew nomogram for acetaminophen toxicity, *508*, 508–509

S
Sacrum fracture, 837t
Sager traction, 839
SAH. *See* Subarachnoid hemorrhage
Salicylate overdose, 505–507
clinical features of, 469t, 505–506
diagnosis and differential of, 506
management of, 506–507
Salivary gland disorders, 725–726
masticator space abscess, 726
sialolithiasis, 726
suppurative parotitis, 725–726
viral parotitis, 725
Salmeterol, for high-altitude pulmonary edema, 580
Salmonella infection, 349t
Salter-Harris fracture classification, *383*, 383–384
SARS. *See* Severe respiratory distress syndrome
SBO (small bowel obstruction), 217–218
SBP (spontaneous bacterial peritonitis), 244
Scabies, 570, 757
Scalp lacerations, *94*, 94–95, 763
in children, 764
pressure dressings for, 118
Scaphoid fracture, 824
Scapholunate dissociation, 824
Scapular fractures, 833
Scapular manipulation technique, for glenohumeral joint dislocation, 832
Scarlet fever, 332, *376*, 376–377
SCD. *See* Sickle cell disease
SCFE (slipped capital femoral epiphysis), 386–387
Schistosomiasis, 435
Schizophrenia, 880
Schizophreniform disorder, 880
SCI. *See* Spinal cord injury
Scleritis, 868
Scopolamine

for herpes simplex conjunctivitis, 716
for herpes zoster ophthalmicus, 717
overdose of, 468t
for vertigo, 691
Scorpion stings, 569
Scrotal abscess, 272
Scrotal injuries, 810, 813
Scuba diving complications, 581–583
SDH. *See* Subdural hematoma
Sea cucumbers, 576
Sea snakes, 576, 577
Sea stars, 576
Sea urchins, 576
Sedation
conscious, 67
for delirium, 680
minimal, moderate, and deep, 67
of pediatric patients, 67, 766
procedural, 67–71
dosing for, 69t
indications for, 67
medications for, 691
preparation for, 67–68
of violent patients, 884
Sedative-hypnotic toxicity, 489–493
barbiturates, 489–490
benzodiazepines, 490–491
nonbenzodiazepines, 491–493
Seizures, 693–698. *See also* Status epilepticus
absence, 693
in children, 344–347
breakthrough seizures in known epileptic, 346
clinical features of, 344
diagnosis and differential of, 344–345
febrile seizure, 347
first seizure, 346
head trauma and, 347
infantile spasms, 347
management of, 345–347
neonatal, 347
posttraumatic, 766
risk factors for, 344
status epilepticus, 345–346
classification of, 693, 694t
clinical features of, 693–694
diagnosis and differential of, 694–696
drug-induced, 470t–471t
in eclampsia, 693
generalized, 693
management of, *696*, 696–698, 697t
in meningitis, 708, 709

Seizures (*Cont.*)
  partial, 693–694
  posttraumatic, 779
    in children, 766
  in pregnancy, 290
  primary, 693
  psychomotor, 694
  secondary, 694, 695t
  vs. syncope, 138
  temporal lobe, 693
Seldinger technique, 8
Selective serotonin reuptake inhibitor
    (SSRI) toxicity, 482–483
Sellick maneuver, 6
Senile gait, 687
Sensory ataxia, 687
Sepsis
  in children, 316–318
    clinical features of, 317
    diagnosis and differential of, 317
    management of, 317–318
    microbiology of, 317t
    neonates, 316–328, 320
  in sickle cell disease, 395
Septic abortion, 294
Septic arthritis, 113, 862–863, 865t
  in children, 387, 862
Septic bursitis, 866
  of foot, 872
Septic shock, 53–56
Sequestration crisis, in sickle cell
    disease, 394
Serotonin syndrome, 469t, 479
  newer antidepressants and,
    481–483
Severe respiratory distress syndrome
    (SARS), 182–183
  clinical features of, 182
  diagnosis and differential of, 183
  etiology of, 182
  management of, 183
Sexual assault, 283, 894–896
  clinical features of, 894
  diagnosis and differential of, 895
  evidence collection for, 895
  follow-up care for, 896
  management of, 895–896
  physical examination for, 894–895
Sexual child abuse, 892
Sexually transmitted diseases (STDs),
    401–406
  chancroid, 405
  Chlamydia trachomatis, 401–402
  genital herpes, 404–405
  gonorrhea, 402–403
  HIV infection and, 416

  lymphogranuloma venereum,
    405–406
  prophylaxis after sexual assault, 896
  reporting of, 401
  syphilis, 403–404
  treatment recommendations for, 401
  trichomoniasis, 403
Shark bites, 575–577
Sharp object ingestion, 210
Sheehan syndrome, 618
Shigella infection, 349t
Shin splints, 843
Shingles, 411–412
Shock, 49–52
  abdominal aortic aneurysm and, 162
  anaphylactic, 60–61
  cardiogenic, 57–59
  in children, 317, 764
  with cyanosis in children, 325–327
  neurogenic, 62–63
  septic, 53–56
  spinal, 62, 780, 785t, 786
Shoulder dystocia, 301
Shoulder injuries, 830–834
Shoulder pain, 860–861
  clinical features of, 860
  diagnosis and differential of,
    860–861
  management of, 861
SIADH (syndrome of inappropriate
    antidiuretic hormone), in cancer
    patients, 661
Sialolithiasis, 726
Sickle cell β-thalassemia disease, 396,
    642
Sickle cell disease (SCD), 641–642
  in children, 391–396
  clinical features of, 641
  diagnosis and differential of,
    641–642
  hematologic crises in, 394–395,
    641
    acute sequestration crisis, 394
    aplastic episodes, 394
    hemolytic crisis, 394–395
  infections in, 395
  intraocular pressure elevation in,
    720
  management of, 395–396, 642
  in pregnancy, 289
  variants of, 396, 642
  vasoocclusive crises in, 391–394,
    641
    acute central nervous system
      events, 393
    acute chest syndrome, 392–393

Sickle cell disease (SCD) (*Cont.*)
  pain crisis, 391–392
  priapism, 393–394
Sickle cell hemoglobin C disease, 396, 642
Sickle cell trait, 396, 642
Silver nitrate cautery, for epistaxis, 731
Silver sulfadiazine
  for burns, 589
  for pemphigus vulgaris, 752
Simple interrupted percutaneous sutures, 87–89, *88*
Sinus bradycardia, 9–10
  in acute myocardial infarction, 130
Sinus dysrhythmia, 9, *9*
Sinus fracture, 787
Sinus tachycardia, 10
  in acute myocardial infarction, 130
  in cardiogenic shock, 57
  in children, 30
Sinusitis, 732–733
  in children, 335–336
  clinical features of, 335, 732
  complications of, 732–733
  diagnosis and differential of, 335, 732
  management of, 336, 732–733
Sit-up test, 200
Sitz baths, 229
Sjögren syndrome, 868
Skin disorders, 745–758. *See also* Rash
  abscesses, 450–451
  acneiform eruptions, 756
  alopecia, 754
  in anthrax, 444
  bullous pemphigoid, 751–752
  contact dermatitis, 753–754
  due to caustic exposures, 530, 531
  erythema multiforme, 748–749
  exfoliative dermatitis, 747–748
  in helminthic infections, 432t
  herpes zoster, 411–412, 756–757
  in meningococcemia, 752
  pediculosis, 571, 757–758
  pemphigus vulgaris, 751–752
  photosensitivity, 753
  psoriasis, 755–756
  scabies, 570, 757
  tinea infections, 755
  toxic epidermal necrolysis, 749
  toxic infectious erythemas, 749–751
Skull fractures, 774–776, 787
  in children, 765

SLE (systemic lupus erythematosus), 867–868
Slipped capital femoral epiphysis (SCFE), 386–387
SLUDGE syndrome, 533
Small bowel injuries, 803
Small bowel obstruction (SBO), 217–218
Smallpox, 453, 454t
Smith fracture, 825
Smoke inhalation, 588
Snakebites, 572–574
  coral snake, 574
  pit vipers, 572–573
  sea snakes, 576, 577
Sodium bicarbonate
  for acute renal failure, 262
  for antipsychotic overdose, 487
  for barbiturate overdose, 490
  for children with altered mental status, 361
  for cocaine toxicity, 502
  for diabetic ketoacidosis, 356, 609
  for hyperkalemia, 36, 852
  for hypermagnesemia, 40
  for metabolic acidosis, 43, 43t, 52, 56
  for metformin-induced lactic acidosis, 556
  for neonatal resuscitation, 31
  for pediatric resuscitation, 29
  for poisoning, 473t
  for rhabdomyolysis, 852
  for salicylate overdose, 506
  for selective serotonin reuptake inhibitor overdose, 483
  for tricyclic antidepressant toxicity, 480
Sodium nitrite, 472t
  for cyanide poisoning, 551, 552t
Sodium nitroprusside
  for aortic incompetence, 146
  for cardiogenic shock, 58
  for hallucinogen intoxication, 504
  for hypertension in hemorrhagic stroke, 677
  for hypertensive emergencies, 160
    in children, 161
  for mitral incompetence, 144
  for monoamine oxidase inhibitor overdose, 485
  for pulmonary edema, 140
  for right ventricular infarction, 136
  for stimulant toxicity, 502
  toxicity of, 519–520

Sodium polystyrene sulfonate
  for hyperkalemia, 37, 38, 852
  for hyperphosphatemia, 852
  for lithium overdose, 488
Sodium thiosulfate, 472t
  for cyanide poisoning, 551–552,
    552t
Soft tissue foreign bodies, 109–111
  clinical features of, 109
  delayed removal of, 111
  diagnosis and differential of, 109
  fishhooks, *110,* 110–111, *111*
  imaging evaluation of, 111
  indications for removal of, 109–110
  metallic needles, 110
  post-removal treatment, 111
  wood splinters and organic spines,
    110
Soft tissue infections, 447–451
  cellulitis, 448–449
    in children, 336–337
    facial, 724–725, 734–735
    periorbital and orbital, 337, 717
  cutaneous abscesses, 450–451
  erysipelas, 449–450, 724
  gas gangrene, 447–448
  necrotizing fasciitis, 253–255,
    408–409, 448
  of oral cavity, 735–736, 743
  sporotrichosis, 451
Sonoran coral snake bite, 574
Sorbitol, for constipation, 238
Sotalol, for wide-complex tachycardia,
    17
Specific phobia, 881
Spectinomycin
  for gonococcal infection, 402
  for gonococcal pharyngitis, 333
Sphenoid sinusitis, 732
Spherocytosis, hereditary, 643
Spider bites, 567–568
Spinal cord compression, 859
  in cancer patients, 656–657
Spinal cord injury (SCI), 780–786. *See
    also* Cervical spine injury
  in children, 765, 767
  clinical features of, 780
  complete vs. incomplete, 780, 782
  diagnosis and differential of,
    780–782
  management of, 786
  mechanisms of, 780, 781t
  neurogenic shock and, 62–63
  spinal shock and, 780
Spinal cord syndromes, 782, 785t
Spinal fractures, 780–786

cervical spine, 782, 783t–784t
  in children, 765
  management of, 786
  radiographic evaluation of,
    780–782, 781t
  thoracic, 856–858
Spinal immobilization, 786, 795
Spinal shock, 62, 780, 785t
  management of, 786
Spinous process fracture of cervical
    spine, 784t
Spironolactone toxicity, 518
Splenic injury, 803
  in pregnancy, 771
Splenic sequestration crisis, in sickle
    cell disease, 394
Splinters, removal of, 110
Spontaneous bacterial peritonitis
    (SBP), 244
Sporotrichosis, 451
Spurling sign, 856
SSRI (selective serotonin reuptake
    inhibitor) toxicity, 482–483
Staphylococcal scalded skin syndrome
    (SSSS), 749–751
  clinical features of, 749–751
  diagnosis and differential of, 751
  management of, 751
Staphylococcus infection
  from dog bites, 116
  S. aureus
    antibiotic prophylaxis for, 113
    bullous impetigo, 374, 724
    cellulitis, 336, 337, 724–725
    gastroenteritis, 349t
    impetigo contagiosum, 374–375
    infective endocarditis, 419
    otitis externa, 728
    otitis media, 728
    pneumonia, 179, 180
    from puncture wounds, 112
    toxic shock syndrome, 407–408,
      749–751
  S. saprophyticus, urinary tract
    infection, 269
  scalded skin syndrome, 749–751
Staples for wound closure, 92, *92*
Status epilepticus, 693. *See also*
    Seizures
  in children, 345–346
  management of, *696,* 697
  in pregnancy, 290
STDs. *See* Sexually transmitted
    diseases
Sternal fractures, 796
Sternoclavicular joint injuries, 830

Stevens-Johnson syndrome, 376, 510, 748
Still murmur, 325
Stimson technique, for glenohumeral joint dislocation, 832
Stimulant toxicity, 500–502
  clinical features of, 500–501
  diagnosis and differential of, 501
  management of, 501–502
Stingrays, 576
Stomach injuries, 803
Stomas, complications of, 256
Stool tests
  in diarrhea, 235–236
  in helminthic infections, 431
Streptococcal toxic shock syndrome (STTS), 408–409, 749–751
  clinical features of, 408–409, 749–750
  diagnosis and differential of, 409, 409t, 751
  management of, 409, 751
Streptococcus infection
  from dog bites, 116
  group A
    acute rheumatic fever, 389
    erysipelas, 375, 449–450
    impetigo contagiosum, 374–375
    necrotizing fasciitis, 448
    peritonsillar abscess, 740
    pharyngitis, 332–333, 740
    pneumonia, 179
    reactive arthritis after, 390
    scarlet fever, 376
  S. pneumoniae
    cellulitis, 337, 724
    otitis media, 330, 728
    pneumonia, 179, 180
    sinusitis, 335
  S. pyogenes
    cellulitis, 336, 724–725
    erysipelas, 724
    nonbullous impetigo, 724
    toxic shock syndrome, 408–409, 749–751
Streptokinase, 654
  for acute coronary syndromes, 132t, 135
  for pulmonary embolism, 158
Streptomycin
  for plague, 446
  for tuberculosis, 185, 186t, 417
  for tularemia, 442
Stridor
  in bacterial tracheitis, 371
  in croup, 369
  due to foreign body aspiration, 371
  in epiglottitis, 370
  neonatal, 322
Stroke, 673–678
  brainstem, 673
  clinical features of, 673–674
  diagnosis and differential of, 674–675, 675t
  hemorrhagic, 674, 674t
  with hypertension, 160
  ischemic, 655, 673, 674t
  lacunar infarcts, 673
  management of, 675–678, 676t
Strongyloides stercoralis infection, 433
STTS. *See* Streptococcal toxic shock syndrome
Stye, 715
Subacromial bursitis, 860
Subacromial tendonitis, 860
Subarachnoid hemorrhage (SAH), 667–668
  clinical features of, 674
  complications of, 668, 677
  diagnosis of, 668
  headache from, 667, 674
  management of, 668, 677, 779
  traumatic, 776, 779
  xanthochromia and, 668
Subclavian artery injuries, 801
Subclavian steal syndrome, 138
Subconjunctival hemorrhage, 718
Subcutaneous emphysema, 795–796
Subdural hematoma (SDH), 777
  end-stage renal disease and, 264–265
  headache from, 667
  management of, 670
Subfalcial herniation, 777
Submersion injuries, 584–585
Substance-induced disorders, 499–505, 879. *See also* Drug abuse
Substance withdrawal, 879
Subtrochanteric fractures, 837
Subungual hematoma, 104
Succimer
  for arsenic poisoning, 540
  for lead poisoning, 538
  for mercury poisoning, 541
Succinylcholine, for rapid sequence induction, 5
  in children, 28
Succussion splash, 212
Sucking chest wounds, 795
Sucralfate, for peptic ulcer disease, 213

Sudden cardiac death, in children and
adolescents, 363
Suicidal patients, 882–884
acetaminophen overdose, 467
aspirin overdose, 467
caustic ingestion, 530
wrist lacerations, 100
Sulfacetamide, for conjunctivitis, 715
Sulfadiazine, for toxoplasmosis, 417,
458
Sulfasalazine
for Crohn disease, 222
for ulcerative colitis, 224
Sulfhemoglobinemia, 553–554
Sulfonamides, use in pregnancy, 291t
Sulfonylurea overdose, 555–557, 607
Sumatriptan
for cluster headaches, 670
for migraine, 668, 671t
use in pregnancy, 292t
Sunburn, 753
Superior orbital fissure syndrome, 790
Superior vena cava syndrome,
658–659
Superwarfarin ingestion, 535, 536t
Supracondylar fractures, 826–827
Supraspinatus tendonitis, 860
Supraventricular tachycardia (SVT),
14, 14–16, *15*
in children, 29
paroxysmal, 14
in Wolff-Parkinson-White
syndrome, 25
Sutures, 87
timing for removal of, 119
Suturing techniques, 87–91
continuous "running" percutaneous
sutures, 89, *89*
deep dermal sutures, 89–90, *90*
delayed closure, 91
mattress sutures
horizontal, 91, *91*
vertical, 90, *91*
simple interrupted percutaneous
sutures, 87–89, *88*
for specific wounds
cheek and facial lacerations, 98,
98
dorsal hand lacerations, 102
ear lacerations, *97,* 97–98
extensor tendon lacerations, 102,
102
eyelid lacerations, 95
finger and finger tip injuries, 104,
104
foot lacerations, 108

forearm and wrist lacerations,
100, *101*
intraoral mucosal lacerations,
738
lip lacerations, *96,* 96–97, 738
nasal lacerations, 96
palm lacerations, 100–101
scalp and forehead lacerations,
94–95
tongue lacerations, 738
SVT. *See* Supraventricular tachycardia
Swallowing
difficulty with, 206
of foreign bodies, 209–211
"Swimmer's ear," 728
in children, 331–332
Swinging-light test, 787, 790
Sympathomimetic overdose, 468t
Syncope, 137–139
cardiac, 137, 138
in children and adolescents,
363–365
causes of, 364t
clinical features of, 363
diagnosis and differential of,
363–364, 365t
management of, 364–365
sudden cardiac death and, 363
clinical features of, 137–138
convulsive, 138
diagnosis and differential of, 138
drug-related, 138
in geriatric patients, 768
heat, 565
hypertrophic cardiomyopathy and,
137, 151
management of, 139
near syncope, 689
orthostatic, 137, 138
vasovagal, 137
Syndrome of inappropriate antidiuretic
hormone (SIADH), in cancer
patients, 661
Synovial fluid analysis, 862, 864t
Synovitis, crystal-induced, 863
Syphilis, 403–404
clinical features of, 403–404
diagnosis and differential of, 404
management of, 404
stages of, 403–404
Systemic lupus erythematosus (SLE),
867–868

T
TAC (tetracaine adrenaline cocaine),
73

Tachycardia
 in children, 29–30
 multifocal atrial, *11,* 11–12
 sinus, 10
 supraventricular, *14,* 14–16, *15*
 ventricular, 19, *19*
 wide-complex, 16
 in Wolff-Parkinson-White
  syndrome, 25
Tacrolimus, 459t
Taenia saginata infection, 435
Taenia solium infection, 435–436
Talus fractures, 847
Tapeworms, 435–436
Tarantulas, 569
Tarsal fractures, 847
Tarsal tunnel syndrome, 873
TBI (traumatic brain injury), 774–779.
 See also Head trauma
TCAs. *See* Tricyclic antidepressant
  toxicity
TCT (thrombin clotting time), 625t
Teardrop fracture
 extension, 784t
 flexion, 783t
Teeth. *See* Tooth
Teething, 734
Telecanthus, 788
Telogen effluvium, 754
Temporal arteritis, 671–672, 723, 868
Temporomandibular joint
 dislocation of, 791
 dysfunction of, 672, 726–727
TEN (toxic epidermal necrolysis), 749
Tendon lesions
 Achilles tendon, 107, 842, 844, 873
 of foot, 873–874
 of forearm and wrist, 100, 100t,
  101t
 of hand, *102,* 102–103, 822
 of lower extremity, 106, 107t
 patellar tendon rupture, 841–842
 quadriceps tendon rupture, 842
Tendonitis
 in hand, 871
 patellar, 843
 rotator cuff, 860
 subacromial, 860
 supraspinatus, 860
Tenecteplase, 654
 for acute coronary syndromes, 132t,
  135
Tenosynovitis
 De Quervain, 871
 in foot, 873–874
 in hand, 869, 870t, 871

Tensilon test, 705
Tension headache, 667
 management of, 669
Tension pneumothorax, 188, 762, 793,
 796–797
Terazosin toxicity, 519
Terbinafine, for onychomycosis, 755
Terbutaline
 for asthma, 193, 341
 for priapism, 273, 393
Testicular injuries, 813
Testicular torsion, 271
"Tet spells," 326
Tetanus, 422–423
 cephalic, 422
 clinical features of, 422
 diagnosis and differential of, 422
 management of, 422–423
 neonatal, 422
Tetanus immune globulin, 423, 590
Tetanus prophylaxis, 86, 118–119,
 763
 for burn injuries, 590
 for cat bites, 117
 for dog bites, 116
 for extremity lacerations, 99, 106
 for human bites, 115
 in pregnancy, 773
 for puncture wounds, 112–113
Tetracaine, 71
Tetracaine adrenaline cocaine (TAC),
 73
Tetracycline
 for dog bite prophylaxis, 115
 for ehrlichiosis, 443
 for *Helicobacter pylori* infection,
  213
 for Rocky Mountain spotted fever,
  377, 440
 use in pregnancy, 291t
Tetralogy of Fallot, 326
Theophylline toxicity, 512–513
 clinical features of, 512
 diagnosis and differential of, 512
 management of, 512–513
Thermal burns, 586–590
 burn unit referral criteria for, 589,
  590t
 calculating size of, *586,* 586–587,
  587, 587t
 classification of severity of, 588
 depth of, 587–588
 diagnosis and differential of, 588
 to ear, 729–730
 with inhalation injury, 588
 management of, 588–590

Thiabendazole, for *Strongyloides stercoralis* infection, 433
Thiamine
  for alcoholic ketoacidosis, 613
  for alcoholic liver disease, 245
  for ethanol intoxication, 494
  for ethylene glycol poisoning, 497
  for patient with ataxia, 687
  for patient with hypoglycemia, 556, 607, 697
  for poisoned patient, 473t, 474
  for tricyclic antidepressant toxicity, 480
Thiazolidinediones, 555, 607
Thiopental, for rapid sequence induction, 5
  in children, 28
Thomas splint, 839
Thompson test, 107, 844, 873
Thoracic duct injuries, 802
Thoracic trauma. *See* Cardiothoracic trauma
Thoracolumbar pain, 855–859
Thoracotomy
  for cardiac injury, 799
  for hemothorax or pneumothorax, 797
Threadworm, 433
Thrombin clotting time (TCT), 625t
Thrombin inhibitors, 654
Thrombocytopenia
  heparin-induced, 168, 630
  idiopathic thrombocytopenic purpura, 628
  thrombotic thrombocytopenic purpura, 628, 643–644
Thromboembolic disorders
  acute arterial occlusion, 168–169
  antithrombotic therapy for, 653–655
  in cancer patients, 659
  cavernous sinus thrombosis, 734–735
  deep venous thrombosis and thrombophlebitis, 166–168, 167t
  dilated cardiomyopathy and, 149
  disseminated intravascular coagulation, 630
  postoperative thrombophlebitis, 254, 255
  in pregnancy, 288–289
  in prosthetic heart valve patients, 146, 148
  pulmonary embolism, 156–158
Thrombophlebitis, 166
Thrombotic thrombocytopenic purpura (TTP), 628, 643–644

Thrush
  in HIV infection, 416
  management of, 417
  neonatal, 323
Thyroid storm, 614–615
  clinical features of, 614
  diagnosis and differential of, 614
  management of, 614–615, 615t
  in pregnancy, 288
TIA (transient ischemic attack), 673–678
Tibial fractures, 841
Tibial plateau fractures, 840
Tibial spine fractures, 840
Tic douloureux, 672
Ticarcillin-clavulanate
  for cirrhosis and liver failure, 245
  for diverticulitis, 226
  for Ludwig angina, 734
Tick paralysis, 441–442
Tilt-chin lift maneuver, 3
Timolol, for intraocular pressure elevation, 720, 722
Tinea capitis, 754
Tinea cruris, 755
Tinea infections, 755
Tinea manuum, 755
Tinea pedis, 755
Tinel sign, 871, 873
Tinnitus, 730
Tinzaparin, for deep venous thrombosis, 168
Tirofiban, 654
  for acute coronary syndromes, 132t, 136
Tissue adhesives, 92–93, 106
  eye exposure to, 721
Tissue plasminogen activator (tPA), 654
  for acute coronary syndromes, 132t, 135
  for pulmonary embolism, 158
  for stroke, 675–677, 676t
TLS (tumor lysis syndrome), 660
TMP-SMX. *See* Trimethoprim-sulfamethoxazole
TOA (tubo-ovarian abscess), 305–306
Tobramycin
  for conjunctivitis, 335, 715
  for corneal abrasion, 718
  for diverticulitis, 226
  for septic shock, 55
  for tularemia, 443
Tocolytics, 296, 773

Toe injuries
  digital blocks for, 72–73
  hair tourniquet syndrome, 108
Tolazoline, for clonidine toxicity, 519
Tongue lacerations, 738
Tooth
  alveolar osteitis after extraction of,
    735
  avulsion of, 737
  bleeding after extraction of,
    738–739
  concussion of, 737
  decay of, 734
  eruption of, 734
  luxation of, 737
Toothache, 734
Topical anesthetics, 73
Topiramate, for seizures in children,
  346
Torsades de pointes, 20, *20*, 480, 487
Torsemide toxicity, 518
Total body water deficit, calculation
  of, 35
Toxic epidermal necrolysis (TEN),
  749
Toxic infectious erythemas, 407–409,
  749–751
Toxic megacolon
  Crohn disease and, 221
  ulcerative colitis and, 223
Toxic shock syndrome (TSS),
  407–409, 749–751
  clinical features of, 407, 749–750
  diagnosis and differential of, 407,
    408t, 749–750
  management of, 407–408, 751
  streptococcal, 408–409, 749–751
Toxicology and pharmacology,
  465–557
  alcohols, 494–498
  analgesics, 505–511
  anticholinergic toxicity, 476–479
  antimicrobials, 549–550
  cardiac medications, 514–520
  caustic agents, 530–532
  cyanide, 551–552
  drugs of abuse, 499–504
  dyshemoglobinemias, 553–554
  hazardous materials, 542–545
  herbals and vitamins, 546–548
  hydrocarbons and volatile
    substances, 527–529
  hypoglycemic agents, 555–557,
    607–608
  insecticides, herbicides, and
    rodenticides, 533–534

iron toxicity, 524–526
  metals and metalloids, 538–541
  phenytoin and fosphenytoin toxicity,
    521–523
  poisoning, 467–475
  psychopharmacologic agents,
    479–488
  sedatives and hypnotics, 489–493
  theophylline, 512–513
Toxidromes, 467, 468t–469t
Toxoplasmosis
  in HIV infection, 415
  management of, 417, 458
  in transplant recipients, 458
tPA. *See* Tissue plasminogen activator
Tracheitis, bacterial, 371
Tracheobronchial injuries, 797–798
Tracheostomy tube, 7
Tranexamic acid, for bleeding, 639
Transfusion therapy, 646–652
  for abdominal trauma, 805
  administration of, 652
  for anemia, 627
  for bleeding in liver disease, 629
  blood products for, 646–648
    albumin, 648
    antithrombin III, 648
    coagulation factors, 649t
    cryoprecipitate, 647
    fresh-frozen plasma, 647
    intravenous immunoglobulins,
      647–648
    packed red blood cells, 646
    platelets, 647
    whole blood, 646
  blood type and crossmatch for, 646
  complications of, 648, 650t–651t
    delayed reactions, 648–649
  for disseminated intravascular
    coagulation, 630–632
  emergency transfusion, 649–652
  for hemolytic anemia, 644
  hemolytic reactions to, 643
  for hemophilia, 635
  for hemoptysis, 191
  for iron poisoning, 525
  massive transfusion, 652
  platelet transfusion, 628
  for ruptured abdominal aortic
    aneurysm, 163
  for shock, 52
    septic shock, 56
  for sickle cell disease, 393, 396, 642
  for thrombolytic-induced
    hemorrhage, 135
  for toxic shock syndrome, 408

Transfusion therapy (*Cont.*)
  for trauma patients, 762–763
    children, 766
    geriatric patients, 770
  for von Willebrand disease,
    639–640
Transient ischemic attack (TIA),
  673–678
Transient synovitis of hip, 388
Transillumination, 8
Translaryngeal ventilation, 8
Transplantation
  cardiac, 460–461
  complications related to
    immunosuppressive agents for,
    459–460, 459t
  infectious complications after,
    456–459, 457t
  liver, 462–463
  lung, 461–462
  renal, 462
Transposition of great vessels, 326
Transtentorial herniation, 777
Transverse myelitis, 704
Trapezium fracture, 825
Trapezoid fracture, 825
Trauma, 759–815
  abdominal, 803–806
  approach to patient with,
    761–763
  cardiothoracic, 795–802
  chemical burns, 590–592
  clinical features of, 761
  diagnosis and differential of,
    761–762
  ear, *97*, 97–98, 729–730
  electrical injuries, 593–595
  genitourinary, 810–814
  geriatric, 768–770
  head, 774–779
  intimate partner violence and abuse,
    894–897
  laryngeal, 744, 792
  lightning injuries, 595–597
  management of, 762–763
  mandibular dislocation, 727
  maxillofacial, 787–791
  nasal, 732, 787, 788
  ocular, 719–721, 787
  orofacial, 736–738
  orthopedic, 819–847 (*See also*
    Dislocations; Fractures;
    Musculoskeletal disorders)
  pediatric, 764–767
    child abuse, 891–892
    fractures, 383–386

penetrating injuries of extremities,
  814–815
penetrating injuries of flank and
  buttock, 807–809
in pregnancy, 771–773
sexual assault, 894–896
spine and spinal cord, 780–786
thermal burns, 586–590
wound care for, 83–86 (*See also*
  Lacerations; Wound care)
Traumatic brain injury (TBI),
  774–779. *See also* Head trauma
Trazodone toxicity, 481
Trematodes, 435
Trench foot, 561–562, 874
"Trench mouth," 735
Trephination, for increased intracranial
  pressure, 779
Treponema pallidum infection,
  403–404
Triamterene toxicity, 518
Triceps rupture, 828–829
Trichinella spiralis infection, 434
Trichomonas vaginalis infection, 303,
  403
  prophylaxis after sexual assault,
    896
Trichuris trichiura infection, 434
Tricyclic antidepressant (TCA)
  toxicity, 479–481
  clinical features of, 479–480
  diagnosis and differential of, 480
  management of, 480–481
Trifluorothymidine, for herpes simplex
  conjunctivitis, 716
Trifluridine, for herpes simplex
  conjunctivitis, 335
Trigeminal neuralgia, 672
Trigeminy, 16
Trigger finger, 871
L-Triiodothyronine, for myxedema
  coma, 616
Trimethoprim
  for urinary catheterization, 275
  for urinary tract infection, 269
  use in pregnancy, 291t
Trimethoprim-polymyxin B, for
  conjunctivitis, 715
Trimethoprim-sulfamethoxazole
  (TMP-SMX)
  for brain abscess, 712
  for diarrhea, 236, 349t, 350
  for diverticulitis, 226
  for foot wound prophylaxis, 108
  for frontal sinus and frontal bone
    fractures, 790